PSYCHIATRIC NURSING
Promoting Mental Health

Ann Wolbert Burgess, CS, DNSc, FAAN
*van Ameringen Professor of Psychiatric
Mental Health Nursing
University of Pennsylvania School of Nursing
Philadelphia, Pennsylvania*

Appleton & Lange
Stamford, Connecticut

Copyright © 1997 by Appleton & Lange
A Simon & Schuster Company

97 98 99 00 01 / 10 9 8 7 6 5 4 3 2 1

Prentice Hall International (UK) Limited, *London*
Prentice Hall of Australia Pty. Limited, *Sydney*
Prentice Hall Canada, Inc., *Toronto*
Prentice Hall Hispanoamericana, S.A., *Mexico*
Prentice Hall of India Private Limited, *New Delhi*
Prentice Hall of Japan, Inc., *Tokyo*
Simon & Schuster Asia Pte. Ltd., *Singapore*
Editora Prentice Hall do Brasil Ltda., *Rio de Janeiro*
Prentice Hall, *Upper Saddle River, New Jersey*

Psychiatric nursing : promoting mental health / [edited by] Ann W.
    Burgess.
       p.   cm.
    ISBN 0-8385-8087-4 (case : alk. paper)
    1. Psychiatric nursing.   I. Burgess, Ann Wolbert.
    [DNLM: 1. Mental Disorders—nursing.   2. Psychiatric Nursing—
    methods.   3. Nurse–Patient Relations.   WY 160 P9729 1996]
RC440.P766   1996
610.73'68—dc20
DNLM/DLC
for Library of Congress   96-8408
                                                                 CIP

ISBN 0-8385-8087-4

Editor-in-Chief: Sally J. Barhydt
Development Editor: Barbara Severs
Production Editor: Maria T. Vlasak
Designer: Libby Schmitz

9 780838 580875

90000

Contents

Preface

Psychiatric nursing took a giant leap forward with Hildegard Peplau's 1952 book, *Interpersonal Relations in Nursing.* Until that time it was frowned upon, if not outright forbidden, for a nurse to talk with patients in most health care institutions. Peplau's text argued that the patient was a subject, not an object for "spectator observation" by nurses. It suggested that in nurse–patient relationships, nurses first ought to notice their own behavior, then note the patient's behavior, and finally grasp the relationships (i.e., the patterns, linkages, and connections) that go on within the nurse–patient relationship. The text also provided a structure for phases in the relationship, and it proposed concepts and personality development theory applications (Peplau 1996).

This advance enabled psychiatric nursing to begin to look at the human process from many perspectives: sociocultural, philosophical, and behavioral, as well as psychological. We are now at a point where assumptions about the underlying neurobiology of behavior can be intricately related to the domains of comprehensive patient care.

Psychiatric nursing in the twenty-first century will present exciting challenges to students and practitioners as changes continue in the delivery of mental health services. In addition to traditional hospital settings, psychiatric nurses now practice in homes, in jails and prisons, in domestic abuse shelters, in respite care facilities, with emergency department triage teams, on crisis hot lines, and in 23-hour psychiatric holding centers. The authors of this textbook, *Psychiatric Nursing: Promoting Mental Health,* have had an opportunity to write about contemporary mental health care issues facing the profession and to describe the traditional clinical skills and the values held by psychiatric nurses that have met the test of time.

■ THE HUMAN FACTOR

This text focuses on the relationship dimension in psychiatric nursing originally described by Hildegard Peplau. Patients matter as people. They must be seen as individuals who are suffering in their behaviors, thoughts, and especially in their feelings. Mental illness represents a patient's attempt to cope with overwhelming experiences; it is the patient's way of making the best of a bad situation.

In our focus on humanness, we also say that nurses matter as people. Students need to understand that strong reactions to patients represent both potential diagnostic clues to the patient as well as an awareness of their own vulnerabilities. In relationships with patients come this complex interaction between one's own vulnerabilities and the emotional messages from interaction. Student discomfort with patients does not represent a treatment failure, but rather a diagnostic clue that a subtle, complicated situation needs to be understood. For example, a student in class discusses a case example from Chapter 27 about child maltreatment in class and describes her outrage that an adolescent boy would hurt young babies. The instructor helps the student step back from her feelings to understand that the origin of the youth's sadistic behavior stems from his own father's abandonment of the family and his subsequent sadistic abuse at the hands of his mother's paramour.

■ THE STRESS–CRISIS CONTINUUM

A contemporary aspect of this text is its presentation of a framework based on developmental crisis theory that has been part of the editor's paradigm for more than a decade. This paradigm is coming of age with increased knowledge regarding the linkage of stress, trauma, and behavioral health problems to neurobiological function and immune system depletion. Part III of the text, Clinical Disorders on the Stress–Crisis Continuum, is based on that theory. The framework is particularly useful in this period of managed care and focused, time-limited treatment. It gives precision to assessment and selection of intervention strategies, for example, how to combine counseling with medication to manage depressive symptomotology in a primary health care setting.

■ OTHER NURSING FRAMEWORKS

It is prudent for students to understand how several nursing models and systems theories are used in psy-chiatric nursing. Traditional psychiatric nursing places a primary emphasis on theoretical frameworks, systems of therapy, and the process of communication within the therapeutic alliance of the nurse–patient relationship. In this text, we have presented an overview of nursing models in psychiatric nursing practice as well as examples of how some of the contributing authors apply various theoretical frameworks in their practice. Contemporary psychiatric nursing practice adds research to the equation for a closer link of mind and brain to behavior to help answer the question of causality or why patients think, feel, and act as they do.

This text, of course, is written for students of psychiatric nursing, but also for nurse practitioners who care for patients with a secondary condition of behavioral or emotional distress. The emphasis in the beginning of the twenty-first century will be on primary health care and extending care into various community-based programs. In these settings the professional nurse will be required to assess, manage, and monitor the overall care, including physical, of persons who have emotional and psychiatric problems. This is a basic text that provides a background of strategies and techniques for nursing practice at a general level. It is also a resource for nurses in primary care.

■ TEXT AIMS AND OBJECTIVES

Psychiatric Nursing: Promoting Mental Health has two aims: first, to meet the growing need in psychiatric nursing for an undergraduate literature that clearly demonstrates how nurses use neurobiological, behavioral, and social science theories and research in the care of patients, and second, to develop a foundation for preparing nurses for a major role in primary mental health care. The author team is comprised primarily of psychiatric nurses who teach psychiatric nursing, have a clinical practice, or conduct clinical research.

This text is a tool for preparing students to practice contemporary psychiatric nursing. To practice effectively, students will need to achieve the following:

- A basic, theoretical, research-based understanding of the neurobiology of behavior and the relationship between the behavioral and biomedical sciences in maintaining mental health and preventing or limiting psychiatric dysfunction
- Communication skills

- An entry level of practice with various treatment modalities for individuals and families including psychopharmacology
- Knowledge of psychiatric and psychiatric nursing language
- An understanding of the standards and procedures for ethical and legal psychiatric nursing practice

The objectives of *Psychiatric Nursing: Promoting Mental Health* are to:

- Explain stressful and troubled human behavior as it presents itself in patient behavior
- Help students understand the biology of mental illness and its relationship to psychopharmacological interventions
- Identify factors that facilitate the therapeutic alliance and the communication process
- Assist students in conducting assessments for various conditions underlying mental health and mental disorder
- Provide a DSM-IV diagnosis and a psychiatric nursing diagnosis to a patient condition within the context of the nursing care plan

To achieve those objectives, the content addresses developing skills at essentially four levels: *cognitive,* to present a theoretical framework for clinical psychiatric nursing; *conceptual,* to provide the framework for understanding patient problems and developing strategies for change; *communications,* to enhance information exchange in the therapeutic relationship and to facilitate creation of a nonthreatening, open relationship; and finally, *clinical,* to facilitate implementation of effective therapeutic strategies.

In summary, the emphasis of this text is communicating with patients, understanding the biopsychosocial components of their illness, and appreciating their humanism within a stress–crisis continuum. Psychiatric nursing's commitment to a theoretical model that supports the healing processes of the individual, family, and community, and to raising the human dimension of patienthood provides a solid basis for optimal treatment to be possible in the delivery of mental health case services.

I especially wish to acknowledge the contributions of Colleen Powell MacLean and graduate students at the University of Pennsylvania School of Nursing. I appreciate the support and advice of Appleton & Lange's Editor-in-Chief Sally Barhydt, Senior Development Nursing Editor Barbara Severs, and Production Editor Maria Vlasak. Above all, I owe a special debt to Allen G. Burgess for computer programming design and assistance through all phases of the manuscript preparation.

—*Ann Wolbert Burgess*

The Artwork in this Text

The artwork in this textbook was contributed by patients at Stamford Hospital in Stamford, Connecticut, and by patients whose artwork appeared in the journal Psychosocial Nursing and Mental Health Services, *January 1990.*

Ann Wolbert Burgess and Appleton & Lange express their sincere appreciation to those individuals for their generosity. Judith Nicit Tota, who was instrumental in arranging for use of the art, describes art therapy in the following paragraphs.

The therapeutic use of art materials encourages creativity as a tool to stimulate problem-solving skills. The most immediate problems to overcome in art sessions are often the blank page and the patient's inhibitions. Through art, patients are encouraged to help themselves get "unstuck" and have a more spontaneous, creative experience. Feeling "stuck" in life's problems is the experience of most people seeking mental health treatment. The art process can provide an empowering experience of gaining control and using creativity to get beyond a personal impass. The patient works to gain control of materials or technical skills and learns to master impulse, strengthen weakness, and positively influence his or her world. In this way, the artmaking process becomes meaningful and therapeutic.

The product, or art, that results from an art therapy session, is also a valuable tool for the patient; it enhances the individual's skills in relating to others. For some patients, their art may be a powerful tool for expressing hidden strengths, and through this expression, individuals are able to relate to others more easily. For other patients the artwork may help the therapist and patient understand aspects of the patient's personality and coping skills in ways that words alone cannot.

—Judith Nicit Tota, BFA, MS, ATR
Activities Therapy Coordinator
The Stamford Hospital
Stamford, Connecticut

Contributors

Kathleen M. Andolina, RN, MS, CS-P
The Center for Case Management
South Natick, Massachusetts

Laureen McAvoy Burgess, MBA
PixelVision, Inc.
Acton, Massachusetts

Verna Benner Carson, RN, CS-P, PhD
National Director of Behavioral Health for Staff
    Builders
Baltimore, Maryland

Paul T. Clements, Jr., RN, MSN
PhD(c) University of Pennsylvania
Philadelphia, Pennsylvania

Rockford Center
Newark, Delaware

Linda S. Cook, RN, PhD, CF
Temple University
Philadelphia, Pennsylvania

Theresa M. Croushore, BSN, MHA, CIC
Behavioral Health Services of the Wyoming Valley
    Health Care System
Wilkes-Barre, Pennsylvania

Elizabeth B. Dowdell, RN, PhD
Thomas Jefferson University
College of Allied Health Sciences/
    Department of Nursing
Philadelphia, Pennsylvania

Jacqueline Fawcett, PhD, FAAN
Professor
University of Pennsylvania School of Nursing
Philadelphia, Pennsylvania

Regina D. Gavlick, RNC, MS
Middletown Psychiatric Center
Middletown, New York

Associate Director of Nursing
Orange County Department of Residential Health
    Care Services
Goshen, New York

Carol A. Glod, RN, CS, PhD
Assistant Professor
Northeastern University College of Nursing
Boston, Massachusetts

Lecturer in Psychiatry
Harvard Medical School
Cambridge, Massachusetts

Nurse Researcher
McLean Hospital
Belmont, Massachusetts

Christine A. Grant, RN, CS, PhD
Associate Professor (Faculty of Nursing)
The Royal Melbourne Institute of Technology
Melbourne, Australia

Carol R. Hartman, RN, CS, DNSc
Professor Emeritus
Boston College School of Nursing
Chestnut Hill, Massachusetts

June Johnston-Wolff, RN, CS, PhD
Private Practice
Newton, Massachusetts

Lifespan Associates
Brighton, Massachusetts

Susan J. Kelley, PhD, FAAN
Director of Research and Professor
College of Health Sciences
Georgia State University
Atlanta, Georgia

Joan S. Kings, RN, MSN
Doylestown Hospital
Doylestown, Pennsylvania

Margaret Knight, RN, CS, MS
Regis College
Weston, Massachusetts

Joyce K. Laben, JD, MSN, CS, FAAN
Vanderbilt University School of Nursing
Nashville, Tennessee

Pamela E. Marcus, RN, MS, CS-P
Private Practice
Upper Marlboro, Maryland

Maureen P. McCausland, DNSc, FAAN
Vice President for Nursing
The Mount Sinai Hospital
New York, New York

Victor A. McGregor, MSN, RNCS, NPP
PhD(c) Union Institute Graduate School
Columbia University

Critical Time Intervention Mental Health Program
Columbia Presbyterian Medical Center
New York, New York

Wanda K. Mohr, RNC, PhD
University of Pennsylvania
Philadelphia, Pennsylvania

Freida Hopkins Outlaw, RN, CS, DNSc
University of Pennsylvania School of Nursing

The Visiting Nurse Association of Philadelphia
Philadelphia, Pennsylvania

Mary Pickett, RN, PhD
Research Assistant Professor
University of Pennsylvania School of Nursing
Philadelphia, Pennsylvania

Carole-Rae Reed, RN, MSN, CS
PhD(c) University of Pennsylvania School
of Nursing
The Graduate Hospital
University of Pennsylvania School of Nursing
Philadelphia, Pennsylvania

Denise J. Ribble, RN, MPA
Middletown Psychiatric Center
Middletown, New York

Albert R. Roberts, MA, DSW
Graduate School of Social Work
Rutgers—The State University of New Jersey
New Brunswick, New Jersey

Sandra L. Rosen, RN, MSN, CS
Private Practice
Philadelphia, Pennsylvania

Margaret P. Shepard, RN, PhD
University of Rochester School of Nursing
Rochester, New York

Shirley A. Smoyak, PhD, FAAN
Professor and Director of Public Health
Rutgers—The State University of New Jersey
The Bloustein School of Planning and Public Policy
    Program in Public Health
New Brunswick, New Jersey

Burton Thelander, RN, MS, CS
Middletown Psychiatric Center
Middletown, New York

Sharon Valente, PhD, FAAN
Assistant Professor, Clinical Specialist in Mental Health
University of Southern California Department of
    Nursing
Consultant, Department of Veterans Affairs
Los Angeles, California

Doris C. Vallone MSN, RNC
Assistant Professor
Allentown College of St. Francis de Sales
Center Valley, Pennsylvania

Barbara E. Wolfe, RN, CS, PhD
Instructor in Psychiatry
Harvard Medical School
Cambridge, Massachussets

Clinical Nurse Specialist
Beth Israel Hospital
Boston, Massachusetts

Reviewers

Nola Cottom, RNC, MSN
Clinical Instructor
School of Nursing
University of Texas at Austin

Benna E. Cunningham, RN, MSN, FNP
Assistant Professor of Nursing
Medical College of Georgia

Janice M. Dyehouse, RN, PhD
College of Nursing and Health
University of Cincinnati

Laura Dzurec, PhD
Associate Dean
Oregon Health Sciences University

Sarah P. Farrell, PhD, RN, CS
Assistant Professor
University of Virginia

Gloria Fazio, RN, MSN, CS
Norwalk Community College

Janice Cooke Feigenbaum, BSN, MSN, PhD
Coordinator of Graduate Program in
  Community Addictions Nursing
D'Youville College

Laura Meeks Festa, EdD, RNCS
MCV–Virginia Commonwealth University

Dorothy M.B. Johnson, EdD, RN
Assistant Professor
West Virginia University

Judith Lynch-Sauer, PhD, RN
Lecturer
University of Michigan

Linda Nance Marks, RN, EdD
Associate Professor
School of Nursing
University of Texas at Arlington

Leonie Pallikkathayil, DNS
Associate Professor
School of Nursing
University of Kansas

Patricia A. Slater, RN, MSN
Assistant Professor
College of Mount St. Joseph

Barbara Montgomery Stewart, PhD, RN
Professor
Lienhard School of Nursing
Pace University

George Stricker, PhD
Distinguished Research Professor
Adelphi University

Gale R. Woolley, EdD, ARNP
Professor
Miami–Dade Community College

Foreword

The past 50 years have witnessed psychiatric nursing leadership accomplish two goals: to assess, diagnose, and manage mental illness and to integrate psychiatric nursing principles into general nursing practice to foster recovery from physical illnesses. The accomplishment of these initial goals established the credibility of psychiatric nursing practice with patient populations and as a method of intervention.

The legitimization of psychiatric nursing as a practice domain is well recognized through nursing research and practice expertise in state statutes and courts of law. Psychiatric nursing investigates not only long-standing clinical problems but breaks new ground in such practice areas of child, adolescent, and geropsychiatric nursing as well as criminal victimology and forensic evidence collection. The legitimization has occurred within an understanding of public health needs. There has always been an understanding of practice based on primary, secondary, and tertiary interventions; consequently psychiatric nursing in many ways led specialized nursing into the community. Public health nursing early recognized the need for mental health consultation with the complex problems derived from the behavior of patients who resided in the community.

The early professionalization of psychiatric mental health nursing emphasized not only the direct practice role but the consultative role. These efforts gave a foothold to psychiatric nurses carrying out independent research. The evolution of the research role in psychiatric nursing coupled with the direct and indirect practice role now defines the broad scope of psychiatric nursing practice. With the modernization of the delivery system, psychiatric nursing is gaining leverage on the accounting and documentation of program outcomes addressing a wide range of mental illness. Nurses have been key in developing path evaluations of patient hospital stays, identifying criteria for meeting therapeutic outcomes, and defining units of care from the least to the most restrictive settings. They now challenge corporate parameters for outcome by demanding that standards of practice, severity of illness, and functional ability be the criteria by which managed care is structured and within which it operates.

While psychiatric nursing has been at the forefront of linking theoretical understanding to practice, maintaining such a cutting edge needs to move beyond "fixing" health care problems to an understanding of the "why" of the problem. A twenty-first century goal is to continue to expand and carry out a program of psychiatric nursing research as the vehicle to explain the multiple causalities of psychiatric illness.

In *Psychiatric Nursing: Promoting Mental Health*, Ann Burgess and her contributing authors take on this contemporary challenge of applying scientific information about how troubled people think and behave to design psychiatric nursing interventions and strategies for a basic entry level text.

—Hildegard Peplau

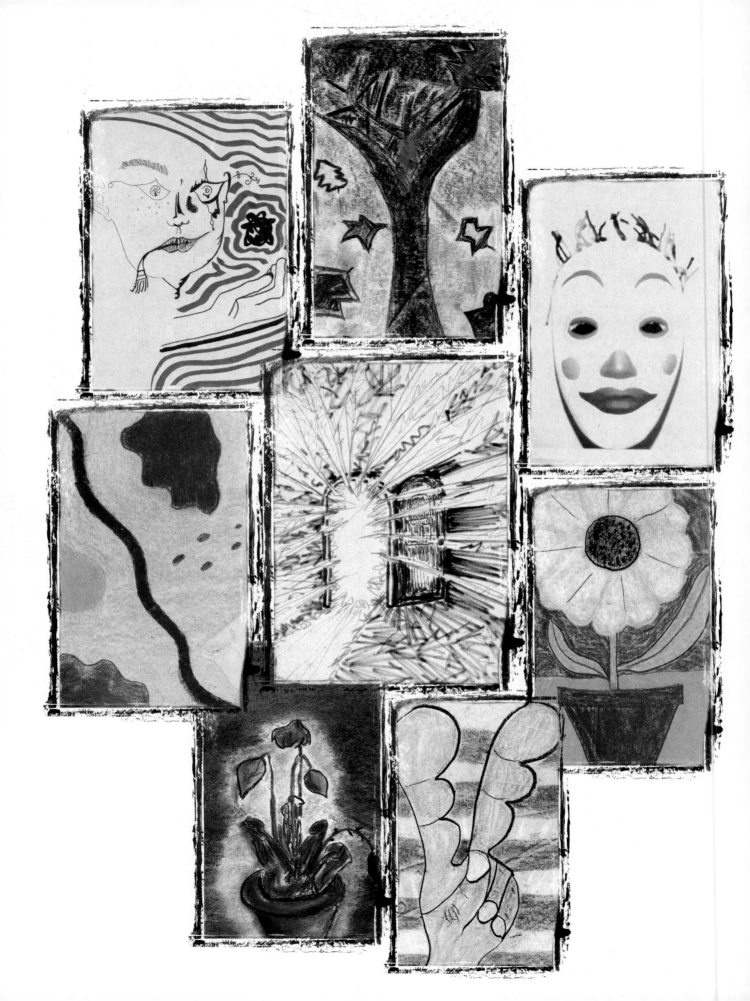

ENTERING THE 21ST CENTURY

Psychiatric nursing involves subtle, complicated clinical situations. To prepare to practice in this field, students are schooled in the biopsychosocial and cultural aspects of mental illness. Student self-examination is another focus of preparation. Students strive to recognize their own feelings—the uncertainties associated with caring for individuals with a mental illness. Their preparation is the foundation for effective therapeutic nurse–patient relationships.

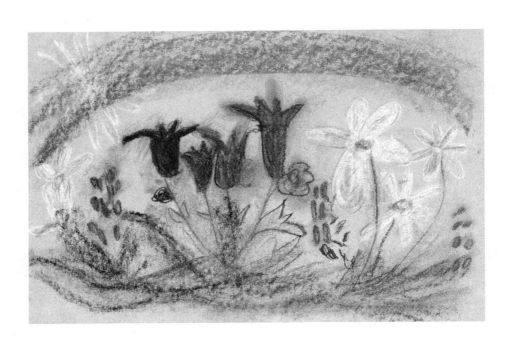

Keep strong, if possible. In any case, keep cool. Have unlimited patience. Never corner an opponent, and always assist him to save his face. Put yourself in his shoes—so as to see things through his eyes. Avoid self-righteousness like the devil—nothing so self-blinding.

Sir Basil Henry Liddell Hart 1895–1970

Deterrent or Defense (1960) *Advice to Statesmen*

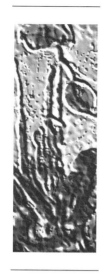

1

Beginning the Psychiatric Nursing Experience

Carol R. Hartman / Ann W. Burgess

Understanding the human dimension is critical in psychiatric mental-health nursing. To accomplish this task, students need to perceive patients as they really are, regardless of the setting in which they are found, and to understand their own reactions to these patients. This chapter identifies common concerns and anxieties of students in the psychiatric mental-health nursing experience, and outlines ways in which they can increase their self-awareness through self-inventory.

■ SELF-INVENTORY

The first step in becoming a psychiatric nurse is to take a personal or **self-inventory.** A personal inventory is based on one's capacity to reflect as objectively as possible on thoughts, feelings, and behaviors. The importance of this inventory is to make a distinction between self and others in order to identify and empathize with what is unique to the patient without projecting one's own misconceptions and emotions onto the patient.

How do we begin to increase our capacity for self-awareness and self-observation? The first exercise is to reflect on your thoughts and feelings in the weeks before your psychiatric nursing experience. Role-play a reporter interviewing yourself, asking questions that relate to beginning and practicing in the psychiatric nursing rotation.

INTERVIEW YOURSELF

Do you have any strong feelings or emotions that come to your awareness when you think of walking into a psychiatric hospital or unit? What are they? Once you know what they are, what images come to mind? For example, a student may say, "I'm frightened!" and then ask, "When I'm frightened, what am I frightened of or about?" The answer may be, "Someone may try to hurt me." The next question to ask is "Who is the person I am afraid will hurt me?" The answer might be, "A male patient." Then ask, "What makes me frightened of a male psychiatric patient?" The answer might be, "I just read of a man who became enraged in court when he was picked up for vagrancy."

The next set of questions to ask include: "What has been my experience with people who have been mentally ill?" The answer might be, "I haven't had any, but I have read stories and my mother is concerned for me."

These responses can be analyzed. The student's feelings are connected with images of situations that could or might have occurred, and the feelings are associated with certain thoughts and information both valid and invalid. Some thoughts and feelings are influenced by what other people think and believe. This leads to the statement, "I'm scared of beginning the psychiatric nursing rotation."

It is common for students to feel frightened and inadequate before beginning a new venture, and to have fantasies and images about the best and the worst experiences. These thoughts can come from stories, past experiences, or stereotypes. It would be unusual for a student to feel calm and assured when beginning the psychiatric nursing experience. To manage such fears and anxieties, factual information must be sought. Mental illness is not contagious, and most mentally ill patients are not violent. Patients' behaviors may differ from the usual norm and may not always fit within a social context, but that difference does not spell violence.

One may argue that there is the possibility of injury in a psychiatric setting. This is true, just as is the possibility of injury or of being assaulted in any other setting. One needs to be oriented to the precursors of aggressive behavior and instructed in behavior directed toward personal safety.

Situations that are strange and different can be frightening and produce stress and anxiety. Yet, at the same time, they may evoke curiosity. There can be a mixture of feelings. The response to self-inventory at this initial stage of the psychiatric nursing experience is to recognize that the situation is strange and different and to acknowledge the feelings of anxiety. This acknowledgment helps you to step back and observe what is going on before moving forward. Is the patient threatening? Is he or she afraid? What is the patient saying that makes you afraid? Can you break the patient's words or behavior down to some sensible understanding of what is presenting you with risk? Is the patient talking in an angry or aggressive tone or using frightening gestures? Or is it that the patient can't modulate his or her tone of voice and tends to be excitable? Is it the tone rather than other aspects of the patient's speech content that is alerting you? As time goes on, you will find that you are more comfortable addressing the behaviors that upset you and communicating this to the patient. For example, you may tell the patient: "When you speak to me in a loud voice and shake your fist, I feel uncomfortable, and I don't know whether to tell you how I feel or to walk away." As time passes and you get to know yourself and others more deeply, you might say, "I notice that you do this with me and other people. Are you frightened? Is this the only way you know in which to tell people not to get too close to you?" A less direct manner may be, "Well, it looks like you don't want to talk at this time; I'll come back later."

PSYCHIATRIC NURSING PRACTICE

In the early clinical days of their psychiatric nursing rotation, students describe feeling awkward, useless, and appearing like beginners. As one student said, "I can't figure out what to do." While some students worry about whether a patient will talk, others wonder what to say or not say to the patient. They wonder about what to

E CASE EXAMPLE

▶ A CONVERSATION

The following interaction initially sounds strange, but understanding the patient's history provides the interpretation for it. A 49-year-old Irish woman, separated from her family for many years because of psychiatric hospitalizations, is visiting her home for the first time in a number of years. She says to the nurse, "Oh, hello. The barbed wire is around me and it's been there for a long time." The nurse responds, "It has been a long time and you have been cut off from seeing me and other people." The patient smiles shyly and says, "Yes, it has been very hard. I'm now in a halfway house."

The nurse knew this mother and wife in earlier phases of the woman's illness. The nurse was familiar with the woman's identification with the liberation causes of her family of origin in Ireland, and she was familiar with the pain and loss experienced by the woman through her years of illness and hospitalizations. Among the tragic experiences was her recovery from a suicidal experience in which the woman threw herself in front of a train and suffered near fatal injuries. When the nurse heard the woman express that "barbed wire" had been around her for a long time, the theme of bondage and pain inflicted by her illness and the terrible loss was partially acknowledged in the nurse's response.

do if they upset the patient. They believe that they have no understanding of how people behave and of the nature of psychological problems.

In one sense, students are beginners; they do not know what to do in many situations, and must learn to deal with the uncertainty of a first experience. In another sense, however, they are not beginners, because they have spent years talking with and listening to people. Friends, patients, and family members, for example, have asked them for psychological help in times of trouble. Moreover, at some time during the students' lives they have undoubtedly experienced their own stresses and problems, and have sometimes shared them with others. Although students do have a great deal to learn during the psychiatric nursing experience, they already have a good start.

Students have questions about how to be a real person to psychiatric patients. Psychiatric patients have their own thoughts and feelings, as well as their own lives. They are frightened by what has happened to them. They feel ashamed, defensive, and misunderstood. They have the basic worries that all people have. They wonder if they can manage their lives and get through a current crisis. They wonder how they appear to other people, and whether they will ever fit in with society. They worry about what others would say if they knew about the patient's mental illness.

Sometimes beginning students feel they cannot talk with a patient until they have read a chart and talked with everyone who knows the patient. This quest for knowledge beyond a comfortable feeling of being able to say "Hello" should be a clue that the student is afraid or blocked in some way from moving forward. This gives students the opportunity to appreciate experienced nurse supervisors. Supervision, a process whereby student and supervisor review the student's clinical work, is not done to analyze the student, but to help with the student's self-inventory assessment.

IDENTIFYING WITH THE PATIENT

Students in any nursing rotation sometimes think they have developed symptoms similar to those of patients. If a patient is depressed and the student begins to feel depressed, the student's feeling may center around the student's belief that he or she should be able to alter the patient's depressed state. Sometimes students are depressed by what they have heard from a patient. Patients sometimes reveal very painful life events so overwhelming that they have come to the hospital for help in coping with them. What becomes clear is that these life events are also overwhelming to anyone hearing about them. This is evident in the case of a woman who has delivered a baby and has also just heard that she has breast cancer. The patient is upset, the doctor who had

to tell her that she has cancer is upset, and the nurse attending the patient is upset. These are natural interactive responses. These strong emotions in relationships with patients often reflect the initial underdeveloped capacity for empathy, an initial phase of identification. This phase leads to the ability to hear such events as part of the life of the patient, for whom the nursing student can have empathy and sympathy; however, the student is simultaneously aware of being a separate person, and need not feel guilty or responsible for the patient's experiences. This becomes the ever-evolving practice and process of developing a capacity for self-awareness. This self-appraisal is essential for any nurse, but is particularly emphasized in psychiatric mental-health nursing because the primary tool for intervention in such nursing is the therapeutic relationship and alliance.

In some situations a student may feel angry, embarrassed, or overwhelmed by a patient. Although such situations are initially uncomfortable, as time passes they become the basis for a true understanding of the interactive human process between the nurse and a patient. These strong emotions can be insights into defensive behavior on the part of the patient as well as self-insight into one's own defensive behavior and prejudices.

Additional questions for self-inventory include:

- Are strong emotions coming from your expectations of appropriate behavior in a particular situation?
- Do you believe that persons who demand much or who keep describing the severity of their depression are simply self-centered and indulging themselves? Asking such questions challenges you to examine your thoughts about self-centeredness and what is wrong with it. If patients are demanding, you are challenged to examine how much you yourself are able to speak up for what you want. Once you have defined your beliefs, you can talk with patients about their repeated depressive thoughts and find out what they are thinking. More importantly, you can ask them if their own behavior can make them more depressed, and if so, what kinds of thoughts and images might have that effect. If they can make themselves more depressed, what would help them to have an image that would make them feel less depressed? What stops them from focusing on images and thoughts that reduce their depression?

What these questions begin to develop in the patient is a capacity to observe internal processes, such as repeated thoughts and images that are associated with either feeling depressed or less depressed. This is a first step in introducing the patient to how their own patterns of thinking influence their emotional responses. Special techniques have been organized in cognitive/behavioral modalities to capitalize on the therapeutic benefits of patients becoming aware of and attending to internal processes which contribute to negative emotional states.

THE DEMANDING PATIENT

The demanding patient can be interesting, complicated, and exasperating. Exasperation comes from some sense of having to take over the patient's own responsibilities. This presents a good example of the need to know yourself and to be able to step back and say, "Look, is this something the patient can do for him- or herself? What is it that I am doing that keeps leading the patient to demand the same thing?" An example involves a patient who telephoned her psychotherapist at 10:45 P.M. and said, "Is it too late to be calling?" The therapist said, "Yes, it is." The patient became angry, swore at the therapist, and slammed down the telephone receiver. The phone rang again two minutes later and the patient complained bitterly that the therapist didn't want to hear that there was an emergency, and then again slammed down the phone. The phone then rang a third time and the patient said that the emergency was about another patient. Three days later, the patient came to the therapist's office with a rose and apologized. It had taken many years to help the patient with these emotional storms of extreme demand, and to help her reflect and regain some balance and focus on her behavior. The point of the vignette is that this patient's major problem was that she wanted people to do things for her even if she could do them for herself. The emotional pain she felt when someone did not attend immediately to what she wanted done for her resulted in many emergency situations for her. She felt so abandoned, unloved, and deserted when she perceived she was not getting what she wanted that she reacted with strong emotion and a deep sense of needing an immediate response. When it was not forthcoming she would go into a defensive rage. This caused great difficulties in her personal relationships and marriage. She would criticize her husband for not bringing water in the correct cup or not brewing the tea the right way. The woman had somehow connected her personal sense of self-worth to what other people did for her. Moreover, she believed that if they really loved her, they would know what she wanted without her asking for it. To do things for herself made her feel separate from others, which she experienced as terrifying rather than as accompanied by a sense of competency and mastery. This is a complicated example of demanding behavior, but one that creates curiosity about some of the most annoying behaviors that psychiatric nurses experience in working with patients.

ON THE SPOT

Students who observe interactions on a psychiatric unit will note that patients say things to staff members that put the latter "on the spot." Such statements seem to elicit embarrassment, guilt, or excessive self-consciousness on the part of the staff members. In general, these are responses that show discomfort and social distress. When a student becomes the focus of this patient strategy, it can be rather perplexing and overwhelming. An example involves a young attractive graduate student, who was also a nun and was interviewing her first male patient in a psychiatric service. Not more than five minutes into the initial interview, this elderly man began detailed discussions of sexual encounters and sexual problems. With each statement, the young nun became increasingly blushed. When she discussed this with her instructor, she was distressed, and as she attempted to repeat what was said to her, her distress was noted in her deep, intense blushing. Reading about this episode probably arouses anxiety in students as they realize that the same thing could happen to them.

How are this interaction and patient to be understood? When two persons sit down to talk with one another, there transpire various levels of information that are intended to set a level of closeness or distance between the two communicants. If, for whatever reasons, one wishes to be distant or possibly to push away the other, he or she will employ various strategies (behavioral and verbal) and evaluate the other's response to them. Did the strategy work to engage or to distance the other person? Although it is inadvisable to assume the intentions of others, the nurse is not restricted in expressing perplexity over a patient's behavior. A nurse may ask about the patient's intentions, particularly if the nurse feels like withdrawing from the relationship. Clarifying the intentions of the patient can be instructive to both the patient and the nurse, thus aborting distance in the nurse–patient relationship. In the example, bringing forth an open acknowledgment of the sexualized behavior and its potential of driving the nurse away could open up the patient to recognizing how embarrassing it is to have a nun talking with him or his resentment toward women in general. In the example of the nurse-nun given above, we could speculate about the patient's intentions, but the appropriate response would be a frank acknowledgment that the nature of his presentation was eliciting embarrassment on the part of the nurse-nun. What was the patient attempting to convey in discussing these matters with the nurse? This is not simply a question of being prudish about sexual issues, but is rather a question of attending to the context and process in which the issues arose. Could the patient have been angry at the church represented by the nun? Was he attempting to express frustration over possible hypocrisy? Was he nondiscerning and lacking a capacity to monitor his own impulsive experiences and feelings? Was he attempting to embarrass the nun-student because he himself felt embarrassed in the situation? These are all possibilities, and there are many more.

The supervisor assured the student nurse that her reactions had occurred in the context of certain behaviors on the part of the patient. It was suggested to the student that the best approach for her next meeting with patient would be to explore his thoughts of meeting: (1) with the student, (2) with a young woman, (3) with a nun, and (4) with a person younger than he. All of these obvious dimensions could have contributed to his need to detail sexual material. Indeed, when the student did raise these questions during her next session with the patient, he expressed useful information about his feelings and motivations in meeting with her. He acknowledged that her youth and attractiveness had caught him by surprise, and he wondered how she could be sufficiently experienced to understand him. He then asked why she had become a nun. The student then felt "on the spot," not only because the material expressed to her remained tainted with sexualized innuendoes, but also because it challenged her motivations. In short, the patient consistently turned the focus of the interview onto the nursing student.

The supervisory process reveals the defensive and transferential qualities of the patient's reaction to the student. First, he did not wish to focus on himself, second, he sought continually to keep the student in an uncomfortable position. At its roots, the patient's behavior may have reflected long-standing patterns of feeling exploited and retaliating for this by becoming the exploiter. This latter hypothesis might gain potential merit as one learned more about the lifelong history of the patient's interaction patterns. Again, what is important is that through supervision and being "put on the spot," students learn how to separate themselves and their personal reactions from the patient. The student then learns the more complex issue of dealing with repetitive defensive styles on the part of others. This task takes years of experience, supervision, and additional training. For the beginning nurse, it is helpful to operate from the premise that a patient's behavior represents his or her best available patterns of reacting to situations, and that the effectiveness of these patterns is determined by how well the patient is able to function in life. For the man described above, the patient's pattern of behavior was obviously not serving him well.

SAYING THE WRONG THING

Saying the wrong thing puts one in the best position to learn something. Unfortunately, many persons feel that

E CASE EXAMPLE

▶ SAYING THE WRONG THING

A woman in her late fifties comes to an outpatient setting for clinical evaluation. She is extremely distressed, and keeps saying that her heart is being torn apart. Although the patient's point of distress is a current crisis in which her beloved son, who was an accountant, has been accused of taking money from his place of employment, she also has a cardiac disorder and hypertension. Her son's position is that he has not taken the money, and that the company's books had been altered by the employer. Because there was no way of substantiating this in court, the son was sent to prison. His mother is agitated and not sleeping or eating. She worries constantly about him. In the outpatient setting, the nurse responds, "It is very depressing to go through all this." The patient reacts with, "I'm not depressed. There is nothing wrong with me. My heart is being torn apart." The nurse quickly recognizes that her choice of language and understanding of the patient have failed to correspond in any way with what the patient was telling her. The nurse had jumped to a clinical conclusion without sufficiently translating the patient's language and experiences into the clinical picture the patient is presenting. The

nurse quickly recognizes this and immediately says, "Your heart is being torn apart." The woman clutches her chest, tears come to her eyes, and she says "Yes."

The nurse then reconstructs what the patient had said, carefully using the sequence and language that the patient had used in talking about her son and about her reaction to what was going on. As this progresses, the patient becomes calmed, and rapport is re-established. When the patient completes her expression of distress, the nurse, carefully using the patient's own language, talks about depression being a clinical term that relates to the patient's lack of sleeping and eating, weight loss, inability to concentrate, and preoccupation. This opens the door to a more thorough clinical evaluation of the patient, who is basically looking for someone to free her son from prison. This reality and the limitation of the nurse in the clinic have to be faced and shared with the patient. The resources available at the clinic could assist her in getting legal assistance to help clarify her son's situation and what she could do about it. The nurse is able to convey to the woman that her son would be concerned that her worrying might make her ill.

they must be right all the time, which keeps them from learning anything. On page 7 is an example of an experienced nurse who spoke wrongly in the context of a particular situation.

HURTING THE PATIENT

While assessing patients, students often become concerned about hurting them. What in the assessment concerns or frightens the student? Often it is the fundamental questions posed during the initial assessment; those that seek to ascertain the kind of control the patient has over impulses and whether he or she is oriented to reality. Such questions may include: "Have you ever thought of hurting yourself? When did you think about it? How you would do it? Do you feel that you would do it? What stops you? Can you agree not to hurt yourself?" A student's concern with this kind of question is: "Am I suggesting an action?" The answer is basically "No."

Such questions become a normal, expected part of an assessment, to the extent that you can understand self-destructive behavior as an option that some people consider but that not all are aware of considering. The ability to comfortably ask about self-destructive thoughts and behaviors conveys the insight that suicidal ideation is not a foreign experience in people who are emotionally upset, and makes it easier for the patient to open about such thoughts, actions, and personal commitments to either life or death. Exceptions, of course, are found. Some persons do not think that suicidal ideation is something that comes consciously to mind. The nurse must be alert to this kind of thinking and to some of the reasons why people are not aware of self-destructive thoughts. Religious teachings about suicide, for example, might cause such guilt in a person (e.g., one who has a loving family) that the person could not admit having such thoughts. In more complex situations, aggression and self-destructive behavior are so repressed in an individual's experiential and behavioral response that the individual is totally unaware of this potential behavior. The fear of hurting the patient arises for some students in asking patients about their sexual behavior, or about punching, hitting, kicking, or fighting. Students think that direct questions about sex and aggression may encourage a guilty response or in some way cause embarrassment or shame. Another sensitive interview area involves asking about previous interpersonal traumatic events in the patient's life. In this type of inquiry, the nurse must again be comfortable realizing that these events are possibilities in any person's life, and that someone is not unique in having experienced such events. When the nurse inquires about such events, using detailed descriptive behaviors, rather than labels such as physical or sexual abuse, patients can more easily respond to such traumatic events as life experiences. For example, a young woman undergoing an evaluation conveyed she had a deviated septum from a broken nose. The nurse asked how her nose had been broken. The young woman said that when she had been an adolescent, her father, during a verbal altercation, had punched her in the nose and broken it. The nurse and patient then talked about the hitting and punching that went on between the patient and her father. It turned out that the patient had been brutally spanked, restrained, screamed at, and beaten by her father on many occasions. The nurse did not say anything at the time, but in later sessions raised the question of whether that patient's father had physically abused her. The patient replied that that could not have happened. The nurse asked why and the patient replied: "Because we're Jewish and Jewish fathers aren't physically abusive." There was a moment of silence, and a profound shock of awareness, as well as curiosity, came over the patient. She said, "I had never really thought of it as abuse but it does make some sense." At the next session the patient reported to the nurse that she had discussed the various incidents of beating with her father and that he had confirmed them. He had also apologized.

■ INCREASING SELF-AWARENESS

How do nurses enhance their self-awareness as a clinical tool? They may increase self-awareness through involvement in relationships with others and by reading and writing.

INVOLVEMENT IN RELATIONSHIPS

Communication with others and involvement in relationships are important ways to learn about oneself. One's first **social network**—the family—is a primary learning arena. Family relationships provide some of the most enduring lessons in self-awareness. The second social network system—the school—provides additional lessons relating to authority figures. One can learn through relationships with teachers and mentors. Teachers usually assume positions of influence to the degree that the student allows the influence process to develop. In nursing, the student–supervisor relationship can be an influential avenue for self-awareness. Another valuable influential relationship is that with a mentor. A mentor is a guide who supports, facilitates, and promotes the intellectual and career development of another person. Sometimes an instructor or supervisor becomes a mentor. The mentor's expertise and caring are a powerful combination in guiding the nurse's growth in self-knowledge. Lessons learned in these various relationships are modified by subsequent life experiences that usually include other deep and lasting relationships.

Counseling and therapy are additional ways to learn about oneself. A nurse who is in therapy or counseling can learn self-inventory. Alternatively, nursing students may elect to work with a therapist to learn how to be more effective in therapeutic relationships with patients. Through this exchange, the nurse creates an opportunity to gain greater self-awareness, a more positive regard for self, and personal characteristics that increase effectiveness in working with patients.

READING

Reading is a second route to self-awareness. Through the formal study of psychiatric mental-health nursing, students are exposed to written ideas about clinical practice. The habit of reading should always be encouraged. Reading fiction and nonfiction helps one learn about human nature as well as about oneself. Books portray human lives in terms of human struggles and emotions and the ways in which people relate themselves to others. Autobiographies are rich sources of detail about personal experiences.

WRITING A DIARY

A third route for enhancing self-awareness is writing a diary, journal, or log. The student can write completely unstructured notes as sporadically or regularly as desired to gain the most benefit from personal experience.

Process recording is a more formal method of writing that helps students deal more effectively with clients. Process recordings are descriptions and analyses of interactions with patients. Various formats may be used, but the record usually includes a verbatim account of nurse–patient communication. Process recordings contribute to the effectiveness of clinical supervision. Over time, at regular intervals, they can be reviewed and summarized to document major patterns or themes and the overall progress of the nurse–patient interaction.

O AN OVERVIEW

- Nursing students must learn to appreciate the value of self-inventory.
- Lack of self-awareness may result in transgression and error in practice.
- Self-awareness affects the therapeutic relationship—the major vehicle for therapy.

TD TERMS TO DEFINE

- patient reactions, demands
- routes toward self-awareness
- self-inventory
- social networks

Q STUDY QUESTIONS

1. List all of the thoughts you have concerning your knowledge that you will use in your work with psychiatric patients. Examine how these thoughts and expectations have come to you.

2. List five ways you can deal with your fearful thoughts.

3. List experiences that have increased your sense of awareness of your own behavior.

4. List situations in which your lack of self-awareness caused difficulties for you and others.

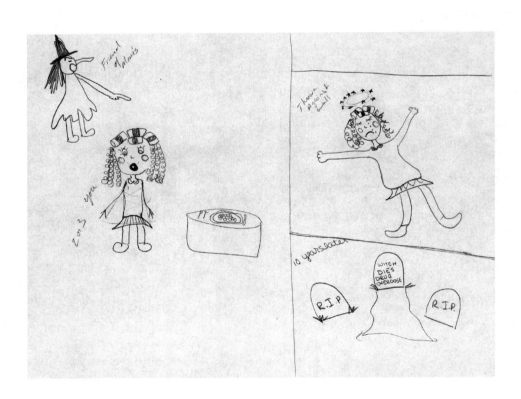

The poets and philosophers before me discovered the unconscious; what I discovered was the scientific method by which the unconscious can be studied.

Sigmund Freud
On his seventieth birthday
(1926); from Lionel
Trilling's *The Liberal Imagination*
Nicomachean Ethics Bk. I, ch. 1

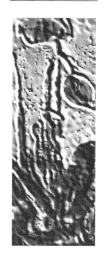

2

Psychiatric Nursing

Ann W. Burgess

The field of psychiatric mental-health nursing is on an expanding, productive trajectory as we approach the 21st century. Influenced by the rapid expansion of biological sciences and technology, psychiatric mental-health nurses are in an advantageous position to address the re-integration of physical and psychosocial care for persons with mental illness (McBride, 1993). Psychiatric nursing practice is being revitalized with the emphasis on the connections among brain, spirit, mind, and body.

Rapid change in the delivery of mental-health services has resulted in the need for psychiatric mental-health nurses to provide primary mental-health care. Nurses remain alert to opportunities to promote mental health and detect and intervene in situations of increased stress, developmental crises, family crises, and traumatic and catastrophic stress, which often predispose people to mental illness (ANA, 1994).

■ DEFINITION

The **Statement on Psychiatric Mental Health Clinical Nursing Practice** defines psychiatric mental health nursing as the diagnosis and treatment of human responses to actual or potential mental-health problems. Psychiatric mental-health nursing is a specialized area of nursing practice employing neurobiological principles and theories of human behavior as its science and purposeful use of the self as its art (ANA, 1994).

■ PHENOMENA OF CONCERN

Psychiatric mental-health nursing is particularly focused on 12 areas called **phenomena of concern,** as follows:

- The maintenance of optimal health and well being and the prevention of psychobiological illness.
- Self-care limitations or impaired functioning related to mental and emotional distress.
- Deficits in the functioning of significant biological, emotional, and cognitive systems.
- Emotional stress or crisis components of illness, pain, and disability.
- Self-concept changes, developmental issues, and life-process changes.
- Problems related to emotions such as anxiety, anger, sadness, loneliness, and grief.
- Physical symptoms that occur along with altered psychological functioning.
- Alterations in thinking, perceiving, symbolizing, communicating, and decision making.
- Difficulties in relating to others.
- Behaviors and mental states that indicate the client is a danger to self or others, or has a severe disability.
- Interpersonal, sociocultural, spiritual, or environmental circumstances or events that affect the mental and emotional well-being of the individual, family, or community.
- Symptom management, side effects and/or toxicity associated with psychopharmacological intervention and other aspects of a treatment regimen.

Legislation has changed the level of skills employed by an advanced practice specialist in psychiatric nursing. For example, prescriptive authority is now granted in many states. Although it is exciting to know about the many advances in the field, it is important to review the history of psychiatric nursing and acknowledge the leaders in the profession whose efforts have brought us to this juncture.

■ THE ROOTS OF TREATING THE MENTALLY ILL

THE SUPERNATURAL MODEL OF HEALING

The earliest known method of treating the mentally ill may be described as the supernatural or mystical model of healing. Since the beginning of humankind, behavior has been in part explained by supernatural powers. It was a normal consequence of this method of thinking to interpret the behavior of the mentally ill as being caused by demons, malevolent gods, witches, werewolves, vampires, the movement of planets, and changes in the atmosphere. In Babylon, more than three thousand years ago, the power of spirits and how they could possess a person was central to the writings of the Akkadians. Similar notions are revealed in the mythologies of the Far East. For example, it was believed that the fox could re-create itself as a supernatural power, enter the body of a man or woman, and induce madness. Other cultures also had their feared animals. The most feared and widely acknowledged power, even today, is that of the devil. The devil is also known by such names as Satan and Lucifer.

Demonology was the primary causal premise in the study of mental illness during the Middle Ages. Out of this literature and within the context of religious practices came the ritual of exorcism. An example of a pseudomedical procedure in some cultures, such as the ore in Egypt, was trephining. In this procedure, a portion of the skull was removed, thus allowing evil spirits to escape. Evidence of this practice was noted when skulls with holes drilled in them (trepa) were found far from city limits.

In 1257, St. Mary of Bethlehem Hospital was founded in London. Its principal function was to incarcerate a diverse group of social misfits: vagrants, prostitutes, criminals, feeble-minded persons, and the mad. The hospital became known as "Bedlam" and its residents were known as "Bedlamites." Their treatment included chaining of the hands and ankles, beatings, forced nakedness, bleedings, isolation, and public ridicule and mockery. To outsiders, Bedlam was a circus, a place of entertainment where people could spend a Sunday afternoon laughing and teasing the Bedlamites, and all for the price of a shilling (Bromberg, 1975).

The purpose for pointing out the inhumane conditions that existed in these times is to help students appreciate the significance of the reforms the conditions eventually provoked. Inhumane and unethical practices still persist, and even today court cases are attempting to deal with the constitutionality of involuntary commitment and forced treatment.

In 1486 the Handbook for Witch-Hunters was published as *The Malleus Maleficarum*. This was a sinister guide to inhumanity and terror written by two respected scholars of the time, Johann Sprenger, Dean of Cologne University, and Heinrich Kraemer, who held high offices in the church. There were three sections of the book, each dealing with a specific task for the judge or hangman. The first section stressed the enormity of witchcraft and sought to raise in the reader a sense of fear and hatred toward witches. Biblical quotes and commandments demonstrated that God strongly opposed witches and wished for their extermination. The second section included methods of identifying possession by a witch and counteracting its effects. The third section concerned itself with procedures for examining and passing sentence on the witch. To be absolutely sure that the person was a witch, the prosecutors always had to get a confession. The confession was obtained by torture (e.g., thumb screws, whipping, or pressing the accused into a spiked chair). After the confession the person was burned alive with green firewood, causing a slow and agonizing death. Between 1603 and 1628, it is estimated that this practice took the lives of about 70,000 people in England, 100,000 people in Germany, and 200,000 people throughout the rest of Europe (Robbins, 1959). No wonder this period of time was called the Dark Ages.

THE CUSTODIAL MODEL OF HEALING

A model of healing the mentally ill that replaced the mystical mode was described as the custodial method. The decline of demonology began when the Greek physician Hippocrates suggested that mental disorders probably had their origin in some brain dysfunction. In turn, he proposed that the brain might be affected by various imbalances of body fluids such as bile and blood. Hippocrates developed one of the early classification systems for mental disorders, which included encephalitis, then called phrenitis, as well as mania and melancholia. He advocated therapeutic procedures quite apart from the magical procedures used for expelling spirits. For example, rest, a good diet, exercise, and other therapies unusual for this time were prescribed. Hippocrates' classification system represented advanced thinking as well as humane treatment methods for the mentally disturbed. After this period ended, however, two major trends emerged in which there was vigorous use of the supernatural to explain mental disturbances and an increase in inhumane treatment for the mentally ill.

In response to some of the cruel aspects of such treatment, there emerged *moral management* through the efforts of Philippe Pinel in France, William Tuke in England, and Dorothea Dix in the United States. Morality was conceived in terms of the practices of treating people, and humane treatment for the mentally disturbed was emphasized.

Pinel's "Memoir on Madness" was read to the Society for Natural History in Paris on December 11, 1794, soon after the fall of the Jacobean dictatorship in the French Revolution. It is therefore a political document, an appeal to the Revolutionary government to build asylums where the mentally ill could be decently treated. Pinel (1745–1826) served as "physician of the infirmaries" at Bicetre, the public hospital for men from 1773–1775. In his paper, he explains the principles of the humane treatment that made him the founder of psychiatry in France. Pinel states that mental illness is often curable. To arrive at a diagnosis, he instructs the clinician to carefully observe a patient's behavior, interview the patient, listen carefully, and take notes. The natural history of the patient's disorder and the precipitating event are needed in order to write an accurate case history, following which diagnosis and prognosis can be made. Pinel's assistant, Jean Baptiste Pussin, removed the chains from the insane men at Bicetre and replaced them with straightjackets. Pinel followed suit at the Salpetriere, the public hospital for women, in 1801. Later, Pinel states that one must "dominate agitated madmen while respecting human rights" (Weiner, 1992).

William Tuke (1732–1822) was a Quaker tea merchant who devoted much of the latter part of his life to bringing humanitarian reform to the lunatic asylums of England. In 1792 Tuke founded the Retreat at York, which provided care to about 30 mentally ill patients. The patients were treated as guests, and manual labor and occupational therapy were considered beneficial.

Dorothea Lynde Dix (1802–1887), a former schoolteacher, began her humanitarian work in mental health care in America in 1841. After observing the suffering of jailed "lunatics," she advocated proper care of the mentally ill. Rather than working with patients, she went directly to legislators and the President. As a result of her efforts, over 30 mental hospitals were changed and a new wave of concern followed. Dix has been credited with being one of the greatest social reformers in American history.

■ NURSING CARE OF THE MENTALLY ILL

During the 18th century, most persons now identifiable as mentally ill were cared for in their own homes or boarded out with families at private or public expense. Others were housed in jails, poorhouses, workhouses, and houses of correction. Indiscriminate segregation of the mentally ill among groups who were socially unacceptable and for the most part economically dependent reflected the level of understanding of the nature of emotional disorders (Deutsch, 1949).

In the 19th century, the mentally ill were collected into groups and someone was paid to keep watch over them. Thus developed the model of custodial care, supported financially by private and community efforts.

This particular model developed from necessity because families could not bear the full responsibility for managing the care of their mentally ill members. At this time, mental difficulties were considered irreversible, so protecting society from the mentally disturbed therefore took precedence over other treatment models. Thus, mental institutions operated on the concept of detention rather than treatment.

State institutions soon became overcrowded. The goal of the custodial role was to keep patients safe, guard them, and manage them. The premise was that they were incapable of managing their own lives.

Mental hospitals during this era functioned autocratically, rendering patients helpless by their treatment. Patients were seen as defective, incompetent, and potentially dangerous. Rights were denied them and they were considered incapable citizens in society. The patient was forced into an institutional mode of behavior. Families were discouraged from taking an active role in treatment, and were often discouraged from visiting patients in state institutions. The stigma of mental illness was communicated to the patient. Social isolation and forced conformity to the needs of the institution prevailed.

The institution did provide custodial care of shelter, food, and rest. Mentally ill patients increasingly lost their options, interacted mainly with other mentally ill patients, and dealt with an untrained and frequently punitive staff. Consequently, patients became more institutionalized, more chronically ill, and less able to return to their families and communities.

The introduction of organized nursing into hospital settings initiated major change in the care of the mentally ill. The Nightingale model of training was brought to America from England in 1873. In May of that year the Bellevue Hospital School of Nursing in New York City began to train nurses in the Nightingale method of nursing; in October the Connecticut Training School opened; and in November the Boston Training School began. Linda Richards, one of America's first trained nurses, believed that the mentally ill person also needed nursing care. This belief led to her initiative to create schools of nursing in state hospitals. In 1882, Richards worked with Edward Cowles, the med-

ical director at the McLean Hospital in Belmont, Massachusetts, to begin the first psychiatric nurse training school in the United States. By 1890 this two-year program had graduated 90 nurses. The value of this school was so quickly appreciated that within 10 years 19 American institutions were providing psychiatric nurse training programs.

In 1886, McLean Hospital took another step forward and established an affiliation with the Massachusetts General Hospital whereby credit for a full nursing course was given upon completion of a student's senior year at McLean Hospital. In England a similar program was in effect, and a certificate was given to the nursing graduates by the Medico-Psychological Association.

Despite these promising beginnings, by the end of the 19th century the vast majority of professional nurses who worked in psychiatric hospitals had little or no training in psychiatry. For the most part, they adapted their training in the physical care of psychiatric patients, helping to administer medications and hydrotherapy and to maintain hygiene. Their effectiveness was enhanced by their kindness and understanding, but there was no systematic program of psychiatric nursing care.

The greatest problem in the development of psychiatric nursing in America was that there seemed to be little demand for the so-called "asylum-trained" nurse. By 1916, half of the mental hospitals in the United States still had no schools for their nurses. These hospitals employed attendants at very low wages and provided very poor living conditions for nurses. About 40 mental institutions, however, were operating some sort of training school for their nurses, although the standards for admission and graduation were much lower than those for schools of nursing in general hospitals. During this time nurse educators were working toward establishing psychiatric nursing affiliations for students enrolled in schools of nursing in general hospitals, but this goal was not realized until later in the 20th century. It is no wonder that nursing of the mentally ill was so slow in catching on.

By 1935, only half of the then-existing diploma schools of nursing offered psychiatric nursing in their curriculum. Although the first textbook about psychiatric nursing, Harriet Bailey's *Nursing Mental Diseases*, was published in 1920 by the Macmillan Company in New York, its educational value was largely ignored. Psychiatric nursing was not a requirement for state licensing until as late as 1952.

Until 1946, nursing leaders pioneering in psychiatric care worked primarily with long-hospitalized psychotic patients—the patient population left untreated or even unattended in some institutions. These nurses provided general nursing care for the mentally ill with minimal financial return. Wages were extremely low, and many nurses with advanced academic education had to settle for room, board, and uniforms. This is the heritage and backbone of the kind of nurse who aided mental healing in the first half of the 20th century (Doona, 1978).

Although its historical roots can be traced over a period of several centuries, psychiatric mental-health nursing's current position as a specialty area in nursing and as a mental health profession really started in 1946. That year marked the passage of the Mental Health Act, which provided federal funds for the support of psychiatric nursing at both the undergraduate and graduate levels.

■ DEVELOPMENTS IN PSYCHIATRIC NURSING SINCE 1946

POLITICAL-LEGISLATIVE DEVELOPMENTS

In the 1940s and 1950s, a series of political-legislative developments significantly influenced the advancement of the psychiatric field in general and psychiatric nursing in particular. The Mental Health Act of 1946 provided training funds for psychiatric nurses, psychiatrists, psychologists, and psychiatric social workers. It also provided research funds and grants-in-aid to all of the states for clinic and service components. In 1949, the National Institute of Mental Health was established to begin to identify and promote goals and priorities for the mental-health field. During the early 1950s, public concern for the mentally ill continued to grow as the conditions in state mental hospitals were exposed.

In 1955, President Dwight Eisenhower signed into law the Mental Health Study Act, thus establishing a Joint Commission on Mental Health and Illness. The commission's charge was to analyze and re-evaluate the human and economic problems of mental illness, and to recommend actions. After extensive analysis and evaluation of the needs and resources available to the mentally ill, the Joint Commission published *Action for Mental Health,* a report that laid the groundwork for the further development of national mental-health policy (1961). This report placed a strong emphasis on community-based services and called for a reduction in patient population through the closing of large state hospitals; the development of mental health services in local communities; and the upgrading of quality of care in the remaining state hospitals so that patients could be returned as quickly as possible to their own communities (1961). The recommendations set into motion a major change in the mental-health field and resulted in an emphasis on the development of community-based services as opposed to large, inpatient facilities as the loci of treatment. The main thrust of this change was

prevention-oriented, and federal regulations mandated that mental-health services be provided to specific areas with population-defined, geographic groups. A full range of services was offered, including psychiatric nursing. Within this clinical atmosphere, nurses had considerable opportunities to implement new roles.

In 1963, President John F. Kennedy signed into law the Community Mental Health Centers Act, which authorized money for the construction of community mental-health centers. However, financial assistance to communities for the development of services was not provided until 1965, when Congress amended the Community Mental Health Centers Act to include initial staffing grants for professional and nonprofessional personnel. It was proposed that staffing grants be funded for a relatively short period (51 months). Theoretically, community mental-health centers would be self-sufficient by the end of the staffing grant period. By the late 1960s, however, it was clear that the majority of the nation's community mental-health centers would not be self-sufficient within the 51-month time frame. Therefore, Public Law 91-211 was passed by Congress in 1970 to extend the staffing grants for another eight years. Then, in 1975, Congress amended PL 91-211 with PL 94-63, which authorized funds to create new community mental-health centers and to continue existing centers.

The next major mental health legislation grew out of the 1978 *Report to the President from the President's Commission on Mental Health* (1978). This report recommended the development of mental-health services throughout the country that would be responsive to changing circumstances and to diverse cultural and racial backgrounds, with:

- Adequate funding from the public and private sector to finance services.
- Assurances that appropriately trained personnel would be made available.
- Provision of services for populations with special needs such as children, adolescents, and the elderly.
- Establishment of a national priority to meet the needs of the chronically mentally ill.
- Coordination of mental-health services with other health and human service agencies and with personal and community support systems.
- Extension of the knowledge base of psychiatric care with respect to treatment.
- Focus on the prevention of mental illness.
- Assurances that freedom of choice be guaranteed.

The recommendations of the report were implemented through the Community Mental Health Centers Extension Act, which was signed into law by President Jimmy

Carter in 1978. This law addressed the recommendations of the Commission on Mental Health. In the interim, President Ronald Reagan was elected. His attitudes and policies regarding the funding mechanisms for social programs, including mental health, were vastly different from those of his predecessor. The Reagan Administration was committed to decentralizing the disbursement of funds from a federal to a state level, and to increasing the involvement and financial commitment of the private sector to social programs. Consequently, the Community Mental Health Centers Extension Act of 1978 was never fully implemented.

This bitterly contested issue included extensive lobbying efforts by mental-health professionals and organizations, and the act was finally replaced by the Omnibus Reconciliation Act, which was signed into law by President Reagan in 1981. The Omnibus Reconciliation Act created a block-grant mechanism for direct funding to states for the provision of mental-health services; considerable discretion was left to the states about how the funds were to be spent. In addition, the amount of financial support provided by the government for mental-health services was reduced. This clearly reversed the strong federal governmental role in providing mental-health services for the people of the nation; the intent was to strengthen states' and communities' commitment to their people.

From among these various political-legislative developments between 1946 and the 1980s, one of importance to psychiatric nursing was the recommendations made in the President's Commission on Mental Health (1978) report about who shall provide mental-health services. The report clearly identified psychiatric nurses as members of the interdisciplinary mental-health team, and stated that they should be eligible for third-party reimbursement for services.

EDUCATION OF NURSES IN PSYCHIATRIC NURSING

The Second World War profoundly affected psychiatric nursing. Nurses returning from service were eligible under the GI Bill for advanced education. The three existing graduate programs leading to a masters degree in nursing were unable to meet the demand. The passage of the National Mental Health Act of 1946, enacted in response to the overwhelming numbers of psychiatric casualties encountered both in the type of person entering the service and in response to combat, provided funds for graduate education in nursing, psychiatry, psychology, and social work. The funding influenced the scope and direction of nursing and psychiatric nursing education (Critchley, 1985). The legislation encouraged nurses to fill a wide variety of roles, especially because of the shortage of staff to care for the mentally ill. Psychiatric nurses Theresa G. Muller and Hildegard

Peplau were instrumental in shifting the physician-directed psychiatric nursing practice toward a theory-based nursing practice. Muller was influential in obtaining recognition of nursing as the fourth professional discipline in mental health. She established four of the early programs leading to a masters degree in psychiatric nursing at Catholic University in Washington, D.C., Boston University, Indiana University, and the University of Nebraska. She emphasized the need for graduate education and interdisciplinary preparation as a means of establishing collaborative practice. Clinical practice, rather than functional specialization, was a clear emphasis in these programs (Muller, 1950; Johnston and Fitzpatrick, 1982).

Another major impetus for psychiatric nursing resulted from a study by the National League for Nursing in 1950, which concluded that special training was required for psychiatric nursing. This report coincided with the renewed interest in psychiatric care precipitated by the Second World War.

DOCTORAL NURSING EDUCATION

Doctoral education in nursing gained momentum in 1955 when the United States Public Health Service, through the National Institutes of Health (NIH), initiated the Special Pre-doctoral Research Fellowships, which could be used to finance doctoral education. Fellowships were awarded directly to students. A second program, the Nurse Scientist Training Program, provided grants to schools of nursing. These funds were used to finance doctoral (Ph.D.) education for nurses in disciplines related to nursing. One intent of the program was to help build a core of faculty who would be prepared to develop doctoral programs in nursing. In 1960 there were only four doctoral programs, making opportunities for nurses to pursue doctoral study truly scarce. Teachers College at Columbia University in New York City offered a doctorate of education (Ed.D.) in nursing; this program was the oldest and most well established, having been started in the 1920s. The University of Pittsburgh established a Ph.D. program in 1954. In 1960, Boston University established a program that awarded the doctorate in nursing science (D.N.Sc.) in psychiatric mental-health nursing, and New York University began offering a Ph.D. in nursing. As predicted, the Special Pre-doctoral Fellowships and the Nurse Scientist Training Program were successful, since both provided opportunities for education and financial support that had not been available previously. It is estimated that more than 500 nurses received support through these programs. Nicoll (1986) observed two indicators of the success of these training programs. First, many nurses who received support through these programs have continued to be very active in nursing, contributing through research, practice, and publication. Second, a core of scholars were prepared to take on the task of developing doctoral programs in nursing. These programs have been implemented in many colleges and universities.

■ CONTEMPORARY DIMENSIONS OF PSYCHIATRIC NURSING

THE PSYCHIATRIC NURSE AS A CLINICIAN

From the sensitivity and exploration that are parts of the one-to-one relationship between today's psychiatric nurse and a patient, the nurse has gained both depth and scope in exploring the power of relationship and communication in the total healing and health-maintenance processes. The psychiatric nurse engages not only in interesting and compelling collaboration with individuals and their problems, but with individuals and larger groups involved in maintaining and protecting positive mental health. Psychiatric nurses are actively involved in innovative efforts at the three levels of nursing practice: (1) primary preventive intervention to educate about mental health risks before illness occurs; (2) secondary preventive intervention to treat mental illness as quickly as it is diagnosed; and (3) tertiary preventive intervention to minimize the effects of long-term or chronic psychiatric illness.

In primary preventive intervention, psychiatric nurses may be involved in all types of educational programs, such as violence prevention. The scope of psychiatric nursing involvement in secondary preventive intervention is extensive, ranging from setting up crisis teams for natural disasters to using home visits to help family members cope with illness or devastating tragedy. In the tertiary area, nurses are active in such community projects as arranging for the homeless and working with self-help groups to pass active legislation to protect the interests of severely mentally ill and retarded people. A major advance has been the participation by psychiatric mental-health nurses in the psychiatric home-care, case-management, and private practice models of health-care delivery. In many states, psychiatric nurses are now reimbursed through the patient's insurance benefits.

THE PSYCHIATRIC NURSE AS A RESEARCHER

Nursing research, which has long been considered an integral part of nursing practice, is critical to all subspecialties. An era of intense research and theory development is unfolding. The specialty of psychiatric mental-health nursing has contributed significantly to the present maturity of the nursing profession, and there is every reason to believe that it will continue to be on the cutting edge of progress in nursing. Practice-based research has been a dominant method of psychiatric nursing research. The 1950s witnessed dramatic progress. In 1952 psychiatric nurse Gwen Tudor Will reported her study on psychosocial nursing in an inpatient hospital setting. The thesis of the Tudor article was that the social milieu of a psychiatric ward operated to maintain deviant patient behavior. While working with sociologists over a six-month period exploring the social dimension of psychiatric care, Tudor observed that a discrete pattern of mutual avoidance emerged between the staff and a female patient. After making notes of her observation, Tudor initiated her intervention. Gradually she began to disrupt the pattern of withdrawal by initiating conversation with the patient, moving closer to her, and eventually engaging her in activity. Not only did Tudor's pattern with the woman change, but so did the response of other staff members and patients. To test her concept of "mutuality" with regard to social withdrawal, Tudor supervised a nursing student's intervention with the patient and the pattern of withdrawal was reversed. The study's importance was to challenge the notion that social withdrawal was a sign of mental illness. It was seen instead as a behavior sensitive in its development and maintenance to the social context. The study that emphasized the critical role of the nurse in managing the social milieu of the ward environment was conducted before psychotropic drugs had been initiated for the treatment of psychiatric illness (Tudor, 1952).

Gertrude Schwing's *The Way to the Soul of the Mentally Ill* became available to nurses (after translation) in 1954 in the United States. Her work and Sechehaye's *Symbolic Realization* (1951) are important for their contributions to a different focus on the nurse's therapeutic potential with patients. Both Schwing and Sechehaye were European nurses trained in psychoanalysis and who worked with psychotic patients. Schwing emphasized the mother-surrogate role and corrective nurturing experience in the rehabilitation of severely disturbed patients. Sechehaye also addressed the symbolic meaning of language and nonverbal behavior with patients. The works are important as precursors to drug therapy, demonstrating the power of human communication in treating the mentally ill.

Reviewing psychiatric nursing's clinical contributions, beginning with the one-to-one relationship, we discover how the presence of psychiatric nurses took on a meaning that helped people come together with themselves and their lives. One milestone was Hildegard Peplau's work defining the importance of interpersonal relations in nursing. The work emphasized how a nurse worked with a client to gain reasoned control and flexibility over unreasonable thoughts and experiences (Krauss, 1987). Other nurses expanded these concepts, including psychiatric nurse Dorothy Gregg, who discussed reassurance (1954) and the role of the psychiatric nurse (Gregg, 1954).

In an excellent analysis and report on the development of a conceptual base for psychiatric nursing, nurse-clinician Suzanne Lego cites the following as the three most influential theoretical frameworks: the works of Hildegard Peplau, June Mellow, and Ida Jean Orlando (Lego, 1995). Peplau's interpersonal relations framework has had the most far-reaching impact. It draws heavily from Harry Stack Sullivan's interpersonal theory and, to a lesser degree, from learning theory. In essence, the framework provides a system within which the nurse helps the patient to examine situational factors, with the focus on improving interpersonal competencies that have been lost or never learned. Peplau emphasizes the following nurse–patient steps: observing patient behavior, describing and analyzing the patient's behavior with the patient, formulating the connections noted, testing, and integrating new behaviors of the patient. In addition Peplau describes the importance of the nurse assessing her own interpersonal behavior as it affects the therapeutic relationship, the work roles of the psychiatric nurse, and the phases of the nurse–patient relationship (Peplau, 1952).

JUNE MELLOW

Nurse-therapist June Mellow's theoretical framework, called nursing therapy, was derived from work with schizophrenic patients in an intensive one-to-one relationship (Mellow, 1966). Nursing therapy as a clinical specialty within psychiatric nursing was introduced into the professional literature in 1953. This approach in psychiatric treatment involves the intensive therapeutic work of a graduate nurse with an emotionally disturbed patient. The concern of nursing therapy is with giving the patient an opportunity to participate in a corrective emotional experience in order to facilitate the integration of the patient's overwhelmed ego.

The work of nursing therapy has two phases: experiential and clinically investigative. Initially, the work of nursing therapy took place in the experiential phase. It incorporated and emphasized the advantages of the traditional aspects inherent in the role of the psychiatric nurse. Specifically, the concern was with such factors as living through highly charged emotional experiences with the patient, sharing an everyday human interchange, setting limits, providing controls, satisfying regressive needs, providing an identification figure, and providing therapeutic punishments. Sharing experiences was emphasized, not hearing about them from the patient after they occurred. The goals were aimed at resolving the acute phase of the patient's illness in preparation for long-term psychotherapy with a psychiatrist.

The work of nursing therapy was then broadened to include the clinically investigative phase. In this phase, the patient's needs shift to gaining insight into his or her personality structure and to developing mastery over conflicts. The nurse must be prepared to cope with the intense patient feelings that develop (transference), manage his or her own feelings that develop during the relationship (countertransference), and use skills similar to those needed for psychoanalytic psychotherapy. Mellow's work articulated the process in which the nurse participates and creates an experiential mode of restoring people who are terrified, alone, and lost to their internal processes. The Mellow framework was also used as the core clinical component of the first Doctor of Nursing Science program at Boston University from 1960 to 1966. During that period, over 20 nurses graduated as the first cadre of nurse-psychotherapists.

IDA JEAN ORLANDO

Ida Jean Orlando's theory of the dynamic nurse–patient relationship appeared in the literature in 1961. Orlando describes her theory in terms of the nurse observing the patient's need or distress and helping the patient to "express the specific meaning of his (her) behavior in order to ascertain the help he (she) requires so that (the patient's) distress may be relieved" (Orlando, 1961). In addition, the nurse is encouraged to explore with the patient the nurse's observations or reactions.

DISSEMINATING RESEARCH FINDINGS

The belief is well experienced in psychiatric mental-health nursing that the quality of care will improve with strengthening the scientific base for practice. Part of the research movement in psychiatric nursing is to disseminate research findings in scientific journals to other nurses and this method of reporting has advanced in two areas. First, research writing has been strengthened. A study by McBride (1986) compared the scientific rigor of published psychiatric and mental-health nursing research between 1970 and 1985. The results suggest the following:

- Research articles are more likely to be published in clinical rather than research journals.
- A study is more likely to be conducted to fulfill an academic degree.
- The author is more likely to be a nurse with higher academic degrees.
- The article is written with clarity of presentation and sophistication in study design and execution (McBride, 1986).

Second, research is no longer reported only in general research journals (e.g., *Nursing Research, Research in Nursing and Health, Western Journal of Nursing Research*), but is becoming an integral part of specialty journals (*Journal of Psychosocial Nursing, Issues in Mental Health, Perspectives on Psychiatric Care, Archives of Psychiatric Nursing,* and *Capsules and Comments in Psychiatric Nursing).*

With the research process strengthened, McBride (1986) predicted a shift in focus, over time, from isolated pieces of research to a research program. The nurse researcher will build on his or her own work, and faculties will build on the strengths and resources of their institutions. The Division of Nursing of the U.S. Department of Health and Human Services supports this change in its concept of cluster grants.

In 1986, McBride recommended changes in the character of the research done by psychiatric mental-health nurses. First, the development of large data bases should be a focus. In addition, evaluation research and the connection between research and policy-making should be of concern. According to McBride, there is need for an emphasis on the phenomena of concern (e.g., human response to mental health problems). To this end, McBride and Austin (1995) published a text on nursing research focusing on integrating the behavioral and biological sciences. With programs of research implemented, state-of-the-art conferences developed in which the findings of several nurse-researchers converged.

■ A COALITION FOR PSYCHIATRIC NURSING ORGANIZATIONS

Efforts are coalescing to make psychiatric nursing stronger within the overall field of nursing. At the invitation of Patricia C. Pothier, chairperson of the American Nurses Association (ANA) Council on Psychiatric and Mental Health Nursing (PMHN), the leadership of each of the four national psychiatric nursing organizations met in Kansas City at ANA headquarters on June 10, 1987. The purpose of the meeting was to explore how the ANA Council on PMHN, American Psychiatric Nursing Association (APNA), Society for Education and Research in Psychiatric Nursing (SERPN), and Advocates for Child Psychiatric Nursing (ACPN) could work together to advance psychiatric and mental-health nursing. Objectives were to identify common goals, areas of overlap, and specific differences in the organizations' goals and interests, and to explore mechanisms for continued collaboration with the National Institute on Mental Health (NIMH). Each group affirmed the need and desire for cooperative efforts, and through discussion they were able to identify common overlapping and differing areas of concern.

The APNA was recognized for its focus on providing continuing education to its members. In addition, the APNA regularly distributes its comprehen-sive psychiatric nursing publication, the *Journal of the American Psychiatric Nurses Association.* The SERPN concentrates on activities related to the interface of education and research in psychiatric nursing, and works in the area of political advocacy. ACPN emphasizes practice issues related to children, adolescents, and their families. ACPN also addresses advocacy concerns for professional education of child psychiatric nurses.

These major goals were viewed at the 1987 conference as separate, yet complementing the needs of psychiatric nursing. It was also recognized that each group could engage in policy activity and political advocacy related to their unique goals, but that each group would apprise and seek the support of the others so that psychiatric nursing could speak with "one voice" on issues of common concern and thereby gain strength from the support of collective numbers.

The leaders determined with their memberships that an annual meeting be held of the four psychiatric nursing organizations' leaders (with two representatives from each organization), in conjunction with a regularly scheduled annual meeting of one of the participating organizations; and that this collaborative mechanism be designated the **Coalition of Psychiatric Nursing Organizations (COPNO).**

The goal of COPNO meetings is to explore issues of mutual concern and to plan jointly sponsored initiatives. The responsibility for these meetings rotates among the organizations on an annual basis. In addition, ongoing communication between the groups is implemented by telephone conference calls as issues arise during the year. The coalition shares informational materials such as newsletters, publications, and minutes on a regular and timely basis.

One of the outcomes of this collaborative alliance was the formation in 1992 of a Task Force to Revise the Statement on Psychiatric Mental Health Nursing Practice and Standards of Psychiatric Mental Health Nursing Clinical Practice. Critical parts of this report are a discussion of primary mental-health care and the scope and basic level of psychiatric mental-health clinical nursing practice.

■ PRIMARY MENTAL-HEALTH CARE

Psychiatric–mental-health nurses deliver **primary mental-health care.** This care is initiated at the first point of contact with the mental-health-care system. Primary mental-health care is defined as the continuous and comprehensive services necessary for the promotion of optimal mental health, prevention of mental illness, health maintenance, management of and/or referral of mental- and physical-health problems, diagnosis and treatment of mental disorders and their sequelae, and rehabilitation. Because of its scope, psychiatric mental-health nursing is necessarily holistic and considers the needs and strengths of the whole person, the family, and the community.

Diagnosis of human responses to actual or potential mental-health problems involves the application of theory to human phenomena, through the processes of assessment, diagnosis, planning, intervention or treatment, and evaluation. Theories relevant to psychiatric mental-health nursing are derived from various sources, including those from nursing as well as the biological, cultural, environmental, psychological, and sociological sciences. These theories provide a basis for psychiatric mental-health nursing practice.

An assessment, derived from data collection, interview, and behavioral observations, provides information upon which a diagnosis is based and, when appropriate, validated with the client. The psychiatric mental-health nurse uses nursing diagnoses and standard classifications of mental disorders such as *The Diagnostic and Statistical Manual of Mental Disorders* of the American Psychiatric Association (American Psychiatric Association, 1994), or the *International Classification of Diseases* (World Health Organization, 1993) to develop a treatment plan based on assessment data and theoretical premises. The nurse then selects and implements interventions directed toward a client's response to an actual or potential health problem. The nurse periodically evaluates the client outcome and revises the plan of care to achieve optimal results.

■ LEVELS OF PSYCHIATRIC MENTAL HEALTH CLINICAL NURSING PRACTICE

Psychiatric–mental-health nurses are registered nurses (RNs) who are educationally prepared in nursing and licensed to practice in their individual states. Registered nurses are qualified for specialty practice at two levels, basic and advanced. These levels are differentiated by educational preparation, professional experience, type of practice, and certification. In addition, these levels can differ based on the nurse's focus on clinical, administrative, educator, and research roles.

BASIC LEVEL

Psychiatric–Mental-Health Registered Nurse

The Psychiatric–Mental-Health Nurse is a licensed R.N. who has a baccalaureate degree in nursing and demon-

strated clinical skills within the specialty of psychiatric mental-health nursing, exceeding those of a beginning R.N. or a novice in this specialty. The designation Psychiatric–Mental-Health Nurse applies to those nurses who are certified within the specialty and who meet the profession's standards of knowledge and experience. Certification is the formal process that validates the nurse's clinical competence. The letter "C," placed after the letters R.N. (i.e., R.N., C.), designates basic-level certification status.

Many professional nurses who contribute to the basic level practice of psychiatric–mental-health nursing and care for mental-health patients are either entry-level R.N.s or novices in the specialty. These nurses practice in conjunction with psychiatric–mental-health nurses and are responsible for adhering to the specialty practice standards as designated by the profession.

ADVANCED LEVEL

Psychiatric Mental-Health Advanced Practice Registered Nurse

At the advanced level of practice, the Psychiatric-Mental-Health Advanced Practice Registered Nurse (A.P.R.N.) is a licensed R.N. who is educationally prepared at the master's level, at a minimum, and is nationally certified as a clinical specialist in psychiatric and mental-health nursing. This preparation is distinguished by a depth of knowledge of theory and practice, supervised clinical practice, and competence in advanced clinical nursing skills. The psychiatric–mental-health A.P.R.N. has the ability to apply knowledge, skills, and experience autonomously to complex mental-health problems.

The doctorally prepared psychiatric–mental-health nurse in advanced practice has both a master's degree in nursing and a doctorate in nursing or a related field. Academic programs in nursing leading to a doctorate follow one of two traditions: (1) advanced development of the clinical nursing role with a research component directed toward the investigation of specific clinical problems (D.N.Sc.); or (2) research and theory development in the science of psychiatric–mental-health nursing (Ph.D.).

The scope of practice in psychiatric–mental-health nursing is expanding as the context of practice, the need for patient access to holistic care, and the various scientific and nursing knowledge bases evolve. Many state legislatures and Congress have acknowledged the unique role of advanced-practice psychiatric nurses in the delivery of mental-health services by passing legislation that makes them eligible for prescriptive authority, admission privileges, and third-party reimbursement.

Historically, the psychiatric–mental-health nurse in advanced practice has been called a clinical nurse specialist (C.N.S.). The term *advanced-practice registered nurse* (inclusive of the terms *clinical nurse specialist, nurse anesthetist, nurse midwife,* and *nurse practitioner*) has emerged in response to the need for uniform titling within the nursing profession. The appropriate credential for advanced clinical practice in this specialty is that of the Certified Specialist in Psychiatric and Mental Health Nursing (R.N., C.S.).

■ SUBSPECIALIZATION

Subspecialization in a specific area of practice occurs during master's and doctoral degree preparation in nursing, and/or through continuing professional education. Subspecialization is focused on the development of additional knowledge and skills for providing services to a population. Subspecializations within psychiatric–mental-health nursing are based on current and anticipated societal needs for specific specialty nursing services. This subspecialization may be categorized according to a developmental period (e.g., child and adolescent, adult, geriatric), a specific mental/emotional disorder (e.g., addiction, depression, chronic mental illness), a particular practice focus (e.g., community, group, couple, family, individuals), and/or a specific role or function (e.g., forensic nursing, psychiatric consultation/liaison). These categories are not mutually exclusive but provide a matrix within which the parameters of subspecialization are defined.

Some psychiatric–mental-health nurses in advanced practice seek certification in subspecialty areas as a means of obtaining recognition in a particular practice focus. At this time, not all subspecialties are coupled with a certification process, nor is subspecialty certification essential for practice. It is graduate preparation, additional training and experience, and the individual nurse's judgment about readiness to work with a particular situation or patient population that constitute appropriate practice.

Given this additional preparation, a nurse who is certified as a specialist in an area of psychiatric mental-health nursing can appropriately practice in a subspecialty area with or without certification in that area. In other words, subspecialty certification in a particular category of psychiatric mental-health nursing does not confine the certified specialist to the area of subspecialization. For example, nurses certified as specialists in adult psychiatric and mental-health nursing also work with children as part of a family approach either to family therapy or adjunctively in the treatment of adult parents. Similarly, certified specialists in child and adolescent psychiatric–mental-health nursing see adults (e.g., parents) in therapy.

■ PSYCHIATRIC MENTAL-HEALTH NURSING CLINICAL PRACTICE FUNCTIONS

BASIC LEVEL FUNCTIONS

There are basic level functions provided by the psychiatric–mental-health nurse. The nurse works with individuals, families, groups, and communities to assess mental-health needs, develop diagnoses, and plan, implement, and evaluate nursing care. **Basic level psychiatric mental-health nursing practice** is characterized by interventions that promote and foster health, assess dysfunction, assist clients to regain or improve their coping abilities, and prevent further disability. These interventions focus on psychiatric mental-health clients and include health promotion and health maintenance; intake screening and evaluation; case management; provision of a therapeutic environment (i.e., milieu therapy); tracking of clients and assisting them with self-care activities; administering and monitoring psychobiological treatment regimens (including prescribed psychopharmacological agents and their effects); health teaching; crisis intervention and counseling; and outreach activities such as home visits and community action.

Health Promotion and Maintenance

As a primary health-care provider, the psychiatric mental-health nurse emphasizes health promotion and health maintenance, reflecting nursing's long-standing concern for individual, family, group, and community well-being. The psychiatric–mental-health nurse conducts health assessments, targets at-risk situations, and initiates interventions such as assertiveness training, stress management, parenting classes, and health teaching, in addition to targeting potential complications related to symptoms of mental illness and adverse treatment effects.

Intake Screening and Evaluation

Psychiatric mental-health nurses function at the point of an individual patient's entry into the mental-health system, performing intake screening and evaluation including physical and psychosocial assessments, rendering diagnostic and dispositional judgments, and facilitating the patient's movement into appropriate services. Data collection at the point of contact involves observational and investigative activities that are guided by the nurse's knowledge of human behavior and the principles of the psychiatric interviewing process. The nurse considers biophysical, psychological, social, cultural, economic, and environmental aspects of the patient's life situation to gain an understanding of the problem as it has been experienced and to plan the kind of assistance that is indicated. The nurse is responsible for recognizing areas in which additional clinical data are needed and referring the patient for more specialized testing and evaluation.

Case Management

Case management is a clinical component of a nurse's role in both inpatient and outpatient settings. Nurses who are case managers support the patient's highest level of functioning through culturally relevant interventions designed to enhance self-sufficiency and progress toward optimal health. These can include supportive counseling, problem solving, teaching, medication and status monitoring, comprehensive care planning, and linkage to and identification and coordination of various other health and human services.

Milieu Therapy

In the practice of milieu therapy, the nurse utilizes the human and other resources of institutional and supervised community-based residential or day-treatment settings to foster the restoration of individual patients' previous adaptive abilities and their acquisition of new ones. A key idea in milieu therapy is that virtually all aspects of the therapeutic community, comprising staff and patients, can exert a major influence on behavior, facilitating or impeding the individual's potential for growth and change. On behalf of individual patients, the psychiatric–mental-health nurse assesses and develops the therapeutic potential of a given setting by attending to a wide range of factors such as the physical environment, the social structure and interaction processes, and the culture of the setting.

Similarly, the nurse may practice the use of self as a therapeutic resource through interactions at a one-to-one or group level, in structured or informal sessions, and in the physical as well as the psychosocial aspects of care. Formulation and implementation of the nursing-care program proceed from individualized assessments of client needs, and involve the client and the client's family and significant others to the fullest possible extent.

Self-Care Activities

A major dimension of direct nursing-care functions within the therapeutic milieu involves self-care activities of daily living. Examples of nursing care that takes advantage of the learning potential inherent in the daily life cycle are personal hygiene, feeding, recreational activities, and socialization in practical skills of community life, such as shopping and using public transportation. By comforting, guiding, and setting limits, the nurse can make use of patients' experiences of daily living to help them move from dependent to more independent modes of behavior.

Psychobiological Interventions

Another dimension of psychiatric mental-health nursing derives from the understanding and application of psychobiological knowledge bases for psychiatric mental-health nursing care. The nurse's distinctive contribution rests in the ability to evaluate patients holistically and treat their responses to actual and potential health problems. The psychiatric mental-health nurse employs psychobiological interventions that include various emergency procedures and standard nursing measures, such as relaxation techniques, nutrition/diet regulation, exercise and rest schedules, and other somatic treatments, including monitoring of the patient's responses to psychobiological interventions and the overall treatment program. Psychobiological interventions also include such activities as the interpretation and implementation of prescriptions related to medication, electroconvulsive therapy, and other treatment regimens.

Nurses in a variety of mental-health settings plan and implement services to meet patients' needs for a stable emotional and social support system. A frequent component of these support services is the nurse's support and surveillance of the patient's pharmacologic treatment. These services may be provided on an individual or group basis. The aim is to teach patients about their medications and assist them in dealing with practical problems related to side-effects and other difficulties encountered in continuing a prescribed medication regimen while maintaining residence in the community setting.

An essential aspect of the patient's response is the right to exercise personal choice about participation in proposed treatments. The nurse's responsible use of authority respects the patient's freedom to choose among existing alternatives, and facilitates awareness of resources available to assist with decision making.

Health Teaching

Another aspect of the psychiatric mental-health nurse's work with individuals, families, and community groups is health teaching. In performing this function, the nurse integrates knowledge of the principles of teaching and learning with knowledge of health and illness. The need for health teaching may relate to biological, pharmacological, physical, sociocultural, or psychological aspects of the patient's care. Selection of particular formal and informal learning methods depends on identified needs and learning outcomes. Nurses recognize that experiential learning opportunities are particularly important in developing understanding of mental-health problems and skills for coping with them. Constructive role modeling by the nurse is an inherent part of the teaching function.

Crisis Intervention

Psychiatric mental-health nurses provide direct crisis intervention services to persons in crisis, and serve as members of crisis teams. Crisis intervention is a short-term therapeutic process that focuses on the resolution of an immediate crisis or emergency through the use of available professional personnel, family, and/or environmental resources.

Counseling

In nursing, the aim of counseling is to focus, specifically and for a limited period with a patient, family, or group, on a problem representing an immediate difficulty related to health or well-being. The difficulty is investigated through a problem-solving approach, so that the experience may be understood more fully and integrated with other life experiences.

Home Visits

Psychiatric mental-health nurses utilize the home visit as an effective method of responding to the mental-health needs of an individual or family. In this context, the term "home" refers to private residences or substitute dwellings (e.g., prisons, halfway houses, homes for the disabled, nursing homes, foster care residences, or shelters for the homeless). In some instances, the nurse's insight into a mental-health problem and the resources available to cope with it depend on the assessment data available in the home setting. The nurse may also select the home visit as the most efficacious means of intervention by promoting the potential helping responses of family members or other significant persons. Efforts to help the family adapt to the re-entry of a discharged psychiatric patient into the home environment is another example of the nurse's function within the home setting.

Community Action

Psychiatric mental-health nursing involvement includes community action in the form of concern for sociocultural factors that adversely affect the mental health of population groups and the design of activities that can ameliorate these problems. The psychiatric–mental-health nurse who functions in the life of the community itself may often deal with problems that occur at a wide variety of different points on the health–illness continuum. The practices of these community-oriented nurses vary in the emphasis given to consultation and education aimed at enhancing others' mental-health capabilities on the one hand, and direct therapeutic involvement with patients on the other hand. Involvement with community planning boards, advisory groups, paraprofessionals, and other key people is an important means by which nurses can mobilize the community's resources and bring about changes that address the mental-health needs of particular population groups.

Advocacy

A particularly important dimension of the clinical role of psychiatric mental-health nurses is that of the advocate and policy influencer/maker. These nurses have a long history of supporting the cause of one of the most neglected constituencies—the population with mental illness. However, there is a need for new energy and political activism in this work. Some nurses are influencing policy by assuming leadership positions in government agencies at the local, state, and federal levels, and by running for legislative office.

Others are joining in consumer and professional groups' campaigns to demystify mental illness, abolish the stigma so often attached to it, and achieve parity between health-care coverage for mental and physical illness. To accomplish this, nurses are engaging in public speaking, writing articles for the popular press, and lobbying their congressional representatives on behalf of better mental-health and psychiatric care for all Americans. In clinical practice, the nurse-advocate vigilantly protects the rights of patients and speaks for those who, for whatever reason, cannot speak for themselves. Because of nursing's strong commitment to the health, welfare, and safety of the patient, the nurse must be aware of and speak for individuals, groups, and families; therapists and counselors for suicide prevention and crisis intervention; clinical specialists for special populations, supervision, consultation, and education; and researchers to study human responses to mental-health problems.

As psychiatric nursing has moved from its historical custodial function to the widespread challenges described above, it has enjoyed the opportunity to improve the care of the psychiatrically ill and the emotionally distressed, while at the same time advocating the optimal level of mental health for all people, strengthening the knowledge development in nursing, and enhancing the professional growth of the psychiatric nurse.

As a result of these challenges posed both to nursing and psychiatric nursing, and as we enter the

21st century, we note that nursing has emerged with clear and distinct statements as to its domain, its scope of practice, its art, and its science. The research and theory-development movement in nursing has had a powerful effect on advancing the profession. Now, the critical task is to maintain nursing's productivity, and the challenge is to expand and advance its knowledge base.

O AN OVERVIEW

- Innovative psychiatric nursing issues to be studied include case management; seriously mentally ill persons; short-term hospitalization; and work with children, adolescents, and the elderly.

- Since the advent of the Mental Health Act, psychiatric nurses have developed expertise as managers of the patients' hospital environment; psychotherapists for individuals, groups, and families; therapists and counselors for suicide prevention and crisis intervention; clinical specialists for special populations and for supervision, consultation, and education; and researchers of human responses to mental-health problems.

- In moving from their historical custodial function, psychiatric nurses now have the opportunity to improve the care of psychiatrically ill and emotionally distressed patients and to advocate the optimal level of mental health for all people.

- A critical task of nursing is to maintain the profession's productivity; a challenge is to advance and expand its knowledge base.

TD TERMS TO DEFINE

- advanced-level psychiatric nursing
- ANA Statement on Psychiatric Mental Health Clinical Nursing Practice
- basic-level functions
- Coalition of Psychiatric Nursing Organizations (COPNO)
- phenomena of concern
- primary mental-health care
- subspecialization

Q STUDY QUESTIONS

1. Psychiatric mental-health nursing is the:
   a. the assessment of psychiatric problems.
   b. the diagnosis and treatment of psychiatric problems.
   c. the management of psychiatric problems.
   d. the care of psychiatric patients and their families.

2. The earliest known method of treating the mentally ill was
   a. humanistic care.
   b. custodial care.
   c. mystical healing.
   d. psychotherapeutic care.

3. An early social reformer who used a legislative approach to impact humane treatment for the mentally ill was:
   a. Hildegard Peplau.
   b. Dorothea Dix.
   c. June Mellow.
   d. Florence Nightingale.

4. The first American psychiatric nurses training school was started at
   a. Bellevue Hospital.
   b. St. Elizabeth's Hospital.
   c. Pennsylvania Hospital.
   d. McLean Hospital.

5. The Mental Health Act of 1946 provided funds to
   a. treat psychiatric patients.
   b. train psychiatrists.
   c. train in the 4 psychiatric disciplines.
   d. research mental illness.

6. What two psychiatric nurses have contributed to practice-based research?

7. What are three influential conceptual bases for psychiatric nursing?

8. List three national psychiatric nursing organizations.

9. What does COPNO stand for?

10. Define primary mental health care.

■ REFERENCES

American Nurses Association: *A Statement on Psychiatric–Mental-Health Clinical Nursing Practice and Standards of Psychiatric–Mental-Health Clinical Nursing Practice.* Washington, D.C.: American Nurses Publishing, 1994.

American Psychiatric Association: *Diagnostic and Statistical Manual of Mental Disorders, fourth edition.* Washington, D.C.: American Psychiatric Press, 1994.

Bromberg W: *From Shaman to Psychotherapist.* Chicago, Henry Regnery, 1975.

Colliton C: The history of nursing therapy. *Perspect Psychiatr Care* 1965; 3.

Cook F: *Life of Florence Nightingale.* London, 1913.

Critchley DI: Evolution of the role, in Critchley DL, Maurin JT (eds): *The Clinical Specialist in PMHN.* New York, John Wiley & Sons, 1985.

Deutsch A: *The Mentally Ill in America: A History of Their Care and Treatment from Colonial Times.* New York, Columbia University Press, 1949, pp 1–58.

Doona ME: *Travelbee's Intervention in Psychiatric Nursing,* ed 2. Philadelphia, F. A. Davis, 1978, p 261.

Gregg D: The psychiatric nurse's role, *Am J Nurs* 1954; 54: p.

Gregg G: Reassurance, *Am J Nurs* 1955; 55:171.

International Classification of Diseases, 9th revision, Clinical Modification (ICD-9-CM), Third edition, (March, 1989). U.S. Department of Health and Human Services, HCFA, DHHS, Publ. No. PH-S 89-1260.

Johnston R L, & Fitzpatrick, J J: Relevance of psychiatric mental health nursing theories to nursing models. In J Fitzpatrick, A Whall, R Johnston, & J Floyd (eds.), *Nursing Models and their Psychiatric Mental Health Applications.* Bowie, Md.: Brady, 1982, pp. 1–15.

Joint Commission on Mental Health and Illness: *Action for Mental Health.* Washington, DC, US Government Printing Office, 1961.

Lego S: Psychiatric nursing: Theory and practice of the one-to-one client-nurse relationship. Paper presented at an invitational conference, The State of the Art of Psychiatric Nursing, April 1974. Also published in conference proceedings: *Psychiatric Nursing: 1946-1974: A Report on the State of the Art,* C. A. Anderson (ed): St. Louis: Mosby, 1995.

Matheney RV, Topalis, M: *Psychiatric Nursing.* St. Louis, CV Mosby, 1950.

McBride AB, Austin JK (eds): *Psychiatric-Mental Health Nursing: Integrating the Behavioral and Biological Sciences.* Philadelphia, Saunders, 1995.

McBride AB: Theory and research: Present issues and future perspectives on psychosocial nursing. *Journal of Psychosocial Nursing,* 1986; 24: 28–33.

McBride AB: Psychiatric nursing: Coming of age at NIMH. *Hospital and Community Psychiatry,* 1993; 44:(1).

Mellow J: Nursing therapy as a treatment and clinical investigative approach to emotional illness, *Nurs Forum,* 1966; 5:64.

Muller TG: *The Nature and Direction of Psychiatric Nursing: The Dynamics of Human Relationships,* Philadelphia, Lippincott, 1950.

Nicoll LH Three landmark symposia. In LH Nicoll (Ed), *Perspectives on Nursing Theory.* Boston: Little, Brown, 1986, pp 91–92.

Nightingale F: *Notes on Nursing: What It Is and What It Is Not* (facsimile of 1859 ed). Philadelphia, J.B. Lippincott, 1946.

Orlando IJ: *The Dynamic Nurse-Patient Relationship.* New York, GP Putnam's Sons, 1961.

Peplau H: *Interpersonal Relations in Nursing.* New York, GP Putnam's Sons, 1952.

Pothier PC: Coalition of psychiatric nursing organizations proposed, *Pacesetter,* 1987; 14:1.

President's Commission on Mental Health: *Report to the President,* Vol 1. Washington, DC, U.S. Government Printing Office, 1978, pp 9–10.

Robbins RH (ed): *The Encyclopedia of Witchcraft and Demonology.* New York, Crown, 1959.

Sechehaye MA: *Symbolic Realization.* New York, International University Press, 1951.

Schwing G: *A Way to the Soul of the Mentally Ill.* Edstein R, Hall BH (trans). New York, International University Press, 1954.

Sullivan HS: *The Interpersonal Theory of Psychiatry.* New York, WW Norton, 1953.

Tudor GE: A sociopsychiatric nursing approach to intervention in a problem of mutual withdrawal on a mental hospital ward. *Psychiatry,* 1952; 15:193.

Weiner DB: Philippe Pinel's "Memoir on Madness" of December 11, 1794: A fundamental text of modern psychiatry, *Am J Psychiatry,* 1992; 149:725.

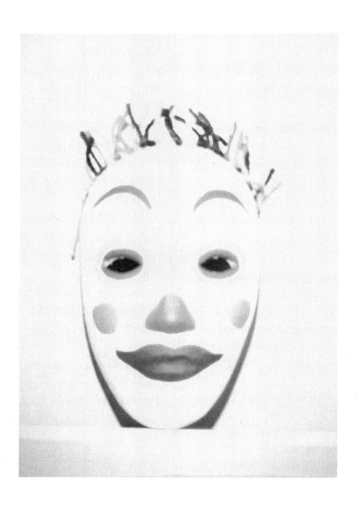

A modern poet has characterized the personality of art and the impersonality of science as follows: *Art is I; Science is We.*

From *Bulletin of New York Academy of Medicine*

Vol IV, 1928, p. 997

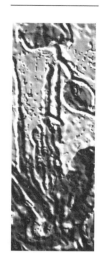

3

Patterns of Psychiatric Nursing Practice: Integrating the Arts with the Science

Wanda K. Mohr

Despite much talk about holism, in nursing; many nursing courses continue to categorize and count, divide, and subdivide. For example, the focus of nursing—the person of flesh, bone, and spirit—may be referred to as having a physical versus a mental illness, a matter of either-or. It is problematic when nursing courses reduce the patient to abstractions and teach students how to practice learned interventions on individuals, each intervention being neatly linked to a desired outcome. Similarly, in nursing subspecialties (e.g., maternal/child health and community health), students are not served well when courses functionally define humans as part of a network of concepts that are drained of individual identity and smothered beneath labels.

Although it is convenient, and sometimes necessary, to use labels, it is also paramount that nurses not lose touch with the richness and depth of the human self. With this in mind, the framework developed by nurse-educator Barbara Carper in the late 1970s has been woven into the text of this chapter. Carper (1978) wrote that nursing knowledge comes from formal as well as common, everyday forms of knowing. She said that nursing knowledge is founded on patterns of knowing that include empirics, personal knowledge, ethics, and esthetics.

◼ THE PATTERNS OF KNOWING

Empirics as a pattern of knowing is concerned with the traditional idea of science. Some of the methods used are observation and experimentation. Description, prediction, and control are involved. It can readily be seen why this pattern alone is inadequate to deal with very human issues such as love, spirituality, caring, and psychic pain. **Personal knowledge,** the second pattern of knowing, has to do with the process of knowing ourselves, our values, where we are in life, and how, by reaching deep into our own well of experience, we can be helped to interact on some meaningful level with another human being. Although personal knowledge helps to develop awareness of others' selves, it does not help much in the acute treatment of disregulated diabetes.

Ethics, the third pattern of knowing, concerns moral knowledge in nursing. From its earliest times the profession of nursing has maintained that nurses' primary responsibility is to their patients. The professional code of ethics and the profession's social policy statements reflect and affirm the idea that the nurse is an autonomous professional who assumes responsibility and accountability for his or her individual nursing judgments and actions. Both the code of ethics and the policy statements take strong stands on the "profound regard for humanity" (ANA Social Policy Statement, 1980, p. 18) and "respect for human dignity and the uniqueness of the (individual) client" (ANA Code, 1980, p. 1). Again, moral knowledge, while important, is only a single aspect of approaching nursing in its entirety.

Esthetics, the final pattern of knowing, concerns the art of nursing. Esthetics concerns beauty and the understanding and expression of what is possible in the practice of nursing. Carper wrote that each creative and esthetic act that nurses employ is unique, just as any other work of art is unique. Esthetic acts come from deep within the nurse, much as a beautiful painting comes from deep within a visual artist. In addition, esthetics reflects the use of cultural art forms in nursing practice. Some artistic media, such as literature, poetry, painting, and music, can be used by nurses and patients in learning and for diagnosis, therapy, and expression.

The four patterns of knowing are interrelated and dynamic, which is to say always changing and shifting. This is because we and our world are always changing. What we know, therefore, changes as well. Chinn and Kramer (1991), who expanded on Carper's work, wrote that although each pattern of knowing is a separate entity of nursing knowledge, one should not stand alone or take precedence over the others. This text emphasizes integration of the patterns.

◼ THE CHALLENGE OF CHANGE

Undergraduate learning experiences are being reexamined in light of shorter hospital stays and greater emphasis on community and home care. In the past, learning experiences focused on chronic and severe mental illness, and involved clinical placements within patient facilities. Now students do not have the opportunity to establish long-standing therapeutic relationships with patients because they are frequently discharged after the initial encounter. State hospitals enable a longer stay for chronically mentally ill patients, but in many areas of the United States, state hospitals are becoming obsolete. The challenge is how to teach what is needed for empirical practice without reducing the description of clinical conditions to a laundry list of symptoms for students to memorize. However, we must go beyond facts and communicate the elements and the patterns of knowing that seem neglected in this new world of health care.

◼ CORE CONTENT

The core content of psychiatric mental-health nursing is included in the grid presented in Figure 3–1. The grid, consistent with the recommendations of the Society for Education and Research in Psychiatric Nursing, is the framework for a model undergraduate curriculum in psychiatric–mental-health nursing. The core content is the starting point of the curriculum. It reflects the phenomena of nursing concern and includes key and up-to-date content in the areas of mental health and mental illness. In addition, the curriculum is community oriented, and the clinical portion includes a significant community practicum. The key assumption underlying the curriculum is that mental-health practice is fundamental to everything that happens to the patient, whether this is in a psychiatric hospital or critical-care unit.

EMPIRICS

To achieve the assessment and diagnostic skills essential in psychiatric–mental-health nursing practice, it is necessary to have a broad knowledge base. The various areas essential for study include the brain, neuroanatomy, neurophysiology, neuroendocrinology, and neuroimmunology, as well as recent findings about the growth and development of the adult and child/adolescent. Such content is also necessary to understanding the rationales behind nursing interventions. For example, students of mental health nursing may become discouraged in trying to communicate with

FIGURE 3–1.   CORE CONTENT OF BASIC PSYCHIATRIC MENTAL-HEALTH NURSING

Core Content	PMH Course Content	Competencies
Nursing: historical and contemporary	Psychiatric nursing: historical and contemporary	Describe models of treating the mentally ill
Growth and development	Age-appropriate care for psychiatric clients	Plan and implement age-appropriate care
Neuroanatomy, neurophysiology, neuroendocrinology, neuroimmunology	Neurocognitive alterations in mental illness, neurobiological alterations in mental illness, stress	Demonstrate basic assessment skills to include: a. sensory perception, cognitive deficits b. information processing resulting in alterations of behavior and social functioning and bio-psycho-neuroimmunologic changes
Diagnostic thinking; Inductive, deductive, and retroductive reasoning; syntactical thinking	Major psychiatric diagnostic classifications according to the *Diagnostic and Statistical Manual;* mental-health alterations and nursing diagnosis; patient in context.	Identify symptoms of each category. Describe what data are present and demonstrate how conclusions were reached
Basic management principles	Referral processes	Ability to participate in case management and management of psychiatric care.
Case management	Expected outcomes of psychiatric treatment	Plan for a continuum of care. Mobilize resources to provide safety, structure, and support for the mentally ill.
Critical pathways	Critical pathway related to major mental illness	Implement critical pathways related to patients with major and minor mental illness
Interdisciplinary roles	Roles of various mental-health-care providers, including roles of psychiatric nurses with various levels of education	Demonstrate ability to work with various members of the interdisciplinary team.
Health care promotion and illness prevention	Principles of teaching smoking cessation; exercise; nutritional aspects of mental health; sobriety	Plan and facilitate a mental-health promotion plan for a patient with serious mental illness.
Principles of learning and learning theories	Psychoeducational approaches to working with individuals, families, and consumers	Demonstrate ability to develop and implement a teaching project related to mental-health illness issues.
Community health	Community mental health; community support initiatives for at-risk populations; social policy regarding care of mentally ill	Participate in delegating care and making appropriate referrals for psychiatric patients. Identify at-risk populations and major policy governing mentally ill.
Stress and crisis	Stress-crisis continuum	Assess seven levels of stress-crisis for intervention strategy.
Ethical and legal principles; values clarification	1. Nurse Practice Acts 2. Standards of Practice for PMHN 3. Confidentiality 4. Least restrictive treatment	Clarify personal values continuously with regard to mental illness. Facilitate others to clarify values and attitudes related to self and mental illness
Person as consumer; family/significant other	Principles of collaborative relationships with individuals and families, consumer and advocacy groups	Demonstrate ability to partner with individuals and families in developing and implementing care plans for psychiatric patients.
Basic pharmacology	Major psychotropic agents for identified psychiatric illness that include: a. action and expected effects b. side effects and toxicity c. potential interactions with other medications	Evaluate effects of medication on patients, including symptoms, side effects, toxicity, and potential interactions with other medications/substances. Teach patients and families medication management. Evaluate outcomes of medications.
Communication theory and skills	Therapeutic use of self a. understanding, using, and controlling affective responses b. integrating affective and cognitive responses with appropriate intervention c. continuing clarification and maintenance of professional boundaries d. evaluating interventions with psychiatric clients	Demonstrate therapeutic use of self, self-inventory
Crisis intervention in violence and suicide	Principles of anger and aggression. Crisis intervention with psychiatric clients.	Assess potential violence; suicidality; intervene in acute agitation
Cultural and ethnic differences Spiritual needs	Compare and contrast psychiatric symptoms and cultural and spiritual self-expression	Provide culturally and spiritually competent care that meets client needs

continued

FIGURE 3–1—CONT'D.

Core Content	PMH Course Content	Competencies
Child/adolescent development	Recognition of major child/adolescent disorders. Contrast with adult disorders	Articulate interventions that might be used with children/adolescents who have behavioral deviations
Chronic illness	Symptom management in seriously and persistently mentally ill patients Relapse care/prevention	Establish therapeutic relationship with seriously and persistently mentally ill patients.
Advocacy	Consumer advocacy groups	Observe functioning of advocacy groups. Become acquainted with support groups and articulate their role
Concepts of risk and screening	Risk factors, screening, and referral related to psychiatric illness and social problems a. suicide/homicide b. substance abuse c. violence/abuse	Screen for substance use/abuse Screen for victim violence/abuse Screen for suicide and homicide
Group process	Therapeutic factors in group intervention	Demonstrate beginning group participation/leadership skills.

profoundly ill schizophrenic patients if they do not understand that blood flow to key regions of the brain is curtailed in these individuals. These patients may take twice as long as others to respond to their care-givers. If it is not known that the patient's blood supply is diminished, the patient's behavior becomes easy to dismiss as noncompliance or obstinacy. Similarly, if the principles underlying the effects of medications given in psychiatric–mental-health settings are not understood, a patient may be caused more suffering.

ETHICS

During the late 1980s, laws were passed that would further ensure patients' rights, leading to a significant restructuring of the legal environment of mental-health care. In seeking patient protection from undue restraint, commitment laws were strengthened, and in some hospital systems where abuses had existed, patients and their families enjoyed greater autonomy, confidentiality, and self-direction. Much of the content in this book stresses a deep respect for patients and their autonomy. As illustrated in figure 3–1 special concern is paid to ethics.

Changes occurred for more than legal reasons. For example, it was found that nurses who have a healthy respect for a patient's right to self-determination are much more successful in their practice than nurses who try to dictate to patients.

Health care has a moral core, and this core, which underlies each chapter in this book, should be an integral part of the structural practice of nursing. The structural practice of nursing includes the following elements:

- Tasks of caring.
- Patients' rights and responsibilities, including legal status, the right to treatment, the right to refuse treatment, and the right to be treated in the least restrictive environment possible.
- Nurses' rights and responsibilities, guided by the Standards of Nursing Practice and the Code of Ethics.

Ethical issues will be of particular importance as health care becomes increasingly profit driven. During the 1980s, a major investigation of investor-owned psychiatric hospitals found fraud, patient abuse, and other unethical conduct. A study was conducted of Texas nurses employed in for-profit psychiatric hospitals from 1985 to 1991 to determine how they experienced their professional situations in these deviant environments (Mohr, 1995). The researcher found that nurses felt poorly prepared for their roles; failed to recognize and deal with deviance; were subjected to intimidation tactics; bracketed off their feelings about the inappropriate conditions; and focused on tasks. The results of this study have implications for policy, research, education and practice, insofar as health care is becoming increasingly management controlled.

Ethics are only principles. They are not carved in stone, and exceptions do come up in practice. Concentrating excessively on the pattern of ethics can result in inflexibility and a lack of sensitivity in the face of changing contexts and circumstances. Moreover, ethics cannot help to treat a patient with diabetes, except perhaps to underscore that he or she is a self-determining person who cannot be forced to adhere to a diet or to take prescribed insulin.

PERSONAL KNOWLEDGE

Many experienced nurses know the value of personal knowledge—the knowledge that comes from deep within us when our intuitive whiskers begin to twitch. It is an asset that is fine-tuned through experience; however, each student has personal knowledge to bring to practice. Personal knowledge is particularly helpful in assessment and diagnostic reasoning, and in the sensitivity of the nurse's communication. Communication theory and the skills that enable nurses to talk with patients and families as well as listen to them are the keys to all nursing practice. On the grid (Figure 3–1), a rather large portion of the curriculum is devoted to communication theory.

Although communication theory is important, sometimes, in the therapeutic use of the self, a finely tuned understanding of a patient's plight based on personal experiences or the experiences of friends can bring a special dimension to a therapeutic encounter. Sometimes a nurse does not have time to think about theory, such as in a crisis situation. In these instances, personal knowledge and a deep gut-level reaction of how to handle the crisis can be significant. Case studies in this textbook are a means of illustrating another care-giver's personal knowledge.

ESTHETICS

Understanding certain human experiences, such as the nature of self, anguish, guilt, and love, is central to nursing. Opportunities for nursing students to learn firsthand about the entire range of human conditions are difficult to find. The grid (Figure 3–1) indicates that achieving considerable knowledge about the human condition and psychiatric nursing is important for students. They must understand the condition of humanness, not simply know that people suffer, or that they have joy, or that they get better.

Esthetics may be used to approach some aspects of human-ness. Many chapters in this text include beautifully articulated examples from the literature that might help to explain or illustrate how people experience those feelings and thoughts that patients sometimes cannot express. Within the text's chapters, drawings created by patients also illustrate the human struggle.

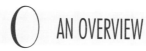

ART THERAPY

Art therapy combines the disciplines of psychology and art. There are two principal approaches to the therapeutic value of using art to facilitate healing. One school of thought posits that the making of art itself is healing, the *process* is emphasized rather than the product. The other school believes that creating images helps to make "the unconscious conscious." The content, its meaning, and the patient's associations to the image may be explored with the therapist. Adults may need a directive—to be invited to draw a particular event or feeling—to help them engage in the creative process. On the other hand, when working with children, a nondirective approach may be favored because children tend to be less inhibited, more spontaneous in their expression.

There is a psychology of art material: pencils foster control, painting invites a freer form of expression. Depending on the treatment goals and ego strengths of the individual, the art therapist presents the appropriate choice of mediums to the client. A psychotic patient would benefit from an intervention that emphasizes reality testing. A person who is depressed or has experienced trauma in life can use the art as a safe container for repressed or early nonverbal feelings. In work with trauma victims, the patient selects the medium for expression.

Art therapy can address the needs of individuals or groups seeking support because of medical or psychological difficulties as well as clients seeking to explore their true selves.

Elizabeth Baring, MS
Art Therapist
Stamford Hospital
Stamford, Connecticut

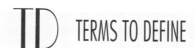 AN OVERVIEW

- The approach taken by the writers of this textbook integrates Barbara Carper's concept that nursing knowledge is built on empirics, personal knowledge, ethics, and esthetics.

- Employing the Carper concept is a strategy that encourages syntactical thinking and ensures that the student's educational experience goes beyond the sterile recitation of micro-facts.

- The 21st century appears to hold increased threats of dehumanization and particularization within the health-care system.

- Psychiatric nursing must reflect holistic practice that focuses on the human-ness of patients.

TD TERMS TO DEFINE

- empirics
- esthetics
- ethics

- personal knowledge
- syntactical learning

■ REFERENCES

American Nurses Association: *Code Book for Nurses with Interpretive Statements*. Kansas City, MO, American Nurses Association, 1985.

American Nurses Association: *Nursing: A Social Policy Statement*. Kansas City, MO, American Nurses Association, 1980.

Carper BA: Fundamental patterns of knowing in nursing, *Adv Nurs Sci,* 1978; 1:13–23.

Chinn PA, Kramer MK: *Theory and Nursing: A Systematic Approach*. St. Louis, CV Mosby, 1991.

Mohr WK: *The Nature of Nurses' Experiences in for-Profit Psychiatric Hospital Settings*. Unpublished doctoral dissertation. University of Texas at Austin, Austin, TX, 1995.

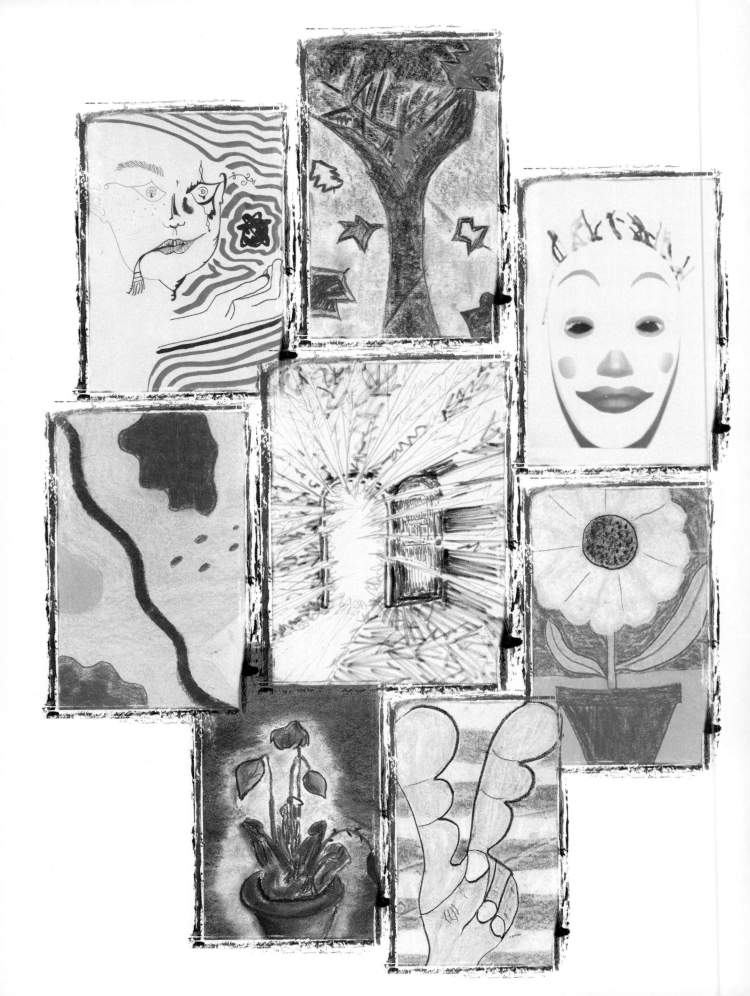

II

BASIC PROFESSIONAL CONCEPTS

Nurses work in therapeutic relationships with an extraordinary variety of individuals. In their professional role, nurses do well to understand the intricacies and recognize the mysteries of human growth, behavior, and relationships. To be most effective, nurses must appreciate the potential for individual learning and the confining influences of illness, and at the same time integrate the social realities that come into play. Such concern and understanding are of particular consequence for psychiatric nurses in their relationships with individuals experiencing emotional disorders.

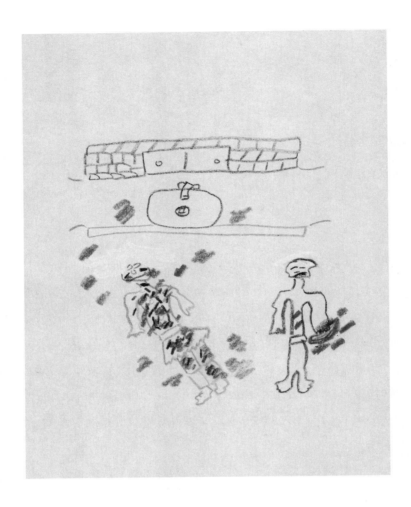

Volumes are now written and spoken upon the effect of the mind upon the body. Much of it is true. But I wish a little more was thought of the effect of the body on the mind.

Florence Nightingale
1820–1910

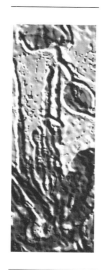

4

The Brain and Behavior

Barbara E. Wolfe

Today, practitioners, researchers, teachers, and students are faced with the challenge of integrating rapidly expanding information about the brain and behavior. At the transition to the 20th century, Adolph Meyer (1866-1950) introduced the concept of "psychobiology," noting that psychology and biology are not mutually exclusive aspects of mental illness. Scientists continue to explore the relationships among physiological functions and anatomical structures, and their association with mental processes, including consciousness, memory, and emotions. Similarly, studies explore ways in which mental processes influence both the internal and external response patterns of an individual. Advances in psychopharmacology, neurophysiology, molecular biology, and technology have greatly expanded the knowledge of both the brain and behavior, while an understanding of the clinical significance of their connections remains in its infancy.

Supported in part by USPHS grant K07 MH00965 from the National Institute of Mental Health.

■ THE NEURON

Neurons are nerve cells, the most fundamental units of the nervous system. Approximately ten-billion neurons are in the average human brain. Neurons are non-reproducing cells and, after an individual reaches adulthood, die at an estimated rate of 1,000 per day.

The role of most neurons is to send and receive impulses (messages) within and outside the brain. The brain relies on these impulses to assist in the regulation of many behaviors, including breathing, eating, body movement, and emotional states. Upon receiving these impulses, the brain sends signals to elicit, inhibit, or maintain a certain response. Neurons are extremely interactive; one cell may network with more than 10,000 other neurons.

COMPOSITION AND CELL STRUCTURE

Neurons are composed of some of the common structural components found in other types of cells (Figure 4–1). The nucleus of the cell is its control center. It contains the genetic materials deoxyribonucleic acid (DNA) and ribonucleic acid (RNA), and is responsible for regulating the cell's functioning. Also within the cell are organelles (e.g., mitochondria) that produce proteins necessary for energy production and expenditure. Both the nucleus and organelles are surrounded by cytoplasm, the intracellular fluid composed largely of water. The cytoplasm also contains nutrients needed to maintain cellular functioning, as well as ions integral to the conduction of impulses that signal information to and from the brain. The nucleus, organelles, and cytoplasm are all contained within the cell membrane, which serves as a "gatekeeper." The cell membrane is permeable, allowing certain materials to flow in and out of the cell (e.g., ions, nutrients, waste).

Unlike other types of cells, the neuron is characterized as having specific anatomical and functional structures, described as the soma, axon, dendrites, and terminal bouton (Figure 4–1). Intracellular structures, including the nucleus, are contained within the soma (cell body). Additional organelles are found in other regions of the neuron. Nissl substance, important for protein synthesis, is present in the dendritic processes. Mitochondria, sources of cellular energy, are concentrated in the terminal end of the axon (terminal bouton area).

Each neuron consists of a single axon that extends out from the cell body or dendrite. Axons are cylindrical structures, varying in diameter (from 0.001 to 0.10 mm) and length (up to 1 m) in humans. The role of the axon is to relay information away from the cell body to the terminal bouton of the neuron. The wider the axon diameter, the faster the transmission of information (signal transmission, or a nerve impulse) from the cell body to the terminal bouton. Some axons also have a protective covering, or sheath, called myelin. This sheath consists of a thin blanket of cells wrapped around the axon to create an insulating effect, which assists in the rate of signal transmission. The clinical importance of myelination in regulating the rate of signal transmission is illustrated by multiple sclerosis, in which degenerative demyelination leads to slowed conduction and subsequent behavioral impairments.

At the end of the axon is the terminal bouton, which contains thousands of vesicles. The vesicles store chemicals called neurotransmitters, which are released into the synaptic cleft when the cell is excited or stimulated. The synaptic cleft is a gap (approximately 20 nm wide) between the terminal bouton of the pre-synaptic cell and dendritic process of the post-synaptic cell. Storage of the neurotransmitters in vesicles prevents their degradation by enzymes located in the terminal area of the neuron.

While the main function of the axon is to transmit information *from* the cell body, dendrites relay information *to* the cell body. Dendrites, which are branched processes extending from the cell body, receive signals from numerous neurons. The extending branches of each dendrite are called *dendritic spines*. Thus, axons, cell bodies, and dendrites form an ongoing system to transmit impulses in the nervous system.

STRUCTURAL CLASSIFICATION

Neurons are classified in different ways depending on their structure, function, and association with specific neurotransmitters. Structural classification may be determined by the number of processes extending from the cell body (i.e., unipolar, bipolar, or multipolar). Most neurons are multipolar (Figure 4–2). Neurons

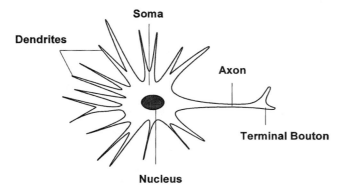

Figure 4–1. Cell Structure.

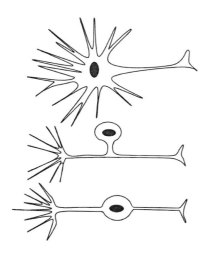

Figure 4–2. Cellular structural classification according to processes: multipolar (top), unipolar (middle), bipolar (bottom).

may also be structurally classified according to their axonal length. Neurons having long axons are classified as Golgi type I, and those with short axons as Golgi type II. A majority of neurons are type II.

Functional classification of neurons may be motor, sensory, or interneuron. Motor neurons transmit signals to muscles, glands, and blood vessels. Sensory neurons receive stimuli from internal and/or external environments. Interneurons are nerve cells that interconnect other neurons; they are generally Golgi type II neurons.

Neurons may also be classified according to their specificity for releasing a particular neurotransmitter. For example, neurons that release the neurotransmitter **acetylcholine** are called *cholinergic* neurons. Similarly, those that release serotonin or dopamine are referred to as *serotonergic* or *dopaminergic* neurons, respectively.

■ THE DELICACY OF DYNAMIC COMPLEXITY

The body's environment substantially influences neuronal functioning. Environmental considerations include oxygenation, nutritional adequacy, external toxins, internal structural changes, and stress. For example, normal nerve-cell functioning requires a large amount of energy and is therefore particularly reliant on the availability of oxygen. Up to 25% of the body's oxygen consumption occurs in the brain. Any compromise in the brain's oxygen supply leaves nerve cells extremely vulnerable to damage or cell death, potentially impairing associated behavioral functions. Impaired brain oxygenation resulting from a cerebral vascular accident (stroke), for example, causes neuronal

damage that may result in paralysis, slurred speech, unconsciousness, and even death. In carbon monoxide poisoning the brain is deprived of oxygen as a result of excess carbon monoxide in the blood. The resulting decrease in transport of oxygen to the brain poses the potential for cell damage or cell death.

Another environmental influence on neuronal functioning is nutrition. Inadequate nutritional intake and subsequent nutrient deprivation can result in behavioral manifestations of clinical significance (e.g., depressed mood). The essential amino acids are necessary for the synthesis of neurotransmitters that, for example, influence mood. Cells are also sensitive to vitamin deficiencies. Neuritis is a possible consequence of deficient vitamin B_6 intake. Change in mental status may occur with inadequate niacin intake. Wernicke's encephalopathy, characterized by mental confusion and ataxic gait, results from vitamin B_1 (thiamine) deficiency.

Nerve cells are sensitive to environmental toxins and internal structural changes. Lead poisoning, most frequently occurring in children, can result in lead encephalopathy, and potentially permanent damage to the central nervous system. Internal structural changes, such as tumors and hemorrhage (e.g., from head trauma), can raise internal pressure, leading to cellular dysfunction, with possible behavioral impairment.

Stress, internal or external, can result in adaptive or maladaptive physiological responses. Stressors commonly trigger increased neuronal activity, leading to excitatory electrical firing and subsequent intracellular responses. The subsequent chemical responses can stimulate a chain of physiological responses (e.g., enzymatic phosphorylation), which alter biological responses. Enzymatic phosphorylation of proteins involved in gene regulation may lead to altered gene expression. These effects may last only minutes or persist for days, possibly resulting in permanent structural changes within the nerve cell itself.

■ SIGNALING IN THE CENTRAL NERVOUS SYSTEM: HOW DOES IT WORK?

A distinctive feature of the neuron is that it is excitable. Neuronal firing allows for the transmission of impulses from one nerve cell to another. In the synapse, the terminal bouton of one neuron is within close contact to the axon, dendrites, or cell body of another neuron. The actual synapse involves the membrane of the presynaptic cell (the sender), the synaptic cleft, and the membrane of the post-synaptic cell (the receiver) (Figure 4–3).

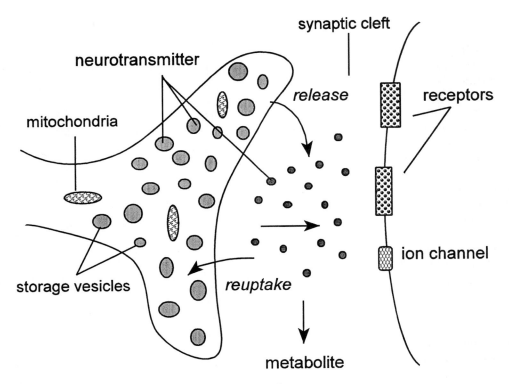

Figure 4–3. Components of synaptic activity.

PRE-SYNAPTIC ACTIVITY

Pre-synaptic cells are activated by electrical impulses. Most cells are polarized, meaning that there is a difference in the ionic balance between the cell's internal and external environment. Many different events can change the intra- and extracellular ionic balance. When the neuron is at rest, the extracellular concentrations of sodium are much higher than its intracellular concentrations. This disequilibrium in ionic distribution results in a negatively charged internal cellular structure. Some of the intracellular negative charge is balanced by positive ions in the form of internally high concentrations of potassium; however, the cell remains negatively charged.

The ionic disequilibrium between the internal and external environments results in an electrical potential known as the *resting membrane potential*. At rest, the cell membrane is more permeable to potassium ions than to sodium ions, leading to the high intracellular potassium concentration (hyperpolarized state). This resting state results in the cell's inhibition or inability to transmit impulses. A stimulus that decreases the resting polarization causes a change in the membrane permeability, leading to an intracellular influx of sodium ions (depolarized state). The influx of sodium results in a rapid increase in positively charged ions within the cell.

A sudden change in ionic balance can (although not always) cause the initiation of an action potential, or cell firing. When the cell fires, it generates an impulse that travels down the axon at a constant rate known as an *all-or-none* effect; thus, the impulse does not lose velocity as it travels. After firing, the cell quickly returns to its resting potential (repolarization) prior to the next depolarization. The recovery period, referred to as the *refractory period,* is quite short, given that many cells can fire more than 1,000 times in a single second.

Cell-membrane permeability to specific ions is influenced by specific proteins embedded in the cell membrane, and known as *ion channels.* Ion channels are selective for particular ions according to the diameter and ionic characteristics of the channel. Larger channels are likely to be more permeable to larger ions than are smaller channels. Channels with positively charged linings are more selective for anions, whereas those with negatively charged linings are likely to attract cations.

Ion channels can be open or closed. In order for ions to pass through a membrane, the ion channels must be open. The availability of the channel (its openness) is regulated by *gates.* The ion-channel gates may be electrically controlled, through changes in the membrane potential (voltage-gated channels), or chemically controlled, such as by neurotransmitters (ligand-gated channels).

SYNAPTIC ACTIVITY

Although electrical impulses cannot jump across the synaptic cleft, they can induce a chemical signal that allows for communication between nerve cells. After travelling down an axon, the action potential causes neurotransmitter-containing vesicles in the terminal bouton to move toward the cell membrane. Subsequently, neurotransmitters contained in the vesicles are released into the synaptic cleft. Once released, the neurotransmitter molecules can cross the synapse and communicate signals by attaching to receptor sites on the post-synaptic membrane. The combined effect of multiple pre-synaptic action potentials is more likely to influence activity in the post-synaptic neuron than is a single firing. Multiple pre-synaptic firing can occur from a single cell (temporal summation) or from simultaneous action potentials occurring in discrete pre-synaptic neurons (spatial summation).

Following the release of a neurotransmitter into the synaptic cleft, some neurotransmitter molecules are taken back into the terminal of the pre-synaptic cell (reuptake) for storage and subsequent release. Others are broken down into metabolites (by-products) in the intracellular space. The metabolites are eventually excreted into cerebrospinal fluid, blood, and urine. Laboratory analysis of metabolite levels in these fluids may provide an indirect measure of neurotransmitter function.

POST-SYNAPTIC RESPONSE

Once a neurotransmitter molecule occupies a post-synaptic neuronal receptor site, a series of events occurs. Some receptors are coupled (paired) to an ion channel in the membrane. Binding of the neurotransmitter to these receptors can induce a direct change in cellular permeability or ionic balance, thus altering the resting potential of the post-synaptic neuron. Other receptors, which are not coupled to an ion channel, rely on intracellular *second-messenger* systems to transmit the chemical signals generated by a nerve impulse. In second-messenger systems, chemical processes are initiated by the binding of a neurotransmitter to a receptor that is coupled to either an inhibitory or stimulatory G protein (guanosine triphosphate-binding protein). Second-messenger systems elicit a chain of chemical and physiological reactions that influence behavior. Three important second-messenger signalling systems—involving calcium, adenylate cyclase, and inositol triphosphate (IP$_3$)/phospholipase-C—are described below. In general, different receptor subtypes use one of these second-messenger systems to influence cellular activity.

Calcium (Ca^{2+})

Binding of neurotransmitter to the receptor–G protein complex can alter the permeability of calcium-ion

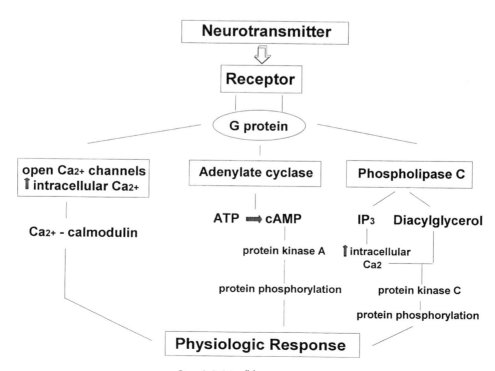

Figure 4–4. Intracellular messenger systems.

(Ca^{2+}) channels, resulting in increased intracellular Ca^{2+} (Figure 4–4). Increased availability of Ca^{2+} allows for the binding of this ion to calmodulin (a calcium-binding protein located in the dendritic area of many neurons).

Adenylate Cyclase

Adenylate cyclase is an enzyme that catalyzes the synthesis of cyclic-AMP (adenosine 3′,5′-cyclic monophosphate) from ATP (adenosine triphosphate) (Figure 4–4). Cyclic-AMP plays a key role in metabolic responses to cellular signaling. When a neurotransmitter binds to a receptor that is coupled to an *inhibitory* G protein, the complex inhibits the ability of adenylate cyclase to convert ATP to cyclic AMP. When a neurotransmitter binds to a receptor coupled to a *stimulating* G protein, adenylate cyclase converts ATP to cyclic-AMP. The production of cyclic-AMP activates an enzyme known as protein kinase-A, resulting in the phosphorylation of intracellular proteins. Cyclic-AMP is inactivated when it is broken down into 5′-AMP by yet another enzyme known as phosphodiesterase. Substances such as caffeine and theophylline inhibit the breakdown of cyclic-AMP by phosphodiesterase, and thus might be expected to enhance the signalling effects of an increased intracellular concentration of cyclic AMP.

Inositol Triphosphate (IP₃)/Phospholipase-C

Activation of the enzyme known as phospholipase-C by a neurotransmitter–receptor–G-protein complex results in the release of diacylglycerol and IP_3 from lipids bound to the membrane (Figure 4–4). IP_3 increases Ca^{2+} availability inside the cell and, together with the diacylglycerol, triggers protein kinase-C. Activation of protein kinase-C leads to the phosphorylation of intracellular proteins.

Other Messengers

Phospholipase-A_2 is the key component of a fourth, more recently identified second-messenger system, although its role in intracellular signalling is not well understood at present. In addition, the steroid hormones constitute another group of intracellular chemical messengers. Steroids can diffuse across cell membranes and bind to receptors in the cytoplasm and/or cell nucleus. By binding to specific receptors, steroid hormones can influence the rate of DNA transcription and translation of messenger RNA (mRNA).

As noted above, neurotransmitter-induced activation of second-messenger systems results in the phosphorylation of proteins, which leads to a cascade of bio-logical responses. The specificity of the biological responses to second-messenger systems, and their relationship to psychiatric illnesses, is currently an area of increased research in molecular biology.

■ THE NERVOUS SYSTEM

The following review of the major anatomical and functional aspects of the nervous system will help provide a contextual understanding of the environment in which neurons operate. The nervous system consists of two main interactive organizations: the **central nervous system** (CNS), including the brain and spinal cord; and the peripheral nervous system (PNS), concerned with the transmission of brain signals to and from areas outside the CNS.

STRUCTURE AND GENERAL FUNCTION OF THE CNS

The brain, also referred to as the encephalon, is a small organ relative to its complexity. The human adult brain weighs approximately 1,350 grams and is made up of neurons and neuroglia (support cells). Structurally, nerve cells form gray and white matter. Gray matter, found in areas including the cerebral cortex (outer layer of the brain) and spinal cord, is composed of nerve-cell bodies. White matter is made up of myelinated nerve-cell processes that form connective tracts joining various brain structures. The corpus callosum, the largest commissure (band of nerve fibers that cross the midline of the brain) in the brain, consists of white matter that connects the right and left hemispheres.

Three lining membranes (meninges)—the pia mater (inner membrane), arachnoid (middle membrane), and dura mater (outer membrane)—encapsulate and protect the brain. The brain is also protected by the layer of endothelial cells that form the inner lining of cerebral blood vessels, and which characteristically have tight junctions between one another. These junctions, which limit access of blood constituents to the CNS, create a protective barrier known as the *blood–brain barrier.*

The brain is subdivided into areas that arise from embryonic divisions (Table 1). Major structures within the brain include the cerebrum, thalamus, hypothalamus, cerebellum, brainstem, limbic system, and ventricles.

CEREBRUM

The cerebrum includes the cerebral hemispheres (structures in the telencephalon) and the structures associated with the diencephalon (Table 4–1). Each of

TABLE 4–1. MAJOR ANATOMICAL SUBDIVISIONS OF THE BRAIN

Divisions	Associated Structures
I. Telencephalon	Cerebral hemispheres, cortex, olfactory structures, basal ganglia, and lateral ventricles
II. Diencephalon	Epithalamus, thalamus, hypothalamus, subthalamus, and third ventricle
III. Mesencephalon	Cerebral aqueduct and substantia nigra
IV. Metencephalon	Pons and cerebellum
V. Myelencephalon	Medulla oblongata

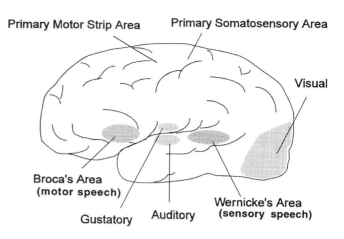

Figure 4–6. Functional localization in the cerebral cortex.

the two cerebral hemispheres include the frontal, parietal, temporal, occipital, insular, and limbic lobes (Figure 4–5). Two lobes are not shown in the figure: the insular lobe, tucked underneath the frontal and temporal lobes, and the limbic lobe, in the medial region of each hemisphere of the brain. Several prominent gray areas within the medial area of the brain include the caudate nucleus, lentiform nucleus, amygdaloid nucleus, and claustrum. Collectively, these areas are known as *basal ganglia,* and play a role in motor activity.

The cerebrum is the brain center responsible for intellectual functions, including learning, judgment, reasoning, and memory. It plays a primary role in processing emotions and processesing sensory input and impulses from the voluntary muscles of the body. The surface of the brain has many folds and grooves, known as *gyri* (ridges), *sulci* (shallow grooves), and *fissures* (deep grooves). The *cortex* (the Latin for *rind* or *bark*) forms the outer layer of the cerebral lobes, and consists of the neocortex (six layers) and the allocor-

tex (three layers). The cortex has a major role in processing sensory information. Figure 4–6 illustrates the activities associated with the frontal, parietal, temporal, and occipital lobes of the cortex. Functional studies have identified two central regions that play a major role in verbal communication. **Broca's motor speech area** is located on the left side of the brain (it is named after French surgeon Pierre Paul Broca, 1824–1880). Wernicke's sensory speech area is located in either the right or left hemisphere, according to which of the two is dominant in a particular individual (it is named after German neurologist Karl Wernicke, 1848–1905).

THALAMUS

The largest structure of the diencephalon is the thalamus. Its primary function is to receive sensory impulses (excluding olfactory impulses) from throughout the body (Figure 4–7). It is involved in relaying sensory impulses primarily concerned with pain, visual, auditory, temperature, and tactile sensations to the cerebral cortex. To a lesser extent, motor information, related primarily to reflexes, is also processed in the thalamus. A major function of the thalamus is integrating sensory and motor stimuli. The thalamus also plays a role in regulating mood and memory, and is involved in relaying input to and from the hypothalamus, as well as input to the amygdaloid nucleus. Near the thalamus lies the epithalamus, a structure of the diencephalon that contains the pineal gland. The pineal gland, which lies outside the blood–brain barrier, is the structure in which the hormone melatonin is synthesized. Melatonin is thought to play a role in the regulation of circadian rhythms.

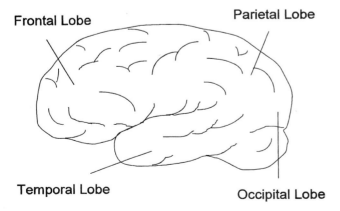

Figure 4–5. Cerebral lobes.

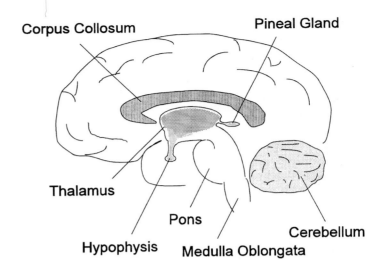

Figure 4–7. Additional anatomical structures of the brain.

HYPOTHALAMUS AND PITUITARY GLAND

Beneath the thalamus lies the hypothalamus, an integral component of the limbic system, **autonomic nervous system** (the nervous system that regulates automatic functions), and endocrine system. The hypothala-

mus plays a primary role in maintaining bodily homeostasis, including the regulation of body temperature, water balance, circadian rhythms, and food intake. The hypothalamus is also involved in the expression of mood (a function of the limbic system), stimulation of the autonomic nervous system, and release of an array of hormones (Table 4–2). Release of these hormones can have a stimulating or inhibiting effect on target-gland activity, depending on the hormone released. Trauma to or destruction of particular hypothalamic areas can result in functional disturbances including, for example, hyperthermia, diabetes insipidus, and loss of appetite.

Linked to the hypothalamus is the pituitary gland, also referred to as the hypophysis. The pituitary gland has two lobes, an anterior lobe (adenohypophysis) and a posterior lobe (neurohypophysis). The pituitary gland is controlled by the hypothalamus, and plays a key role in hormone synthesis (Table 4–2). Impaired pituitary functioning is associated with several endocrine disorders. Patients with abnormal hormonal functioning may present with what may initially appear to be psychiatric symptoms. For example, fatigue, decreased libido, and slurred speech are manifestations of acromegaly, an endocrine disorder involving hypersecretion of growth hormone.

TABLE 4–2. HYPOTHALAMIC AND PITUITARY HORMONES

Hypothalamus	
Corticotropin-releasing hormone	CRH
Gonadotropin-releasing hormone	GnRH
Growth hormone-inhibiting hormone (somatostatin)	
Growth hormone-releasing hormone	GHRH
Prolactin-inhibiting factor (dopamine)	PIF
Prolactin-stimulating factor	PSF
Thyrotropin-releasing hormone	TRH
Pituitary (Anterior)	
Adrenocorticotropic hormone	ACTH
β-lipotropin	
Follicle-stimulating hormone	FSH
Growth hormone	GH
Lutenizing hormone	LH
Melanocyte-stimulating hormone	MSH
Prolactin	PRL
Thyroid stimulating hormone	TSH
Pituitary (Posterior)	
Antidiuretic hormone (vasopressin)	ADH
Oxytocin	OT

LIMBIC SYSTEM

The **limbic system** includes a number of brain structures thought to play an important role in regulating emotions. Major components of the limbic system are the hippocampal formation (including the hippocampus) and the amygdaloid complex (amygdala). Functions of the hippocampal formation concern memory and learning. The amygdala (Greek for *almond shape*) is involved in feeding, sexual, and aggressive behaviors.

Neuronal damage in these structures can produce a range of behavioral or emotional alterations, including overeating (hyperphagia), hypersexuality, rage, or passivity. The thalamus and hypothalamus are also components of the limbic system. Other key structures of this system include the cingulate gyrus and the limbic midbrain nuclei (the origins of noradrenergic, dopamine, and serotonin neurotransmitter pathways). Damage to the cingulate gyrus can result in mutism, akinesia, and alteration in pain intolerance. Damage to the neurotransmitter nuclei may result in symptoms reflecting abnormalities in the regulatory influence of the particular neurotransmitter affected by the damage.

CEREBELLUM AND BRAINSTEM

The cerebellum is located in the posterior area of the brain and is connected to the brainstem. The cerebellum functions to maintain balance and muscle tone, and to coordinate voluntary muscles. Behavioral manifestations of cerebellar impairment include loss of balance, muscle in-coordination (dyssynergia), and decreased muscle tone (hypotonia). Impaired gait associated with alcohol intoxication is an example of dyssynergia secondary to cerebellar dysfunction.

Major structures of the brainstem include the pons and medulla oblongata. The brainstem contains the reticular formation, a structure controlling sleep and wakefulness. It is also the area directing visual and auditory reflexes. The medulla oblongata controls respiration, gastrointestinal motility, and circulation. Both the medulla oblongata and pons contain nerve-fiber pathways relaying information to other areas of the CNS, and from the CNS to peripheral tissues.

The brainstem contains nuclei that play a key role in neurotransmitter functioning, including the substantia nigra, locus ceruleus, and raphe nuclei. The substantia nigra contains the cell bodies of neurons specific for the neurotransmitters **dopamine** and **gamma aminobutyric acid (GABA).** The locus ceruleus contains the largest number of neuronal cell bodies specific for the neurotransmitter **norepinephrine.** The raphe nuclei contain the cell bodies of neurons specific for the neurotransmitter **serotonin.**

From the brainstem emerge ten of the twelve cranial nerves (III to XII). Injury to an individual cranial nerve is likely to produce symptoms specific to the area innervated by that cranial nerve (Table 4–3).

Extending down from the brainstem is the spinal cord, which continues to the first lumbar vertebra. The spinal cord includes 31 pairs of nerves divided into five areas: cervical (8 nerves), thoracic (12 nerves), lumbar (5 nerves), sacral (5 nerves), and coccygeal (1 nerve). A transverse cross-section of the spinal cord shows a butterfly-like appearance (gray matter) surrounded by white matter (Figure 4–8). The gray matter on each

TABLE 4–3. CRANIAL NERVES AND CLINICAL CORRELATES

Cranial Nerves	Area of Innervation	Clinical Correlates Reflective of Impairment
I. Olfactory Nerve	Smell	Anosmia
II. Optic Nerve	Vision, pupillary reflexes to light	Blunted pupillary light reflexes, papilledema, ipsilateral blindness
III. Oculomotor Nerve	Eye movement, pupillary constriction	Ptosis (upper eyelid drooping), diplopia (double vision), fixed dilated pupil
IV. Trochlear Nerve	Superior oblique muscle (inward and downward eye movement)	Eye extorsion, difficulty with downward eye movement, vertical diplopia
V. Trigeminal Nerve	Mastication muscles, facial sensations (skin, mouth, nose, eyes), tympanum	Loss of jaw movement and facial sensations, diminutive corneal reflex, low-pitch deafness
VI. Abducens Nerve	Lateral rectus muscle (eye abduction)	Convergent strabismus (eye turns inward); horizontal diplopia
VII. Facial Nerve	Facial muscles, taste buds (salty, sweet, sour), lacrimation, salivation	Facial paralysis and spasm, mouth droop, loss of corneal reflex (blinking), loss of taste, difficulty closing eyes; associated with Bell's palsy
VIII. Vestibulochochlear Nerve	Auditory, balance	Loss of hearing, tinnitus, disequilibrium, vertigo; associated with Meniere's syndrome
IX. Glossopharyngeal Nerve	Gag reflex, swallowing, bitter taste buds	Loss of gag reflex, loss of taste (posterior third of tongue)
X. Vagus Nerve	Gag reflex, swallowing, phonation, mucous membranes and internal organs of the thoracic, abdominal and neck cavities	Loss of gag reflex, hoarseness, dysphagia, and dysphonia (related to ipsilateral drooping of soft palate)
XI. Accessory Nerve	Shoulder and head movement, larynx muscles	Drooping shoulder and difficulty in turning head (related to paralysis of sternocleidomastoid and trapezius muscles)
XII. Hypoglossal Nerve	Tongue movement	Hemiparalysis of the tongue; associated with brainstem lesions

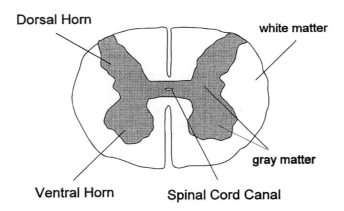

Figure 4–8. Transverse section of the spinal cord.

side of the spinal cord consists of three regions: the dorsal horn, lateral horn, and ventral horn, which are integral to peripheral nervous system (PNS) functioning described below.

VENTRICLES

Cerebrospinal fluid (CSF) is produced by the choroid plexus and found within the four fluid-containing, inter-connecting ventricles (cavities) of the brain. CSF is produced at a rate of 500 ml/day, with the total steady-state volume ranging from 100 to 140 ml in an adult. CSF functions to cushion the brain, deliver hormones, and transport waste products. Waste products in the

CSF are removed through the arachnoid villi, which are finger-like processes projecting into the subarachnoid space. CSF is transported out of the ventricular system into the subarachnoid space via the cerebral aqueduct (aqueduct of Sylvius). Blockage of the cerebral aqueduct results in hydrocephalus, an enlargement of the head secondary to increased CSF volume.

■ STRUCTURE AND GENERAL FUNCTION OF THE PERIPHERAL NERVOUS SYSTEM

Spinal nerves relay information *to* (afferent) and *from* (efferent) the CNS. The *visceral afferent neurons* send stimuli to the CNS from peripheral organs and smooth muscles. The *somatic afferent neurons* send signals from voluntary muscles and skin to the CNS. In general, the dorsal horn (composed of neurons that receive sensory impulses) and the lateral horn (composed of neurons receiving viscerosensory impulses) are associated with the afferent neurons.

The ventral horn is primarily involved in efferent signaling (efferent neurons) (Figure 4–8). From a functional perspective, the efferent division of the peripheral nervous system (PNS) can be further divided into the somatic nervous system and the autonomic nervous system (Figure 4–9). The somatic nervous system innervates the skeletal muscles and is responsible for voluntary movement. Because of its complexity and its frequent involvement in symptoms of psychiatric dis-

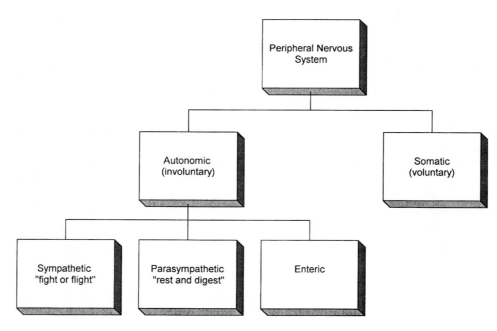

Figure 4–9. Peripheral nervous system.

orders, the autonomic nervous system is discussed in more detail below.

AUTONOMIC NERVOUS SYSTEM

The autonomic nervous system is responsible for a wide spectrum of involuntary, automatic functions. For example, a person breathes without actively contemplating inhalation. The heart beats without a person's consciously considering the action of cardiac contractions. Peristalsis occurs without a person's thinking about intestinal movement. All of these functions are controlled by the autonomic nervous system. The autonomic nervous system transmits signals through two types of efferent fibers: preganglionic and postganglionic neurons. Preganglionic neurons have their cell bodies located within the CNS and carry signals from the CNS to cell bodies grouped together in the periphery, and known as ganglia. Postganglionic neurons, whose cell bodies are located in the ganglia, then relay these signals to the targeted tissue. The autonomic nervous system is divided into the sympathetic, parasympathetic, and enteric divisions.

Sympathetic Division

The sympathetic division of the autonomic nervous system (involving preganglionic neurons that arise from the thoracic and lumbar areas of the spinal cord) is often referred to as the *adrenergic system* or *fight or flight* stress-response system. Stress can be physiological (e.g., exercise), emotional (e.g., fear), or both. In a stressful situation, a person is likely to confront the situation (fight) or remove him- or herself from the immediate threat (flight). The body needs to be prepared to handle either response. Stimulation of the sympathetic nervous system results in increased blood flow to skeletal muscles, increased heart rate, increased blood pressure, sweating, and dilation of the pupils to prepare for the stress. Functions less critical to the immediate need of fight or flight (e.g., gastrointestinal motility and skin blood flow) are slowed by sympathetic stimulation.

Two neurotransmitters are primarily involved in the transmission of sympathetic signals: acetylcholine (released from preganglionic sympathetic neurons), and norepinephrine (released from postganglionic sympathetic neurons). (Activation of the adrenal medulla results in the release of epinephrine.) Secretion of norepinephrine and epinephrine increases tissue response in organs that have receptors specific for these adrenergic hormones.

Parasympathetic Division

Sympathetic activity is counterbalanced by the parasympathetic division of the autonomic nervous system (involving preganglionic neurons that originate from the cranial and sacral regions of the body). The parasympathetic division is often referred to as the *rest and digest* division or *cholinergic system*. Unlike the sympathetic system, the parasympathetic system fosters a normal homeostatic state. Rather than mobilizing and expending resources, the parasympathetic system functions to conserve energy. Thus, this division serves to decrease the heart rate and blood pressure, and to constrict the pupils. Acetylcholine is the primary neurotransmitter involved in both pre- and postganglionic parasympathetic signaling.

Enteric Division

A third division of the autonomic nervous system is the enteric division, which is chiefly concerned with regulating gastrointestinal motility. Its function is influenced by both the sympathetic and parasympathetic divisions. Sympathetic activity commonly results in inhibition of gastrointestinal functions, whereas parasympathetic activity has an excitatory effect.

■ NEUROTRANSMITTER REGULATION AND PSYCHIATRIC ILLNESSES

In contrast to neurological disorders, which are often associated with structural lesions in the CNS, psychiatric disorders are thought to be influenced by abnormal patterns of interaction between neurochemical messenger systems in the brain. The role of the major neurotransmitter systems in behavior, emotion, and cognition is reviewed in the following sections.

NEUROTRANSMITTERS

Neurotransmitters typically are synthesized, stored, and released by the neuron. Recent research suggests that nerve terminals are capable of storing multiple neurotransmitters. Secretion of neurotransmitters often follows a circadian rhythm, and these substances may therefore be secreted at different rates at different times of the day. The classification of neurotransmitters is based on their chemical structure, and includes the cholinergic, monoamine, amino acid, peptide, and nitric oxide groups of neurotransmitters (Figure 4–10).

Although neurons generally follow the same process of neurotransmitter storage and synaptic release, different neurotransmitters are synthesized in different ways. For example, in the production of acetylcholine, extracellular choline is transported into the cytoplasm of the neuron, where it undergoes an enzymatic reaction that forms the neurotransmitter acetylcholine. The synthesis of some neurotransmitters de-

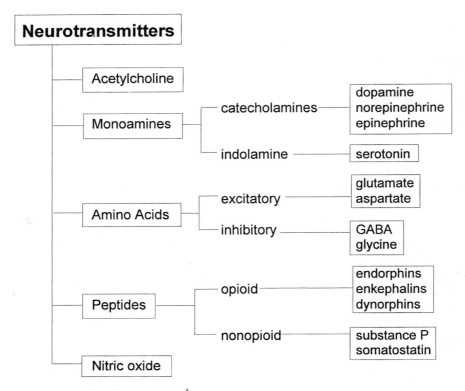

Figure 4–10. Classification of neurotransmitters.

pends on amino acid precursors obtained from dietary intake. For example, dopamine is synthesized from the amino acid tyrosine. Following transport into a dopamine-producing neuron, tyrosine is chemically transformed (by hydroxylation) into dihydroxyphenylalanine (DOPA), which is subsequently converted (via decarboxylation) into dopamine (Figure 4–11). Since the neurotransmitter norepinephrine is synthesized from dopamine, it also depends on the availability of tyrosine (Figure 4–11). Other examples of neurotransmitters derived from amino acids include serotonin, which originates from tryptophan (Figure 4–12); hista-

mine, formed from histidine; and GABA, formed from glutamate.

NEUROTRANSMITTER RECEPTORS

Receptors are located on the pre-synaptic (autoreceptors) and post-synaptic cell membranes. The different subtypes of receptors for neurotransmitters differ in their binding affinity for their respective neurotrans-

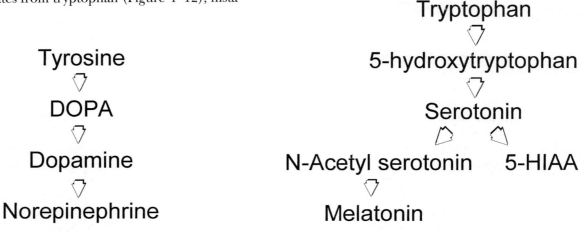

Figure 4–11. Synthesis of dopamine and norepinephrine.

Figure 4–12. Synthesis of serotonin.

mitters, and also in their binding affinity for drugs related to a particular neurotransmitter. Receptor subtypes are often located in different functional areas and mediate different behavioral or therapeutic effects. Major types of receptors are those that serve the cholinergic, dopaminergic, noradrenergic, and serotonergic systems.

Cholinergic receptors are characterized as either muscarinic or nicotinic. Muscarinic receptors bind to acetylcholine as well as muscarine (an alkaloid). Five known muscarinic receptor subtypes (M_1 to M_5) are currently known. Nicotinic receptors bind to acetylcholine, but also bind to nicotine. Dopaminergic receptors are characterized as D_1 through D_5, and adrenergic receptors are identified as α_1, α_2, β_1, and β_2. Receptors that are specific for serotonin are divided into two types: 5-HT_1 and non-5-HT_1. (5-HT is the abbreviation for 5-hydroxytryptamine, the chemical name for serotonin). Serotonin receptors are also further divided into additional subtypes, including 5-HT_{1A} through 5-HT_{1F}, and 5-HT_2 through 5-HT_7. Thus, there is the potential for great specificity in neurotransmitter receptor activity. Classification of the subtypes of neurotransmitter receptors is in a continued phase of evolution.

The stimulation or inhibition of neurotransmitter receptors results in biological and behavioral responses that include both desired and unwanted effects. For example, administration of a neuroleptic/antipsychotic medication that blocks the dopamine D_2 receptor may result not only in relief of psychotic symptoms, but also in extrapyramidal symptoms (EPS), e.g. tremors, dystonia, akathisia and dyskinesia. This appears to occur because D_2 receptors, according to current thought, are involved in mediating both psychotic symptoms and extrapyramidal symptoms. Tricyclic antidepressants often cause side effects in addition to intended antidepressant effects; blockade of muscarinic receptors by these drugs results in the commonly observed anticholinergic effects of blurred vision, dry mouth, and constipation.

HOW ARE NEUROTRANSMITTERS RELATED TO PSYCHIATRIC SYMPTOMATOLOGY?

Although the specific roles of neurotransmitters in psychiatric illnesses are not known, most evidence suggests that none of the major psychiatric disorders is a result of abnormalities in a single neurotransmitter system. Rather, psychiatric illnesses are associated with alterations in several neurotransmitters. Alterations in neurotransmitter functioning could result from problems at one or more sites in the system. For example, neurotransmitter synthesis, the availability of neurotransmitter precursor, pre-synaptic release mechanism function, receptor sensitivity, and re-uptake capability can alter neurotransmitter action and influence nervous-system function and behavior. The following section illustrates some of the postulated associations between specific neurotransmitter functioning and illnesses seen in the psychiatric setting.

Schizophrenia

Research and clinical observations suggest that increased dopamine, increased norepinephrine, and the balance between dopamine and serotonin in the CNS may play a role in schizophrenia. Recent attention has focused particularly on the role of dopamine. Several lines of evidence are consistent with a *dopamine hypothesis* of schizophrenia, which proposes that psychotic symptoms associated with this illness result from excessive dopamine activity in areas of the CNS associated with cognitive functioning. Pharmacologically related support for this hypothesis derives from observations that prolonged self-administration of high doses of stimulant drugs (e.g., amphetamines) can result in psychotic symptoms. Research has shown that amphetamine can increase dopamine function by augmenting pre-synaptic dopamine release and blocking pre-synaptic re-uptake of this neurotransmitter. Biological studies involving post-mortem studies and dopamine metabolite levels in CSF have not provided consistent evidence for alterations in dopamine activity in schizophrenia. Recent studies have, however, shown that antipsychotic medications with the ability to block D_2 receptors produce a therapeutic behavioral response, suggesting a role for post-synaptic dopamine receptors in the course of schizophrenia. Although this evidence suggests that patients with schizophrenia may have an increase in the number of D_2 receptors in the CNS, other etiologies for schizophrenia cannot be ruled out at the present time.

Excessive concentrations of the excitatory amino acid glutamate in the CNS may also contribute to psychotic symptomatology. Observations of psychosis, hallucinations, and disorganized thought content after the administration of drugs (e.g., the hallucinogen phencyclide [PCP]) that block glutamate receptors provide supportive evidence for this hypothesis. Additionally, impaired memory and cognitive functioning may be related to functional disturbances of glutamate neurons that project into the cerebral cortex and hippocampus.

Mood Disorders

Major depression has been associated with the *norepinephrine hypothesis*, which suggests reduced norepinephrine functioning in the CNS as a cause for depression. Monoamine oxidase inhibitors (MAOIs) prevent the breakdown of norepinephrine. This pharmacologic effect increases norepinephrine concentrations available for interacting with receptors, and appears to contribute to the therapeutic response to MAOIs in many patients with depression.

Affective illnesses are thought to also involve the serotonin system. A serotonin hypothesis in major depression is supported by findings of reduced levels of the serotonin metabolite 5-HIAA (5-hydroxyindoleacetic acid) in cerebrospinal fluid, and a pharmacologic response to antidepressant medications that augment serotonin availability in the synaptic cleft (e.g., serotonin reuptake inhibitors [SSRIs]).

Anxiety Disorders, Eating Disorders and Impulse-Related Disorders

Anxiety disorders and mania have been linked to increased norepinephrine concentrations in the CNS. More than 50% of the cell bodies of neurons that produce norepinephrine as a neurotransmitter are located in the locus ceruleus, and stimulation of this area can result in an anxiogenic behavioral response. Treatment of anxiogenic symptoms with anti-anxiety medications tends to decrease nerve-cell firing in the locus ceruleus, potentially contributing to the therapeutic effect of anti-anxiety agents. Behavioral symptoms of arousal sometimes noted in cocaine-abusing patients may be related to cocaine's interference with the normal reuptake of norepinephrine (as well as dopamine), which results in the presence of increased quantities of this neurotransmitter in the synaptic cleft.

Serotonin is thought to play a role in regulating eating behavior, particularly satiety (how satiated or full one feels after a meal). Because of this functional role, and evidence from clinical studies, altered serotonin regulation is suspected in some patients with eating disorders, including bulimia nervosa. Reduced levels of serotonin have been implicated in bulimia nervosa and also in impulsive and aggressive behaviors. Current investigations are examining the relationship between serotonin and obsessive-compulsive disorder.

Other Disorders and Neurotransmitter Systems

More recent investigations have begun to explore the potential psychiatric correlates of alterations in amino acids, acetylcholine, neuropeptides, and nitric oxide neurotransmitters.

In addition to norepinephrine, the inhibitory neurotransmitter GABA, derived from glutamate, may also be involved in anxiety disorders. Many anti-anxiety medications are indirect GABA agonists (augment GABA function), suggesting that GABA plays an important role in anxiety disorders.

Impaired memory may involve a number of neurotransmitters including acetylcholine, somatostatin, and nitric oxide. Alzheimer's disease has been associated with impaired brain function in areas with high concentrations of acetylcholine-producing neurons. Drugs that block muscarinic receptors for acetylcholine can induce memory impairment. Concentrations of the neuropeptide somatostatin in the neocortex and hippocampus have been shown to be reduced in Alzheimer's disease. Reduced norepinephrine levels have also been linked to Alzheimer's disease, which has been related to a loss of noradrenergic neurons in the locus ceruleus. Nitric oxide, a recently identified neurotransmitter, is thought to play a role in memory formation.

Abnormalities in neurotransmitter functioning are believed to contribute to certain neurological conditions as well as to psychiatric disorders. Kindling-induced seizures may be related to a dysregulation of glutamate. Migraine headaches are thought to be associated with abnormalities in serotonin function, particularly in light of their frequent therapeutic response to medications that enhance serotonin function, including a drug that is a 5-HT1$_d$ receptor agonist. Substance P (a nonopioid neuropeptide) and enkephalins (opioid neuropeptides) play a role in pain transmission and pain suppression, respectively. Huntington's chorea has been linked to a loss of GABA neurons in the striatum. Parkinson's disease, involving the degeneration of the nigrostriatal tract, is associated with altered dopamine functioning. The nigrostriatal tract is a concentrated area of dopaminergic neurons, and insult to this area is thought to contribute to reduced levels of dopamine in the CNS in patients with Alzheimer's disease.

■ CLINICAL ASSESSMENT OF BRAIN FUNCTIONING: LABORATORY TECHNIQUES

Several laboratory techniques involving brain imaging and electrophysiology are currently available to assess the relationship between the structure and function of the brain and behavior. A basic medical evaluation, however, is important to rule out the potential contribution of underlying medical illness to psychiatric symptomatology, since behavioral problems can have multiple etiologies.

BRAIN-IMAGING TECHNIQUES

Techniques for imaging the brain include **computed tomography (CT), positron emission tomography (PET), single-photon emission computed tomography (SPECT), magnetic resonance imaging (MRI), electroencephalogram (EEG), polysomnography,** and **evoked potentials (EP).**

Computed Tomography (CT)

CT imaging produces a series of X-rays that are processed by a computer to construct an image of the brain. Integration of the individual X-ray images results in a cross-sectional picture of the brain. Computer compilation of many consecutive cross-sectional images produces a three-dimensional image. Clinically, CT is used to assess suspected organic brain disorders, and is helpful in assessing bone structures. Research using CT with various psychiatric populations has led to the finding of ventricular enlargement in some patients with schizophrenia. This abnormality has been correlated with a poor response to medication.

Positron-Emission Tomography (PET)

PET, another brain-imaging technique, involves the administration of a small amount of a radioactive compound (radioligand), which is delivered via the circulatory system into the brain. Fluorodeoxyglucose (FDG) is an example of such a radioligand. Once in the brain, the radioligand emits gamma rays, which can be recorded by an array of detectors placed around the head, and can be analyzed by a computer. Like CT, PET produces cross-sectional images of the brain and transforms them into a three-dimensional image. Glucose utilization, blood flow, and neurotransmitter-receptor activity in the brain can be examined with PET. Although PET is a helpful research tool for studying the relationship between brain function and psychiatric conditions, its clinical use requires further exploration.

Single-Photon-Emission Computed Tomography (SPECT)

SPECT is a brain-imaging technique similar to PET, but it uses a longer-acting radioligand. The long-acting radioligand allows computer detectors to rotate around the head and make additional planar images of the brain. Although it images the same structures as PET, SPECT has less resolution yielding images with less detail than those produced by PET. Its clinical use needs further investigation.

Magnetic Resonance Imaging (MRI)

MRI, a relatively recent brain-imaging technique, uses a magnetic field projected onto the brain; energy from brain activity is detected by sensors to produce an image. In comparison to CT, PET, and SPECT, an advantage of MRI is the lack of patient exposure to ionizing radiation. With MRI, the clinician can distinguish between white and gray matter. Thus, MRI is clinically useful in identifying areas of demyelination in the brain, e.g. multiple sclerosis. A disadvantage of MRI is that patients must lie still in an enclosed, confined space for the procedure to be done. This experience provokes anxiety for some individuals, particularly those with a history of claustrophobia.

Electroencephalogram (EEG)

The EEG measures electrical activity in the brain. Electrodes are placed on designated areas of the scalp and detect electrical activity resulting from electrical potentials in the neurons. The amplitude and frequency of this electrical activity is recorded and transcribed into a wave recording with separate tracings for delta, theta, alpha, and beta waves. Delta and theta waves occur during sleep, alpha waves when one is in a relaxed, awake state with eyes closed. Beta waves are commonly observed during alert states. Clinically, EEGs help to differentiate organic and functional disorders of the central nervous system.

Polysomnography

Polysomnography uses an EEG to obtain electrophysiological measurements of brain activity during sleep. It is also used to record eye movement during sleep, which is characterized as rapid eye movement (REM) and non-rapid eye movement (non-REM). There are four stages of non-REM sleep; stage one reflects light sleep and stage four a deep sleep, characterized by slow waves. When REM occurs, the slow waves of stage-four sleep are replaced with rapid activity similar to that of an awake state. Abnormal patterns of REM sleep have been observed in patients with depression.

Evoked Potentials (EP)

EP are EEG measurements recorded in response to an external stimulus (visual, auditory, or somatosensory). The timing of peaks in the wave recording provides an index of cognitive processing, and has been used in research studies to compare cognitive processing in psychotic and nonpsychotic patients.

COMPUTERS AND THE HUMAN BRAIN

—Ann Wolbert Burgess

Following the Second World War and the advent of digital computers, computer engineers pushed science technology to its limits using traditional computer architectures. To achieve more complex computers, engineering researchers began to investigate how the brain processed data. This research has followed two paths: biological, based on the neuronal model; and artificial intelligence. The most difficult part of this research thus far has been to develop the rules that govern human thought, that is, the discipline of artificial intelligence.

Neuronal Model

Warren McCulloch and Walter Pitts, in 1943, showed that the operation of a nerve cell and its connection with other nerve cells (a so-called neural network) could be modeled in terms of logic. Nerves could be thought of as logical statements. This thought led to the model of the human brain as a system operating via the principles of logic, and thus as a powerful computer. Rather than trying to build machines that mimicked the physiology of the brain, analogies could be pursued at a higher level in terms of the kinds of thinking that go on in the human brain. Logical constructs for human problem-solving might then be converted into logical and mathematical propositions to be embodied in a computer program (Heimes, 1980).

In the 1940s, mathematician Norbert Weiner, at the Massachusetts Institute of Technology (MIT), put forth the then-radical notion that it is legitimate to describe machines that exhibit feedback as "striving toward goals," as calculating the differences between their goals and their actual performance, and as then working to reduce these differences. Machines were purposeful. Wiener's thinking was applied to the CNS as follows:

> The central nervous system no longer appears as a self-contained organ, receiving inputs from the senses and discharging into the muscles. On the contrary, some of its most characteristic activities are explicable only as circular processes, emerging from the nervous system into the muscles, and re-entering the nervous system through the sense organs, whether they be proprioceptors or organs of the special senses. This seemed to us to mark a new step in the study of that part of neurophysiology which concerns not solely the elementary processes of nerves and synapses but the performance of the nervous system as an integrated whole (Wiener, 1948).

This critical contribution of such a *feedback loop* led to a concept of mind as more than physiology and response. In 1961, Wiener introduced his neologistic science as follows: "We have decided to call the entire field of control and communication theory, whether in the machine or in the animal, by the name Cybernetics" (Weiner, 1961). In his book, Weiner set down an integrated vision that linked developments in understanding the human nervous system, the electronic computer, and the operation of other machines. He underscored his belief, as well as that of John von Neumann and MacCulloch, and Pitts, that the functioning of the living organism and the operation of the new communication machines exhibited crucial parallels (Gardner, 1985).

Information theory

Another key progenitor of cognitive science was Claude Shannon, an electrical engineer at MIT who is credited with devising information theory. He stated that all information can be represented with binary codes. His basic theory was that any analog signal such as sound, can be encoded with a minimum number of codes. This made possible computer processing of natural phenomena such as the voice and music. The new digital networks of the telephone companies are one result of his research. Shannon's work led to the notion that information can be thought of in a way entirely divorced from specific content or subject matter; that is, simply as a single decision between two equally plausible alternatives. According to information theory, the basic unit of information is the bit (binary digit), or the amount of information required to select one message from two equally probable alternatives.

In the human system, on the other hand, a unit of information is not equivalent to all other information. Value orientation, or weighting of the information, must occur. A theory of information processing is emerging. It is another way of thinking about mind and behavior, and ultimately about how people learn. Unlike the computer, which is capable of doing only what a program tells it to do, individuals are capable of doing what they have learned to do. Table 4–4 compares the personal computer system and the human system.

TABLE 4–4. PERSONAL COMPUTER SYSTEM AND HUMAN EQUIVALENTS

Information Processing	
COMPUTER ⇔ HUMAN INTERACTION	**HUMAN ⇔ HUMAN INTERACTION**
Power on	Neurotransmitters activated
Load program	Associative cues
Password to use program	
Input data (human)	Sensory inputs
Process data (computer)	Sensory processing
Output data (computer)	Verbal, and/or physical responses
Input data (human response to output)	Sensory inputs

System Failures	
COMPUTER PROBLEMS	**PSYCHIATRIC MENTAL HEALTH PROBLEMS**
Program error	Trauma, physical or chemical imbalance
Input corruption	Impaired thought processes; perceptual processing physical impairment; (e.g., hearing, sight)
Memory failure	Short-term memory error: forgetting
Disk failure	Long-term memory error: amnesia, dementia

O AN OVERVIEW

- The interface between the brain and behavior is complex and endlessly intriguing.

- Physiological aspects of the brain can influence behavior, behavior can similarly influence basic physiological processes.

- Increased understanding of the dynamic interplay between brain function, current environmental influences, and an individual's past experiences can lead to a greater appreciation and understanding of the person.

- Understanding the individual facilitates the practitioner's ability to assess the individual and to plan interventions to enhance that person's physical and emotional well being.

TD TERMS TO DEFINE

- acetylcholine

- autonomic nervous system

- Broca's area

- central nervous system

- computed tomography (CT)

- dopamine

- electroencephalogram

- gamma aminobutyric acid (GABA)

- limbic system

- magnetic resonance imaging (MRI)

- norepinephrine

- positron emission tomography (PET)

- serotonin

- single-photon emission computed tomography (SPECT)

Q STUDY QUESTIONS

Multiple Choice Questions:

1. Stress stimulates all of the following events EXCEPT

   a. enzymatic phosphorylation.
   b. norepinephrine secretion.
   c. electrical cellular firing.
   d. pupillary constriction.

2. Mrs. Lenz has been diagnosed with multiple sclerosis. Which of the following statements does NOT reflect her condition?

   a. Mrs. Lenz may experience behavioral impairments resulting from interrupted cellular signalling.
   b. Mrs. Lenz is experiencing degeneration of gray matter in the central nervous system.
   c. Magnetic resonance imaging (MRI) is more likely to detect Mrs. Lenz's condition than is computed tomography (CT).
   d. Mrs. Lenz's condition involves impaired myelination.

3. Mr. Parker, 38 years old, is suffering from a chronic history of schizophrenia. He currently exhibits delusional symptoms and is experiencing extrapyramidal side effects (EPS) from his antipsychotic medication. Which of the following statements does NOT reflect a current understanding of possible biological underpinnings related to schizophrenia?

   a. Mr. Parker may have biological vulnerability to excessive dopaminergic activity in the central nervous system.
   b. Mr. Parker's extrapyramidal symptoms (EPS) are likely to be exacerbated by traditional antipsychotic drugs (e.g., haldol) than by antipsychotics with weak D_2 affinity.
   c. Mr. Parker may have impaired functioning in the substantia nigra and/or cingulate gyrus of the brain.
   d. Mr. Parker's chronic illness is most likely a result of neuronal death secondary to external toxins incurred during experimental use of marijuana at age 16.

4. Neurons are similar to many other types of cells EXCEPT that they:

   a. are dependent upon adequate nutrition.
   b. require proteins for energy production and expenditure.
   c. are not capable of cellular division.
   d. rely on the cell membrane for transporting nutrients.

5. The brain-imaging technique that does NOT increase a patient's exposure to ionizing radiation is
   a. computed tomography (CT).
   b. positron emission tomography (PET).
   c. single-photon emission computed tomography (SPECT).
   d. magnetic resonance imaging (MRI).

6. Each of the following substances is primarily involved in second-messenger signaling EXCEPT
   a. guanosine triphosphate-binding proteins (G proteins).
   b. Ca^{2+}.
   c. glutamate.
   d. adenylate cyclase.

7. Which of the following is NOT a protective mechanism of the brain?
   a. Meninges
   b. Blood brain barrier
   c. Cerebrospinal fluid
   d. Sulci

8. The following is a list of brain structures and their associated function(s). Which grouping is INCORRECTLY matched?
   a. Basal ganglia: motor activity
   b. Reticular formation: melatonin synthesis
   c. Broca's area: speech
   d. Hypothalamus: temperature, water balance, food intake
   e. Cerebellum: coordination, balance
   f. Hippocampus: memory

9. Mr. Sachs presents with the following symptoms: diminished gag reflex, hoarseness, and dysphagia. He is otherwise healthy, does not take medications, and has no known active medical or psychiatric illness. His presentation suggests possible impairment of the
   a. vagus nerve.
   b. accessory nerve.
   c. trigeminal nerve.
   d. abducens nerve.

Short Essay Questions:

1. Describe a synapse and include a discussion of the antecedents and consequences of cellular firing in the central nervous system.

2. Discuss three areas in which understanding the relationship between brain and behavior has the potential for beneficially influencing patient care.

3. Discuss the role of serotonin in mental illness. Describe the synthesis of serotonin, potential influences on its availability at the synaptic site, and the role that medications may play in manipulating its concentrations in the brain.

■ REFERENCES AND SUGGESTED READING

Fischbach GD: Mind and brain. *Sci. Amer.* 1992; 267:48–57.

Gardner H: *The Mind's New Science.* New York; Basic Books, 1985.

Griffen JE, Ojeda SR (eds): *Textbook of Endocrine Physiology,* ed 2. New York, Oxford University Press, 1992.

Cooper JR, Bloom FE, Roth RH: *The Biochemical Basis of Neuropharmacology,* ed 6. New York, Oxford University Press, 1991.

Hales RE, Yudofsky SC (eds): *Textbook of Neuropsychiatry,* ed 2. Washington, DC, American Psychiatric Press 1992.

Heimes SJ: *John von Neuman and Norbert Weiner.* Cambridge, MA, MIT Press, 1980; 211.

Hunter R, Macalpine I: *Three Hundred Years of Psychiatry: 1535–1860.* New York, Oxford University Press, 1963.

Siegel GJ, Agranoff BW, Albers RW, Molinoff PB (eds): *Basic Neurochemistry,* ed 5. New York, Raven Press, 1993.

Schatzberg AF, Nemeroff CB (eds): *Textbook of Psychopharmacology.* Washington, DC, American Psychiatric Press, 1995.

Weiner N: *Cybernetics, or Control and Communication, in the Animal and the Machine,* ed 2. Cambridge, MA, MIT Press, 1961; 8. Original work published in 1948.

V VOCABULARY

acetylcholine—a neurotransmitter synthesized from choline; decreased acetylcholine is thought to play a role in Alzheimer's disease and memory impairment.

action potential—cell firing often initiated by a sudden change in cellular ionic balance.

adenylate cyclase—a second-messenger system involving the stimulation and inhibition of formation of cyclic-AMP from ATP.

amygdala—Greek for "almond shape"; a brain structure involved in regulation of feeding, sexual, and aggressive behaviors.

autonomic nervous system—a division of the peripheral nervous system primarily concerned with involuntary functions; divided into the sympathetic, parasympathetic, and enteric systems.

autoreceptors—neurotransmitter receptors located on the membrane of the presynaptic cell.

axon—a cylindrical structure that is part of the neuron, varying in diameter and length; it relays information away from the cell body to the terminal bouton of the neuron.

blood-brain barrier—a protective system, consisting of the lining of blood vessels and comprising endothelial cells with tight junctions, thus limiting access of blood constituents to the CNS.

brain—also known as the encephalon; comprised of nerve cells; it weighs approximately 1,350 grams (human adult).

Broca's area—a motor speech area located on the left side of the brain (after French surgeon Pierre Paul Broca, 1824–1880).

Calcium (Ca^{2+})—a second messenger that activates calcium ions within the cell.

cell membrane—a permeable membrane that allows the flow of materials into and out of the cell.

central nervous system (CNS)—the brain and the spinal cord.

cerebellum—a brain structure responsible for balance, muscle tone, and voluntary muscle coordination.

cerebral cortex—the outer layer of the cerebral lobes; it plays a major role in the processing of sensory information.

cerebrum—a brain structure that includes the cerebral hemispheres and structures associated with the diencephalon; the center for intellectual functions including learning, judgment, reasoning, and memory; it plays a primary role in the processing of emotions and sensory input and impulses from voluntary muscles.

cerebrospinal fluid—a fluid produced by the choroid plexus in the ventricles to cushion and protect the brain; it is produced at a rate of 500 ml/day; it transports hormones and waste products.

choroid plexus—the brain structure that produces cerebrospinal fluid; it is contained in the ventricles of the brain.

computed tomography (CT)—an imaging technique using X-rays for the construction of a three-dimensional image.

cranial nerves—twelve nerves, each associated with specific areas of functioning; these nerves arise from the brainstem.

cytoplasm—an intracellular fluid composed largely of water; it contains nutrients needed to maintain cellular functioning.

dendrites—branched processes extending from the cell body that relay information to the cell body and receive signals from numerous neurons.

dendritic spines—extending branches of dendrites.

depolarization—a change in the neuronal membrane permeability resulting from a decrease in resting polarization; it begins with the intracellular influx of sodium ions.

dopamine—a monoamine (catecholamine) neurotransmitter synthesized from tyrosine; it is thought to play a role in schizophrenia.

electroencephalogram (EEG)—a measure of electrical activity in the brain using electrodes placed on the scalp; it detects the amplitude and frequency of electrical activity transcribed into wave recordings characterized as delta, theta, alpha, and beta waves.

enkephalin—an opioid peptide neurotransmitter thought to play a role in pain suppression.

enteric—a division of the autonomic nervous system primarily concerned with regulating gastrointestinal motility.

evoked potentials (EP)—EEG measurements recorded in response to an external stimulus (visual, auditory, or somatosensory).

fissures—deep grooves observed on the surface of the brain.

gamma aminobutyric acid (GABA)—an inhibitory amino acid neurotransmitter synthesized from glutamate; it is thought to play a role in anxiety disorders; loss of GABA neurons is associated with Huntington's chorea.

glutamate—an excitatory amino acid neurotransmitter and precursor to GABA; it is thought to play a role in psychosis and kindling-induced seizures.

Golgi type I neurons—neurons having long axons.

Golgi type II neurons—neurons having short axons.

gray matter—CNS tissue consisting of nerve cell bodies; it is found in areas including the cerebral cortex and spinal cord.

gyri—ridges observed on the surface of the brain.

histamine—a neurotransmitter synthesized from histidine.

histidine—an amino acid; precursor to histamine.

hyperpolarization—the cellular resting state, characterized by high intracellular potassium concentrations.

hypothalamus—the brain structure involved in homeostasis, including the regulation of body temperature, water balance, circadian rhythms, and food intake; a component of the limbic system, autonomic nervous system, and endocrine system.

inositol triphosphate (IP_3)/phospholipase-C—a second-messenger system .

interneurons—nerve cells that interconnect other neurons.

ion channels—proteins along the cell membrane that are selective for particular ions according to the diameter and ionic characteristics of the channel.

continued

V VOCABULARY Continued

ligand-gated channels—ion channels that are chemically controlled by substances including neurotransmitters and second messengers.

limbic system—the regulatory center of emotion; it plays a role in memory and learning; structurally it includes cingulate gyrus, limbic midbrain nuclei, hippocampus, amygdala, thalamus, and hypothalamus.

locus ceruleus—the area of the brainstem containing the largest number of neurons specific for the neurotransmitter norepinephrine.

magnetic resonance imaging (MRI)—an imaging technique that uses a magnetic field projected onto the brain, allowing energy from brain activity to be detected and an image produced.

medulla oblongata—a region of the brain stem; it controls respiration, gastrointestinal motility, and circulation.

meninges—three protective membranes (pia mater, arachnoid, and dura mater) surrounding the brain.

mitochondria—organelles providing cellular energy.

motor neurons—neurons that transmit signals to muscles, glands, and blood vessels.

myelin—a protective covering or sheath of cells wrapped around the axon to create an insulating effect; it assists in the rate of impulse transmission; its degeneration is observed in multiple sclerosis.

neurons—nerve cells; the fundamental units of the nervous system; non-reproducing cells that send and receive impulses within and outside of the central nervous system.

neurotransmitters—chemical substances that relay messages between pre-synaptic and postsynaptic cells or autoreceptors; typically synthesized, stored, and released by the neuron.

Nissl substance—a substance present in the dendritic processes of the neuron; it is important for protein synthesis.

nitric oxide—a gaseous neurotransmitter thought to play a role in memory impairment.

norepinephrine—a monoamine (catecholamine) neurotransmitter synthesized from dopamine; it is thought to play a role in schizophrenia, anxiety, and mood disorders, and in Parkinson's disease.

nucleus—the cell structure responsible for regulating cell functioning; it contains the genetic materials deoxyribonucleic acid (DNA) and ribonucleic acid (RNA).

parasympathetic nervous system—a division of the autonomic nervous system; it is also known as the cholinergic system; it is responsible for the "rest and digest" response and functions to conserve energy.

peripheral nervous system (PNS)—the nerve network that is concerned with the transmission of brain signals to and from areas outside the CNS; it is divided into the somatic and autonomic divisions.

phospholipase-A$_2$—a second-messenger system.

pineal gland—the brain structure that synthesizes melatonin; it lies outside the blood–brain barrier.

pituitary gland—the hypophysis; comprised of an anterior lobe (adenohypophysis) and posterior lobe (neurohypophysis); it plays a key role in endocrine physiology, including the synthesis of hormones.

polysomnography—electrophysiological measurements using an EEG to assess brain activity during sleep; it is also used to record eye movement during sleep.

positron emission tomography (PET)—an imaging technique involving administration of a radioligand and resulting in the emission of gamma rays that can be recorded by detectors placed around the head and analyzed by computer; it produces three-dimensional images.

raphe nuclei—area of the brainstem containing cell bodies of neurons specific for serotonin.

receptors—components of the cell membrane having the capacity to bind to a specific neurotransmitter.

refractory period—the recovery period for a nerve cell to return to its resting potential prior to the next depolarization.

repolarization—the process in which a nerve cell returns to resting potential after firing.

resting potential—the electrical potential that occurs when the cell membrane is more permeable to potassium ions than sodium ions, leading to a high intracellular potassium concentration (hyperpolarized state); a state resulting in the cell's inhibition, or inability to transmit impulses.

reticular formation—a midbrain structure controlling sleep and wakefulness; it is also involved in visual and auditory reflexes.

re-uptake—the process of taking back released neurotransmitter molecules into the terminal of a pre-synaptic nerve cell for storage and subsequent release.

second messengers—secondary chemicals produced by the binding of a neurotransmitter to a receptor coupled to a G protein.

sensory neurons—neurons receiving stimuli from internal and/or external environments.

serotonin—a monoamine (indolamine) neurotransmitter synthesized from tryptophan; it is thought to play a role in the regulation of mood, eating behavior, impulsivity, aggression, and migraine headaches.

single photon emission computed tomography (SPECT)—an imaging technique involving the use of a longer-acting radioligand than does PET, to allow for rotating detectors to make additional planar images.

soma—the cell body of the neuron.

spatial summation—multiple pre-synaptic cellular firing produced by simultaneous action potentials of different pre-synaptic neurons.

spinal cord—a continuous extension of the brainstem; it consists of 31 pairs of nerves divided into five areas: cervical, thoracic, lumbar, sacral, and coccygeal.

somatic nervous system—a division of the peripheral nervous system; it is responsible for voluntary movement and the innervation of skeletal muscles.

somatostatin—a non-opioid peptide neurotransmitter thought to play a role in memory formation.

V VOCABULARY Continued

substance P—a non-opioid peptide neurotransmitter thought to play a role in pain transmission.

substantia nigra—an area of the brainstem containing cell bodies of neurons specific for the neurotransmitters dopamine and gamma aminobutyric acid (GABA); it is involved in the control of motor behavior.

sulci—shallow grooves observed on the surface of the brain.

sympathetic nervous system—a division of the autonomic nervous system; also known as the "adrenergic system" or "fight or flight" stress response system; it mobilizes and expends resources in response to stress.

synapse—the area involving the membrane of a pre-synaptic neuron (the sender), the synaptic cleft, and the membrane of the post-synaptic neuron (the receiver).

synaptic cleft—a gap between the cellular membranes of the terminal bouton of the pre-synaptic neuron and dendritic processes of the post-synaptic neuron; it is approximately 20 nm wide.

temporal summation—multiple pre-synaptic cellular firing produced by a single cell.

terminal bouton—the area of the neuron containing thousands of vesicles that store neurotransmitters.

thalamus—a brain structure having a primary role in receiving sensory impulses and relaying sensory impulses concerned with pain, visual, auditory, temperature, and tactile sensations; it integrates sensory and motor stimuli; it is part of the limbic system.

tryptophan—an amino acid; a precursor in the synthesis of serotonin.

tyrosine—an amino acid; a precursor in the synthesis of dopamine and norepinephrine.

ventricles—four cerebrospinal fluid-containing, inter-connecting cavities of the brain; they contain choroid plexus.

voltage-gated channels—ion channels that are regulated electrically by changes in the membrane potential.

Wernicke's area—a sensory speech area located in the dominant hemisphere of the brain (after German neurologist Karl Wernicke, 1848–1905).

white matter—CNS tissue consisting of myelinated nerve-cell processes.

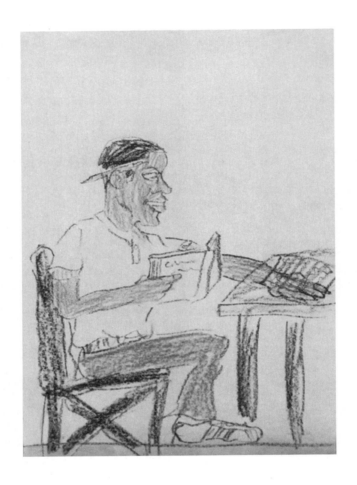

*Learning without thought is labor lost; thought without learning is
perilous.*

Confucius

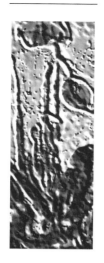

5

Learning and Mental Health Teaching

Ann Wolbert Burgess

Teaching patients, families, and communities is a major nursing intervention. The American Nurses Association (ANA) Standard of Care describing health teaching states that "the nurse, through health teaching, assists (patients) in achieving satisfying, productive, and healthy patterns of living. Health teaching is based on principles of learning. It includes information about coping, interpersonal relations, mental health problems, mental disorders, treatments and their effects on daily living, as well as information pertinent to physical status or developmental needs. The nurse uses health teaching methods appropriate to the (patient's) age, developmental level, gender, ethnic/social background, and education. Constructive feedback and positive rewards reinforce the (patient's) learning. Practice sessions and experiential learning are used as needed."

This chapter discusses the learning theory upon which health teaching is based, the patient's processing of information that is taught, and finally, the actual process of health teaching.

■ LEARNING THEORY

MOTIVATION

Abraham Maslow's (1970) theory of psychological health presents a hierarchy of needs underlying human **motivation,** starting with basic physiological needs and extending to the highest order of spiritual and esthetic needs. In treatment, Maslow focused on increasing self-knowledge and understanding, and mobilizing the resources of the person toward greater self-realization.

Motivation is a critical issue in health teaching. The question of how to motivate people can be outlined into two motivational approaches: content and process. These approaches and major theories are summarized in Table 5–1.

TABLE 5–1 MAJOR APPROACHES TO MOTIVATION

Approach	Theories	Primary Concern
Content	Need-hierarchy theory	Concerned with *what* motivates people
Process	Reinforcement theory	Concerned with *how* people are motivated

Content Approach

The content approach to motivation is concerned with *what* within people motivates them to behave in a certain way. What forces prompt people to behave as they do? Following this approach, to understand what motivates people, you must identify their needs. The needs for security and recognition are only two examples of forces that may motivate people and determine their actions. Abraham Maslow's theory of need hierarchy is one of the most popular and widely known theories of motivation (Maslow, 1970). According to Maslow, people are motivated to satisfy five categories of needs:

- Physiological needs, including food, water, air, and sex.
- Safety needs, or security, stability, and freedom from fear of threat.
- Social needs, including friendship, affection, acceptance, and interaction with others.
- Esteem needs, including both personal feelings of achievement (self-esteem) and recognition (respect from others).
- Self-actualization needs, a feeling of self-fulfillment, or the realization of one's potential.

Maslow held that these needs are arranged in a hierarchy of ascending importance, from low to high. He contended that a "lower" need must be satisfied before the next "higher" need could motivate behavior. For ex-

ample, a person's safety needs would have to be satisfied before the next level of need (social) could motivate behavior. Thus, the strength of any need is determined by its position in the hierarchy and by the degree to which it and all lower needs have been satisfied. Satisfaction of a need, however, triggers dissatisfaction at the next higher level. This sequence of "increased satisfaction, decreased importance, increased importance of the next higher need" repeats itself until the highest level of the hierarchy (self-actualization) is reached.

Maslow suggested that a person could progress down as well as up the various need levels. If a lower-level need (safety, for example) were threatened at some later time, it would again become dominant and assume an important position in a person's total motivational system. Thus, sudden unemployment or loss of a loved one could shift one's concern from a pursuit of personal recognition to a preoccupation with providing for home and family.

Critics of Maslow's theory focus their comments in two areas. First, research has been unable to reproduce the five need levels Maslow proposed, suggesting instead no more than two or three levels. Second, although people do generally place a great deal of emphasis on satisfying their lower-level needs (e.g., hunger, thirst, sex), research suggests that once these needs are satisfied, most people do not climb Maslow's need hierarchy in the proposed manner. Indeed, no particular pattern appears to govern which needs will become dominant once a person's lower-level needs are satisfied.

Implications for Patient Teaching

Despite criticism of it, Maslow's need-hierarchy theory continues to exert a significant influence on current thinking about motivation. Perhaps its greatest value lies in its nursing implications, especially for patient teaching.

- Motivation is generally determined by multiple needs. The belief that one, and only one, factor accounts for motivation is usually an oversimplification.
- A patient's need for satisfaction can be linked to desired outcome. For example, symptom reduction (less anxiety) or function improvement (clearer thinking) can be built-in incentives. Thus, recognition of the patient who successfully completes a health-promotion course could be achieved by listing the patient's name with others.
- What motivates one person may not motivate another. Different people want different things. Nurses must be sensitive to differences in reward preferences.

Process Approach

In contrast to the content approach, the process approach to motivation is concerned with *how* people are motivated, and focuses on the direction or choice of behavioral patterns (Skinner, 1953).

The theories of **learning** that have accumulated over the years have followed a traditional research protocol that begins with a systematic set of observed events, the development of hypotheses, and experimentation to confirm or refute hypotheses. Ultimately, as a theory matures, laws are defined. A characteristic of a good theory, however, is that it is modifiable and testable, and can accommodate new information and challenges.

With the advances in learning theory, it remains true that the fundamental bases of learning theory are, in large measure, rooted in systematic theoretical formulations based on long experimental investigations by a relatively small group of scholar scientists: Hull, Skinner, Pavlov, and Thorndike.

Learning theorists differ over the definition of learning. One group relates learning to measurable, observable events in the physical world, whereas a second group is concerned with describing basic processes that the theorist believes are necessary for learning to take place. Regardless of the approach, however, there appears to be general agreement that learning is a change in behavior that results from practice, whether the practice reflects encoded neural pathways or a strengthening of certain responses. Moreover, learning is viewed as an intervening process that links an organism's states before and after a change in behavior occurs. There is also a general assumption that learning represents a long-term change in behavior, different from changes induced by such factors as fatigue and maturation.

Learning, then, may be defined as a change in behavioral potential resulting from reinforced practice. Reinforcement, so considered, is basic to much of contemporary learning theory.

CLASSICAL CONDITIONING

Many theorists accept two types of **conditioning:** classical (Pavlovian) and instrumental (operant). The pioneer in classical conditioning, the Russian physiologist Ivan Pavlov, observed in his work with gastric secretions in dogs that stimuli that were often present at the time the dogs were offered food came to evoke salivation in the dogs, even though the dogs could not see or smell food. Pavlov assumed that the stimulus of footsteps came to be associated with food. His research was directed toward an analysis of this event, which he called the "conditional reflex"—the reflex that would occur under certain, specific conditions.

OPERANT CONDITIONING

Edward Thorndike in 1913 postulated the *law of effect:* the consequences of a behavior determine the frequency of that behavior. Burrus Skinner (1953), a central figure in the development and exposition of behavioral theory, is known for his work in operant conditioning and reinforcement theory.

APPLICATION OF LEARNING THEORY TO HEALTH TEACHING

Although various revisions have appeared in recent years, the basic concept behind behavior modification remains quite simple. Health behaviors that lead to desirable consequences are likely to be repeated. Health behaviors that lead to undesirable consequences are less likely to be repeated. This reasoning involves three components.

- Stimulus—an event that leads to a response.
- Response—a unit of behavior that follows a stimulus.
- Reinforcement—a consequence of a response.

The relationship between these components is that a **stimulus** (event) leads to a **response** (behavior) that is reinforced by a consequence. Note that none of the components involves thinking. Behavior modification holds that current behavior is solely determined by a person's history of reinforcement. Thus, according to behavior modification, if a particular stimulus and response (or stimulus–response pair) is followed by a desirable consequence, the stimulus will be more likely to prompt the same response in the future. Conversely, if the consequence is undesirable, the response is less likely to recur. In sum, the consequences of a person's behavior are dependent upon his or her response to a stimulus.

REINFORCEMENT

From a nursing perspective, at least four types of reinforcement are available for modifying patient behaviors, as summarized in Table 5–2. Of these four types of

TABLE 5–2 TYPES OF REINFORCEMENT

POSITIVE REINFORCEMENT: Strengthens behavior by providing a desirable consequence when a desirable behavior occurs.

AVOIDANCE LEARNING: Strengthens behavior by teaching individuals to respond in ways that avoid undesirable consequences.

EXTINCTION: Weakens behavior by withholding a desirable consequence when an undesirable behavior occurs.

PUNISHMENT: Weakens behavior by providing an undesirable consequence when an undesirable behavior occurs.

reinforcement, two strengthen or increase behavior, whereas the other two weaken or decrease it.

Positive Reinforcement

A means of strengthening behavior, **positive reinforcement** increases the likelihood that a desired behavior will be repeated. For example, a nurse will praise an adolescent for consistently returning to the ward at the scheduled time. Positive reinforcers can include time off, bonus credits, and other benefits.

Avoidance Learning

A second means of strengthening behavior is **avoidance learning,** which occurs when individuals respond in ways intended to avoid undesirable consequences. The nurse does not engage in intense questioning of the adolescent who returns to the ward at the scheduled time, and the adolescent in turn learns that being on time diminishes the likelihood of being interrogated about his or her activities.

Extinction

As a means of weakening behavior, **extinction** attempts to eliminate an undesirable behavior by withholding a desirable consequence when the behavior occurs. Under such conditions, the undesirable behavior will diminish and eventually become "extinct" as a result of not being positively reinforced. For example, withholding a ward pass may prompt an adolescent to maintain a consistent on-time schedule. Presumably, the adolescent will eventually realize that chronic lateness is not producing a desired consequence.

Punishment

A second means for weakening behavior, **punishment** provides an undesirable consequence when an undesirable behavior occurs. For example, punishments for an adolescent who is late for a scheduled meeting could include withholding of privileges, probation periods, or restrictions in other life areas.

In 1932, Thorndike modified his law and indicated that rewarded responses are always strengthened but that punished responses do not always diminish in strength, thus leading to an emphasis on reward as a primary determinant of behavior. According to Skinner (1953), punishment has the effect of reducing the tendency to act in a given way, at least in the short run. Many consider punishment to be one of the least understood and most abused aspects of behavior modification.

■ MEMORY AND LEARNING

Although learning theory provides a major contribution to nursing practice in offering a basis for health teaching, the roles of neural pathways and memory are also critical. Building on the memory concept, it is theorized in psychology that learned experiences form the basis of much human and animal behavior. Experiences, stored as memory, determine much of current perception and performance.

PROCEDURAL (IMPLICIT) AND DECLARATIVE (EXPLICIT) MEMORY

The notion that memories affect behavior, both in the presence and absence of conscious awareness, appears in theories of implicit and explicit memory, or **procedural** and **declarative memory** (Mandler, 1983; Willingham, Nissen, and Bullemer, 1989). In cases of implicit and explicit memory, behavior is affected by prior experience, but only explicit (declarative) memory is subject to conscious assessment (Squire, 1987). Table 5–3 lists the procedural and declarative memory networks.

Implicit, or procedural, memory represents the earliest, genetically based neural system organized into constructive patterns of learning and memory. The implicit memory system is strongly developed through genetics, and is the basis of structure and function in experience. These patterns are essential to survival, growth, and development, and persist in their importance even through advanced levels of memory and learning (e.g., imprinting). Different subtypes of memory are being studied within the broad constellation of implicit memory.

A great deal of the learning that is stored in memory is not within conscious awareness, and is not

TABLE 5–3 IMPLICIT AND EXPLICIT MEMORY NETWORKS

Procedural (Implicit)	Declarative (Explicit)
Genetically based neural system	Developmental neural system
Located in brainstem/hippocampus	Rooted in brainstem/neocortex
Patterns of learning and memory	Associative learning
Priming and imprinting	Working memory
Simple classical conditioning	Operant memory
Out of awareness	Remembering events
No spontaneous recall	Spontaneous recall possible
Skills	Domain of learning
Observed through behavior and symptoms	Language and meaning networking
Hard to alter or change	Linked to associative stimuli

amenable to free recall. Implicit memory is totally out of awareness and nonretrievable. However, memory can be seen as operating at the level of priming, imprinting, and classical conditioning.

Priming experiments have dealt with people who have amnesia from organic lesions, particularly damage to sections of the hippocampus, a structure important in early brain organization. People with this amnesia, who cannot remember events from one moment to the next, can be presented with visual stimuli such as words or aspects of words, and will be able to identify the patterns and structures of these words even though they do not remember the setting in which they were presented with the words. Furthermore, this learning persists over time. Priming experiments have raised great interest among investigators working in the area of memory disruption in trauma victims. Research suggests that trauma causes biochemical shifts in the brain systems that are integrally involved with learning, memory, and the information processing of experience; in overwhelming trauma, morphological changes occur in these structures (Squire, 1987, 1993).

Explicit memory is subject to spontaneous recall. It is the major domain of learning with language and meaning networks, and has a developmental neural pathway rooted in the brainstem and neocortex. Explicit memory is the more familiar basis for associative learning that incorporates the organization of experience by language and meaning. It is a working memory. For example, you hear a graduation speaker; five years later, when talking to a friend about graduations, you are able to recall this speaker and what was said.

MEMORY DEVELOPMENT

One is not born with memory; it develops. The neural pathways of implicit and explicit memory need to mature. Nancy Perry (1992) reviews memory development from infancy through adolescence, when it is believed that the neurobiological development needed for memory is completed. Perry presents an organizational scheme for examining children's memory, consisting of: memory processes (acquisition, storage and retrieval); types of memory (recognition, reconstruction, and free recall); and strategies for and deficiencies in remembering. See Table 5–4.

Memory Processes

Children who can pay attention so as to remember events acquire information. Although the perception and encoding of events begin early in the life of atten-

tive children, they do have difficulty in conceptualizing complex events, identifying relationships such as cause and effect, recognizing feelings, and attributing intentions (Fantz, 1965; Perry and Tephy, 1984–1985). The ability to order and interpret perceptions is seen as an acquired skill that does not reach the standard of adult reliability until the age of 12 years (Collins et al., 1978; Flapen, 1968).

Storage of information in memory does not change greatly with age. Therefore, preschoolers are believed to remember as well as adults (Werner and Perlmutter, 1979). It is the retrieval of information that determines its storage.

Retrieval of information through the recall and reporting of events by children is compromised by their effectiveness in communicating the content of the event from which the information was retrieved. Although children may effectively perceive, encode, and store an event accurately, other domains of development need to be sufficiently sophisticated for them to communicate their memory of the event.

TABLE 5–4 MEMORY DEVELOPMENT

Memory Process	Definition
Acquisition	Perception of information
Storage	Encoded data/event
Retrieval	Recall
Types of Memory	
Recognition	Sensory system cue
Reconstruction	Restating context
Free recall	No cues or prompts
Strategies for Remembering	
Rehearsal	Repeat/memorize
Categories	Organize data
Associative cues	Conduct memory search

Types of Memory

Recognition is the simplest form of memory, and is within the capacity of the infant (Piaget and Inhelder, 1973). Within the first 2 weeks of life there is olfactory recognition of mothers' milk (Cernoch and Porter, 1985) and preferences for visually perceived shapes. Children's recognition memory improves rapidly. Children 2 years of age correctly recognize 81% of the objects presented to them, and 4-year-old children recognize 92%. There is some indication that recognition memory varies, being very good in the early elementary years (ages 6 to 10), then declining (ages 11 and 12) and then again improving at 13 and on (Carey 1978; Goodman and Reed, 1986). Skill in identifying faces increases with age. Children under 10 years old have difficulty in identifying faces that are observed only briefly or are disguised. But even with the improvement after 10 years of age, facial recognition lacks consistency, even in adulthood (Ceci, Toglia, and Ross 1987; Chance and Goldstein, 1984).

Recognition memory is very good among children beginning school, and 5-year-old children have been as proficient as adults in recognizing common places and objects (Nelson and Kosslyn, 1976). However, children do not do well in scanning and registering complex information (Perlmutter, 1984).

Reconstruction memory involves reinstating the context in which an original event occurred (Piaget and Inhelder, 1973). The requirements for accuracy are that there be a match between encoding a situation and the retrieval of environmental features. Consequently, the greater the number of cues shared at the time of acquisition of information, the better the retrieval. Two- to 3-year-old children demonstrate 75% accuracy in simple reconstructions (Perry et al., 1987).

Free recall memory is the most complex form of memory. It is the retrieval of previously observed events from storage with few or no prompting cues. Free recall is strongly age-related. Infants are poor recallers; preschoolers can aid recall as they begin to organize memories around concepts. These organizational skills develop gradually and depend on the development of language and higher levels of thought organization. Although the number of facts recalled about an event increases with age (Marin et al., 1979; Perry et al., 1987), the facts that are recalled by younger children tend to be correct (Lepore, 1991).

Children can answer simple direct questions about an event (Goodman and Helgerson, 1985). Six- to 7-year-old children recall a story with as much accuracy as adults (Kail and Hagen, 1977). Moreover, memory for core aspects of events tends to be stronger than for peripheral aspects of events, and in some cases children are more accurate in their memory than are adults (Lindberg, 1991).

STRATEGIES FOR AND DEFICIENCIES IN REMEMBERING

Children have limited ability to use memory strategies. Strategy development is closely akin to language development and the use of internal processes such as visualization. Clearly, increased use of strategies enhances recall.

Rehearsal is almost automatic for adults, but its use has been noted among 10-year-old children. Young children have not mastered it (Harris and Liebert, 1991). Although mental picturing develops later in children,

younger children can use imagery when instructed through context reinstatement (i.e., the showing of photographs, asking the child to draw a picture, or demonstrating with dolls).

Organization of memories according to themes, categories, and common elements does not occur as proficiently in pre-school-aged children as it does in older children.

The use of external and internal cues to conduct consistent searches of memory is not as developed in pre-school-aged children and 6 year olds as it is in 9-year-old children (Chi and Koeske, 1983); however, younger children can be taught how to use these cues, which can result in phenomenal memory with some children.

Howe and Courage's (1993) review of the empirical and theoretical literature on neurological, perceptual, and memory development in very young children establishes that the fundamental processes that comprise memory are relatively sophisticated even in infancy, and that although clear developmental shifts in memory occur throughout the early years of development, they are probably not the primary source of later failures to recall early childhood events before the age of 3 or 4 years. Researchers argue that the emergence of the infant's sense of self is the cornerstone in the development of autobiographical memory.

■ INFORMATION PROCESSING

What is meant by human information processing? Consider a behavioral act, such as listening and retaining a professor's hour lecture for a future test. What terms or definitions are used to describe the hour transaction? First, the professor speaks from lecture notes. These are auditory stimuli. The professor is beginning a chain of events and processes that link the presentation of auditory stimuli and the student's response to them. In this case, it is to write key themes on paper, and that entails a large number of stages and controlling or modifying processes between the stimulus and the response.

STAGES OF PROCESSING

What processing is involved in the example of remembering key ideas from the professor's lecture? This initial processing stage is called sensory registration; in the auditory case, it is called echoic memory. The physical energy of the professor's speech is translated (converted) into electrical impulses in the student's nervous system. Specifically, the auditory vibrations of the professor's words stimulate the student's ear and thus generate electrical impulses in the student's acoustic nerve. These sensory impulses are transmitted to the cortical level, where they are perceived as a simple sensory message, namely, a phonetic sound. At this sensory stage, however, the sound is not necessarily categorized, but remains as a sound without an informational signal or symbol value.

If no further processing is to be done to the auditory stimulus, such as ascribing meaning to it by labeling it as a letter or number (pattern recognition), then the sensory memory for the sound decays and the sound is not remembered. A large number of auditory stimuli to which people are subjected are not processed beyond sensory registration. Persons are constantly bombarded by many more stimuli than they can respond to, and these stimuli are ordinarily regarded as noise.

If the words heard are not those expected, then not much attention would be given to them. This fact illustrates the importance of attentional factors in information processing. Attention has a major influence on what is or is not processed, as well as on how it is processed.

In the example of the professor's lecture, because the students are anticipating a test, they would presumably process the sensory memory of his words. The next stage of processing is perceptual and called *pattern recognition*. When phonetic sounds are given meaning by a listener, auditory pattern recognition has occurred. Recognition is accomplished by a process of comparing the stimulus pattern to be identified with patterns previously stored by the listener as part of the listener's long-term or short-term memories.

The next stage of processing is *short-term memory*, a cognitive process. This memory must last long enough for the student to write key words on a piece of paper. To help students remember, the professor usually repeats key terms during a lecture. This *rehearsal* (hearing the professor's repeated statements) is one of several ways students can facilitate memorization. Without rehearsal, the sensory memory of words following pattern recognition would rapidly decay.

THE NATURE OF PROCESSING

In any processing experiment, the only elements that can be directly observed and measured are the initiating stimulus and the resulting end-response. The intervening processes are hypothetical constructs; they cannot be directly measured, but must instead be inferred. Processing may be analyzed in terms of several general questions discussed in the following sections.

What is Being Processed?

The *what* question refers to whether the primary influence of the stimulus is physical energy or information. Is it energy or information that is being processed?

Across the three domains of processing—sensory, perceptual, and cognitive—the relative emphasis given

to energy and information differs. For example, the response to a word presented visually may entail first the sensory processing of contrast and color; next the perceptual processing of lines, angles, and letter forms; and finally the cognitive processing of the word's meaning.

In general, both energy and information are processed in the three domains (sensory, perceptual, and cognitive) because energy is the carrier of information. Energy stimuli are defined completely with reference to their physical characteristics (e.g., wave frequency or light intensity). The description of informational stimuli is more complicated because the term *information* is used loosely to mean stimulus complexity or the amount of stimulus patterning. In addition, the quality of information processing depends on the individual.

Where Does Processing Occur?

The *where* of processing introduces questions about physiology. One approach considers whether the processing occurs more peripherally or centrally in the nervous system. A second approach considers the hemisphere of the brain in which processing is most likely located.

When Does Processing Occur?

The sequence of processing stages takes place between the presentation of a stimulus and the subsequent response. The stages are generally described as:

- Input, when energy and information components of the stimuli are incorporated.
- Classification of components.
- Organization of the classified components.
- Interpretation of what has been processed.
- Output, which culminates in a response.

The types of information processing may differ, depending on the type of sensory stimuli, the processing task, and the person's stage of practice or experience.

THE THREE PROCESSING DOMAINS

The schema, or mental codification of experience that is made possible by the three levels of information processing influences how and what a child can learn and remember from personal experiences, and how that learning and the resulting memory can be demonstrated at different ages and stages of development.

Sensory

Sensory information is processed within the peripheral nervous system (PNS), brainstem, basal ganglia, and amygdala. The neural system within these areas develops and strengthens as the child develops physically (e.g., the child learns to hold a bottle, eat with a spoon, roll over, crawl, and walk).

Conditioned learning is first noted at this stage of processing; for example, the child associates and anticipates events in his or her experience, such as the routines of feeding, diapering, and playing games such as peek-a-boo. Repetition of the neural stimuli attached to these events strengthens the neural pathways involved in sensory processing. The strengthened pathways lead to an automatic, conditioned response to a specific sensory stimulus. Children demonstrate learning and memory when they open their mouths for food or cry when it is taken away. In addition, the child cries when awakened, anticipating the pattern of parental response of someone coming to pick it up.

Perceptual

Processing **perceptual information** involves the neurological ability to retain aspects of perceptual experience as memory. Perceptual processing allows us to remember what rain felt like on our faces or what grass felt like on our bare feet. With the development of specialized cortical areas, the child can retain aspects of sensory experience as perceptual representations in the form of remembered sights (iconic memory) or sounds (echoic memory). Children demonstrate iconic memory when they draw an event or spontaneously sing a song they have learned at school.

Cognitive

Processing **cognitive information** requires the development of neural systems that permit response and retention, as well as cognitive interpretation and the description of internal and external perceptions, using words as symbols for experience. This is what allows the child to ask for a favorite bedtime story.

APPLICATION TO PATIENT CARE

Research suggests that information processing in psychiatric patients may differ from that in mentally healthy individuals. For example, Emil Kraepelin described schizophrenic patients as having difficulty in shifting their attention from some trivial portion of the environment, a perseverative behavior.

A theory proposed for depression, which has an information-processing premise, suggests that depression is a defense reaction intended to cope with anxiety arising from a defect in the patient's information-processing mechanisms. Because of increasing anxiety, the patient stops analyzing incoming sensory information and becomes lethargic and unresponsive to stimuli.

Information processing is the focus on learning deficits in children and organic conditions in the elderly. The cognitive sciences have also aided in the un-

derstanding of post-traumatic symptoms. Beginning work in this area was by Mardi Horowitz (1976), Figley (1978), van der Kolk (1984), and Hartman and Burgess (1988). When trauma occurs, as in child abuse, biological alterations lead to the reproduction of molecular cells engineered for survival. Indeed, these stress hormones may reduce the flexibility and continued growth of the memory systems and thus interfere with new learning. The adaptation is made for survival and stimulates a powerful level of learning to protect the organism; such learning is not easily altered and undone. It is believed that this is why some behavioral traits persist into adulthood.

■ THE HEALTH-TEACHING PROCESS

Components of the health-teaching process include assessment of the patient, planning what is to be taught and how, and the skill and style of teaching.

PATIENT'S LEARNING PROFILE

Assess the patient's age, sex, position in his or her family, marital status, occupation, educational level, sociocultural background, ethnic values, past health history, and mental-health status. These profile variables influence the style and technique of teaching.

In addition, assess the patient's cognitive and psychological levels, memory capacity, perception of health, understanding of illness, level of stress, number of stressors present, personality style, motivation to learn, and level of comprehension. These profile variables influence the level of teaching.

PLAN FOR TEACHING AND IMPLEMENTATION

As individualized patient needs and goals are identified, the information to be taught is planned. The patient's motivation and learning pace are also considered. The teaching plan needs to include preparation of the environment so that it is conducive to learning. Content must be organized and relevant. Goals are written in the nursing plan.

NURSE'S TEACHING SKILLS AND STYLE

Teaching skill includes several principles:

- Using an organized plan.
- Presenting content in small segments.
- Using language that is free of jargon.
- Routinely asking questions and seeking feedback.
- Maintaining eye contact.
- Using audiovisual aids when possible.

- Requesting a return demonstration from the patient when appropriate.
- Offering positive reinforcement (praise) when learning occurs.

Teaching style involves:

- Knowing the information content to be taught.
- Being aware of one's own security in teaching.

- Being flexible in approach.
- Listening carefully to the patient.
- Presenting content calmly, unhurriedly, and in an interesting way.

To evaluate whether learning has occurred, changes in the patient's behavior are assessed, as is the patient's ability to answer or ask questions. Test questions may be completed. (See Figures 5–1, 5–2, and 5–3.)

Figure 5–1 MEDICATION TEACHING TOOL

Patient:
Provider:
Date:

PROZAC FACT SHEET

Drug Name: Prozac
Generic Name: Fluoxetine

Purpose: This drug is used to treat depression.

Warnings:
- This drug can take as long as 5 to 6 weeks to work.
- Take Prozac in the morning. It can interfere with sleep.
- Tell your doctor if you have history of seizure or eating disorders.
- Do not drive or operate machinery until you know how you'll react to this medication.
- Always tell your doctor the medicines you are taking.
- See your doctor regularly for check-ups.
- Do not stop taking this medication without talking to your doctor.
- Ask your doctor for advice about drinking alcoholic beverages.
- Women who are pregnant, plan to become pregnant, or are breast-feeding should inform their doctor about this.
- Do not allow anyone else to take this medication.

Common Side Effects	What To Do
Anxiety; nervousness; insomnia; apathy; fatigue; loss of appetite; nausea; diarrhea; headache; drowsiness; weakness; tremor; lightheadedness; sweating; decreased ability to concentrate; abnormal dreams; agitation; indigestion; joint or muscle pain.	If these effects are severe and do not lessen with time, contact your doctor. Your dose may have to be adjusted. You may need medication for insomnia.
Skin rash; hives; itching; flu symptoms; seizures.	Stop taking drug immediately. Contact your doctor.
Dry mouth.	Suck sugarless hard candy or chew sugarless gum.

As with any anti-depressant, this medication can precipitate a manic episode.

- You are taking _____ mg Prozac _____ times a day. Your schedule is _____
  _____

- If you miss a dose and remember within 2–3 hours, take it. Otherwise, skip it and take remaining doses as scheduled. DO NOT double up.

Source: Bay Area Health Care, Developed by Dr. Verna B. Carson, 1991. Reprinted with permission.

Figure 5–2 MEDICATION PRE AND POST TEST

PATIENT:
NURSE:
DATE:
Score:

1. I am taking _____ (name medications) _____ .
2. I am taking _____ mg _____ times per day.

3. My schedule is _____

4. My medication helps me:
    a. Feel less sad.
    b. Feel less nervous.
    c. Feel less bothered by bad thoughts I can't control.
    d. Other (list any other benefits).

5. If I miss a dose of my medicine, I should:
    a. Double up on the next dose.
    b. If I remember to take it close to the regularly scheduled time, I should take it and stay with my normal schedule.
    c. If it is several hours from when I should have taken it, I will forget the missed dose and get right back on my normal schedule with the next dose.

6. My medication may make me feel drowsy and even clumsy. When I first begin taking the medicine it is a good idea to:
    a. Stay at home all the time until I feel more alert and sharper in my thinking.
    b. Avoid driving a car or operating machinery until I know how I will react to this medicine.
    c. Avoid taking the medicine right before I need to be alert in my actions and thinking.
    d. Tell my doctor I want another medication.

7. If I am going to have surgery, even dental surgery, I should:
    a. Stop taking the medication the day before the surgery.
    b. Tell my surgeon all the medications I am taking.
    c. Take more of my medication right before surgery to put me in a better state of mind.

8. Before drinking any alcohol, whether in beer, wine, whiskey, wine coolers, or over-the-counter medications, I should:
    a. Stop taking my medication.
    b. Talk to my doctor about whether it is safe or not to mix alcohol with this medicine.
    c. Read the label on the bottle or package containing the alcohol to see what I should do.

9. If I am taking this medicine, there are certain things that I should tell my doctor or nurse. Please check off at least three things from the following list:
    _____ a. I have a history of an eating disorder.
    _____ b. I have a history of seizures.
    _____ c. I am pregnant or want to become pregnant.
    _____ d. I am breast-feeding.
    _____ e. I am taking other medications.
    _____ f. I have certain allergies.
    _____ g. I have a history of heart problems, high blood pressure or have had a recent heart attack.
    _____ h. I have a history of kidney disease.
    _____ i. I am a diabetic.

10. A friend asks me for a dose of my medicine to help him/her feel better. I should:
    a. Refuse and explain that the medicine may make him/her sick.
    b. Give one dose away just so the friend can see if it helps or not.
    c. Freely share my medicine with other people who have the same symptoms as me.

If you are taking a medication to make you feel less sad, please answer the next four questions.

11. My medication can produce some side effects that are bothersome but not serious. These include (please, choose at least two from the following list):
    a. Drowsiness, feeling tired, weak.
    b. Excitement, insomnia, blurred vision.
    c. Lightheadedness when I get up too quickly from a lying down or sitting to a standing position.
    d. Sensitive to sunlight.
    e. Dry mouth.
    f. Constipation, blurred vision, difficulty urinating.

12. My medication does not make me feel better right away. It may take as long as:
    a. Two to three weeks.
    b. Three to four weeks.
    c. Five to six weeks.

13. Most of the side effects that my medication produces can be dealt with easily. Column A lists the side effects and Column B lists the common remedies. Please match the remedy with the side effect.

        Column A   Column B

    a. Drowsiness   1. Take medicine with meals.
    b. Excitement, insomnia   2. Wear sunblock and hat.
    c. Sensitive to sunlight   3. Chew sugarless gum and suck on sugarless hard candy.
    d. Dry mouth   4. Eat more bulk foods, drink more water.
    e. Constipation   5. Take medicine at bedtime.
    f. Nausea   6. Take medicine in morning.

14. There are some side effects that I should immediately tell my doctor about. Which of the following falls into that category (check all that apply)?
    _____ a. High fever, chills, sore throat
    _____ b. Change in skin color
    _____ c. Any unusual bleeding
    _____ d. Swelling of feet and lower legs
    _____ e. Headache
    _____ f. Diarrhea

If you are taking a drug that is an MAO inhibitor, please answer the next two questions.

15. My medication can react with certain foods containing tyramine to make my blood pressure go dangerously high. Please check off three foods from the following list that contain tyramine.
    _____ a. Alcoholic drinks, especially wine (chianti and champagne) and beer, and nonalcoholic beer
    _____ b. Aged or processed cheeses
    _____ c. Chicken liver
    _____ d. Hamburgers
    _____ e. Hot dogs
    _____ f. Peaches
    _____ g. Bananas
    _____ h. Chocolate-covered raisins
    _____ i. Sour cream
    _____ j. Yogurt
    _____ k. Milk
    _____ l. Ice cream

16. Even after I have stopped taking the MAO inhibitor for my depression, I need to avoid these foods:
    a. Forever.
    b. For two weeks.
    c. For one month.
    d. For one year.

If you are taking a medicine to make you feel less nervous, please answer the next three questions.

17. My medication can be habit forming. I should:
    a. Take the medication exactly as prescribed.
    b. Only take the medication when I feel desperate.
    c. Stop taking the medication as soon as I feel better.

18. When I feel better, I should:
    a. Stop taking the medication.
    b. Work with my doctor on a schedule to wean me off the medication.

19. Stopping the medication abruptly can cause me to:
    a. Have a heart attack and other coronary complications.
    b. Have seizures and experience withdrawal.
    c. Need more of the medication.

Continued

If you are taking a medicine to help you feel less bothered by troublesome thoughts you cannot control, please answer the following four questions.

20. My medicine can cause some unpleasant side effects that involve unusual movements. If I notice that I can't sit still (I have dancing feet) and I feel jittery inside, or I am experiencing spasms of my muscles in my face or other places in my body, I probably need to take some cogentin, benadryl, artane, or amantadine as ordered by my doctor. If I do not have any of these medicines available, I should:
    a. Stop taking my medicine.
    b. Call my doctor immediately or go to an emergency department.
    c. Take a double dose of my medication.

21. My medication can cause tardive dyskinesia, a more serious movement disorder with jerky movements of the face and extremities. If this happens to me, my doctor will probably:
    a. Increase the dose of my medicine.
    b. Decrease the dose of my medicine.
    c. Stop my medication immediately.

22. Because of the side effects of my medicine, my doctor my have also prescribed another medication for me, such as benadryl, cogentin, artane, kemedrin, akineton, or amantadine. These medications are used to control:
    a. The movement problems that come with my medicine.
    b. The dry mouth and constipation that come with my medicine.
    c. The blurred vision that comes with my medicine.

23. These additional drugs also have side effects. These include:
    a. Dry mouth, blurred vision, constipation.
    b. Fast heartbeat.
    c. Seizures.
    d. Parkinson's disease.

If you are taking Tegretol or Dilantin please answer the following question.

24. Frequently the dose of my medicine must be adjusted. Because of this it is important that I:
    a. Get a sample of my blood taken so that my doctor can monitor how much of the medicine is in my system.
    b. Eat a balanced diet with 8 full glasses of water a day.
    c. Collect my urine for 24 hours to see that I am urinating the right amount.

Source: Bay Area Health Care, Developed by Dr. Verna B. Carson, 1991. Reprinted with permission.

Figure 5–3 PSYCHIATRIC CARE PLAN

Patient's Name: _____ Date: _____

Nurse's Signature: _____

Patient Outcomes/Orders/Interventions	Dates of Interventions and Resolution

PG = Patient Outcomes	PO = Orders	Letters = Interventions

_____ PG.0 Patient will have thorough assessment

_____
_____ PO1 Skilled nursing visit frequency = _____
_____ PO2 Assess vital signs
_____ PO3 Assess medications
    _____ A. Assess medication effectiveness
    _____ B. Assess medication side effects
    _____ C. Assess medication supply
    _____ D. Assess medication compliance
_____ PO4 Assess Mental Status
    _____ A. Complete mini mental status examination
    _____ B. Complete global assessment form
    _____ C. Complete affective scale
    _____ D. Complete anxiety scale
    _____ E. Other
_____ PO5 Assess social support system
    _____ A. Complete social support tool
    _____ B. Assess who is a support
    _____ C. Assess what kind of support is given
_____ PO6 Assess nutrition/hydration
    _____ A. Have patient do 24-hour diet recall
    _____ B. Assess food likes/dislikes
    _____ C. Assess budgetary restraints on food purchasing
    _____ D. Assess nutrition knowledge
    _____ E. Assess cultural and/or religious impacts on diet
    _____ F. Assess physiological impacts on
    _____   intake/elimination
    _____ G. Assess adequacy of diet
_____ PO7 Assess Sleep Pattern
    _____ A. Assess quantity of sleep
    _____ B. Assess quality of sleep
    _____ C. Assess for presence of sleep routines
    _____ D. Assess for problems that interfere with restful sleep

_____ PG.1 Patient/caregiver and nurse will develop a therapeutic relationship

_____ PO8 Develop a therapeutic nurse–patient relationship
    _____ A. Demonstrate trustworthiness at every visit
    _____ B. Listen attentively to patient/care provider concerns
    _____ C. Demonstrate empathy by reflecting patient's feelings and reactions to situations
    _____ D. Demonstrate therapeutic communication skills to assist the patient to self-disclose
    _____ E. Teach the patient about the boundaries of the relationship
    _____ F. Teach the patient about the importance of discussing thoughts and feelings honestly and openly
    _____ G. Demonstrate acceptance of patient with affirmation and consistency
    _____ H. Teach the patient the impact of patient's behaviors on others
    _____ I. Teach the patient the need for limits on inappropriate behavior
    _____ J. Confront the patient with discrepancies in behavior
    _____ K. Summarize the accomplishments of the relationship
    _____ L. Teach the patient the value of terminating the relationship in a planned way that allows open discussion of feelings and thoughts
    _____ M. Other
    _____ N. Other

_____ PG.2 Patient/caregiver will demonstrate criteria for MD alert and on-call nurse

Continued

_____ PO9   Teach patient how to use 911 and on-call nurse
  _____ A. Teach how to use 911
  _____ B. Teach what situations warrant use of 911
  _____ C. Teach how to contact on-call nurse
  _____ D. Teach what situations warrant contacting on-call nurse

_____ PG.3   Medication Regime as indicated by a passing grade as a medication post-test and at least 75% rate of compliance with medication use.

_____ PO10   Teach patient purpose for medications, side effects of medications, and importance of adhering to schedule
  _____ A. Teach importance of taking medication according to schedule
  _____ B. Teach the major effects of each medication
  _____ C. Teach major side effects of each medication
  _____ D. Teach strategies to alleviate side effects
  _____ E. Teach what side effects require medical intervention
  _____ F. Teach how to obtain medication
  _____ G. Teach patient how to use compliance packs
  _____ H. Obtain return demonstration on all information that is taught and/or demonstrated
  _____ I. Give homework assignment to patient related to medication issues
  _____ J. Provide positive reinforcement for desirable behavior in relationship to managing medications appropriately

_____ PG.4   Patient/caregiver will understand S/S of illness exacerbation by

_____ PO11   Teach patient/care provider characteristic signs and symptoms of illness exacerbation
  _____ A. Teach patient strategies of early recognition of illness
  _____ B. Teach patient ways of dealing with symptoms before re-hospitalization becomes necessary
  _____ C. Teach patient causes of depression/anxiety/delusional thinking
  _____ D. Teach physical effects of depression/anxiety
  _____ E. Teach emotional and spiritual effects of depression/anxiety
  _____ F. Teach effects of depression on interpersonal relationships/anxiety
  _____ G. Teach inter-relationship of thoughts and feelings in producing sadness/anxiety
  _____ H. Teach effects of guilt
  _____ I. Teach problem solving
  _____ J. Teach biochemical causes of illness
  _____ K. Teach grief process
  _____ L. Other
  _____ M. Other

_____ PG.5   Patient will have reduced anxiety to optimize functional independence

_____ PO12   Teach strategies to reduce anxiety
  _____ A. Teach deep breathing as an anxiety-reducing technique
  _____ B. Teach imagery
  _____ C. Teach progressive relaxation
  _____ D. Teach benefits of physical exercise
  _____ E. Teach benefits of hobbies, reading, television, and radio as distraction techniques to lower anxiety
  _____ F. Teach benefits of spiritual activities such as prayer and meditation
  _____ G. Teach benefits of interpersonal relationships to decrease anxiety
  _____ H. Teach cognitive strategies of anticipating and asking "What if?"
  _____ I. Defuse patient's anxiety through verbal means as well as strategies to relax patient
  _____ J. Use crisis intervention techniques to calm patient and restore control so that patient does not progress to a panic level of anxiety
  _____ K. Teach management of headache and other physical symptoms of anxiety and/or stress
  _____ L. Other
  _____ M. Other

_____ PG.6   Patient will demonstrate reduced hopelessness to optimize functional independence

_____ PO13   Teach strategies to reduce feelings of hopelessness
  _____ A. Teach cognitive strategies to reframe negative thoughts
  _____ B. Teach patient thought stopping techniques
  _____ C. Teach patient value of self affirmation
  _____ D. Teach patient through case examples of strategies others have used to work through depression
  _____ E. Other
  _____ F. Other

Source: Bay Area Health Care, Developed by Dr. Verna B. Carson, 1991. Reprinted with permission.

O AN OVERVIEW

- Patients must be motivated to learn in order for health teaching to be successful.
- Positive reinforcement produces a better learning outcome than negative reinforcement.
- Declarative (explicit) memory is subject to recall.
- Information processing occurs at the sensory, perceptual, and cognitive levels.

TD TERMS TO DEFINE

- avoidance learning
- cognitive information
- conditioning
- declarative (explicit) memory
- extinction
- learning
- Maslow's hierarchy of needs
- motivation
- perceptual information
- positive reinforcement
- procedural (implicit) memory
- punishment
- rehearsal
- response
- sensory information
- stimulus
- types of memory
- free will
- recognition
- reconstruction

Q STUDY QUESTIONS

1. T F Motivation is a critical component of learning theory.
2. T F Learning involves a change in behavior.
3. T F Behavior modification holds that current behavior is determined by past behavior.
4. Give examples of four types of behavior reinforcement.
5. T F Implicit memory is genetically developed.
6. T F Implicit memory is subjected to spontaneous recall.
7. T F Humans are born with memory.
8. Health teaching includes assessing the patient's learning profile. Identify the profile variables that influence teaching.
9. List six principles of teaching related to the nurse's teaching style.
10. Prepare a health-teaching module about a psychotropic medication.

■ REFERENCES

Carey S: A case study: Face recognition, in Walker E (ed): *Explorations in the Biology of Language.* Montgomery, VT, Bradford Books, 1978, pp 175–201.

Ceci SJ, Toglia MP, Ross DF: *Children's Eyewitness Memory.* New York. Springer-Verlag, 1987.

Cernoch JM, Porter RH: Recognition of maternal axillary odors by infants. *Child Dev.* 1985; 56:1593–1598.

Chance JE, Goldstein AG: Face-recognition memory: Implications for children's eyewitness testimony. *J Soc Iss* 1984; 40:69–85.

Chi MTH, Koeske RD: Network representation of a child's dinosaur's knowledge. *Deve Psychology* 1983; 19:29–39.

Collins WA, Wellman H, Keniston A, Westby S: Age-related aspects of comprehension and inferences from a televised dramatic narrative. *Child Dev.* 1978; 49:389–399.

Davis M: *Computability and the Unsolvability.* New York, McGraw Hill, 1950.

Fantz RL: Visual perception from birth as shown by pattern selectivity. *Ann NY Acad of Sci* 1965; 118:793–814.

Figley CR (ed): *Stress Disorders Among Vietnam Veterans.* New York, Brunner/Mazel, 1978.

Flapen D: *Children's Understanding of Social Interaction.* New York, Teachers College Press, 1968.

Freud S: Three essays on the theory of sexuality, in Strachey J. (ed): *The Standard Edition of the Complete Psychological Works of Sigmund Freud,* Vol 7. London, Hogarth Press, 1953, pp 135–243) (original work published in 1905).

Freud S: Introductory lectures on psychoanalysis, in Strachey J (ed): *The Standard Edition of the Complete Psychological Works of Sigmund Freud,* Vols 15–16. London, Hogarth Press, 1963, pp. 243–496 (original work published in 1916–1917).

Gardner H: *The Mind's New Science,* New York, Basic Books, 1985.

Goelet P, Kandel E: Taking the flow of learned information from membrane receptors to genome, *Trends Neurosci* 1986; 9:492–499.

Goodman GS, Helgeson VS: Child sexual assault: Children's memory and the law. *Univ Miami Law Rev* 1985; 40:181–208.

Goodman GS, Reed RS: Age differences in eyewitness testimony. *Law Hum Behav* 1986; 10:317–332.

Harlow HF: The development of affectional patterns in infant monkeys, in B. Foss (ed): *Determinants of Infant Behavior.* London, Tavistock Institute of Human Relationship, 1961; pp 75–100.

Harris J, Liebert R: *The Child.* Englewood Cliffs, NJ, Prentice Hall, 1991.

Hartman C, Burgess A: Information processing of trauma. *J Interpers Violence* 1988; 3:443–457.

Hays BJ, Norris J, Martin, KS, Androwich J: Informatics issues for nursing's future. *Adv Nurs Sci* 1994; 16:71–81.

Heimes SJ: *John von Neuman and Norbert Wiener,* Cambridge, MA, MIT Press, 1980, p 211.

Hess EH: Imprinting. *Science* 1959; 130:133–141.

Horowitz MJ: *Stress Response Syndromes.* New York, Jason Aronson, 1976.

Howe ML, Courage ML: On resolving the enigma of infantile amnesia, *Psychol Bull* 1993; 113:305–326.

Hull CL: *Principles of Behavior: An Introduction to Behavior Theory.* New York, Appleton-Century-Crofts, 1943.

Isakower O: A contribution to the patho-psychology of phenomena associated with falling asleep, *Int. J. Psa 1938;* 19:331–345.

Jacobs AM, dela Cruz FA: The informatics education needs of graduate nursing students, in Arnold JM, Pearson GA (eds): *Computer Applications in Nursing Administration and Practice.* New York, National League for Nursing, 1992, p 335.

Jeffress LA (ed): *Cerebral Mechanisms in Behavior: The HixonSymposium,* New York, John Wiley & Sons, 1951, p 135.

Kail RV Jr, Hagen JW: *Perspectives on the Development of Memory and Cognition.* Hillsdale, NJ, Lawrence Erlbaum Associates, 1977, pp xi–xiii.

Lepore SJ: Child witness: Cognitive and social factors related to memory and testimony, *Iss Child Abuse Accus* 1991; 3:65–89.

Lindberg M: An interactive approach to assessing the suggestibility and testimony of eyewitnesses, in J Doris (ed): *The Suggestibility of Children's Recollections: Implications for Eyewitness Testimony.* Washington, DC, American Psychological Association, 1991, pp 47–55.

Lorenz K: *On Aggression.* New York, Harcourt, Brace and World, 1966.

Mandler JM: Representation, in Mussen P (series ed) and J Flavell & E Markman (vol eds): *Handbook of Child Psychology,* Vol 3: Cognitive Development. New York, John Wiley & Sons, 1983, pp 420–494.

Marin BV, Holmes DL, Guth M, Kovac P: The potential of children as eyewitnesses. *Law Hum Behav* 1979; 3:295–306.

Maser JD, Seligman MEP (eds): *Psychopathology: Experimental Models,* San Francisco, WH Freeman, 1977.

Maslow AH: *Motivation and Personality,* ed 2. New York, Harper & Row, 1970.

Nelson K, Kosslyn SM: Recognition of previously labeled or unlabeled pictures by 5-year olds and adults, *J Exp Child Psychol* 1976; 21:40–45.

Pearlmutter M: Continuities and discontinuities in early human memory paradigms, processes, and performances, in Kail RV. Spear NE (eds): *Comparative Perspectives on the Development of Memory,* Hillsdale, NJ, Lawrence Erlbaum Associates, 1984, pp 253–287.

Perry NW: How children remember and why they forget, *Advisor* 1992; 5:1,2,13–16.

Perry NW, Nielsen D, Burns D, Cunningham E, Jenkins S: Young children's ability to provide accurate testimony following a witnessed event. Paper presented at the spring meeting of the Nebraska Psychological Association, Lincoln, Nebraska, 1987.

Perry NW, Teply LL: Interviewing, counseling and in-court examinations of children: Practical approaches for attorneys, *Creighton Law Rev* 1984–1985; 18:1369–1426.

Piaget J, Inhelder B: *Memory and Intelligence.* New York, Basic Books, 1973.

Pynoos RS, Nader K: Children's memory and proximity to violence. *J Am Acad Child Adolesc Psychiatry* 1989; 28:236–241.

Rainey J, Aleem A, Ortiz A, Yaragani V, Pohl R, Berchow R: Laboratory procedure for inducement of flashbacks. *Am J Psychiatry* 1987; 144:1317–1319.

Simpson RI: *Technology: Nursing the System, a Collection of Articles on Nursing Informatics.* Atlanta, HBO and Company, 1992.

Skinner BF: *Science and Human Behavior.* New York, Free Press, 1953.

Squire LR: *Memory and Brain.* New York, Oxford University Press, 1987.

Tiecher MH, Glod CA, Surrey J, Swett C Jr: Early childhood abuse and limbic system ratings in adult psychiatric outpatients. *J Neuropsychiatr Clin Neurosci* 1993; 5:301–306.

van der Kolk B: The trauma spectrum: The interaction of biological and social events in the genesis of trauma response. *J Traum Stress* 1988; 1:274.

van der Kolk B: The compulsion to repeat the trauma: Re-enactment, revictimization, and masochism. *Psychiatr Clin North Am* 1989; 12.

van der Kolk BA (ed): *Post-traumatic Stress Disorder: Psychological and Biological Sequelae,* Washington, D.C., American Psychiatric Press, 1984.

Walker PH, Walker JM: Nursing informatics: Opportunities for administrators, clinicians, and researchers. *J Am Psychiatr Nurs Assoc* 1995; 1:22–29.

Weiner N: *Cybernetics, or Control and Communication in the Animal and the Machine,* ed 2. Cambridge, MA, MIT Press, 1961, p. 8. (Original work published in 1948).

Werner JS, Perlmutter M: Developments of visual memory in infants, in Reese HW, Lipsitt LP (eds): *Advances in Child Development and Behavior,* Vol 14. New York, Academic Press, 1979, pp 1–56.

Willingham DB, Nissen MJ, Bullemer P: On the development of procedural knowledge. *J Exp Psychol: Learning, Memory, Cognit* 1989; 15:1047–1060.

Yuhuda R, Resnick H, Kahana B, Giller EL: Long-lasting hormonal alterations to extreme stress in humans: Normative or maladaptive? *Psychosom Med* 1993; 55:287–297.

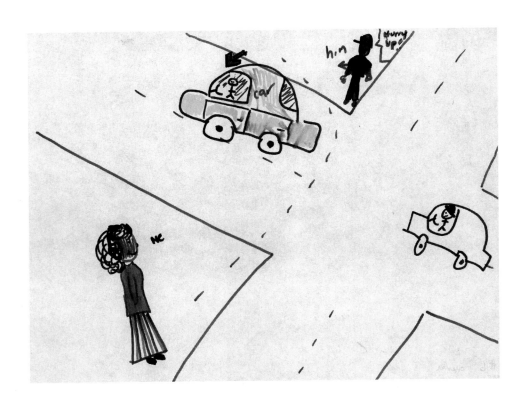

Like one that on a lonesome road
Doth walk in fear and dread,
And having once turned round walks on,
And turns no more his head;
Because he knows a frightful fiend
Doth close behind him tread.

Samuel Taylor Coleridge, 1772–1834
The Ancient Mariner, pt.VI, st. 10

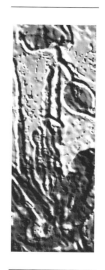

6

Stress, Coping, and Defensive Functioning

Ann W. Burgess / Paul T. Clements, Jr.

For many, students, the concept of mental health is abstract, and they are therefore afraid of being unable to grasp its many dimensions. There is an obvious difference between the assessment of a medical-surgical patient, for whom data are often quantifiable, and assessment of a psychiatric patient, for whom data take on a qualitative, subjective character. When a person's mental health is "out of balance," it is not easily measured and quantified. The patient does not demonstrate readily interpretable physical symptoms. The mainstays of psychiatric nursing, therefore, are subjective input from the patient, an analysis of the patient's behavior, and the nurse's interpretation of this information to appropriately determine the treatment issues and subsequently plan and implement effective nursing care.

As discussed in Chapter 1, a key factor in dealing with a patient's anxiety is to be aware of one's own feelings about mental illness. Students must explore their feelings of apprehension or fear for personal safety, preconceived notions that little or no hope exists for a person with mental illness, or firsthand exposure to the mental-health system through family members' experiences. This chapter introduces the concepts of stress, coping, mental health, mental illness, and psychological defensive functioning.

■ STRESS

In recent years, stress and its possible effect on mental health have become increasingly important in nursing generally and in psychiatric nursing in particular. Moreover, the public has become more aware of the potential effects of stress on their lives, as research proliferates and new understandings are disseminated.

Stress can be defined by two separate but related meanings. First, it is a stimulus that upsets an individual's balance or homeostasis. Used in this general sense, stress refers to any stimulus that creates such upset, including general life stressors and those associated with illness or trauma. Second, stress is an individual's response to a stressful stimulus. In this textbook, the word *stress* will refer to an identified stimulus that creates upset in an individual (Lowery and Houldin, 1995); however, the primary focus of the book is stress with the second definition. That is, the major emphasis is on the biological, psychological, social, and cultural reactions of an individual to a stressor (or activator), and the consequences of those reactions with respect to psychiatric illness. This latter definition is addressed in the American Nurses' Association's (ANA) definition of nursing. The ANA (1994) defines nurses as dealing with human stress response, as follows: "Nursing is the diagnosis and treatment of human responses to actual or potential health problems; . . . assisting sick and well people, individually and in groups, in the promotion, maintenance, and restoration of health."

Because human response to a stressor may be complex and interactive, the concept of stress as used within this textbook is global and includes emotions such as fear, anger, anxiety, depression, or a combination of these, as well as the wide range of human responses to stressful events. A framework for studying the stress-stressor phenomenon combines two models: one reported by the Institute of Medicine study of Stress and Human Health (Elliot and Eisdorfer, 1982) and the second representing a continuum of stress-crisis (Burgess and Roberts, 1995). Figure 6–1 illustrates this continuum.

ELEMENTS OF THE FRAMEWORK

The model resulting from the Stress and Human Health study has three primary elements: the activators/stressors, the reactions, and the consequences, which are referred to as the x-y-z sequence (Eliot and Eisdorfer, 1982). Activators/stressors may be internal or external events or conditions that are sufficiently intense or frequent to evoke some change in the individual, such as the death of a family member. The stress may be assessed on a continuum of seven levels (Burgess and Roberts, 1995).

The consequences are the prolonged and cumulative effects of the aforementioned reactions, such as psychiatric illness. The model attends to individual differences and variations throughout the sequence by means of its conceptualization of mediators, which are the filters and modifiers in the sequence (Elliot and Eisdorfer, 1982). This model suggests a dynamic, interactive process across the stress continuum between an individual and the environment.

■ MENTAL HEALTH

The term **mental health** encompasses a broad, abstract concept. The past decade has heightened public awareness and focus regarding "good mental health." What is the measure of sound mental health and emotional equilibrium?

In the broadest definition of mental health, normality may be conceptualized as an individual's ability to successfully cope with stress and conflicts in a capacity that permits optimal functional ability. The conflicts may be stressors that are encountered by everyone (work, school, parenting, etc.), and the traumatic crises that are seemingly increasing in our society (e.g., crime, rape, earthquakes, and airplane disasters).

Mental health follows a continuum, and permits varying levels of stability throughout the life-span of an individual. Everyone experiences stress; it is a necessary motivating factor. Individuals perceive and manage stressors differently, however. For example, a woman with a productive career and two young children, who is generally in psychological equilibrium, may encounter a period of depression during a marital divorce and require short-term crisis management during the child-custody component of the divorce.

■ MENTAL ILLNESS

Although many psychiatric nurses spend a great deal of time assisting patients to adjust to anticipated life experiences, the main reason for psychiatric assessment and evaluation is to identify mental disorders and illness. To do this effectively, students must develop an understanding of what constitutes "abnormal" behavior.

In the nursing care of adults and children, students learn to differentiate a normal condition from the abnormal. They learn normal ranges of pulse, respiration, and blood pressure. Laboratory tests list ranges within and outside the normal range; certain findings indicate abnormality. For example, skin lesions and bleeding are abnormal; chest rales are absent in healthy individuals.

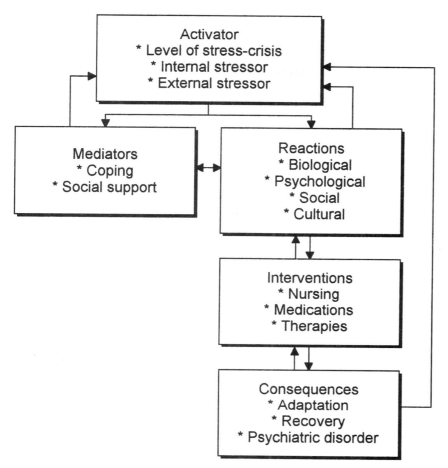

Figure 6-1.   An interactive stress-crisis framework: mediating individual and environmental reactions.

What, however, constitutes normal thoughts, emotions, and behavior? Although there is diversity about what constitutes "normality," most texts define it as behavior that falls within a commonly recognized "standard" within a given culture. Aberrant behavior can be identified by this method, although the reliability of such an approach is limited by cultural diversity (ethnic: white, black, Asian; religious: Hare Krishna, Jehovah's Witness, fundamentalist; organizational: Ku Klux Klan, motor-cycle gangs) and by the cultural background, personal biases, and norms of the nurse performing the assessment. Essentially, what is deemed "normal" ends up being that which is not too different from the accepted cultural and behavioral norms of the evaluator (Yates, Kathol, and Carter, 1994).

Mere recognition of "abnormal" behavior is insufficient for diagnosing a psychiatric disorder. That would be equivalent to calling a jockey who races horses and a person who plays center on a basketball team medically ill because they fall at the extremes of a bell-shaped curve for height.

Despite the difficulty in specifying abnormal emotions and behaviors, there are clearly individuals who are functionally impaired as a result of thoughts, feelings, or behavior. Few would argue that a person with dementia or a patient profoundly depressed represents a variant of normal behavior. Rather, it is impaired functioning that distinguishes eccentric behavior from psychiatric illness. As with all other medical disorders, psychiatric illness includes conditions associated with pain, disability, death, or an increased liability to these states (Robins and Guze, 1970; Yates, Kathol and Carter, 1994).

Assessment and understanding are necessary to correctly identify the person who is suffering from **mental illness,** as it is embodied in a wide variety of symptoms and behaviors. In general, mental illness is identified by a person's inability to adaptively cope with psychological conflict, thereby weakening self-esteem and eventually interfering with the ability to effectively accomplish the necessities of daily living.

EPIDEMIOLOGY

Many families have had a family member affected by mental illness. The percentage of the population who are mentally ill or who require treatment for maintaining mental health or for substance abuse has risen significantly in recent decades. According to estimates from the National Institute of Mental Health (NIMH), 20% of adults in the United States suffer from an active mental disorder within a given year, and 32% can be expected to have such an illness at some time during their lives (Robins and Regier, 1991).

The nature and type of mental disorders vary according to age. It is estimated that about 12% of the nation's 63-million children and adolescents suffer from one or more mental disorders, including autism, attention deficit hyperactivity disorder (ADHD), severe conduct disorder, depression, and alcohol and psychoactive substance abuse and dependence (DHHS, 1991; IOM, 1989). Toward the other end of the life-span are the 4-million older Americans who, according to a National Institute on Aging estimate, are likely to be suffering from Alzheimer's disease (Evans et al., 1990). Dementia symptoms, some argue, are part of the normal aging process. This amount of mental illness in the population has contributed significantly to the need for health-care professionals who can accurately assess and intervene with persons requiring psychiatric treatment.

PSYCHIATRIC DIAGNOSIS

Mental disorders are clinically significant behavioral or psychological syndromes or patterns that occur in an individual and that are associated with present distress (e.g., a painful symptom) or disability (e.g., impairment in one or more important areas of functioning), or with a significantly increased risk of suffering death, pain, or disability, or with an important loss of freedom (APA, 1994). These syndromes, or patterns, are not expected and culturally sanctioned responses to a particular event, such as the death of a loved one. Instead, they are manifestations of behavioral, psychological, or biological dysfunction in the individual (APA, 1994, p. xxi).

■ COPING

Coping, the mediating behavior between stress and anxiety, influences whether the individual will maintain homeostatic balance (e.g., sustain positive mental health) or experience disorganized or negative thinking, feeling and behaving in response to a stressor. Coping refers to activities that modify the negative effects of social or psychological strain (Solomon & Draine, 1995).

A major component of mental health maintenance is the ability to effectively cope with stress and anxiety. Stress is an ever-present state that affects an individual both physically and emotionally. It varies in intensity relative to internal and external stimuli. The stimuli are physical (temperature, sound, light), chemical (pollutants, drugs), microbiological (bacteria, viruses), emotional, situational, and environmental. Stressors may be individual, usually existing in combination with one another. A person will respond to eliminate or master the stressor and attempt to effectively maintain his or her activities of daily living.

ANXIETY

When a stressor overwhelms a person's ability to resolve or cope with it, **anxiety** results. Anxiety is a ubiquitous emotional state that is experienced when the self-identity or essential values of a person are threatened; however, it has no specific object. Anxiety is an uneasiness or fearfulness stemming from anticipated threat. It is, however, differentiated from fear, in which there is an identifiable stressor. The feeling state is characterized by a subjective sense of dread, apprehension, threat, failure, helplessness, or impending disaster; by a sense of losing control, becoming disoriented, or committing a destructive act; or by fear of sudden death.

The feeling of discomfort in anxiety, which ranges from mild levels to panic, may be acute or chronic. Without an etiology, treatment is difficult. There is a seemingly natural propensity to eliminate or at least avoid the discomfort of anxiety.

The anxiety response is generally characterized by a feeling of impending disaster. Listed below are the common physical or somatic alterations in body systems associated with anxiety.

- Circulatory system: perspiration, clammy hands, flushing, blushing, feeling hot or cold.
- Respiratory system: heavy breathing, sighing respirations, hyperventilation, dizziness.
- Gastrointestinal system: abdominal pain, anorexia, nausea, dry mouth, diarrhea, constipation, "butterflies" in the stomach.
- Genitourinary system: urinary frequency, various interferences with sexual function.
- Cognitive functioning: impaired attention span, poor concentration, impairment of memory, changes in outlook and future planning.
- Emotional reaction: irritability, mood fluctuations, dream disturbances, changes in relationships with family and friends.

ANXIETY LEVELS

Anxiety occupies a focal position in the dynamics of all human adjustment, and serves as the driving force for most of our adjustments in life. Peplau's (1952) classic levels of anxiety are mild, moderate, severe, and panic. Each stage has its particular effect on the sensory perception of the individual.

Mild anxiety can motivate learning and stimulate growth and creativity in the individual. A person's sensory field increases, and he or she is alert to the environment and able to sharply discern the anxiety-producing experience, thereby maximizing the options for decision-making.

Moderate anxiety tends to narrow the perceptual field and block out peripheral stimuli. The patient does not attend to the factors operating in the environment, but is able to focus if another person so directs. The choices available to a person at this level are restricted.

Severe anxiety drastically reduces a person's perceptual field. The primary goal of the individual is to get relief from the feeling. With much direction from another person, the severely anxious individual is able to attend to a specific area. Self-awareness is greatly diminished and choices are severely limited.

Panic levels of anxiety result in the individual's loss of control. He or she becomes disorganized and needs help from another human being in order to function. The perceptual field is blocked and self-awareness is almost absent. The feelings associated with this level of anxiety are dread, terror, awe, and danger. If such a state continues over a long period, exhaustion and death may result because of the strain of such an overwhelming experience.

When assessing a patient's anxiety level, nurses need to try to ascertain whether they comprehend the situation that the patient is experiencing. They may then assess whether the anxiety level seems appropriate to the situation. Does the patient's anxiety level stimulate or facilitate personal growth, happiness, and satisfaction, or does it inhibit and thwart attainment of these goals? These questions need to be addressed by the nurse prior to formulating a diagnosis and developing an appropriate nursing intervention.

■ DEFENSIVE FUNCTIONING

Having knowledge of an individual's personality style is important for understanding that person's psychological strengths and vulnerabilities. One way to understand personality styles is to study the defensive functioning and structure of a person by observing their use of **defense mechanisms.** Defensive functioning is part of the coping process. Knowledge of this is essential for students of human behavior as they begin to work with the defensive styles of persons under stress from a physical and/or mental-health problem.

Since Sigmund Freud, Anna Freud, and Erik Erikson began to report in the first half of the 20th century about ego development and the mechanisms of defense, studies of the ego have taken two major directions. Each has considerable clinical importance. In one direction, have been studies of various ego functions (including defensive functioning) that are primarily conflict-free and result from maturational aspects of intellectual functioning. In the second direction have been studies of the major mechanisms of ego defense.

EGO FUNCTIONS

What is ego? Freud's concept of three agencies of the mind outlines the id, superego, and ego. The id, a primitive instinctual drive, is a major source of psychic energy and provides fuel for the ego and superego. The superego strives for morality, internalizing values and beliefs as right or wrong. The **ego** is the reality balance; it mediates the pressures of the environment and the pressures of instinctual satisfaction, and preserves the integrity of the individual.

One of the earliest studies on the role of the ego was by Bellak, Hurvich, and Sheehy (1976). They described 10 major functions of the ego. Psychiatric nurses benefit from being able to assess ego functioning as it relates to defense mechanisms, which are important in patient evaluations (*DSM-IV,* 1994). The assessment may be part of a mental-status examination. Ego functions may also be used as a checklist to focus on deficient areas of functioning that are troublesome for the patient (Figure 6–2).

Ego development is involved with individual coping and adaptation—processes highly relevant for understanding impairments and gains in the maturational process. Loevinger and Wessler (1970), in an early study of ego development, presented the concept that ego development assumes that each person has a customary orientation to the self and the world, and that these frames of reference are ordered along a continuum. Loevinger and Wessler (1970) delineated stages of ego development defined by age. Each stage (early, middle, and later) differs from the others in impulse control, conscious concerns, and interpersonal and cognitive styles.

MECHANISMS OF DEFENSE OF THE EGO

The hypothesis underlying the psychodynamic model of the human mind is that all human behavior makes sense; that is, whatever comes from the mind of a person is subject to rational explanation. The explanation is to be found in further information about that person. Thus, the psychodynamic model places the psyche (ego, self, mind, soul) in the center of the active consciousness with the goal of making sense of an individual's behavior. The absence of ego places the individual under the control of instinctual drives. The presence of ego gives personality its boundaries and its direction (Binstock, 1979).

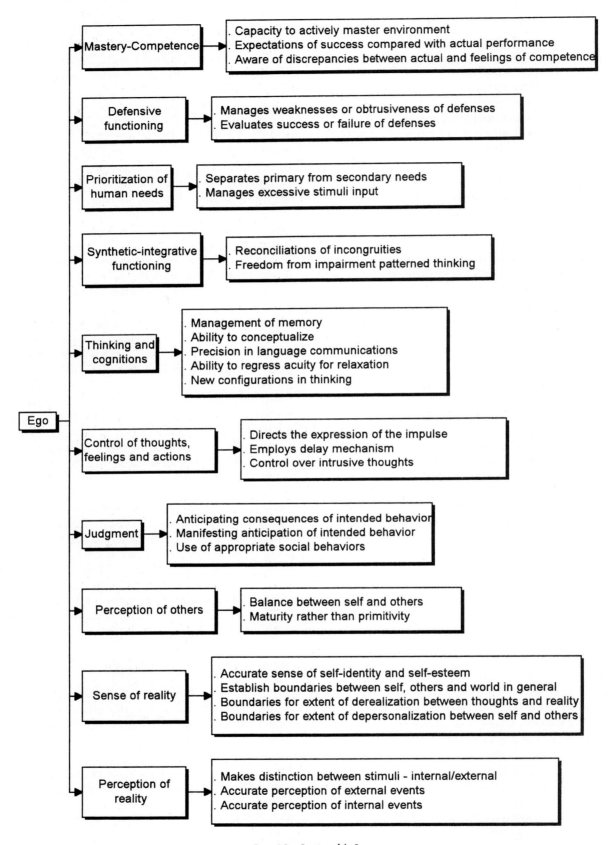

Figure 6-2. Functions of the Ego.

The psychodynamic view of mental health posits that mental symptoms arise when conflicting emotions, such as love or hate, or assertiveness or passivity, produce unmanageable distress. Sigmund Freud (1926) suggested that psychological conflict created an energy imbalance in the psychological apparatus. Anxiety warned a patient of this imbalance. This psychological alert, called signal anxiety, induced the psychological apparatus to relieve distress by transferring awareness of the conflict beyond conscious awareness. The mechanism that assigns such information to the unconscious is called **repression.** Repression, however, often fails to bury the conflict totally. Elements of the awareness leak into consciousness and again cause anxiety. Then, in an attempt to diminish distress, the psychic apparatus further disposes of the anxiety by transforming it into a psychological symptom. Freud (1926) suggested that psychic defenses (**defense mechanisms**) developed to protect against intrapsychic conflict and anxiety. He considered symptom formation largely a consequence of failed mechanisms of defense (Preven and David, 1995; p. 6).

Defense mechanisms, then, are adaptive functions of the personality and are specific intrapsychic processes, operating unconsciously. Defense mechanisms are employed when an individual seeks relief from emotional conflict and freedom from anxiety. Defenses are considered successful if they abolish the need for immediate gratification or if they find substitute gratification.

Several questions need to be answered by the nurse during an assessment of defense mechanisms.

- Are the defense mechanisms used by the patient effective in decreasing the patient's anxiety level?
- What is the psychological price of this relief?
- Do the mechanisms interfere with perception of reality, isolate the patient from others, immobilize creative energies?

■ DEFENSE LEVELS AND INDIVIDUAL DEFENSE MECHANISMS

DEFENSE LEVELS

The concept of stress, coping, and adaptation has received major attention in the health-care literature. Methods of defense or coping have been studied in the area of physiology, including their role as a response to invading organisms or physical trauma. In the psychological literature, coping is discussed in terms of activities or a style of coping. Defenses are part of coping.

Psychiatrist George Vaillant (1976) initiated research on categorizing defense mechanisms. His study of a sample of men selected for psychological health

showed that they tended to progress through ego-function levels throughout their life-span, and that each level was associated with a different level of adaptation to life. His 12-year follow-up study of heroin addicts suggested that patients tended to recover sequentially through these same levels (Vaillant, 1976).

Sigmund Freud, Anna Freud, Otto Kernberg, George Vaillant, and Elvin Semrad are recognized clinicians and researchers who defined and developed methods to categorize defense mechanisms. Studies have supported a hierarchy of defense mechanisms related to levels of health and illness. Battista's (1982) testing of Vaillant's hierarchy of ego functions on a clinical population of 78 patients provided empirical support for a four-category system, ranging from psychotic defenses to mature and healthy defenses. In a nursing study of coping and adaptation following traumatic crisis, Burgess and Holmstrom (1986) conducted a follow-up study of 81 rape victims years after the rape incident. They found that victims recovering fastest used more adaptive strategies than those not recovered in 4 to 6 years. Further advancement in the field of categorizing defenses is noted in the *DSM-IV* (1994).

By understanding a patient's defense level, psychiatric nurses can assess the patient's potential for recovery from an illness and thereby determine appropriate interventions. For example, the recovery of a patient with acute anxiety, whose habitual defense is reaction formation, may be facilitated by providing the patient with work that he or she views as useful, while at the same time giving medication and psychotherapy. Conversely, someone who uses higher-level adaptive defenses (i.e., humor, sublimation, and suppression) might recover best through the creative arts, as in occupational therapy, as an adjunct to medication and supportive psychotherapy. Appendix B of the *Diagnostic and Statistical Manual,* Fourth Edition *(DSM-IV)* contains a number of proposals for diagnostic criteria and axes that were suggested for further study. Although the *DSM-IV* Task Force believed that these categories needed further empirical study, they were included in an Appendix (1994) to stimulate further study. One such category is a defensive functioning scale (Table 6–1). The following sections list the various defense levels with examples of defense mechanisms.

High-Adaptive-Level Defenses

Defenses in the **high adaptive level** are clearly associated with good coping skills. This level of defensive functioning results in optimal adaptation in handling stressors. These defenses usually maximize gratification and allow the conscious awareness of feelings, ideas, and their consequences. For example, suppression allows an anxiety-producing conflict to be put out of awareness until one is ready to deal with the issues. Hu-

TABLE 6–1 DEFENSE LEVELS AND INDIVIDUAL DEFENSE MECHANISMS

1. High Adaptive Level	5. Major Image-Distorting Level
Anticipation	Autistic fantasy
Affiliation	Projective identification
Altruism	Splitting
Humor	
Self-assertion	
Self-observation	
Sublimation	
Suppression	

2. Mental Inhibitions Level	6. Action Level
Displacement	Acting out
Dissociation	Apathetic withdrawal
Identification	Help-rejecting complaining
Intellectualization	Passive aggression
Isolation of affect	Regression
Reaction formation	Conversion
Repression	
Undoing	

3. Minor Image-Distorting Level	7. Level of Defensive Dysregulation
Compensation	Delusional projection
Devaluation	Psychotic denial
Idealization	Psychotic distortion
Introjection	
Omnipotence	
Substitution	
Symbolism	

4. Disavowal Level	
Denial	
Projection	
Rationalization	

mor reflects a capacity to accept a situation while taking the edge off its painful aspects. Sublimation, on the other hand, uses an anxiety-provoking impulse in the service of a creative response. These three defenses are associated with a constructive mastery of conflict by temporarily putting it aside, making a joke of it, or transforming it into a creative product.

The defense mechanisms in the high adaptive level are defined below, and an example is given of each.

Anticipation: Emotional reactions are thought about and experienced in advance.

Example: A nursing student, anticipating presenting a case study to a treatment team, believes she will do the best she can, and that comments and criticisms will help her to learn.

Affiliation: The individual deals with emotional conflict by turning to others for help or support. Problems are shared with others, but this does not imply trying to make someone else responsible for them.

Example: A 28-year-old teacher who has lost her pet is able to talk with friends who have pets and can appreciate her loss.

Altruism: The individual deals with emotional conflict by meeting the needs of others. Unlike the self-sacrifice sometimes noted in reaction formation, the individual receives gratification either vicariously or from the response of others.

Example: During the holidays, a 19-year-old student, home on vacation, is notified that a family friend has just been hospitalized. She cancels a movie date and visits the friend.

Humor The amusing or ironic aspects of a stressor or conflict are emphasized.

Example: A graduate student gets a D on an examination and says, "How dare I get a D when I was out partying the night before the exam!"

Self-assertion Feelings are expressed directly in a way that is not coercive or manipulative.

Example: A teacher has been irritable and yelling at students during a semester. The students confront the teacher and ask if she can change the tone of her voice because it is upsetting to them.

Self-observation One's own thoughts, feelings, motivation, and behavior are reflected upon, yielding an appropriate response.

Example: A 45-year-old mother was unable to find a particular compact disk, and sharply asked a young clerk for help. The clerk angrily picked it out from the shelf. The woman, realizing her own impatience, complimented the clerk on her attractive outfit, said that she appreciated the help, and apologized for her abrupt manner. The clerk's demeanor changed quickly to smiles.

Sublimation Unacceptable instinctual drives are diverted into socially and personally acceptable channels.

Example: A 35-year-old lawyer whose early life was emotionally barren becomes a successful prosecuting attorney. His anger and rage are channeled into prosecuting suspected criminals.

Example: A 13-year-old junior-high-school student has an intense crush on her science teacher. She does outstanding work in his class and receives an A+ in the course.

Suppression: Unacceptable ideas or impulses are voluntarily relegated from the conscious to the unconscious mind.

Example: A college student is angry at his friend for not calling. He goes to the library and puts it out of his mind.

Example: An accountant in a large business organization feels a strong sexual attraction to her boss. When at work she consciously puts the feelings out of her mind.

Mental Inhibitions (Compromise-Formation)-Level Defenses

Defensive functioning at the **mental inhibitions level** keeps potentially threatening ideas, feelings, memories, wishes, or fears out of awareness. The defense mechanism of **reaction formation** reflects a need to perceive oneself as good, kind, helpful to others, and never angry. For example, a person with such a formation would say, "If someone mugged me and stole my money, I'd rather he be helped than punished."

Patients often come to the attention of clinicians when they suffer a loss and their characteristic pattern of response to stress cannot synthesize their anger and anxiety. They then become depressed. The defense mechanisms at this level are also called self-sacrificing defenses.

Defense mechanisms at the mental inhibition level include the following:

Displacement: The redirection of an emotion from one idea, object, or person to another.

Example: A 5-year-old girl who was angered by her teacher in school yells inappropriately at her mother.

Dissociation: The detachment of emotional significance from an idea, situation, object, or relationship.

Example: A rape victim describes her rape experience with a bland, flat affect.

Identification: The unconscious adoption or patterning of personality characteristics on an admired other.

Example: A young soldier begins to socialize with his friends, just like his sergeant.

Intellectualization: The excessive use of abstract thinking or the making of generalizations to control or minimize disturbing feelings.

Example: A 43-year-old man says, "I don't need to brood about the death of my child. I know children die of disease and the doctors were competent and knew what they were doing. Life goes on."

Isolation of affect: Separation of ideas from the feelings originally associated with them.

Example: A father calmly talks about the total loss of his home in the aftermath of a hurricane.

Reaction formation: The direction of overt behavior or attitudes in the opposite direction to the individual's underlying motives, feelings, or wishes.

Example: A 35-year-old woman has unconscious feelings of anger and hatred for her father; but when he visits, she is polite and sweet-mannered.

Repression: The involuntary banishment of unacceptable or painful thoughts, feelings, and impulses into the unconscious.

Example: A 17-year-old parent has no recollection of hitting his infant son.

Example: A 55-year-old European businesswoman has no memory of the frequent air raids she experienced as a young child.

Undoing: An endeavor to actually or symbolically erase a previously consciously intolerable experience.

Example: A husband and wife have an intense emotional argument at breakfast. The husband brings her flowers when he comes home from work.

Example: Lady Macbeth's ritualistic handwashing was an attempt to undo the crimes she and her husband had committed.

Minor Image-Distorting Level Defenses

Defenses at the **minor image-distorting level** are characterized by distortions in the image of the self, body, or of others that may be employed to regulate selfesteem. The essence of these defenses is to split the image of self and other into good and bad and strong and weak. This defense level could interfere with interpersonal relationships, but not necessarily with achievement and accomplishment. These defenses could be invoked in the service of constructive adaptation in situations of stress by persons who do not use them habitually (e.g., one way of dealing with severe physical illness may be to trust in the omnipotence of the physician).

Examples of minor image-distorting defenses include:

Compensation: A conscious or unconscious attempt to overcome real or imagined inferiority or inadequacies.

Example: An underweight, short 15-year-old boy joins the weight-lifting club at school.

Devaluation: Attributing exaggerated negative qualities to oneself or others.

Example: A student states, "The teacher really doesn't know what she is talking about. Why should I pay any attention to what she is saying?"

Idealization: Attributing exaggerated positive qualities to others.

Example: A patient says, "I think the nurses are so good; they are always there for you; they know so much; they would never upset me." Or, "I always feel that someone I know is like a guardian angel."

Introjection: The symbolic assimilation (taking into self) of loved or hated attitudes, wishes, ideals, or persons.

Example: A 16-year-old girl decides not to participate in her friend's stealing expedition. (She has introjected her parents' values.)

Example: A young boy walks and talks like his father.

Omnipotence: Acting or feeling as if one possesses special powers or abilities and is superior to others.

Example: An elderly depressed man says, "I don't see any reason for seeing a psychiatrist. He can't understand the human mind like I do."

Substitution: The replacement of an unattainable or unacceptable need, emotion, drive, or goal by one that is attainable or acceptable.

Example: Instead of becoming a class-office candidate, a young woman college student becomes a campaign manager.

Symbolism: A mechanism by which an external object is used to represent an internal idea, belief, attitude, wish, or feeling.

Example: During the late 1960s, the hair and dress style of young people symbolized their feelings and attitudes toward authority and the prevailing values of the culture.

Disavowal Level

The **disavowal defense level** is characterized by keeping unpleasant or unacceptable stressors, impulses, ideas, affects, or responsibility out of awareness, with or without their misattribution to external causes. Nursing intervention seeks to assist the person with such defenses to deal with reality. For example, the intervention for a projecting person who puts the blame and responsibility on others instead of accept-ing his own impulses would be to review the issue at hand in order to determine responsibility for specific events.

Disavowal level defenses include the following:

Denial: The unconscious disavowal of thoughts, feelings, wishes, needs, or external reality factors that are consciously unacceptable.

Example: A 65-year-old man continues to plan future projects within his work environment even though his retirement is imminent.

Projection: The attributing to another person or object of thoughts, feelings, motives, or ideas that are unacceptable to oneself.

Example: A 30-year-old college professor accuses a colleague of wanting to be the chairperson of the department.

Example: A 50-year-old psychiatric patient is certain that the hospital food is poison and that the staff wants to kill her.

Rationalization: An attempt to modify unacceptable motives, feelings, needs, or impulses into ones that are acceptable.

Example: A 37-year-old man who was passed over for a job promotion says the new position was not challenging enough.

Example: A young college graduate who did not get accepted into graduate school says he did not really need more schooling.

Example: A 13-year-old girl has a crush on her 17-year-old neighbor; but when she sees him, she talks about how much he annoys her with his mannerisms.

Major Image-Distortion Level

The **major image-distortion level** of defense is characterized by gross distortion or misattribution of the image of oneself or others. These image-distortion defenses differ from minor image-distortion defenses in that they are habitually used. Use of these defenses guarantee problems in interpersonal relationships, since persons who use such defenses have difficulty in viewing themselves realistically.

Major image-distortion defenses include: autistic fantasy, projective identification, and splitting of self-image or image of others.

Autistic fantasy: The individual deals with emotional conflict by excessive daydreaming as a substitute for human relationships, more effective action, or problem solving.

Example: A 35-year-old woman daydreams about her ideal boyfriend and going on a romantic vacation, rather than dealing with the fact of losing her job.

Projective identification: The false attribution to others of one's own unacceptable feelings, impulses, or thoughts.

Example: A young mother tells her infant son to stop screaming and yelling; that the baby is a bad child.

Splitting: This compartmentalizes opposite affect states and fails to integrate the positive and negative qualities of the self into cohesive images. Self and object images tend to alternate between polar opposites: exclusively loving, powerful, worthy, nurturing, and kind—or exclusively bad, hateful, angry, destructive, rejecting, or worthless.

Example: A patient screams and accuses one nurse that she does nothing right; that she is stupid. She complements a second nurse, saying that that nurse is perfect. Or, "There's no such thing as finding a little good in everyone. If you're bad, you're all bad."

Action-Level Defenses

Defenses at the **action level** are characterized by defensive functioning that deals with internal or external stressors by action or withdrawal. The common feature determined for this level is that all of an individual's behaviors indicate the inability to deal with impulses by taking constructive action on his or her own behalf. Nursing interventions seek to correct this inability. The acting-out person requires controls. The withdrawn or inhibited person needs to be actively drawn out. The passive-aggressive person acts to provoke anger in the person with whom he or she is involved. The regressed person requires someone to take over and do something for him or her.

Action-level defenses include the following:

Acting out: The individual deals with emotional conflict by actions rather than reflection or feelings. Defensive acting out is not the same as "bad behavior" because it requires evidence that the behavior is related to internal or external stressors.

Example: Forgetting an appointment or coming late to a dinner party given by someone with whom you are angry.

Conversion: Elements of intrapsychic conflict are disguised and expressed symbolically through physical symptoms.

Example: A patient currently involved in a divorce situation cannot move her legs, although no organic basis for her symptoms can be found.

Apathetic withdrawal: Behavior that is avoidant and lacks energy, suggesting a depressed mood.

Example: A hospital patient who is denied a request to go home retreats to her room and refuses to eat or attend meetings or social events.

Help-rejecting complaining: Making repeat requests for help that disguise overt feelings of hostility or reproach toward others, and then rejecting the suggestions, advice, or help that they offer.

Example: An elderly woman asks her children for advice about buying real estate and does just the opposite of the advice given.

Passive aggression: Indirectly expressing aggression toward others.

Example: A young woman tells her friend, "I didn't know you didn't want me to tell John that you went out with Jimmy. I'm so sorry." Or, "If my boss bugged me, I might make a mistake in my work or work more slowly so as to get back at him.

Regression: The return to an earlier and subjectively more comfortable level of emotional adjustment.

Example: A 5-year-old girl, the week before starting kindergarten, becomes clinging and fearful of leaving her mother.

Example: A 28-year-old career woman cries uncontrollably when confronted with negative feedback from her boss.

Defensive-Dysregulation Level

The defense level of **defensive dysregulation** is characterized by an individual's failure to contain his or her reaction to stressors, leading to a pronounced break with objective reality.

Delusional projection: Projected thoughts are false, fixed ideas.

Example: A patient believes that the hospital staff are FBI agents in disguise.

Psychotic denial: An assertion that something that is obviously true is neither true nor part of reality.

Example: A patient denies that his mother died 3 years ago, but instead says that she is alive and going to poison him.

Psychotic distortion: A belief that has no grounding in reality.

Example: "If I get in the elevator, it will take me to hell."

E CASE EXAMPLE

Mr. and Mrs. Jackson, in their eighties and married 60 years, had lived in a modest apartment despite increasing health problems. Mr. Jackson had severe emphysema and intermittent cardiac arrhythmia, and was becoming forgetful. Mrs. Jackson had mild hypertension and senile dementia. On the evening of his 85th birthday, Mr. Jackson became short of breath and anxious that he was going to die. He was taken to the hospital and further testing revealed he had inoperable lung cancer for which only palliative treatment could be offered.

While Mr. Jackson was hospitalized, Mrs. Jackson went to live with their daughter and son-in-law. At night she wandered the rooms of the house, looking for her husband. She was confused and argumentative. Her family had been aware of her increasing mental problems, but she was more disturbed than they had realized or perhaps had wanted to realize.

Mrs. Jackson's behavior could be explained in two ways: (1) she was undergoing a period of acute situational stress; and (2) her deteriorated functioning had not been obvious when she was part of a functioning couple. Her husband, who had helped her at home and covered up her deficits, was no longer there. Plans were made to discharge Mr. Jackson to a nursing home, where he could live with his wife in a double room. Although he was depressed, he adjusted to the nursing home, accepting the fact that he would live out his days there. He lived to see his grand-daughter married and then he died. Mrs. Jackson never adjusted and her mental condition continued to deteriorate. She continued to expect her husband to come home each evening from the hospital, and concluded that she never saw him because he left early in the morning before she awoke and returned home after she was asleep.

---

*Goldman, H. (1995) Case adapted and printed with permission.

This case illustrates an interaction of biomedical and psychosocial stressors. Mr. Jackson's illness precipitated a change in the delicate balance of the couple's independence. Mrs. Jackson needed nursing care but Mr. Jackson's illness kept him from providing it. Many people become ill or die upon achieving certain milestones. Mr. Jackson's 85th birthday had had special significance. His driver's license, the key to his independence and his ability to care for his wife, expired on his birthday. He had been preparing for his driving test and was afraid he would not pass it. Going to a nursing home gave him the comfort of knowing that when he died his wife would be cared for and not be a burden to the family. His cancer had been developing for a long time, but clinically obvious illness began on his birthday. His defensive functioning allowed a positive coping style. Mrs. Jackson was unable to cope without him.

Assessing patients from a biopsychosocial perspective and as they interact with their environment provides a holistic perspective on their behavior. Human responses must be viewed in terms of their precipitating factors, in terms of humans' perceptions of themselves and the events within and around them, as well as their perceptions of any consequences of these events.

O AN OVERVIEW

- The psychodynamic investigation is a search for signs of conflict and the "missing link." Why is an individual under stress?

- The intrapsychic component, or what is carried inside the mind, is one cause of a patient's stress.

- When the mind is in conflict with itself, it has mechanisms to defend itself; these are called ego defenses.

- To assess the defensive structure of a patient, the psychiatric nurse should list the patient's specific defenses or coping styles, indicating the prominent defense level that is exhibited.

- Assessment should reflect the defenses or coping style that an individual employs at the time of evaluation, as well as whatever supplemental information is available about the individual's defenses or coping patterns during the recent time period preceding evaluation (*DSM IV*, 1994).

- Nothing is learned about an individual's state of health from the fact that he or she is employing mechanisms of defense.

- A great deal can be learned about an individual's personality style and general state of health or illness by noting which mechanisms of defense the individual most prominently employs and how well they are working.

TD TERMS TO DEFINE

- action-level defenses
- coping
- defense mechanism
- defensive dysregulation
- disavowal defense mechanisms
- ego
- high-adaptive defense mechanisms
- major image-distortion defense mechanisms
- mental health
- mental illness
- mental-inhibition defense mechanisms
- mild anxiety
- minor image-distorting defense mechanisms
- moderate anxiety
- panic
- reaction formation
- repression
- severe anxiety
- stress

Q STUDY QUESTIONS

1. T F Subjective input is the only valid interpretation of whether a situation is stressful.

2. T F There is no difference between coping style and defensive functioning.

3. T F Stressful life events have been directly linked to physical and mental illness.

4. T F Social support has been found to be a critical mediator in the management of life stresses.

5. Define and give examples of coping styles and defensive functioning.

6. Discuss the critical aspects of George Vaillant's categorizing of defense mechanisms.

7. Mrs. J. has never liked Mrs. G., but when she sees Mrs. G., Mrs. J. always smiles sweetly. One day, Mrs. J. says, "How are you, my dear? You look so nice in black. Why don't you wear it more often?" This is an example of the following defense mechanisms:
   a. Denial
   b. Projection
   c. Reaction formation
   d. Rationalization

8. Sally has received a D in her clinical evaluation in Introduction to Nursing. While in conference with her teacher she says, "The instructor never told me what I should be doing. She always paid attention to the other students and never answered my questions. If I had had more help from her, I could have done better." Sally's statement illustrates which of the following defense mechanisms?
   a. Denial
   b. Projection
   c. Reaction formation
   d. Rationalization

9. Mrs. O came with her therapist for an evaluation with a consultant. As they sat down and prepared for the interview, Mrs. O turned to the consultant, looked at him sternly, and said, "I didn't think you would even want to see or talk to me!" The consultant responded, "How could that be, since I do not even know who you are?" Mrs. O's thinking is an example of which of the following defense mechanisms?
   a. Denial
   b. Projection
   c. Reaction formation
   d. Rationalization

10. Mrs. A is terrified and says to the nurse, "Don't stick me with that needle. It has radium in it and you are trying to poison me." Which of the following replies by the nurse would be most effective?
    a. "This isn't radium. It is haldol."
    b. "What makes you think I would try to hurt you?"
    c. "You're not allergic to haldol, are you?"
    d. "You are frightened and may think I am trying to hurt you, but I am not. Let me give you the medicine."

■ REFERENCES

American Psychiatric Association: Diagnostic and Statistical Manual of Mental Disorders, ed 4, APA, 1994.

Battista JP: Empirical test of Vaillant's hierarchy of ego functions, *Am J Psychiatry* 1982; 139:356–357.

Binstock W: The psychodynamic approach, in A Lazare (ed.) *Outpatient Psychiatry.* Baltimore, Williams & Wilkins, 1979.

Burgess AW, Holmstrom LL: *Rape: Crisis and Recovery.* West Newton MA: Awab, Inc., 1986.

Burgess AW, Roberts AR: Levels of Stress and Crisis Precipitants, *Crisis Intervention* 2(1):31–47. 1995.

DHHS (Department of Health and Human Services). Healthy People 2000. Washington, DC: Government Printing Office; DHHS Pub. No. (PHS) 91–50212, 1991.

Elliot G, Eisdorfer C: (eds.): *Stress and Human Health.* New York: Springer, 1982.

Evans DA, Scherr PA, Cook NR, et al: Estimated prevalence of Alzheimer's disease in the United States. *Milbank Q* 1990; 68:267–289.

Erikson E: *Childhood and Society.* New York: Norton, 1963.

Freud S: Inhibitions, symptoms and anxiety, In The Complete Psychological Works. J. Strachey (trans.) London, Hogarth Press, 1926. vol. 20.

Goldman HH: *Review of General Psychiatry.* Norwalk, CT, Appleton & Lange, 1995, pp. 1–3. Adapted and reprinted with permission.

Institute of Medicine (IOM): *Research on Children and Adolescents with Mental, Behavioral, and Developmental Disorders.* Washington, DC, National Academy Press, 1989.

Loevinger J, Wessler R: Measuring Ego Development San Francisco, Josey-Bass, (vol. 1).

Lowery BJ and Houldin AD: From stressors to illness: The psychological-biological connections. In AB McBride and JK Austin (eds.) *Psychiatric–Mental-Health Nursing,* Philadelphia: W.B. Saunders, 1995.

Peplau H: *Interpersonal Relations.* New York: Putnam, 1952.

Preven D, David J: Theoretical foundations of psychiatry. In Goldman HH (ed): *Review of General Psychiatry,* ed 4. Stamford, CT: Appleton & Lange, 1995.

Robins E, Guze SB: Establishment of diagnostic validity in psychiatric illness: Its application to schizophrenia. *Am J Psychiatry* 1970; 126:983–987.

Robins LN, Regier DA (eds): *Psychiatric Disorders in America: The Epidemiologic Catchment Area Study.* New York, Free Press, 1991.

Solomon P, Draine J: Subjective burden among family members of mentally ill adults: Relation to stress, coping, and adaptation, *Am J Orthopsychiatry* 1995; 65(3):420.

Vaillant G: Natural history of male psychological health: The relation of choice of ego mechanism of defense to adult adjustment, *Arch Gen Psychiatry* 1976; 33:535–545.

Yates WR, Kathol RG, Carter J: Psychiatric assessment, DSM IV, and Differential Diagnosis, in Stoudemire A (ed): *Clinical Psychiatry for Medical Students,* ed 2. Philadelphia, JB Lippincott, 1994 pp. 2–3.

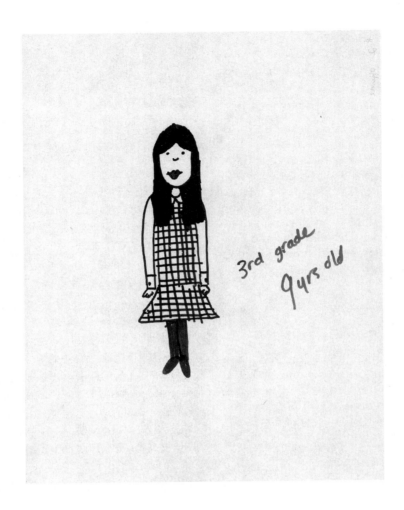

3rd grade
9 yrs old

In our springtime every day has its hidden growth in the mind, as it
has in the earth when the little folded blades are getting ready to
pierce the ground.

George Eliot, 1819–1880

Felix Holt, the Radical (1866) Ch. 18

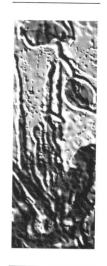

7

Human Growth and Developmental Tasks

Lauren M. Burgess / Ann Wolbert Burgess

Understanding human development and the emotional reactions that might be expected at various stages of the life-cycle helps us to support ill individuals and their families. The life-cycle is a sequence of milestones. Each life-cycle stage has specific developmental challenges and opportunities that are reached at a unique time for each individual. A person's innate developmental process should not, under most circumstances, be hurried or imposed upon by external factors.

The stages are identified by specific tasks, conflicts, and viewpoints occurring during relatively stable periods. Some of the stages, such as childhood and maturity, are universal, and others, such as the 30- and 40-year transitions, are influenced by culture. Each developmental line (love, work, play) proceeds at its own pace, and a person may advance rapidly in some areas and remain the same or regress in others.

The timing differences in the stages of the life-cycle arise from the individual's unique biological, psychological, and social conditions. Healthy psychological development, which also proceeds on a uniquely individual basis and at a variable rate, is dependent on culture and gender factors.

Carl Jung was the first mental-health researcher to focus on the life-cycle. His belief that the personality had developed by adolescence assisted people to begin living as adults and to assume the responsibilities required of them by family, work, and community. He suggested that the next major opportunity for personal growth, following adolescence, was around age 40, a mid-life phase.

Life change generally occurs through the sequence of preparation (transition), rapid change (normal development, or normative crisis, such as childbirth, mid-life, or marital crisis), and finally, consolidation (achievement of a new stage or plateau).

Transitions are important in the process of responding to the demands of successive stages of the life-cycle. People need time to adjust to each new stage and to determine what to retain from the previous stage. Rites of passage serve a function similar to transition, as they, too, can be the vehicle that carries someone from one stage to another. Transitions involve repetitious acts or re-assessing and re-experiencing the past while planning for the future. Repetition can be beneficial, as it allows an individual to re-work tasks and conflicts of earlier areas, particularly those of separation-individuation.

The primary characteristic of a normative crisis is turmoil. Turmoil can arise from external factors, such as illness or another misfortune, or from internal conflicts between opposing alternatives, such as self versus others and living versus dying.

Some regression tends to be experienced during the developmental process. Regression is the revival of earlier, more childlike behavior that usually occurs in response to stress. It is expected behavior during normative crises or transitions.

■ DEVELOPMENTAL FRAMEWORK

Using a **developmental framework,** this chapter focuses on evolving communication skills as well as physical growth and affective development. The variability that characterizes these developmental tasks (Table 7–1) may be based on cultural and gender differences. The stage framework for tracking childhood development is not as useful for tracking adult development, owing to the variability of development from one adult to the next. (Adult development is not detailed in Table 7–1.)

INFANCY: 0 TO 12 MONTHS

The two developmental tasks in infancy include regulation of bodily states and emotions, and attachment.

Regulation of Bodily States and Emotions

The 1-minute Apgar score is the first formal assessment of the infant (Apgar, 1953). The Apgar score assesses five physical signs—heart rate, respiratory effort, reflex irritability, muscle tone, and color—as 0, 1, or 2. The to-

TABLE 7–1. DEVELOPMENTAL TASKS

Infancy	Attachment
	Assistance in the regulation of bodily states, emotion
Toddlerhood	Development of symbolic representation and further self–other differentiation
	Problem-solving, pride, motivation for mastery
Preschool	Development of self-control; the use of language to regulate impulses, emotions; and store information; ability to predict and make sense of the world.
	Development of verbally mediated or semantic memory
	Gender identity
	Development of social relationships beyond immediate family, and generalization of expectations about relationships
	Moral reasoning
Latency age	Peer relationships
	Adaptation to school environment
	Moral reasoning
Adolescence	Re-negotiation of family roles
	Identity issues (sexuality, future orientation, peer acceptance, ethnicity)
	Moral reasoning
Young adult	Continued differentiation from family
	Refinement and integration of identity with particular focus on occupational choice and ultimate partners
	Moral reasoning

Source: National Psychological Maltreatment Consortium, (1995) Office for the Study of the Psychological Rights of the Child, School of Education, Indiana University-Purdue University at Indianapolis. Reprinted with permission.

tal score ranges from 0 (none of these signs present) to 10 (a completely healthy infant). Assessment of the 1-minute score begins 55 seconds after complete emergence of the infant at birth. Infants rarely score 10 at 1 minute. With a score of 5 or less the infant should receive resuscitation. A 1-minute score of 7 or more means the infant is making a good transition into the world.

The newborn infant has remarkable sensory abilities. In just one day, the infant can fixate on a complex pattern such as the human face. By the second day the infant will look at its mother's face longer than that of another woman. Within the first month the infant uses visual information to influence motor responses such as grasping and reaching. The visual acuity of a 4-month-old is generally believed to be as good as that of an adult.

During an infant's first week, it will learn to distinguish the smell of its mother's breast milk from another woman's, and be able to identify its mother's voice from others. Contrary to earlier beliefs that infants did not perceive pain, they can sense pressure, body position, and touch from birth. In fact, infants have been found to be at least as sensitive to pain as adults. This information has led to a dramatic reduction in the number of circumcisions and major surgeries performed on infants without the benefit of anesthesia.

At birth, gross motor abilities are primitive, since newborns are unable to deliberately reach or grasp at objects. By 16 weeks they can hold up their heads, and sit without support at 28 weeks. At 40 weeks infants sit without aid, creep, and pull up into a standing position. At 1 year they are able to walk with support (cruising).

At 6 to 9 months, most infants sleep through the night. Half of all infants have irregular sleep patterns and occasional night awakening through the first year.

In the first year there is rapid physical growth, with a weight increase of approximately 300%.

Piaget's (1977) sensorimotor phase of development encompasses the first 2 years. Initially, motor reflexes are centered on an infant's own body (thumb sucking), but they become more complex as the infant tries to accomplish a task over and over again.

From 4 to 10 months the infant uses the external environment to produce interesting chance events, and by 10 to 12 months can overcome simple obstacles.

Infants cry to communicate fatigue, pain, hunger, fear, discomfort, anger, or a wish for contact. They also participate in a non-communicative form of crying that is also known as "3-month colic". This tension-relieving activity generally occurs in the afternoon and evening when the infant is between the ages of 3 and 10 weeks. Although all normal infants demonstrate this type of crying, a wide variation exists in its duration and intensity. This crying is particularly perplexing to parents, as it has no apparent cause, and comforting the colicky infant is very difficult.

Along with crying, the infant has other ways to communicate such as smiling, reaching, and looking away from an object or person. At 1 year, most children use two or more words besides "Mama" and "Dada," and understand simple commands.

Attachment

Attachment, a key developmental task of infancy, is an emotional or affective tie formed between one person and another that lasts over time and in infants leads to seeking physical closeness to the care-giver (Bowlby, 1969). It specifically describes the infant's thoughts, feelings, and behaviors toward the care-giver. Infants may form attachments to more than one person, and generally form an attachment to the mother and the father at the same time. An infant's attachment behavior induces contact from these significant figures and supports the ability of infants to dramatically influence adult behavior.

The process of attachment begins as early as the infant's first few hours of life, and by 6 to 8 weeks the infant can distinguish its mother's smile from others, and respond to her with a smile. This interaction produces a strong affective response in the mother. Other behaviors that strengthen attachment are crying, looking, clinging, greeting, and vocalizing.

Appropriate levels of attachment occur over a period of time, and can be halted or delayed under certain adverse conditions. Illness of the child, physical or mental illness of the parent, or parental lack of sensitivity to the infant can negatively affect the attachment process. Furthermore, attachment may not occur if the infant is abused or neglected. This could result in serious consequences for future personality development and the formation of meaningful relationships.

The first year of life is a crucial period for attachment to a care-giver figure. Such factors as parental abuse or illness can impair attachment formation (Dulcan, 1994). The particular level of attachment achieved can be used as a indicator of developmental problems that may occur later in childhood. Problems with attachment formation have had lasting effects on personality, and can lead to increased vulnerability to childhood and adult psychiatric illness.

The four types of attachment are:

- **Secure attachment.** The child experiences a normal phenomenon called separation anxiety when in a new situation or when afraid, and wants to be close to its parent.
- **Insecure attachment.** The parent does not properly respond to the infant's needs or responds inappropriately, which has negative implications for future development of trust and healthy relationships.
- **Anxious resistant attachment.** This phenomenon is brought on by parental inconsistency, such as frequent separations or controlling the child through threats of abandonment, which manifests itself in the form of excessive separation anxiety.
- **Anxious avoidant attachment.** The parent regularly rebuffs the infant when it seeks comfort—an extreme case of abuse or neglect.

In the second half of the first year of life, the infant shows the most discriminate forms of attachment. Behavioral observations made of 3½- to 6-year-old children can be linked to the degree of attachment achieved during the first year.

Children who have problems in developing secure attachments may also have difficulty forming intimate, lasting relationships later in childhood, adolescence, and adulthood. Poor attachment promotes an expectation of rejection that leads to a defensive posture of maintaining emotional distance and avoiding intimacy and commitment.

Attachment behavior is exaggerated under stress from discomfort or separation from the parent. Traumatic, prolonged separation can result in **anaclitic depression** (the child does not eat, becomes withdrawn, and sometimes becomes mute) or death. Later symptoms may indicate an inability to form meaningful relationships, show empathy, develop post-traumatic stress disorder, and show decreased intelligence.

TODDLERHOOD: AGES 1 TO 3 YEARS

The developmental tasks of toddlerhood include development of symbolic representation and further self–other differentiation; and problem-solving skill, pride, and motivation for the mastery of skills.

Toddlers, who are able to run by 30 months of age and rapidly increase their abilities in other areas, sleep an average of 12 hours daily.

Much slower physical growth and an increasing interest in other activities leads to a marked decrease in appetite. Parent management of this change can greatly influence whether a power struggle over feeding will ensue. Young toddlers show a desire to feed themselves, first with their fingers and then with utensils.

At 18 to 30 months of age the child develops the pre-requisites for toilet training: a sense and control of the bladder/sphincter muscles; psychological ability to delay urination and bowel movements; a desire to imitate and please parents and other adults; and the ability to communicate the need and coordination to perform toilet tasks. Positive re-enforcement, not punishment, can facilitate learning of toilet needs. Most children can control urination during the day by 2½- years and at night by 3½- years of age. Ten percent of all 6-year-olds, usually boys, still occasionally wet their beds, which tends to be seen as a familial pattern. Bowel control is usually achieved by age 4.

At 18 months, toddlers recognize themselves in mirrors and pictures. As a precursor to further language development, they also begin to retain and use mental symbols. They still have a gap in their understanding of consequences, and with their increased desire to explore, the result is often a greater frequency of accidents and injury.

For children who by age 3 years, do not meet the communication milestones of achieving a vocabulary of about 300 words and speaking in short sentences, hearing tests and language assessments are performed. Although delayed talkers can be normal, the delay may in some cases indicate deafness, aphasia, mental retardation, autism, or a developmental language disorder.

Social referencing is a common phenomenon that begins in the first half of the second year of life. This involves looking to the parent for emotional cues about a new event. The child moves away from the parent to explore, only to return regularly to re-establish emotional contact. Securely attached children use the mother as the base from which they venture out to explore the environment.

At 16 to 24 months, the rapprochement sub-phase of development begins. The child realizes separateness and feels ambivalence about attachment and dependency needs (Mahler, 1972). Tantrums, thumb/finger sucking, transitional objects, and increased clinginess to parents are common from this point to about 36 months of age.

As children approach the last half of the third year of life, they become comfortable with brief separations as they struggle with psychological autonomy and separateness. Often described as the "terrible twos," this period of negativism is critical to the development of a sense of mastery, pride, individuality, and independence. Parents' need to set limits on the negative behaviors is common during this period. Time-out periods are often used. In this method, children are placed in a chair, by themselves, for a specific length of time. The period of time is recommended to be one minute per year of the child's age.

From 24 to 36 months of age, children understand their emotions and can verbally identify them. They also begin to identify with a gender role. In addition, they develop an ability to empathize with others. They also develop defense mechanisms to respond to stressful situations. For example, reaction formation is common in previously toilet-trained children who become

excessively upset when they soil their pants. Common fears are of loud noises, animals, the dark, and separation from the parents.

Piaget's (1977) pre-operational stage of intellectual development is from ages 2 to 7. In this phase, children learn to classify, place objects in order, and construct sets of objects equivalent in number by matching one to one. Problem solving is still by trial and error rather than as a planned process. Children in the pre-operational stage of development are normally egocentric, believing that everything relates to themselves. They are unaware that others have different points of view or knowledge. During this period, symbolic play begins and children play to dramatize roles or stories that symbolize real objects or persons.

PRE-SCHOOL: AGES 3 TO 6 YEARS

Developmental tasks for children of pre-school age include:

- Development of self-control: the use of language to regulate impulses, emotions, store information, and predict and make sense out of the world.
- Development of verbally mediated or semantic memory.
- Gender identity.
- Development of social relationships beyond the immediate family, and generalization of expectations about relationships.
- Moral reasoning.

During these years children refine their gross-motor and fine-motor skills. For example, 5-year-olds should be able to copy a square and a triangle, draw a recognizable human figure with basic body parts, and plan sometimes elaborate drawings in advance.

Identification with a gender role is firmly established during the pre-school period. This identity is largely determined by biological gender, but can be greatly influenced by temperamental factors, parent modeling, and psychological and sociocultural factors. Males are generally more aggressive than females from age 2 through adolescence. The 3-year-old can identify tasks and possessions as masculine or feminine.

By 3 years, children are aware of sex differences. Boys become increasingly aware of sensation in the penis. Children may begin to demonstrate behavior that seems to indicate that they have thought about or heard sounds associated with parental sex (Dulcan, 1994). Sex education about pregnancy should be provided at the level of the child's curiosity and understanding.

Early in the second year of life the child becomes curious about other children. Parallel play is solitary play occurring in pairs. As the child approaches the end of the third year, more associative play occurs. This involves pairs or small groups of children doing the same thing side by side. Most of this play involves sensori-motor activities such as opening, shutting, emptying, and filling objects.

Moral reasoning begins to develop during this period. The young child believes that all events can be explained by the action of some other force that wills things to happen for its own purposes. Moral development involves development of a sense of justice, the inevitability of punishment, and the belief that guilt is determined by the amount of the damage caused by an act rather than the motivation or intent behind it.

Children of pre-school age are impressionable, and seek to be like people they admire. Children whose parents are loving, fair, and honorable are more likely to grow up with the same characteristics.

Through improved communication ability, the child learns to better control impulses and delay gratification. Its vocabulary is expanding rapidly as the child learns an average of nine new words a day until age 6. The specific language milestones are:

- Age 3—Asks many questions just to talk and plays with words.
- Age 4—Context of speech is quite intelligible, although not very articulate.
- Age 5—More articulate, with language development running ahead of the ability to understand concepts.

The pre-school period initiates development of the ability to predict and make sense of the world. Beginning at 3 years of age, the child believes in object constancy. This involves maintaining a positive inner image of an important person even when the person is not present. The child continues to have fears, similar to those in the toddler years, and they may now also include fears of ghosts, monsters, and death.

Some children who are creative develop imaginary friends with names, appearances, and characters. This being is sometimes the child's scapegoat, playmate, or protector.

During this period, children also often show some signs of romantic behavior to the parent of the opposite sex, along with rivalry with the same-sex parent. Later, this turns into a healthy, balanced relationship with both parents and allows the child the freedom to develop relationships with its peers.

Play is critical in development, since it allows children to act out scenarios over which they previously had no control. Four-year-olds participate more in group play, which necessitates the onset of sharing with others. A 5-year-old will plan and implement group projects that can result in elaborate dramatic play.

LATENCY/MIDDLE CHILDHOOD: AGES 6 TO 12 YEARS

Developmental tasks in middle childhood, also called **latency,** include peer relationships, adaptation to the school environment, and moral reasoning.

As children begin to attend elementary school, they develop their cognitive and motor capacities to allow for their gradual independence from the family. Significant maturation of the child's central nervous system is evident, since it can now perceive and understand more complex sensory stimuli. It can distinguish right from left and handedness is determined along with eye and foot dominance.

The skills a child needs to engage in sports improve greatly between the ages of 7 and 10 years. Balance, equilibrium, large muscle control, and timing are all essential to this period.

Sexual development can also begin during the latency period. Girls are the first to show signs of puberty. By age 12, a girl's growth spurt has peaked. She will have more rounded hips, an accentuated waist, and early pubic hairs. Ten or 11-year-old boys have a slight growth of the penis and testes, followed by a growth spurt in height about a year later.

The development of moral reasoning continues. Piaget's (1977) stage of concrete operations occurs when children begin to consider more than one spatial dimension simultaneously. They also develop the ability to reverse operations mentally, a basic skill needed to allow them to add and subtract. The understanding that changes in the shape or size of a substance do not change its properties also develops during this period.

During the middle childhood period, morality becomes less objective and more subjective as children become able to evaluate motivation as a factor in judging right and wrong. A greater understanding of the feelings of others, and of how the child's own actions affect others, is also established.

Adaptation to school is a critical task. In general, girls are better students than boys (Dulcan, 1994). At 8 years of age children read for pleasure, but their ideas exceed their ability to communicate in writing. Nine-year-olds can plan and finish a task. They may enjoy school very much, but have a real fear of failure.

Ten year olds can memorize easily, but cannot fully understand abstraction; can count indefinitely forward by ones, twos, fives, and tens, and backwards by ones; can add and subtract easily; and can identify similarities and differences in objects.

By age 11, children can multiply and divide. Although they can interpret proverbs, they generally do not understand sarcasm and irony. A more realistic understanding of death occurs at this age, but many children still do not fully understand the irreversibility of death, and believe that it is punishment for bad behavior.

Children eventually comprehend how they learn, and use this knowledge to improve their academic performance. Six- to 8-year-olds begin to think privately in attempting to solve problems, and by 11 have developed this private speech to improve their level of learning. Children who have problems with learning, with conduct, or with attentiveness will generally have trouble developing learning skills unless they have the appropriate intervention and tutoring.

During latency, children become better able to control their drives and inhibit certain behaviors to postpone gratification. The 8- to 10-year-old child can differentiate between right and wrong, along with being truthful and honest. The child's internalized values are stronger determinants of behavior than is the seeking of reward or avoidance of punishment (Dulcan, 1994).

Common occurrences for boys in middle childhood are sexual exploration, including comparing of genitals. Pre-pubertal boys have a renewed interest in scatological humor, often using sexual or excretory terms as expletives. Sex education continues, although children may be afraid to ask questions through fear of appearing ignorant about the subject. As puberty nears, the child finds that school activities are no longer sufficient to gratify its needs for excitement, and turns to sports and teen-age activities. Children of this age can worry about their competence and appearance.

Peer relationships develop during this period. An 8-year-old has a good grasp of rules, and can cooperate when playing games. The 9- and 10-year-old is more cooperative, but also learns to become more competitive. This can lead to more frequent disagreements when playing games. Eleven- and 12-year-old children can spend the entire day setting up a game: making rules, choosing teams and leaders, and negotiating how the game will be played. They may become so involved in the organizational process that they do not get to play the game. This behavior promotes social interaction and strengthens the barrier against regression. Children are viewed as popular when they follow the rules and cooperate, although athletically or academically achieving children can be even more popular at this age. Children who are bossy, hyperactive, or uncontrolled are likely to be rejected, even after treatment corrects this behavioral problem.

Children in the latency age period tend to gravitate toward single-sex groupings for play, sports, and other events. This becomes a time of extreme peer pressure to exhibit culturally appropriate gender-related behavior, especially for boys. By this age, children already have a firm sense of stereotypically male or female behavior. Girls tend to develop closer and more intense friendships with one or more peers. They sometimes even develop a normal admiration on a slightly older female who represents an ego-ideal.

Children ages 6 to 12 years of age are far more exposed to and led by their external environment than they were at an earlier age. A subculture that does not involve adult influence develops among children of this age, and they create rhymes, jokes, chants, superstitions, and secret codes of their own. Hero worship is common, often involving movie or television stars and sports or music figures.

Becoming part of a group or club, whether formal or informal, is important, albeit these groups often evolve to exclude certain children. Children also seek peer acceptance, adopting certain characteristics such as loyalty, the ability to compromise, being good sports, and not "tattling" on others. This social competence teaches the child how to adapt to social situations and take on more mature qualities, such as a more indirect, process-oriented approach to social goals.

Unfortunately, not all group behavior is positive. Substantial peer pressure can lead to dangerous and immoral behavior, especially for boys. Teasing is common, and may continue to be cruel and unrelenting. Girls can become obsessed with physical appearance and express unrealistic expectations about obesity and diet. This may lead to the development of bulimia or anorexia nervosa.

ADOLESCENCE

Developmental tasks during adolescence include renegotiating family roles; identity issues such as sexuality, future orientation, peer acceptance, and ethnicity; and moral reasoning.

By adolescence, neurologic development is mature. Dendritic connections have attained their adult level, and 14-year-olds show mature alpha rhythms on electroencephalograms. The adolescent reaches puberty, with the attainment of reproductive capacity. An early onset of sexual activity (at 10 to 15 years of age) has been linked to lower contraceptive use. Sexual activity of early onset is likely to lead to more frequent sexual activity and a greater number of sexual partners (Centers for Disease Control, 1992). Very little is known about the circumstances of early adolescent sexual activity (Paikoff, 1995).

Through the effect of pubertal changes in anatomy and physiology, the adolescent focuses more attention on his or her body. Hormonal changes and social and cultural factors tend to increase interest in sexuality and sexual experimentation. Teenagers may engage in sexual activity before they are emotionally mature.

Piaget's (1977) stage of **formal operations** is attained during puberty, and young persons in this stage can use abstract thought in order to consider theories and devise and test hypotheses. In late adolescence, the teenager understands metaphor and complex, abstract subjects such as algebra and calculus. Some teenagers reach this stage as early as 12 years of age, while only 35% achieve it by 16 or 17 years of age. Many adults never attain this level of abstract thinking, preventing them from fully dealing in a flexible and rational manner with abstract concepts such as religion, morality, philosophy, politics, and ethics. Occasionally, because of peer pressure, teenagers regress temporarily to the level of concrete operations.

The renegotiation of family roles is a critical developmental task in puberty. Adolescents experience many stressors and pressures. This creates adolescent turmoil, a ubiquitous but necessary experience in order to form an adult identity and separate from one's parents. Adolescent turmoil, described as psychological upheaval leading to disruption in personality organization, with disequilibrium and disturbances in mood behavior, can be brought on as the teenager moves to high school, where less supervision, greater academic requirements, and a larger, more diverse peer group are the norm.

Adolescents become more independent as they prepare mentally for leaving home. Many exhibit an increase in the frequency with which they argue with their parents and deliberately behave provocatively. Most American adolescents are not necessarily financially or emotionally prepared to leave home, even though they may be biologically prepared to do so.

Adolescents are acutely interested in their peers, and often form intense friendships with a youth of the same sex. Early adolescents seek to conform with their peer group, and are very self-conscious about their behavior and appearance.

In early adolescence, many normal teenagers undergo a transient disturbance of self-esteem, experience depression, and are oversensitive to humiliation. Boys have more behavioral and emotional disorders than girls prior to adolescence, although with adolescence such disorders become more frequent in girls in the form of eating disorders and depression.

Some adolescents show a temporary increase in less mature defense mechanisms, such as projection, denial, reaction formation, repression, and externalization, as well as the onset of more advanced defense mechanisms such as rationalization, identification, and sublimation. Most adolescents have a greater capacity than earlier age groups to use mature defenses, tolerate frustration, and delay gratification (Dulcan, 1994).

Unfortunately, the common adolescent belief in personal omnipotence may lead to dangerous, risk-taking behavior. The three leading causes of death among teenagers are accidents, homicide, and suicide. To most teenagers, death is not accepted as a possibility, although it is cognitively understood.

Adolescents frequently fluctuate between unrealistic positive and negative views of themselves. They are more inclined to attribute responsibility for their failures to others, while taking appropriate credit for their successes. Late adolescence brings an acceptance of some hardship in life and reduced thoughts of omnipotence.

Personal decision-making is tested through experimentation with tobacco, alcohol, and drugs. Also, sexual activity usually begins during this time, with masturbation as a way to reduce anxiety and discharge tension. Adolescent sexual activity is becoming more the norm than the exception. Risk factors for early sexual activity include weak religious affiliation, early/frequent dating, lack of educational ambition, and lack of parental support. Teenagers with these characteristics run a greater risk of pregnancy, acquired immune deficiency syndrome (AIDS) and other sexually transmitted diseases.

The awareness of having a gay or lesbian identity is particularly disturbing to the adolescent. Teenagers are generally more homophobic than adults, and often, tease, reject, or become physically aggressive to peers who they believe are gay. Those parents of such teenagers who are unwilling to discuss their children's concerns about gender identity can alienate their children and increase the latters' thoughts about or attempts at suicide.

■ ADULT AND LATER-LIFE DEVELOPMENT

TRANSITION TO ADULTHOOD

Adult development has been difficult to analyze and report owing to the absence of biologic demarcations, the tendency for major tasks to overlap, and the limited research available about the adult development process (Table 7–2). Many researchers have believed that much of the relevant human development of individuals occurs prior to their becoming adults. Indeed, Sigmund Freud felt that much of personality was fixed by the age of 6.

The transition to adulthood is a transition to an occupation, which often includes trying out different styles, roles, and techniques of living. Experimentation also occurs with intimate relationships. In this period, the young adult learns about relationships, and thoughts about an ideal mate must be tested against reality.

Problems in early adulthood are often associated with a delay in initiating adult tasks, with the most frequent cause of this being an inability to fully separate from the parents. Two difficult pre-adult problems are pseudo-adulthood and precociousness. The pseudo-adult tends to remain, in some way, attached to the parents and create an adult "false self." The true internal identity of such an individual is in fact still that of a child who has never grown up. The precocious adult has somewhat of the opposite problem. He or she detaches himself from his parents at an early age and may have resorted to self-parenting, possibly due to earlier deprivation of parental care. These individuals are usually seen as highly competent, but at the same time as stilted and lifeless. Many become workaholics and repeat the deprivation pattern with their own children.

THE CONSOLIDATION OF ADULTHOOD

At about the age of 30, the young adult begins a stage of consolidating personal and occupational identity. This stage comes with some amount of inner struggle over the new "fixity" of adulthood, its associated commitments, and the loss of other options. Table 7–2 outlines the stages of adulthood including transitional issues, rites of passage, symptoms of crisis, and pathologic outcome.

The term *consolidation* is sometimes synonymous with occupational/professional identity to the exclusion of personal identity. This involves seeing work as the vehicle for obtaining not only income, but also status, self-esteem, and a social life. This type of personality often becomes a workaholic, who can later experience a traumatic mid-life crisis, be faced with the alienation from friends and family, and have difficulty in facing retirement.

One rite of passage into adulthood involves a grad-uation or certification ritual. The old student identity is canceled as a new title and identity are conferred on the young adult. Generally, this public ritual completes a process that has already been accomplished in private by the young adult.

MARRIAGE

Courtship, the precursor to marriage, is the transition to a committed partnership. Dating is a rite of passage into the courtship phase of life. The joining of two individuals into a couple indicates that this phase has been achieved. Today, more people are living together and experiencing "trial marriage." Although this arrangement serves as something of a laboratory for experiencing what marriage may be like, it does not necessarily model a true marital relationship. The couple may inevitably postpone consideration of the more contractual aspects of marriage.

Psychological marriage does not always coincide with the marriage ceremony. This post-courtship transition ideally occurs between two personally mature individuals who see each other as whole, individual persons. Ideally, each has his or her own identity and appreciates the other's characteristics.

When couples marry before they have consolidated their own adult identities, they may continue to exhibit infantile or adolescent dependence on each other. This can further prevent the relationship from developing to a more mature level. This type of marital problem is also evident when one partner's professional development or education is ahead of the other's. Often a marital crisis occurs at a particular stage in the life-cycle such as childbirth, mid-life or after children leave their parents (the "empty nest"). Healthy mar-

TABLE 7–2. ADULT LIFECYCLE: TASKS AND STAGES

Stage	Transitional Issues	Rite of Passage	Symptoms of Crisis	Pathologic Outcome
Pre-adulthood	Novice, student	Matriculation	School/work phobia	Agoraphobia
Consolidation of adulthood	New title	Graduation	Repeated career changes	Pseudo-adult
Courtship	Experimentation	Dating, "trial marriage"	Premature or delayed commitment	Schizoid character, precocious adult
Marriage transition	Contract with spouse	Marriage ceremony	Boredom or constant warfare	Separation or divorce
Pregnancy	Physical change	Baby shower, childbirth education	Hypochondriasis, detachment	Denial
Childbirth	Pregnancy	Labor and delivery	Excessive anxiety: prepartum and during labor	Postpartum depression
Parenting	Primary maternal preoccupation	Naming ceremony	Marital unrest, developmental delay in child	Parental deprivation or overstimulation of child
Midlife transition	Mourning, loss of youth	Midlife crisis	Withdrawal, sudden life change	Depression, substance abuse
Transition to old age	Repository of cultural values	Retirement, illness, death of spouse/friends	Regression	Depression, pseudodementia

riages usually experience a sequence of growth, plateauing, stagnation, reassessment, and new growth. The time-frame for these sequences can vary from weeks to months or years.

The 9 months of pregnancy offer expectant parents a period of transition prior to childbirth and parenting. The soon-to-be parents have the opportunity to make room for a new person in their lives and adjust their relationship accordingly. The resultant changes in a woman's body direct her attention inward to the child growing within her. She often becomes preoccupied with herself (maternal preoccupation), and rapidly forms a strong attachment to her infant.

Pregnancy creates demands on both marital partners' senses of adult identity. Those who do not have a solid sense of themselves may be at greater risk of experiencing postpartum depression or other psychiatric disorders.

The pain of impending childbirth causes anxiety for the expectant mother and her spouse. Childbirth classes, which facilitate this rite of passage into parenthood, help to diffuse this anxiety by teaching parents about pain management and working together as a cohesive unit.

Although expectant parents have 9 months in which to prepare for the birth of a child, childbirth is viewed as a normative crisis in life. The transition to parenthood arrives so rapidly that it causes many couples to experience an emotional shock. Often, weeks or even months are required for the reality of parenthood to be realized.

Parenting skills are greatly influenced by two factors: the strength of the parental partnership and the experience each parent has had with his/her own parents. Usually, new parents modify and re-allocate roles and tasks to fit with their new responsibilities. This new orientation may worsen previous problems and negatively affect intimacy between the partners in a parental couple. Parenting can be used to mask these problems, and the couple must work hard at continuing their personal communicating and preserving their private relationship.

When an infant is born, the parents create a "holding environment." This environment literally includes the holding of the infant, as well as a stable psychological and physical home life. As the mother's empathy for her infant grows, the father "holds" or emotionally embraces and protects the mother and child so that they can devote themselves to each other.

Even if both parents of an infant have achieved emotional adulthood, which is not always the case, they will both be prone to certain parental stresses. In the case of the newborn, the parents may find that its extreme dependency brings on a variety of emotional re-actions ranging from stoic non-dependency to resentment. As the child grows older, the holding environment must remain strong yet flexible enough to endure later developments such as sibling rivalry and adolescent rebellion. The parents must continue to function as a team and not let their children drive them apart.

Parenthood affords the opportunity for growth and development. It brings awareness of the importance of being reliable and consistent, along with the opportunity to re-experience or re-work some of the parent's own childhood experiences. At this time, a connection to the childhood stage of the life cycle is made even though the parent is moving further away from this stage.

CHILDLESSNESS

A major crisis occurs in the lives of many women in their mid- to late thirties if they do not have children. This crisis often affects their future decisions about work and marriage. Feelings of guilt or questioning of their female identity are common occurrences. Some seek a male partner primarily on the basis of his willingness to have children with them. Others consider becoming a single parent through adoption, artificial insemination, or other means.

A couple that decides not to have children can still have a deeply satisfying marriage as long as their decision is truly a mutual agreement. Problems do arise for couples when only one wants to have a child or the couple is infertile. This situation produces a greater likelihood of divorce unless the partners reach a compromise about how to resolve their problem. The incidence of infertility has risen dramatically in the United States, and women who have put other issues ahead of attempts at conception may experience age-associated physiologic infertility.

SINGLE PARENTING

For a single parent, raising a child poses many challenges. Women more often than men are single parents, and they may find themselves in this situation by their own choice or from a divorce or unplanned pregnancy. However they came into this role, they generally experience the additional stresses of trying to meet their own needs without negatively affecting the needs of their child.

Some single parents have difficulty in coping with these challenges, and resent their child or attempt to delay the child's independent development. Both situations create an unhealthy environment for both the parent and the child, and can be prevented through support networks and other child-care arrangements.

MID-LIFE TRANSITION

Before the mid-point of their lives, most adults enjoy steady progress toward their professional and personal goals and have little time for introspection. This changes between the ages of 35 and 55 as they realize that they have reached the mid-point of life. Life's end is now visible and life may be seen as having boundaries and limits. This readjustment of the adult self is usually brought about by a crisis or trauma such as a medical illness, physical aging, career plateauing, or the death of a peer.

During this mid-life transition, adults often reassess their lives and review what they have and have not done in light of their mortality. This internal adjustment generally affects relationships with others while the new self is integrated into the adult's life.

This particular developmental stage is currently receiving major attention, with a special focus on studying the mid-life transition on a gender basis. Men and women are being studied independently in order to prevent generalizations about one group being transferred to the other. A classic mid-life study of men was completed by psychologist Daniel Levinson and his colleagues in 1978 (Levinson et al., 1978). Levinson and his associates studied men between the ages of 35 and 45. Their findings propose a universal human life cycle consisting of specific eras and periods in a set sequence from birth to old age, constituting a psychosocial theory of adult development.

An era is the basic unit of the life cycle, and lasts roughly 20 years. The eras are: preadulthood, 0 to 20 years; early adulthood, 20 to 40 years; middle adulthood, 40 to 60 years; late adulthood, 60 to 80 years; and late, late adulthood, 80 years to death. Each era has its own distinct character. The character and structured life changes from one era to the next, and the change is profound. The transitional period for this change takes about 4 to 5 years. The mid-life transition links early and middle adulthood, and normally lasts from about age 40 to 45.

The developmental tasks in the mid-life transition are to question one's current life structure, terminate early adulthood, and create a basis for entering middle adulthood. The individual confronts various polarities such as young–old; masculine–feminine; destructiveness–creativity; and attachment–separateness. In this period, the individual may begin a process of individuation and genuine flowering of the personality, or a process of spiritual and psychological decay.

Research on the mid-life crisis in women was pioneered by Beatrice Neugarten (1968) in a study of men and women that stressed the importance of certain characteristics of middle age for this group. The theme of reassessment of the self is most salient, and the concept of time is established in relation to the time since birth. One important finding was that men and women use different criteria on which to base their sense of middle age. Married women in this study identified their middle-age status in terms of launching their children into the adult world.

Women psychologists and social scientists are studying the effects of work and motherhood on the life cycle of the family. Additional research is examining the importance of biologic functioning for women, and such issues as menopause, which has long been stereotyped as dominating the mid-life phase of the life cycle for women.

Psychiatrist Malkah T. Notman (1978) argues that it is important to distinguish a woman's concerns about individual fulfillment and self-realization because the traditional stereotype is that a woman's role is focused on motherhood rather than on a broader view of womanhood. In reality, Notman continues, many women have not found their children or their role as mothers to be predominately gratifying, but have rather found the child-rearing process to be stressful, draining, and conflict-producing. Thus, the traditional stereotype imposes stress if a woman finds conflict in her role as a mother, rather than experiencing her larger role as a woman.

Some women view the mid-life period as a time for self-expression. The potential for autonomy; for changes in relationships; and for the development of their occupational skills, contacts, and self-image provide the opportunity to begin anew after childbearing and -rearing are completed. The life issues of separation and autonomy, however, need to be kept analytically distinct from the feeling states of aloneness and isolation.

The entry into adulthood confronts the individual with many choices, such as selecting one job over another or one relationship over another, which lead to a specific life path. Committing oneself to a particular choice often means changing the direction of one's entire life, and in some cases altering one's destiny and sense of identity. However, with the wide range of choices in adult life, those made in mid-life or later do not necessarily involve dramatic changes in behavior. Thus, individuals making radical changes in life-style after mid-life are rare. Often the changes are symbolic and reflect a decision to become more health conscious by stopping smoking or exercising, or more family oriented by visiting one's family more often or spending more time with one's spouse.

In later life, some individuals feel that they have been deprived of having the idealized life of which they had always dreamed. This often provides them with a catalyst for real change and allows them to have a "second chance at life." Unfortunately some believe that they cannot control their lives and will continually be subject to failure. These persons may minimize the influence of their choices in molding their lives.

BEREAVEMENT

Loss plays a necessary role in every life transition. The forward progression of life inevitably leads to the release of important elements of the earlier phases of life. In experiencing this growth, the individual needs to work through his or her reactions to loss, whether real or imagined. During a period of loss, the adult must commit psychological resources to the task of reviewing and reliving the lost relationship, whether with a spouse, a child, a relative, or even a body part. This painful, protracted, and time-consuming task allows the gradual, natural resolution of grief.

When first told about a sudden loss, most people respond with some form of denial. Some react emotionally and others do not. For the latter, the absence of outward emotion is generally due to shock or psychic numbing. This can result in postponement or failure to ever reach the grief experience.

Coming to terms with ambivalence about a deceased person is an important part of resolving grief. Bereavement tends to exaggerate mixed feelings of frustration and caring. As a result, this ambivalence can lead to problems with feelings of guilt. Some bereaved individuals believe that ambivalence of feeling is not permitted. Instead, they turn their ambivalence into an over-idealized image of the lost person while creating scapegoats to blame for the loss. With time, most persons realistically see the good and bad in the lost person and develop a lasting, meaningful memory of that person in their minds.

The ability to finally detach from a deceased person is facilitated by a series of reality tests. This includes the awareness that, whenever the bereaved individual's thoughts turn to the deceased, they are accompanied by the realization that the other is no longer alive. This gradual detachment enables the bereaved to "bury the dead" and go on living life.

The rites of passage in the grieving process involve funerals, vigils, eulogies, fasts, wakes, and burial rites. Such rituals provide the bereaved with much-needed support during this difficult time. Often, it is easier to relinquish attachments to the dead in unison with others who also have attachments to their own deceased persons.

TRANSITION TO LATER LIFE

A major task in old age is to enhance and maintain a sense of inner emotional integrity in the face of increasing risks to health and well-being. Throughout life, the sense of identity is supported by a variety of external factors, including family and social network, work-place authority, healthy body, and productivity. The loss of these with aging causes stress and requires a calling upon inner resources to deal with the resulting identity confusion and depersonalization.

Fortunately, not all of this loss occurs at the same time; usually, each threat to emotional integrity can be met separately. At retirement, the older person experiences a loss of authority and power, and subsequently needs to find new sources of productivity and creativity. With the reduction in work-place demands, the older person can explore new interests and deepen old ones.

Older age generally requires the construction of a new social network to replace what has changed through retirement and the growth of one's family.

Many older individuals re-engage in society in a new way. The wisdom they have gained from years of experience can be passed to grandchildren, employees, and other younger members of society. One important social role in aging is to convey the traditions of the past to those who will carry them into the future.

Unfortunately, not everyone can do these things; some individuals become caught up in the belief that the end of work signifies the end of growth and development. The most common threat to the older person's integrity is isolation. Like infants, the elderly are more prone to having a negative reaction to stimulus deprivation. A positive sense of personal identity can generally be maintained by surrounding the older person with familiar people and objects.

The elderly tend to see some type of illness as a rite of passage into old age. This kind of normative crisis often forces the older person to overcome passivity and helplessness, and to fight what Erik Erikson called the battle between "integrity and despair."

DEATH AND DYING

At the end of the life-cycle, individuals may experience a greater intensity of awareness of the present moment, and a greater depth of self-awareness. The elderly often express an increased involvement with religious concerns and important social issues.

The awareness of one's own impending death is an emotionally traumatic event, whose impact often exceeds even that of bereavement. This is due largely to three factors:

- Death threatens our need to control our destiny. Many persons continue to harbor the fantasy of immortality even into old age, and can't grasp the idea of non-existence;

- The awareness of death reignites personal infantile fears and fantasies about itself.
- The past century has produced a substantial denial of death in Western culture. This denial places death outside the realm of the normal life-cycle, and attempts to exclude it from everyday awareness.

The classic work of Elizabeth Kubler-Ross (1969) has led to awareness of the encounter with death as a developmental process not unlike other life transitions. Kubler-Ross describes the working-through of death-related tasks—denial and isolation, anger, bargaining, depression, and acceptance—as roughly analogous to the stages of bereavement. As one develops, their relationship with death takes on a new meaning. It may be viewed as a new journey, culminating one's life, a profound rest, and/or a life transition.

AN OVERVIEW

- In infancy and childhood, the care-giver–child relationship is best considered within a developmental framework, which takes into account the primary developmental task of the child and the related tasks of the care-giver.
- An infant's two primary developmental tasks are to form a secure attachment with an adult care-giver, learning in the process to trust others, and to regulate bodily states and emotions.
- A caregiver who predominantly rejects a child's bids for attention (for comfort, play, or assistance) negatively shapes a child's sense of self, worthiness, competence, efficacy, and trust in others.
- Childhood dependence on the parents must be shed for a more mature, independent relationship.
- Young adults are generally in a learning phase as students or apprentices, with the freedom to explore opportunities without full responsibility.
- The student–mentor relationship helps to bring about adult mutuality and modifies idealistic beliefs.
- The modification that occurs in a student–mentor relationship bridges the gap between childhood fantasies and adult aspirations.
- The developmental tasks of adulthood are identified by transitional issues, rite of passage, symptoms of crisis, and outcome.

TD TERMS TO DEFINE

- anaclitic depression
- anxious avoidant attachment
- anxious resistant attachment
- attachment
- consolidation
- developmental framework
- formal operations stage
- insecure attachment
- latency
- life-cycle stage
- mid-life transition
- normative crisis
- regression
- secure attachment
- social referencing
- transition
- 3-month colic

Q STUDY QUESTIONS

1. When diagnosing and treating mental illness in adults, why is it important to understand childhood and adolescent development?

2. Which statement is an INACCURATE description of infant development?
   a. A weight increase of approximately 300% occurs within the first year.
   b. Infants are at least as sensitive to pain as adults.
   c. After a week of life, the newborn can distinguish the smell of its mother's breast milk and distinguish its mother's voice from others.
   d. The 4-week-old newborn has visual acuity as good as that of an adult.

3. Why is attachment to a mother or mother figure so important in the first year of life?

4. Why are toddlers prone to accidents and injury? Give a physical and cognitive explanation.

5. Describe the play patterns of a toddler, young child, and middle child.

6. The text describes the adolescent period as longer than it was a century ago. Why is that? What impact does this have on today's teenager?

7. The process of repetition during a life-cycle stage is
   a. the revival of earlier, more child-like behavior.
   b. usually in response to stress.
   c. often beneficial to the individual, as it permits the attainment of mastery of earlier, highly conflicting issues.
   d. similar to a rite of passage, a vehicle for bringing someone to the next life-cycle stage.

8. Describe the adulthood consolidation stage of the life cycle and what its consequences may be for married couples who have not reached this stage.

9. Discuss the changes in the mid-life period for women today versus women several decades ago.

10. In what order are the common phases of bereavement, as described by Dr. Elizabeth Kubler-Ross, experienced?
    a. Denial, bargaining, anger, depression, and acceptance
    b. Denial, anger, bargaining, depression, and acceptance
    c. Regression, transition, depression and consolidation
    d. None of the above

■ REFERENCES

Apgar V: Proposal for a new method of evaluating the newborn infant, *Anesth Analg* 1953; 32:260–267.

Bowlby J: *Attachment, in Attachment and Loss.* New York, Basic Books, 1969, vol 2.

Centers for Disease Control: Sexual Behavior among High School Students. *JAMA* 1992; 267:628.

Dulcan MK: Childhood and adolescent development, in Stoudemire A, Kluman B (eds): *An Introduction to Medical Students*, ed 2 Philadelphia, JB Lippincott, 1994.

Erikson EH: *Childhood and Society.* New York, WW Norton, 1963.

Fagot BI: Beyond the reinforcement principle: Another step toward understanding sex role development. *Dev Psychol* 1985; 21:1097–1104.

Freud A: The concept of developmental lines. *Psychoanal Study Child* 1963; 8:245–265.

Freud S: Mourning and melancholia. 1917, in Strachey J (ed): *The Standard Edition of the Complete Psychological Works*, London, Hogarth Press, 1958, vol 14.

Gilligan C: *In a Different Voice: Psychological Theory and Women's Development.* Cambridge, MA, Harvard University Press, 1982.

Jung CG: The stage of life, in Read H, Fordham M, Adler G (eds): *Collected Works.* Princeton, NJ, Princeton University Press, 1960, vol 8.

Koenig HG, Cohen HJ, Blazer DG, et al: Religious coping and depression among elderly, hospitalized medically ill men. *Am J Psychiatry* 1992; 149:1693–1700.

Kubler-Ross E: *On Death and Dying.* New York, Macmillan, 1969.

Levinson DJ, Darrow CM, Klein EB, et al: *The Seasons of a Man's Life.* New York, Alfred A Knopf, 1978.

Lewis M, Volkmar F: *Clinical Aspects of Child and Adolescent Development*, ed 3. Philadelphia, Lea & Febiger, 1990.

Mahler MS: The rapprochement subphase of the separation-individuation process. *Psychoanalysis* 1972; 41:487–506.

Miller JB: *Women's Psychological Development: Theory and Development.* Women's Mental Health Occasional Paper Series. Rockville, MD, National Institute of Mental Health, 1986.

Neugarten B: The awareness of middle age, in Neugarten B (ed): *Middle Age and Aging.* Chicago, University of Chicago Press, 1968.

Notman MT: Women and mid-life: A different perspective. *Psychiatric Opin* 1978; 15:12–18.

Paikoff RL: Early heterosexual debut: Sexual possibility situations in the transition to adolescence, *Am J Orthopsychiatry* 1995; 65:389–401.

Piaget J: *The Development of Thought.* New York, Viking Press, 1977.

Spitz RA: Anaclitic depression. *Psychoanal Study Child* 1946; 2:313–342.

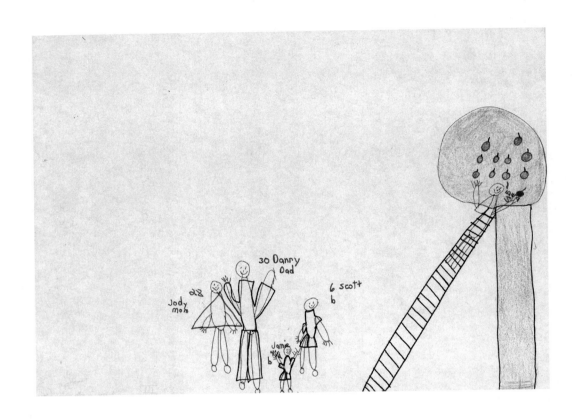

Broad-streeted Richmond . . .
The trees in the streets are old trees
used to living with people,
Family trees that remember your grandfather's name.

Stephen Vincent Benet, 1898–1943

John Brown's Body (1928) Bk. IV

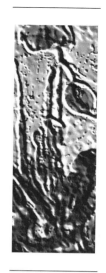

8

Systems Theory as a Model
for Understanding Families

Shirley A. Smoyak

Scientists who attempt to study the family are faced with a peculiar dilemma: Something that is very familiar to most of us somehow eludes the grasp of the scientific method. Because most of us have experienced childhood and adolescence in some kind of family setting, and because most of us, as adults, create families of our own, the temptation is very great to view our experiences as normal and to use them as a standard for understanding, and sometimes judging, others. This ethnocentric tendency leads to assumptions that the familiar must be the correct way, or the better way, and that other styles or patterns at best are strange and at worst wrong or deviant. The family is an elusive concept; its shape, character, and functions have been interpreted very differently by historians, sociologists, psychologists, and anthropologists. Economists cannot even agree on what to name and how to describe a family economic unit; instead, they focus on individuals and study the changes over time as individuals move in and out of family settings and relationships. (Smoyak, 1991)

Nurses must be knowledgeable about families, because no matter what the area of their practice or specialization, they will encounter families as contexts or supporters of the individual patients for whom they are caring, and at times will deliver care for entire families. At other times, nurses will experience families *as barriers to the care that they are trying to arrange and deliver for specific individuals. These barriers may not always be obvious, but may be discovered only when the best laid plans are disrupted or sidetracked.*

This chapter provides basic sociodemographic and historical material about families, and describes the systems approach to understanding family structures and psychodynamics. It describes how nurses work with family systems and explains paradigms for assessing families. The genogram, an assessment tool, is outlined, and examples of its use are presented.

■ BACKGROUND FOR STUDY OF THE FAMILY

Privacy about matters of family life has produced what sociologists call pluralistic ignorance. Each of us knows what goes on in our bedrooms and bathrooms, and how we handle a misbehaving 2-year-old at bedtime, or an adolescent who comes home drunk or bleary-eyed from drugs, but we do not know how the neighbors do it. Systematic, rigorous research on the intimacies of family life is still in its infancy, although the interest of scholars in the study of marriage and the family can be traced back several centuries. Until recently, most family research was conducted by academicians who saw the family as one specialization among several that they pursued. Thus, the research literature on the family developed slowly (Spanier, 1981). In the past quarter of a century, scientists who have a primary interest in the family have emerged in large numbers and the literature has expanded dramatically. Today in the United States there are more than two-dozen professional family journals, some dealing only with theory and research, some with family issues and policy matters, and many focused on clinical and therapeutic concerns. Family agendas are addressed at conferences convened by prominent professional associations in the major social-science disciplines, and the field is not lacking in newsletters, monographs, audio and videotapes, and books.

"The trouble with the origin of the family is that no one knows". Gough (1986) follows her compelling opening statement with evidence that it is not known when the family originated (probably between two million and 100,000 years ago, nor whether some kind of embryonic family came before, with or after the origin of language. Some kind of family exists in all known human societies, although varying a great deal in terms of structures and functions.

"Family" implies that several universals are operating.

- Sexual relations between close relatives are forbidden (note: husbands and wives are not relatives; they are strangers who marry).
- Men and women cooperate through a division of labor based on gender.
- Marriage is a durable, though not necessarily life-long arrangement.

Another universal—that men generally have higher status than and authority over the women in their families—has generated much controversy between feminist scholars and other historians. Although feminist writers have persuasively demonstrated the long-standing, erroneous bias of earlier male scholars (Gilligan, 1982), they disagree among themselves about the exact nature of past relationships among men and women in families.

The exact nature of family structure and gender relationships is shrouded in layers of conjecture and scientific guesswork. Since the beginning of recorded history, no fixed pattern across cultures has been found (Hareven, 1986). Culture, not biology, determines the rules of organization within families. Different cultures had different rules regarding dominance of family lines and descent. In most primitive, nomadic cultures or communal societies, family descent was traced through the mothers, possibly because maternity could be verified, but paternity was many times a mystery. About 5,000 year ago, when agricultural development so drastically changed how people lived and organized themselves, patrilineal groups emerged. As the concept of private property developed, the transfer of such property from father to son influenced not only economic patterns, but social ones as well.

Historians of the family, notably Phillipe Aries (1962), have taught us that much of what we take as familiar and commonplace is a relatively recent invention. Childhood as a concept is very real to us, yet Aries maintains that it did not exist as an idea before the Middle Ages. In medieval days, a child was accorded adult status as soon as it could live without the constant attention of its mother. Leonard Sagan (1989) states that no institution has been changed so remarkably by modernization as has the family. Until the late 18th century, families were primarily economic units. Marriages were arranged to preserve property, and children were a cheap source of labor.

Historically, all the work needed for the safety and survival of individuals was done within the family. Within the boundaries of the family, functions performed were educating the young, ensuring safety from invaders, praying to God or a superior being, providing nurturance, clothing and shelter and caring for the sick, infirm, young or disabled. Every family textbook includes a discussion of the "erosion of family functions", and it has become quite popular from time to time to predict the eventual demise of the family as we know it today, since all of the reasons for its existence have been reassigned to institutions outside of the family, such as schools, hospitals, welfare boards, churches and the like. There actually have been several experiments in alternative forms of living in human groups, but none has survived. The fact is that while there is no general societal law that people must live in families, most do.

An historical perspective is immensely useful when one is attempting to understand social contexts and institutions. Present day patterns, when the observer can view their past roots, take on richer meaning and make more sense. More importantly, such understanding eliminates or dampens the tendency toward emotionality over issues of intimacy, closeness and human relationships.

Perceptions of American family life are full of myths, such as the belief that a three-generational household was the norm at the beginning of this century. Such beliefs create a "false nostalgia," a longing for what never was the case. Norman Rockwell enjoyed the positive regard and high esteem of millions of Americans for his paintings of families and household/farm scenes. In so masterfully popularizing this notion that families lived together in three-generational households, he actually did a disservice to the American public. Folks looking at the lovely families on the covers of the Saturday Evening Post often negatively compared

their own families, who fell short of that standard. Such negative comparisons, founded on inaccurate data, lead to unnecessary agonizing about one's own shortcomings. Such nostalgic beliefs also led to conclusions about generalized family breakdown, which is not the case at all.

At the turn of the century in America, the expected life-span was only 49 years; most grandparents could not possibly have lived with their grandchildren.

Today, the life expectancy for Americans is 75 years. In 1920, the chance of a 10-year-old having two living grandparents was 40%; today it is 75%. Children today may not only have living grandparents, but great-grandparents and great-great-grandparents as well. This increased longevity, with families having four and five generations alive at one time, produces great dilemmas for family systems. There are no religious, philosophical, or pragmatic guides for families as they face multiple demands for care-taking and strains on scarce resources. Many middle-aged couples see the years ahead of them not as golden, but as burdened by financial and social-support obligations for several elders, as well as for their adult children.

Family life cycles can no longer be described as they were just a generation ago: courtship, marriage, childbearing and child rearing, emptying the nest, retirement, and the death of one or both spouses. Today, according to Ahluburg and DeVita (1992), "Family patterns are so fluid that the U.S. Census Bureau has difficulty measuring family trends. Most large-scale, nationally representative surveys cannot readily tell us what proportion of husband–wife families are step-families; how adopted or foster-care children are faring; distinguish roommates from cohabiting couples; or measure the extent of family support networks for elderly persons who live alone." Today families most likely have two or fewer children. Mothers are likely to be employed outside the home, even when children are under 6 years of age. Young people are marrying at older ages. Men and women alike continue to delay marriage, with the median age at first marriage rising in 1993 to 26.5 years for men and 24.5 years for women (*New York Times*, 1994). Many people are exercising the option of never marrying. While marriage is less permanent today (the number of divorced persons tripled to 16.7 million in 1993, from 4.3 million in 1970), it is still highly likely that it will be the future of better than 90% of Americans. (*New York Times,* 1994) A very drastic recent trend is that more births are occurring outside of marriage, and that more children are being raised in single-parent homes.

The high divorce rates in the United States have been viewed by some as symptomatic of an erosion of the American family and its associated value systems. An alternative view, however, is to interpret these statistics as indicating that Americans today place a higher value on forming successful marriages than did earlier generations. The new requirement that marital partners "love each other" carries with it the expectation that irreconcilable differences can be settled by divorce. The consequences of divorce for children is a separate issue (Smoyak, 1996).

To build an enduring marriage, family researcher Judith Wallerstein (1994) argues that couples must address and resolve seven psychological tasks during the early years of marriage and again at the milestones of adult life. These tasks are described as follows:

- Consolidating separation from parents and establishing new connections.
- Building the marital identity: togetherness vs. autonomy.
- Establishing a sexual life.
- Establishing marriage as a zone of safety and nurturance.
- Making psychological room for children.
- Building a relationship that is fun and interesting.
- Maintaining a vision.

■ FAMILY SYSTEMS THEORY

INTRAPSYCHIC AND INTERPERSONAL THEORIES

The first scientific theories to explain human behavior appeared in the literature at the turn of this century. Earlier textbooks for nurses working in psychiatric settings synopsized the work of Freud and his followers and actually provided very little practical help in the day-to-day management and care of acutely and chronically ill psychiatric patients. Freud's theories were rooted in very early developmental moments of infants and children, and were deterministic in their design. The operative ideas suggested that specific early trauma produced specific later, troubled outcomes. Further, the nature of the concepts was abstract and not directly observable, thus requiring interpretation, inference and judgment on the part of the observer. Freud's theories were read and quoted widely in the Western world, and were almost the only available source of understanding and theorizing about human behavior for the first half of this century.

Libido, superego, ego and id, while not visible directly, were presumed to be the foundation of clinical knowledge about human actions. Families were not seen as relevant, since these theories were about what was happening inside individual human systems, not outside of them. Mothers were considered important, but only in very early infant and child development, not later.

In the early 1900s, when psychoanalytic concepts were the only available rational explanations for human behavior, no one scrutinized the behavior of nurses or other professionals in terms of its impact on the course of the client's illness. The illness was presumed to have had its roots in the far past of the patient's life; psychoanalytic techniques and strategies merely made these early traumas available to recall and reconsideration. No one, for the first half of this century, thought that nurses or others could actually create or maintain an illness in a patient, or make matters worse, by what the care provider said and did. The only requirement of the nurse was to provide an environment in which natural healing might occur. No cures were known for any mental illness.

Families were kept apart from patients, who were housed in large state hospitals, usually very far from their homes. The thinking was that the patients needed to have some distance and respite from their relatives to abate whatever noxious forces had been operative in causing their illness. If family members were consulted, it was only to provide a history of the patient's illness. Families were implicated as causes of current problems, but usually in historical, not current, ways.

In non-psychiatric settings, families were also excluded from care. Even pediatric patients were separated from their families, and visiting hours were very strict. For children who had asthmatic attacks, a clinical approach popular in the fifties was to do a "parentectomy" by removing the child entirely from the family system. With asthmatic children, the thinking was that parents somehow caused and perpetuated the attacks.

The Second World War provided the impetus for some very practical changes in the way military men were treated when they succumbed to the stresses of war. Interpersonal strategies, such as group therapy, were used. Grinker and Spiegel, in *War Neuroses*, described their discovery that commanding officers were precipitants of psychiatric casualties, and that group processes could help ferret out the connection of immediate problems to past faulty learning in handling stressful situations. The search for causes of psychic distress or mental illness shifted from the very distant past to the immediate present.

The National Institute for Mental Health, a United States federal government agency, was created in 1946. Through this agency, scientists were funded to pursue the study of the causes of schizophrenia and other severe mental disorders. Gregory Bateson, Don Jackson, Paul Watzlawick, Jay Haley and Virginia Satir are recognized names in the arena of scientists who developed interpersonal theories to explain dysfunctional human behavior. The double-bind hypothesis emerged in the 1950s as a very popular idea and was used widely by clinicians for the next two decades. The work of Harry Stack Sullivan was also widely quoted and used as a framework to teach psychiatric professionals to work with the mentally ill.

Interpersonal theories focused on dyads; mothers were significant others in these theories about how interactions were formed and led to various outcomes. Mothers were implicated as causes of illness, just as they had been in Freud's theories, but the thinking in the era following the Second World War was that mothers operated in the here and now, not the past, to maintain an illness in a son or daughter. Frieda Fromm-Reichmann coined the term *schizophrenogenic mothers* for mothers who had sons and daughters with one of the diagnosed patterns of schizophrenia.

When interpersonal theories were the basis for treatment strategies for patients, professionals' behaviors were also examined. The new thinking was that the professionals engaged in therapeutic interactions with patients were significant others, and were as influential in labeling and defining behavior as the patients' earlier significant others, such as the patients' mother, father, relatives, and authority figures. The focus was not on the family as a system, but on dyads—the patient and one significant other—examined in sequences.

Psychiatric nurses used interpersonal theories in inpatient and community settings, and published reports of their work in journals and books. The most often quoted and most highly regarded work of this period was published in a book edited by Smoyak and Rouslin (1982); it was *A Collection of Classics in Psychiatric Nursing Literature.* Hildegard E. Peplau is recognized as a key figure in the development of the clinical practice of psychiatric nurses; her analysis of the historical developments in psychiatric nursing appear in the collection.

THE EMERGENCE OF SYSTEMS THINKING

The theories explaining human behavior before the emergence of systems thinking limited the view to intrapsychic or interpersonal dynamics. Systems thinking expanded this view considerably, by taking in more of the surrounding context of the problem identified in a patient. Rather than seeing an individual as sick or disturbed, the system itself was viewed as the patient. Traditional symptoms, formerly seen as "owned by" or existing within individual patients, underwent a transformation and began to be considered as "signals of system distress." The causes of psychiatric illness were not seen as linear, but rather as cyclical and interactive at many levels of systems.

The new language for clinicians working with this new viewpoint was developed by Ludwig von Bertalanffy, who was born in Austria in 1901. von Bertalanffy was a leading biologist, with wide-ranging scientific and cultural interests. In the first issue of the journal *General Systems,* published in 1956, von Bertalanffy states that "General systems theory is a new discipline whose subject matter is the formulation and derivation of those principles which are valid for systems in general."

He defines a system as sets of elements standing in interaction with one another. The **general systems theory** is a logical-mathematical concept that deals with scientific doctrines of wholeness, dynamic interaction, and organization.

The general systems theory was not formulated by von Bertalanffy all at once, but rather emerged from a long and interesting evolution of views. The concept of a general systems theory (referred to by von Bertalanffy as general system theory [1968]) was not published until 1945. von Bertalanffy's work was seen as providing a bridging framework that permitted specialists in diverse fields to communicate with one another. Some referred to his work as a language rather than a theory. Others called it a meta-theory, since it provided a way to think about theories.

In the 1950s, psychiatrists began to involve total family systems in their treatment plans. A spirit of openness and collegiality replaced the closed, private ambiance of the earlier psychoanalytic approach. Videotaping of family sessions became very popular, and conferences sometimes included watching and analyzing live family sessions. Probably the best known application of general systems theory to psychiatry has been the collected work of Gray, Duhl and Rizzo (1969), where contributors, including Menninger, Arieti, Miller and others described their particular uses and elaborations of the original work. In 1975, Smoyak provided *The Psychiatric Nurse as a Family Therapist* for clinicians using systems concepts in their work with families and the mentally ill.

PRINCIPLES OF SYSTEMS THEORY

Five concepts within systems theory are built around the topics listed below. They are discussed in the paragraphs that follow.

- The whole as greater than the sum of its parts.
- Rules of organization.
- Janus effect and hierarchical order.
- Depth and breadth of hierarchies.
- Adaptation.

The Whole Is Greater Than the Sum of Its Parts

Probably no systems principle has been repeated more often than the one about the whole and its parts, or is so poorly understood by lay people and professionals alike. What it means is that there is an entity, quality, or abstract essence in a system that cannot be understood as simply an additive, mechanistic property. The key to understanding this principle is to see the "greater than" as symbolizing "organization." Parts of anything, without organization, remain just parts. They become an identifiable system only when they are organized.

Rules of Organization

Systems theorists and clinicians working with troubled human systems have found it useful to describe the concept discussed above as a set of rules by which the parts of a system—consisting of family members or other players, or both—arrange themselves. Rules of organization are not directly visible, nor are they generally written down. They can, however, be relatively easily detected by asking or observing. A family's rules of organization are determined by their culture, which embodies ethnic, religious, and social factors. Tradition is a ritualized, remembered, and enacted set of rules of organization that serve to place people in their proper roles by age, gender, and generational rank in the family or community. Everyone in a particular social group or family system understands these rules, and also understands how violations of them will be perceived, tolerated, dismissed, or punished.

Each human social system takes its identity from these rules of organization. A system is recognized by what it "stands for"—an operative knowledge of its rules of organization and values. Family systems remain identifiable across time, surviving the entries and exits of individual members and subsystems by birth, death, marriage, moving to distant locations, and other changes. The family name carries this embodiment of the family's operative rules. Beyond family systems, work systems also carry their identities through time. For example, hospital departments remain constant in the eyes of others because they can be relied upon to respond to others in particular ways, living out the interactive codes set for them in the system's rules of organization. Throughout the world, any ethnicity is understood as a set of expectations that can be relied upon to produce particular responses. Adjectives such as strong-willed, determined, goal-oriented, and future-directed come immediately to mind for the Germans, for instance. Individual German families modify these identity markers through religious and regional differences. Practitioners in the field of family therapy pay considerable attention to how family systems develop and modify their rules of organization; ethnicity provides very useful benchmarks for this approach.

Janus Effect and Hierarchical Order

A system is a set of interacting parts, organized by rules. The boundaries, or parameters, of various systems vary in size and complexity. The system may be as small as a cell nucleus and its environment, or it may have thousands of parts, scattered geographically, as in a nation. *Holon* is the term used to capture the essence of the system under analysis; it means the interacting parts that make up the system, and their boundary. Janus refers to the Roman god who both looks to the past and contemplates the future, and whose name is captured in the month we call January.

The analyst, theoretician, or clinician determines what constitutes a particular holon; there are no formalized methods for defining such an entity. In a family, for example, a holon might be the marital pair or it might be the nuclear family unit. A holon might also be a five-generation family unit, depending on the goals and aims of the analyst.

A system, or holon, has subsystems or parts. The subsystems are arranged hierarchically, and are inferior (beneath, in complexity) to the system and to suprasystems (larger entities above the system level). For example, a nuclear family might be considered as the system, with marital dyads and siblings the subsystems. A nuclear family system would have its larger, extended family as the suprasystem.

The concept of the Janus effect reminds the systems theorist that any given holon has subsystem components and, on the other hand, is a part of a larger suprasystem. For example, Frederick may be considered a holon for the moment, and his subsystems might be his superego, ego, and id, or they might be his thoughts, feelings, and actions, or they might be his respiratory, excretory, circulatory, digestive, neurological, and reproductive subsystems. Frederick, as a holon, might become a subsystem of a suprasystem of a marriage, nuclear family or family of origin. Another way to think of this analysis would be to view Frederick's place of employment as the system for study. He would then be the subsystem worker in that unit. The decision to view one or another level of a system as the primary unit depends entirely on the purposes for which the analysis is being conducted.

Subsystems, systems, and suprasystems are arranged hierarchically. For family systems, it is tempting to think of a generation as being a hierarchy, but this is not necessarily so. An entire two- or three-generational system may be a holon, or a particular sibling system may be a holon. The notion of hierarchies becomes clearer when exchanges are discussed later in this chapter.

Depth and Breadth of Hierarchies

The arrangements of systems, in terms of the breadth and depth of the hierarchies that form them or of which they are a part, yield a clue to their complexity. For example, a system that is the governance structure of a city or nation may have only one unit at a particular level and hundreds at another. Most hospital-governance systems are seven layers deep, with most work units arranged laterally and having fewer than 20 subsystems each. Classrooms typically have one teacher, at a superior level, and perhaps a hundred or more students at a lower level, for a large lecture class. A nuclear family may have two parents and only one child, or a dozen or more children.

The concept of breadth and depth of hierarchies is generally used more in organizational, agency, and institutional analyses than in family therapy or other kinds of psychodynamic treatments. However, these ideas may be salient in an analysis that includes families interacting with school systems, or governments, or legal systems.

Adaptation

In common usage, *adaptation* means that an object, or an act, or a process is measured or brought to bear against an external standard of some sort. For example, a two-pronged electrical plug may need an adaptor to fit a wall receptacle that has three prongs, one prong being a ground connector. Alternatively, an entire electrical box may be needed to convert or adapt appliances to different forms of electricity in different countries. Or a nursing action may be evaluated or measured against an accepted standard for nursing practice set by the profession. Procedure manuals in hospitals are standards against which care is measured, and when the judgment is that the care does not "measure up," then the care must be adapted to fit the measure. This commonly used sense of adaptation presumes that the standard or measure is correct or right.

When used in systems thinking, however, the meaning of adaptation is very different from that given above. The context is that of two units or subsystems interacting with each other by exchanging matter, energy, or information. Subsystem A and Subsystem B, in order to be adapted to each other at the outcome of their exchanges, need to make the exchanges in a specific way. This paradigm for subsystem exchanges was developed by Harry C. Bredemeier at Rutgers University in the course of his theory-building in the area of social interaction, beginning in the 1960s. It has been adapted as part of the strategies used by family therapists working with systems that they meet in very varied settings.

Let us consider, for example, subsystem A and subsystem B, which might be a husband and wife, or two siblings, or any two members of a system engaged in a social interaction. The matter, energy, and information are the substances of their exchange. This substance (matter, energy or information) must be considered both in terms of quantity and of timing. The quantity of what is exchanged might be excessive, just right, or too little. The timing might be late, on target, or too early. In order for A and B to be adapted to each other, the following eight transactions must take place:

- A needs to obtain matter, energy, or information from B in order to survive.

- A needs to keep out (to prevent from entering its subsystem) those things from B that A does not need or want (that would strain or overload A).
- A needs to retain those things within itself that it cannot afford to give to B.
- A needs to dispose of certain products or wastes to B. (Likewise, B needs to engage in the same types of exchanges with A.)
- B needs to obtain matter, energy, or information from A in order to survive.
- B needs to keep out those things from A that it does not want or need.
- B needs to retain those things within itself that it cannot afford to give to A.
- B needs to dispose of certain products or wastes to A.

When the matter, energy, and information that A and B each need to obtain and to dispose of, or to keep out or retain, are exchanged in the quantities and timeframe suited for the exchange, the two subsystems A and B are understood to be adapted to each other. Maladaptation occurs when any or several of the exchanges does not occur, or is blocked, or a transaction is attempted that either subsystem does not desire. In this type of analysis, neither subsystem is considered as "doing something wrong" or "doing something right." Rather, the focus is on the negotiated order created by an adaptive transaction. When clinicians use this type of analytical device, they are more likely to manage a no-fault or non-blaming exploration of a maladaptive difficulty, and to design strategies for its resolution or for intervention.

Social Exchange Paradigm

Subsystem A   Subsystem B
(matter . . . energy . . . information)

OBTAIN   OBTAIN
CONTAIN OUT[- - - - - - - - - - -]CONTAIN OUT
RETAIN IN) - - - - - - - - - - (RETAIN IN
DISPOSE OF   DISPOSE OF

A and B might be a husband and wife in a traditional marriage, who are at first adaptive to one another and engage in transactions familiar to their respective, original family systems. A, as husband, obtains from B, his wife, expressions of love and loyalty, and of energy directed at child-bearing and child-rearing. (These are what B disposes to A.) A contains out of his subsystem news of bad behavior of the children, or trouble with tradesmen, or complaints of malaise on the part of B. (These are what B agrees to retain within her subsystem.) A retains within his subsystem fears of losing his job and also any clues that he might be attracted to his secretary. (These are what B agrees to contain out in her interchanges with A.) A disposes to B a weekly paycheck, expressions of admiration, and public acknowledgment of her household-management capabilities. (These are what A seeks to obtain from B.). Thus, the two subsystems are adapted to each other. Maladaptation may occur when either of them decides to change these adaptive interactions by demanding more or less of something, or changing the timing, or moving something from a not-demanded to a demanded category (A "contain out" item is shifted to a "dispose." For instance, B might decide that she wants information which she previously did not demand.) The system would now be maladapted and in need of re-equilibration.

Decision-Making

The rules of organization described above may be thought of as a regulator of a system's functioning. However, when the system is maladapted, or confronted with a new or different situation, decision-making functions are called into play. In human systems, decision-making is closely related to power issues. Cultural norms are also guides to understanding the kinds of power which would be called upon in given social situations.

■ MODES OF TRANSACTION

The **social exchange paradigm** is a framework for analyzing the substance of exchanges between two subsystems. An associated paradigm, which has as its focus the modes or ways in which the exchanges might be handled, and is entitled **modes of transaction** was also developed by Bredemeier. The social-exchange paradigm dealt with the substance of an exchange. The *modes of transaction* paradigm deals with the "how" of the exchange.

Each of two interacting subsystems tries to persuade the other to comply with its wishes, needs, or requests. In order to gain compliance, each engages in a series of tactics or strategies to convince the other that non-compliance with its needs will reduce the other's gain or profit from the continued relationship, and that compliance will improve the relationship and guarantee future fruitful interchanges. Each needs to know what the other values and respects in order for these persuasive moves to go well. These tactics or strategies—modes of transaction—are categorized into five groups: bargaining, legal-bureaucratic, gemeinschaft, team cooperative, and coercion.

The **bargaining mode of transaction** is frequently used in market-place exchanges, with a market being considered an applicable metaphor for a workplaces or home environment. If A says to B: "I want you to do X,"

B's question would be: "Why should I?" A persuasive bargaining response could be: "Because it will be well worth your while in the long run. You will decrease your costs and increase your benefits."

The **legal–bureaucratic mode of transaction** is formalistic and relies on the two interacting subsystems valuing the notion of rules, duties, and job descriptions associated with a designated status or office, as in the philosopher Max Weber's sense of bureaucracy. If A says to B: "I want you to do X," B's question of "Why should I?" would be answered in legal–bureaucratic terms, suggesting that a duty be performed. A might say: "Because it's your job. You agreed to do this as part of your work."

The **gemeinschaft mode of transaction** is a familistic one in which warmth, affection, and interpersonal bonding are relied upon. If A says to B: "I want you to do X," B's question of "Why should I?" would be answered by a reminder that B shares the family bonds and well-being. For instance, A might say: "Because you love me and I love you," or "Because we're husband and wife."

The **team–cooperative mode of transaction** suggests that the interacting members are part of a group or team effort to accomplish a task, which won't be completed unless the members pull together to get the work done. If A says to B: "I want you to do X," B's question of "Why should I?" would be answered in terms of a common goal being at stake. For instance, A might say, "Without you, we'll never win this," or "I need you to help because I can't get there (goal) without you."

The fifth mode of transaction is **coercion.** It operates when two subsystems do not belong to a larger system that has an available and operative set of rules for interacting, short of force, fraud, deception, and violence. It is a default category, called into play when the other four modes of transaction fail to operate. If A says to B: "I want you to do X," B's question, "Why should I?" would be answered with some type of force. A might say: "Do it or I'll hurt you if you don't" or even, "Do it or I'll kill you."

Families tend to prefer one of the modes of transaction more than the others, but rarely use one of them exclusively. Rather, depending on the nature of the interaction and where it is taking place, one or another of the modes would be used. For example, within the family's home, parents of teen-agers might be willing to bargain, but in public would rely on the gemeinschaft or team-cooperative modes of interaction. In some cultures, married couples rely on gemeinschaft interactions, while in others, legal–bureaucratic tactics might be more commonly found.

For use in systems analysis, the modes of transaction are placed on a grid (see Figure 8–1), with the five choices of A across the horizontal rows and B's expectations about what mode A ought to be using on the vertical columns. If A and B agree on the mode to be used,

	Bargaining	Legal–bureaucratic	Sub-system A Gemeinschaft	Team-cooperative	Coercion
Bargaining	X				
Legal–bureaucratic		X			
Gemeinschaft			X		
Team-cooperative				X	
Coercion					X

Figure 8–1. Modes of transaction.

then they are adapted to each other. When in B's view A is using an inappropriate mode, the system becomes maladapted.

On the grid used for analysis, there appear to be only 5 chances out of 25 that the two interacting subsystems will be adapted to each other. However, it is important to remember that these interactors have probably been socialized to the same set of values and norms, including the appropriateness of the rules for conducting their interchanges. Conflicts do occur, but the normative order is maintained more often than not.

The social transaction and modes of transaction paradigms are very useful tools for clinicians both for the assessment and treatment phases of work with patients in the context of systems, whether the latter be family, school, or work systems. While the clinician would not necessarily use the same language modes or exchanges that have been used here for the two paradigms, the system framework, translated to an agreeable level of understanding, is invaluable.

■ A FRAMEWORK

In a brief chapter such as this, it is impossible to describe all of the variants in given systems, how they operate, and the nature of the dysfunctions that occur within them. What can be made clear, however, is that using systems theory as a framework for understanding what people do and why and how they do it provides a rich, non-judgmental approach to clinical work. Symptoms used as markers in psychiatric diagnoses can no longer be viewed as belonging to an individual, but rather become statements about system maladaptation or signals of distress for the system.

These concepts are broad enough to be applicable to systems of any size, in any context. Their use is determined by the purposes of the systems analyst, whether a student, an advanced professional, or simply someone trying to understand the complexities of human beings interacting with each other in daily life.

The foregoing concept of system maladaptation is less pejorative and blame-laying than diagnostic systems

such as the International Classification of Diseases, Ninth Edition (ICD-9) or the Diagnostic and Statistical Manual of Mental Disorders, Fourth Edition (DSM-IV), which are popular assessment devices in psychiatric practice. These more familiar diagnostic tools place the dysfunction within the individual; systems analysis instead focuses on violations of rules and failed expectations.

In work with families, the use of a picture to diagram all of the members makes the systems framework easier to implement. Rather than recording data about significant relationships among the family members in the usual paragraph or sentence notation pattern, a figure representing family members can be used. It is a straightforward tool, and easily learned.

■ CLINICAL ILLUSTRATIONS

The case examples in this chapter describe seven families in terms of their genograms, rules of organization, and maladaptations (violations of system rules).

Families often view work as a normalizing dynamic. So long as a person works, his or her faults, shortcomings, or illnesses are handled and/or tolerated with less disruption than when the person does not, or cannot, work. Whether a mental illness prevents work or not working precipitates a mental illness is a chicken-and-egg issue over which many families agonize. "Is he lazy or is he sick?" is a question frequently asked of clinicians. For many families struggling to live with a mentally ill family member in a home setting, the failure of that person to work is often more distressing than the person's symptoms, even such bizarre ones as talking to voices, strange gesturing, or rituals.

Work is one of the crucial roles performed by people in any society. Although the structure and nature of work vary immensely within and between societies over time, production through work remains central. Not only does work serve as a basic function of economic production, but in many societies, success and achievement in the occupational sphere are intertwined with

CASE EXAMPLE

▶ THE JOHNSON FAMILY: WORK AS A NORMALIZING DYNAMIC

The Protestant work ethic and the Scandinavian—American family ethic advocate similar values to one another.

The Johnsons are a two-generation, Norwegian—Swedish Methodist family. Dick and Doris, both 57 years old, share their household with Tim, a 28-year-old first-born son, in whom schizoaffective disorder was diagnosed 5 years ago. Tim's younger sister, Sally, is married and has two small children. The Johnsons sought help from a community mental health center (CMHC) because of difficulty in handling Tim's behavior at home.

Tim graduated from college with a bachelor's degree in 1983. After graduation he moved about 700 miles away, taking a job at a research institute in Virginia. Within 6 months he had his first psychotic episode, which was associated with alcohol abuse. Since then Tim has been hospitalized several times for short periods, and has been referred to partial care. His attendance at the partial-care program is intermittent. Every few months he manages to find a job, works briefly, and is then fired or quits. At the present time he seems to be compliant with taking the antipsychotic medication, and attends Alcoholics Anonymous meetings twice weekly.

Tim's parents, Dick and Doris, are both employed, Dick as a construction worker and Doris as a secretary. They deny any problems at home or within their marriage, and see Tim's illness as having been caused entirely by his move away from home to Virginia. They believe that the move from an urban area to a rural one was not good for Tim, and verbalize this as the reason for his illness. Their voiced concerns are more about his seeming inability to hold a job than about his psychiatric symptoms. Dick and Doris focus on work as their chief concern, and seem unable to grasp the fact that their son has a chronic mental illness. They have shared, in family sessions, their belief that if a person works hard and goes to church, then that person is doing everything that he or she can do; and conversely, if one doesn't work, then one cannot lead a normal life.

The following is an excerpt from a tape-recorded dialogue during a family session.

Therapist: Work seems important to you.

Dick: It is. Tim with his problem holding a job. . . . I've always felt that if a person stays away from work, they lose their desire to work. . . . How's Tim going to make it in life if he doesn't work? You know, we're not going to be around forever.

Doris: I don't understand why this happened to Tim. . . . He had a happy childhood. He was always a hard worker. He's been attending a program here because they said they would find him a job (referring to the partial-care program).

For the Johnsons, work is a normalizing dynamic. Despite the fact that Tim is delusional from time to time, they believe that he would be normal if he would just get a job and stick with it. It is not quite accurate to view the family as being in denial; rather, they seem unable to realize the implications of a diagnosis of mental illness. So far, the therapist has not succeeded in getting them to consider an alternative explanation for his not working. Tim's being at home again has drastically altered the life-style of his parents: they are at a stalemate in what some authors call the launching phase of their family development. Because this family insists so strongly on focusing on Tim's

employment, the degree to which other family issues may or may not serve as stressors is unclear.

▶ THE FOLATYS: MAINTAINING A SERIOUSLY MENTALLY ILL SON AT HOME

The Folatys are a Ukrainian—American family struggling with the burden of trying to maintain a seriously mentally ill member at home. Both parents are professionals; Steven is a physician and Anna a music teacher.

The Folatys value both work and education; work, in their family system, has to be of a professional nature. Maria is a graphic artist, with a dual degree in architectural design. Rosa is a musician with a master's degree in fine arts. The identified patient and son, John, with a diagnosis of schizophrenia, earned a bachelor's degree in political science at a highly respected university. Maria, the Folaty's daughter, believes that her father's interference in the lives of his children is a considerable negative influence on all of them, but particularly on John. Maria states, "I guess I saw the trouble starting with John earlier than anybody. He began to be lazy—to space out, even without drugs— in his sophomore year in college. However, the trouble was that he was living at home and commuting, and my father would get on his case and keep at it until he turned in papers and did the work. My father earned that bachelor's degree, not my brother; the wrong name is on the diploma!

By the time he had graduated, John was sleeping most of the day, avoiding family members, and listening to music in his room at night. He has not worked since graduating from the university, other than at some temporary jobs that were below his status and embarrassing to his parents. When he occasionally gets violent and pushes his mother about, his father takes steps to hospitalize him involuntarily, in private settings. The father, Steven, who is a general practitioner, is ambivalent about what his psychiatrist colleagues have told him. He says, "I hear their words; I don't believe them. John needs reputable work. That would fix everything. I just don't know what went wrong. We are all hard-working, God-fearing, respectable people. I have no explanation for this, It doesn't make any sense". The father is able to state how schizophrenia is described in the *DSM IV,* and acknowledges that John's symptoms match the descriptions, but then states, "Show me the organism. Show me the damaged tissue. Show me something I can see with my own eyes, and I'll understand it." John's mother Anna, who has had surgery and is undergoing continued treatment for her cancer, is very tearful whenever John is mentioned. Her view is that she failed as a mother because she didn't insist on his continuing to go to church when he started college. She says, "I'm very worried about what God is going to do to me. Steven doesn't quite see it this way, but he's a scientist and I'm an artist."

These families' rule of organization placed work first, as a normalizing, stabilizing focus. Maladaptation occurs when the ill member cannot fulfill the expectations. Referring to the paradigm of social exchange, the identified patient is not producing what the parents and siblings want of him. Further, the patient wants to be left alone and not badgered about finding and keeping jobs. More stress occurs when family members differ in their opinions about how to manage the maladaptation. Continuing therapeutic dialogue is possible when the family is invited to see the issue as one of conflicting views and expectations, rather than as a right-wrong situation.

The Johnson Family

indices of personal worth. Moreover, work often has religious and moral value.

The work ethic consists of beliefs that: (1) people have a moral and religious obligation to fill their lives with heavy, physical toil; (2) men and women are expected to spend long hours at work, with limited time for leisure; (3) workers should be highly productive; and (4) workers should take pride in their work.

■ THE GENOGRAM

The **genogram** provides a succinct picture of family structures and relationships that includes all family members and shows their generational context (Smoyak, 1982, 1987). It can be drawn quickly, using only plain white paper and a sharp pencil. Recently, computerized versions have been attempted (Chan et al., 1987), but they are still unwieldy to operate and not yet very adaptable to wide clinical use.

There has been increasing interest among clinicians in ways in which to assess and use psychosocial data in the diagnosis and treatment of psychiatric disorders. Journal articles repeat the message about the importance of psychosocial and family data in diagnosis and treatment, yet are usually not clear about how the clinician is to collect these data, nor about how to analyze and use them. The point has been made (Like, Rogers, and McGoldrick, 1988) that genograms are diagnostic tests, and that diagnosis is more than the simple process of labeling. Like and colleagues say that the use of genograms facilitates "the elucidation of the contributing causes of the patient's distress or complaints in such

The Folaty Family

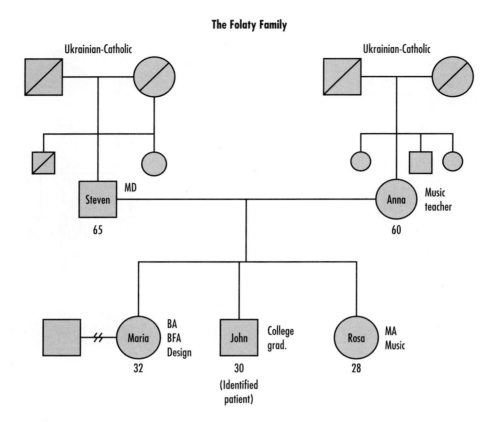

a manner that the clinician will be able to understand more about the way in which a patient is ill, the mechanisms by which the illness is produced, and the reasons why the patient is ill at this particular time so that an appropriate therapeutic intervention can be initiated."

Rogers and Durkin (1984) suggest that most physicians would agree on the importance of taking a family history, yet note the general lack of information about the relative utility of different methods of collecting this information. They conducted a study to test the efficacy of using the genogram, compared with informal interviews, on first visits of patients to a university family practice center. The average time for constructing the genogram was 20 minutes, and its use quadrupled the information gathered.

A growing body of research provides evidence for seasoned practitioners' long-held notion that family function is related to patterns of illness. How a family functions is tied to the physical and emotional well-being of its members. An ill family member does not exist in a vacuum, but rather clearly influences those around him or her, and in turn is influenced by them. Family dynamics, as causal, contributory or simply correlational have been examined in recent studies. For example, family stresses have been related to the frequency of a variety of illnesses, as well as the severity and duration of respiratory illnesses in children (Boyce, T. et al 1977).

Constructing a genogram provides benefits for both clinicians and families beyond the data gathered. The device signals the clinician's interest in the family, and establishes a firmer rapport with them. Families are more likely to remember contributory events more clearly, and to become more actively involved in discovering relevant factors and historical events, when a genogram is used. Because simple paper and pencil are used to create the genogram, families do not feel subjected to the sometimes frightening high-technology machinery and materials now associated with scientific medicine. They can see what is being drawn and understand what the clinician is trying to discover. Clinicians can teach as they draw, pointing out areas for further inquiry and asking questions in a more focused manner. If, for example, a child has been seen repeatedly for upper respiratory infections or asthma, the smokers in the family could be highlighted on the genogram in color, thus more graphically illustrating the family's role in the child's illness. Handled as information, this is more likely to seem like concern rather than guilt-induction or preaching. Admonitions to "quit smoking" in the absence of a graphic portrayal of its effects are likely to be less effective.

Another use of genograms is to assess the risk of familial disease and future illness. Thus, an obese child in a family in which one parent and two of the four grandparents are diabetic needs careful monitoring and strategies for preventing diabetes.

DRAWING THE GENOGRAM

As noted above, the only tools needed to create a genogram are plain, white paper and a sharp pencil with an eraser. The clinician should sit in such a way that the family members can watch what is being drawn. At the outset, it is useful to tell the family that the genogram is a diagnostic device, much like blood test-

ing or an X-ray. It also helps to allay anxiety by pointing out that the genogram is not a "test," such as one encounters in school, and that the eraser is handy and is almost always used, since most people remember more accurately and see the need to make corrections as the figure is being developed.

Males are placed on the genogram in boxes, and females in circles. Marriages are indicated by a straight horizontal line, connecting the husband and wife, with the husband on the left and the wife on the right. Dotted horizontal lines indicate cohabitation without mar-

E CASE EXAMPLE

▶ THE GIOVANNI FAMILY: STRUGGLE WITH VIOLENCE

In the wake of de-institutionalization, many families find themselves struggling to manage a seriously mentally ill individual at home. The family's coping strategies are challenged to the maximum when the mentally ill member is a young adult, with chronic illness, and is very strong, very ill, and resists attempts to manage troublesome symptoms with psychopharmacological agents.

The process of public education has somewhat succeeded in changing people's minds about the mentally ill and their dangerousness. Yet it remains true that untreated mental illness, especially in the community, is associated with a greater frequency of violence. Families need training in techniques for recognizing warning signals of dangerous behavior, diffusing patients' anger, protecting themselves from physical harm, and knowing when to seek shelter with neighbors and relatives. Families who care for young, chronically mentally ill relatives at home feel ill-prepared to deal with the potential for violence.

The Giovannis are an Italian–American family with a mentally ill son living at home, where his violent outbursts have become a frequent occurrence and a primary concern of his care-givers. His father John and mother Angie are both retired, and are the care-givers for Eddie, their first-born son, who is 35 years old; Maria, Eddie's recently divorced younger sister also lives at home. Eddie's psychiatric history is fairly typical of the young adult, chronically mentally ill, population described in the literature. He began having overt behavioral problems in late adolescence and was hospitalized numerous times at different public and private institutions. He has been variously diagnosed as having paranoid schizophrenia, an antisocial personality, and bipolar disorder with psychotic features. He has always lived at home, and has never been able to maintain employment other than for short periods. He frequently abuses drugs and alcohol, and is non-compliant with his medication regimens. He refuses to attend family-therapy sessions but insists that his parents go. Excerpts from a family session capture the sense of the family's frustration:

Angie: Eddie tells me what to do. I want to be left alone to do what I want to do.

John: I feel threatened, intimidated by Eddie. I'm not the head of the house-

hold; he assumes the responsibility. I want to get to the source of our problems. I want to have the role of the father.

Maria: Eddie is an alcoholic and a drug addict. I would like to make living normal and pleasant. Not like a nightmare. No more violence; there's been a lot of that. My parents can't handle him. When he acts up, they say, "This is it!" and they take him back to the hospital.

The hospital stays, however, are short, and the family repeatedly has Eddie back home, with little change in his behavior. Prior to one hospitalization, Eddie tried to choke his mother. Although his parents went to court and a restraining order was issued, Eddie returned home within days. He was furious at the court's intervention, and when his father asked him to leave the house, Eddie punched him in the eye, causing permanent loss of vision.

When Eddie is at home, the family has adapted to the fear of his outbursts by avoiding confrontations. Although John is upset that his role as head of the household has been usurped by Eddie, he chooses most of the time to avoid head-on confrontations with him about power or authority. For instance, if Eddie is upset and demanding his mother's attention, even though it is dinner time, she pays attention to him and ignores her husband. Eddie stays in the kitchen with his mother, and John eats alone in the dining room. This is a particularly disturbing situation, since it is a clear violation of the expected gemeinschaft mode in an Italian household and interrupts the solidarity of the marital dyad, leaving the possibility for continuing coalitions (of mother and son) across the generational boundary. Infants and children, because of their pressing physiological and psychosocial needs, have a built-in license to engage in such interruptions. However, the expectation for older children, and certainly for adult children, is that the marital dyad's needs are honored.

Within several months, Eddie had again decompensated and was hospitalized involuntarily, after he threatened to "ice" (kill) his father. He was outraged at his family for its action, and voiced the belief that things that their comments about him in family-therapy sessions had contributed to his involuntary status. The dilemma for families is how to take action for self-protection, while convincing the ill member that they are not doing so as an attack or an insult, but rather from fear.

The Giovanni Family

riage; these lines can also be used to connect members of a homosexual couple. Children are drawn by suspending them on a sibling line, which is a horizontal line below the parents, connected with the parents' line by a vertical line. Boxes are drawn for boys and circles for girls, with the oldest child to the left. Pregnancies are indicated as triangles in the appropriate place on the sibling line. If there is only one child, or a first pregnancy, only the vertical line from the parent's (marriage) line is drawn. Adoptions are shown by using a dotted line as the vertical line to the marriage line. Divorces and separations are noted by drawing "//" in the middle of the marriage line, with "m" for the date of marriage, "d" indicating divorce, and "s" indicating separation. People who are not family members but are closely involved in family life can be shown on the genogram and connected by dotted lines where appropriate. For instance, a female au paire would be a circle, connected by a dotted line to the parent(s). Companions, home health aides, and very frequent visitors can be shown similarly as needed.

Genograms may include only the basic data about a family, or may have data added to suit the goals of the clinician, such as prevention or hypothesis-testing. For most purposes, the following data should be noted for each person on the genogram.

- The birth date, preceded by "b" and noted under the box or circle.
- Education, noted by whatever shorthand system the clinician likes to use, (e.g., h.s., 4th gr., M.S.).

- Occupation (e.g., acc't., stu.).
- A "/" (slash) is indicated across the box or circle for someone who dies, with the death date placed below the birth date.

The ethnic/religious origin is noted for the family members of the oldest generation, above the oldest person in that generation; a shorthand system can be used for this (e.g., Irish RC, Ger.-Luth., Russ. Jew). Additional information that may be noted includes health and illness status, risk factors, and geographical location of the family members.

A practical technique is to copy the genogram on a photocopier. The family may be given a copy, and clinicians may use another to circle currently ill family members or to design hypothetical drawings of alliances, cutoffs in relationships, or problems. Color coding can be used to track illnesses, such as diabetes or depression. For example, in one family in which three adolescents were seriously overweight, the family designed a color code to indicate exactly how much overweight each of the family members was, including those of other generations.

■ FAMILY THEORY AND RESEARCH

While there has been a voluminous addition to the family literature in recent decades, clinical theory about dysfunctional families has not kept pace with the dramatic changes which have occurred in family structures

E CASE EXAMPLE

▶ THE FLANAGAN FAMILY: RETIREMENT PLANS DERAILED

The Flanagans, Joe, 65, and Mary, 60, had been planning for many years for their retirement, looking forward to increased leisure and fulfillment of their travel dreams. Their four daughters, ranging in age from 35 to 25 years, have not been living at home for 5 years. Mary planned to retire at the age of 62. Joe had retired at 62 and has been spending his time doing household repairs that had been neglected. He also watches his grandchildren—pre-schoolers of his daughter Maura who is finishing graduate school. Maura and her husband John live 10 miles from the Flanagans. The two younger daughters moved to San Francisco, where they share an apartment with two other young women. The Flanagans' oldest daughter Sheila, lives in Washington, DC, with her political-scientist husband, Michael, and three children.

As Mary describes their family: "We were a typical family, fun-loving, family-centered, Irish, happy. We were atypical only in that no one had any serious drinking problems. Then the bomb struck."

The "bomb" was a telephone call from Sheila, who said that her husband Michael had called her from Japan and told her that he wasn't coming home from a business trip for "a while" because he had fallen in love with a woman Japanese business associate. When Sheila began to assess her financial status, she discovered that Michael had remortgaged their home, and that their second mortgage was three months in arrears. Moreover, because of Michael's gambling, the family's car payments were past due and their two cars were in the process of being repossessed. Sheila asked her parents to let her and the children come and stay with them, and Joe and Mary now have a six-person household, as well as Maura's two children for most of the week.

Families' views of the origin and needed treatment for an illness may be in direct opposition to professional care-providers' views of the situation. Professionals often disagree among themselves and with families about the plausible explanation for behavioral events, as well as the most efficient course of action to bring disturbances under control. For instance, some family theorists would view the organizational structure of a family as creating a dilemma, while others would see the family member's illness as creating anomalies in the family structure. In the United States, the National Alliance for the Mentally Ill, a voluntary group, challenges the four mental-health professions (psychiatry, psychology, psychiatric nursing, and social work) to justify their statements about the origins of a patient's illness and the best treatment available for it. The group takes particular issue with untested theories that implicate families as the causes of illness. Another position of the group is that illness behavior can most effectively be understood as a complex interaction of both biological or organic causes with organizational or structural variables.

It is particularly difficult to correct hierarchical maladies and put parents back in charge of a family when the family system includes a mentally ill adult child who frequently precipitates violent interchanges or threatens to do so. Clinicians, who have available help for in-patients, including chemical and physical restraints, are sometimes at a loss to help families design strategies that will work in home settings. The police are often called upon in community settings to help control a family disturbance. However, they are largely reluctant to do so because they are ill-prepared to judge the nuances of the family's interchanges. Police refusing to respond to family violence calls have often said, "We're enforcement officers, not social workers!" A police chief, asked to come to a community mental health center meeting to discuss plans for alternative strategies in dealing with family problems in an inner-city area, stated, "I see it as rather futile; family violence and the weather are the same. Everybody talks about it, but nobody can change it." Such demoralization unfortunately dampens the efforts to seek solutions to this pressing need.

The maladaptations presented in this study include:

1. Michael and Sheila's sub-system, with most communication managed by lawyers and long-distance telephone calls.
2. Joe and Mary's sub-system, with serious disagreement between them about how long they should "endure" this new complexity.
3. Sheila's children, who are belligerent, tearful, and showing many other signs of distress, such as lying and stealing, bed-wetting, renewed thumb-sucking, and frequent night awakening.
4. Sheila and Maura, who are in conflict with each other and in competition for their parents' resources (particularly regarding child-care).
5. Michael and John, who were college classmates but now exchange heated international phone calls. John is convinced that if Michael went into treatment for his gambling, the old normative order of that nuclear family would be restored.

The family was referred for therapy when Sheila's son Michael, Jr., was caught with money for a fourth-grade class trip hidden in his backpack. The family therapist, a clinical specialist in psychiatric nursing, has prepared a genogram, incorporating all of the family members in problem-defining and problem-solving sessions. Her primary work is on the mutual expectations of the adults for one another.

At the intake session, the therapist asked Michael, Jr., if he had had a plan for the stolen money. He said that he had planned to send it to his father in Japan so that the latter could "pay all his debts and not be ashamed and be with us again." Michael Jr. earned the designation "Signaler of System Distress", and at subsequent family sessions often voiced what the adults were reluctant to mention. As Wallerstein and Blakeslee (1989) have shown, divorce is a shock, and often a prolonged one, to both nuclear and extended family systems. To the extent that Michael, Jr., and his siblings are not helped in their coming to grips with the loss of their father (and uncle), more acting out can be expected. Sheila's two younger sisters may have reservations about entering marriage. Joe and Mary may find that the increased demands being made on them exacerbate physical ailments such as Joe's hypertension or Mary's arthritis. The adults in the family disagreed with the therapist's suggestion that they spend time grieving for their various losses (of husband, of marriage, of father, of cherished dreams), although Joe says that "Our dreams aren't dead yet; they just need a little resuscitation," and that "When Sheila gets herself together . . . we'll go on as we wanted to."

The Flanagan Family

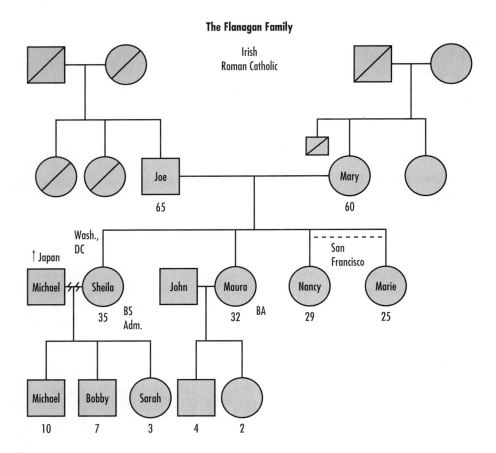

Irish
Roman Catholic

and associated functions and ways of living. As Walsh (1987; p. 497) points out, "Most clinical theory explicitly or implicitly upholds the ideal model of the family as intact, with father as primary wage-earner and instrumental leader, and mother as primary parent, homemaker, and socioemotional caretaker." The fact is, however, that fewer than 20% of American families fit this pattern (Rossi, 1993). Still, deviation from this standard is regarded in much of the clinical literature as unquestionably pathogenic. Some current textbooks used in clinical training virtually ignore alternative arrangements as possibly being more normative. Even when divorce and/or separation are acknowledged as occurring in half of all marriages in the United States, the normal sequence of dissolution of ties, emotional upset, management of stress, and adaptations to community demands are not given appropriate consideration.

Walsh (1987) states that clinicians thus lack knowledge about what is normal and what is not in family life. She describes two types of frequent errors, the first being to mistakenly identify as pathological a family pattern that is normal, and the second to fail to recognize a pattern as dysfunctional by assuming that it is normal. An example of the first type of error occurs when a clinician, reared in a family in which adults were not very demonstrative of affection and in which children were supposed to follow the directions of adults, encounters a family that is noisy, affectionate, and very open about their expressions of both joy and anguish. The clinician, seeing the solicitous concern of a mother for her child, even to the point of her bringing homemade lasagna for a hospitalized child, would see this as enmeshment or symbiosis instead of normal caring.

Some clinicians see their own upbringing as departing from normal, and apply that view to the families they see. When they encounter a family similar to their own, they view it suspiciously and diagnose it as pathological.

An example of the second type of error described by Walsh is acceptance of the myth that healthy families are free of conflict. Such a view would preclude the clinician's exploring an assertion by a couple that they have not disagreed in 20 years of marriage. In addition, what is common may also be accepted as normal. For example, noncustodial fathers are so frequently cut off from their children after a divorce that clinicians may see this as normal, and thus fail to explore ways in which the father and his children might be together.

If nurses feel uncomfortable about exploring the psychosocial aspects of their patients' families, they miss opportunities to suggest beneficial measures and to prompt the families to re-think their animosities and cut-offs. Recent research demonstrates a positive association between continued supportive contact by a non-custodial divorced parent and the long-term adjustment of children. Such contact also has a positive effect on custodial mothers. Even when previous contact was negative, continuing cut-offs produce poorer functioning and more symptomatic behavior, especially with boys. Fathers who had negative father–child relationships before divorce have been found in many cases to be able to develop improved relationships with their children following divorce. Walsh, citing several long-term studies, concludes that a clinical imperative in cases of cut-off parents is to assess and build a co-parenting alliance in post-divorce family systems. In doing this, systems analysis allows non-judgmental discussions to take place, and encourages the development of better solutions to troublesome situations.

The degree to which nurses feel comfortable in adding psychosocial exploration to their intake evaluations or to their ongoing assessments of the course of treatment or monitoring depends on the messages they received from their mentors, or the subsequent pushes to change practice habits, which might come from colleagues, or the families, themselves. Some are reluctant to suggest that psychiatric consultation should be sought, even when there is clear-cut evidence of the need, either in the child or the parent. Some are reluctant to discuss behavior which might be seen as willful, or as part of a lifestyle, rather than illness. Drug abuse and alcohol abuse are examples of problems which, even when noticed, are not mentioned by many clinicians.

Early research in the field of family studies tended to over-represent white, Anglo–Saxon, Protestant, middle-class families. Recent, comparative studies are including the differences in structures and styles of relating in various ethnic groups (McGoldrick et al., 1982). Other research studies alternate family forms, such as single-parent and blended family systems. Wallerstein (1989) has contributed an insightful and clinically relevant study of the children of divorced parents, following families 5 and 10 years after a marital break-up. Rossi

E CASE EXAMPLE

▶ THE DANIELS FAMILY: ADOLESCENT CARETAKER SISTERS

Familial rules of organization about inter-generational obligations have many different variations. The Daniels represent a situation in which adolescent sisters become the caretakers for their younger female siblings, which can lead to dysfunctional relationships when these women reach adulthood. In such a relationship, reciprocity does not exist; loyalty is entirely from the caretaker to the recipient, in contrast to care-giving, which includes both loyalty and reciprocity (Bank and Kahn, 1982).

The nature of the caretaker–recipient relationship among siblings is qualitatively different from many other familial patterns of care. Bank and Kahn (1982) observe that the parental role is of such great importance to the healthy development of children that family researchers have focused almost exclusively on parents' organizational functions. Families with a dysfunctional parent sub-system have difficulty in coping with developmental changes and life stresses. In such family systems, role expectations are often poorly defined.

The Daniels are three-generational, white, Anglo-Saxon family. The mother, Robin, now 76, has had three husbands, all alcoholics, and is herself an alcoholic. Pat, her daughter and only child from her first marriage, was the adolescent caretaker sibling for Robin's younger daughter Diane, now 35, and Diane's older brother, who died from a drug overdose. Currently married to an alcoholic, Pat, as an adolescent caretaker, was very autocratic in her disciplining, and Diane describes her as somewhat erratic in her behavior generally.

When Diane sought treatment, she presented herself as highly anxious, needy, disorganized, and unsure of herself, with thoughts that were negative and obsessive. Issues of differentiation from her family of origin, unresolved grief, and failed role negotiations in her marriages quickly became apparent. Diane's daughter Robin, witnessed much of the abuse of Diane by her first husband and Robin's father, who abused drugs and died of AIDS in 1987. Robin's childhood appears to have been as chaotic as her mother's; with her often having been the champion of her mother against her father's abuse.

Diane has expressed concern about her inability to sleep alone at night. She has sought treatment for her recently, this time with worries about her obsession with homework, her general negativity, her lack of friends, and arguments between mother and daughter. She has recently re-married (within nine months of her husband's death from AIDS) and moved to a new town. Both she and her daughter continue to express fear about possible contagion from her former husband's illness.

Diane's inability to differentiate normal adolescent struggle from pathological levels of disturbance can be understood in the light of her own experience as an adolescent, with a harsh, unyielding caretaker sister. She often succumbs to Robin's demands but with accompanying negativity and anger. Bank and Kahn (1982) assert that the recipient of care from an inflexible and compulsive caretaker, who answers non-compliance by inducing guilt and making threatening stances, often responds passively, but with underlying hostility and anger. Diane and her daughter are re-living an earlier familiar pattern. Limit-setting and the warm expression of love elude Diane as a mother.

The Daniels Family

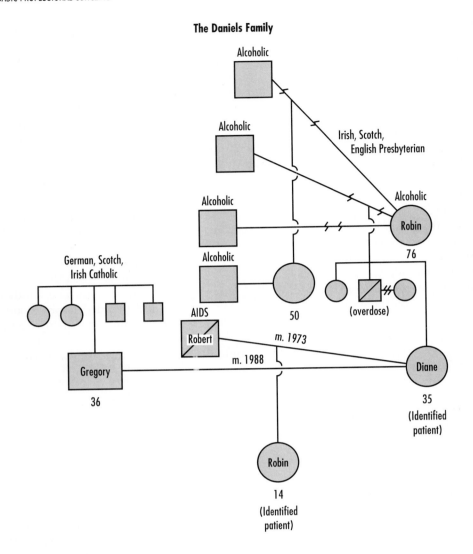

(1993) reviews demographic trends in family life and gender roles in terms of the work–family interface.

An emerging theme is that no single pattern distinguishes well-functioning families from pathological ones. Something that seems like intrusiveness to a less-than-careful observer may simply be caring expressed in a particular ethnic style. Also, no specific family structure is healthier than any other arrangement. Children in single-parent families, or those raised by a homosexual couple, can do as well as those in families in which two biological parents are present, when the stresses and the available resources are more or less equivalent.

Walsh cautions that "Too often, families with the same presenting problem are presumed to have a similar dysfunctional style, when research, albeit limited to date, reveals a good deal of diversity among families with similarly diagnosed members." (Walsh, 1987, p. 499) Clinicians need to remind themselves that there is

no one-to-one correspondence between symptom and system. Just as no single pattern clearly demarcates a normal family, it is equally true that families cannot be typed by the diagnosis of a family member, whether the latter is asthma, alcohol dependency, or cancer.

Faulty conclusions can be avoided by keeping in mind that families are tremendously complex and that a wide array of variables is operative at any moment in the interactions of their members. A better stance is forming tentative hypotheses and then engaging the family in a mutual exploration of these.

■ CHANGING SOCIALIZATION NORMS

As functions formerly performed by families were transferred to agencies and institutions outside the home, the remaining functions of childbearing, child rearing

E CASE EXAMPLES

▶ THE SHAH FAMILY: MIXED CULTURES/SIBLING CARETAKER/PARENTING CHILD

The Shah family is a three-generational system of mixed cultures. Sam Shah, age 26, is the third son of Egyptian/Moslem parents who value education highly and are themselves white-collar professionals. His wife Antoinette, age 29, is the fourth-born daughter of an Italian Roman Catholic family, whose parents were blue collar workers and did not finish high school. Sam is Antoinette's first husband. They were married three years ago. However, Antoinette has a daughter, Grace, age 9, who is the product of a prior, short-lived relationship.

Antoinette's family of origin was highly chaotic, violent, and dysfunctional. When she was seven, she witnessed the killing of her mother by her father, through multiple stabbings. Following the murder, she was raised by her second oldest sister, Theresa, then 17 years of age. An older sister had already married and left home. Antoinette spent some time in a Catholic boarding school, but was expelled for arguing with the nuns. Because of constant arguing, turmoil, and severe disciplining from Theresa, Antoinette had also been expelled from the house on several occasions and sent to live with other relatives. Nevertheless, over the years she had developed strong bonds with her younger siblings, establishing loyalties to them, but harbored continued animosity toward Theresa.

Grace, age nine and the identified patient in this family system, was born when Antoinette was 19 years old. Grace never knew her biological father, who departed shortly after her birth. She has had multiple caretakers and has also served as a companion to her mother in struggles with loneliness and poor relationships with men. Grace becomes inappropriately demanding and controlling of Antoinette, who is ineffective as a parent and very inconsistent in her attempts at limit-setting. When counselors expressed concern about her sexual acting out and assertions of sexual abuse by a baby-sitter and her step-grandfather from Egypt, Grace was referred by her school system for treatment. The allegations of sexual abuse were investigated and not sustained.

Daughters are socialized to be women primarily by their mothers. When the primary socialization of the mother has been defective, the result is an inability of the daughter to become an effective parent, particularly with female children. When the mother as a child has experienced conflicting messages about femininity and the expectations of women, and has had disturbing sexual experiences or poor role modeling from a same-sex parent or caretaker, she will be unable to function normally as a mother. Frequently, when the parental dyad is dysfunctional, a child (often the oldest or most responsible female) emerges to protect the dyad by assuming child-care responsibilities. The unspoken hope of such children is that relieving their parents of some child-care tasks will enable the parents to resolve problems and return to their normal tasks. Unfortunately, the hope is often not fulfilled, particularly when the parents are abusing drugs and/or alcohol. Caretaker siblings often also provide parenting directly for their parents, such as by preparing meals, doing laundry, and in other ways.

The youngest caretaker sibling discovered by a university community mental health center in New Jersey was an 8-year-old boy who successfully cared for 6-, 4-, and 2-year-old siblings after his parents deserted the family. His caretaking went undiscovered for more than 2 months, coming to light when school officials investigated his frequent absences from school. He had been feeding his family by taking discarded food from fast-food outlets. He ultimately had a very difficult time in returning to third grade and being raised by foster parents, feeling deprived in having his former significant role taken away from him.

Clinicians have noted that in adulthood, caretaker siblings often seem sad if not clinically depressed. Having not experienced the joys of childhood, they seem unable to experience anything joyful in adulthood. The outcomes of caretaker versus care-giver siblings have not been fully studied. In family systems with a chronically ill child, the family's social class, resources, and support systems appear to influence outcomes. Smaller families with fewer people to rely upon for help seem to experience more stress and disruption.

▶ THE SMITH FAMILY: MULTIPLE SYSTEMS STRESSES

Rob and Lisa Smith, married for 22 years, have struggled to maintain a degree of family normality, avoiding serious discussions of differences, including Rob's war experiences in Vietnam, his many extramarital affairs, alcohol problems in both families, obesity in both families, and life-threatening cardiac disease in Rob. One very problematic family rule is that Rob decides what he's willing to discuss and no one can persuade him to change his mind. Lisa complains that she is living with a changed person, that a different man came back from Vietnam, but she feels helpless to push past his no discussion rule. They have been referred for therapy because Rob is a candidate for heart transplantation but is alcoholic and has serious obesity that has resulted in his having a low priority score in a donor review. They agreed to family sessions only with the understanding that his might improve Rob's chances of a transplant.

Rob's extended family includes four living generations. His maternal grandfather, 88, is thought to have Alzheimer's disease, and is cared for by his wife, aged 82. Rob's parents continue to endure a long-conflicted marriage made more difficult by problem drinking and a diagnosis of emphysema for Rob's father. His parents argue bitterly about responsibility for the care of elders and what they owe Rob, who has financial worries, in addition to physical and emotional ones. Lisa's father, although an invalid throughout most of her life, controlled his family from his sick-bed. Lisa's older sister was a caretaker sibling in her family. Lisa fails to negotiate well with Rob, and does just as poorly with their daughter, Rita.

Over the years, Lisa has attempted to get Rob to accept the need for counseling for his alcoholism, as well as marital counseling and medical help for his obesity and heart disease. As she tearfully states, "My life is just one long frustration; if I pushed too hard, he'd just walk out and leave—and have another affair. Then things would be no better, and usually just get worse." She acknowledges her own obesity, but seems puzzled that clinicians list her children as obese (both are more than 60 pounds overweight). She says, "Well, they just need to be more active. Exercise or work would help. But I guess they eat when they're troubled, just like I do."

The Shah Family

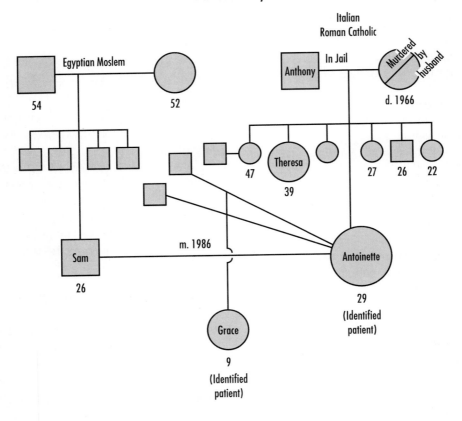

The Smith Family

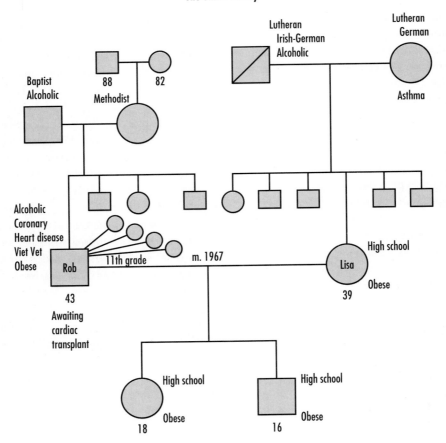

and primary socialization assumed more importance. Generations ago, parents simply bore children and raised them, with almost no inputs from strangers, and generally few, depending on the ethnicity, from extended family members. Today there are specialists in every dimension of individual and family functioning—from how to be healthy in pregnancy to how to respond to an adolescent's bad manners.

Depending on their social class and culture, people choose to consult different authorities. The appropriate resource for questions is very much determined by an individual's social group, level of education, and general sense of assuredness about his or her abilities. Most people do not measure advice against a standard of good research, but whether the advice-giver is trustworthy, or in the past has given sensible advice.

Fifty years ago, no profession identified as one of its functions to teach parents how to be parents. Parents were supposed to know what to do with their children either intuitively or from having grow up in large, extended families. Today, advice, counseling, and teaching about parenting are considered part of the work of nurses, physicians, psychologists, social workers, clergy, and members of new fields, such as health educators. Courses on effective parenting can be found in the curricula of high schools, colleges, and graduate schools, as well as on public television. Failure of socialization might be treated in an educational course or by a stay at a psychiatric hospital; some parents still see the military as a positive solution for offspring who fail to adopt parental values and norms. When a younger child behaves badly in the classroom or resists going to school entirely, the tendency today is to treat this as a system difficulty and to use a range of strategies to involve the parents in some type of parenting program. Programs are also held for parents whose teenagers abuse drugs or alcohol, with support groups for the teenagers' siblings.

Children do not become well-adjusted adults unless nurtured in some type of close, continuing social unit, in which norms are clearly set, self-esteem is fostered, and issues of separateness and connectedness are worked on openly and directly. The most important work of parents as socializing agents is to inspire each succeeding generation to want to advance in life. In one way or another, parents have to help their children become "hooked" on the idea of continuity. Simply put, parents must make it pleasant to be alive and to suggest that one's "debt" for such pleasure is to pass it on to the next person or next generation. Warmth and tenderness must be experienced before they can be valued and shared with others. Too many people have had traumatic experiences, with love turned to hate, warmth to cold, and tenderness to hostility. They fear being vulnerable and fear trusting others.

A large dimension of parenting is to protect children from developing distrust and hostility, and to predispose them to enjoy working and to appreciate tenderness. In other words, parents must convince children that they live in a just world. Otherwise, "behaving," achieving, and going on would make no sense.

More children today are being reared in an androgynous fashion. Boys are being invited to explore dimensions of experience previously totally associated with the female sex. Boys in nursery school, for example, now cuddle baby dolls or offer to cook; girls learn how to operate dump trucks. Boys in junior high school learn how to sew; girls study woodworking. Most gym classes are no longer sex-segregated; rather, each child is challenged to perform to his or her physical potential. Doomsayers see this as producing mass confusion over sexual identity in the next generation. Optimists rejoice at the creation of more fully human persons.

■ THE FUTURE

The future of the family cannot be predicted without placing it squarely in its social context. The trend toward equality of the sexes within families and the larger society certainly has increased self-esteem for women, but may cause new stress for men. The careful study of morbidity and mortality data will provide a clue to the impact of this important social trend. Divorce rates have leveled, and marriage is again gaining popularity (Ahrons and Miller, 1993). Dual-career or dual-job marriages and unions are gaining ground each year. While such arrangements do improve a family's economic assets, child care becomes a complex and costly issue, especially in the pre-school years.

Considering recent trend analyses and surveys, it seems likely that the following future directions for families might be possible:

- There will continue to be increasing value placed on human potential, tenderness and warmth, and the fulfillment of psychosocial needs, rather than on material pursuits, as a primary goal for families.
- The trend toward decreasing numbers of children per family will continue. Consequently, greater attention will be paid to parent–child relationships, and professionals will find increased use as parenting advisers.
- Neighborhoods will be reinvented, along with community support centers.
- Extended families will gain the attention of researchers, as will grandparent–grandchild relationships.

- A new ideal—strength without domination—will gain impetus and influence in family socialization patterns.

The challenge will be to keep abreast of changes in family patterns and dynamics, and to use this knowledge in providing humanistic and enlightened patient care. In this context, systems-oriented thinking should prove to be an asset.

O AN OVERVIEW

- Although families may differ in structure and function, marriage is desired in most; close relatives are forbidden to marry; males have higher status than females; and work tasks are defined by gender.°
- Traditional frameworks for understanding families are based on intrapsychic and interpersonal theories.
- von Bertalanffy's systems theory emerged from organismic biology and open-systems theory.
- Six basic principles frame general systems theory.
- Genograms provide a visual picture of family structure and relationships.
- Clinical nursing research could yield important information about providing care to dysfunctional families.
- For children to grow up well adjusted, they need to be nurtured in a close, continuing social unit.

TD TERMS TO DEFINE

- bargaining mode of transaction
- coercion
- gemeinschaft mode of transaction
- genogram
- legal/bureaucratic mode of transaction
- modes of transaction
- social exchange paradigm
- systems theory
- team—cooperative mode of transaction

Q STUDY QUESTIONS

1. Families may generally be described as
   a. diverse, and only understood one case at a time.
   b. best understood by using intrapsychic theories.
   c. best understood by applying systems paradigms.
   d. atheoretical and chaotic.

2. A genogram is a
   a. multidimensional representation of patterns and dynamics.
   b. multifactorial analysis system.
   c. device used for genetic analysis.
   d. multigenerational analytical tool.

3. Which of the following elements would be required to complete a useful genogram?
   a. Pencil and paper and less than one hour
   b. A data manager system using "Genograx"
   c. A data manager system using SPSS or SAS
   d. A clinician who has a masters degree in statistics

4. Explain the dis-utility of using nursing diagnoses when the nurse works in settings in which there is close interaction among diverse professional groups. Provide the alternative case for using a systems model.

5. Describe how the use of the genogram and a systems perspective keeps ethnocentrism in check and provides a clear understanding of family problems.

■ REFERENCES

Ahrons CR, Miller RB: The effect of postdivorce relationship on paternal involvement, *Am J Orthopsychiatry* 1965; 63:441–450.

Ahluburg & DeVita: New realities of the american family. *Population Bulletin* 1992; 47(2):2–44.

Aries P: *Centuries of Childhood.* New York, Vintage Books, 1962.

Bank & Kahn: *The Sibling Bond.* New York: Basic Books, 1982.

Bredemeier HC: Social Systems Integration and Adaptation. Doctoral Seminars, Rutgers University, New Brunswick, NJ, 1968.

Chan D, Donnan, S, Chan N, Chow G: A microcomputer-based computerized medical record system for a general practice teaching clinic, *J Fam Pract* 1987; 24:5, 537–541.

Gilligan C: *In a Different Voice: Psychological Theory and Women's Development.* Cambridge, Harvard University Press, 1982.

Gough K: The origin of the family, in Skolnick A Skolnick J. (eds): *Family in Transition: Rethinking Marriage, Sexuality, Child Rearing and Family Organization.* Boston, Little, Brown, 1986.

Gray W, Duhl F, Rizzo N. (eds): *General Systems Theory and Psychiatry*. Boston: Little, Brown, 1969.

Grinker R, & Spiegel J: *War Neuroses*. Philadelphia, PA, 1945.

Hareven T: American families in transition: historical perspectives on change, in Walsh, F (ed): *Normal Family Processes*. New York, Guilford Press, 1982.

Like R, Rogers J, McGoldrick M: Reading and interpreting genograms: a systematic approach, *J Fam Pract* 1988; 26:4, 407–412.

McGoldrick M, Pearce J., Giordano J (eds): *Ethnicity and Family Therapy*. New York, Guilford Press, 1982.

Rogers J, Durkin M: The semi-structured genogram interview: I. protocol, II. evaluation *Fam Syst Med* 1984;2:2, 176–187.

Rossi AS: The future in the making: Recent trends in the Work-Family Interface, *Am J Orthopsychiatry* 1993; 63(2):166–176.

Sagan L: Family ties: the real reason that people are living longer, in *Annual Editions: Health, '89/'90*. Connecticut, Dushkin Press, 1989.

Spanier G: The changing profile of the American family. *J Fam Pract* 1981; 13:1, 61–69.

Smoyak S: Family systems: use of genograms as an assessment tool, in Clements J, Buchanan D (eds): *Family Therapy in Perspective*. New York, John Wiley & Sons, 1982.

Smoyak, S: Assessing aging caretakers and their families, in Wright L, Leahey, M (eds): *Families and Chronic Illness,* Springhouse, PA., Springhouse Corporation, 1987.

Smoyak, S: Changing American families, in Hoekelman R, and Friedman S (eds): *Primary Pediatric Care*. St. Louis, MO, Mosby, 1996.

von Bertalanffy L: General System Theory in General Systems 1956 vol. 1., No. 1

von Bertalanffy, L: *General System Theory*. New York, George Braziller, 1968.

Wallerstein J, Blakeslee S. *Second Chances: Men, Women and Children a Decade After Divorce*. New York, Ticknor & Fields, 1989.

Wallerstein J: The early psychological tasks of marriage, *Am J Orthopsychiatry* 1994; 64:640–650.

Walsh F: The clinical utility of normal family research. *Psychotherapy* 1987; 24:35, 496–503

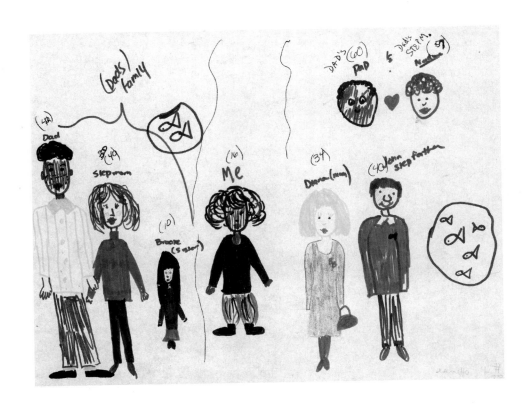

Thus the sum of things is ever being renewed, and mortals live dependent one upon another. Some races increase, others diminish, and in a short space the generations of living creatures are changed and like runners hand on the torch of life.

Lucretius, 99–55 BC

De Rerum Natura, bk. II, 1 75

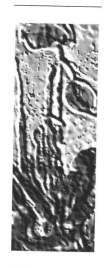

9

Culture, Ethnicity, and Race in Mental Health and Illness

Freida H. Outlaw

The study of the relationship between the provision of psychiatric services and culture, race, ethnicity, and socioeconomic status is not new (Hughes, 1993). According to Berry and colleagues (1994), the discussion of the relationship between psychological theory and culture began in limited, organized fashion just after the Second World War. A proliferation of literature in the past three decades has focused on the ways in which culture, race, ethnicity, and socio-economic status influence the therapeutic process when the therapist and the client differ in these respects. Many clinicians, however, remain unaware of this body of knowledge (Boyd-Franklin, 1989). In order to avoid misdiagnosis, inappropriate treatment, and noncompliance with treatment, the therapist needs to have knowledge of such influences on psychotherapeutic care (Andrews, 1992; Hughes, 1993).

Like many other disciplines, such as psychology and social work, nursing has for at least three decades been concerned with providing sensitive and competent care to culturally, racially, and ethnically diverse patient populations (Outlaw, 1994). The formal area of study called "transcultural nursing" was developed by Leininger during the 1950s, and the study of transcultural nursing was further supported during the 1960s by nurse leaders in the Division of

Nursing who funded nurses for doctoral study in anthropology (Brink, 1990). This cadre of nurse anthropologists was primarily responsible for introducing knowledge about racial, ethnic, and cultural diversity into nursing curricula. (Brink, 1990). Mirroring other disciplines, however, nursing has not consistently embraced the content concerned with cultural diversity because, according to Brink (1990), many nurses have shared the predominant belief in American society that understanding culture, race, and ethnicity is unimportant.

Current migratory patterns and increased birth rates among particular racial and ethnic groups are rapidly changing the demographics of the United States, and will necessitate a change in thinking and behavior among health-care providers about the importance of the cultures of different races and ethnic groups. Clearly, these demographic shifts have already begun to change the characteristics of many patient populations being seen by health-care providers. Moreover, nurses will be called upon with increasing frequency to care for patients who are very different from themselves culturally, racially, and ethnically. The U.S. Bureau of the Census has projected that by the year 2000, one quarter of the United States population will be ethnically non-European persons of color (Andrews, 1992). The following groups will be prominently represented: people of African descent, including African-Americans and African-West Indian Americans; Hispanics, including Mexican-Americans, Cubans, Puerto Ricans, and other Spanish-speaking people; Asian-Americans, including Japanese, Chinese, Filipinos, Koreans, Pacific Islanders, and people of East Indian descent such as Indonesians; and Native Americans, Native Alaskans, and Native Hawaiians (Andrews, 1992; Hacker, 1992).

This chapter examines the rich, complex meanings of culture, race, ethnicity, and socio-economic status in the context of mental health and mental illness. Clinical guidelines are provided for psychiatric nurses and other clinicians to enrich the psychiatric treatment of all patients by increasing the therapist's sensitivity and competence about diversities, while ensuring that the uniqueness of each individual client and family is recognized.

■ DEFINING CULTURE, RACE, AND ETHNICITY

The terms used to address cultural diversity have not been clearly defined and are seldom used in a consistent manner. *Culture* is often used to speak about race, and *minority* is often used to describe persons of low socio-economic status. McAdoo (1993) postulated that these terms are often used interchangeably, with their meanings often confused, or are used as insidious short-hand terms to connote inferiority.

CULTURE

Culture is defined by Chrisman (1991; p 45) as "a learned, shared, and symbolically transmitted design for living." Culture has been determined to be socially acquired and socially transmitted by means of symbols, including customs, techniques, beliefs, institutions, and material objects.

Most definitions of culture support the notion that it is learned, rather than transmitted biologically. This is particularly salient because there is a widely held belief that all members of a particular culture naturally have the same cultural orientations. This belief may be attributed to a misunderstanding about how culture is transmitted. Berry et al. (1994) identified three definitive ways in which culture is transmitted. The passing on of cultural characteristics from one generation to another is called **vertical cultural transmission,** and involves the teaching of values, beliefs, behaviors, and motives by parents to their children. **Horizontal cultural transmission** occurs when individuals learn from their peers. In the United State's society, horizontal transmission is especially evident during the adolescent years. The third type of cultural transmission discussed by Berry et al. (1994) is **oblique cultural transmission,** which takes place when cultural norms are learned from other adults and from institutions either in the individual's culture of origin or from other cultures. If all of a body of teaching and learning takes place within an individual's original culture, the individual is deemed encultured and socialized. When societies were more segregated by race, three or four decades ago, individuals were more likely to be more encultured and socialized than in today's society. However, groups such as the Amish, who for religious and philosophical reasons create more self-contained communities, may be thought of as highly encultured and socialized.

In contrast to enculturation and socialization, acculturation and re-socialization refer to cultural and psychological changes brought about by contact with persons who belong to different cultures and exhibit different behaviors (Berry et al., 1994). Most of us have been acculturated and re-socialized into broader world views, complete with a variety of beliefs, values, behaviors, and motivations. Even in the most isolated, economically deprived communities, television has been responsible for the acculturation and re-socialization of many individuals. It is important to note, then, that members of a particular racial group may not share the same cultural beliefs, values, behaviors, and motivations because of many factors, including their different levels of acculturation and re-socialization. Therefore, when broad statements are made about the impact of culture on one's behavior, beliefs, and values, the important factor to remember is that cultural orientation has to be determined by careful assessment, and should not be assumed simply on the basis of an individual's race or ethnicity.

ETHNICITY

Ethnicity is frequently but inappropriately interchanged with the terms *minority, race,* and *socioeconomic status* (Barthwell, Hewitt, and Jilson, 1995; McAdoo, 1993). McGoldrick (1993) has suggested that people in general have been conditioned to think of ethnicity as referring exclusively to minorities, which makes minorities even more marginalized and peripheral to the dominant social groups within the society. For example, in nursing it is rare to have ethnicity considered as a variable when the patient is white. Ethnicity is defined as "a consciousness of group belonging that is differentiated from others by symbolic markers (culture, biology, territory), that is rooted in bonds of a shared past and perceived ethnic interest" (Spott, 1993; p. 270). Racial groups may comprise a number of ethnic groups who have among themselves relatively distinct cultures. Ethnic groups have been determined to be socially distinguishable by virtue of their cultural orientation, heritage, and distinct sense of difference (Barthwell et al., 1995). For example, what is commonly refered to as the white race of European descent can be distinguished further as consisting of a number of ethnic groups, such as Irish, German, and Italian.

RACE

Race is usually thought of as a more straight-forward concept. Popular definitions of race categorize people by skin color as the marker of difference; white, black, yellow, and red commonly describe divergent groups of people. Race and ethnicity are also used interchangeably, which illustrates the common misconception about these concepts. Race, in the broadest sense, is primarily biologically determined. Ethnic difference, however, can be observed among groups of people who are considered to constitute a single racial group (Hufford, 1994). For example, Gopaul-McNicol (1993) argued that African-Americans and African-West Indian Americans share the same biological/racial African heritage, with skin color as its most obvious marker. However, she strongly suggests that for a care-giver to fail to understand that a black African-West Indian in America has a different ethnic identification and divergent cultural experiences from a person of African descent born in the United States may prevent the formation of a therapeutic alliance. The outcome of a lack of therapeutic alliance in psychiatric care is "mistrust of the therapeutic process, communication difficulties, and ultimately therapeutic resistance" (Gopaul-McNicol, 1993; p. 51). According to Gopaul-McNicol (1993), the most salient difference between the African-American and African-West Indian groups of black people is that 82% of the black population in the West Indies, by the preponderance of their numbers, have been able to retain much of the element of their African culture, which has served to empower them. In contrast, persons of African descent native to the United States have been viewed as a minority group who, in part because of minority status, have had to live and contend with racism.

Important to black West Indian people is that their migration to the United States was voluntary; thus, they can truly be considered immigrants, unlike African-Americans, who are descendants of persons primarily brought to this country as slaves (Gopaul-McNicol, 1993). In order to be able to provide culturally competent care, nurses need to be cognizant that a myriad of ethnic and cultural differences can exist among the members of groups who have been considered as constituting a single race (Hufford, 1994).

The notion of any single race has been refuted by some scientists, who instead define race as a social grouping based on arbitrarily selected physical characteristics (Barthwell, 1995), with socially constructed characteristics established by law and/or social conventions, rather than by anthropologists or biologists (Davis, 1991). The argument about the "social construction" concept of race has further been fueled by those who point out that black people, as well as all races in America, are becoming more racially mixed. According to Davis (1991; p. 29), "from 75 to well over 90 percent of all American blacks apparently have some white ancestry, and up to 25 percent have Indian background."

■ GENERALIZING AND STEREOTYPING

Cookbook approaches to racial, social, or cultural identity based on the structural/functionalism of anthropology can serve to stereotype the group that is being described and cause the caregiver to think about the ethnically, racially, and culturally specific patient in fixed generalizations that are too often reductionistic and negative (Brink, 1990; Browning and Woods, 1993; Outlaw, 1994; Tripp-Reimer and Fox, 1990).

One of the crucial tasks facing nursing has been identified as the development of methods that focus on eliminating racism, racial prejudice, and invidious discrimination from nursing practice (Barbee, 1993; Alleyne, Papadopoulos, and Tilki, 1994). Racism is based on prescribed notions of inferiority and negative behaviors, through attributes assigned to certain groups primarily because of the connection of these beliefs to skin color. According to Barbee (1993), the discussion of race and, concomitantly, the social dimension of racism in nursing is avoided by emphasizing that nurses need to understand cultural diversity and ethnocentrism. Nursing may then avoid racism as a structural and insidious phenomenon supporting, creating, and maintaining the inequalities often experienced by black people and other minorities in all facets of their lives, including their health care. What is important about this is that ethnocentrism implies a cultural bias based on unfamiliarity (Barbee, 1993), which can be eliminated in part by learning about the customs, beliefs, and values of divergent groups, a position often taken in nursing and exemplified by teaching cultural diversity and trans-cultural nursing.

Studies such as those conducted by Flaherty and Meagher (1980) and by Chung, Mahler, and Kakuma (1995) have revealed differences in the in-patient treatment of black and white patients. Flaherty and Meagher (1980) found that black patients were less likely to receive recreational and occupational therapy, receive more medication *pro re nata* (p.r.n.), be placed in seclusion and restraints more often, and receive fewer privileges than white patients. They concluded that these findings could result from a "subtle stereotyping of black patients and a greater familiarity with and preference for white patients by white caregivers, who tend to outnumber black caregivers in most psychiatric settings" (Flaherty and Meagher, 1980).

Chung, Mahler, and Kakuma (1995), replicating the study by Flaherty and colleagues, tried to ascertain whether racial differences and bias continue to exist in in-patient psychiatric units. Although they found that many of the differences in treatment attributed to race as cited in the study by Flaherty and colleagues (1980) were not substantiated, they did find that "African-Americans with high socio-economic status, regardless of diagnosis, were more likely to be tested for use of alcohol or drugs through urine screens, and were more likely to receive a diagnosis of alcohol or substance abuse disorders than comparable whites, despite similar rates of positive urine drug screens in the two racial groups" (Chung, Mahler, and Kakuma, 1995; p. 590). Chung, Mahler, and Kakuma also found that African-Americans with non-psychotic disorders were discharged earlier than white patients with similar disorders, and were more likely to be diagnosed as having a substance-abuse or drug-abuse disorder, whereas non-psychotic white patients were more likely to be diagnosed as having personality disorders. They suggested that many clinicians may view a diagnosed substance-abuse disorder as less treatable than a personality disorder, explaining the earlier discharge of African-American patients (Chung, Mahler, and Kakuma, 1995). Finally, they found that white patients were more likely to be put under one-to-one observation than African-American patients. This has implications for the safety of black patients, since one-to-one observation is an intervention that is usually reserved for suicidal patients.

Subtle stereotyping or negative racial counter-transference on the part of the psychiatric nurse is a factor that will influence the treatment process. Negative racial counter-transference feelings are engendered or aggravated by the exposure of nurses and other health-care providers to newspapers, television, and other media. For instance, because a disproportionate number of media stories report negative events involving black males, a common negative stereotype among nurses may be that black males are more dangerous than other types of patients. It is not uncommon to note that nurses and other clinicians harbor a subtle fear of black male patients (Boyd-Franklin, 1989; Outlaw, 1994). On in-patient psychiatric units, this irrational fear may result in more restrictive treatment of the black male patient, including avoidance of the patient by the nurse and premature seclusion and restraint of the patient.

Giger and Davidhizar (1991), McGoldrick (1984), and Valente (1989) argue that generalizations about ethnic, racial, and cultural patterns serve to familiarize the nurse and other clinicians about the need for expanding their knowledge about a particular racial or ethnic group Guidelines and generalizations are to serve only as "road maps" with which to organize one's thoughts about individuals belonging to various ethnic, racial, and cultural groups. They are not to be inappropriately used as fixed truths (McGoldrick, 1984). McGoldrick (1984) posits that the only effective way in which nurses and other clinicians can expand their knowledge about culturally, racially, and ethnically diverse groups is to create a simple paradigm about each group. The essential factor to remember about such simple paradigms is that they are only guides, and that the nurse must therefore, remain open to new experiences and new information when working with racially, culturally, or ethnically diverse patients, groups, or families. To think of diverse groups in stereotypical ways is counterproductive to treatment, but failure to understand the importance of race, ethnicity, and culture to the individual's or family's understanding of the meaning of and response to the patient's illness is equally counterproductive.

The concepts of race, ethnicity, and culture, and the mitigating concept of socio-economic status, must be understood systematically because they are related in very rich and complex ways. For example, black people in the United States can be racially linked with their African ancestry, yet vary considerably in their ethnicity, culture, and socio-economic status. Most, if not all, however, have been affected by racism at some time in their personal lives, and institutional racism is an ongoing reality for many black people (Barbee, 1993; Billingsley, 1992; Boyd-Franklin, 1989; Pierce, 1975).

■ THE REALITY OF RACISM

Nurses who are racially, culturally, ethnically, and, frequently, socio-economically different from the black patients they are working with need to first accept that racism is an ongoing constant stressor in the lives of their black patients (Barbee, 1993; Outlaw, 1994). When the nurse is white and the patient is black, psychiatric nurses, who are arguably more focused than any other nurses on the establishment of a therapeutic relationship with the patient, must learn to make the subject of racial difference part of the discussion when forming a therapeutic bond. According to Boyd-Franklin (1989), to omit this discussion of racial difference will impede the development of an open, trusting relationship between the white therapist and the black patient. In psychiatric nursing practice, it is imperative that the nurse understand that race, although a factor, does not necessarily determine the patient's ethnic identification or cultural beliefs and values. The first step in providing competent care is to use broad understandings about race, ethnicity, and culture, and to begin to think about the most therapeutic ways in which to approach diverse patients. The psychiatric nurse, however, must move beyond broad guidelines about race, ethnicity, and culture and assess what is reality for the individual patient.

■ THE CHRISMAN MODEL: CULTURE-SENSITIVE CARE

The Chrisman (1991) **culture-sensitive care model** is a parsimonious conceptual framework that takes into account racial, ethnic, and cultural diversity. This model is based on three principles: knowledge, mutual respect, and negotiation. The knowledge that the clinician needs about the racial, ethnic, and cultural identity of the patient is based on information about the patient in his or her cultural context (Chrisman, 1991). According to Chrisman (1991), respect for the patient's beliefs, values, and behaviors is more likely to develop when the nurse becomes knowledgeable about these features of the patient. Negotiation is interdependent with knowledge and mutual respect: the nurse with crucial knowledge about cultural diversity will be able to make cultural assessments the patient that facilitate promotion of those cultural factors that are helpful to the patient while encouraging him or her to accept treatment interventions that may have *previously* been rejected by the patient (Chrisman, 1991). A map or guideline describing African Americans, one of America's largest culturally, racially, ethnically diverse groups, will be highlighted. Nurses can use this and other models for gathering knowledge about culturally and ethnically diverse groups with whom they come into contact in their clinical work.

GAINING KNOWLEDGE

Chrisman (1991) suggests that knowledge about patients in their cultural contexts can be obtained by reading books and articles about particular cultural groups. More specific information about the patient's ethnicity and cultural beliefs and values can be learned from talking and listening to patients and their family members. Boyd-Franklin (1989) invites white therapists to avoid thinking of black patients in stereotypical ways by encouraging their black patients to share their experiences of being black in American society. The following case study illustrates this point:

The key to gaining specific knowledge about the patient in this case study is that the young nurse introduced the subject of an obvious difference between herself and the patient, and then listened to the patient's response The intervention opened a dialogue about racism and invidious discrimination, about which she had no first-hand knowledge, but which had been a very painful part of the patient's life experiences. The outcome was that the patient benefited from talking about a painful subject with a young white woman, and the nurse learned something about the patient's racial experiences that helped her to understand him better. Another case study in which knowledge about a particular racial and ethnic group benefited both the patient and the nurse is the following:

Failure to understand how African-Americans in general have been influenced by religious beliefs in the development of their psyches is a serious mistake that therapists often made when treating them for psychiatric problems (Boyd-Franklin, 1989). She has postulated that the deep-rooted spirituality of the majority of the black population across socio-economic classes in the United States stems from the African tradition, in which spirituality and religion are an integral part of the culture. The black church has historically been an institution that serves many functions in the black community, including religious teaching and leadership development, while also serving as a cultural and economic resource (Aponte, 1994; Billingsley, 1992; Boyd-Franklin, 1989). The black church remains the institution of connecteness and validation for many black people regardless of their socio-economic status or position in society, thereby serving a vital social function for black people in America.

Knox (1985) views spirituality as a coping mechanism that needs careful assessment in terms of its use in therapeutic work with black patients and their families. In working with black patients and their families, she uses a spiritual reframing, in which the patients and families employ statements such as "The Lord will give me no more than I can bear" as a coping mechanism. This type of coping was found to be used extensively by black patients in a qualitative study recently done by Outlaw and Johnston Taylor (1996), in which cancer patients were asked about their prayer beliefs and behaviors as evidenced in statements such as "God will take care of me no matter what the outcome of this illness." Boyd-Franklin (1989) argues that failure to recognize such statements as reflecting a generalized spiritual orientation and representing a legitimate method of coping that is almost universally used by black people may be detrimental to the therapeutic process.

ESTABLISHING MUTUAL RESPECT

The importance of the nurse's knowledge about the patient as a basis for the development of mutual respect is illustrated by a case study in which the nurse learned about the pain and suffering a black patient had endured as a result of racist and discriminatory practices. She demonstrated caring by asking questions about their differences and listening to the patient describe his experiences. Boyd-Franklin (1989) suggests that listening to the patient is the most important function of the clinician who is working with a racially and culturally specific patient. It is counterproductive to the establishment of a mutually respectful relationship to try to minimize the patient's experience or to try to identify with that experience on the basis of similar experiences.

Simple appropriate behaviors such as how the clinician greets a patient often foster respect from racially and ethnically distinct patients. The initial greeting is the beginning of the joining process, which Minuchin and Fishman (1981) believe is the foundation from which the rest of the therapeutic process will develop. Often, nurses call patients by their first names in an effort to appear more informal, believing that such demonstrations of familiarity will foster an atmosphere of trust and put the patient and the family at ease. For most black patients, especially the elderly, this type of informal greeting can impede the joining process. The greeting is seen as disrespectful, and is symbolic of a time when the patient was not treated with dignity. The

following excerpt illustrates the magnitude of this feeling among many black people:

Boyd-Franklin (1989) writes extensively about the role of respect, which is crucial to the establishment of a therapeutic relationship when the therapist is white and the patient and family are black. She cautions that clinicians both black or white who presume to know about the experiences of black people may have their behaviors resulting from their perceptions interpreted by the patient as disrespectful. Instead, she advises that the clinician assume that each black patient and family is unique and let them teach the clinician about their particular ethnic and cultural beliefs and values. Therefore, prior general knowledge about the meaning of race, ethnicity, and culture (the first step of the Chrisman model) is used as a guideline for what needs to be explored in therapy sessions specifically pertaining to patients and their families. Patient respect for the clinician is earned when clinicians can actively listen to patients and their families without assuming that they know the patients' or families' experiences. Boyd-Franklin (1989) has found that black families in particular are constantly evaluating the therapist's credibility.

Boyd-Franklin (1989) advises that the nurse or therapist refrain from trying to "save the patient and his/her family" or to being over-zealous about taking care of "these poor people," since these behaviors are patronizing and insulting. Such behaviors are very detrimental to the establishment of a personal connection, which has been identified as necessary when working with all families, but especially with black patients and their families because of their frequently negative experiences with the health-care system (Aponte, 1994; Boyd-Franklin, 1989).

The clinician's respect for the racially, culturally, and ethnically different patient has to spring from an examination of his or her own culture and ethnic ori-

E CASE EXAMPLE

After several non-productive visits to a long-term care facility to see an elderly black male patient who had been diagnosed as depressed, a student nurse presented the case in a clinical seminar. After a lengthy discussion, the suggestion was made that perhaps the differences between the patient and the nurse needed to be addressed. The student was encouraged to begin with a sentence such as "You may be wondering what interest a young white woman has in you." The statement was enough to open up the dialogue

and subsequently the relationship between the nurse and the patient. In later meetings the patient was able to share many past instances of being discriminated against. He was also able to describe his initial discomfort about being in a room alone with a young white woman, a situation that would have been unthinkable in the segregated South where he grew up.

E CASE EXAMPLE

A black patient presented for her appointment at a psychiatric clinic, stating that "while praying at church on Sunday the Lord had told her what to do" about a decision she had to make. The psychiatrist who saw the patient was immediately alarmed and wanted to increase the psychotropic medications the patient was taking. After a consultation with the nurse-clinical specialist, who was African-American, it was decided that a more detailed assessment of the patient's mental status would be done before her medication was changed. It was determined upon further assessment that the patient was not experiencing an exacerbation of symptoms, but was describing a religious experience.

---

gins, including beliefs, values, and prejudices. Clinicians' examination of their own ethnocentric beliefs will help them to develop insight into how their personal beliefs, values, and prejudices influence their therapeutic responses.

NEGOTIATING TREATMENT

According to Chrisman (1991) adherence to the tenets of knowledge and mutual respect—the first two tenets of his model for working with ethnic, racial, and culturally distinct patients—will facilitate the third and last step in the model: negotiation between the patient and clinician about the patient's treatment plan. The ability to maintain a non-reactive, non-judgmental posture when negotiating with patients about their health- and illness-related beliefs, values, and practices has been noted by Valente, (1989) to encourage patients' to disclose their cultural beliefs and practices. The clinician can use broad knowledge and respect for the patient's culture, racial identity, and ethnicity to make the provision of care more culturally sensitive and competent. The following example illustrates a negotiation process between a clinician and a patient about an issue of treatment:

In this example, the patient had been assessed as being very depressed as well as having many family problems with a husband who was unavailable emotionally, and with a daughter who presented a behavioral problem. The patient also had many financial problems and lived in substandard housing. In order to relate to the patient, the nurse had to be careful not to be critical of the patient's situation, and to be respectful of her statement that she would use her religion to solve her problems. The nurse was also mindful of having to demonstrate respect for the patient's home and religious beliefs in order to establish a therapeutic relationship.

The Chrisman model for providing culturally sensitive and competent care is useful for psychiatric nurses because it provides broad guidelines that are simple to follow and can be used by novices and experienced psychiatric nurses alike. It also can be used by psychiatric nurses who are working with groups, as well as individuals or families. In addition, the model can be linked with other conceptual frameworks that guide the nurse's practice, such as family systems theory or psychoanalytic theory. Finally, it can be operationalized without adding to the nurse's work-load.

E CASE EXAMPLE

I don't remember my mother ever calling my father by his first name, Henry. He was always "Mr. Delany" or "Your Pa." Now, I do recall that my father would call my mother "Miss Nan" in private moments, but he usually called her Mrs. Delany in front of everybody, including us children. Now you might think this seems a bit formal. But the reason they did this is that colored people were always called by their first names in that era. It was a way of treating them with less dignity. What Mama and Papa were doing was blocking that. Most people never learned their first names. (Delany, Delany, and Hearth, 1994; p. 9).

E CASE EXAMPLE

A psychiatric nurse had been asked to make a home visit to a 46-year-old obese, black woman with multiple physical problems who had been described by the medical-surgical nurse as possibly depressed. When the nurse arrived at the patient's home, she found the patient in a very dark, unkempt house, with the religion cable-television channel playing very loudly. When the nurse explained to the patient that her primary nurse had thought that she might benefit from talking with the psychiatric nurse, the patient responded by saying that "all her problems she talked over with God and therefore she did not need further help." The nurse, using her knowledge about the role that religion might play in this poor black patient's life, and being aware that demonstrating respect for the patient's beliefs was very important if a nurse-to-patient connection was to be made, acknowledged that "it was important that she felt connected to God since it sounded as if that was a source of constant comfort." The nurse reminded the patient that "God works in mysterious ways and that perhaps she could also benefit from working with the psychiatric nurse who was available to listen and assist her to solve problems. After further discussion, the patient agreed that talking with the nurse might be helpful. She also decided that the nurse might be someone with whom her daughter would like to talk.

O AN OVERVIEW

- Culture is learned, not biologically transmitted.
- Culture can be learned and transmitted vertically, horizontally, or obliquely.
- Ethnicity is defined as group membership that is differentiated by biology, culture, and territory and solidified by a shared past and common interest.
- Racial groups are comprised of many distinct ethnic groups.
- Cook-book approaches to culturally, racially, and ethnically diverse patients can serve to stereotype them.
- Subtle stereotyping of the patient on the part of the nurse negatively influences the treatment process.
- Guidelines and generalizations can be useful, but become stereotypes when they are accepted as fixed truths.
- Nurses must remain open to new experiences and new information when working with diverse groups of patients.
- Personal and institutional racism is an ongoing reality for people of color.
- Nurses need to be cognizant of the racism that is a constant stressor in the lives of the black patients for whom they care.
- The Chrisman culture-sensitive care model is a parsimonious framework to guide nursing practice when the nurse and the patient are racially, culturally, or ethnically different.

TD TERMS TO DEFINE

- Chrisman Model
- culture
- ethnicity
- race
- racism
- stereotyping

Q STUDY QUESTIONS

1. Discuss the three principles of the Chrisman culture-sensitive model. Discuss clinical examples in which these three principles may be used to provide more culturally competent care to diverse groups of patients.

2. Discuss the differences in the concepts of race, ethnicity, and culture.

3. In a recent health-care publication, race was defined as: African-American, Puerto Rican, Cuban, Mexican American. Discuss the use of race in this context. Us-

ing the information in this chapter, how would you describe these groups of patients?

4. Discuss the rationale for discussing race with the patient when the patient belongs to a racial group different from that of the nurse.

5. Discuss at least one factor that the nurse must consider in order to provide culturally sensitive care to a patient who is racially, ethnically, or culturally different from the nurse.

■ REFERENCES

Alleyne J, Papadopoulos I, Tilki M: Antiracism within transcultural nurse education. *Br J Nurs* 1994; 3 (12):635–637.

Andrews MM: Cultural perspectives on Nursing in the 21st century. *J Prof Nurs* 1992; 8 (11):7–15.

Aponte HJ: *Bread & Spirit: Therapy With the New Poor: Diversity of Race, Culture, and Values.* New York: WW Norton Company, 1994.

Barbee E: Racism in US Nursing. *Med Anthropol Q* 1993; 7:346–362.

Barthwell A, Hewitt W, Jilson I: An introduction to ethnic and cultural diversity. *Pediatr Clin North Am* 1995; 42 (2):431–451.

Berry JW, Poortinga YH, Segal MH, Dasen PR. (eds): *Cross-cultural Psychology: Research and Applications.* Cambridge University Press. 1994.

Billingsley A: *Climbing Jacob's Ladder: The Enduring Legacy of African-American Families.* New York: Simon and Schuster, 1992.

Boyd-Franklin N: *Black Families in Therapy: A Multisystems Approach.* New York, Guilford Press, 1989.

Brink P: Cultural diversity in nursing: How much can we tolerate?, in McCloskey JC, Grace HK (eds): *Current Issues in Nursing.* St. Louis, CV Mosby, 1990, pp. 521–527.

Browning M, Woods J: Cross-cultural family-nurse partnerships, in Feetham S, Meister S, Bell J, Gilliss C. (eds): *The Nursing of Families: Theory, Research, Education, Practice* Newbury Park, California, Sage Publishers, 1993, pp. 177–187.

Chrisman NJ: Cultural systems, in Baird S, McCorkle R, Grant M (eds): *Cancer Nursing: A Comprehensive Textbook.* Philadelphia, WB Saunders, 1991, pp. 45–53.

Chung H, Mahler JC, Kakuma T: Racial treatment differences in treatment of psychiatric inpatients. *Psychiatr Serv* 1995; 46 (6):586–591.

Davis JL: *Who is Black? One Nation's Definition.* University Park, Pennsylvania: The Pennsylvania State University Press, 1991.

Delaney S, Delaney A, Hearth A: *Having Our Say: The Delaney Sisters First 100 Years.* New York: Kodansha International, 1994.

Flaherty J, Meagher R: Measuring racial bias in inpatient treatment. *Am J Psychiatry* 1980; 137 (6):679–682.

Giger J, Davidhizar R: *Transcultural Nursing: Assessment and Intervention.* St. Louis, Mosby-Year Book, 1991.

Gopaul-McNicol SA: *Working With West Indian Families.* New York, Guilford Press, 1993.

Hacker A: *Two Nations: Black and White: Separate, Hostile, Unequal.* New York, Ballantine Books, 1992.

Hufford D: Terms central to the discussions of folk medicine: Notes on culture and ethnicity. *Behav Sci* 1994; 2:1–5.

Hughes C: Culture in clinical psychiatry, in Gaw AC (ed): *Culture, Ethnicity and Mental Illness.* Washington, DC, Psychiatric Press, 1993 pp. 3–41.

Knox DH: Spirituality: A tool in the assessment and treatment of Black alcoholics and their families. *Alcohol Treat Q* 1985; 2(3/4):31–44.

McAdoo HP: *Ethnic Families: Strengths That Are Found in Diversity.* Newbury Park, California, Sage Publications, 1993.

McGoldrick M: Normal families: An ethnic perspective, in Walsh F (ed): *Normal Family Processes.* New York, Guilford Press, 1984, pp. 399–421.

McGoldrick M: Ethnicity, cultural diversity and normality. In Walsh F. (ed): *Normal Family Processes.* 2nd edition. New York, Guilford Press, 1993, pp. 331–360.

Minuchin S, Fishman C: *Family Therapy Techniques.* Cambridge, MA, Harvard University Press, 1981.

Outlaw FH: A reformulation of the meaning of culture, and ethnicity for nurses delivering care. *MEDSURG Nurs* 1994; 3 (2):108–111.

Outlaw FH, Johnston Taylor E: Prayer among persons with cancer: A phenomenological investigation. Unpublished raw data. 1996.

Pierce C: The mundane extreme environmental stress: The case of black families in white America, in Brainard SG (ed): *Learning Disabilities: Issues and Recommendation for Research.* Washington, DC: Institute of Education, 1975, pp. 1–23.

Spott J: (1993). The black box in family assessment: Cultural diversity, in Feetham S, Meister S, Bell J, Gilliss C (eds): *The Nursing of Families: Theory, Research, Education, Practice.* California, Sage Publications, 1993, pp. 189–199.

Tripp-Reimer T, Fox S: (1990) Beyond the concept of culture, in McCloskey JC, Grace HK (eds): *Current Issues in Nursing.* St. Louis, CV Mosby, 1990, pp. 542–546.

Valente S: Overcoming cultural barriers. *Calif Nurse* 1989; 85 (8):4–5.

Yancey WL, Ericksen EP, Juliani RN: Emergent ethnicity: A review and reformulation. *Am Sociol Rev* 1976; 41 (3):391–403.

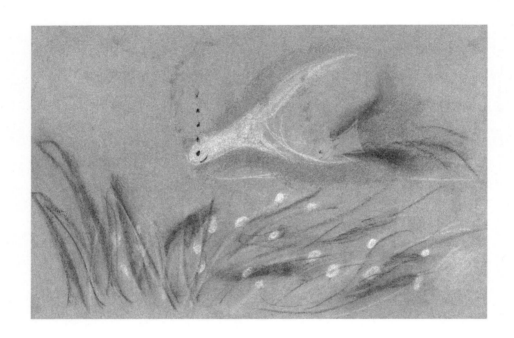

Man found that he was faced with the acceptance of "spiritual" forces, that is to say such forces as cannot be apprehended by the senses, particularly not by sight, and yet having undouted, even extremely strong, effects.

Ernest Jones
Life and Works of Sigmund Freud, vol. 1 (1953) ch. 1

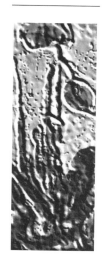

10
Spirituality and Patient Care
Verna Benner Carson

Humankind has traditionally debated and philosophized about the purpose of life. In the opening line of his best-selling book, *The Road Less Traveled*, Peck (1978) wrote, "Life is difficult." The success of Peck's book seems to suggest that the need for a personal spirituality, for finding meaning and purpose in life, and for reconciling its injustices is both universal and ongoing. Sidney Jourard, author of *The Transparent Self*, is quoted as saying:

> Man needs reasons for living and if there are none, he begins to die . . . man is incurably religious. What varies among men is what they are religious about. Whatever a person takes to be the highest value in life can be regarded as his God, the focus and purpose of his time and life. *(Stoll, 1979)*

With Jourard's observations in mind, it seems easy to understand the common practice, among both lay persons and professionals, of using the terms religion and spirituality interchangeably. To avoid obscuring the more vital, central, and universal issues of concern to patients—those related to meaning and purpose—and other human experiences—several terms are defined below.

■ SPIRITUALITY: DEFINITION

For some people, religion provides the structure within which they express their spirituality; for others, there is little connection between the two. Individuals may not embrace a formal faith tradition, yet may be very spiritual; or they may be regular church attendees with little spiritual development.

For the purposes of this text, **spirituality** is the umbrella under which religion and religiosity stand. Spirituality encompasses a personal relationship with a higher being. It involves transcendent values such as truth, beauty, and love, and a commitment to spiritual principles for one's life, such as truthfulness, caring, and affirming others in what they do. Spiritual qualities include attributes of gentleness, tolerance, patience, forbearance, and forgiveness (Carson, 1989).

Religiosity encompasses a chosen religious belief system, active participation within a church, adherence to religious principles, and embracing the principles and values of one's church.

■ SPIRITUAL WELL-BEING

The National Interfaith Coalition on Aging (NICA) defines **spiritual well-being** as "the affirmation of life in a relationship with God, self, community, and environment which nurtures and celebrates wholeness." Spiritual well-being implies spiritual and psychological health, expressed through the experience of feeling alive, purposeful, and fulfilled.

The benefits of spiritual well-being include a sense of inner peace, serenity, and harmony within one's person. There is an expressed belief in a God, and a reverence for and sense of purpose to one's life. There are feelings of compassion and concern for others, a deep sense of gratitude, and acceptance of one's experiences and relationships as being meaningful and enriching.

■ PROFESSIONALS' AMBIVALENCE

Over time, a disparity has developed between the importance attached to spirituality and religiosity by patients as compared with mental-health professionals. Many patients use mental-health professionals concurrently with a religious advisor (i.e., priest. minister, rabbi) to help meet their needs. Patients report that they use prayer and scripture as a source of support, and that religious services, practices, and beliefs give them something to hang onto when their situations appear hopeless.

Some mental-health professionals have either ignored or disparaged the spiritual and/or religious realm, which perhaps has roots in Freud's belief that religion was a panacea for the masses. Sometimes, mental-health professionals dismiss issues of spirituality and religious belief as irrelevant to the care of an individual who is struggling with a psychiatric illness. This approach ignores a major source of strength and integration in the patient. Holistic care deals with more than broken minds, it addresses broken bodies, hearts, and souls.

Some mental-health professionals, however, have specifically focused on or addressed patients' spiritual values. Victor Frankl and Carl Jung recognized the importance of spiritual issues. Moreover, many mental-health professional organizations support and recognize the religious and spiritual needs and concerns of patients, (e.g., the American Nurses Association [ANA] and the American Psychiatric Association). For years there has been a group of psychologists in the American Psychological Association who have supported the notion of integrating spirituality and/or religious belief into therapy, and have advocated research into this area.

■ PSYCHIATRIC NURSES AND SPIRITUAL CARE

The importance of spiritual care is stated in the ANA 1994 *Standards of Psychiatric Mental Health Clinical Practice*, which lists phenomena of concern as: "interpersonal, systemic, sociocultural, spiritual, or environmental circumstances or events which affect the mental and emotional well-being of the individual family, or community."

The importance of spiritual care is also stated in the ANA *Standards of Care on Assessment*. These standards state, that "data may include but are not limited to spiritual or philosophical beliefs and values," and the *Standard on Diagnosis* states that "diagnoses identify actual or potential psychiatric illness and mental health problems of (patients) pertaining to interpersonal systemic; sociocultural, spiritual or environmental circumstances; or events which have an effect of the mental and emotional well-being of the individual family, or community."

Spiritual issues are mentioned in the ANA *Code for Nurses* (1985) with regard to respecting human dignity, recognizing everyone's equal right to health care regardless of national, ethnic, religious, racial, cultural, political, economic, developmental, role, and sexual differences. Nurses enable the patient to live with as much physical, emotional, and spiritual comfort as possible, and they support the values that the patient has treasured in life. NANDA lists two diagnoses, spiritual distress and potential for enhanced spiritual well-being. (See Appendix A.)

Research supports the importance of spiritual and religious issues to psychiatric patients. Lower rates of hospitalization were noted among patients with schizophrenia who either attended church or were given supportive after-care by religious care-givers and ministers. In fact, participation in religious worship resulted in significant reductions in a wide variety of psychiatric symptoms including depression and anxiety. A lack of religious commitment was documented as a risk factor for substance abuse (Larson and Larson, 1991).

A growing body of nursing research supports the nurse's role in promoting spiritual well-being, especially with regard to the promotion of prayer and its effects. Also, repeated Gallup surveys indicate that over 90% of Americans pray daily and believe that prayer affects their lives. In addition, the *Journal of Psychology and Theology,* published by Biola University in California, explores the integration of mental health and religion.

SELF-ASSESSMENT

One basic obstacle to effectively dealing with spiritual needs arising from within the self or others is that the exploration and resolution of such needs require an individual to confront his or her limitations. Fish and Shelley (1978) observe that "illness, suffering, and death serve to remind us that we are not very sufficient unto ourselves, but are, indeed, very human and very helpless."

It seems obvious that a primary requisite for effectively managing one's own spiritual needs or those of others is to acknowledge the legitimacy and universality of these needs for all persons. Self-assessment, the process of getting in touch with one's own spiritual beliefs and values, is thus essential for the clarification and integration of such beliefs and values into one's own life. It is also important for the resolution of underlying, dormant conflicts that might otherwise become manifest within the context of the therapeutic relationship.

Nurses can assess their individual attitudes and beliefs about religion and spirituality. Consider the following story.

A believer and a skeptic went for a walk. The skeptic said, "Look at all the trouble and misery in the world after thousands of years of religion. What good is religion?" His companion noticed a child, filthy with grime, playing in the gutter. He said, "We've had soap for generation after generation and yet look

---

1. MALE ___ FEMALE ___
2. AGE ___
3. MARRIED ___ SINGLE ___ WIDOWED ___ DIVORCED ___
4. WOULD YOU RATE YOUR OVERALL HEALTH AS
   EXCELLENT ___ GOOD ___ FAIR ___ POOR ___
5. PLEASE CHECK YOUR RELIGION OR BELIEF SYSTEM:
   CATHOLIC ___   OTHER RELIGION ___
   PROTESTANT ___   AGNOSTIC OR SKEPTIC ___
   OTHER CHRISTIAN ___   ATHEIST ___
   JEWISH ___
6. DO YOU HAVE A PERSONAL RELATIONSHIP WITH GOD?
   YES ___ NO ___ NOT SURE ___
7. HOW IMPORTANT TO YOU IS ATTENDING RELIGIOUS SERVICES?
   VERY IMPORTANT ___   IMPORTANT ___
   SOMEWHAT IMPORTANT ___   NOT IMPORTANT ___
8. HOW OFTEN WOULD YOU ATTEND RELIGIOUS SERVICE IF ABLE?
   NOT AT ALL ___ ONCE A YEAR ___ SEVERAL TIMES A YEAR ___
   ONCE A MONTH ___ ONCE A WEEK ___
9. HOW OFTEN DO YOU USUALLY ATTEND RELIGIOUS SERVICE?
   NOT AT ALL ___   ONCE A YEAR ___
   SEVERAL TIMES A YEAR ___ ONCE A MONTH ___
   ONCE A WEEK ___   MORE THAN ONCE A WEEK ___
10. I WOULD DESCRIBE MYSELF IN RELATION TO SPIRITUAL WELL-BEING AS FOLLOWS:
   _____
   _____

Figure 10–1. Demographic survey on spirituality.

DIRECTIONS. Please insert the choice that best describes how much you agree with each statement. There is no right or wrong choice.

    1. Strongly agree   4. Disagree
    2. Moderately agree   5. Moderately disagree
    3. Agree   6. Strongly disagree

1. PRAYER IS AN IMPORTANT PART OF MY LIFE ___
2. I BELIEVE I HAVE SPIRITUAL WELL-BEING. ___
3. AS I GROW OLDER, I FIND MYSELF MORE TOLERANT OF OTHERS' BELIEFS. ___
4. I FIND MEANING AND PURPOSE IN MY LIFE. ___
5. I FEEL THERE IS A CLOSE RELATIONSHIP BETWEEN MY SPIRITUAL BELIEFS AND WHAT I DO. ___
6. I BELIEVE IN AN AFTERLIFE. ___
7. WHEN I AM SICK I HAVE LESS SPIRITUAL WELL-BEING. ___
8. I BELIEVE IN A SUPREME POWER. ___
9. I AM ABLE TO RECEIVE AND GIVE LOVE TO OTHERS. ___
10. I AM SATISFIED WITH MY LIFE. ___
11. I SET GOALS FOR MYSELF. ___
12. GOD HAS LITTLE MEANING IN MY LIFE. ___
13. I AM SATISFIED WITH THE WAY I AM USING MY ABILITIES. ___
14. PRAYER DOES NOT HELP ME IN MAKING DECISIONS. ___
15. I AM ABLE TO APPRECIATE DIFFERENCES IN OTHERS. ___
16. I AM PRETTY WELL PUT TOGETHER. ___
17. I PREFER THAT OTHERS MAKE DECISIONS FOR ME. ___
18. I FIND IT HARD TO FORGIVE OTHERS. ___
19. I ACCEPT MY LIFE SITUATIONS. ___
20. BELIEF IN A SUPREME BEING HAS NO PART IN MY LIFE. ___
21. I CANNOT ACCEPT CHANGE IN MY LIFE. ___

Figure 10–2. Jarel spiritual well-being scale. (Hungelman, Kenkell-Rossi, Klassen, 1989.)

1. THE INDIVIDUAL'S NEED FOR A MEANINGFUL PHILOSOPHY OF LIFE
   (A challenging object of self-investment is being met)
   a. What is important to you in life right now?
      If the person responds with nothing . . .
      Ask: What was important to you?
   b. What does "being old" mean to you? Do you consider yourself old?
2. SOURCE OF HOPE
   a. Do you think your life has become better or worse as you have grown older? Why?
   b. Do you foresee your life as better or worse in the future?
   c. When you're discouraged or feeling hopeless, what keeps you going? Where have you found strength in the past?
3. TRUSTING RELATIONSHIPS WITH GOD, PEOPLE AND NATURE (Your relationship with God, People and Nature: How do you keep it together? What is the person's image of God?)
   a. Do you believe in a power greater than yourself? Can you tell me about that power (i.e., Who or what it is?)?
   b. Do you feel more like being alone or with other people right now?
4. SELF ACTUALIZATION
   a. How much control do you believe you have over what happens to you in life?
   b. To what extent do you believe other forces play a role in what happens to you in life?
   c. Do you have a personal means for meeting your inner spiritual needs? Describe it.
   d. What do you believe about death?
   e. What are your special creative abilities?
   f. Tell me what beauty means to you? What is there in the world that you consider beautiful?

Figure 10–3. Assessment of spiritual awareness.

how dirty that child is. Of what value is soap?" "But soap cannot do any good unless it is applied," protested the skeptic. "Exactly," replied the believer.

In considering their own spiritual and religious beliefs, do nurses view themselves as believers or skeptics? If they are believers, then in what do they believe? If they are skeptics, what are they skeptical about?

In implementing their role in assisting patients with spiritual care psychiatric nurses have a two-fold responsibility: they must be willing to discuss spirituality with the patient and to discuss the patient's relationship with God.

■ ASSESSING PATIENTS' SPIRITUAL AND RELIGIOUS NEEDS

The nature of a patient's spiritual and religious beliefs, as well as the reciprocal relationship between the beliefs and the patient's current illness or life situation, can be systematically assessed as part of the nursing admission history. Such an assessment includes more than inquiry into the patient's religious group affiliation. The assessment could range from implementing a religiogram (see Chapter 14 on In-Patient Assessment) to the use of a brief assessment survey on spirituality (Figure 10–1).

Other assessment tools designed to more comprehensively assess the spirituality needs of patients are shown in Figures 10–2, 10–3, and 10–4).

For each of the following statements, circle the choice that best indicates the extent of your agreement or disagreement as it describes your personal experience.

SA = Strong Agree   D = Disagree
MA = Moderately Agree   MD = Moderately Disagree
A = Agree   SD = Strong Disagree

1. I don't find much satisfaction in private prayer with God.
   SA   MA   A   D   MD   SD
2. I don't know who I am, where, I cam from, or where I'm going.
   SA   MA   A   D   MD   SD
3. I believe that God loves me and cares about me.
   SA   MA   A   D   MD   SD
4. I feel that We is a positive experience.
   SA   MA   A   D   MD   SD
5. I believe that God is impersonal and not interested in my daily situations.
   SA   MA   A   D   MD   SD
6. I feel unsettled about my future.
   SA   MA   A   D   MD   SD
7. I have a personally meaningful relationship with God.
   SA   MA   A   D   MD   SD
8. I feel very fulfilled and satisfied with life.
   SA   MA   A   D   MD   SD
9. I don't get much personal strength and support from my God.
   SA   MA   A   D   MD   SD
10. I feel a sense of well-being about the direction my life is headed in.
    SA   MA   A   D   MD   SD
11. I believe that God is concerned about my problems.
    SA   MA   A   D   MD   SD
12. I don't enjoy much about life.
    SA   MA   A   D   MD   SD
13. I don't have a personally satisfying relationship with God.
    SA   MA   A   D   MD   SD
14. I feel good about my future.
    SA   MA   A   D   MD   SD
15. My relationship with God helps me not to feel lonely.
    SA   MA   A   D   MD   SD
16. I feel that life is full of conflict and unhappiness.
    SA   MA   A   D   MD   SD
17. I feel most fulfilled when I'm in close communion with God.
    SA   MA   A   D   MD   SD
18. Life doesn't have much meaning.
    SA   MA   A   D   MD   SD
19. My relation with God contributes to my sense of well-being.
    SA   MA   A   D   MD   SD
20. I believe there is some real purpose for my life.
    SA   MA   A   D   MD   SD

Source: Ellison, C. (1983) Spiritual well-being: Conceptualization and measurement. *J Psychol Theology* 11(4), 330–340.

Figure 10–4. Assessment of spiritual well-being.

SPIRITUAL AWARENESS TOOL

The spiritual awareness tool developed by Hopkins, and colleagues (1994) is derived primarily from the work of Ivy (1985), who based his assessment on the works of James Fowler, Robert Kegan, and the constructivist/developmental model of psychology. This model recognizes that people construct meaning from their experiences. The model is developmental in that it recognizes

E CASE EXAMPLES

Although it is beyond the scope of this chapter to present a detailed discussion of nursing interventions relevant to spiritual and/or religious needs, three case excerpts are offered to assist the reader in this aspect of nursing practice.

▶ CASE 1

Patient: Since John died I have no reason to go on. It's just no use.

Nurse: I hear how hopeless you feel now about your loss. What about John do you miss the most?

Patient: I guess the way that he made me feel important and special.

Nurse: I can see how you would miss such a feeling. What are some of the ways he did that?

Patient: He would tell me how much he enjoyed my cooking, and he would just look at me with such love in his eyes.

Nurse: It is hard to realize that neither of these things will happen again and that no one can exactly take his place.

Patient: It really is. We were married thirty years.

Nurse: I wonder what it would take for you to allow what he gave you to become part of you so you could continue to feel that way.

Patient: I guess I would have to admit to myself that I really am important and special. Though I miss him a lot, I can go on.

Nurse: You and I can talk again about what you received from him that you will never lose, what you still need and will have to find other ways to get, and maybe what you need to let go of that only he could give.

Patient: I think John would have wanted me to do that. It won't be easy, but I am willing to try.

This discussion highlights an important issue in terms of spiritual care and that is that much spiritual care is done without overt mention of God or religion. In this example, the nurse is assisting the patient to examine the source of her feelings that her life lacks purpose and meaning. Without her spouse, John, there seems to be no overreaching "why" that motivates her to continue living. John, through his love, made her feel important and special. Without John, the patient's challenge is to re-define her purpose and meaning and to recognize that her specialness and importance did not cease to exist when John died.

▶ CASE 2

Patient: Even God doesn't care anymore. I used to think I could count on Him.

Nurse: What happened to change your being able to count on God?

Patient: I feel so useless. Since my son left home and got married, I don't feel needed.

Nurse: You said God doesn't care anymore. I wonder whether you also think your son doesn't care because he does not need you in the same way he did.

Patient: I guess so. My son used to tell me how he could not get along without me.

Nurse: I wonder whether your feeling that God does not care could be related to your feeling useless and thinking that your son does not count on you anymore.

Patient: Gosh, maybe. I don't really want my son to continue to need me. I want him to grow up, but it is hard to let him go.

Nurse: It is. Maybe it would help if you and I talk again about the changes that have taken place, what your beliefs are about them, and what you can do to get your needs met.

In this example, the patient's feelings of uselessness are related not only to her son's growing independence from her but also to beliefs about God. The patient's initial comment, "Even God doesn't care anymore. I used to think I could count on Him" is not an uncommon response from people who are hurting. They conclude that He is as much a part of the problem as what ever the actual source of suffering is. In this case, the sense of separation the patient is feeling from her son is mirrored by a sense of separation from God. One of the challenges facing this patient is to recognize that separation and independence are not synonymous with cessation of love, concern, or a broken relationship either with a significant other or with God.

▶ CASE 3

Patient: I really feel guilty for the way I treated my mother.

Nurse: What did you do?

Patient: She asked me to continue with the same church she went to and I didn't. When I married my husband I changed to his church.

Nurse: Talk about how it happened.

Patient: I learned what his beliefs were and I found that they fit with my experience of God. I really feel this is where I belong.

Nurse: It sounds like you feel guilty because you did not meet your mother's expectations. However, you acted courageously on your own beliefs.

Patient: Yes, I do not feel guilty about that—only because my mother does not understand. So I just avoid the issue with her.

Nurse: What do you think you could do to relieve your guilt?

Patient: Now that I think about it, what I feel the most guilty about is that I now don't talk about religion to her at all, and that was important to both of us. I would feel better if I could talk over with her how I came to believe the way I do and how it feels right to me. Even if she still does not understand, I will feel relief.

Nurse: That sounds like a helpful plan. Let me know how it goes.

that people change over time, and that the way in which they use criteria to construct meaning also changes. This developmental approach helps to understand patients' spiritual awareness in a way that respects their evolving integrity. Trained staff are intended to administer the interview, which takes at least 20 minutes.

The spiritual awareness assessment has four parts:

- Philosophy of life
- Source of hope
- Trusting relationships
- **Self-actualization.**

It focuses on the individual's main concerns at the present time. It is helpful to ask individuals who are more alert and oriented, to reflect on how the important things and relationships in their lives have changed over time. It is also helpful to ask why the individual finds specific things in life important. Some questions help reveal how the individual perceives "being old." For example, people might say that loss of independence is the main criterion for being old, or that loss of health signals the onset of old age.

In Part 2 of the assessment, the focus on the source of hope, gives the participant an opportunity to talk about his or her concept of spirituality. One question (2.a) identifies the wisdom/despair challenge identified by Erik Erikson. Question 2.b is designed to explore the individual's fears and anxieties, and question 2.c helps the participant to recall times in the past when he or she had found spiritual strength.

Part 3, of the assessment, on trusting relationships, specifically speaks to the participant's image of God. The critical questions are: How is the subject experiencing God at this time in his or her life? How has this changed over time? Does the subject feel an increase in isolation, or is he/she at peace with increasing aloneness? Does the subject withdraw into isolation through feeling unwanted or unloved? Does the subject seek companionship because he/she is lonely?

Finally, in Part 4, of the assessment, the degree of self-actualization is explored to get a sense of the individual's view of his or her personal agency. What is the balance that the individual has achieved between acceptance and change? How does the individual maintain his or her spiritual identity? Questions 4.e and 4.f are designed to conclude the interview on a positive and hopeful note. Often the participant will spend a considerable amount of time talking about his/her creative abilities and personal sources of beauty.

This spiritual awareness assessment is given to selected participants when staff members feel that additional information about these participants' spiritual needs is indicated, or in situations in which staff members believe that systematic exploration of spiritual issues would benefit the participant. Most of the questions used in the spiritual awareness assessment have been incorporated into themes used in spiritual awareness group.(Hopkins, Woods, Kelley, et al, 1995.)

O AN OVERVIEW

- Psychiatric nurses have a role in promoting spiritual well-being.
- Nurses, it is believed, have the capability to inspire those whose spirits are low because of physical, emotional, or spiritual pain.
- The nurse who continues to reach out with love, hope, and concern is offering a spiritual safety net to individuals who are in need.
- The spirituality of the nurse may keep the patient from drowning in the black waters of depression or flying too high in the face of a manic episode.
- The failure to address a component of holistic care—physical, emotional, or spiritual—constitutes providing fragmented and incomplete care to psychiatric patients.

TD TERMS TO DEFINE

- religiosity
- self-actualization
- spirituality
- spiritual well-being

O STUDY QUESTIONS

1. Identify three aspects of spirituality.
2. Identify two aspects of religiosity.
3. What does the *DSM IV* say about spiritual/religious concerns and problems?
4. Describe two methods to assess spiritual needs.

5. Identify two nursing strategies to provide spiritual care.

6. What was Freud's position on religion?

7. What was Victor Frankl's position on religion?

8. What do current psychiatric standards of practice say about spiritual issues?

9. Define spiritual well-being.

10. Identify three benefits of spiritual well-being.

11. Discuss the results of repeated Gallup surveys and Paloma's research regarding prayer.

■ REFERENCES

American Nurses Association: A Statement on Psychiatric Mental Health Clinical Nursing Practice and Standards of Psychiatric-Mental Health Clinical Nursing Practice. Washington, D.C.: American Nurses Publishing, 1994.

Carson VB: Spiritual Dimensions of Nursing Practice, Philadelphia, WB Saunders, 1989.

Erikson E: Childhood and Society. New York: Putnum, 1953.

Fish, S, Shelley JA: *Spiritual Care: The Nurse's Role.* Downer's Grove, IL: Intervarsity Press, 1978, p. 22.

Fowler J: *Stages of Faith: The Psychology of Human Development and the Quest for Meaning.* New York, Harper and Row, 1981.

Hopkins E, Woods Z, Kelley R, Dently K & Murphy J: Working with Groups on Spiritual Themes, Vol 2, Deluth, MN: Whole Person Press, 1995.

Hungelman J. Kenkel-Rossi E, & Klassen L, Development of the JAREL Spiritual Well-Being Scale In Classification of Nursing Diagnoses: Proceedings of the Eighth Conference, Edited by RM Carroll-Johnston, Philadelphia, Lippincott: 393-398.

Kegan R: *The Evolving Self: Problem and Process in Human Development.* Cambridge, MA, Harvard University Press, 1982.Ivy SS: *The structural Developmental Theories of James Fowler and Robert Kegan as Resources for Pastoral Assessment.* Ann Arbor, University Microfilms International, 1985.

Larson DP, & Larson SS: Religious Commitment and Health Valuing the Relationship Second Opinion 1991; 17: 27-40.

National Interfaith Coailition on Aging, Spiritual Well-Being-Definition, Athens, GA, 1975; 1.

Peck MS: *The Road Less Traveled: A New Psychology of Love, Traditional Values, and Spiritual Growth.* New York, Simon & Schuster, 1978, p. 15.

Stoll RI: Guidelines for spiritual assessment, *Am J Nurs* 1979; 79:1574–1577.

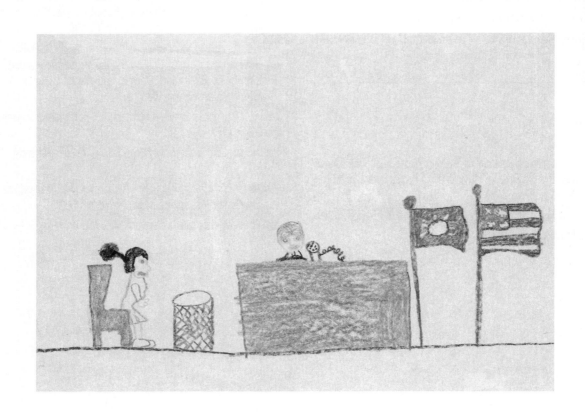

The people's safety is the highest law.

Legal and political maxim

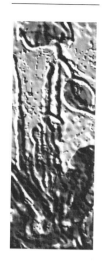

11
Legal Issues in Psychiatric Nursing

Joyce K. Laben

In the past thirty years, legal issues related to care of the mentally ill have become a major consideration in providing therapeutic interventions. Litigation has been related to challenging patient commitments, the right to treatment, the right to refuse treatment, and the duty to protect. "Law and mental health care are now so interconnected that it is difficult to remember a time when they did not interact."[1]

There are special legal issues involved with the provision of care for individuals who manifest symptoms that are indicative of mental illness. Nurses who provide care for the mentally ill should be conversant with current legal and ethical problems in order to ensure adequate care for patients. There has been a dramatic increase in the number of mental-health-related lawsuits in the last 25-30 years, which makes it imperative for mental health professionals to keep current with the law. Only those legal areas specific to the treatment of the mentally ill will be discussed in this chapter.

■ HISTORICAL PERSPECTIVE

Because few institutions for the mentally ill had been established in the United States before the middle of the 19th century, few statutory provisions relative to conditions for institutional admission were enacted before 1860. Persons confined were generally those who were clearly "deranged" and violent. The decision to admit a patient to a facility was wholly within the discretion of the hospital administrator, who would often be under great pressure to admit indigent or dangerous persons in view of the lack of alternatives for their support and care in the community.

If a person exhibited dangerous behavior, however, English common law and the early colonies in America allowed for his removal from society. These individuals were generally placed in jails along with the criminals. This authority to remove dangerous people from society was based on the state's police power, which embraces all authority used by the states for the protection of health, safety, and the general welfare of citizens.[2] It is important to remember the concepts of *parens patriae* and *police power* because the justification for involuntary hospitalization today rests upon these doctrines.[3]

In the United States, there were few institutions for the mentally ill until the middle of the nineteenth century. Because of lack of resources, those confined were generally only those who were clearly "deranged" and violent. Therefore, until 1860, there was a dearth of statutory provisions relative to conditions for and limitations upon admission to mental institutions. The decision to admit to a facility was wholly within the discretion of the hospital administrator, who would often be under great pressure to admit indigent or dangerous persons in view of the lack of alternatives for support and care in the community.[4]

The movement toward the creation of state mental health institutions was stimulated by the crusading of individuals such as Dorothea Lynde Dix. From 1840 to 1880, Miss Dix conducted a personal crusade to expose the conditions existing in poorhouses and local jails where many mentally ill persons were ultimately placed. She effectively lobbied in many states for the creation of public institutions.[5] The increase in the availability of institutions focused attention on the need for rational and fair admission procedures, particularly for persons who refused to voluntarily admit themselves to hospitals.

The efforts of Dorothea Dix and other activists also brought reforms in the admission process, principally in the form of statutes requiring that no one could be involuntarily committed without a jury trial by his or her peers. The common law requirement for dangerousness was changed and by the end of the 19th century, many states permitted commitment based upon a wide range of showings of mental illness and did not require dangerous behavior. Forms of these statutes remain in effect in most states.[6]

From the 1930s through 1950s, there was a trend away from strict procedural commitments and hearings. The power to commit was entrusted to one or two physicians, sometimes with hearings conducted after the original commitment had taken place and only at the instigation of the patient.[7] From the beginning of the 20th century until the early 1960s, the population in state and county inpatient facilities continued to increase. With the passage of the Community Mental Health Centers Act of 1963, a movement began to treat individuals in the community rather than in hospitals.[8] During the beginning of the 1970s, attorneys began to assist individuals in asserting their rights, especially in relation to their long term treatment in inpatient facilities.

There was a trend toward viewing the commitment process as one to be administered by the judiciary rather than left to the medical decisionmakers.[9] At this time, laws were rewritten to include the criteria of dangerousness or likelihood of serious harm to self or others as the guidelines for the involuntary commitment to hospitals.

The movement toward patients' rights led to the release of large numbers of individuals into the community, and concerns were raised that facilities and services were inadequate to care for these persons. The mentally ill in jails is a major problem which has drawn growing attention in recent years. Torrey and associates conducted a study which represented 41% of the jails and 62% of the inmates in the United States. They found that 7.2% of the inmates were identified as having a severe mental illness.[10] Because of the increasing number of mentally ill persons on the street and the appointment of more conservative judges, who were reluctant to become involved in the running of hospitals, recommendations for expanding the mental health commitment laws emerged. A tendency developed in some jurisdictions—such as in the state of Washington—individuals were committed in greater numbers under the gravely disabled, unable to care for self, rather than the dangerousness criteria.

Appelbaum comments that in the 1970s statutes in the United States were changed to dangerousness criteria because it was thought that the definition, "need for treatment" was too vague. He writes that dangerousness definitions are often "circular", unclear and vague and that mental health professionals have great leeway in making commitment decisions.[11]

He also points out that in studies that have been conducted, the term **"gravely disabled"** is used in about one third of cases. This latter terminology means that the person is unable to provide basic personal needs such as shelter, food and clothing for him or herself.

Appelbaum writes about the changes in the commitment laws in the 1970s. It was thought that there would be great difficulty in having persons committed. This has not turned out to be the case. Poythress undertook a program to work with attorneys. In Texas, a group of lawyers was identified, based on their representation of patients at commitment hearings. Seminars were conducted including how to cross examine mental health professionals at commitment proceedings. In the final analysis of the project, behavior of the lawyers did not change, not one participant attorney attempted to challenge a witness incorporating the teachings. In interviews with the participants afterwards, the focus, as the lawyers saw their roles, was to help people get needed treatment.[12]

Appelbaum states that judges, clinicians, attorneys and family members developed common sense models. If an individual needed treatment, methods were found to have the person hospitalized.[13] He believes that commitment statutes that need to be enacted are "simultaneously fair, reasonable and compassionate."[14]

Many states have developed programs using crisis mobile teams to prevent hospitalization. Respite stabilization units and short-term inpatient facilities are available in some areas so that a person does not have to be hospitalized. Managed care is now decreasing the hospital length of stay.

■ COMPETENCY

There is a misconception that persons admitted to an inpatient psychiatric facility lose their civil rights and are incompetent to handle their own affairs. Under current law as it applies to voluntary as well as involuntary patients, this is inaccurate. Unless a court has found an individual incompetent to manage personal matters and a guardian has been appointed, the individual does not lose the right to make decisions relating to personal or business matters when admitted to a hospital. Until the 1960s, an individual was generally found incompetent at the time of commitment to the hospital.

A person who is 18 or older is permitted to manage his own property and health in any way he or she chooses. A person who appears to be "incompetent," is still legally **competent** until a court declares him or her to be incompetent and appoints a guardian or conservator to act on his or her behalf. Currently, most states have laws that authorize the court to find a person to be totally competent or incompetent. There is a trend, however, to amend state laws to authorize courts to declare individuals disabled only in those areas of their lives in which the individual is unable to manage and to appoint a limited guardian for those areas.[15]

In an inpatient or outpatient setting, a nurse should assess as to whether the person being treated has been declared incompetent. If this is the case, a copy of the court order should be obtained for the record and documentation established as to who has authority to consent to treatment of the patient or authorize release of records.

■ LEAST RESTRICTIVE ALTERNATIVE ENVIRONMENT

One of the concepts in the delivery of mental health care is that of the **least restrictive alternative.** In planning mental health care, professional care givers should plan a treatment program that can be implemented in the least restrictive environment. If a person can be treated in a halfway house, or in his or her own home, this is a preferable alternative to that of involuntary commitment on a locked ward in a psychiatric hospital. A case that discussed this issue extensively is *Dixon v. Weinberger (1975).*[16]

This doctrine of least restrictive alternative for care is based on the principle that the state may have a legitimate reason for wanting to treat an individual, but that treatment must be provided in the least restrictive manner that can provide sufficient care for the patient's needs. Some states have enacted statutes that explicitly state this requirement. It is an important point to consider when planning care. Each person's specific needs at a particular time should be assessed. These needs should be reevaluated at frequent intervals to determine whether the patient might need a more or a less restrictive environment.

■ INPATIENT HOSPITALIZATION

Generally, there are three types of admission to inpatient psychiatric hospitals: voluntary, emergency involuntary, and indefinite involuntary (judicial commitments).[17] Any person who is mentally ill, in need of inpatient care, and is willing to seek admission can be admitted to a psychiatric hospital as a voluntary patient. Because of recent trends toward managed care, permission from the managed care organization might have to be obtained for a voluntary patient. A voluntary patient must consent to all treatment and must be released upon request within a reasonable period of time, which will be specified by state law and may be from 8 hours to several days after receipt of the request for release. If an individual refuses treatment or requests release at a time when he or she is a danger to others, the staff must look to state law to determine whether the individual must be released or if a petition for judicial commitment should be initiated.

In a New York case, an individual was admitted to a psychiatric center in May 1984 as an involuntary patient.[18] He became a voluntary patient after having been continuously hospitalized from 1984 to December 1987. This patient refused to have electroconvulsive therapy (ECT) for an atypical bipolar disorder. The hospital attempted to convert his status to that of an involuntary patient and two examining physicians signed certificates. In New York, however, these certificates must be accompanied by a third physician's confirmation, and this was not done. The hospital began proceedings to arrange for the patient to receive ECT and also to convert his status to an involuntary one. The patient moved to dismiss both proceedings because the hospital had not compiled with the law. The hospital contended it didn't need the third signature except when a patient was initially committed. The court ruled in the patient's favor because the proper procedures had not taken place.

Historically, parents have been allowed to authorize the "voluntary" admission of juveniles under the age of 18. This practice, however, has been challenged in court in a number of states such as Georgia and Pennsylvania, and attorneys for juveniles have requested that no juveniles be admitted to a psychiatric facility without court approval.[19]

Other states, both through court decisions and amendments in state law, have recognized that at a certain age minors are "mature" enough to determine their own admission.[20] Under certain circumstances, this would still allow parents to authorize the admission of younger juveniles to psychiatric facilities. The Supreme Court authorized this practice in *Parham v. J. R. et al. (1978)* and stated that it was not a requirement that court approval be given for all juveniles admitted to psychiatric facilities.[21] It did find, however, that some kind of inquiry should be made by a "neutral fact finder" to determine whether statutory requirements for admission are satisfied in such cases. The Court clarified that a formal or quasiformal hearing is neither required nor has to be conducted by a law-trained or judicial or administrative officer for the hospitalization of juveniles.

Most states provide for emergency involuntary admission to a psychiatric facility when an individual is thought to pose an immediate threat of serious self harm or harm to others as a result of mental illness, and is willing to seek treatment. This type of involuntary commitment differs from indefinite judicial commitment because it usually permits commitment, for a few days, without a court hearing.

State statutes have been narrowed in the past few years to require a threat of actual physical harm before

an emergency involuntary admission can take place. When this occurs, a law enforcement official or more usually a licensed physician is authorized to take the individual into custody for the purpose of an initial evaluation and eventual transportation to a psychiatric facility if this is determined appropriate. The individual can then be detained for a brief period before a court hearing to determine whether emergency admission standards have been met and to authorize short-term hospitalization of the individual. Normally, aversive therapy such as ECT is not allowed during the initial detention. When the period authorized for the emergency commitment ends, the individual must be released; a petition must be initiated for an indefinite judicial commitment; or the individual must agree to voluntarily remain in the health care facility.

The only instance in which someone may be detained in a psychiatric facility for an indefinite period against his will is through the judicial commitment process. Most state statutes allow this process to be initiated when an authorized official, mental health professional, or family member files a petition for such commitment along with certification by two physicians or other mental health professionals that the individual is mentally ill, poses a likelihood of serious harm because of his or her mental illness, and suitable community resources for treating the individual are unavailable. Generally, the standard for "likelihood of serious harm" is broader for indefinite judicial commitment than for emergency commitment, and includes both immediate danger to self or others as well as more passive types of danger that can result from a person's inability to avoid or protect him or her from harm because of mental illness. More recently, as mentioned earlier, the term gravely disabled is utilized by some jurisdictions to commit individuals who cannot manage themselves.

In Alabama, an individual with paranoid schizophrenia challenged his commitment into a psychiatric hospital because he had not committed dangerous acts in the recent past. A psychologist testified that the patient had not been taking the prescribed medication, had threatened to injure others including a woman with whom he had had a relationship in the past. The court issued a ruling, based on clear and convincing evidence, that the individual needed continued hospitalization.[22]

Numerous court decisions during the past three decades reflect the severe attack that has been made on the judicial commitment process. Some people believe because commitment results in deprivation of liberty, the procedures required for it should parallel those provided in a criminal trial.

The Supreme Court of the United States reviewed the indefinite commitment statute of the state of Texas as well as a variety of procedural issues related to involuntary commitment. The Court ruled that the proof needed for involuntary commitment must be greater than a preponderance of evidence and that "clear, un-equivocal and convincing" evidence is constitutionally adequate for such commitment. The Court determined that the standard of "beyond a reasonable doubt" is not required, indicating that it based its' decision on a standard higher than that required for civil cases, preponderance of the evidence, but lower than that required for criminal prosecution.[23]

The Court also stated that the substantive standards and procedures for civil commitment may vary from one state to another, as long as they meet the constitutional minimum. The opinion further held that the state has a legitimate interest under its *parens patriae* power in providing care for its citizens who are unable to care for themselves as the result of mental illness, and that the state has the authority under its police power to protect the community from dangerous tendencies of those who are mentally ill.

■ PREVENTIVE OR MANDATORY OUTPATIENT TREATMENT

Many mental health professionals have been perplexed about how to intervene with patients that are continuously noncompliant. Because of the recent tendency to hospitalize for shorter periods of time, there has been a movement toward mandatory outpatient treatment also called preventive or involuntary outpatient treatment.

In a recent study of outpatient commitment, Torrey and Kaplan found that 35 states and the District of Columbia have laws permitting outpatient commitment. Georgia, Hawaii, and North Carolina use different criteria for outpatient than for inpatient commitment. In only 12 states was outpatient commitment commonly utilized. Reasons for not using it were violations of civil liberties, liability and fiscal burden. Some states did not have enforceable consequences for noncompliance or had criteria for noncompliance that were thought to be too restrictive. Other states use mechanisms such as conditional release or guardianship rather than outpatient commitment.[24]

■ LEGAL RIGHTS

An individual admitted to a psychiatric hospital maintains certain legal rights although the individual may be deprived of the freedom to leave the hospital. Because the rights are sometimes defined by state laws, mental health professionals should be familiar with patients' rights as defined by statute in the jurisdiction in which they practice. As stated earlier, unless declared incompetent, an individual maintains the rights of any citizen such as the right to vote, to manage financial affairs, and to execute legal documents.

Because of the restrictive nature of confinement of a patient to an inpatient psychiatric facility, certain rights are given special focus. These include the right to communicate with an attorney in person, by letter, and by telephone. The patient also has a right to receive mail without interference or censorship, the right to receive visitors, and the right to the basic necessities of life in the name of treatment. Although these rights may be temporarily restricted (under certain circumstances), a mere claim by the staff that interference with these rights is necessary for treatment purposes is not sufficient to deny a patient these rights.[25]

A patient right that emerged in the late 1960s and early 1970s was a right to treatment when hospitalized. A landmark case for the right to treatment doctrine was *Rouse v. Cameron (1967)*,[26] which involved a person found not guilty by reason of insanity and was committed to a federal mental health facility. This case was the first to hold that society has a legal duty to provide adequate treatment for the mentally ill and to ensure that confinement for purposes of treatment does not degenerate into punishment. The court did not characterize the right to treatment as a constitutional right, but instead relied upon a District of Columbia statute that specifically cited this right. The court stated that the right to treatment would be satisfied by bona fide efforts of the staff to provide treatment consistent with present medical knowledge.

The most publicized case in the area of right to treatment is *Wyatt v. Stickney (1971)*.[27] This Alabama case involved a district federal judge who threatened to sell state property to ensure that the state would have enough money to provide adequate treatment to its mental patients. The importance of this decision was that it established a constitutional basis for the right to treatment for the involuntarily committed patients by analyzing the nature of the commitment process itself. The basis of this process is that justification of the involuntary commitment restriction of the individual's freedom, requires the provision of treatment must be provided once the individual is hospitalized.

Wyatt v. Stickney states that treatment must provide realistic opportunities to be treated and established three necessary categories for treatment: (1) humane psychological and physical environment; (2) qualified staff personnel in sufficient numbers; and (3) individualized treatment plans. The court came to this conclusion after extensive expert testimony was provided in the case.

Another case that has received widespread publicity is *O'Connor v. Donaldson (1975)*, decided by the United States Supreme Court. This case involved a Florida patient who was not considered dangerous but had been hospitalized against his will for over 15 years without treatment.[28] In *O'Connor v. Donaldson* the court stipulated that a state cannot constitutionally confine without treatment a nondangerous individual who is capable of surviving safely in the community alone or with the help of willing and responsible family members or friends. To do so, the Court held, would be a deprivation of liberty.

A subsequent United States Supreme Court decision, *Youngberg v. Romeo (1982)*, further reviewed the issue of "right to treatment."[29] This case concerned a person involuntarily committed to an institution for the mentally retarded. In a concurring opinion by Justice Warren Burger, who also wrote the *O'Connor* decision, it specifically states that there is no constitutional right to "habilitation or training for social adaption."[30] The concept of "habilitation" for the mentally retarded individual is parallel to the concept of "treatment" for a mentally ill individual; therefore, this case is pertinent to the issue of "right to treatment." However, the majority of the Court held that a committed mentally retarded person has a right to minimally adequate or reasonable training to ensure safety and freedom from undue restraints. Ultimately, the Court again declined to rule on whether an individual involuntarily committed to a state institution has some general constitutional right to training per se.

■ INFORMED CONSENT

Adults who are of sound mind, that is, mentally competent, have the right to determine what will be done to their own bodies,[31] moreover, a person must have enough information or knowledge to provide an informed consent to an anticipated procedure or treatment to be performed by health professionals.

When an individual is admitted to a hospital for a mental illness, the right to consent to a treatment is not abdicated. A *voluntary* patient should have the right to refuse any kind of treatment.[32] An attempt should, however, be made to explain to the individual the various kinds of treatments and alternatives that might be available. Once the possible treatments and alternatives are presented to the patient along with relevant facts, it is up to the patient to make the decision about the treatments. When a decision is made, even though it might differ from the mental health professionals' preferred choice, the patient should be allowed to pursue the course chosen without repercussions from the hospital staff. For example, if a patient chooses not to have electroconvulsive therapy (ECT), other alternatives should be explored, and the staff should not withdraw their support from the individual even though the patient's treatment choice differs from the decision recommended by a therapeutic team.

The real difficulty seems to arise when a procedure recommended for an involuntarily committed patient

is refused. In many instances, the patient although involuntarily committed, has not been found incompetent to manage his or her affairs. According to Roth, even committed patients must be given adequate information on which to base informed consent to intrusive procedures such as ECT.[33] If such a patient is not thought competent to make this decision, then a court should make the finding of incompetency, and an appropriate consent should be obtained from a formally appointed substitute for the patient such as a guardian.

■ THE RIGHT TO REFUSE MEDICATION

In the past years there have been some lawsuits that have pertained to a patient's right to refuse psychotropic medication. Two major cases on this issue are *Rogers v. Okin*, later entitled *Mills v. Rogers*, which originated in the State of Massachusetts, and *Rennie v. Klein* which originated in New Jersey.[34] Both of these cases were appealed to the Supreme Court, which sent them back to lower courts for resolution.

Both cases concerned the rights of involuntarily hospitalized patients to refuse the taking of psychotropic medication. Because of the potential for incurable side effects from this medication such as tardive dyskinesia, patients in both cases were motivated to file suit to protect their right to refuse medication.

In a recent Wisconsin case, Virgil D. requested a review of a prior decision whereby a circuit court granted a petition to allow his involuntary treatment with psychotropic drugs because of mental illness. Based on testimony at a hearing, he was found not competent to exercise informed consent.[35]

Virgil was diagnosed as having chronic paranoid schizophrenia for a period of time. He had been treated on prior occasions with Prolixin. During the first hearing, the examining psychiatrist testified that Virgil could communicate an understanding of the advantages and disadvantages of, and alternatives to psychotropic medication, however, he was not competent to exercise informed consent about its use because he did not recognize that he was mentally ill. The circuit court found that Virgil was competent to refuse medication. Three months later, the county again filed a motion to give him the medications involuntarily. Virgil stated that the medication hindered him, slowed down his thoughts and "tortured" him. He also stated that he had been committed even though he had been taking Prolixin at the time. This time the circuit court concluded that he was not competent to refuse medication. The Court of Appeals upheld this decision.

The Supreme Court reversed the Court of Appeals decision. It wrote that nowhere in the Wisconsin statute was it written that Virgil had to have an appreciation of his mental illness in order to refuse medication. There was only one standard, did he know the risks, benefits and the alternatives to the medication? The court went on to say, "even if Virgil's decision to refuse to take Prolixin is a poor choice, it is his to make as long as he understands the implications of that decision."[36]

The guidelines for managing an incompetent involuntary patient seem to follow several courses: appointment of a court-ordered guardian who will make a decision on the basis of one or two guidelines or a combination of both. The first is what treatment is in the best interests of the patient? The second is a "substituted judgment" decision. What would the patient want if he or she were competent? Some states use administrative procedures such as bringing in an outside psychiatrist consultant to examine a drug-refusing patient or establishing a specially appointed treatment team to evaluate the necessity for giving forced medications to an incompetent mentally ill person.[37]

In a one year study completed in Louisiana, it was found that of 1,949 patients, 40 patients had to be medicated involuntarily. In this particular state, administrative and not judicial review is required before involuntarily medicating refusing patients.[38] The Louisiana procedure for this includes the psychiatrist discussing with the patient the reasons for the medication including the anticipated results and possible side effects. If the patient continues to refuse the medication, an inquiry is made about the reason for the refusal. A second psychiatrist then examines the patient and endorses or modifies the proposed treatment. After informing the patient of the results of the consultation with the second psychiatrist, the patient is seen by an advocate if the refusal continues. Legal rights are explained to the patient.

Following this dialogue, the patient can appeal to the medical director for an administrative review of his or her case. After a careful assessment of all the facts, including the reason for the refusal of medication such as delusional thinking, the medical director makes the final decision.

Sixty-seven percent of the refusing patients were admitted involuntarily. The primary reasons for medicating against the patients' will was potential violence and delusional thinking. The major reason for refusing medication was not the presence of side effects, unlike other studies that have been completed, but severe delusional thinking or personal reasons. Most of the administrative reviews took place within five days. This compares well, with the average time for judicial review of 4.5 months.

In a study of 24 involuntarily medicated patients at Beth Israel Medical Center in New York City, 71% felt that the refusal of medication had been correctly overruled and that they should be treated against their wishes in the future.[39] Certain steps that state systems or individual facilities can currently take when managing the care of a refusing patient are, first, procedures should be established on how to intervene with a drug-refusing patient. Additionally, guidelines on how to manage the involuntarily hospitalized patient who refuses medication should incorporate state law, case decisions, rules and regulations, and consent decrees of the particular jurisdiction in which the facility is located.

There is, however, no substitute for a therapeutic relationship between a patient and a mental health professional to resolve issues about medication. An ongoing dialogue during several sessions can assist in assessing the patient's reason for refusing medication. Continuing inservice education about medication and its side effects is an important mechanism for keeping professionals informed about the current literature on the subject.[40]

■ AVERSIVE THERAPIES

It is especially important to be careful and thorough in obtaining valid consent for certain intrusive procedures. Electroshock treatments (ECT) are still given to psychiatric patients throughout the country. The competent patient should be fully informed of all the facts about the treatment, including its side effects. The patient can refuse the treatment. In at least one jurisdiction, only a court can consent to ECT for a minor.[41] The parents cannot give such an authorization. According to Ennis and Emery, all jurisdictions allow substituted consent for incompetents.[42] Nurses should know what the law is concerning ECT in the state in which they are practicing, and the hospitals should have policies and procedures for obtaining consent from patients for its' use.

In one study it was reported that ECT use is decreasing. More women than men receive ECT, but age and diagnosis are the most important factors in selecting to undergo the treatment. It is primarily used by white voluntary patients in private psychiatric facilities.[43] Recently, *USA Today* reported that the elderly account for more than 50% of all ECT administered. There is some question as to the safety of administering this treatment to the elderly, especially those with multiple health problems.[44]

■ SECLUSION AND RESTRAINT

The use of seclusion and restraint of the mentally ill has been the subject of much clinical and legal debate for three decades. In two legal cases, *Wyatt v. Stickney* and *Rogers v. Okin*, seclusion and restraint were major issues in the treatment of patients in Alabama and Massachusetts. Recently two studies have found that rates of seclusion and restraint vary greatly, even within the same state.

A survey of the incidence of seclusion and restraint in state psychiatric hospitals throughout the United States elicited 101 responses from 44 states. The study found that smaller hospitals had higher rates of seclusion and restraint than did larger ones. The authors attributed this result to the fact that larger state hospitals are treating a more chronic rather than acutely ill psychiatric patients.[45]

A study conducted in New York state found that the use of restraint and seclusion varied among psychiatric settings.[46] The authors recommended that in future studies such variables as staffing patterns and policy mandates for seclusion and restraint be analyzed.

In a recent ruling concerning the consent decree in *Wyatt v. Stickney,* a federal judge in Alabama mandated the revision of seclusion and restraint guidelines.[47] The numbers of staff members were greatly reduced who could authorize nonemergency seclusion and restraint. Only a psychiatrist or qualified physician with specialized training can issue such an order. Currently, only eight hours is allowed for seclusion and restraint time from the time it is originally ordered. Moreover, the patient must be monitored every 15 minutes instead of the previous 1 hour. In emergency situations, a qualified registered nurse is authorized to issue a seclusion and restraint order if no doctor is available. The nurse must personally evaluate the situation and chart the observations in the patient's record. This authority extends to only one hour. A physician must see the patient within 4 hours, preferably sooner, but can extend the emergency seclusion to only 4 hours. These are the guidelines for Alabama; the original guidelines in the *Wyatt* case were adopted throughout the country.

■ GENERAL ISSUES IN MENTAL HEALTH CARE

DOCUMENTATION

Practicing psychiatric/mental health nursing in the community or hospital setting requires attention to adequate and careful documentation. Treatment plans should be up-to-date and written in behavioral terms. An in-depth assessment of the patient including any physical problems that might be problematic in providing mental health care should be addressed. Careful documentation of all recommendations including the basis for such recommendations should be included, as well as the follow-up on whether or not they were implemented. The nurse should be familiar with relevant law in the state that applies to documentation as well as requirements for documentation in relation to reimbursement from third party payers for services provided.

There should be an accurate recording of the treatment process. It is better to describe a patient related event in detail than to label the patient's behavior. For example, it is more delineative to record that a patient was visited at home and refused to come out of the bedroom for 30 minutes, while the nurse was there, than to simply note that the patient was withdrawn.

Another important issue to document is a patient's crisis episode and the therapeutic intervention provided for it. The nurse's assessment of the crisis and the intervention should be recorded not only for the protection of the patient, but also for the protection of the nurse, especially if the patient later responds to the crisis situation with self-inflicted injury or follows through on other threats that were made. Although only a small percentage of patient records are subject to public scrutiny as the result of subpoena by a court or review by the patient, it is good practice to always document events as though the record were going to be reviewed by a third party.

MEDICATION

With the introduction of phenothiazines for the treatment of persons with schizophrenia in the 1950s, the population of mental hospitals declined, and the majority of patients are now treated in community settings through the use of medication. All medications that are prescribed for a psychiatric patient must be documented, including the period of their use throughout the treatment process.

Concern has been raised about the long-term effects of medication on individuals who are mentally ill. Nurses caring for patients in the community should be particularly sensitive to individuals who are on drug therapy and patients who complain of difficulties. It is imperative that any complaints of side effects from medication be immediately and accurately recorded and reported to the prescribing physician or nurse.

Nurses should be particularly aware of the symptoms of neuroleptic malignant syndrome which can be fatal. Persons younger than 20 and older than 60 seem to have a higher mortality rate from this syndrome.[48] In addition, use of the newer Serotonin-Reuptake Inhibitors (SSRI) with other serotonergic agents can cause "serotonin syndrome." Nurses should be alert to the symptoms of these syndromes in order to intervene quickly when appropriate.[49]

MALPRACTICE

A matter about which all nurses and mental health professionals should be educated is that of **malpractice.** Malpractice is a form of **negligence** and is a legal issue that comes within the field of tort law. A person who feels injured as the result of the actions of a nurse could bring suit in a civil court for money damages for malpractice.

There are certain elements that must be proven in order to win a case for malpractice. The court will analyze all of the elements of malpractice in relationship to the facts of the case before determining whether malpractice in fact exists.

STANDARDS OF CARE

There is a legal fiction called the reasonably prudent person. Courts over a period of many years have relied on this concept to require nurses to function at a minimum standard of care that is equivalent to that of a reasonably prudent nurse delivering care in the same circumstances.

LEGAL DUTY

Once a nurse initiates a professional relationship with a patient, a nurse-patient relationship is established, and the nurse is obligated to provide care in an appropriate manner. In addition, if the nurse observes an action by another professional that he or she thinks breaches the standard of care and can predict or foresee from this action possible harm to the patient, the nurse has the responsibility to intervene and prevent the injury.

CAUSATION

In order for a nurse to be found liable for negligence, the person bringing the lawsuit must demonstrate that there is a causal relationship between the nurse's acts and the alleged injury, however it is often difficult to establish such a causal link.

INJURY

It must be established that an injury was incurred by the plaintiff from the acts of the professional and that the injury can be recompensed with money damages. An example of a potential malpractice issue often involving mental health professionals relates to the suicide of a patient after discharge from a facility or during off-the-ward activities. Courts generally have ruled in the following manner: If the staff has carefully observed the patient and suicidal behavior has not been exhibited, verbally or nonverbally, the mental health team will not be held liable for the patient's injury; however, if the patient has exhibited current suicidal tendencies and is discharged or given a pass, it is conceivable the ruling would not be in favor of the mental health staff.[50] It is imperative that communication about a patient's condi-

tion be reported verbally and also be written in the record.

In a personal injury claim against the state by a patient who had leaped from a third-floor window of a psychiatric facility, the court ruled that the patient did not prove by a preponderance of the evidence that the state had been negligent. The patient had been "demanding, restless, hostile and easily agitated," but had not indicated in any manner that he was suicidal. He had been friendly to staff members and other patients. Even though he told a staff member that he planned to leave the center, he did not indicate any suicidal intent.[51]

Although the facility was not found responsible in this particular case, suicide is a frequent cause of litigation for malpractice. Hughes writes that in reviewing studies of suicides it is not clear that suicide prevention centers and educational efforts are effective deterrents.[52] One study has suggested that with the trend toward fewer inpatient days that has come with managed care the risk of suicide may increase. The results of this particular study indicated significant clustering of suicides during the four weeks post hospitalization.[53] Hughes observes that at present, suicide cannot be effectively predicted, however, that does not relieve the mental health practitioner from assessing the risk of its occurrence.

CONFIDENTIALITY AND PRIVILEGE

Two often misunderstood concepts, vitally important to a relationship with the patient, are **confidentiality** and **privilege.** Confidentiality relates to the responsibility of the care providing agency and professional to keep confidential and private all information, records and correspondence relating to the patient and to allow third parties to have access to these records only under specifically defined circumstances. Privilege refers to the relationship of a particular professional to a patient and provides protection of the information obtained from the patient as a result of this relationship. Each state defines by law the professionals who have privilege and whether the privilege is absolute. The professionals who most often are given privilege are ministers, psychiatrists, psychologists, and lawyers. Privilege can be asserted only by the client and does not exist unless there is a patient-therapist relationship. When someone other than the patient and the therapist is present when the information is conveyed, privilege is unlikely to exist.

A mental health professional should investigate in the state in which he or she is practicing which professionals are granted privilege and under what circumstances information about the patient and their records should be released. Usually, records may be released only with the written permission of the patient or by court order. There may also be specific statutory exceptions to confidentiality, such as mandatory child-abuse-reporting laws or laws relating to emergency situations.

DUTY TO PROTECT

Although litigation in the mental health field has been increasing, much of it has been directed at state mental health inpatient facilities and has focused on such issues as appropriate standards and procedures for involuntary hospitalization, provisions for treatment in the least restrictive alternative, and the patient's right to treatment and to refuse treatment. The results of this litigation, however, have directly influenced the practice of community mental health. Most states have now amended their commitment laws to allow only the most dangerous persons to be hospitalized against their will, to limit the period of hospitalization, and to mandate that services be provided in the least restrictive setting whenever possible.

This has led to an expansion of the range of patients that are now served at the community level. Fewer persons can be referred to hospitals when problems arise. More *potentially* dangerous clients must continue to be served at the community level and more severely and persistently mentally ill patients must be supported in the community. Thus it is particularly important for all mental health professionals to have a working knowledge of the mental health laws in the state in which they are practicing. This is particularly important when they determine that an individual must be referred for inpatient care.

It is at this point that the concept of voluntariness becomes critical. The treatment deemed appropriate for a patient should be discussed with the patient so that he or she can make an informed decision about being hospitalized, if possible, however, if the individual is unwilling to either seek inpatient care or poses an immediate threat of harm to self or others, a decision must be made concerning involuntary commitment to a psychiatric facility. If the individual does not pose a threat of causing serious harm as a result of mental illness, it may not be possible or desirable to force the person to be hospitalized involuntarily. The professional should always determine whether all alternatives for treatment in the community have been exhausted before attempting involuntary hospitalization.

Another issue involving the care of individuals in the community setting is their potential danger for being dangerous to third parties and the responsibility of the therapist to warn those third parties of this danger. *Tarasoff v. Regents of the University of California (1974)* is a case in California that has generated anxiety among mental health professionals.[54] In this particular decision, an individual who was in treatment with a psychologist confided in the course of therapy that he intended to kill a young woman whom he knew. The university police were notified by the psychologist and they briefly detained the patient but decided to release him. The psychologist did not see the patient again, nor did the psychologist attempt to warn the victim or her family of the patient's statements. When the patient subsequently killed the young woman as he had threatened to do, her family filed a lawsuit. The Supreme Court of California held that a duty to warn third parties existed when a therapist determines, or according to the standards of the profession or who should determine, that a patient presents a serious physical danger to another person. The Court stated that this situation created an exception to the confidential relationship of therapist and patient and that a potential victim can be warned of danger since "the protection of privilege ends where the public peril begins." Other states have adopted the Tarasoff concept to require that professionals notify third parties about dangerous individuals.[55] Kjervik maintained that although nurses have not been defendants in a lawsuit of this kind, they had the duty to warn when serving in a therapeutic capacity.[56]

In a recent case concerning the duty to protect, survivors of a victim of a motor vehicle accident in Missouri who was killed in a collision with a car being driven by a patient, brought an action for wrongful death. The patient had gone to the community psychiatric rehabilitation center where she was seen by two social workers. The patient told them that she was going to leave the facility and kill herself by wrecking her car. The social workers and a medical doctor were consulted and "failed to stop her departure from the facility." The patient had been hospitalized on 15 prior occasions and was on a "critical intervention plan" that included a 96 hour hold if the need were to arise. The question in the court case was, whether the facility and its employees owed a duty to the motorist who was killed. The court ruled that the facility had no duty to the general public. "In the absence of a duty, there could be no breach and thus no liability for the death."[57]

It is important for the mental health practitioner to know the law in the state where practicing, not only when it is required to report conduct of a patient/client that might harm a third party, but when to commit a patient to prevent harm. Appelbaum writes that the duty to protect now looks like a reasonable step in the evolution of mental health law.[58]

BOUNDARY VIOLATIONS

One of the bases for health care, the helping process, has special significance in providing mental health care. There has been a great deal written in recent years about **boundary violations.** Surveys have been done exploring boundary violations of psychiatrists, social workers and psychologists. Although it is known that nurses have also violated patient boundaries, no major study of this topic appears to have been completed.

What is meant by a boundary violation? According to Pilette (1995) and associates, boundaries mark territory.[59] As humans we mark out territory with gates, fences, doors, walls, personal space while interacting with others and borders between nations. Gutheil and Gabbard (1993) have defined boundary violations as "boundary crossings" that are injurious to patients.[60]

Hankins and colleagues report from 7 to 10% of male therapists and from 1 to 3% of female therapists disclose having had sexual intercourse with one or more patients.[61] Reports of violations by female therapists have been infrequent and most have been for homosexual involvement.[62] According to Russell, the profile of an offending therapist is one who is male, has probably had some personal therapy, and is accredited by a professional body.[63] Bouhoutsos found that 90% of these individuals reported feeling lonely, vulnerable, and needy at the time of the incidents. Most were separated, divorced, or unhappily married. Their average age was 43.5.[64] Once a therapist has had sexual relations with a patient, the behavior is likely to recur. Epstein in a review of the literature reports that many authors have focused on the role of narcissistic pathology. He points out that "middle-aged clinicians in their prime may become blinded to their patient's boundary needs because they have become overconfident and intoxicated by success, recognition and power they have achieved." Finally at the end of the therapist's career, thoughts of diminishing options can lead to feeling "rejuvenated" by a relationship with a younger patient.[65]

Russell reports that offending therapists tend to rationalize their behavior, deny the behavior and assert that the client, patient agreed to sexual contact. If the incidents take place outside therapeutic hours, they allege that the relationship is one of love.[66]

When a therapist transgresses the boundaries of professional care, the patient in most instances, finds it difficult to establish his or her own boundaries because of transference. Simon defines transference as, "the unconscious assignment to others of feelings and attitudes that were originally associated with important figures (parents, siblings) in one's early life."[67] Simon writes that initially the relationship is like a high from a drug but when the relationship is terminated the patient "crashes". The therapist also is an impaired person, whether or not she or he is apprehended.[68]

Basic information on ethical prohibitions should be made available to all trainees in the helping professions. This should include information about abuse of power and breach of trust including with the theory of victimology. Issues relating patients to identity, self-esteem and self-image are imperative. Managing countertransference is highly important and attraction to a patient should be openly discussed with supervisors without fear. Keeping the patient's/client's welfare should be the driving force. Dealing with the patient's sexual feelings and acting out by the patient should also be discussed in the supervisory sessions.[69] Epstein reports the following teaching methods: reviewing the code of ethics, using case histories of sexual misconduct, and using small-group training to help establish a group frame for ethical norms.[70]

At least seven states have adopted statutes making therapist-patient sex a criminal offense. In at least one state, the sentences imposed were brief.[71] The down side of this approach is that practitioners would be reluctant to report a colleague if they knew that the person could go to prison. The same may be true for the patient.

AMERICAN WITH DISABILITIES ACT

The American with Disabilities Act, effective in 1991, includes protection for individuals with mental health problems that limit them in one or more major activities.[72] When an individual is employed, he or she cannot be asked about prior mental health treatment as a part of the pre-employment evaluation process. Once the individual is hired, it is expected that the employer will make reasonable accommodations for him or her.

Persons who are considered to be dangerous to others by virtue of their behavior are not considered as being in the protected group. Persons who are taking prescription drugs without supervision from a health care professional are also not included.

In a recently reported case, the first of its kind in the United States, an arbitrator ruled that the Pacific Gas & Electric Company had to make a reasonable accommodation for a staff attorney who had been diagnosed with major depression, and awarded him over one million dollars.[73] The attorney had asked for a 90 hour limit for a 2 week period to accommodate to his disability. The arbitrator ruled that the attorney's proposals deserved a "fair try."

FORENSIC SERVICES

Mental health professionals can be asked by the courts to evaluate individuals who have emotional problems and have been charged with crimes. The first issue in such matters that must be addressed is the competency of the individual to stand trial. This is a limited concept that relates to the mental condition of the defendant at the time of the trial. Competency can be defined as a defendant's ability to advise counsel, understand the charges against him or her, and understand the nature, object and consequences of the proceedings.[74]

The second issue that the courts usually request the mental health professional to address is an evaluation of the individual that relates to the insanity defense (criminal responsibility). An insanity defense plea relates to the defendant's mental status at the time of the alleged crime.

Competency to stand trial is raised more often than the insanity defense and is an important concept, since the court and prosecuting attorney, as well as the defense attorney, have an obligation to ensure that the defendant is competent in order to receive a fair trial. Most evaluations for competency to stand trial can be done on an outpatient basis. If a patient needs to be hospitalized, every effort should be made to enable him or her to become competent to stand trial as quickly as possible so that he or she may proceed through the criminal justice system expeditiously.

Until the 1970s, pretrial defendants could be institutionalized for years before being brought to trial or committed under the same standards as those of civil patients. The United States Supreme Court, in the decision of *Jackson v. Indiana (1972)*, mandated a change in this process.[75]

In this case, a retarded deaf-mute resident of a maximum security unit was awaiting trial on criminal charges. Because of his disabilities, it was impossible for him to ever become competent to stand trial. Therefore, he had essentially been given a life sentence without trial. The Court held that Mr. Jackson was denied equal protection of the law because he had been subjected to a "more lenient commitment standard and to a more stringent standard of release" than other patients in psychiatric hospitals.[76] The court also pointed out that persons with criminal charges against them who are hospitalized because of their incapacity to stand trial cannot be "detained more than a reasonable period of time necessary to determine whether there is a substantial probability that they will attain competency in the foreseeable future."[77]

As a result of this decision, patients cannot be kept for long periods in a mental institution for determination of their competency to stand trial unless they are committed according to the same standards that are applied to all civil patients. In order for a pretrial defendant to be detained in a mental hospital for more than a reasonable period of time, the person must be evaluated according to the civil commitment standards of that state. An individual may still be confined in a mental hospital with charges pending for a long period of time, but only if he or she meets the standards of commitment for any patient. The treatment goal is to assist the individual to become competent to stand trial.

Several states have recently adopted a Guilty But Mentally Ill Statute (GBMI). This statute does not abolish the insanity defense but provides an alternative plan for those defendants who were mentally ill, but not insane, at the time of committing the crime.[78]

Since most states are already required to provide services to mentally ill persons who are convicted of crimes, it would appear that the main purpose of this statute is to reduce the successful use of the insanity defense and to label these individuals "mentally ill offenders."

In Tennessee, a psychiatric mental health nurse clinical specialist is considered qualified, after a training course, to testify on the issue of a defendant's competency to stand trial. Qualified nurses may be involved in this aspect of care in increasing numbers. In most jurisdictions, it is still considered necessary to have a psychologist with a doctoral degree or a psychiatrist testify on the issue of an individual's insanity or criminal responsibility.

O AN OVERVIEW

- Litigation related to the care of mentally ill patients has been related to challenging commitment, the right to treatment, the right to refuse treatment, and the duty to protect the patient.

- In an in-patient or out-patient setting, a nurse should assess whether the patient being treated was declared incompetent by a court of law; if so, a copy of the court order should be obtained and documentation established about who has authority to consent to the patient's treatment or authorize release of the patient's records.

- In planning mental-health care, professional care-givers should develop a treatment program that can be implemented in the least restrictive environment.

- Admission to in-patient psychiatric hospitals may be voluntary, involuntary on an emergency basis, or involuntary and indefinite (judicial commitments).

- Preventive or mandatory out-patient treatment has been invoked in a large number of states to address the dilemma of what to do with individuals who, when discharged from an in-patient treatment facility, discontinue their medication, deteriorate, and exhibit dangerous behavior.

- An individual admitted to a psychiatric hospital maintains certain legal rights (e.g., the right to treatment or to refuse medication), although that individual may be deprived of the freedom to leave the hospital. These rights are sometimes defined by state law, enabling mental-health professionals to be familiar with patients' rights as defined by statute in the jurisdiction where they practice.

- Boundary violations, or boundary crossings, involve abuse of the professional's power and breach of the patient's trust, in the relationship between the professional and patient. This may occur, for example, in the form of a sexual relationship between the two.

TD TERMS TO DEFINE

- boundary violations
- competency (patient)
- confidentiality
- gravely disabled
- least restrictive alternative
- malpractice
- negligence
- privilege

Q STUDY QUESTIONS

1. The evidentiary standard for committing a mental-health patient to a hospital is
   a. beyond a reasonable doubt.
   b. preponderance of the evidence.
   c. clear and convincing evidence.
   d. vicarious liability.

2. In the decision in *Tarasoff v. Regents of the University of California*, the Supreme Court of California ruled that
   a. the therapist was under no duty to report patient assault threats to a potential victim.
   b. the therapist had a duty to keep information elicited in therapy sessions confidential.
   c. only psychiatrists and psychologists had privileged communication in California.
   d. based on the facts, "the protection of privilege ends where public peril begins."

3. Competency to stand trial means that a person
   a. can be found not guilty by reason of insanity or guilty but mentally ill.
   b. must know of the charges, be able to advise counsel and be aware of the consequences of the charges.
   c. can be committed for an indefinite period to a mental hospital until competency returns.
   d. must be evaluated by a psychiatrist before proceeding with the charges.

4. The typical profile of a mental-health provider who violates boundaries is
   a. a female with an advanced degree who has been sexually abused.
   b. a divorced single mother who has an advanced degree.
   c. a male who is nationally credentialed and divorced or not happily married.
   d. a young male who is uncertain and inexperienced with providing treatment.

5. Informed consent involves
   a. giving a brief description of the proposed procedure, including its risks and benefits.
   b. giving a description of the proposed procedure, including its risks and benefits, and the alternatives with their risks and benefits.
   c. giving a comprehensive description of the proposed procedure, listing every possible risk and benefit.
   d. allowing any relative to sign for the patient upon a brief description of the procedure.

6. Discuss the procedure in your jurisdiction that applies to psychiatric units in state, county, and private facilities for patients who refuse psychotropic medication.

7. Describe the difference between confidentiality and privilege, and how it would influence your practice as a nurse.

■ END NOTES

[1] Sales, B. D., & Shuman, D. W. (1994). Mental health law and mental health care: Introduction. *American Journal of Orthopsychiatry, 64*(2), 172–179, p. 172.

[2] Ennis, B. J., & Emery, R. D. (1978). *The Rights of Mental Patients: The Revised ACLU Guide to a Mental Patient's Rights.* New York: Avon, pp. 43–48.

[3] Saphire, R. B. (1976). The civilly committed public mental patient and the right to aftercare. *Florida State University Law Review, 4,* 255.

[4] Ibid., pp. 229–242.

[5] Ibid.

[6] Ibid.

[7] Appelbaum, P. S. (1994). New York: Oxford University Press.

[8] LaFond, J. Q. (1994). Law and the delivery of involuntary mental health services. *American Journal of Orthopsychiatry, 4*(2), 209–222.

[9] Ibid., p. 211.

[10] Torrey, E. F., Stieber, J., Ezekid, S., Wolfe, M., Sharstein, S., Noble, J. H., & Flynn, L. M. (1992). *Criminalizing the Seriously Mentally Ill. The Abuse of Jails as Mental Hospitals.* A joint report of the National Alliance for the Mentally Ill and Public Citizen's Health Research Group.

[11] Appelbaum, P. S., op. cit., p. 45.

[12] Poythress, N. G. (1978). Psychiatric expertise in civil commitment: Training attorneys to cope with expert testimony. *Law & Human Behavior*, (2), 1–23.

[13] Appelbaum, op. cit., p. 48.

[14] Ibid., p. 57.

[15] Legal issues in state mental health care: Proponent for change. *Mental Disability Law Reporter*, 2(1), p. 68. (1977).

[16] *Dixon v. Weinberger*, 405 F. Supp. 974 (D.C. Cir. 1975).

[17] Hemelt, M. D., & Mackert, M. E. (1978). *Dynamics of Law in Nursing and Health Care*. Reston, VA: Reston Publishing Co., pp. 101–102 and; *Tennessee Code Annotated* 33–6–102 to 33–6–104.

[18] *In re Pilgrim Psychiatric Center*, 610 N.Y.S. 2d 962 (NY App. 1994).

[19] *Bartley v. Kremens*, 402 F. Supp. 1034 (E.D. Pa. 1975), vacated and remanded 97 S. Ct. 1709 (1977); *J. L. and J. R. v. Parham*, 412 F. Supp. 112 (M.D. Ga. 1975).

[20] *Tennessee Code Annotated* 33–6–102.

[21] *Parham v. J. L. and J. R.*, 442 U.S. 584 (1978).

[22] *Mink v. Alabama Department of Mental Health and Mental Retardation*, 620 So 2d 22 (1993).

[23] *Addington v. Texas*, 441 U.S. 418 (1979).

[24] Torrey, E. F., & Kaplan, R. S. (1995). A national survey of the use of outpatient commitment. *Psychiatric Services*, 46(8), 778–784.

[25] Ennis & Emery, op. cit., p. 154.

[26] *Rouse v. Cameron*, 373 F. 2d 451 (D.C. Circuit, 1967).

[27] *Wyatt v. Stickney*, 325 F. Supp. 781 (M.D. Ala. 1971), on submission of proposed standards by defendants 334 F. Supp. 1341, enforced 344 F. Supp. 373 (1972), affirmed in part, remanded on other grounds sub nom; *Wyatt v. Aderholt*, 503 F. 2d 1305 (Fifth Circuit, 1974).

[28] *O'Connor v. Donaldson*, 422 U.S. 563 (1975).

[29] *Youngberg v. Romeo*, 102 Sup. Ct. 2452 (1982).

[30] Ibid.

[31] *Schloendorff v. Society of New York Hospital*, 211 N.Y. 128–129, 105 N.E. 92–93 (1914).

[32] Report of the task force panel on legal and ethical issues. *Task Force Panel, Reports Submitted to the President's Commission on Mental Health* (Vol. 4, Appendix), p. 1434, Washington, D.C. 1978.

[33] Roth, L. (1977). Involuntary civil commitment: The right to treatment and the right to refuse treatment. *Psychiatric Annals*, 7(5), 50–244.

[34] *Rogers v. Okin*, 478 F. Supp. 1342 (D. Mass. 1979), *Rogers v. Okin*, 634 F. 2d 650 (1st Cir. 1980), *Rennie v. Klein*, 462 F. Supp. 1131 (N.J. 1978) at 1135, *Rennie v. Klein*, 476 F. Supp. 1294 (D.N.S. 1979).

[35] *In re Virgil D.*, 524 N.W. 2d 894 (Wis. Sup. 1994).

[36] Ibid., p. 900.

[37] Parry, J. (1987). A unified theory of substitute consent: Incompetent patients right to individualized health care decision-making. *Mental and Physical Disability Law Reporter*, 11(6), 378–385.

[38] Urrutia, G. (1994). Medication refusal—Clinical picture and outcome after use of administrative review. *Bulletin of the American Academy of Psychiatry and the Law*, 22(4), 595–603.

[39] Schwartz, H. I., Virgiano, W., & Perez, C. B. (1988). Autonomy and the right to refuse treatment. Patients attitudes after involuntary medication. *Hospital and Community Psychiatry*, 39(10), 1049–1054.

[40] Laben, J. K., & MacLean, C. P. (1989). *Legal Issues and Guidelines for Nurses Who Care for the Mentally Ill*. Second Edition. Owing Mills, Maryland. National Health Publishing.

[41] *Tennessee Code Annotated* 33–6–320.

[42] Ennis & Emery, op. cit., p. 139.

[43] Thompson, J. W., & Blaine, J. D. (1987). Use of ECT in the United States in 1975 and 1980. *American Journal of Psychiatry*, 144, 557–562.

[44] Couchon, D. Controversy and questions: Shock therapy: Patients often aren't informed of full danger. *USA Today*, December 6, 1995, 1A–2A.

[45] Crenshaw, W. B., & Francis, P. S. (1995). A national survey on seclusion and restraint in state psychiatric hospitals. *Psychiatric Services*, 46(10), 1026–1031.

[46] Ray, N. K. (1995). Use of restraint and seclusion in psychiatric settings in New York State. *Psychiatric Services*, 46(10), 1032–1037.

[47] News & Notes. (1992). Recent court ruling in Alabama's Wyatt case modifies 20 year old patient care standards. *Hospital and Community Psychiatry*, 43(8), 851–852.

[48] Maxmen, J. S. (1991). *Psychotropic Drugs: Fast Facts*. New York: W. W. Norton & Company.

[49] Bexchlibnykbutler, K. Z., Jeffries, J. J., & Martin, B. A. (1994). *Clinical Handbook of Psychotropic Drugs*. Seattle: Hogrefe and Huber.

[50] *Cohen v. State of New York*, 382 N. Y. 2d 128, (1976); *Torres v. State of New York*, 373 N.Y.S. 696 (1975).

[51] *Johnson v. State*, 603 N.Y.S. 2d 852 (A.D. 1 Dept. 1993).

[52] Hughes, D. H. (1995). Can the clinician predict suicide? *Psychiatric Services*, 46(5), 449–451.

[53] Goldacre, M., Seagroatt, V., & Hawton, K. (1993). Suicide after discharge from psychiatric inpatient care. *Lancet*, 342, 283–286.

[54] *Tarasoff v. Regents of the University of California*, 592 P. 2d 553, (1974).

[55] California court reaffirms Tarasoff ruling, finds duty to warn third parties. *Mental Disability Law Reporter*, 1976, 129.

[56] Kjervik, D. (1981). The psychiatric nurse's duty to warn potential victim of homicidal psychotherapy outpatients. *Law, Medicine and Health Care*, 9(6), 11–16.

[57] *Matt v. Burell, Inc.*, 892 S.W. 2d 796, (1995), p. 801.

[58] Appelbaum, op. cit., p. 102.

[59] Pilette, C. P. C., Berck, C. B., & Achber, L. C. (1995). Therapeutic management of helping boundaries. *Journal of Psychosocial Nursing and Mental Health Services*, 33(1), 40–47.

[60] Gutheil, T. G., & Gabbard, G. O. (1993). The concept of boundaries in clinical practice: Theoretical and risk-management dimensions. *American Journal of Psychiatry*, 150, 188–196.

[61] Hankins, G. C., Vera, M. I., Barnard, G. W., & Herkov, M. J. (1994). Patient-therapist sexual involvement: A review of clinical and research data. *Bulletin of the American Academy of Psychiatry and Law*, 22(1), 109–126.

[62] Mogul, K. M. (1992). Ethics complaints against female psychiatrists. *American Journal of Psychiatry, 149*(5), 651–653.

[63] Russell, J. (1993). *Out of Bounds: Sexual Exploitation in Counselling and Therapy.* London: Sage Publications.

[64] Bouhoutsos, J. C. (1985). Therapist-client sexual involvement: A challenge for mental health professionals and educators. *American Journal of Orthopsychiatry, 55*(2), 177–182.

[65] Epstein, R. S. (1994). *Keeping Boundaries: Maintaining Safety and Integrity in the Psychotherapeutic Process.* Washington, D.C.: American Psychiatric Press, Inc.

[66] Russell, op. cit.

[67] Simon, R. I. (1994). Transference in therapist-patient sex: the illusion of patient improvement and consent, Part I. *Psychiatric Annals, 24*(10), 509–515, p. 510.

[68] Ibid., p. 512.

[69] Blackshaw, S. L., & Patterson, P. G. R. (1992). The prevention of sexual exploitation of patients: Educational issues. *Canadian Journal of Psychiatry, 37*(5), 350–353.

[70] Epstein, op. cit.

[71] Strasburger, M. D., Jorgenson, L., & Randles, R. (1991). Criminalization of psychotherapist-patient sex. *American Journal of Psychiatry, 148*(7), 859–863.

[72] USC§ 12101–12102.

[73] Arbitrator awards lawyer with disability $1/1 Million. *Mental and Physical Disability Law Reporter, 19*(5), 560, 1995.

[74] National Institute of Mental Health. (1973). *Competency to Stand Trial and Mental Illness,* (Crime and Delinquency Issues Monograph Series, DHEW Publication No. HSM 730–9105). Washington, D.C.: U.S. Government Printing Office, p. 20.

[75] *Jackson v. Indiana,* 406 U.S. 715 (1972).

[76] Ibid., p. 716.

[77] Ibid.

[78] Laben and MacLean, op. cit.

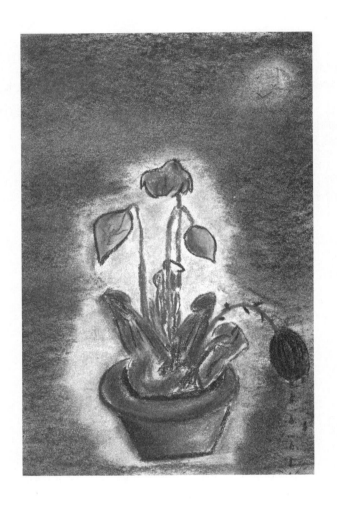

Speech was made to open man to man, and not to hide him. . . .

David Lloyd, 1635–1692

The Statemen and Favorites of England Since the Reformation vol. 1, p. 503

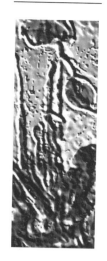

12
Therapeutic Communication

Christine A. Grant /Carol R. Hartman

What is communication? It is a continuous activity of information generation, information exchange, and information processing.

The concept of communication directs attention to the processes involved in generating, exchanging, and interpreting information. Delving into the intricacies of communication provides critical information about how life is influenced and changed during an individual's growth and development. Not only does the concept of communication organize our thinking about patterns of maintenance and change, it also broadens our scope to recognize that, in human terms, communication goes beyond the spoken and written word.

It is understandable, then, that when two people meet for the first time, such as a nurse meeting with a patient at home, they exchange at least 2,000 bits of information within the first few seconds of meeting. The spoken and unspoken behaviors of both people, and the arrangement of clothing and other inanimate objects in the environment, become part of the information exchange. In addition, the process of exchange engenders for both parties experiences that increase the amount of new information available to both. What is consciously attended to in the interchange is only a small part of all that takes place.

■ WHAT INFLUENCES COMMUNICATION?

Many factors influence communication in a health-care setting: culture, gender differences, socio-economics, social distance, power relationships, the number of participants, language, internal state, past experiences, the level of the nurse's expertise, and the patient's medications. Many other influences are involved. For example, early studies of inherited characteristics of human language and expression have focused on congenitally blind and deaf children belonging to different cultures. The congenital defects are viewed in these studies as factors that control or reduce culture influences on the expression of certain behaviors that can be assumed to be universal. Similarities in crying, coughing and being surprised are examples of behaviors more controlled by inborn traits than by culture. Rather than a polarized argument between nature and nurture, we learn that the biological basis for universal behavior such as learning a language is innate, whereas its presentation is mainly factored by cultural differences.

CULTURE VARIATIONS

Rules governing intimacy vary from one culture to another and from one class to another. There are, for example, cultural rules for status who should speak to whom, rights of questioning, and order of speaking. Certain unspoken gestures take on cultural meaning and are emblems. For example, raising the middle and index fingers to form a V for victory has a special meaning in the United States. A circle made by joining the index finger and the thumb represents perfection, and is another example of an American emblem. In Russia, raising one's hands over one's head and clasping them is a means of graciously acknowledging the recognition of a group; whereas in the United States it is interpreted as a gesture of triumph and superiority. When one thinks of Italian or French movies, many of the actors' gestures depict cultural variations in meaning and expression.

The cultural backgrounds of nurses and patients can profoundly affect therapeutic communication. One's customs, beliefs, values, and knowledge guide behavior and communication. Successful interactions depend on the nurse's ability to appreciate the norms, traditions, customs, and shared values of the patient. These cultural influences can either directly or indirectly affect the therapeutic process. The nurse who is aware of his or her own deficiencies and limitations in appreciating a patient's culture will be willing to learn from others. Increased awareness and enhanced understanding of the patient's background are essential.

GENDER DIFFERENCES

In the United States there are many assumptions about gender differences in expressive behavior, such as the belief that women express more emotion than men both verbally and facially. Research has not always upheld such specified differences. Research has demonstrated that there are gender biases in observers' interpretation of tonal qualities in speech determined by the gender of the speaker. In a study of tonal breathing characteristics (Addington, 1968), more judgments were made about female speakers than about male speakers. Thinness of voice in women led to attributions of immaturity and sensitivity, but had no effect on the judgments concerning male speakers. Males with deeper voices were described as mature, sophisticated, and well adjusted, whereas deep-voiced women were seen as boorish, ugly, lazy, and sickly (Addington, 1968).

Again, the relative influence of gender on communication characteristics is debated: do differences arise from cultural determinants or innate determinants?

SOCIO-ECONOMIC BACKGROUND

"The rain in Spain is mainly on the plain . . . I think she's got it!" says Professor Henry Higgins in the musical *My Fair Lady*. This delightful musical, based on George Bernard Shaw's play *Pygmalion,* underscores class differences with regard to speech patterns and syntactical variations, as well as semantic differences, to say nothing of non-spoken behavior. Education, vocabulary, personal experiences, and relative status positions all influence variations in patterns of communicating, and provide an experiential basis for differences in the interpretation of spoken and non-spoken behavior. In addition, other implicit aspects of social structure generate rules of communicating and both expectations and privileges not readily recognizable but clearly manifested in communication behavior.

SOCIAL DISTANCE

Age, status, and, at times, gender dictate the degree of familiarity with and of receptivity to the communications of another. For example, a worker on an assembly line is overheard stating, "Gee, I'm surprised the boss knew me and stopped and spoke." Similarly, in hospital settings, patients are often reluctant to ask anything of the physician because of a sense of social difference (distance). Patients may feel that they have nothing of value to say, or that the physician would not understand what they would say. In the mental-health field, the concept of social distance and its relationship to a free flow of communication was recognized in the mid 1950s and 60s as contributing to nontherapeutic care in state hospitals. Premises concerning the damaging effects of social distance carried over to the self-help movement efforts. These propositions are an important dimension in Alcoholics Anonymous, as well as other group movements today.

What is important is that each individual varies in what they consider appropriate and comfortable degrees of physical closeness in selected social and interpersonal situations. The number and types of verbal and nonverbal behaviors and values varies in each individual.

POWER RELATIONSHIPS

Ascribed and prescribed power in interpersonal relationships is most evident in the type, direction, frequency, and content of the material that is communicated. Relative levels of power are ascribed according to the tone of the speaker's voice and the speaker's body posture, as well as the speaker's phrasing. Power is ascribed in a specific manner to people regardless of their social position. Based on an individuals personal view of the social world, strength and weakness are inferred from these communication behaviors.

For example, a patient may be admitted to a ward believing that he is a king, and may in fact attract a relatively greater degree of attention from the staff and perhaps greater privilege by his bearing in relation to other patients. Alternatively, a physician who is unsure of himself may find that neither patients nor nursing personnel attend to his requests as they do to those of other physicians.

The notion of power is expressed and played out in many ways in human interactions. Because social position alone does not establish power in a relationship, it is important to assess how it is interpreted with each individual.

NUMBER OF RECEIVERS

Based on personal criteria, the size of a group determines how often some participants or speakers will speak and what is said. Some people are shy in small groups and one-to-one relationships, but have little difficulty lecturing before a large audience. Small-group participation often provokes anxiety because of the personal processing required by an individual who does not want to compete or be compared with others. The number of people involved in a particular communication sphere influences one's patterns of initiating, confirming, and negating information and one's willing-

ness to speak freely. Again, this sense of personal power in relationships is influenced by an individual's personal criteria for control and effectivness as it relates to closeness to others.

LANGUAGE

Language is the tool for communication, and it is essential that in therapeutic communication, the nurse recognize the patient's level of language comprehension. The nurse will need to clarify how the patient interprets words, validate the patient's meanings, and search for shared thoughts. The nurse's awareness of non-verbal communication is also critical, particularly when the nurse and client do not share a common language.

PAST EXPERIENCES

People's backgrounds influence their ability to communicate. For example, children who were supported and encouraged to verbalize their thoughts, ideas, and feelings within their family will have different communication abilities than persons whose upbringing endorsed the common saying that children should be seen and not heard. One's own experiences with self-disclosure, freedom of expression, and feelings of self-esteem will affect communication.

Nurses' attitudes and perceptions affect their abilities to perceive and interpret communication. Nurses' beliefs about others result from their own experiences and the influences of people and events important to them in their lives.

Nurses must be aware of their attitudes about clients and examine their behavior and thinking about the following terms: stereotypical, labeling, accepting, caring, judgmental, open-minded, closed-minded, opinionated, decisive, and prejudicial. All of these terms are ill-defined. When nurses sets forth their criteria to define each term, they can examine how inclusive or exclusive their perceptions are of others. For example, in careful examination of a response to someone the nurse lables as "closed-minded," she discovers that agreement is a primary criteria for concluding that a person is not closed-minded while another nurse attends to whether the individual attends to what is being said to determine if he is "closed-minded" (not attending) or "open-minded" (attending) to what is being said by repeating the conversation using the words of the sender. Nurses' abilities to examine their attitudes and perceptions will enhance their therapeutic communication.

LEVEL OF EXPERTISE

The level of nursing expertise can influence the process of therapeutic communication. Nurses who have a good understanding of self, of communication theories, and of the principles of interpersonal communication may have the advantage of being more effective communicators. Experienced nurses generally feel comfortable when relating to clients, as well as having a relaxed and self-assured style. The beginning nurse is encouraged to practice the communication techniques presented in this chapter, and to remember that therapeutic communication skills are improved through practice.

INTERNAL STATE

How one feels greatly influences one's patterns of communication. One may infer much about another's feelings from how that person communicates. Yet because many factors influence communication and the way in which one interprets another's behavior, the observer must take care about being correct in presuming another's internal state on the basis of that person's behavior. Nevertheless, it is valid to note that emotions, such as fear, anxiety, sadness, and elation influence posture, gait, voice, and language. Part of knowing people is learning their behavior in relation to their statements about their internal state. Behavior such as tone of voice, rate of speech, autonomic behavior such as skin tone, verbal phrases, patterns, become repetitive emotional states. We know people by their laugh, their eyes are examples which sharpen our ability to communicate with others.

DRUGS

Drugs affect the various forms of communication, including the transmission of information, its receipt, and its processing. Although nurses are familiar with the influence of drugs on message transmission, as in cases of intoxication, continued research in this area is needed. It is particularly needed in the area of drug use over a long period. Considerable clarification is also needed about the influence of drugs on learning, (e.g., storing, using, and communicating information). For example, we need to understand whether antidepressant drugs facilitate or inhibit an individual's use of positive thinking strategies when dealing with loss.

OTHER CONSIDERATIONS

Other factors that may alter communication behavior at all levels include loss of sensory acuity caused by sensory-organ disease, and other forms of ill health. Indeed, variations in communication behaviors may indicate underlying disease processes. For example, distraction, slurred speech, and problems in recalling immediate events could indicate interference with brain functioning.

Another important factor already suggested but worthy of underscoring is age. Attending to differences in the communication processes of young children and adolescents will facilitate better relationships between adults and children. The same is true of older people.

■ HOW DO WE COMMUNICATE?

Two broad categories of how humans communicate—spoken and nonspoken (nonverbal) behavior—are the subjects of research and theory.

SPOKEN BEHAVIOR

Spoken behavior is basic to communication. Words, their use and emphasis, are tools or symbols to express ideas and feelings. Speech can be studied from the following perspectives.

Phonology

Phonology is the study of how sounds are put together to form words. Investigations of the developing speech of children often focus on the evolution of sounds to words.

Syntax

Syntax refers to how sentences are formed from words. Implicit in the study of syntax is grammar. Syntactical patterns have been associated with different ages and different psychological states.

Semantics

Semantics is concerned with the interpretation and meaning of words. Considerable emphasis has been placed on the thematic aspects of language in the practice of different types of psychotherapy and in the development of nursing practice. Investigations and analyses of verbatim transcripts of interviews have focused on theme development and have led to concepts about psychological conflict and motivation. Thematic aspects of language refers to the metaphorical dimensions of speech references. When these are repeated in communication, assumptions have been made as to the psychological significance of these references and their meaning at the route of psychological conflict and motivation. For example, the constant degrading comments of a man toward women is interpreted as representing deep conflicts in early life with caretakers, which now results in an inability to have a close relationship with a woman and to intense expressions of anger if challenged by a woman. The themes are represented in speech and behavior, however the dynamic interpretations are based on models of intrapsychic life and its development within the context of certain types of interpersonal relationships, i.e. loving relationships or demeaning relationships. Underscored in this area of study has been the distinction between private and shared meaning. **Denotation** refers to the general meaning of a word. **Connotation** refers to the particular meaning of a word to a particular person. Confusion about meaning can be seen in a small child who objects when a woman introduces her own mother to the child. The child may object because to the child, the word *mother* connotes the child's own mother. As yet, the denotative meaning of mother—a type of relationship—is not clear to the small child. That words have this twofold potential for meaning (private and public), and that the choice of words is influenced by the context in which a person exists at a particular time, suggests a great potential for misunderstanding.

Pragmatics

Pragmatics is the investigation of how we participate in conversations with one another. In verbal communication, particular attention is paid to the ways in which the participation of those in conversation either confirm or deny the experiences of another person. Consequently, the language that is used is assessed in the context of non-verbal phenomena, such as intonation, pauses, rate, amplitude, and pitch (paralanguage).

Paralanguage

Paralanguage consists of nonverbal aspects of speech, such as tone or tenor of voice. Many researchers in paralinguistics believe that these aspects of speech convey emotion. Consequently, it is felt that studies of paralanguage are important in personality research as well as in the study of psychopathology. Variables such as intonation, pitch, volume, rhythm, voice quality, and frequency of pauses convey information about affective states.

NONSPOKEN BEHAVIOR

A wide variety of nonspoken behaviors may be observed, such as body language, writing, spatial behavior, autonomic nervous system responses, clothing style, and use of symbols.

Body Language

In studies of behavior, body language is often a focus. Unfortunately, many interpretations attempt to generalize what is happening within another person from their posture, gait, mannerisms, gestures, and facial ex-

pressions. Although it is often true that stooped shoulders, a slow gait, and slowed speech are associated with depression, it is not universally true. Information communicated in body language is most useful if interpreted within the total context of an individual.

Handwriting

Little research has been done on handwriting. Graphology and handwriting analysis, however, have been pursued by lay people for many years. Some graphologists claim that they can interpret emotional distress and other personal problems by analyzing handwriting. They develop categories of handwriting styles, and relate them to personality traits and characteristics. These efforts to draw definitive conclusions about an individual's behavior from his or her handwriting have a high risk of error. In semantics, suicide notes have been studied and attempts made to relate their content and themes to variables that might predict suicidal behavior.

Diaries, journals, and biographical sketches require more in-depth study for diagnostic and treatment purposes. The trials of assassins and persons who attempt to murder prominent people sometimes disclose the premeditation of such behavior recorded in personal journals. Forensic nurses are involved in research on threat communication.

Spatial Behavior

Spatial behavior (proxemics) concentrates on the psychological implications of the use of space. When the nurse walks through a psychiatric ward, it is interesting to observe who sits where, and how close these positions are to other people, activities, and strategic aspects of the ward, such as the nursing station. Anthropologists pioneered in the study of space, noting how tribal living arrangements were set up and how space related to other aspects of tribal life, as well as how it influenced patterns of communication.

Sommer (1965) studied the connection between spatial arrangements and group tasks. He found that competing pairs sat opposite one another, conversing pairs sat diagonally, and cooperating pairs sat side by side.

Autonomic Nervous System Responses

The responses of the autonomic nervous system constitute a large area within the study of communication. Tearing, blushing, crying, pallor, gastrointestinal sounds, and breathing patterns have always been the province of expert clinicians. One such clinician, Dr. Milton Erikson, the father of hypnotherapy, used autonomic responses such as breathing to pace his use of language, and induced hypnotic states through this technique.

Calibrating (visually measuring) tics and other non-spoken mannerisms to specific topics under discussion often provides the clinician with clues that a topic has more significance than might be consciously apparent to the patient. Of particular significance in this area are studies that correlate patterns of verbal behavior and thought with changes in physiological states, such as blood pressure. A model neuro-linguistic programming, links eye movements with certain linguistic patterns (Diltz, et al., 1980).

Clothing and Symbols

Clothing and the use of symbols are other forms of nonspoken behavior that are integral to the process of communicating. In clinical practice, observing the care and appropriateness of dress are part of patient assessment. Inferences about psychological organization and social responsiveness are examples of information drawn from dress and clothing.

Styles and customs reveal information about an individual's group life, such as the habit of a nun or the uniform of a policeman. The dress of adolescents may indicate their social group and conformity. Certain aspects of grooming, such as makeup, beards, and hairstyles, may also communicate information. The wearing of jewelry, such as wedding rings or special amulets, also conveys information.

THE RELATIONSHIP BETWEEN SPOKEN AND NONSPOKEN BEHAVIOR

Much of what individuals communicate is beyond their awareness. Nurses need to recognize the potential for confusion and be sensitive to feedback in order to adjust their communication patterns. Adjustment is facilitated in realizing that one's tone of voice, facial expression, and posture may present another person with information that is experienced as incongruent with the words used by the speaker. The point is to now view the communication process and the deriving of meaning between people as being forged by more personal constructs than an agreement on the meaning of a word. Meaning is shaped not just by the sender but also by the receiver who has very personal criteria for drawing conclusion regarding meaning. When the nurse recognizes that the meaning of her/his communication is the response she/he elicits, adjustments can be made more quickly to work toward understanding rather than misunderstanding. Following this proposition, the nurse can learn to suspend judgment and work toward taking on the perspective of another for purposes of understanding. Knowing that meaning is derived from

nonspoken as well as spoken information, gives the nurse the capacity to listen with the "third ear," that dimension of human awareness that leaves one open to new possibilities.

Besides understanding how these two dimensions of communication (spoken and non-spoken) converge in interpersonal exchange, it is important to understand how they operate intrapersonally. Research is revealing an internal system of communication that has physiological consequences, and that physiological experiences can have psychological consequences. Attending to speech as well as body movement in a more comprehensive manner opens a window into how behavior is maintained and changed both by the individual and through interaction with others.

■ THEORETICAL MODELS OF HUMAN COMMUNICATION

A GRADATION OF THEORETICAL COMPLEXITY

A brief historical review of theories of communication demonstrates how we have moved to a more complex understanding of the communication process and the derivation of personal meaning. Theories are statements of logical propositions designed to give order to experience, to allow for prediction, and to clarify a specific area of study. Among other characteristics, theories contain suppositions about cause and effect. General theories of communication are closely related to theories of learning, since learning is concerned with the intake, storage, and use of experience. Consequently, theories about learning will to some extent be represented in theories of communication, because the communication process is essential for learning. The theories of communication summarized here focus on the dyad, or communication between two entities.

SENDER AND RECIPIENT

The most simplistic theory of communication emphasizes the sender and the recipient. This is based on Hullian's (1952) notions of drive reduction and stimulus-response phenomena. In this model of the world, subjective meaning was discouraged. Rather, behavior resulted from a stimulus (reward, punishment) and internal drives (hunger, sex, aggression). Messages were learned cues that demanded certain behaviors. Skill in communicating was learning the demand characteristic of a stimulus and its association with a specific behavior that would either gain reward or avoid punishment. Briefly, A is the initiator of a communication; the communication is designated the *message;* and B receives the message. Understanding occurs if B accepts, without interference, A's message. This theory assumes that there is a "correct" message and that the sender and recipient are relatively independent of one another, having little influence on the meaning of the message but great responsibility for sending it and the skills needed to receive it. Emphasis is placed on the denotative aspects of words, syntax, and semantics; and skill is based on the selection and appropriateness of words.

Belief in this model typifies many interpersonal arguments that carry both an overt and a covert message of blame. For example, A says, "I told you not to put the car in the garage." B replies, "You told me that you weren't sure you were going to use the car." In the example, the sender and the receiver respond with a sense of blame and criticism. Neither recognizes the limits of their own interpretation of what they said, how it was limited in specific meaning, nor how the receiver was limited in the conclusions drawn as to the meaning of the message. The receiver assumes a consequence and the sender presumes an understanding of options and possibilities.

RECIPROCITY IN INTERACTION

The next level of theory about the communication process emphasizes reciprocity in interaction. Basically, this theory assumes that communication is an interactive process, and that communication is effective when reciprocity is achieved through the process of feedback to ensure agreement about the meaning of a message. The emphases of this theory are that each person has a perspective and that it is important that each step into the other's meaning "framework." What this theory omits is the complexity of the communications exchanged and how interpretation occurs and becomes part of the communication process. This example does not explain how meaning is derived or how it influences communication behavior.

In clinical practice and in interpersonal relationships, adherence to a theory that assumes there is agreement as to meaning in terms of words as concrete stimuli leads to the personal expectation that one person can know the experiences of another in a direct way. A presumption is made that we can truly understand the experiences of another. Patterns of expectations are set up regarding the capacities of oneself and others to understand one another, and with expectations, disappointment and a search for blame. Difficulties arise when the recipient assumes that his impression of and response to what the sender says are the same as the experience being conveyed by the sender. This assumption implies that someone can know the thoughts and experiences of another by putting themselves in the other's position. Failure to "understand" continues to create a pattern of blame in miscommunication.

TRANSACTION

The next level of communication theory incorporates the pragmatics of conversing (environmental influences) and the complexity of meaning. This moves communication from the levels of action and interaction to the level of transaction. What is meant here is that theories of communication moved from understanding that each person has their own symbolic map that shapes meaning and that these are expressed in interpersonal interactions. The communication processes are complex patterns of transaction where meaning is constantly negotiated and, when it is not, there is a breakdown in the process. This breakdown reflects a return to a less complex accounting of what is going on and a reliance of assumptions of concrete agreements to the idiosyncratic thinking of those involved in the process. In short, one becomes committed to only that which one thinks and experiences.

In the mid- and late-1960s, we see in the writings of various people this evolution of communication theories.

The growth in complexity of a two-person conversation has been presented by Laing, Phillipson, and Lee (1966). They see behavior as the result of the personal perception of experience. Perceptions serve a decisive functional role in the behavior generated from experience. The following set of perceptions, during a dyadic exchange, demonstrate the complexity that perception engenders in the communication process.

- How does B think of me?
- How does B think I think of him?
- How A thinks of himself or herself.

These same three perceptual considerations are operant for B. This means that at any point during an interaction between A and B, six dominant perceptual dimensions can be in process. Consequently, the request to garage the car, although shared between A and B, will have decidedly different experiential meaning for each.

PERSONAL PSYCHOLOGICAL CONSTRUCTS

The most complex theory of communication is that meaning is derived from personal psychological constructs (Kohler, 1947). Examples of these personal constructs are assumptions of cause and effect; time orientation (personal); self-concerns versus the needs of others; perception of control from within versus control from without; decision criteria for determining both internal stimuli and stimuli from the outside. This theory has resulted in a model called the **symbolic interactionist model** of communication. Basically, the model attempts to explain communication on an inter-

and intra-personal level while incorporating the tenets of the transactional model set forth earlier. The symbolic interactionist model was first proposed by sociologist J. E. Hulett, Jr. (1966). It is a rapid process in which a person, in his or her mind, plays out personal perceptions of possible consequences of actions on another person. Sometimes the actual outcome is a match and sometimes it isn't. When there is not a match, the sender reacts without realizing that she or he set up the expectations that were not fit for the recipient. A simple example is the child who cries and cringes expecting to be yelled at by the parent because the child lost her mittens and imagined that when the father was told, he would start yelling. Its structure contains input and covert rehearsal. Input refers to any stimulus, external or internal, that engages an individual in an interpersonal interaction for some specific goal. Covert rehearsal is the filter through which personal meaning is derived for the individual. This cognitive map is a source of information, and contains the stored resources for filtering and interpreting messages from without and from within. Covert rehearsal also includes the processes that generate behavior: (1) the message generation, which is the actual act of delivering the message; (2) the environmental event, which in part refers to the new information generated by the delivered message; and (3) the goal response. Covert rehearsal is a phrase to summarize the complex processes that generate behavior. Each of the three points involves its own complex set of processes. What Hulett's thinking did is force those interested in communication to realize that action is not simply reflexive nor is it simply explained by one motivation model of causality. Further, that once behavior is generated, there are consequences that now enlarge the management of the communication process. We can go back to the example of putting the car in the garage. A asks B "Are you going to use the car today?" B replies, "I'm not sure I'm going to use the car today."

The areas of covert rehersal represent phases in the communication process. Communication can be examined both from the viewpoint of the unique functions of each of its phases and as a total process. Critical to this model are the phases of covert rehearsal and the recognition of the environmental event (B confronting A) that emanates from the message generation. A, prior to asking B about the car, has rehearsed in his own mind a personal scenario regarding the car and a goal—let's assume it is to put the car in the garage. B now responds to A's comments about the car from his internal map of possibility and expectation—let's say with the goal of keeping his options open. B replies, "I am not sure." A receives the message and this generates his behavior to put the car in the garage. A goes to get the car, which is in the garage and he concludes that B did not follow his instructions. This generates behavior that now has B confronting A.

This model generates relevant assumptions about communication. Messages are organized by running internal processes that select behaviors reached in response to the perceptions of the individual. There is a trial run of these behaviors, and the individual selects those perceived as being most successful in conveying meaning. Success is a function of the person's criteria. To repeat, criteria are the subjective and objective informational cues that allow a person to select and act. For example, what has to be in a situation for one person to scream at another person for stepping in front of him while in line at the bank? What has to be there for a girl to accept a request for a dance from a young man? What has to be there for a man to speak up to his boss about a raise? In all of these situations, does each person have the same criteria? Our criteria are forged from personal experience and our ideas of anticipated experiences. Criteria are generated from interactions between our self and our external and internal environments. Whatever is communicated at a point in time can never be repeated. Communication is complex and ongoing. Meaning is not transferred; rather it is inferred and negotiated.

■ THERAPEUTIC COMMUNICATION INTERACTIONS

Interactions between a nurse and a patient have specific guidelines and boundaries. When communicating therapeutically with a patient, the nurse is focused on exploring the patient's feelings, experiences, and ideas. Therapeutic communication differs from a social encounter (a topic such as gardening or the weather), and from intimate encounters (where role boundaries blur).

The use of therapeutic communication involves well-planned, patient-focused, and goal-directed interactions. These interactions can be brief and spontaneous, such as discussing a patient's experience at a recreational activity, and well-planned, such as discussing a patient's feelings about returning to the community.

COMPONENTS OF THERAPEUTIC COMMUNICATION

The therapeutic use of self entails a complex, skilled, and active process of communication. The psychiatric nurse brings to it a knowledge of both self and communication theory, and the ability to interact with the patient in a manner that focuses on the patient rather than

TABLE 12–1. ACTIVE LISTENING BEHAVIORS

Facilitate Communication	Hinder Communication
Direct eye-to-eye contact	Avoiding client's eyes
Comfortable physical distance	Too close or too far apart
Leaning toward client to listen	Sitting way back in chair
Open body posture	Folding arms tightly
Gentle nodding, gesturing	Bored appearance
Relaxed manner	Fidgeting, nervousness
Looking concerned	Non-responsiveness
Gentle, reassuring touch	Aggressive physical contact

the nurse. The nurse engages the patient in meaningful communication, and focuses on the patient's needs and ability to disclose feelings by gently guiding and structuring the patient's disclosures. The nurse provides the patient with a feeling of security and is involved in ascertaining the patient's level of comfort. Therapeutic use of self is directly related to the nurses' ability to engender in the patient a sense of trust, or the ability to allow communication to move beyond the superficial and to the personal level. Establishing trust allows the patient to share information in a confidential manner. Trust requires the nurse to keep promises and be reliable, consistent, and truly interested in what the patient says, as well as accepting of the patient's behavior.

Empathy, an essential component of therapeutic communication, involves the nurse's ability to place him- or herself in the patient's position without losing objectivity. The nurse conveys empathy when he or she shares the patient's frame of reference and can respond to the patient's language and mood in a reflective, sensitive manner. The empathetic nurse conveys an understanding of the patient's emotional pain by using active listening skills (Table 12–1) and communicating to the patient an understanding of the patient's perspective.

Respect is conveyed to a client through unconditional positive regard (Rogers, 1961), and is an essential component of therapeutic communication. Respect is the valuing of another person for who they are, not for what they have or can do. Nurses who have respect for their patients value them as individuals, and demonstrate this respect through their actions and words. Respect allows the patient to have positive feelings about him- or herself, to maintain dignity, and to be valued as an individual. Respect, conveyed to a patient through privacy, confidentiality, and dignity, includes the following:

- Introducing oneself and asking how the patient wishes to be addressed.

- Clarifying one's role and duties with the patient.
- Establishing a time frame for interactions, including the length and location of meetings.
- Creating a secure and private environment.
- Reviewing issues of confidentiality with the patient.
- Discussing the patient only with other staff members.
- Protecting the patient's rights, including written records and the sharing of information.
- Advocating the patient's dignity by explaining procedures, policies, and activities.

Genuineness is the ability to convey true interest to a patient, in both the patient and the information the patient shares with the nurse. Genuineness is openness, authenticity, and the ability to be sincere. The patient who perceives genuineness will be more likely to trust the nurse, thus increasing the opportunity for further therapeutic interactions. The components of the therapeutic relationship—respect, trust, genuineness, empathy, confidentiality and the use of self—are reciprocal components, each building on the other.

STRATEGIES TO ENHANCE THERAPEUTIC COMMUNICATION

Nonverbal skills that facilitate therapeutic communication include simple actions that reassure patients that the nurse is listening and attending to them, such as smiling at the patient when appropriate; maintaining an interested and concerned facial expression; assuring that one's own physical proximity to the patient is close enough to express interest but not so close as to create anxiety; making gentle gestures with the hands and arms; maintaining good eye contact; and shifting one's body weight toward the patient in a gesture of active listening. Additional techniques include shaking hands with a patient upon meeting, gesturing to a chair for the patient, and the use of touch. The nurse must use extra caution when utilizing the non-verbal technique of touch. Some patients, like some nurses, do not like to be touched or to touch. The use of a hand upon a patient's shoulder or hand must be carefully assessed in advance, and if a patient rebukes the touch, careful evaluation and processing of the experience must be initiated. The use of touch, as a human interaction, develops with experience and consultation.

Silence is another nonverbal technique of communication. Some nurses are uncomfortable with silence and make every attempt to fill gaps in conversation with questions and/or comments. Yet silence allows the nurse time to think, allows the patient the space in which to respond, and communicates patience. Silence can also convey acceptance of the patient.

Several facilitative communication techniques, designed to assist in gathering information, can be adapted to the needs of the patient.

ACKNOWLEDGMENT

Acknowledging the patient for who he or she is conveys a readiness to interact, portrays a self that is warm but not effusive or too friendly, and affords the patient the respect and dignity needed to facilitate interpersonal interaction. Acknowledgment involves addressing the patient by his or her preferred name, using appropriate distance and touch, and maintaining an attentive stance toward the patient. Thus, "Good morning, Mr. Sherwin. It's nice to see you again. I am Ms. Grant and I will be your nurse today. How did your first evening in the unit go for you?"

OPEN-ENDED QUESTIONS

Open-ended questions allow the patient to respond in a variety of ways, including description, the sharing of information, and changing the topic if necessary. Open-ended questions give the patient the opportunity to choose how to answer a question. Examples of open-ended questions include the following:

"How do you feel about your admission to the hospital?"

"Tell me about your family meeting last evening."

"How did the medication affect your sleep?"

Closed-ended questions are those that require at least a one-word response, and at most a brief and specific response. Most often they seek "Yes" or "No" responses (e.g., "Did you have your medications today? Are you hallucinating?")

PROVIDING INFORMATION

Psychiatric nurses are intricately involved in health promotion and teaching. Providing information in a responsible manner requires good screening questions about what the patient wants to know and why. Specificity and clarification are important when giving information and evaluating a response. They offer the patient data that he or she may need in order to experience growth. Being straight-forward with the patient is preferred to probing, such as "Why do you ask?" Other examples of clarifying or focusing the patient before giving information include:

Client: "What does the doctor say about my treatment?"

Nurse: "Can you be specific about what you would like to know about your treatment?"

Client: "I'd like to know the name of my medication."

Nurse: "Of course. You are on two medications, Mr. Johnson, lithium carbonate and haldol."

Patients may seek personal information about the nurse. Nurses should not hesitate to give information about themselves that is considered public knowledge (e.g., their marital status, school of nursing, etc.). Questions such as "What do you think of my doctor?" are complex, and the patient's intent has to be determined. Clearly, this is a provocative question, (e.g., intended to reveal the nurse's nonverbal response), but it may be genuine in that the patient wants to know the educational level and training of the doctor. A neutral response is indicated, such as, "Dr. Jones has been on this unit for two years (or "is just beginning a residency" or "is a graduate of City Medical School"), why do you ask?" It is helpful to briefly answer the patient's question with a known fact, and to then explore the intent underlying the question.

FOCUSING

Concentrating on eliciting details (focusing) to facilitate communication has elements that are both open-ended and closed-ended. Focusing encourages the patient to answer with more than a simple word or phrase. It assists the patient to pursue an idea or emotion, and eliminates peripheral communication that prevents the discussion of specific information. Examples of focusing questions are:

"You mentioned a sister just briefly. Could you tell me more about your entire family?"

"You stated that you were very depressed last week. How has it been for you since then?"

"Tell me what you did in recreational therapy this morning."

PROBING

Probing includes questions and statements that encourage the patient to express additional information. Probes are focused questions, but can be interpreted by the patient as invasive or insensitive. Skill is necessary to use probes effectively. Examples of probes are:

"Tell me more."

"Can you say more about that?"

"It sounds like there is more to what you are feeling. Can you expand on your thoughts?"

"Go on . . ." (followed by silence).

PARAPHRASING

Paraphrases give the patient a translation of what the nurse thinks the patient is communicating. Paraphrasing is reflective of something the patient says without distorting its meaning. It is a facilitative method for capturing the entire meaning of the patient's statements, not simply a response to an expression.

Paraphrasing requires assimilating and interpreting patients' statements in their own words. It is useful for ascertaining the meaning of a communication and furthering the discussion. Useful prefatory statements in paraphrasing are:

"I hear you saying . . ."

"In other words . . ."

An exchange might be:

Client: "I can't sleep. I get up 3 or 4 times in the night. I am always so tired in the morning."

Nurse: "When you get up, what do you do?"

CLARIFYING

Clarifying ensures understanding of a communication. It is a difficult element of communication to master. When clarifying, it is important not to blame the patient, such as by saying, "Your getting up at night might be the reason you can't go back to sleep."

Requests for clarification are essential, convey a sense of genuine interest in the nurse's interaction with the patient, and can be expressed with warmth and sincerity.

"I'm not sure I understood what you were saying. Could you repeat it for me?"

"I wasn't able to follow you. Can you tell me in another way?"

"Could you go over that once more. I am confused."

EXPLORING AND QUESTIONING

Exploring and questioning are intricately related and should not be confused with simple open-or closed-ended questions that seek to obtain information. The nurse can only explore personal issues with a patient when a therapeutic relationship has been established. In an atmosphere of trust and acceptance, the patient will be able to respond to questions that are personal, highly sensitive, and emotionally charged. Exploration of sensitive issues promotes patients' healing and growth. The patient will respond in a positive manner if the setting is one of mutual respect, confidentiality, and genuineness. The timing of exploration through questioning is critical, and is premature in the early stages of the therapeutic relationship. Many lead-in questions will be essential in order to assess the patient's anxiety level. An example of an exploratory interaction might be as follows:

Nurse: "You told me you were having difficulties in your relationships with women. Could you tell me more about your social life?"

Patient: "Well, I don't go out much."

Nurse: "Go on . . ." (gentle reassurance for the patient to continue).

Patient: "I met this one woman at group, she was really nice, but I'm not sure. I didn't talk to her."

Nurse: "Sounds like you were interested in her."

Patient: "Yes, but I didn't even talk to her. There were too many people around."

Nurse: "Do you remember how you felt when you were in the group with her?"

Patient: "I was really nervous, but a nice kind of nervous. I wished I could have talked to her."

Nurse: "Describe for me what you would have said to her if you had not been in the group setting.

CONFRONTING

Confrontation demonstrates to patients incongruencies, discrepancies, or inconsistencies in their communication and behavior. Confrontation should not be mistaken for aggressiveness, nor is confrontation an attack on a patient. It is rather a skilled and elaborate method of pointing out the underlying truths in a patient's feelings or behavior. The positive aspect of confrontation is expanded self-awareness and behavioral change. Confrontation involves feedback to the patient about how the patient's behavior and actions affect the nurse. Feedback is not advice-giving, but rather an honest response to the patient's behavior and should be explorative, descriptive, content-specific, patient-focused, and time-limited. Constructive confrontations include the following elements:

- Active listening with special attention to non-verbal behaviors.
- Use of "I" statements.
- Acknowledgment that the changing of behavior is difficult.
- Focused feedback statements that point up incongruence and inconsistencies in the patient's feelings, thoughts, and behaviors.
- Supportive statements that challenge the patient to action, including responsibility for his or her behavior and accountability for his or her feelings.
- Integration of patient-identified adaptive coping responses in order to foster confidence that change is possible.

REFLECTING

Reflecting helps the patient to explore his or her own feelings. Responding to the patient's emotional tone or affective statements explores the meaning of a communication. Reflection allows the nurse to state the implied and to remain in the immediate present with a patient; it encourages the patient to explore feelings and, in turn, is an opportunity for the nurse to genuinely respond to those feelings. The following is an example of a reflective interaction.

> Nurse: "You seem very anxious. I will stay with you."
> Patient: "My family was supposed to be here with me. Not you."
> Nurse: "It sounds like you are angry at your family for not being here on time."
> Patient: "They don't know what it is like to be in here!"
> Nurse: "You're feeling alone and uncomfortable about being admitted to the unit."
> Patient: "Yes, I am really very scared."

SUMMARIZING

One of the most important facilitative techniques is summarizing. At the appropriate juncture in an interview, or at the end of a formal session, the nurse verbally captures the essence of the transaction that has taken place. The summary should reflect the main content of the session, the feelings, the facts, and the discrepancies that were discussed. Summarizing allows the patient to hear what is recalled about the conversation and to experience "being heard." It is also an opportunity for the patient to ask questions, seek clarification, provide information, and continue to build rapport for the next meeting. Summarization focuses on the main themes of the session and sets the tone for the next meeting. It is a means for the nurse to terminate an interaction and set the time for the next meeting. Summarizing is not an abrupt end to a conversation, but rather a thoughtful communication technique that demonstrates willingness to work with a patient by being available and interested in the patient as a person. For example:

> Nurse: "Let me see if I can summarize what we talked about today. I heard you tell me about your family's reaction to your hospitalization. You have many concerns about their ability to understand your illness, and although they say they will come to see you on a regular basis you fear they may reject you. From what you've said you would like to continue to work on understanding your depression and feelings of hopelessness. I have to leave now, but I will be here tomorrow at the same time. I have learned from our meeting and I would like to continue our discussion then."

INEFFECTIVE VERBAL TECHNIQUES

Just as facilitative techniques enhance communication, so can ineffective verbal responses limit, hinder, or even stop communication.

Blaming

Blaming is an attack on the patient's behavior or actions. Typically it is hostile and involves "finger-pointing." Statements that indicate blame include: "You always," "It's your own fault," "You caused," and "What are you doing?"

Advice-giving:

Advice-giving is to offer the patient an opinion. Giving the patient suggestions about his or her own beliefs includes statements such as. "I think you should . . . ," "My advice to you is . . . ." "In my view you. . . ."

False Reassurance and Approval

False reassurance and/or false approval when the patient does not want to confront the real meaning of an interaction includes such statements as: "Don't worry." "Everything will be all right." "It's not that bad." "There's no need to get angry."

Judging

Judging a patient's behavior as either "good" or "bad" hinders communication. Judging is similar to reprimanding, scolding, and demonstrating a closed posture. The end result may be that the patient feels guilty and angry. Judgemental statements include: "I would never do that." "You don't know how hard it is going to get." "I don't think that you should . . . ." If you weren't so. . . ."

Rationalizing

Rationalizing reduces and minimizes the patient's real concerns and feelings. Rationalization attempts to explain away the patient's feelings. Rationalizing statements include: "It's not important." "Everyone feels like that." "Oh, don't worry." "We all do that once in a while."

Changing Topics

Changing topics without a clear rationale may meet the needs of the nurse while abandoning those of the patient. It may reflect anxiety about subject matter, may indicate embarrassment, or may indicate indecision about how to respond to a patient.

Other Non-Facilitative Actions

Additional actions that are non-facilitative to communication include leading the patient to the response the nurse desires, moralizing, asking multiple questions without waiting for answers, echoing the patient's words by continual repetition; and patronizing the patient by "talking down," using immature language, and posturing. The use of too many "why" questions and too many closed-ended questions may stall communication.

O AN OVERVIEW

- Therapeutic communication is dynamic, reciprocal, multi-dimensional, and very complex.

- Nurses help clients to express their feelings and thoughts through assessment and understanding of their distress.

- Effective, sensitive communication is a basic skill and includes focused listening and empathy.

- The interpersonal dimension of psychiatric nursing has a strong tradition in the care of all patients in all types of setting.

TD TERMS TO DEFINE

- communication
- connotation
- denotation
- empathy
- language
- paralanguage
- phonology
- semantics
- symbolic interactionist model of communication
- syntax

Q STUDY QUESTIONS

1. Which of the following does not describe therapeutic communication?
   a. planning is essential
   b. it is patient-focused
   c. it is goal-directed
   d. it is patient-initiated

2. Therapeutic use of self includes all of the following except:
   a. complex interactions
   b. purposive interactions
   c. active process
   d. passive process

3. T F Empathy is part of the subjective process.

4. T F Nonverbal behavior is the way a person acts.

5. List four ways respect is conveyed to a client.

6. Resistive silence generally occurs during which phase of the nurse-patient relationship?
   a. Beginning phase
   b. Working phase
   c. Ending phase

7. The nurse takes a direct verbal approach when there is concern regarding a patient's:
   a. emotional reaction.
   b. expression of thoughts.
   c. control of behavior.

8. A patient asks a direct question about his condition. The nurse should:
   a. establish what prompted the question.
   b. answer the question.
   c. divert the patient.
   d. refer the patient.

9. List 4 nonuseful communication responses.

10. Give a brief example from clinical practice of the following:
    Acknowledgment
    Giving information
    Focusing
    Clarifying
    Exploring
    Confronting
    Reflecting
    Paraphrasing
    Summarizing

■ REFERENCES

Addington DW: The relationship of selected vocal characteristics to personality perception. *Speech Monogr* 1968; 35, 492–503.

Standards of Psychiatric Mental Health Clinical Nursing Practice. Washington, DC, American Nurses Association, 1994.

Birdwhistell RL: *Kinetics and Context.* Philadelphia: University of Pennsylvania Press, 1970.

Book HE: Is empathy cost effective? *Am J Psychother* 1991; 45(1):21–30.

Diltz R, Grindler J, Bandler R, Bandler LC, DeLozier J: *Neuro-Linguistic Programming: The Study of the Subject of Subjective Experience.* Cupertino, CA., Meta Publications, 1980.

Dittmann AT: *Interpersonal Messages of Emotion.* New York, Springer, 1972.

Eibl-Eibesfeldt I: Similarities and differences between cultures, in Weitz S (ed): *Nonverbal Communication.* London, Cambridge University Press, 1974.

Gottschalk LA: A computerized scoring system for use with content analysis scales. *Comp Psychiatry* 1975: 16, 177–90.

Hulett JG Jr: A symbolic interactionist model for human communication. *AV Commun Rev* 1966; 14:14.

Hull CL: *A Behavior System.* New Haven, Yale University Press, 1952.

Kemper BJ: Therapeutic listening: developing the concept. *J Psychosoci Nurs* 1992; 30:21–26.

Kohler W: *Gestalt Psychology.* New York, Liverwright, 1947.

LaFrance M, Mayo C: *Moving Bodies: Nonverbal Communication in Social Relationships.* Monterey, CA, Brooks Cole, 1978.

Laing RD, Phillipson H, Lee AR: *Interpersonal Perception.* London, Tavistock, 1966.

Liehr P: Uncovering a Hidden Language: The effects of listening and talking on blood pressure and heart rate, *Arch Psychiatr Nurs,* 1992; 6:303–311.

Macrae JC: Nightingale's spiritual philosophy and its significance for modern nursing, *Image* 1995; 27(1):8–10.Olson T: Fundamental and special: The dilemma of psychiatric mental health nursing. *Arch Psychiatr Nurs,* 1996; 10:3–15.

Shelton SB: The doctor-patient relationship, in Stoudemire A (ed): *Human Behavior,* ed. 2. Philadelphia, JB Lippincott, 1994, 3–21.

Sommer K: Further studies in small group ecology. *Sociometry* 1965; 28:337–348.

Weintraub W: *Verbal Behavior: Adaption and Psychopathology.* New York, Springer, 1983.

Davidhizar R, Bowen M: The Dynamics of Laughter, *Arch Psychiatr Nurs* 1992; 6:132–137.

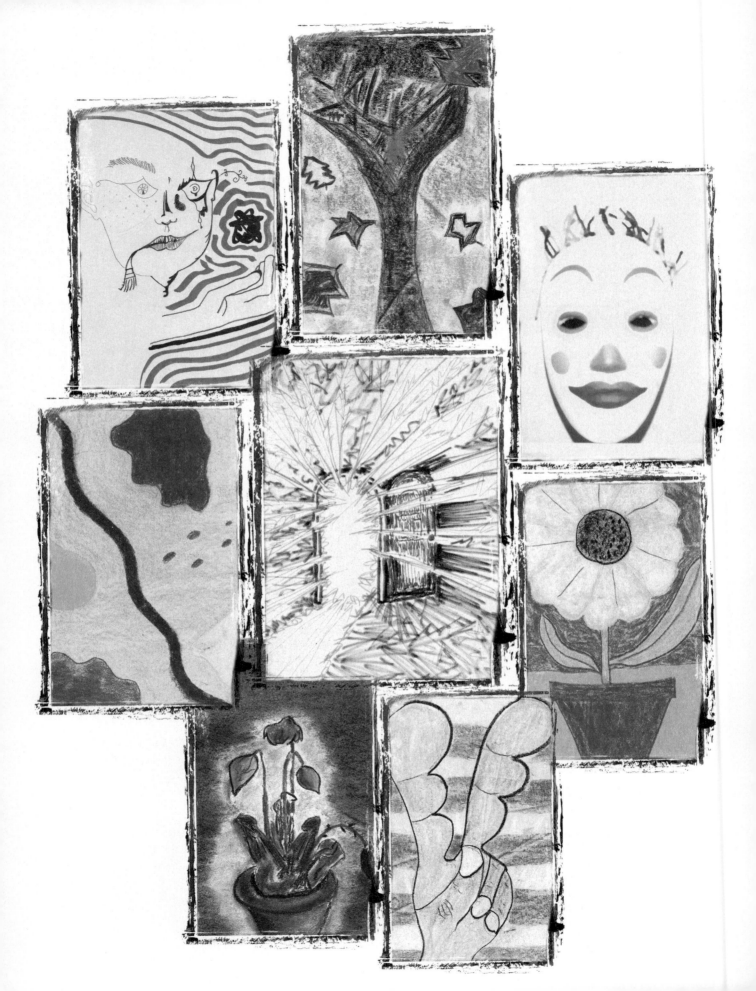

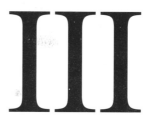
III

CLINICAL DISORDERS ON THE STRESS-CRISIS CONTINUUM

The mental disorders described in Section III are classified on a seven-level stress–crisis continuum. The first levels of the continuum include a high degree of physical symptomatology with a stressful event. The event increases anxiety, which provokes coping behaviors; however, it does not necessarily trigger a crisis state. At the upper end of the continuum is the individual with pre-existing psychiatric conditions that complicate the situation and require intervention for the acute and long-term phases of the patient's care. In advancing from Level 1 to Level 7, the internal biopsychosocial conflicts of the patient and family increase in the expression of progressively more maladaptive coping behaviors. This level-based typology is designed to help in assessing patients, identifying nursing diagnoses, and developing nursing care plans.

Assessing stress in terms of seven levels along a stress–crisis continuum is an adaptation of the work of Peplau (1952), Baldwin (1978), and Burgess and Roberts (1995).

The seven levels are

- *Somatic distress*
- *Transitional stress and altered self-regulatory patterns*
- *Traumatic crises*
- *Relational and family crises*
- *Serious mental illness*
- *Psychiatric emergencies*
- *Cataclysmic stress*

LEVELS OF STRESS-CRISIS CONTINUUM

	1. Somatic Distress	2. Transitional Stress and Altered Self-regulatory Patterns	3. Traumatic Stress	4. Relational and Family Crisis
Defining characteristics:	Physical stress and symptoms with or without stressor, psychiatric symptoms	Disruption of developmental life passage, altered self-regulatory pattern, identified psychological issue	Experiencing, witnessing, or learning about a sudden unexpected stressor, life threatening event	Dysfunctional family
Patient response:	Physical signs and symptoms, pain, fear, anxiety, compulsive behaviors, phobias	Depression and anxiety	Intense fear, helplessness, behavior disorganization, loss of coping skills	Chronic anxiety, inability to protect self and others, interpersonal disruptions
Etiology:	Immune system suppression, physical health disequilibrium, unidentified psychological issue	Interrupted developmental tasks	Neurobiology of life-threatening stress	Undisclosed relationship abuse, divided family loyalty, personality trait rigidity, loss of personal flexibility
Intervention:	Primary health care protocol for physical illness, medication, education, brief group treatment, cognitive/behavioral treatment	Education, brief individual therapy, self-help groups, cognitive-behavioral therapy	Crisis intervention, medication, trauma therapy, relaxation therapy, trauma groups, self-defense classes	Police/state intervention, case management shelters, foster homes, trauma therapy, group work

Burgess, A.W. & Roberts, A.L., Crisis Intervention & Time Limited Treatment, 1995

LEVELS OF STRESS-CRISIS CONTINUUM

	5. Serious Mental Illness	6. Psychiatric Emergencies	7. Cataclysmic Crisis
Defining characteristics:	Mental illness diagnosis, low physical symptoms, high psychiatric issue	Threat or actual harm to self or others	Level 3 (traumatic crises) in combination with level 4, 5, or 6. Community disasters
Patient response:		Social impulse dysfunction	Stress of intense and long duration
Etiology:	Disorganized thinking and behavior	Loss of personal control	Overwhelming grief, Multiple victims
Intervention:	Case monitoring and management, hospitalization or sheltered care, medication, vocational training, group work	Hospitalization, jail, medication, restraint	Supportive therapy, group Community response

1

Level 1

Somatic Distress

A patient seeks help at a primary health-care facility because of physical symptoms. The patient's somatic distress is the result of biomedical illness with or without psychiatric symptoms. A psychological stressor may or may not be clearly identified. The etiology of the stress may be a disequilibrium in physical health (neuroimmunologic) or an underlying psychological issue with psychiatric symptomatology. If a clear medical diagnosis is not identified, the patient may be evaluated for a somatoform, dissociative, or anxiety disorder.

Patients with or without a medical diagnosis can respond with psychiatric symptoms of fear, anxiety, and depression. The stress level of an individual with a medical diagnosis of cancer or diabetes, for example, can easily increase to the point of producing depressive symptoms.

For patients exhibiting somatic distress without a clear medical diagnosis, intervention is focused on symptom reduction. Reducing symptoms has been shown to interrupt the progression of distress to a major psychiatric disorder. Education is the intervention of choice for patients with Level I somatic distress. The health-care provider may teach individual patients or groups of patients about their illness, symptoms, and health care.

Conditions representative of somatic distress are discussed in the following three chapters:

- *Somatoform Disorders*
- *Anxiety Disorders*
- *Dissociative Disorders*

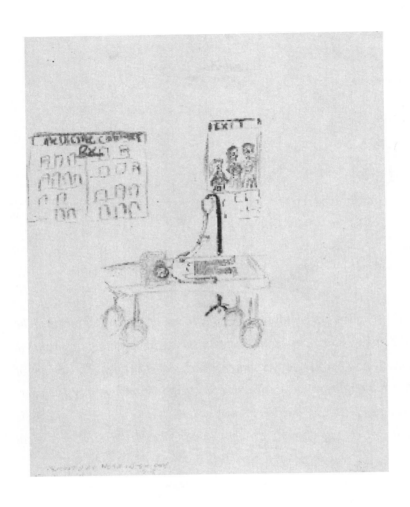

. . . *These troublesome disguises which we wear*

John Milton, *Paradise Lost* (1667)
Book IV, line 739

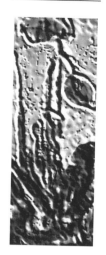

13

Somatoform Disorders

Ann Wolbert Burgess

Somatoform disorders comprise a group of five subtypes of psychological disorder in which symptoms suggest a physical disorder. The symptoms must cause clinically significant impairment or distress in social, occupational, or other areas of functioning. Unlike factitious disorder or malingering, the symptoms are not intentional. Laboratory testing does not confirm the presence of any pathophysiologic processes.

The somatoform disorders are most often encountered in primary-care settings, general medical outpatient clinics, and private medical offices. Patients with somatoform disorder do not perceive themselves as having a psychiatric problem and thus do not seek mental-health care. It is important, therefore, that primary-health-care nurses be familiar with these disorders so that they can be recognized and treated appropriately.

Patients who have persistent and troubling somatic symptoms without an identifiable organic etiology may be expressing psychological distress in bodily terms. The somatoform disorders are more likely to occur among patients with a recent decline in self-esteem, those undergoing serious life stresses, and those whose characteristic coping patterns and defense mechanisms are failing.

■ SUBTYPES

SOMATIZATION DISORDER

A chronic disorder, in which spontaneous remission is rare. A pattern of multiple, recurrent physical symptoms begin most often in the teen years, but by definition before age 30.

CONVERSION DISORDER

Unexplained symptoms or deficits affecting sensory or motor function. The symptoms suggest a neurological or medical condition.

PAIN DISORDER

Characterized by preoccupation with pain that is not attributable to any other mental or physical disorder. Psychological factors are believed to have an important role in the onset, severity, exacerbation, or maintenance of the pain.

HYPOCHONDRIASIS

A preoccupation with the fear of having, or the belief that one has, a serious disease. This belief is based on the patient's misinterpretation of bodily symptoms or functions.

BODY DYSMORPHIC DISORDER

An inordinate preoccupation with an imagined or minor defect in one's physical appearance.

Table 13–1 presents an overview of the features and treatment of the somatoform disorders.

■ SOMATIZATION DISORDER

HISTORY

Patients with persistent physical symptoms in the absence of findings that support the patient's subjective complaints have challenged psychiatric and primary-care practitioners for centuries. In ancient Greek times, somatization disorder was known as *hysteria*, a term meaning uterus. It was believed that many of the dramatic physical symptoms of which women complained were due to the wanderings of the uterus. On the basis of this etiology, the treatment for these symptoms was to place fragrant substances near the vagina so as to attract the uterus back to its proper place.

In Freud's time, hysteria played a major role in the development of psychoanalysis. Freud believed that his female patients with hysterical symptoms suffered from "reminiscences," or emotionally laden, conflictual memories that had been repressed and which then emerged in the form of physical symptoms or loss of function.

Soon after this, physicians began to use the label "hysteria" to describe the state of demanding women with numerous unfounded medical complaints that were impossible or difficult to treat. In an effort to counter this bias, researchers in 1962 proposed Briquet's check-list of signs and symptoms, named for French physician Paul Briquet, who had redefined hysteria in 1859 as a disorder of multiple physical symptoms (i.e., polysymptomatic disorder). Patients who had 13 of the 35 unexplained symptoms in the check-list were given the diagnosis of Briquet's syndrome (LaBruzza, 1994).

TABLE 13–1 SOMATOFORM DISORDERS[1]

	Somatization Disorder	Conversion Disorder	Somatoform Pain Disorder	Hypochondriasis	Body Dysmorphic Disorder
Key Features	Multiple physical symptoms with no organic basis, causing the individual to seek medical care or medications	Loss or change of physical function caused by psychological conflict. Usually single symptom or sign.	Preoccupation with pain symptom in the absence of, or in excess of, physical findings.	The fear of having, or belief that one has, a serious physical disease.	Preoccupation with an imagined body defect
Epidemiology	1-year prevalence: 0.2% women >> men	Rare Women > men	Common Women > men	Common: Men and women	Common: men and women
Treatment	Consolidation of care under single supportive therapist Identification of psychosocial stressors, psychotherapy	Behavioral therapy Psychotherapy	Consolidation of care under single supportive therapist Behavioral therapy, pharmacotherapy with tricyclic antidepressants	Consolidation of care under single supportive therapist Psychotherapy	Seeks out dermatologists or plastic surgeons

[1]Adapted from: MacKay S, Purcell SD: Somatoform and dissociative disorders, in Goldman HH (ed): *Review of General Psychiatry*. Appleton & Lange; Norwalk, CT, 1995

CRITERIA GIVEN BY THE *DIAGNOSTIC AND STATISTICAL MANUAL OF MENTAL DISORDERS,* FOURTH EDITION

The *Diagnostic and Statistical Manual of Mental Disorders, Fourth Edition* (*DSM-IV,* 1994) has greatly simplified the psychiatric criteria for somatization disorder by condensing the 35 items in the Briquet's syndrome checklist into four broad groupings: pain, gastrointestinal, sexual, and pseudoneurological symptoms. The criteria are listed below.

- A history of many physical complaints or a belief that one is sickly, beginning before age 30, persisting for several years, and interfering with social, occupational, and other important areas of functioning.
- Symptoms from the four groupings are:
  Four pain symptoms: a history of pain in at least four body sites (e.g., head, abdomen, back, joints, extremities, chest, rectum, during menstruation, during sexual intercourse, or during urination).
  Two gastrointestinal symptoms other than pain, (e.g., nausea, bloating, vomiting other than during pregnancy, diarrhea, or food intolerance).
  One sexual symptom other than pain, (e.g., sexual indifference, erectile or ejaculatory dysfunction, irregular menses, excessive menstrual bleeding, or vomiting throughout pregnancy).
  One pseudoneurological symptom suggesting a neurological condition not limited to pain, (e.g., conversion symptoms such as impaired coordination or balance, paralysis or localized weakness, difficulty in swallowing, a lump in the throat, aphonia, urinary retention, hallucinations, loss of touch or pain sensation, double vision, blindness, deafness, seizures; dissociative symptoms such as amnesia; or loss of consciousness other than fainting).

A further requirement is that the symptoms cannot be fully explained by a general medical condition or the direct effect of a drug or chemical substance. Or, if there is a medical condition, the symptoms exceed what would be expected from the history, physical examination, or laboratory findings in the patient's case.

CULTURAL FACTORS, GENDER, AND PREVALENCE

The type of physical symptoms in a case of somatization disorder may differ across cultures. For example, burning hands and feet, or the non-delusional experience of worms in the head or ants crawling under the skin, are more common symptoms in Africa and South Asia than in North America. Symptom reviews should be adjusted for the culture in which the disorder occurs. Somatization disorder occurs only rarely in the United States, but its greater reported frequency in Greek and Puerto Rican men suggests that cultural factors may influence the sex ratio of the condition.

Widely variable lifetime prevalence rates of somatization disorder have been reported. Rates range from 0.2% to 2% among women, and below 0.2% in men. Rates of the disorder have been found to differ according to the gender and profession of the interviewer. When non-physician interviewers are used, somatization disorder is much less frequently diagnosed (DSM-IV, 1994; p. 447)

ETIOLOGY

The specific cause of somatization disorder is unknown, but is presumed to be psychological. Pathological identification with a parent, immature efforts to deal with dependency needs, and maladaptive resolution of intrapsychic conflict have all been proposed as mechanisms producing symptoms similar to those seen in somatization disorder (MacKay and Purcell, 1995).

■ CONVERSION DISORDER

Conversion disorder is characterized by a loss of or change in physical functioning that suggests a physical disorder, but which is instead apparently an expression of psychological conflict or need (MacKay and Purcell, 1995). The problem is not under voluntary control, and after careful study, cannot be explained by any physical disorder or known pathophysiological mechanism.

HISTORY

Historically, conversion disorder has also been known as hysterical neurosis, conversion type. Freud's famous patient Dora lost her voice when the man she loved went away on a business trip. There was no medical or neurological explanation for her aphonia. Freud concluded that Dora suffered from conversion hysteria and made the following symbolic interpretation: "When the man she loved was away she gave up speaking; speech had lost its value since she could not speak to him" (Freud, 1955; p. 40).

DSM-IV CRITERIA

The *DSM-IV* criteria for conversion disorder are:

- One or more symptoms of deficits affecting voluntary motor or sensory function that suggest a neurological or other general medical condition.
- Psychological factors are judged to be associated with the symptom(s) because the symp-

E CASE EXAMPLE

A 39-year-old part-time fitness trainer entered a hospital emergency room at 2:00 A.M. complaining loudly that something was wrong with her stomach. She was agitated and tearful, and holding her arms tightly across her abdomen. She said that shortly after her evening meal she had begun to feel nauseated and "bloated," and that she had vomited some undigested food. Within minutes of this vomiting she had begun to feel a dull pain in her periumbilical area, which gradually became sharper and spread throughout her entire abdomen; when the pain became "unbearable," her boyfriend had brought her to the hospital.

A history revealed many prior medical visits for abdominal discomfort over a 19-year period. At age 20 the patient had had a hysterectomy; at age 26 she had had a cholecystectomy, and over the succeeding 10 years she had had three abdominal surgical procedures to correct "adhesions" causing abdominal pain. Additional symptoms that the patient reported included sporadic episodes of dizziness, low back pain, diarrhea, and frequent attacks of indigestion. Various physicians had told her that she had an ulcer or colitis, but despite a variety of medical treatments her symptoms persisted.

When asked about distressing life events, she reported that her grandmother had died 18 months earlier, her grandfather was dying from lung cancer, and her boyfriend had suggested that he and she separate. Figure 13–1 is an example of a critical pathway indicating nursing plan of care for Somatization Disorder.

---

tom(s) are preceded by conflicts or other stressors.

- The symptom(s) is not intentionally produced or feigned (as in factitious disorder or malingering).
- The symptom(s) cannot be explained by a physical disorder, a chemical substance, or a culturally sanctioned behavior.
- The symptoms cause clinically significant distress or impairment in social, occupational, or other areas of functioning.
- The symptom is not limited to pain or sexual dysfunction.

The type of symptom or deficit needs to be specified as conversion disorder with motor symptoms, with sensory symptoms, with seizures or convulsions, or with mixed presentation.

CULTURAL FACTORS, GENDER, AND PREVALENCE

Conversion disorder is reportedly more common in rural populations, among patients in the lower socioeconomic range, and among less psychologically minded patients. Falling, with a loss of or change in consciousness, is a feature of some culture-specific conversion-disorder syndromes. Symptoms of conversion disorder may reflect local cultural ideas about the manner in which to express distress. Assessment is made of whether the conversion symptom is explainable in a particular social context.

Symptoms of conversion disorder in children under 10 years of age are usually limited to gait problems or seizures. Conversion disorder is more common in women than in men, with reported ratios varying from 2:1 to 10:1. Reported rates of the disorder range from 11 to 300 per 100,000 in general population samples. Conversion disorder has been reported to be a focus of treatment in 1% to 3% of outpatient referrals to mental-health facilities (*DSM-IV;* p. 455).

ETIOLOGY

Two mechanisms are used to explain why someone may have a conversion symptom. In one mechanism, the individual achieves a "primary gain" by keeping a psychological conflict out of conscious awareness. For example, after an upsetting experience, an individual may develop a physical symptom, rather than dealing with the inner conflict caused by the experience. Thus, the symptom of blindness might result from viewing a traumatic event, or the paralysis of an arm might follow an argument in which physical violence was witnessed. In the second mechanism, the individual achieves "secondary gain" from the symptom by avoiding a particular, traumatic activity. For example, a "paralyzed" hand can prevent a soldier from entering combat.

PLAN OF CARE

Figure 13–2 is a critical pathway indicating nursing care for conversion disorder.

■ PAIN DISORDER

Pain disorder is essentially the same as conversion disorder except that the symptom involved is limited to

Expected length of treatment:
Nursing diagnosis: Ineffective individual coping
        Altered work role performance
        Altered family role
Related to: (check at least one) identify problem list number.
___ Repressed anxiety   ___ Unmet dependency needs
___ Low self esteem   ___ Focus on self and symptoms
___ Sporadic work performance   ___ Dysfunctional family
___ Other
Outcome: Patient will demonstrate ability to cope with stress by means other than preoccupation with physical symptoms by discharge.
     Patient will verbalize an understanding of the relationship between emotional problems and physical symptoms.
Interventions:

Day Planned	Date Completed	
___	___	1. Monitor ongoing physical assessments, lab data, diagnostic data, etc.
___	___	2. Recognize that physical complaints constitute the symptoms of the psychiatric disorder.
___	___	3. Identify gains that the physical symptom is providing for the patient: increased dependency, attention, distraction from work and family problems.
___	___	4. Prioritize patient's dependency needs.
___	___	5. Gradually withdraw attention to physical symptoms.
___	___	6. Encourage patient to verbalize fears and anxieties. Reduce attention if rumination about physical complaints begins.
___	___	7. Give positive reinforcement to adaptive coping strategies.
___	___	8. Assist patient to identify ways in which to achieve recognition from others without resorting to physical symptoms. Review patient's interpersonal relationships.
___	___	9. Teach patient relaxation techniques and assertiveness skills.
___	___	10. Teach patient how physical symptoms can arise in response to psychosocial stressors. Review patient stressors.

Source: Nursing staff at 1st Hospital of Wyoming under the direction of Theresa M. Croushore

Figure 13–1. Critical pathway for Patient with Somatization Disorder

Expected length of treatment:
Nursing diagnosis: Sensory–perceptual alteration.
Related to: (check at least one) identify problem list number.
___ Repressed anxiety.   ___ Unmet dependency needs.
___ Low self esteem.   ___ Loss/alteration physical functioning without organic pathology.
Outcome: Patient will demonstrate recovery of lost function and verbalize an understanding of relationship of emotional problems by discharge.
     Patient will be able to verbalize adaptive methods of coping with stress and community support systems.
Interventions:

Day Planned	Date Completed	
___	___	1. Monitor physical assessments, lab reports, diagnostic studies.
___	___	2. Identify gains that physical symptom is providing for the patient: increased dependency, attention, distraction from other problems.
___	___	3. Fulfill patient's needs related to activities of daily living with which physical symptom is interfering.
___	___	4. Do not focus on the disability. Allow patient to be as independent as possible.
___	___	5. Encourage patient to participate in therapeutic activities to the best of his/her ability.
___	___	6. Gradually minimize patient's use of the disability; withdraw attention if patient continues to focus on physical limitation.
___	___	7. Encourage patient to verbalize fears and anxieties; teach patient to recognize that physical symptoms appear in times of extreme stress and are coping mechanisms.
___	___	8. Teach patient to identify coping mechanisms that he/she can use when faced with stressful situations.
___	___	9. Teach assertiveness techniques.
___	___	10. Identify community resources and a support system for the patient.

Source: Nursing staff at 1st Hospital of Wyoming under the direction of Theresa M. Croushore

Figure 13–2. Critical Pathway for Patient with Conversion Disorder

physical pain. The major complaint is preoccupation with pain of at least 6 months' duration in the absence of explanatory physical findings.

DSM-IV CRITERIA

The *DSM-IV* criteria for pain disorder are:

- Pain in one or more anatomical sites that warrants clinical attention.
- The pain causes disruption in social, occupational, or other functional areas.
- Psychological factors are judged to have an important role in the onset, severity, exacerbation, or maintenance of the pain.
- The pain is not intentionally produced or feigned.
- The pain is not explained by another disorder.

CULTURAL FACTORS, GENDER, AND PREVALENCE

Various ethnic and cultural groups respond differently to painful stimuli, and express their reaction to pain in different ways. This limits any generalizations that can be made in the evaluation and management of pain. Pain disorder may occur at any age. Females appear to experience headaches and musculoskeletal pain more often than males. Pain disorder appears to be relatively common. It is estimated that 10% to 15% of adults in the United States have some form of work disability due to back pain alone (*DSM-IV*, 1994; p. 460).

E CASE EXAMPLE

A 24-year-old waitress was brought to a clinic with the complaint of total numbness and paralysis in both legs. She had had an episode of bilateral hip pain at age 14 that resolved without medical attention. For the past 2 years she had shared an apartment with two friends, but after a series of arguments, both friends had moved out of the apartment on the day preceding the onset of the patient's symptoms.

On examination, the patient was in no acute distress. Her main worry was how she was going to support herself and pay for the apartment. She was completely unable to move either leg, and there was total anesthesia and lack of response to painful stimuli (pin-prick) in both legs. All deep-tendon reflexes and both plantar reflexes were normal, as was the rest of the examination.

ETIOLOGY

The etiology of the pain in pain disorder is believed to be psychological. One theory is that the pain is a conversion symptom produced by the same mechanisms responsible for the classical symptoms of conversion disorder. A psychological cause of the pain is indicated by: (1) a temporal relationship between an external stressor and pain; (2) the pain enables the avoidance of a distressing activity; or (3) the pain enables the subject to obtain added support from the environment. It is suggested that patients with pain disorder may be less able to experience and verbalize feelings directly; the implication is that emotions are translated into physical pain (MacKay and Purcell, 1995).

PLAN OF CARE

Figure 13–3 is a critical pathway indicating nursing care for a patient with pain disorder.

■ HYPOCHONDRIASIS

Hypochondriasis is the fear of having a serious physical disease.

HISTORY

Hypochondriasis was formerly called hypochondriacal neurosis. A *hypochondriac* is a person who complains of minor physical problems, worries unrealistically about having or developing a serious illness, persistently seeks professional care, and consumes multiple over-the-counter remedies. Minor bodily symptoms are exaggerated. Life-style disruption may be significant in hypochondriasis, with the patient taking to bed and becoming an invalid. In one case, a man so feared that he had heart disease that he developed what was called a cardiac neurosis, in which the unrealistic fear was of heart disease.

E CASE EXAMPLE

A 32-year-old, unemployed college graduate arrived at the emergency room frightened and breathless, complaining of severe substernal chest pain that he characterized as an unbearable "tightness." Except for a slight tachycardia, his vital signs and electrocardiogram were normal. Despite reassurance from the physician, he continued to complain of severe pain and demanded medication. He was medicated with 75 mg of meperidine, after which he felt better.

A history revealed that the patient's father had died suddenly of a heart attack in his son's presence, four years earlier. The patient's first episode of chest pain occurred 1

year after this, when he awakened from sleep on the night before he was to appear in court to testify in a legal proceeding contesting his father's will. Since that time he had had bouts of chest pain, usually requiring narcotic analgesia for relief, about twice a month and occasionally as often as three to four times a week. Examination revealed no organic disease (MacKay and Purcell, 1995).

Expected length of treatment:
Nursing diagnosis: Pain
Related to: (check at least one) identify problem list number.
____ Repeated health visits   ____ Repressed anxiety.
____ Dependency issues   ____ Denial of psychological issue.
____ Other
Outcomes: Patient will demonstrate ability to intervene as anxiety increases, to prevent onset or increase severity of pain.
    Patient will verbalize an understanding of the relationship between pain and emotional problems.
    Patient's normal social and occupational functioning will increase.
Interventions:

Day Planned	Date Completed	
_____	_____	1. Observe and record the precipitants, duration, and intensity of pain.
_____	_____	2. Teach measures to reduce pain related-behavior
_____	_____	3. Use of milieu or group interventions.
_____	_____	4. Assist patient to connect symptoms of pain to times of increased anxiety and to identify specific situations that cause anxiety to increase.
_____	_____	5. Encourage patient to identify alternative methods of coping with stress.
_____	_____	6. Teach patient ways to intervene as symptoms begin to intensify (i.e., visual/auditory distractions, guided imagery, breathing exercises, massage, application of heat or cold, relaxation techniques).
_____	_____	7. Reinforce adaptive coping and behaviors.
_____	_____	8. Refer to an interdisciplinary treatment center for patients with chronic pain, or to support group.

Source: Nursing staff at 1st Hospital of Wyoming under the direction of Theresa M. Croushore

Figure 13–3. Critical Pathway for Patient with Pain Disorder

Hypochondriasis usually begins in adolescence, but may not begin until the fourth decade for men and the fifth decade for women. It is usually chronic, but marked by fluctuation in the intensity with which the belief of illness is held and the degree of functional impairment.

DSM-IV CRITERIA

The *DSM-IV* criteria for hypochondriasis are:

- Preoccupation with the fear of having, or the belief that one has, a serious disease, based on the subject's misinterpretation of bodily symptoms.
- Persistence of the preoccupation despite medical evaluation and reassurance.
- At least 6 months' duration of the disturbance.

As in somatoform disorders, the preoccupation in hypochondriasis causes clinically significant distress or impairment in social, occupational, or other important areas of functioning; the preoccupation cannot be explained by any other disorder, and the belief of having a disorder is not of delusional intensity.

In making the diagnosis, the clinician is to specify if the patient has poor insight (e.g., minimal recognition of the unreasonableness or excessive nature of the expressed symptom). This specification assists in planning care.

CULTURAL FACTORS, GENDER, AND PREVALENCE

In evaluating for hypochondriasis, it is important that the preoccupation with a disease be judged relative to the patient's cultural background. The diagnosis of hypochondriasis must be made cautiously if the patient's ideas about disease have been reinforced by traditional healers who have disagreed with the results of a classical medical examination (*DSM-IV*, 1994; p. 464). The disorder is equally common in females and in males. The prevalence of hypochondriasis in the general population is unknown. Its prevalence in general medical practice has been reported to range from 4% to 9% (*DSM-IV*, 1994).

E CASE EXAMPLE

A 30-year-old computer programmer arrived for a physical examination at a primary care clinic stating that he hoped the physician could "get to the bottom" of his problems. He expressed annoyance that other examiners had refused to perform tests he felt were necessary, and said that he hoped that this health visit would be more helpful.

He stated that he was worried that he had cancer; that 4 or 5 years earlier he had begun to have burning sensations in his upper abdomen after meals. The medical opinion at that time was that he had mild indigestion. He began to scrupulously monitor his diet, keeping records of the frequency and intensity of his gastric symptoms. Over time he began to think he had cancer. He began to feel tired at the end of the workday, and thought that he felt "swollen glands" in his neck which meant that the cancer might be spreading. He cut back on his work in order to increase his rest, and terminated his relationship with his girlfriend.

He had recently become angry when his last physician refused to repeat diagnostic procedures already done, and instead requested records from other clinics.

```
┌─────────────────────────────────────────────────────────────────────┐
│ Expected Length of Treatment:                                         │
│ Nursing diagnosis: Self-care deficit                                  │
│              Impaired physical mobility                               │
│ Related to: (check at least one) identify problem list number.        │
│ ___ Paralysis of body parts      ___ Inability to speak               │
│ ___ Inability to see             ___ Pain, discomfort                 │
│ ___ Inability to hear            ___ Other                            │
│ Outcome: Patient will recover mobility of body part and/or sensory deficit │
│          Patient will maintain optimal of personal care without assistance. │
│ Interventions:                                                        │
│ Day          Date                                                     │
│ Planned      Completed                                                │
│ _____    _____    1. Assess patient's level of disability; note areas of │
│                            strength and impairment.                   │
│ _____    _____    2. Allow and encourage patient to perform normal ac- │
│                            tivities of daily living to his/her level of ability. │
│ _____    _____    3. Encourage independence, but intervene when pa- │
│                            tient is unable to perform.                │
│ _____    _____    4. Convey non-judgmental attitude.            │
│ _____    _____    5. Provide assistance with activities of daily living pro │
│                            re nata.                                    │
│ _____    _____    6. Offer positive reinforcement for activities of daily liv- │
│                            ing performed independently (i.e., verbal praise, in- │
│                            creased privileges). Identify _____).  │
│ _____    _____    7. Encourage patient to discuss feelings about the dis- │
│                            ability and the need for dependency it creates. │
│ _____    _____    8. Teach relationship of physical symptoms to psy- │
│                            chosocial stressors.                       │
│                                                                       │
│ Source: Nursing staff at 1st Hospital of Wyoming under the direction of Theresa M. Croushore │
└─────────────────────────────────────────────────────────────────────┘
```

Figure 13–4. Critical Pathway for Patient with hypochondriasis

ETIOLOGY

Hypochondriasis is believed to have its origin in maladaptive attempts to cope with unmet psychological needs or unconscious psychological conflicts. Some investigators suggest that the hypochondriacal patient merely shows an excessive self-concern; others suggest that hypochondriasis represents a physical expression of low self-esteem (a self-image of being sick, weak, or defective). Still others propose that the subject's self-view protects against destructive impulses toward others; and some view the symptoms of hypochondriasis as resulting from serious defects in the patient's ability to maintain a "sense of self" (MacKay and Purcell, 1995).

PLAN OF CARE

Figure 13–4 is a critical pathway for hypochondriasis.

■ BODY DYSMORPHIC DISORDER

HISTORY

Body dysmorphic disorder has been described for some time in the European, Russian, and Japanese literature under a variety of names, most commonly *dysmorphophonia*, a term coined by Morselli in 1891 (LaBruzza, 1994). The term comes from the Greek *dysmorfia*, meaning ugliness, specifically of the face. It first appeared in the *Histories of Herodotus*, referring to the myth of the "ugliest girl in Sparta," who was taken to a shrine each day by her nurse so that she might be delivered from her homeliness (LaBruzza, 1994).

Janet (1903) described the syndrome as an obsession with shame about the body, and believed it to be a fairly common concern when actively sought. He emphasized the extreme shame felt by patients who feared being ugly and ridiculed. The psychoanalytic literature contains a classic case of dysmorphophobia, the "hypochondriacal paranoia" experienced by the Wolf-Man (Brunswick, 1928). This patient, who had previously had a compulsive neurosis analyzed by Freud, "neglected his daily life and work because he was engrossed, to the exclusion of all else, in the state of his nose (its supposed scars, holes, and swelling). His life was centered on the little mirror in his pocket, and his fate depended on what it revealed or was about to reveal" (Brunswick, 1928). Psychoanalysis suggested that the patient's nose represented his penis and that he desired to be castrated and made into a woman; his symptom was also thought to reflect an identification with his mother, in part because its onset occurred soon after seeing a wart on her nose (Brunswick, 1928).

Patients with body dysmorphic disorder are intensely preoccupied with their imagined defect, regarding it with loathing, repugnance, and shame, sometimes to the point of being tortured by their concern and unable to think of anything else. Patients with this disorder often think that others are looking at, talking about, or mocking their "defect." Consequently, they may try to camouflage it with makeup, their hands, their hair, or with a hat or other clothing.

DSM-IV CRITERIA

The essential feature of body dysmorphic disorder is a preoccupation with some imagined defect in appearance in a person of normal appearance. The most common complaints include facial flaws, such as spots on the skin, wrinkles, the shape of a facial feature, or excessive facial hair. Two diagnostic criteria from *DSM-IV* are listed below.

- Preoccupation with some imagined defect in appearance. If a slight physical anomaly is present, the concern about it is excessive.
- The preoccupation causes clinically significant distress or impairment in social, occupational, or other important areas of functioning.

E CASE EXAMPLE

James, a 19-year-old college student, has been preoccupied with some excess breast tissue since the age of 13 years. He avoids any activity that requires removing his shirt, such as swimming. He has visited three plastic surgeons, all of whom refused to do surgery to alter the appearance of his chest. During his first year in college, he became seriously depressed. After being given an antidepressant drug, he was able to tell his therapist about his concern with his breasts. Medication and psychotherapy helped to resolve the depression, and he has been able to continue with his studies. His psychotherapeutic work focuses on his feelings of inadequacy in relation to a recent break-up with a girlfriend, which heightened his preoccupation with his breasts.

CULTURAL FACTORS, GENDER, AND PREVALENCE

Cultural concerns about physical appearance and one's physical presentation may influence preoccupations about a minor or imagined physical deformity. Body dysmorphic disorder is reported to occur with equal frequency in men and women. Reliable information is lacking, but the disorder may be more common than was previously thought (*DSM-IV*, 1994; p. 467).

ETIOLOGY

Psychological factors are considered a critical etiological factor in body dysmorphic disorder. The disorder usually begins in adolescence, but may not be diagnosed for many years because of the reluctance of the affected individual to reveal his or her symptoms.

Difficulties in social, marital, and occupational functioning can result. One woman with "facial swelling" stopped going to school to avoid being seen by others (Jenike, 1984), and another woman sped dangerously through red lights on her bicycle so that others could not see her "excessive" facial hair (Jenike, 1984). A young man dated only small, slight women, thinking that the "smallness" of his penis would not be noticeable to a woman of smaller build (Hay, 1970).

Uncertainties about the etiology of body dysmorphic disorder are reflected in the diversity of treatments for it, which include medication, psychotherapy, behavioral therapy, and cosmetic surgery (Philips, 1991). Preliminary evidence suggests that antidepressant medications, and particularly the serotonin-reuptake inhibitors, may be helpful in treating the condition. The usefulness of behavior therapy and psychotherapy in treating the disorder is unclear, but de Leon et al. (1989) suggest that attention to psychosocial factors, as well as medications, is essential.

PLAN OF CARE

Figure 13–5 outlines a critical pathway for body dysmorphic disorder.

Expected length of treatment:
Nursing diagnosis: Body-image disturbance
Related to: (check at least one) identify problem list number.
___ Repressed anxiety   ___ Preoccupation with bodily functioning
___ Low self-esteem   ___ Unmet dependency needs
___ Other
Outcome: Patient will verbalize perception of own body that is realistic to actual structure/function.
    Patient will demonstrate acceptance of changes in bodily structure and/or function as evidenced by expression of additional feelings, willingness to perform self-care activities independently, and focus on personal achievements.
Interventions:

Day Planned	Date Completed	
_____	_____	1. Establish trusting relationship with patient.
_____	_____	2. Identify patient's misperceptions/distortions regarding body image. Correct inaccurate perceptions in a matter of fact, non-threatening manner.
_____	_____	3. Withdraw attention when preoccupation with distorted image persists.
_____	_____	4. Assist patient to recognize personal body boundaries.
_____	_____	5. Provide positive reinforcement for patient's expressions of realistic bodily perceptions

Source: Nursing staff at 1st Hospital of Wyoming under the direction of Theresa M. Croushore

Figure 13–5. Critical Pathway for Patient with Body Dysmorphic Disorder

O AN OVERVIEW

- Nurses in primary health-care settings generally see patients with somatoform disorders.

- The essential feature of somatoform disorders is the presence of bodily complaints in the absence of explanatory physical pathology.

- Interpersonal skills are critical to convey understanding and empathy for the patient's distress.

- Focused listening and documentation are essential.

TD TERMS TO DEFINE

- somatoform disorder
- somatization disorder
- conversion disorder
- pain disorder
- hypochondriasis
- body dysmorphic disorder

Q STUDY QUESTIONS

1. All of the following statements are true about Somatoform Disorders EXCEPT
   a. people with these disorders do not perceive themselves as having a psychiatric problem
   b. the symptoms are intentional
   c. significant social and occupational impairments occur
   d. no identifiable organic etiology exists to explain physical symptoms

2. Match the disorder (letter) with its description (number).
   a. somatization disorder
   b. conversion disorder
   c. pain disorder
   d. hypochondriasis
   e. body dysmorphic disorder
      1. preoccupation with imagined or minor defects in physical appearance
      2. preoccupation with fear of having a serious disease
      3. preoccupation with pain that isn't attributable to any other mental or physical disorder
      4. chronic condition involving a pattern of multiple, recurrent physical symptoms
      5. unexplained symptoms or deficits affecting sensory or motor function

3. Why is it important to understand a patient's cultural background when evaluating somatoform disorders?

4. Which somatoform disorder commonly involves multiple physical symptoms?
   a. somatization disorder
   b. conversion disorder
   c. hypochondriasis
   d. pain disorder

5. True or False. Conversion disorder is more common in urban areas among people of a lower socio-economic status who are less psychologically sophisticated.

6. All of the following somatoform disorders are more commonly experienced by women EXCEPT
   a. pain disorder
   b. conversion disorder
   c. hypochondriasis
   d. somatization disorder

7. Which disorder usually involves the involuntary experiencing of pain (for example, a headache) to avoid a distressing activity and gain support from others?
   a. hypochondriasis
   b. conversion disorder
   c. somatization disorder
   d. pain disorder

■ REFERENCES

Brunswick RM: A supplement to Freud's "History of an infantile neurosis." *Int J Psychoanal* 1928; 9:439–476.

de Leon J, Bott A, Simpson GM: Dysmorphophobia; body dysmorphic disorder or delusional disorder, somatic subtype? *Comp Psychiatry* 1989; 30:457–472.

Diagnostic and Statistical Manual of Mental Disorders, ed 4. Washington, DC, American Psychiatric Press, 1994.

Freud S: *The Standard Edition of the Complete Works of Sigmund Freud*, Strachey J (trans.) London, The Hogarth Press, 1955.

Janet P: *Les Obsessions et la Psychasthenie*. Paris, Felix Alcan, 1903.

Jenike MA: A case report of successful treatment of dysmorphophobia with tranylcypromine. *Am J Psychiatry* 1984; 141:1463–1464.

Hay GG: Dysmorphophobia—a long term study. *Br J Psychiatry* 1970; 132:568–570.

LaBruzza AL: *Using DSM-IV: A Clinician's Guide to Psychiatric Diagnosis*, Northvale, NJ, Jason Aronson, 1994.

MacKay S, Purcell SD: Somatoform and dissociative disorders, in Goldman H (ed): *Review of General Psychiatry*, 4/e. Stamford, CT, Appleton & Lange, 1995.

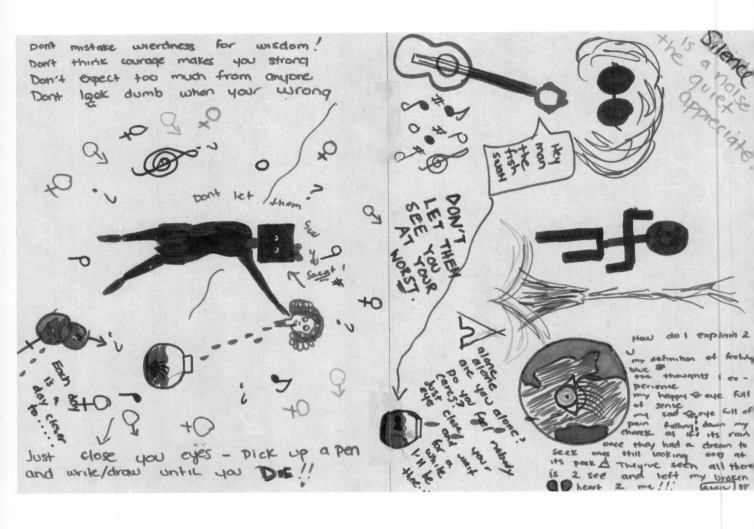

For as children tremble and fear everything in the blind darkness, so we in the light sometimes fear what is no more to be feared than the things children in the dark hold in terror and imagine will come true.

Lucretius 99–55 BC

De Rerum Natura, bk. III, 1. 87

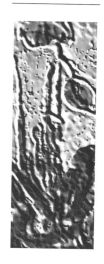

14

Anxiety Disorders

Ann Wolbert Burgess and Laureen M. Burgess

Anxiety disorders, along with mood disorders and substance-related disorders, are among the most common psychiatric disorders in the general population. Many people with an anxiety disorder seek professional help in primary-care settings.

Anxiety commonly occurs as a manifestation of appropriate concern about a medical condition. Illness involving any body system can produce anxiety as a symptom. Also, drugs and dietary factors, particularly alcohol and caffeine, may provoke anxiety.

Nurses will encounter many patients with the symptom of anxiety as well as those with anxiety disorders. This chapter describes the symptom presentation of anxiety and diagnostic categories of anxiety disorders, and suggests nursing diagnoses and planning for patients with these conditions.

■ ANXIETY

Everyone experiences anxiety; however, people vary significantly in their ability to tolerate feelings of anxiety and in their ability to cope with anxiety-producing situations. Because anxiety is both a psychological and physiological experience, individuals will report both psychological and somatic symptoms when they complain of anxiety.

Anxiety and fear are widespread emotions. The two terms have become interchangeable. For example, a phobia is a kind of anxiety that is also defined in the *Diagnostic and Statistical Manual, of Mental Disorders, Fourth Edition (DSM IV)* as a "persistent or irrational fear." *Fear* is defined as an emotional and physiological response to a recognized external threat (e.g., a runaway truck or a sudden airplane descent). *Anxiety* is an unpleasant emotional state, the sources of which are less easily identified (Greist and Jefferson, 1995).

Typical subjective psychological experiences of anxiety include descriptions of apprehension, dread, edginess, fear, fright, inability to concentrate, irritability, nervousness, panic, restlessness, tension, terror, and uneasiness. Typical physiological signs and symptoms of anxiety include anorexia, "butterflies" in the stomach, tightness in the chest, diarrhea, dizziness, dyspnea, dry mouth, faintness, flushing, headache, hyperventilation, light-headedness, muscle tension, nausea, pallor, palpitations, sexual dysfunction, shortness of breath, stomach pain, tachycardia, tremulousness, urinary frequency, and vomiting.

Because the symptoms of anxiety range from psychological to somatic, the understanding of anxiety in a theoretical sense has included both psychological and physiological explanations.

GENETIC THEORY

Genetic studies of twins and first-degree relatives suggest that anxiety disorders are more common among female relatives of patients with anxiety disorders, and familial influences have been found for panic disorder, agoraphobia, and obsessive–compulsive problems. It is also reported some genetic effects can be modified by environmental means (Greist and Jefferson, 1995).

PSYCHODYNAMIC THEORY

Sigmund Freud (1923) reported that anxiety was a signal of threats that could potentially overwhelm the ego; if the threat was actual, the response would be "traumatic" anxiety. Most anxiety, however, reflects unconscious signals of early dangers; for example, separation may trigger a mild form of anxiety. Freud believed that anxiety disorder was the result of unconscious conflict, and this premise was the key to his formulations. He explained that anxiety symptoms are constructed by the ego. Conflict develops between the forbidden, unconscious impulses of the id and the reality strivings of the ego; the superego can side with one or the other.

The ego, which represents the integrity and liaison between the id, superego, and reality of the environment, must control the impulses of the "child-like" id by satisfying them or by manipulating the environment. When this is not possible, the anxiety becomes too much for the ego to tolerate, and defense or coping mechanisms must be used to restore equilibrium. Repression and suppression are the primary coping mechanisms. These processes are unconscious. Such conflicts generate anxiety and threaten psychological stability. Conflicts that cannot be resolved are repressed by the ego. Symptoms of such conflicts include increased anxiety, increased guilt, and depression (Freud, 1943).

INTERPERSONAL THEORY

Anxiety has been explained by Harry Stack Sullivan (1953) as anticipated but unfavorable appraisal of one's current activity. This view of interpersonal theory stresses the importance of interaction or communication. Sullivan's theory has been based on the assumption that human behavior is positively directed toward goals of collaboration and of mutual satisfaction and security, unless anxiety interferes with this. Therefore, the need for relief of anxiety is the need for interpersonal security.

Sullivan believes that anxiety is the chief disruptive force in interpersonal relations and the main factor in the development of serious difficulties in living. In terms of development, Sullivan sees anxiety as being created in the infant by the mother. When the mother experiences tension, possibly because of her own insecurities about mothering, this creates anxiety in the infant. This is also called *malevolent transformation* in which the need for tenderness has, under the impact of anxiety, been replaced by malevolent behavior. This malevolent transformation causes decreased self-esteem and self-respect in the infant (Sullivan, 1953). It is illustrated below in a case example from a community mental health nurse.

Hildegard Peplau (1963) believes that anxiety is one of the key concepts in psychiatric work. Nurses use this concept to help explain and understand behaviors observed not only in patients but also in themselves. Peplau (1963) defines anxiety as "energy; a secondary behavior following an experience, a subjective experience; an emotion without a specific object; anxiety is reaction and fear is expression in objectivated form; inability to achieve self-realization; threat to some value; and danger to self-respect."

Peplau agrees with Sullivan that anxiety is a threat to the security of an individual. This threat can be biologic; anxiety is also always communicated interpersonally. It is important that nurses know what effect anxiety has on observable behavior. These effects—biopsychosocial, cognitive, and perceptual—can be incorporated into the nursing assessment for planning nursing intervention. Nurses also need to remember that anxiety is communicated interpersonally, and they should be aware of their own level of anxiety during interactions with patients.

BIOCHEMICAL THEORY

When compared with normal controls, patients with anxiety disorders have significantly different physiological functioning. Anxiety is experienced by the individual in such physiological functions as increased heart rate and respiration, higher blood lactate levels, increased urinary urgency, dryness of mouth, cold sweat, and fluctuation in blood pressure. The dysfunctional process of increasing stimulus to the midbrain nucleus, which supplies much of the noradrengeric neurons to the central nervous system, is associated with increased anxiety. To further substantiate this theory, antidepressants that down-regulate this function have been effective in treating some anxiety disorders (Greist and Jefferson, 1995).

■ CLINICAL TYPES OF ANXIETY DISORDER

Anxiety is experienced as an apprehension that jeopardizes one's whole existence. It can also be experienced as a "vague discomfort" and feelings of "helplessness" or "impotence." Anxieties can sometimes be differentiated from fears in that the term *anxiety* is applied to states that are diffuse and are without clearly focused targets. Fear can be perceived as coming from a specific object or situation. Three different forms of anxiety exist: spontaneous anxiety, which arises unexpectedly; phobic anxiety, which is predictable in certain situations; and anticipatory anxiety, which is triggered by a thought of a particular situation.

The anxiety disorders are defined in terms of cognitive, somatic, and behavioral symptoms. Cognitive features include fears, worries, intrusive thoughts, obsessions, preoccupations, dissociation, and numbing. Somatic symptoms include motor tension, the startle response, autonomic hyperarousal, and other physical sensations or complaints. The behavioral aspects of anxiety disorders include avoidance of stress stimuli, compulsions, rituals, and compensatory behaviors (LaBruzza, 1994). Four clinical types of anxiety disorder are presented in this chapter.

- Anxiety as the dominant problem, as in generalized anxiety disorder and panic disorder.
- Anxiety experienced if the individual attempts to confront the threatened situation, as in phobic disorders.
- Anxiety experienced if the individual tries to resist thoughts and feelings, as in obsessive–compulsive disorders.
- Anxiety re-experienced after an unusual traumatic event, as in post-traumatic stress disorder.

Anxiety, as a symptom, occurs in varying degrees of intensity, from a vague, constant or intermittent feeling of unpleasantness and preoccupation to extreme panic, and as a constant state of tension. The anxiety state may include sadness, anger, and guilt. Persons experiencing anxiety report physical symptoms of dry mouth, rapid heartbeat, diarrhea, frequent urination, sweating, nausea, hyperventilation, dizziness, faintness, headache, fa-

E CASE EXAMPLE

An 18-year-old married woman came to a community mental health center shortly after delivering her first child, a girl. The woman lived in a two-family house on the second floor with her husband and baby. Her own mother and father lived downstairs. Ever since the new mother had returned home, she had not been able to care sufficiently for the infant, as she had done while in the hospital. She had severe doubts about her ability and competency as a mother. Her husband had been staying home from work to care for the infant. While in the hospital the mother had been adequately able to bathe, change, and feed the infant. The change in the young mother's behavior seemed to have been precipitated by her return home. Upon discussion with the community nurse, the woman began to realize that her own mother had had severe reservations about her having a child because she was so young. The woman began to understand that her fears were generated by her own mother's words and concern about her capability. When the young mother became aware of this, she was able to have more freedom and choice of action to assess her own capabilities in caring for her infant. When her own anxiety decreased, the tension in the infant also decreased. This early intervention by the nurse in the mother–child relationship is an important aspect of prevention.

tigue, insomnia, various aches, and sexual dysfunction. Persons with anxiety also experience chronic irritability and tension, feel insecure, and lack confidence.

The following excerpt from an interview with a patient experiencing symptoms of anxiety illustrates the mental anguish these patients experience.

Nurse: How are you feeling tonight?

Patient: The day has been awful. All I do is worry.

Nurse: What are some of your worries?

Patient: I have pains in my chest and a burning in my stomach and chest. Everyone tells me these symptoms are my "nerves," but I'm worried that it might be cancer or heart disease or an ulcer. I have to be well to care for my sick kids and husband. He can't help me because he's a man and has his job all day.

Then I think about my responsibility at home. I hate the housework part and the kids being sick all the time. I saw my sister at the doctor's office. She used to take care of me when I was little, and I'm afraid I'll be a chronic mentally ill case like her.

Then I worry about the noise, the crowds, and riding in a car. Maybe I should just forget about my kids and the responsibilities. Maybe I'll never be better. Or maybe I should just go home. I'll just have to force myself to do the things I hate to do.

Anxiety disorders are classified by their major presenting symptomatology, epidemiology, etiology, onset/course, impairments, assessment, and treatment. The essential features of each disorder are discussed below.

■ PANIC ATTACKS

A panic attack does not a disorder make (LaBruzza, 1994). Panic attacks are commonly present in several different anxiety disorders, and about 35% of the population experiences one in a year. The primary feature of a panic attack is a distinct period of intense fear or discomfort, in which at least 4 of 13 somatic or cognitive symptoms suddenly develop and peak within 10 minutes. The 13 symptoms are palpitations, trembling, a choking feeling, sweating, fear of losing control, dizziness, feelings of unreality, fear of dying, paresthesias, nausea, chest pain, shortness of breath, and chills or hot flashes (DSM-IV).

The patient usually experiences eight or nine of these symptoms during an attack. These attacks are characterized as being of three different types: unex-pected, situationally bound, and situationally predisposed.

The **unexpected panic attack** occurs without any situational trigger and is required for someone to be diagnosed as having panic disorder.

The **situationally bound panic attack** occurs immediately on exposure to, or in anticipation of, the situational trigger, and is characteristic of social and specific phobias.

The **situationally predisposed anxiety attack** may occur on exposure to a situational trigger, but does not necessarily occur immediately after this exposure. This type is common for panic disorder and occasionally for specific and social phobias.

When the person starts to avoid exposure to a particular stimulus, a phobia may begin to develop.

PANIC DISORDER AND AGORAPHOBIA

Panic disorder and agoraphobia often produce debilitating symptoms that are fairly prevalent in society. Agoraphobia is the most common phobic complaint among psychiatric outpatients.

The Greek meaning of agoraphobia is "fear of the marketplace," and in current psychological terms has come to mean a fear of separation from one's source of security. DSM-IV defines agoraphobia as anxiety about being in a situation from which escape might prove difficult or embarrassing, or where help may be absent should one have a panic attack. Common agoraphobic concerns include being alone and away from home, standing in line at a store, feeling trapped in a small space such as a car or elevator, being in a crowd, or being on a bridge (LaBruzza, 1994).

Panic disorder and agoraphobia are two of the most crippling anxiety disorders because they may lead to severe restrictions on lifestyle and interpersonal functioning. The DSM-IV classifications of these disorders include panic disorder without agoraphobia, panic disorder with agoraphobia, and agoraphobia without a history of panic disorder. Agoraphobia is not a codable disorder, and occurs in the context of panic disorder. Approximately one-third to one-fifth of individuals diagnosed with panic disorder also have agoraphobia (DSM-IV).

Panic disorder includes recurrent and unexpected panic attacks followed by at least 1 month of persistent concern about having another attack, worrying about the consequences of these attacks, or experiencing a significant behavioral change as a result of the attacks.

The person experiencing a panic attack describes a sudden onset of intense apprehension, terror, and fear, accompanied by physiological symptoms of dyspnea, palpitations, chest discomfort, cold and hot flashes, sweating, and other effects. These attack periods generally last for minutes; and more rarely for hours. The attacks are not due to the direct physiological effects of a substance (drug abuse or medication) or a general medical condition, and are not better explained by another anxiety disorder. Attacks involving four or more symptoms are panic attacks; attacks involving fewer than four symptoms are limited symptom attacks.

The frequency and severity of the attacks vary widely. Some individuals have attacks at least once a week for months, others have short bursts of more frequent attacks that can be separated by weeks or months.

Individuals who have had panic attack(s) usually present at a hospital thinking that they are having a stroke, heart attack, or another serious medical problem. Fear is continually present after the first attack, as they wonder what is wrong and when it will occur again. Eventually they may become afraid of situations that they associate with the attack, and become anxious about whether they can flee from the situation, or whether help will be available if an attack occurs. This is known as panic disorder with agoraphobia.

The focus of the fear in this condition is of being in places or situations from which escape might be difficult (or embarrassing), or in which help might not be available in the event of a panic attack. There may be persistent avoidance behavior that originated during an active phase of panic disorder, even if the person does not attribute the avoidance behavior to fear of having a panic attack. As a result of this fear, the person either restricts travel or needs a companion when away from home, or endures agoraphobic situations despite intense anxiety.

In panic disorder with agoraphobia, the individual has a marked fear of being alone, or of being in public places from which escape would be difficult in the face of sudden danger. This individual fears crowds, bridges, tunnels, and public transportation, where escape is limited without assistance. The individual either avoids public places or travels in the company of a family member or friend. Normal activities are usually progressively constricted until the avoidance behavior dominates the individual's life. The individual will describe physiological symptoms of breath-holding or difficulty in breathing, nausea, sweating, weakness, palpitations, and various epigastric sensations when confronted with the feared activity (e.g., flying) (DSM IV).

Agoraphobia without panic disorder includes a fear of developing panic-like symptoms. The disturbance is not due to the direct physiological effects of a substance or a general medical condition. This disorder is similar to panic disorder with agoraphobia, but its focus of fear is on the occurrence of incapacitating or extremely embarrassing panic-like symptoms or limited-symptom attacks rather than full panic attacks.

EPIDEMIOLOGY

Studies from around the world indicate that the lifetime prevalence of panic disorder (with and without agoraphobia) is between 1.5% and 3.5%. Women have a greater likelihood of experiencing agoraphobia and panic disorders, although it is believed that men may under-report the symptoms of these disorders or disguise them with alcoholism. Individuals who are unmarried or have not attended college also experience higher rates of these disorders. Childhood separation anxiety is experienced by 20 to 50% of patients with panic disorders (DSM IV).

ETIOLOGIC FACTORS AND FAMILY PATTERNS

Biological Theories of Familial and Genetic Basis

First-degree biological relatives of individuals with panic disorder have a four- to seven-times greater chance of developing panic disorder. Also, twin studies show a higher concordance of panic disorder for monozygotic twins than for dizygotic twins.

Biochemical Sources

Yohimbine, an alpha-2-adrenergic receptor antagonist, produces increased anxiety, increased blood pressure, and elevated plasma levels in patients with panic disorder. Involvement of the serotonergic autonomic nervous system in anxiety has also been suggested. Caffeine generates more pronounced anxiety symptoms in patients with panic disorder by increasing the firing rates of neurons in the locus cerulus.

Behavioral Theories

A panic attack is derived from an internal rather than external stimulus. Patients associate the somatic sensations as a threat, and respond with fear and anxiety, which leads to more somatic symptoms. This eventually spirals into a marked increase in anxiety and symptoms.

More emphasis has been placed on behavioral causes for the development of agoraphobia. Pairing of associated events, such as a panic attack and being in an airplane, together with operant conditioning, leads to behavior modification that involves avoiding potentially negative events. This panic attack may generalize to other situations and become associated as a negative event, further creating panic attack episodes.

Psychoanalytic Theories

Freud theorized that unconscious psychological conflict is the cause of panic attacks. He believed that anxiety was a signal to the ego that it was in a dangerous situation. Neurotic symptoms then develop to reduce this anxiety and avoid the impending danger. Freud also believed that agoraphobia was due to recalling an anxiety attack along with fearing that a future attack would occur in a situation from which there was no escape.

AGE OF ONSET AND COURSE

The age of onset in panic disorder varies, but is most often between late adolescence and the mid-30s. It is rare for someone to develop this disorder after the age of 40. Seventy-eight percent of patients with panic disorder have a spontaneous initial panic attack; the remainder have the first attack triggered by a phobic stimulus. This disorder often occurs within 6 months of a major life crisis such as separation, pregnancy, or a job change.

The course of panic disorder is generally chronic, sometimes with periods of remission. Panic disorder with agoraphobia usually develops within the first year of recurrent panic attacks. The course of agoraphobia and its relationship to the course of panic attacks are variable. For some individuals the agoraphobia remains constant with or without the presence of panic attacks; for others, agoraphobic anxiety decreases as panic attacks decrease. Little is known about the course of agoraphobia without a history of panic disorder.

The prognosis for these disorders is poor. Studies have shown that from 6 to 10 years after treatment, 30% of patients have recovered, 40 to 50% are better but still symptomatic, and the remaining group is the same or worse.

IMPAIRMENTS AND COMPLICATIONS

The significant changes in behavior that result from panic disorders can have a marked impact on functioning. Individuals who suffer frequent panic attacks often become demoralized and feel discouraged and ashamed that they have difficulty in performing normal, "everyday" activities. As a result, work is often missed or school is skipped, leading to unemployment and dropping out of school. Those who also have an agoraphobic condition may not be able to travel to work or even perform basic housekeeping tasks such as buying groceries or running errands.

Panic disorder is frequently associated with major depression and other anxiety disorders. Those individuals with agoraphobic patterns also experience a higher percentage of additional phobias. Moreover, the affected individual may exhibit a dramatic personality change. A formerly independent and outgoing individual, for example, may become passive, inhibited, and dependent. Such a person may also self-medicate, thus increasing the risk for alcohol and substance abuse.

TREATMENT

The most effective course of treatment for panic disorders often involves a combination of behavioral and pharmacologic therapies. Each is briefly described below.

Behavioral

Exposure. Exposure therapy is utilized to substantially reduce the frequency and severity of panic attacks. This involves actual exposure to the stimulus that evokes the anxiety until the patient can be comfortable. The patient lists all of his or her phobic stimuli from the highest to lowest fear response that each generates. The least phobic stimulus is then gradually introduced, with progression to the highest. Prolonged (2 hours) and frequent (daily) exposure is more effective than brief, spaced sessions. A group-therapy setting may be incorporated.

Panic Control. A form of cognitive behavioral therapy, panic control, involves retraining in breathing, cognitive restructuring, and exposure to cues that trigger the anxiety response. The goal is to desensitize an individual to the symptoms of panic attacks.

Psychoeducation. In patient management, it is very important that the patient with a panic disorder be provided with information about the diagnosis and its symptoms. Awareness of the prognosis and treatment can help the patient to remain emotionally and behaviorally stable. Group therapy is also useful, since it relieves the patient to know that he or she is not the only person suffering from the disorder.

Pharmacological

Many antidepressants will decrease the frequency and severity of panic attacks, often preventing them altogether (See Chapter 42). A combination of pharmacologic and behavioral therapies has been beneficial for many patients with panic disorders, and helps to decrease the relapse rate after withdrawal from medication.

NURSING ASSESSMENT AND PLAN OF CARE

Evaluating panic disorders is difficult, since many other disorders can trigger panic attacks. These disorders include anxiety disorder due to a major medical condition; substance-induced anxiety disorder; social phobia; obsessive–compulsive disorder; post-traumatic stress disorder; specific phobia disorder; and separation anxiety disorder.

E CASE EXAMPLE

▶ PANIC DISORDER

A 21-year-old woman, the eldest of 10 children, has a prior history of good socialization skills as well as dating. She has a strong interest in the mechanics of automobiles as an occupation, and attended a school for this, where she excelled. Soon, however, she developed a fear of being around people, which affected her socializing with friends, and she seeks counseling. Her presenting request is her distress over not being able to leave the house.

In counseling, she gradually reveals that she was having increasing difficulty in getting a job as an automobile mechanic even though she was the top student in her class. She was being discriminated against as a female seeking employment in a male-dominated vocation. She was also receiving major criticism from family and friends for her vocational pursuit.

In the first interview it becomes apparent that she is very depressed about others' social response to her. Her therapy focuses on her sense of low self-esteem, failure, and rejection. As her depressive symptoms are dealt with, her phobia begins to subside. She eventually feels stronger as a woman, and is able to pursue her vocation as an auto mechanic.

NURSING DIAGNOSIS

Anxiety related to panic. See Figure 14-1.

NURSING INTERVENTION

The goal in planning nursing interventions for patients with panic disorders is to help them to be able to identify sources of anxiety and to use coping mechanisms to manage the anxiety. Nursing interventions include the following:

- Encourage the patient to verbalize concerns.
- Allow for the patient's anxiety level when teaching.
- Encourage patient responsibility in the decision process.
- Assist the patient to establish an activity routine.
- Involve the family in the patient's care and treatment process.

Patients having severe panic attacks are flooded with anxiety and cannot close it off. The patient begins to respond to the panic and the emotion or effect escalates. Three interventions are listed below.

- Relax the patient and break the cognitive pattern, particularly the patient's internal dialogue.

PATIENT: I feel my heart racing, my palms sweating. What is the matter with me? I know I am going to have another attack. I know it is going to come. (The result is that the patient's anxiety increases.)

One difficulty for the patient experiencing the anxiety is that he or she is not sure when the attack is going to end. If this were known, the patient would be able to calm down.

- Have the patient put his or her mind on another issue. Suggest taking deep breaths to change the physiological pattern attending an attack.
- Move the patient from an internal to an external focus. This technique draws the patient out of him- or herself, rather than moving into the anxiety. Do not ask about the attack or the anxiety because that will only increase the patient's anxious sensation. In essence, this is a "talking the patient down" approach, moving the patient away from a focused concentration.

EVALUATION

Has the patient demonstrated the following achievement?

- listed anxiety sources.
- gained knowledge about factors that cause anxiety.
- knowing whether increased activity decreased his or her level of anxiety.
- expressed an improved sense of responsibility for his or her own life.

■ PHOBIC DISORDERS

The essential feature of phobic disorders is a persistent, irrational fear of a specific object, activity, or situation that results in a compelling desire to avoid the dreaded object. The individual recognizes that the fear is excessive or unreasonable in proportion to the actual danger of the object, activity, or situation.

DSM-IV: Panic disorder

Nursing Diagnosis: ANXIETY (PANIC).

Related to: (check at least one)

Traumatic experience   Threat to self-concept
Unconscious conflicts   Unmet needs
Situational/maturational crisis   Fears of dying
Phobic stimulus   Other

Treatment Goal: PATIENT WILL LEARN TO DISSIPATE AND CHANNEL ANXIETY APPROPRIATELY.

Treatment Goal Can be Measured Using the Following Expected Outcome:

1. By discharge, the patient will be able to recognize symptoms of onset of anxiety and intervene in it before it reaches the panic level.
2. The patient will be able to maintain anxiety at a level in which problem solving can be accomplished.
3. The patient will demonstrate techniques to be used to halt or displace anxiety prior to reaching a panic level.

Interventions:

Date Initiated	Date Discontinued	
_____	_____	1. Maintain calm, non-threatening manner.
_____	_____	2. Reassure patient of his/her safety and security.
		3. Use simple words and brief messages, spoken calmly and clearly, to explain hospital experience to patient.
_____	_____	4. Assess patient's level of anxiety—try to determine the types of situations that increase anxiety.
_____	_____	5. Keep immediate surroundings decreased in stimuli (dim lighting, few people, simple decor).
_____	_____	6. Administer prescribed medication per physician's orders. Assess for effectiveness/adverse reactions. (Identify _____).
_____	_____	7. When level of anxiety has decreased, explore with patient possible reasons for occurrence.
_____	_____	8. Encourage patient to talk about traumatic experience under non-threatening conditions—offer support and reassurance to alleviate any feelings of guilt.
_____	_____	9. Teach patient to recognize signs and symptoms that increase anxiety and ways to interrupt its progression. (i.e., relaxation techniques, deep breathing exercises, physical exercises, brisk walks, jogging). Document teaching/hospital protocol.

Source: Nursing staff at 1st Hospital of Wyoming under the direction of Theresa M. Croushore

Figure 14–1. Individualized nursing care plan

The phobic individual has an intense fear of objects or places, or even of particular groups of people. The phobia defends against conscious as well as unconscious anxiety generated by a variety of situations. Phobias include the chief defense mechanisms of regression, projection, and displacement. In becoming phobic, the individual fears an external object rather than an internal and unknown source of distress. Phobias are common experiences in childhood, including a fear of animals, darkness, lightning, and strangers. In adulthood, a phobia can become a crippling experience.

An individual may often exhibit an irrational avoidance of such things as certain insects or modes of transportation, but this usually has no major effect on the individual's life. Indeed, certain phobic behaviors (e.g., hiding under the bed during a thunderstorm) derive from childhood and from observing the statements or behavior of one's parents. When, however, the avoidant behavior interferes with the individual's social or role functioning, a diagnosis of phobic disorder is made. The phobic disorders are subdivided into specific phobia and social phobia.

SPECIFIC PHOBIA

The person with a specific phobia (formerly known as simple phobia) has a marked, persistent fear or compelling desire to avoid a focal object or situation, which is not explained by any other anxiety disorder. The individual fears that he or she will be harmed by the situation or lose control during it. The response to the phobic stimulus immediately provokes an anxiety reaction. In fact, the level of anxiety often increases as the phobic stimulus gets closer to the individual. Sometimes a full-blown panic attack can occur if the individual can't get away from the stimulus quickly. Most often the individual chooses to avoid the stimulus completely and less frequently endures it with great distress.

The individual may fear a specific animal or insect (animal type), confined places (situational type), heights (natural environment type), air travel (situational type), simple medical procedures (blood/injury/injection type), and storms (natural environment type). The frequency of specific phobias seen in clinical settings, from most to least common, is situational, natural environment, blood/injection/injury, and animal. Many patients experience more than one subtype.

Epidemiology

The prevalence of specific phobias varies according to the threshold used to determine impairment from this disorder. About a 9% prevalence rate of specific phobia has been reported for 1 year, and a rate of from 10 to 11% over a lifetime. The ratios of males to females are different for the subtypes: From 75 to 90% of persons with animal, natural environment, and situational type phobias are female (except for fear of heights, for which 55 to 70% are women): From 55 to 70% of the blood/injury/injection type of phobia also occur in females (*DSM-IV*).

Etiologic Factors and Family Patterns

Theories relating to a familial link, learned behaviors, and psychoanalytic relationships exist for specific phobias.

Familial. A high degree of familial transmission exists for specific phobias by type. For example, a first-degree biological relative of a person with a specific phobias of the situational type is likely to have specific situational phobia, but not necessarily triggered by the same situation. Blood/injury/injection type phobias have a particularly strong history in families. To further substantiate some genetic connection, a higher concordance for this phobia exists for monozygotic than for dizygotic twins.

Behavioral. It is theorized that operant conditioning may produce a specific phobia. The process of an unconditioned response (e.g., the startle response) to an unconditioned stimulus (e.g., a loud noise) being paired with a conditioned stimulus (dog) leads to a conditioned (fear) response.

Psychoanalytic. Freud believed that phobias are symptoms of some unresolved unconscious conflict.

Age of Onset and Course

The mean onset age for specific phobias varies according to their subtype. Animal, natural environment, and blood/injection/injury types of phobias tend to begin in childhood. The situational type is more bimodally distributed, with a peak in childhood and a second peak in the mid-20s.

Phobias may result from traumatic events, unexpected panic attacks in the feared setting, observing others undergoing fearfulness, and information communicated from parental warnings or disaster coverage in the media. Phobias that result from unexpected panic attacks or traumatic events are particularly acute in their onset and do not appear at any particular age. Many childhood-onset phobias remit spontaneously prior to adulthood. Yet if they persist into adulthood, they infrequently remit on their own.

Impairment and Complications

A phobic individual will suffer greater impairments if exposed to the feared stimulus more frequently. The common problems associated with phobia are difficulties in maintaining a daily routine, occupational issues, and a restricted social life.

Certain medical conditions may be exacerbated by phobic avoidance. Individuals with blood/injection/injury phobia may have additional dental or general physical health problems because they may routinely avoid such preventive and pre-emptive care.

Nursing Assessment and Diagnosis

When assessing an individual for a phobic disorder, certain questions must be raised. Does this phobia signifi-

cantly impair functioning or cause marked distress? Is the fear unreasonable, given the context of the situation (e.g., a fear of being shot in a non-dangerous neighborhood?). If the answer is yes to these questions, the diagnosis of a phobia may be made. Patients with specific phobias don't present with pervasive anxiety since their fear is limited to certain, circumscribed situations.

When differentiating between specific phobia and other anxiety disorders, the following factors should be considered: the focus of the fear; a description of the panic attack and the frequency of attacks; the number of situations that are avoided; and the level of the intercurrent anxiety. For example, an individual who had not previously feared or avoided elevators has a panic attack in an elevator and begins to dread going to work because of the need to take the elevator to his job on the 30th floor. If this individual subsequently has panic attacks only in elevators, a diagnosis of specific phobia may be appropriate. If, however, the individual experiences unexpected panic attacks in other situations and begins to avoid or endure with dread other situations because of the fear of a panic attack, then a diagnosis of panic disorder with agoraphobia is warranted.

Nursing Diagnosis

The most common nursing diagnosis is fear. See Figure 14-2.

Intervention

As with panic disorder, exposure therapy has shown success in treating phobias by helping patients achieve habituation or extinction of the fear response. This behavioral method has been particularly helpful for height, darkness, animal, and blood/injection/injury phobias. Cognitive therapy does not appear to benefit the specific phobic patient.

SOCIAL PHOBIA

The individual suffering from a social phobia avoids situations in which he or she may be exposed to scrutiny by others. A companion fear is that he or she will behave in a manner that will be embarrassing or humiliating. This fear leads to a high level of distress and then to avoidance of the phobia-provoking situation. Examples of social phobias include fears of speaking in public, writing in the presence of others, eating in public, and using public rest rooms. The person with such a phobia is usually aware that the fear will be observed by others (e.g., a hand tremor being noticed while writing), and that it is unreasonable to have such a fear.

Socially phobic individuals also experience physical symptoms such as blushing, sweating, trembling, di-

DSM-IV: Phobic avoidance (agoraphobia),

Nursing Diagnosis: FEAR.

Related to: (check at least one)

Specific phobia (specify)   Performing in public
Being alone in public place   Being the focus of attention of others
Other

Treatment Goal: PATIENT WILL DECREASE ANXIETY AND LEVEL OF FEAR TO BE ABLE TO SUCCESSFULLY FUNCTION AND SUCCESSFULLY CARRY OUT THE ACTIVITIES OF DAILY LIFE.

Treatment Goal Can be Measured Using the Following Expected Outcomes:

1. The patient will be able to demonstrate three adaptive coping techniques to maintain anxiety at a tolerable level.
2. The patient will be able to verbalize three methods to be able to avoid or successfully deal with phobic objects of situations.

Interventions:

Date Initiated	Date Discontinued	
_____	_____	1. Reassure patient of his/her safety and security.
_____	_____	2. Explore patient's perception of threat to physical integrity or threat to self-concept.
_____	_____	3. Discuss reality of the situation with patient in order to recognize aspects that can and cannot be changed.
_____	_____	4. Include patient in making decisions related to selection of alternative coping strategies to foster sense of control.
_____	_____	5. Implement prescribed behavior modification program to work on elimination of the fear. (i.e., systematic desensitization) (Identify _____).
_____	_____	6. Encourage patient to explore underlying feelings that may be contributing to irrational fears.
_____	_____	7. Assist patient to understand how facing feelings, rather than suppressing them, can result in more adaptive coping abilities.
_____	_____	8. Administer prescribed medication per physician orders. Assess for effectiveness/adverse reactions. (Identify _____).

Source: Nursing staff at 1st Hospital of Wyoming under the direction of Theresa M. Croushore

Figure 14–2. Individualized nursing care plan.

arrhea, palpitations, and gastrointestinal distress. In severe conditions, the phobic individual may experience a full panic attack. Socially phobic individuals can fear a single performance situation, several social situations, or most social-interaction and public-performance situations. This last type of phobia, termed *social phobia,* has generalized fears, and involves greater social-skill deficits and functional impairments.

Epidemiology

As with specific phobia, the prevalence rates of social phobia can vary depending on the threshold used to determine impairment. Studies indicate that the life-time prevalence rate of social phobia is from 3 to 13%. Most socially phobic individuals fear public speaking most, while other performance fears, such as eating, drinking, or writing in public are less common. Some studies suggest that social phobia is more common in women than in men *(DSM-IV).*

Etiologic Factors and Family Patterns

As with the other anxiety disorders, familial, behavioral, and psychoanalytical theories exist with social phobia.

Familial. Social phobia is more common in first-degree biologic relatives of those with the disorder than in the general population. Some studies suggest that some phobic traits are inherited, such as fear of strangers, shyness, and fear of social criticism. In addition, a higher concordance for this disorder exists between monozygotic than between dizygotic twins (Nagy, Krystal, Charney, 1994).

Behavioral. Socially phobic individuals appear to have similar difficulties in evaluating their performance in social situations, a hypersensitivity to criticism, or early unpleasant social situations.

Psychoanalytic. Social phobia is explained in a similar manner to agoraphobia, with the individual having rigid ideas of social behavior, exaggerated awareness of minimal somatic symptoms, and a tendency to experience others as critical of them. Whether these traits cause or are a result of this disorder is not yet determined.

Age of Onset and Course

Social phobia typically appears between the ages of 15 and 20, with some individuals reporting onset during childhood. Transient social anxiety is common in childhood and adolescence. The onset of social phobia may occur abruptly after a humiliating experience, or take on a slower developmental track. Most socially phobic individuals have this disorder for their entire lives, but some changes in severity occur during adulthood.

Impairments and Complications

Many of the problems experienced by socially phobic individuals are similar to those experienced in the other anxiety disorders. Difficulties with work, school, and social relationships are consistently experienced. Individuals are likely to be underachievers and have a smaller likelihood of marrying, which can lead to further isolation and may trigger substance-abuse prob-

E CASE EXAMPLE

▶ SOCIAL PHOBIA

A 60-year-old woman seeks counseling because her husband has been offered a new job in another state. She fears moving. Her history reveals the onset of anxiety symptoms 2 years after her marriage at age 25. She became panicked in a bus, requiring

her to get off at the next bus stop. Over the years her phobias have expanded, and in the 15 years before seeking counseling she has been unable to travel by public transportation, in tunnels, or over bridges. She is unable to shop in markets, eat in restaurants, ride in elevators, cross wide highways, or use any public facility. She fears worms and live animals. She has few social friends and avoids social gatherings.

---

lems or the development of significant depressive symptoms.

Nursing Assessment and Diagnosis

As with the other anxiety disorders, initially differentiating between phobic disorders can be difficult, and the wrong diagnosis can delay effective treatment. Social phobia is classically characterized by the avoidance of social situations in the absence of recurrent and unexpected panic attacks. When attacks do occur they are generally situationally bound or situationally predisposed. Avoiding public humiliation is always a key characteristic of this disorder.

Performance anxiety, shyness, and stage fright in social situations that involve unfamiliar people are common and should not be diagnosed as social phobia, unless they bring on clinically significant distress or impairment.

Treatment

While some antidepressant drugs have proven successful in reducing the symptoms of social phobia, most treatment programs focus on behavioral treatment. Although pharmacological and behavioral therapies combined have been effective in treating this disorder, no studies have been performed to determine actual efficacy rates.

Behavior modification is sometimes used alone or in conjunction with psychotherapy. Relaxation exercise is also used for treatment.

■ OBSESSIVE–COMPULSIVE DISORDER

Recurrent obsessions or compulsions are essential features of obsessive–compulsive disorders. Obsessions are repeated, persistent thoughts or impulses that are seen as intrusive and inappropriate, but unavoidable. These thoughts are highly charged with emotional significance. Compulsions are the action components of obsessive-compulsive disorders (i.e., repetitive, purposeful behaviors, recognized as unreasonable, but which are nevertheless performed in order to suppress or neutralize the obsessions).

Obsessive–compulsive disorder is classified under anxiety disorders in the *DSM-IV* because of the prominence of anxiety in this condition. The disorder is viewed as a defense against anxiety. Additional ego defenses used by the individual with an obsessive-compulsive disorder include repression, isolation, reaction formation, and undoing. Commonly described obsessions include:

- Thoughts of violence (e.g., ideas of stabbing, shooting, maiming, or hitting).
- Thoughts of contamination (e.g., images of germs, dirt, or feces.).
- Repetitive doubt and concern that something is not right, that a tragic event may occur, or that perfection was not achieved in some act
- Repeating or counting images or words or objects in the environment.

Commonly described compulsions include:

- Touching, usually repetitively, and often combined with counting.
- Washing, especially of the hands, which seem to come in contact with contaminants.
- Doing and undoing, opening and closing doors, walking backward and forward, and changing the order or organization of things.
- Checking, especially to make sure that no disaster has occurred and that someone has not been injured.

The obsessional person, although under the burden of defenses intended to minimize and deflect anxiety and anger, is nonetheless anxious and angry. Not only do the rituals fail to provide a sense of security, they burden the individual further with the symptoms. Most patients experience both obsessions and compulsions; multiple obsessions and compulsions are common.

People with obsessive–compulsive disorder suffer with obsessions or compulsions. If they have obsessions, they attempt to ignore or suppress such thoughts or impulses, or to neutralize them with some other thought or action. They recognize that the obsessions are the product of their own mind, not imposed from without (as in thought insertion). The thoughts, impulses, or worries are not simply excessive worries about real problems. If the individual has compulsions, the resulting repetitive, purposeful, and intentional behaviors are performed in response to an obsession, or according to rigid rules or in a stereotyped fashion. The affected individual recognizes that his or her behavior is excessive or unreasonable (this may not be true for young children or it may no longer be true for people whose obsessions have evolved into overvalued ideas). The disorder causes marked distress, is time-consuming (consumes more than an hour a day), and/or significantly interferes with normal routine, occupational functioning, or usual social activities or relationships with others.

EPIDEMIOLOGY

The lifetime prevalence of obsessive–compulsive disorder is 2.5%. It is equally common in males and females (DSM-IV).

ETIOLOGIC FACTORS AND FAMILY PATTERNS

The etiologic theories of obsessive-compulsive disorder include familial/genetic, psychoanalytic, cognitive, behavioral, and neurobiologic factors.

Familial/Genetic

Higher rates of obsessive–compulsive disorder occur in first-degree biological relatives of patients with this disorder. Some link may also exist with mood disorders and other psychiatric disorders such as Tourette's syndrome. A much higher concordance in monozygotic (75%) than in dizygotic (32%) twins is present (Nagy, Krystal, and Charney, 1994).

Psychoanalytic

Some theorists suggest that obsessive-compulsive disorder evolves from a disturbance in the anal-sadistic phase of development. This conflict can lead to a regression to earlier defense mechanisms such as reaction formation and isolation. The result is ambivalence and "magical thinking."

Cognitive

Persons with obsessive–compulsive disorder are viewed as having a defect in their cognitive information processing mechanism, producing a mismatch between beliefs and sensory data.

Behavioral

Obsessions result from associating mental stimuli with anxiety-provoking thoughts. The compulsions in obsessive-compulsive disorder were formerly benign behaviors that are now linked to anxiety reduction and are reinforced.

Neurobiologic

Research indicates that a dysfunction of the brain serotonergic neuronal systems exists in obsessive–compulsive individuals. This is largely based on the fact that clomipramine, the serotonin reuptake inhibitor, has been found to have therapeutic efficacy (Nagy, Krystal, and Charney, 1994).

AGE OF ONSET AND COURSE

The onset of obsessive–compulsive disorder is usually between adolescence and adulthood, but it may occur in childhood. Male obsessive-compulsives individuals develop the disorder between the ages of 6 and 15 years, and females between 20 and 29 years of age. Onset is generally gradual.

The course of the disorder is chronic and symptoms are exacerbated by stressful life events. The prognosis is not good, but those persons who experience onset at an early age are more likely to have a better long-term outcome. In some extreme cases, the symptoms can worsen and totally consume the affected individual's time. Obsessive thoughts are the only cognitions that are abnormal for the individual. Most obsessive-compulsive behaviors are recognized as strange and unusual, but some have been part of the patient's life for so long that he or she sees them as normal (Nagy, Krystal, and Charney, 1994).

IMPAIRMENTS AND COMPLICATIONS

The obsessive–compulsive individual experiences significant impairments in occupational and social functioning. Other problems may include sleep disturbances, abuse of alcohol and sedatives, and marital problems as a result of the behaviors accompanying the disorder. Suicide risk is high since this act may be the only perceived way to escape from the troubling thoughts and actions.

E CASE EXAMPLE

▶ CASE EXAMPLE A

Sister Patricia, a 40-year-old nun, is admitted to the psychiatric unit after her community becomes unable to manage her behavior. The patient is a teacher who has not worked for about 6 months because of an increase in her obsessive–compulsive behavior of washing. The patient repeatedly washes her arms, hands, clothes, walls, and furniture. This behavior has increased until she has become unable to sleep because of washing her clothes throughout the night and early morning hours.

The patient's ritualistic behavior has been a long-standing problem. She has behaved in this way for many years. The patient has had no recent stressful events that caused her behavior to worsen. The symptoms have persisted and increased as the patient has matured. The accumulated anxiety has caused a worsening depression and low self-esteem. The chronicity of her behaviors has made resolution and nursing management more difficult.

The patient feels that she must wash the psychiatric unit, especially the bathroom, herself, and her clothes constantly. The behavior interferes with her attendance at therapy and activity groups and private sessions. Preventing all of these behaviors would be ineffective and would increase her anxiety, with the risk that the patient might fail in her treatment. The approach is to give the patient a schedule to follow so that she has to limit her ritualistic behavior but not extinguish it entirely. With this, the patient becomes gradually able to attend more milieu and therapy groups and decrease her ritualistic behavior.

▶ CASE EXAMPLE B

A 23-year-old married woman comes to the mental health clinic because "life is gray."

The story unfolds that there are various secrets in her life, especially that she practices rituals. For example, she is compelled to read everything three times and tap three times before opening anything. She also feels compelled to read the obituaries in the newspaper every day. The rituals are done in the service of protecting the people around her. The patient feels the rituals are a part of her. They frighten her, and she wonders if she is crazy. On the other hand, to explore her rituals in therapy will increase her anxiety. Part of her ambivalence in exploring them is that she believes that they separate her from her two sisters and give her a "specialness."

The nursing intervention in Case Example B is to first identify the patient's rituals; next to determine the purpose of the rituals; and third to identify what the patient will need to give up the rituals. She notes that under stress the rituals increase in intensity. She is able to remember that the rituals began when she was age 7 or 8, and that she was always the "good girl" in the family. Thus, one could speculate that the rituals were a defense against assertiveness, impulses, and instincts that opposed her being a "good girl."

▶ CASE EXAMPLE C

In a third example of obsessive-compulsive disorder, the symptoms have accelerated. A fire chief is at a major fire when a wall collapses and kills some of his men, as well as endangering himself. After recovering from the trauma suffered during the fire, he returns to work, but he begins to doubt his ability. Concurrently, the city budget is cut and his anxieties build. He worries constantly about fire. He is unable to leave his house without feeling the walls, and he soon begins to run back to his house during the day to check the walls. The symptoms force him into early retirement on disability.

NURSING ASSESSMENT AND DIAGNOSIS

Recurrent or intrusive thoughts or behaviors may occur in the context of many psychiatric disorders. Obsessive–compulsive disorder is not diagnosed if the content of the individual's thoughts or activities is related to another disorder such as body dysmorphic disorder, specific phobia, or social phobia.

Nursing Diagnosis

Ineffective individual coping. See Figure 14-3.

NURSING INTERVENTION

The nursing-care plan includes the psychiatric diagnosis and nursing diagnosis of ineffective individual coping as well as interventions, expected outcome, and evaluation. The interventions include treatment, close observation, reality testing, symptom substitution, and goal-oriented interviews.

Treatment

Therapeutic gains have been made in the treatment of obsessive–compulsive disorder through the use of pharmacological and behavioral therapies; however, patients with this disorder do not generally fully recover. As stated earlier, the medication clomipramine helps 40 to 60% of patients experience gradual improvement, with a significant reduction of symptoms and disability. Several behavioral treatments are discussed in the nursing intervention section below (Nagy, Krystal, Charney, 1994).

DSM-IV: Obsessive–compulsive disorders

Nursing Diagnosis: INEFFECTIVE INDIVIDUAL COPING.

Related to: (check at least one)

Situational crisis	Inadequate support systems
Maturational crisis	Fear of failure
Ritualistic behavior	Unmet dependency needs
Obsessive thoughts	Other

Treatment Goal: BY DISCHARGE, PATIENT WILL DEMONSTRATE FLEXIBILITIES IN ACTIVITIES OF DAILY LIVING.

Treatment Goal Can be Measured Using the Following Expected Outcomes:

1. The patient expresses three feelings of self-confidence.
2. The patient demonstrates use of three adaptive coping skills.
3. The patient is able to interrupt obsessive thoughts and avoid vitalistic behaviors as required in order to successfully deal with activities of daily living.

Interventions:

Date Initiated	Date Discontinued	
_____	_____	1. Assess patient's level of anxiety and try to determine types of situations that increase anxiety.
_____	_____	2. Assess patient's mood—observe for suicidal behaviors and report these to physician.
_____	_____	3. Initially meet patient's dependency needs as required.
_____	_____	4. Slowly encourage independence and give positive reinforcement for independent behaviors (i.e., verbal praise, increased privileges) (Identify _____).
_____	_____	5. Allow time for rituals.
_____	_____	6. Support patient's efforts to explore the meaning and purpose of the behavior.
_____	_____	7. Provide structured schedule of activities. (Identify _____).
_____	_____	8. Gradually begin to limit amount of time allotted for ritualistic behavior as patient becomes increasingly involved in unit activities.
_____	_____	9. Offer positive reinforcement for non-ritualistic behaviors. (i.e., verbal praise, increased privileges). (Identify _____).
_____	_____	10. Teach patient to recognize situations that provoke obsessive thoughts and/or ritualistic behavior. Also teach methods to interrupt these thoughts and behaviors. (i.e., thought-stopping techniques, relaxation techniques, exercise, play/diversional activities). Document teaching/hospital protocol.

Source: Nursing staff at 1st Hospital of Wyoming under the direction of Theresa M. Croushore

Figure 14–3. Individualized Nursing Care Plan

Close Observation

Acute and pervasive obsessive–compulsive symptoms are often rapidly evolving states that need careful monitoring. The patient needs to be observed for the intensity and severity of symptoms and for the possible emergence of both depression and psychosis.

Reality Testing

The nurse can provide reality-testing methods for the patient who has exaggerated or grandiose thoughts connected with performance of rituals. Reality limits may be unclear, and the nurse may assist as in the following dialogue:

Patient: I am doing this for my salvation and my family's, and maybe for yours also.

Nurse: Tell me again why you think your ritual is for my salvation?

Patient: Well, when I said that, it may not sound right, but that's what I think when I'm doing it.

Nurse: Do I understand you to mean that while you do the ritual you think it is for your salvation, your family's, and mine?

Patient: I did. But when I hear you say it, it doesn't sound right. I had better think about that again.

Symptom Substitution

At times, it may be helpful for the nurse to suggest a symptom substitution. For example, when a patient has the compulsion to check and re-check something, the nurse can ask the patient to sit and think about what he or she is going to talk about with the therapist at their next appointment. This technique introduces a delay in the performance of a compulsion, and should be followed with a verbal acknowledgment that the compulsion was not acted on.

In 1963, J. G. Taylor wrote of a technique known as *thought stopping* (Taylor, 1963) to interrupt obsessive patterns. This technique has gained wide acceptance. The patient is instructed to yell "stop" as loudly as possible in the middle of obsessive thoughts. Behavioral techniques used without other therapeutic approaches are successful with patients for whom obsessive–compulsive symptoms affect only a narrow range of their functioning and whose personality is relatively healthy.

Goal-Oriented Interviews

The nurse works with the patient, through the contract, on goal-oriented issues. Although one should not ignore the patient's obsessive–compulsive symptoms, neither should the nurse allow the interview to progress in an endless discussion of symptoms. The nurse needs to establish goals beyond the reduction of symptoms in the area of strengthening interpersonal relationships.

■ POST-TRAUMATIC STRESS DISORDER (PTSD)

Post-traumatic stress disorder (PTSD) provides a conceptual bridge linking a wide variety of traumatic events, such as war, terrorism, natural disasters, and rape, to a specific set of symptoms. This disorder was not even recognized as an independent diagnosis until the publication of *DSM-III* in 1980, and has become the focus of intensive research in the past decade. The psychiatric diagnostic criteria for PTSD follow.

The individual with PTSD has experienced a traumatic event that involves a threat of serious injury or death, or a threat to the individual's own or someone else's physical integrity. The individual reacts with horror, extreme fright, or helplessness to the event. The individual repeatedly re-experiences the traumatic event, avoids anything that evokes remembrance of the event, experiences a sense of emotional numbing or unresponsiveness, and has symptoms of hyperarousal. Persons with PTSD commonly have intrusive thoughts or memories of the event, suffer flashbacks, feel emotionally detached and blunted, startle easily, and have trouble sleeping and difficulty in concentrating when awake. PTSD can be further specified by duration, acute PTSD lasting less than 3 months; chronic PTSD lasting (three months or longer), and delayed onset PTSD occurring six or more months after a stressful event (LaBruzza, 1994).

Over the past decade, scientific literature has emerged on the effects of massive psychic trauma on human mental functioning and on the psychosocial development of the survivor. The results of studies conducted with survivors of the atomic bomb at Hiroshima; the 1972 flood at Buffalo Creek, West Virginia; the Nazi persecution in the Second World War; veterans of the Vietnam War; and studies of rape and incest victims have shown that PTSD often develops after the catastrophic stressors have ended. It is now recognized by clinicians, scholars, and others that immersion in the death experience and exposure to profound life-death threats may lead to survivor syndromes in which there persists a lasting psychic residue of the traumatic event.

EPIDEMIOLOGY

Significant variability exists when estimating the prevalence of PTSD in the population. Depending on the method of ascertainment and the population sampled, PTSD has a lifetime prevalence of from 1 to 14%. Studies of at-risk individuals (e.g., combat veterans or victims of criminal violence) have yielded prevalence rates ranging from 3% to 58%. An epidemiological survey of adult women revealed alarmingly high rates of traumatic events, particularly being the victim of a crime;

the lifetime prevalence of PTSD for this group was 13% and the current prevalence was 3% *(DSM-IV)*.

Risk factors for exposure to traumatic events were a family history of psychiatric disorder, male sex, extroversion, a history of conduct disorder problems, and neuroticism. The risk for developing PTSD after experiencing trauma is increased when the individual has a family history of anxiety, has been separated from parents in childhood, is female, or has a pre-existing anxiety or depressive disorder or a family history of antisocial behavior (Nagy, Krystal, Charney, 1994).

ETIOLOGIC FACTORS AND FAMILY PATTERNS

PTSD is a unique disorder that leads to psychological, behavioral, and physiological symptoms. Some theorists believe that this disorder is related to a failure to integrate the trauma that lies at its source with one's world image, self-concept, and view of the meaning of life. Other theories describe a psychobiological or behavioral origin.

Psychobiological Factors

Patients with PTSD have heightened autonomic or sensory nervous system arousal when reminded of trauma. Several processes involving the locus coeruleus, hypothalamus, and hippocampus have shown certain abnormalities in PTSD patients. As mentioned in the previous section, genetic and familial factors have also been associated with a vulnerability to PTSD.

Behavioral Factors

The two-factor learning theory involves aversive conditioning to a neutral stimulus that has been combined with a trauma reaction. Further conditioning leads to instrumental learning, whereby behaviors are acquired that are intended to avoid anxiety from the conditioned stimuli. Additional factors interfere with extinction occurring naturally.

AGE OF ONSET AND COURSE

Since a traumatic event must occur prior to the onset of PTSD, no particular onset age is noted. Even children can succumb to this disorder. Months or years can transpire between a traumatic event and the onset of PTSD. The duration of the disorder varies from a few months to several years. PTSD is often more severe or long-lasting when it originates from an act of human design (e.g., rape). Complete recovery can occur within 3 months for at least 50% of patients. Relapse can also occur.

IMPAIRMENTS AND COMPLICATIONS

Individuals with PTSD often experience painful guilt about surviving when others did not, or about what they had to do to survive. Avoidance of situations that resemble or symbolize the original trauma may interfere with interpersonal relationships and lead to marital discord, divorce, or job loss. A complete personality change may occur, in which a formerly happy and productive person becomes hostile, withdrawn, and self-destructive. A higher risk for impulsive behavior and suicide exists.

In addition, there may be an increased risk for panic disorder, agoraphobia, obsessive–compulsive disorder and major depression. Yet it is not known whether these disorders precede the onset of PTSD or follow it.

NURSING ASSESSMENT

When evaluating an individual for the presence of PTSD, questions are asked about any life trauma that has been experienced. It may be difficult to assess whether or not the individual's trauma reaction is normal or truly represents clinical symptomology. The diagnosis should be based on the level of distress, degree of impairment, and duration of the symptoms.

TREATMENT

Rapid assessment and treatment can help to diminish impairments and dysfunction associated with chronic PTSD. The most effective treatment involves coupling pharmacological and nonpharmacological therapies. The pharmacological treatment alleviates the physiological symptoms so that the other psychological issues can be addressed. The medications that have shown some efficacy against PTSD are antidepressants such as fluoxetine (Prozac). This drug, in particular, has shown efficacy in treating symptom clusters.

Cognitive therapy for PTSD involves relaxation, thought stopping, breathing control, learning communication skills, and cognitive restructuring to reduce symptoms at an early stage. This treatment is more successful over the long term when there has been prolonged exposure to the trauma as in incest or combat.

Co-morbid conditions complicate the treatment of PTSD. If a substance-abuse problem exists, it should be the first focus of treatment. Yet treatment of PTSD should first be addressed to treating co-existing depression.

■ ACUTE STRESS DISORDER

A new disorder, acute stress disorder, has been proposed in the *DSM-IV*. Its symptoms are similar to those of PTSD, with acute distress from trauma and functional impairment, but last only 2 days to 4 weeks. The response must occur within 4 weeks after the trauma in order to be classified as acute stress disorder. It is believed that this disorder is a precursor to PTSD.

■ GENERALIZED ANXIETY DISORDER

Persons with generalized anxiety disorder (GAD) experience persistent anxiety of at least 6 months duration. There are also signs of motor tension (shakiness, jumpiness, trembling, tension, fatigue, twitching eyelids, furrowed brow, sighing respirations, etc.); autonomic hyperactivity (sweating, heart pounding, cold hands, dry mouth, upset stomach, etc.); apprehensive expectation (anxiety, worry, rumination, anticipation of dread); and vigilance and scanning (impatience, feeling on edge, easy distractibility, interrupted sleep, fatigue on awakening). The validity of GAD as a diagnosis distinct from other anxiety disorders or depression is still being evaluated.

Patients with GAD describe unrealistic or excessive anxiety and worry (apprehensive expectation) about several life circumstances (e.g., worry about possible misfortune to one's child, who in reality is in no danger, and worry about finances, for no good reason) for a period of 6 months or longer, during which the affected individual has been bothered on more days than not by these concerns. In children and adolescents, this disturbance may take the form of anxiety and worry about academic, athletic, and social performance. Patients find it difficult to control the worry.

Patients must experience at least three of the following six symptoms in order to be diagnosed as having GAD: muscle tension, restlessness, easy fatigability, difficulty in concentrating or mental blankness because of anxiety, trouble falling or staying asleep, and/or irritability.

The anxiety or worry is not about having a panic attack, as in panic disorder; being embarrassed in public, as in social phobia; being contaminated, as in obsessive–compulsive disorder; gaining weight, as in anorexia nervosa; or having an illness, as in hypochondriasis or somatization disorder; and is not part of PTSD. The anxiety, worry, or physical symptoms in GAD significantly interfere with the affected individual's normal routine or usual activities, or cause marked distress; they are not due to a substance-induced or anxiety disorder or general medical condition, and do not occur only during the course of a mood disorder, a psychotic disorder, or a pervasive developmental disorder.

The worry in GAD is out of proportion to the likelihood that the feared events are going to occur. The

E CASE EXAMPLE

▶ CHRONIC POST-TRAUMATIC STRESS DISORDER

Michael Song, age 37, was born in Taiwan, and is the youngest of 10 children. His mother died from a stroke and his father died from a heart attack. He was educated in Taiwan, with a college major in French. He began working in Taiwan at a charter-car company, and his wife worked as a secretary at the same company. They met and were married in 1984. Soon after the marriage, Mr. Song got his immigration visa and came to the United States. His wife stayed in Taiwan, awaiting her visa.

At that time in his life, Mr. Song described himself, and his wife agreed, as outgoing, responsible, happy, ambitious, and sensitive. He had high hopes for his future in the United States in the high-technology business field. He came to New York, where one of his brothers lived, and began working at a metal company.

On a March morning in 1985, Mr. Song was at work painting a wheelbarrow. He was working in front of a large dumpster. Another employee indicated that he wanted to refuel the dumpster in front of where Mr. Song was working. So Mr. Song gathered his work materials, moved across the room, and resumed painting the wheelbarrow. Mr. Song was bent over his work with his head down when suddenly he heard a squeal of brakes and saw a bright flash of light. He was then struck by a truck. Yellow paint spilled; he felt intense pain; he screamed for help. A friend called the supervisor, an ambulance arrived, and Mr. Song was taken to a hospital emergency room.

Mr. Song was hospitalized for about one month. His injuries included severe pelvic fracture, bilateral iliac artery injuries, venous injury, transection of the membranous urethra, and injury to the corpora cavernosa of the penis.

Mrs. Song received a temporary visa and arrived in the United States in April 1985. Mr. Song was having a difficult recovery in the hospital, and it was arranged to have his wife stay with him in his hospital room. She described her her husband during this period as having severe physical pain, a 50-pound weight loss, sleep disturbance, nightmares, crying spells, mood swings, depression, and difficulty in walking.

Since his accident, Mr. Song has had a series of surgical procedures to repair the extensive vascular, neurological, and urinary damage he sustained. He has also had an implantation of a penile prosthesis. His physical recovery was painful and accompanied by surgical and medical procedures for repeated urinary infections. Through his hospitalizations Mr. Song alternated between feeling sad, anxious, and angry. He had constant thoughts of the accident, and this preoccupation impaired his concentration, his intent to learn English, and his ability to relate to people.

The Songs' experience daily anxieties related to any physical activity that might be injurious to Mr. Song's groin and legs. He lives in constant fear of infection or breakdown of the artificial graft material in his body, which could create a life-threatening hemorrhage if medical care was not promptly available. This fear is constantly in both Mr. and Mrs. Song's minds.

Mr. Song is limited in many normal functions. He is not supposed to do any heavy lifting, bending, or prolonged standing, and is supposed to avoid any situation that might compromise his circulation. His injury has caused permanent damage to his physical and psychological health. It has also caused severe injury to his sexual life. He has permanent damage to his erective functioning, which has created major problems in the Songs' sexual relationship. On a percentage scale, Mr. Song ranked his sexual life at 20% of normal. It is difficult for the Songs to discuss their feelings about their sexual life, primarily because of their fear and anxiety about the fragility of Mr. Song's physical abilities.

The *DSM-IV* diagnosis of Mr. Song's condition is chronic PTSD. Specific symptoms include:
- Intrusive thoughts: "I'm always thinking I'm penned in. The brakes sound like thunder. Then white lights are around me."
- A feeling of estrangement from others: "My friends don't know the extent of my injury. I can't talk with them. I have little to talk to them about."
- Recurrent dreams of the accident: "I wake up at night with a nightmare. I feel panic and it is happening all over again."

There are persistent symptoms of increased arousal that were not present before the accident, and which take the forms of difficulty in concentrating ("Can't study English; can't concentrate"), hypervigilance ("I'm worry about money and my family and my caring for them."), and an exaggerated startle response ("The slightest thing upsets me, like the smell of diesel fuel").

Mr. Song continues to be reminded of the accident when he sees trucks, a dumpster, or junk. He constantly asks himself: "Why me?"

The case formulation of Mr. Song's PTSD is that it has been intensified by the threat of loss of limb and life because of the extent of his physical injuries. There have been attempts to regain some normalcy to his sexual relationship with his wife in terms of the penile implant; however, his frequent infections have created anxiety over the implant.

There has been a total disruption of Mr. Song's life goals and plans, and because of the continuing physical danger to his life and his isolation, this has affected his ability to become acculturated into the main community social system. He has not continued his study of the English language and is limited in securing American friends, as he had hoped to do. The energy required for his acculturation has been drained by the demands of surviving.

Mr. Song's major worry is of the future. He worries constantly about his family and what will happen when he is older. He is afraid to ask the doctor about this. He states, "I have lost years of my life. All my energy went into recovering from this. If I hadn't had this accident, I would be able to work very hard and care for my family." He feels inadequate as a husband in terms of being a family provider and as a father in terms of limited physical activity ("I can't play with my children or their friends because I have to be careful of my legs.") He feels like a person in retirement. His friends do not understand this, and ask him why he stays home all the time.

A supportive counseling program should be initiated, with therapeutic efforts made in two major directions: (1) to maintain Mr. Song's physical health; and (2) to strengthen Mr. Song's self-esteem and self-worth through reduction of his symptoms of PTSD. These therapeutic efforts should be in the form of individual and family counseling, and support and rehabilitation, including education courses for Mr. Song's social integration into the community.

The counseling program should be two pronged: (1) to actively deal with the intrusive symptoms, numbing phenomena, and hyperarousal associated with PTSD, and (2) to deal with Mr. Song's fearfulness about the future. This second area would combine with educational efforts for language acquisition and the identification of other skills and abilities that can be exercised within the limits of Mr. Song's physical condition. The intricate aspect of rehabilitation will involve counseling for both husband and wife, and there may be need for some input for the Song's children, particularly given Mr. Song's limitations in the household. This movement cannot be made, however, until there is some abatement of the symptoms of PTSD.

E CASE EXAMPLE

▶ DELAYED PTSD

The following case involves a clinical situation that reactivated a stress disorder, and illustrates the complex and intricate interplay between events. It also describes therapeutic interventions to assist in the resolution of traumatic conflicts.

Mr. Ormsby, a 55-year-old divorced man, was admitted to a psychiatric ward with severe anxiety, multiple somatic complaints, feelings of hopelessness, self-care deficits, depression, and suicidal ideation. He had required psychiatric hospitalization for "nerves" shortly after his discharge from the service at the end of the Second World War. He subsequently had a good adjustment and stable marriage and work history. Three years before his current admission, Mr. Ormsby left his job as an emergency-room technician and began drinking heavily. Eventually his wife left him, and the actual signing of the divorce papers precipitated the symptoms that led to this hospitalization.

Only after another patient on the ward began talking of his own difficulties during the Second World War did Mr. Ormsby reveal the following history. He had been stationed in the South Pacific and survived two battles in which his ship had been destroyed and many people around him violently killed. Shortly after these events his unit had been instructed that island children were being wired as human bombs, and an or-

der was issued to shoot all children approaching the camp. When Mr. Ormsby was on duty, he had been forced to shoot a 10-year-old boy. After this incident, Mr. Ormsby began having nightmares of exploding shells, violent scenes of people being killed, and scenes of himself killing the boy. The nightmares cleared over a period of a few years.

The onset of Mr. Ormsby's symptoms 3 years previously came after an episode at work in the emergency room, when he was told to clean up a child in one of the rooms. He was unaware that the child (a 9-year-old boy) was dead when brought to the emergency room. When Mr. Ormsby discovered that the boy was dead, he was horrified, left work, and never returned. His nightmares resumed, but he felt unable to discuss his war episodes with his wife. At times he would wake up screaming and throw his wife to the floor to "cover" her from exploding shells. It was this unexplained behavior that forced their separation.

During his hospitalization, Mr. Ormsby was able to talk about his war episodes for the first time in more than three decades. He participated in a therapy group of Second World War veterans who focused on the expression of feelings about traumatic war experiences. Gradually, Mr. Ormsby's depression cleared and he reported being less anxious than at any time since the war. He was able to sleep through the night without nightmares, and resumed working (Christiansen et al., 1981)

---

common worries are about job responsibilities, health of family members, and minor matters such as car repairs and household chores.

EPIDEMIOLOGY

The lifetime prevalence of GAD is 5%. Eighty percent of persons with GAD have had at least one other anxiety disorder in their lifetimes. This disorder is slightly more common in young to middle aged women, non-whites, unmarried persons, and persons in a lower socio-economic class (DSM-IV).

ETIOLOGIC FACTORS AND FAMILY PATTERNS

First-degree biological relatives of persons with GAD have an increased frequency of the disorder, but not of the other anxiety disorders. Behaviorists believe that this disorder involves a conditioned response to a stimulus that becomes associated with danger. Since the stimulus is difficult to identify, it is thought to evolve from the cumulative effect of several stressful events (Nagy, Krystal, Charney, 1994).

AGE OF ONSET AND COURSE

The onset of GAD is variable, but is generally between the ages of 20 and 30. The course is chronic and wors-

ens as stress increases. GAD may begin as a childhood disorder of over-anxiety.

IMPAIRMENTS AND COMPLICATIONS

The individual with GAD experiences impairment in social, occupational, and other functional areas. GAD frequently occurs with mood disorders, other anxiety disorders, and substance-related disorders along with other conditions associated with stress, such as irritable bowel syndrome and headaches.

NURSING ASSESSMENT AND DIAGNOSIS

GAD is commonly diagnosed when another disorder is present, since the symptom of anxiety is present in many conditions, including depression, psychosis, substance abuse, and somatoform disorders. The key factors in diagnosing this disorder involve assessing whether the excessive and uncontrollable worrying causes functional impairment and is out of proportion to the actual impact of the feared event.

TREATMENT

The combined treatment of GAD with biofeedback, relaxation, and cognitive therapy has diminished patients' anxiety. Each of these therapies on its own, how-

E CASE EXAMPLE

▶ GENERALIZED ANXIETY DISORDER

A 21-year-old college student, just before final examinations, experiences a severe anxiety attack accompanied by feelings of panic and impending doom. The day prior to the attack was her birthday and the fourth anniversary of her favorite aunt's death. The symptoms described by the student include fatigue, tension, sweating, cold palms, worrying, a feeling of dread, a racing heart, edginess and nervousness, and an inability to

sleep. The nurse learns that the student's mourning for her aunt had been incomplete, at the time the student felt a sense of responsibility to care for her mother, who was very upset over the death of her sister. The student recalled having been anxious and depressed for several weeks prior to her birthdays for the past several years. She had never connected the anniversary of her aunt's death with her anxiety attacks.

---

ever, has had only limited success in GAD. Most antidepressant drugs are ineffective against the disorder. Valium and lithium have aided recovery, but some of their side effects, such as memory loss, sedation, and dependency on their use—have negatively affected their long-term use. The case example describes the nursing intervention and treatment program.

NURSING INTERVENTION

The nursing care plan for GAD includes the nursing interventions of identifying the precipitant, educating the patient, and cognitive reframing.

Identifying the Precipitant

Antecedents of an episode of GAD should be sought within a few hours prior to the acute onset of the disorder or at the maximum, within a few weeks earlier. These events need not be the original traumatic incidents, but may be related to them. The types of events precipitating severe anxiety are an extension of those precipitating normal anxiety, such as separation, fears of being hurt or injured, and fear of facing new tasks or new ventures.

Educating the Patient

The patient is in need of ego mastery. The anxiety overwhelms the patient's ability to be in psychological and physiological control of his or her life; therefore, most patients will wish to be assisted in strengthening their control over anxiety. One strategy is to provide a diagnosis to the patient. Understanding the attack as one of anxiety reduces the uncertainty of what was experienced. A second strategy is to inform the patient that the anxiety attacks will pass without any specific action on the part of the patient. Anxiety attacks are self-limiting. This information can be anxiety-reducing for the patient.

Cognitive Re-framing

Together with the nurse, the patient can review and rehearse the thoughts that led to the anxiety attack. Speaking these thoughts aloud and in the presence of the nurse helps the patient to gain control over the thoughts. The patient can be asked to pace the attack and actually time the symptoms as a method to shorten the duration of the attack. This strategy assists in putting the patient's mind on another task (timing the symptoms) and concurrently shifts the thinking to a positive action.

The patient's rehearsal of the anxiety-laden thoughts and images may also open up previously suppressed or repressed material, which can be discussed with the nurse. This technique will also reduce the intensity of the anxiety.

O AN OVERVIEW

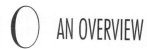

- Anxiety is a common emotion with adaptive value for most people most of the time.

- For some people, anxiety may be a clinical symptom or may develop into a disorder that interferes with daily living.

- Medical conditions and substances can cause and induce anxiety disorders.

- Treatment of anxiety disorders has improved over the past several decades, with behavioral therapy and medications forming the foundation of effective treatment.

- Classification of anxiety disorders is becoming more refined, and understanding of the epidemiologic, genetic, developmental, psychological, behavioral, biochemical, and environmental aspects of anxiety is growing steadily.

TD TERMS TO DEFINE

- agoraphobia
- anxiety
- anxiety disorder
- fear
- malevolent transformation
- obsessive-compulsive disorders
- panic attack
- phobic disorders
- post-traumatic stress disorder
- situationally bound panic attack
- situationally predisposed panic attack
- unexpected panic attack

Q STUDY QUESTIONS

1. Match each of the following disorders with the statement describing how the anxiety is manifested.
   a. obsessive–compulsive disorder
   b. panic disorder
   c. post-traumatic stress disorder
   d. phobic disorder
      1. anxiety is experienced when confronting a threatening situation
      2. anxiety is reexperienced after an unusual trauma
      3. anxiety is the dominant problem
      4. anxiety occurs when resisting thoughts and feelings

2. A panic attack may occur in several different anxiety disorders and is defined as
   a. involving at least 8 of 13 somatic or cognitive symptoms.
   b. developing suddenly and peaking within 10 minutes.
   c. a distinct period of intense fear or discomfort.
   d. all of the above.
   e. B and C.

3. Which type of phobia is most commonly experienced by psychiatric outpatients?
   a. Social phobia
   b. Animal phobia
   c. Agoraphobia
   d. Blood/injection/injury phobia

4. Which patient—one with social phobia or one with panic disorder with agoraphobia—can more comfortably endure a phobic stimulus in the presence of a companion?

5. Describe exposure therapy and give an example of how it can benefit the specific phobic.

6. T F A specific phobic fears being in a place or situation from which escape might be difficult (or embarrassing) or in which help might not be available in the event of a panic attack.

7. T F The obsessive–compulsive individual often recognizes that the obsessive thoughts are abnormal.

8. Are obsessions repetitive, persistent actions or thoughts? Are compulsions repetitive, purposeful actions or thoughts?

9. What is believed to be the precursing condition to most cases of post-traumatic stress disorder?

10. Most anxiety disorders involve some degree of worrying. With respect to that fact, how does generalized anxiety disorder differ from panic disorder?

■ REFERENCES

Diagnostic and Statistical Manual of Mental Disorders, ed 4. Washington, DC, American Psychiatric Association, 1994.

Christiansen RM. et al. Reactivation of traumatic conflicts. *Am J Psychiatry* 1981; 138:984.

Freud S: The ego and the id, in *S. Freud,* Standard Edition. London, Hogarth Press, 1961 (First published in 1923), p. 19.

Freud S: *A General Introduction to Psychoanalysis.* Garden City, NY, Garden City Publishing, 1943, p. 217.

Greist JH, Jefferson JW: Anxiety disorders, in H. Goldman (ed): *Review of General Psychiatry*, ed 4. Norwalk, CT, Appleton & Lange, 1995, pp. 266-282.

LaBruzza, AL: *Using DSM-IV.* Northvale, NJ, Jason Aronson, 1994.

Nagy LM, Krystal JH, Charney DS: Anxiety disorders, in Stoudemire A (ed): *Clinical Psychiatry for Medical Students.* Philadelphia; JB Lippincott, 1994 pp. 233–273.

Peplau H: A working definition of anxiety, in Burd S and Marshall M (eds): *Some Clinical Approaches to Psychiatric Nursing.* New York; MacMillan, 1963 pp. 323–324.

Schweitzer PB, Nesse RM, Fantone RF, Curtis GC: Outcomes of group cognitive behavioral training in the treatment of panic disorder and agoraphobia. *J Am Psychiatr Nurs Assoc* 1995; 1(3):83–91.

Sullivan HS: Interpersonal Theory of Psychiatry. New York: Norton, 1953 p. 113.

Taylor JG: Behavioral interpretation of obsessive-compulsive neurosis. *Behav Res Ther* 1963; 1:237–244.

Turner DM: Panic disorder: A personal and nursing perspective, *J Psychosoc Nurs Mental Health Serv* 1995; 33(4):5–8.

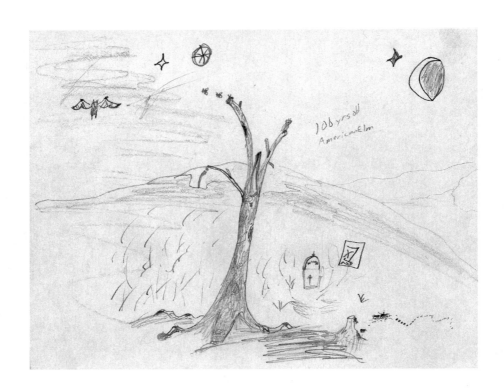

Hide thyself as it were for a little moment, until the indignation be overpast.

The Bible: Isaiah 26:20

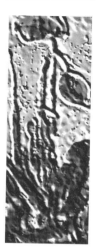

15
Dissociative Disorders

Joan S. Kings

The dissociative disorders are a group of psychiatric syndromes characterized by a sudden, temporary disruption of some aspect of consciousness, identity, or motor behavior. In dissociation, certain mental contents are separated from the usual flow of consciousness. Individuals often mobilize dissociation to protect themselves from being overwhelmed by intense pain and trauma. They split off clusters of distressing thoughts, feelings, and memories from conscious awareness, thereby altering their consciousness. They feel "detached" from their surroundings.

In the 19th century, the French psychiatrist Pierre Janet viewed dissociation as a sign of neurosis, and regarded it as a defect in mental integration. Other psychologists and theoreticians saw dissociation as a universal and basic adaptive ability that if taken to extremes could lead to disordered states of consciousness (LaBruzza, 1994, p. 329).

The functions of memory, personal identity, and motor behavior are critical for an integrated personality— a complex set of mental and behavioral activities. Syndromes of dissociation, which are statistically uncommon, present a dramatic clinical picture of severe disturbance of personality functioning. In their pathology, these disorders are all presumed to share the common defense of dissociation. Table 15-1 presents a decision tree for the DSM—IV diagnosis of the dissociative disorder (MacKay and Purcell, 1995).

■ SUBTYPES OF DISSOCIATIVE DISORDER

The four subtypes of dissociative disorder are:

- *Dissociative amnesia:* Alteration of the memory function of consciousness.
- *Dissociative fugues:* Disturbance in both identity and motor behavior.
- *Depersonalization disorder:* A more limited disruption of identity in which perception of one's own reality is disturbed.
- *Dissociative identity disorder:* Disturbance of personal identity.

Table 15–1 compares these four subtypes of dissociative disorders.

■ DISSOCIATIVE AMNESIA

Amnesia is the loss of memory or inability to recall previously known information. The main feature of **dissociative amnesia** is a loss of memory for significant personal information, often of a traumatic or distressing nature. Such loss of memory is more than simple forgetting, and is not due to dissociative identity disorder, the use of drugs or chemicals, dementia, or a general medical condition. The symptoms of dissociative amnesia cause disruption in social, occupational, or other areas of functioning.

■ DISSOCIATIVE FUGUE

The term, **fugue,** means to flee; it involves actual physical flight from the customary environment or field of conflict. Dissociative fugue is characterized by sudden, unexpected "flights" from work, home, or both, and the assumption of a new identity. It is as if the person is running away from something but is unaware of fleeing. There is an inability to **recall** the past, and when the episode resolves, there is an inability to remember the fugue state. These periods of fugue are very frightening for patients. They may find that they have traveled far in distance, without any memory of doing so. These patients also fear that they may have "done something," during this time of memory blackout.

■ DEPERSONALIZATION DISORDER

Depersonalization disorder is manifested by persistent or recurrent episodes of depersonalization in which there is a sudden, temporary loss of the sense of one's own reality, accompanied by the feeling of being detached from one's self. Patients may describe feeling as though they were mechanical or as though they were in a dream. Depersonalization involves feelings of unreality or strangeness concerning either the environment or the self or both.

TABLE 15–1 DISSOCIATIVE DISORDERS[a]

	Dissociative Amnesia	Dissociative Fugue	Depersonalization Disorder	Dissociative Identity Disorder
Key features	Memory loss following a stressful or traumatic life experience.	Memory loss, travel to new location and assumption of new identity.	Sudden temporary loss of sense of one's reality causing social or occupational dysfunction.	Co-existence of two or more distinct personalities in the same individual.
Epidemiology	Rare More common in adolescents and young adult women.	Rare	Incidence unknown	Exact incidence unknown but may be more common than previously believed. More common in adolescents and young adult women.
Differential	Memory disturbance in organic disorders such as alcoholic blackouts; post-concussion amnesia, transient global amnesia. Dissociative fugue Multiple personality disorder Malingering	Wandering as a result of dementia Dissociative amnesia Multiple personality disorder Malingering	Medication side effects. Neurological diseases, such as epilepsy, brain tumor. May occur as symptom of another mental disorder, such as anxiety and affective disorders, schizophrenia, substance abuse.	Dissociative amnesia Dissociative fugue Schizophrenia Malingering
Treatment	Amobarbital interview Psychotherapy	Amobarbital interview Psychotherapy	Treat underlying condition when present.	Psychotherapy

[a] Adapted from: MacKay S, Purcell SD: Somatoform & Dissociative Disorders, in Goldman, HH (ed): *Review of General Psychiatry.* Appleton & Lange, Norwalk, CT, 1995.

CASE EXAMPLE

▶ DISSOCIATIVE AMNESIA

A 25-year-old woman is admitted to the orthopedic service of a community hospital for treatment of a fractured femur, sustained when the car she was driving left the road and struck a utility pole. Her only child, a two-year-old daughter, was killed in the crash. The ambulance driver reported that when he arrived on the scene, the patient was sitting quietly in the car holding her daughter's body and appearing slightly dazed.

Physical examination reveals no head or neurological injury. It is apparent to the hospital staff that the patient is suffering from amnesia. She provides a history of her past illnesses and life but does not remember the accident. A psychiatric interview on the following day demonstrates that she has no memory of her daughter or of most events subsequent to a vacation trip with her husband about two and one-half years ago. The husband later reports that it was on that trip that the patient first suspected she was pregnant (MacKay and Purcell, 1995).

■ DISSOCIATIVE IDENTITY DISORDER

Dissociative identity disorder, previously known as multiple personality disorder, is the most extreme type of dissociative disorder. As a syndrome, dissociative identity disorder contains all of the principal elements of the three other subtypes of dissociative disorders. Individuals with dissociative identity disorder will, at times, manifest dissociative amnesia, fugue episodes, and depersonalization (Putnam, et. al., 1986a). Dissociative identity disorder presumes the existence of two or more distinct personality states or personal identities that recurrently take charge of the patient's behavior. The patient cannot remember important personal information. The disturbance is not due to the effects of a drug, chemical substance, or a medical condition.

HISTORY

Historically, controversy existed among professionals about whether the condition of multiple personalities actually existed. Cases have been reported since the 17th century. Pierre Janet stands first among clinicians and researchers who have inquired into the nature of dissociation (Putnam, 1989). From the time of its earliest recognition, clinicians have reported unusual physiological changes in dissociative identity disorder patients concurrent with changes in personality. Morton Prince (1906) was the first investigator to attempt to scientifically document physiological manifestations of personality. He noted that the normal individual alternately becomes disintegrated and healthy, changing back and forth from disease to health. He noted that a same patient alternately became a hysteric person and then, a healthy person. He also noted that the same patient looked, talked, and acted altogether like a different person, and that this new consciousness or self claimed to be an entirely different person (Prince, 1906).

Price was soon challenged by other investigators and was accused of having produced the personalities he was observing, and the diagnosis of dissociative identity disorder fell into disrepute shortly thereafter (Putnam, 1986b). From the 18th century through the 1970s, dissociative identity disorder was thought to be nonexistent,

CASE EXAMPLE

▶ DISSOCIATIVE FUGUE

A 32-year-old schoolteacher, after learning of his wife's infidelity, leaves home for work and disappears. Two months later, an acquaintance stops to eat at a small restaurant in the next state and recognizes the man serving the tables. The man does not recognize

him, and does not respond to his name. When the police talk to him, the man claims that he had found himself in the town two months earlier not knowing who he was or what he was doing there. He invented a name and began work at the restaurant. His employer describes him as a quiet and secretive man who nonetheless is a reliable worker (MacKay and Purcell, 1995, p. 298).

E CASE EXAMPLE

▶ **DEPERSONALIZATION DISORDER**

A 38-year-old lawyer tells his therapists that he feels he was "going crazy." He reports having strange "attacks" about once a month for the past several years. These attacks usually occur at work, and on the last two occasions he has had to leave the courtroom in order to gain control of himself. The attacks are accompanied by a general feeling of nervousness, followed by a diminution in size of all objects in his visual field and the perception that his and other people's actions are mechanical and jerky.

---

rare, or an artifact of hypnosis or other iatrogenic mischief (Decker, 1986). Today, the number of individuals diagnosed with dissociative identity disorder has increased markedly (Putnam, 1991). Kluft (1993) holds that this is chiefly because of improvements in the ability of clinicians to identify and treat the disorder.

GENDER, AGE, CULTURE AND PREVALENCE

The demographics of patients with dissociative identity disorder show some interesting trends. In general, there is a high degree of agreement among different sources of data about the gender ratios, age at time of diagnosis, presenting symptoms, and past psychiatric history of the patients who have the disorder (Putnam, 1986a). Most cases of dissociative identity disorder recorded to date have occurred in women, with the female-to-male ratio about five to one (Putnam, et al., 1986). Putnam and Post (1988) found the mean age at diagnosis of dissociative identity disorder to be 28.5 years old. Cross-sectional data on the life course of patients with dissociative identity disorder presented by Kluft (1985b) suggest that the clinical presentation of the disorder varies with age, and that the most floridly "multiple" clinical presentation typically occurs during the third and fourth decades of life. This may explain the remarkable uniformity of age at diagnosis reported across a variety of patient samples (Putnam, 1993).

The ethnic and socioeconomic statistics about patients with dissociative identity disorder are scanty, but sufficient to allow the conclusion that the disorder occurs across all major racial groups, economic, and social settings (Putnam, 1989). Most cases involve Caucasians, African-Americans (Coons and Stern, 1986), and Hispanic persons (Varma, Bouri, and Wig, 1981). Putnam (1989) reported that of the cases he has evaluated, 13% were African-American persons, and about 2% involved Asians. Cross-cultural case reports are scarce, but reported cases of the disorder have occurred in non-Western settings (Varma, Bouri, and Wig, 1981).

ETIOLOGY

The existence of apparently separate and autonomous **alter personalities** exchanging control over an individual's behavior raises questions about the unity of personality and the structure of consciousness (Putnam, 1989). Slowly, the linkage between childhood trauma and dissociative identity disorder has emerged in the clinical literature (Putnam, 1993). Children who are physically and/or sexually abused are at risk for developing the disorder. Dissociation provides a temporary way to cope with the strong emotions evoked by the abuse mechanism, and is a predictable defense for young children, whose natural defense involves fluid role changes as part of fantasy life (Bowman, Blix, and Coons, 1985). In a study of 236 dissociative identity disorder cases, 79.2% of patients experienced extensive sexual abuse and 75.9% experienced physical abuse as children (Ross, Norton, and Wozney, 1989).

Braun and Gray (1986) collected data on whether sexual abuse during childhood in patients with dissociative identity disorder was incestuous. They found indications that more than half of all patients with the disorder are victims of parental incest, and that 25% of all the abusing adults were first-degree female relatives.

THEORIES OF DISSOCIATIVE IDENTITY DISORDER

3-P model

The "3-P" model of dissociative identity disorder (Braun and Sachs, 1985) hypothesizes that predisposing, precipitating, and perpetuating factors are needed to initiate development of the disorder. Two predisposing factors appear necessary to the development of dissociative identity disorder:

- *A biopyschological capacity to dissociate (usually identified with a high degree of responsiveness to hypnosis).*

- *Repeated exposure to an inconsistently stressful environment (e.g., being given love and abuse by the same person or persons at unpredictable times, as one might find in an abusive family environment.)*

The precipitating event in the 3-P model of dissociative identity is almost always one specific traumatic episode to which the predisposed individual responds by dissociating.

Perpetuating phenomena, the third condition needed for the development of dissociative identity disorder, link dissociative episodes through a common affective theme e.g., fear, disgust, or anger; a common neurophysiologic state, or both (Braun 1984a). The accompanying neuropsychophysiologic state may involve a change in heart rate, hormone levels, and other phenomena (Braun, 1983, 1984a). The perpetuating phenomena are typically interactive events, usually involving the abusing and the abused individual.

After continuous exposure to such situations, the affected individual begins to experience unique life "histories" associated with each "file" of memories. One can conceive of these dissociated states, each imbued with a specific sense of self, being elaborated over time as the child repeatedly re-enters a given state to escape from trauma or to execute behaviors that he or she is unable to perform in normal consciousness (Putnam, Guroff, and Silberman, 1986). Each time the child re-enters a specific dissociative state, additional memories, affects, and behaviors become bound to that state, building up a "life-history" for the alter personality. The number of different alter personalities in adult dissociative identity disorder patients is significantly correlated with the number of different kinds of trauma suffered in childhood (Putnam, Guroff, and Silberman, 1986).

Continued unpredictable trauma reinforces the chaining of memories and associated response patterns, with the different adaptive response patterns gradually becoming functionally separated by **amnestic barriers.** Thus, the patient's personality is **"split."** The patient may suspect but not be aware of the extent to which he or she exhibits inconsistent behavior in the form of one of several specific personalities, each with an individual life history. An amnestic barrier more or less prevents each personality from knowing fully about the lives led by the others (Braun, 1984b).

BASK Model

Braun's (1988) BASK model of dissociation suggests that an event can be dissociated into four components: **b**ehavior, **a**ffect, **s**ensation, and **k**nowledge. Dissociation can occur in any one of these components, or in all of them concurrently. Braun (1990b) feels that disso-

ciative identity disorder is the response of a creative mind seeking to escape the saturation of childhood terror and pain, and that the more severe the abuse experienced in childhood, the more fragmented is the patient's personality and thinking. That individuals predisposed to dissociative identity disorder are also usually highly hypnotizable and often artistically creative appears to support the hypothesis that an "ability to dissociate" is important in the pathogenesis of the disorder (Braun, 1990b).

Kluft Theory

Kluft (1984a) put forward a four-factor theory for the etiology of dissociative identity disorder. Simply stated they are:

- Patients with dissociative identity disorder are very adept at dissociating.
- Patients with dissociative identity disorder have used dissociation to cope with severe childhood trauma.
- The form and structure of dissociative identity disorder vary depending on the individual's temperament and nonabuse experience.
- The abuse didn't stop, and the victim did not receive enough consistent love and care to heal his or her wounds. (Ross, 1989).

The genesis of dissociative identity disorder is a little girl or boy imagining that the abuse is happening to someone else. It is a complex biopsychosocial disorder with numerous determinants. It is a strategy for surviving a traumatic childhood (Ross, 1989).

PATIENT PROFILE

A patient profile of dissociative identity disorder is that the patients typically suffer from a profusion of psychiatric, neurological, and medical symptoms; have received a host of diagnoses; and are refractory to the standard treatments for the diagnosed conditions (Putnam, et al., 1986). Unfortunately, this profusion of symptoms, which may be suggestive of a wide range of psychiatric disorders, usually obscures the underlying dissociative pathology, so that patients with dissociative identity disorder often spend years in treatment for conditions they do not have (Putnam, 1991).

As for psychiatric symptoms of dissociative identity disorder, the single most common presenting symptom is depression (Coons, 1986; Bliss, 1986; Putnam et al., 1986). In addition to depressed mood, several other symptoms commonly reported in patients with the disorder would superficially appear to reinforce the diagnosis of a major affective disorder. About three-quarters of patients presenting with dissociative identity disorder describe themselves as having "mood swings," or sudden changes in the way they feel or behave (Putnam et al., 1986). Frequently there is a history of one or more suicide attempts or suicidal gestures (Putnam et al., 1986). The typical **host personality** initially presenting for treatment usually has low self esteem, is overwhelmed, and generally expresses a negative outlook toward life. Patients with dissociative identity disorder may also report difficulty in concentrating, fatigue, sexual difficulties, and crying spells (Putnam, 1989).

The nurse/therapist may be led to suspect dissociative identity disorder by some of the following characteristic signs and symptoms:

- A history of several psychiatric or medical diagnoses (Braun, 1990b).
- Inconsistencies in physical behavior (e.g., changes in voice or facial expression; switching from right to left handedness or vice versa; substantial difference in clothing worn on the first and subsequent visits; or differences in hair style and facial makeup on different visits (Braun, 1990b).
- Psychophysiological manifestations (e.g., headache, anxiety, chest pain, fluctuations in pain threshold (Braun, 1983), or unpredictable responses to medication (e.g., sudden alterations in insulin requirement) (Barkin, Braun, and Kluft, 1986).
- Experiencing voices inside the head talking to one another or to the patient; the schizophrenic patient, by contrast, usually experiences voices originating outside the head (Braun, 1990b).
- A history of dissociative identity disorder or other dissociative disorder; or a history of abuse or of the disorder in the patient's family (Braun, 1985, 1990b).

ISSUES IN TREATMENT

Two issues emerge in the course of therapy for dissociative identity disorder: past and present trauma. Past trauma involves the experience of being abused by parents or other caretakers. Present trauma involves the myriad of difficulties that arise for a person of multiple identities in trying to fit into a society that stresses the continuity of time and self (Putnam, 1991). The treatment of dissociative identity disorder has four primary aims:

- To provide support and safety to the patient.
- To decrease intra-systemic conflict and increase cooperation between the multiple personalities of the affected individual.

- To uncover and work through traumatic memory and affect, with increased informational and experiential sharing between each of the individual's personalities.
- To improve coping skills and reality testing with the gradual relinquishment of dissociative defensive processes in exchange for less distorting defenses (Bloch, 1989).

The treatment of dissociative identity disorder is fraught with difficulty. Although the prognosis is generally good, the actual course of the therapy is long, arduous, and punctuated with crisis (Kluft, 1984b). The goals involve the alleviation of problematic symptoms and character traits, and the achievement of cooperation and stability among the patient's personalities. This may involve the concession of predominance to one personality, the collaborative cooperation of some or all personalities; or their unification or integration. The latter is both the ideal and the most common outcome, but it may be difficult to achieve in patients who are reluctant to work through traumatic events or whose personalities are deeply invested in separateness (Kluft, 1985a).

There has been considerable controversy about the use of hypnosis in the treatment of dissociative identity disorder. Hypnosis is primarily used to gain access to hidden traumatic experiences and memories. It is the means to penetrate the patient's amnesia: once the patient's feelings and memories are conscious, they must be reconciled. This must occur in full consciousness, because it is the patient's conscious mind that must accept the facts of his or her past (Bliss, 1986).

■ THE NURSING PROCESS

ASSESSMENT

It is important in the nursing assessment of patients with dissociative disorders to include questions that will provoke information about the patient's history of abuse. Because many patients will not remember being abused, or will not feel safe in disclosing abuse, it is important to seek hidden signs of it. Patients should be questioned about their earliest childhood memory and what they remember about significant events in their childhood (Lowenstein, 1991). When assessing for amnesiac dissociation it is important to differentiate between knowing about an event and remembering it. Patients can know about events from childhood through stories, photographs, or television viewing without remembering the event (Lowenstein, 1991).

Nurses should inquire about the existence of an imaginary childhood friend, including how long this creation lasted and whether the patient still has interactions with this imaginary companion (Curtain, 1993). The patient should be asked whether he or she has ever had blackouts, or "lost" (forgotten) time, and if he or she ever goes to a "safe place" in the mind to avoid stress (Curtain, 1993). The mental status examination will differentiate between voices heard from within the head and those from outside the head. The nurse should ask the patient to describe these voices in terms of their age; familiarity; names; and the content of the conversations. A child voice is highly indicative of a child alter personality (Curtain, 1993). The nurse who suspects dissociative identity disorder can administer the dissociative experiences scale (Berstein and Putnam, 1986) and/or the dissociative disorder interview schedule (Ross, Heber and Norton, 1989) to help confirm the diagnosis.

NURSING DIAGNOSES

Several nursing diagnoses are related to abuse as follows:

- Low self-esteem related to: a history of abusive relationship(s); feelings of shame or humiliation; or feelings of helplessness.
- Inability to express feelings as the result of: denial of feelings; lack of trust; or fear.
- Helplessness related to: a history of abusive relationship(s); fear; or low self-esteem.
- The potential for self-inflicted injury related to: suicidal ideas or feelings; anger or feelings of hopelessness or despair.
- The potential for injury to others related to: anger or hostility; history of abusive relationship(s); feelings of inadequacy; or substance abuse.
- Difficulty in interpersonal relationships related to: low self esteem; inability to express feelings; feelings of shame or humiliation; or lack of trust.
- Denial of problems or abuse related to: fear of increasing abuse; guilt; fear of having to make life changes; or a grief response.
- Disrupted homeostasis related to: hyperphagia or hypophagia; stress-related physiological problems; injuries; or substance abuse.
- Sleep disturbance related to: stress; a depressed state; fatigue; or substance abuse.

INTERVENTIONS

The general consensus among mental health care providers is that whenever possible, patients with dissociative disorders should be treated on an outpatient basis. Treatment usually extends over years. In a time of

shrinking resources for psychiatric hospitalization, often it is impossible to assume that inpatient treatment represents a viable option for dissociative identity disorder (Kluft, 1991a). Nor is it desirable to reinforce the patient's already diminished autonomy through hospitalization, when community-based treatment can be safely offered.

Hospitalization

The reasons for hospitalizing patients with dissociative identity disorder include suicidal impulses and attempts, self-inflicted injury of a non-suicidal variety, depression, and threats of violence (Putnam et al., 1986). Most admissions of known patients with dissociative identity disorder occur in connection with: (1) suicidal behaviors or impulses; (2) severe anxiety or depression related to the emergence of upsetting alter personalities, or failure of a fusion; (3) fugue behaviors; (4) inappropriate behaviors of alter personalities (including involuntary commitments for violence); (5) procedures or events in therapy during which a structured and protected environment is desirable; and (6) logistics that preclude outpatient care (Kluft, 1984b).

Hypnosis

Hypnosis is a treatment used almost universally with who have dissociative identity disorder (Fike, 1990). Hypnosis may help the patient to recall traumatic information that has been hidden behind amnesiac barriers and to communicate between and with alter personalities (Fike, 1990). Hypnosis may aid the patient in reducing stress, increasing relaxation, and other forms of self-healing, including integration or fusion rituals (Braun, 1984c).

Adapting Kluft's 9 Stages

Kluft (1991b) explains the treatment for the disorder as having a series of overlapping stages since different personalities of the patient may be at very different states at a given moment. In the first stage, known as *establishing the therapy*, the focus is on clarifying the diagnosis and establishing the therapeutic alliance. Kluft (1991b) notes that the patient has often been hospitalized for the symptoms that lead to the diagnosis, or has been overwhelmed by the diagnosis or by a first encounter with traumatic memories, or evidence of the alter personalities' activities.

In the second stage of treatment known as *preliminary interventions*, access is gained to the most available of the patient's personalities, contracts for treatment and against self-harm are established, and attempts are made to enhance communication across the alter personalities (Kluft, 1991b). The patient's priorities, ego strengths, and anxiety tolerance are assessed further and each is addressed in the treatment plan. Efforts are made to offer symptomatic relief.

The focus in the third stage, *history-gathering and mapping the personality system,* is on recognizing the personalities' issues, concerns, and patterns of interaction. During the fourth stage, *the metabolism of the trauma,* previously blocked material is accessed, shared across the alter egos, and **abreacted** (Kluft, 1991b). In the fifth treatment stage, *moving toward intergration/resolution,* the focus is on enhancing internal communication, building on strengths, and working through recovered materials and their implications.

The sixth treatment stage, *intergration/resolution,* involves coming together, or at least achieving of reconciliation, cooperation, and coordination among the alter egos. The seventh through the ninth treatment stages involve *learning new coping skills, solidifying gains and working through, and follow-up.* Looking at these stages and all that they entail, one can see that the treatment of patients with dissociative identity disorder is lengthy and difficult. While working through these stages, a patient with the disorder may have to be admitted to the hospital, even though this is not desirable. This may be in connection with disruptive behaviors (usually self destructive) of alter egos opposing the therapy; of revelations necessary for the treatment to proceed, or because the patient is overwhelmed by the unsettling process of integration (Kluft, 1991b).

EVALUATION

When dissociative identity disorder is diagnosed, the condition is responsive to treatment, even though the treatment is long and difficult. Successful therapies act to prevent further traumatization and harm, accord respect and empathy to the patient's personalities, encourage full expression and the exploration of feelings, facilitate the coalescing of the alter personalities, and provide adequate long-term follow-up. Treatment should not end at the point of reintegration of the patient. Instead, the therapist and patient should work toward stabilizing gains, enhancing non-dissociative defenses and creating conditions under which normal psychological developmental processes can go forward (Kluft, 1985b).

Kluft (1991a) notes that certain goals should be achieved before a patient with dissociative identity disorder is discharged from institutional care. These goals are for the patient to re-establish control over preadmission behaviors that prompted the hospitalization, join disruptive and/or unsuspected alter egos in the

therapy process, and establish a contract for safety and to continue in outpatient therapy (Kluft, 1991a).

■ PHARMACOLOGICAL IMPLICATIONS

When using medication for patients with dissociative identity disorder, one should be cognizant of the symptoms the medication is expected to ameliorate (Putnam, 1989). There is no good evidence that medication of any type has a direct therapeutic effect on the dissociative process as manifested in dissociative identity disorder (Putnam, 1993, Ross, 1989). Medications, however, may at times serve as useful adjuncts in treating the disorder. Putnam (1989) and Ross (1989) both caution that the clinician must be careful not to depend too heavily on the use of medication to treat symptoms that are largely psychosomatic and that usually are important psychodynamic clues to the patient's past trauma.

Kluft (1984b) has developed a number of questions that the clinician should consider before administering medications to a patient with dissociative identity disorder. First, if symptoms such as depression and anxiety are present, are these symptoms causing sufficient distress across the personality system? Would nonpharmacological interventions be equally effective without the risk of potential side effects? Do the potential benefits of medicating the patient outweigh the potential risks?

■ LEGAL/ETHICAL IMPLICATIONS

Patients presenting with dissociative identity disorder create difficult problems for the legal and criminal justice systems. Some questions that arise with regard to such cases are difficult to answer. When one of a patient's alter personalities commits a crime, is it fair to blame and punish the others? What happens when the victim of a crime has dissociative identity disorder? Should a defendant be blamed for harming personalities who were hidden from existence? Should each of a patient's separate personalities be sworn in when the patient testifies? What happens when one personality enters into a contract while the others repudiate it (Saks, 1994)?

The courts are unsure about the legal significance of dissociative identity disorder. For example, in the criminal context, courts have taken several different positions on when the insanity defense is available to persons with multiple personalities (Appelbaum, 1994). The law has formulated tests that focus on an agent's cognitive and volitional impairments at the time of his or her act. Unlike many people with mental illnesses, those suffering from dissociative identity disorder are intact, both cognitively and volitionally, at any given time. What sets them apart is that, over time, they manifest a dividedness that may be inconsistent with viewing them as single agents. The point is that those in the law should not expect much guidance from current doctrine; dissociative identity disorder presses for individualized attention and standards (Saks, 1994, 1995).

The ethical implications for treating a person with dissociative identity disorder are the same as for treating any other person. A person with the disorder is still defined as a living being with physical, cognitive, affective, behavioral, and social dimensions, who interacts with the environment to achieve a chosen life purpose. Nurses, trained to see humans as holistic beings, should have little difficulty conceptualizing and embracing this schema.

■ CLINICAL VIGNETTE*

Mary Thomas is 24 years old and has been diagnosed as having dissociative identity disorder for more than 2 years. She has a history of self-injurious behavior that intensifies when she is under stress. Prior to admission to a specialized facility for treating the disorder, her reported abuser (a member of her extended family) died. Since that time Mary has been using razor blades to superficially cut her arms, legs, and abdomen with increasing frequency. After the admission, the staff noticed the following behaviors: a trance-like state, confusion, isolation from other patients, and switching from childlike behaviors (e.g. asking for candy because she was "good"), to more age appropriate behaviors (e.g. asking about college courses). Mary reports that she is having nightmares, and feels pressure to harm herself, but doesn't want to tell anyone about this. She also verbalizes feelings of anxiety, fear of losing control, anger, sadness and guilt.

CARE PLAN

Mary is given a nursing diagnosis of having a post-traumatic response related to self, secondary to a history of physical/sexual abuse. Subjective criteria include the following statements by Mary: "It's a big release when I cut myself;" "I don't feel any pain;" and "Suzy is the one who likes to cut herself." Objective criteria noted by the interdisciplinary team on the unit include that Mary has numerous superficial lacerations on arms, legs, and abdomen in various stages of healing; often appears confused and acts inappropriate for her chronological age and anticipated psychosocial development; is withdrawn and isolates herself to her room; and is observed by the staff to be **switching** personalities frequently.

The team on the unit defined the following outcome criteria for Mary's treatment plan:

- Patient will tell the staff of desire to cut or otherwise harm herself by discharge.
- Patient will demonstrate alternate coping strategies for her increased anxiety by the end of 2 weeks.

The interdisciplinary team formulated the following interventions specialized for this patient: the mental health technician will have Mary sign a safety contract every hour, and will monitor the patient for any self-injurious behavior; the psychiatrist will meet with the patient daily to assess the need for medications; the nurse will meet with the patient 3 times per nursing shift while the patient is awake in order to discuss the patient's impulses for cutting; the activities therapist and the nurses will engage the patient in groups daily to explore alternative coping strategies; and the social worker will meet with the patient daily to ensure that the appropriate outpatient therapy will be in place by discharge. In the evaluation it was found that the patient did sign in every hour with the mental health technician; was able to verbalize her impulsive feelings to hurt herself; did not engage in any self-injurious behavior on the unit; started a journal which the patient identified as an alternative coping strategy; and formulated a follow-up discharge plan of intensive outpatient therapy 3 times a week.

The rationale for the foregoing interventions is to ensure the patient's safety, increase verbalization of the patient's feelings, help the patient to assume increasing responsibility for her behavior, and ensure effective communication of alternative coping strategies.

■ CLINICAL VIGNETTE*

Lauren Smith is 43 years old, married, and has had a diagnosis of dissociative identity disorder for 7 years. She has had a history of multiple in-patient hospitalizations and has been in outpatient therapy for 12 years. Over the past month, she has had a decreased ability to function in her normal activities of daily living; poor concentration; a decreased attention span; interrupted sleep cycles; and frequent loss of memory of time. She has been irritable and agitated, with verbalizations of her feelings out of control. Today, she became enraged with her husband and physically assaulted him with a knife. Upon admission to the hospital unit, she began pacing and was hostile to the admitting nurse. When she was told that she had been restricted to the unit and would not be allowed outside to smoke, she threw a chair across the room.

CARE PLAN

Lauren is given a nursing diagnosis of a high risk for violence directed at others in relation to a history of physical/sexual abuse, manifested by physical attacks on significant others and poor impulse control. Subjective criteria verbalized by Lauren include, "I'm so angry I could just kill him," and "I sleep with a knife under my pillow to ward off attacks." Objective criteria noted by the staff include that Lauren has a tense facial expression, a rigid posture, walks with clenched fists, paces frequently, has frequent agitation, and has been making verbal threats to other patients and staff involving property destruction and personal harm.

The team on the unit defined the following outcome criteria for Lauren's treatment plan:

- the patient will remain focused on the immediate present for a least 10 minutes of group therapy by the end of the week
- the patient will increase her impulse control as measured by a decrease in property destruction by the end of the current nursing shift, and by a decrease in verbal threats by the end of the week

The interdisciplinary team formulated the following interventions for this patient: all staff will reality test the patient during episodes of dissociation; the activities therapist will provide a safe environment during group sessions; the psychiatrist will limit discussions of the past to 5 minutes; the mental health technician will teach the patient signs and symptoms of increase agitation; the nurse will teach the patient relaxation strategies (e.g., deep breathing and imagery); and the social worker will schedule a family meeting with the patient's husband and formulate appropriate follow-up care. In the evaluation it was found that the patient was able to respond to reality testing during episodes of dissociation; was able to feel safe about talking in group sessions by the end of the week; did learn the signs of escalating agitation, and became adept at self-monitoring her own signs and symptoms; was able to use deep breathing when she recognized her increasing agitation; and was receptive to a family meeting with her husband and the social worker.

The rationale for the foregoing interventions is to: re-orient the patient to the present; teach that safety is a prerequisite to personal disclosure; increase the patient's awareness of loss of impulse control; decrease explosive episodes of threats and property destruction; and to allow the patient to recognize the emotions associated with her behavior.

---

*Clinical vignettes coauthored by Jane Jedwabny, BA, RNC.

O AN OVERVIEW

- People dissociate to process information.
- Trauma may trigger pathological dissociation.
- The dissociative disorders include dissociative amnesia, dissociative fugue, depersonalization and dissociative identity disorder.
- Dissociative identity disorder is not rare, as once thought, but its exact incidence is not known.
- Dissociative identity disorder is often misdiagnosed, with about 7 years as the average time for the patient to be in the mental health system before accurate diagnosis.
- The psychophysiological and neurophysiological correlates of the separate personalities in dissociative identity disorder can be studied.
- Dissociative identity disorder is highly correlated with traumatic experiences in childhood; usually, but not inevitably, child abuse.

TD TERMS TO DEFINE

- abreaction
- alter personality
- amnestic barrier
- dissociation
- dissociative amnesia
- recall
- fugue
- host personality
- split personality
- switching

Q STUDY QUESTIONS

1. What are the key factors in Braun's theory of dissociative identity disorder?

2. What are the key factors in Kluft's theory of dissociative identity disorder?

3. T F A patient who has only two alter personalities does not have dissociative identity disorder.

4. T F A patient can have a fragment of a personality that lasts for a limited time.

5. T F Patients with dissociative identity disorder are usually very intelligent and creative.

6. T F Dissociative identity disorder is rare.

7. T F Children who are physically and/or sexually abused may develop dissociative identity disorder.

8. T F Dissociative identity disorder is unresponsive to therapy.

9. T F A nurse could suspect dissociative identity disorder if a patient has had several psychiatric diagnoses.

10. T F A patient with dissociative identity is usually re-integrated within a short period of time.

▪ REFERENCES

Appelbaum PS: Who's on trial? Multiple personalities and the insanity defense. *Hospital & Community Psychiatry;* 1994; 45(1):965–966.

A Psychiatric Glossary, 4th ed. Washington, DC: American Psychiatric Association: 1975.

Barkin R, Braun BG, Kluft R.P: The dilemma of drug therapy for multiple personality disorder, in Braun, BG (ed): *Treatment of Multiple Personality Disorder.* Washington, DC: American Psychiatric Press, 1986; 109–132.

Berstein EM, Putnam FW: Development, reliability, and validity of a dissociation scale. *J Nerv Ment Disord* 1986;174: 727–735.

Bliss EL: *Multiple Personality, Allied Disorders, and Hypnosis.* Oxford, Oxford University Press, 1986.

Bloch JP: Treatment of multiple personality and dissociative disorder, in Keller PA, & Heyman SR (eds): *Innovations in Clinical Practice: A Source Book, vol. 8.* Sarasota, FL: Professional Resource Exchange, Inc., 1989; 55–67.

Bowman ES, Blix S, Coons PM: Multiple personality in adolescence: relationship to incestuous experiences. *J Am Acad Child Psychiatry* 1985; 24(1):109–114.

Braun, BG: Psychophysiologic phenomena in multiple personality and hypnosis. *Am J Clin Hypnosis* 1983; 23(2): 124–137.

Braun BG: Towards a theory of multiple personality and other dissociative phenomena. *Psychiatr Clin North Am* 1984a; 7: 171–194.

Braun BG: The role of the family in the development of multiple personality disorder. *Int J Fam Psychiatry* 1984b; 5(4): 303–313.Braun BG: Uses of hypnosis with multiple personality. *Psychiatr Ann* 1984c; 14: 34–40.

Braun BG: Dissociation: behavior, affect, sensation, knowledge, in Braun BG (ed): *Proceedings of the Second International Conference on Multiple Personality/Dissociative States.* Chicago, Rush University, 1985, 6.

Braun BG: The BASK model of dissociation. *Dissociation* 1988; 1: 4–23.

Braun BG: Multiple personality disorder: An overview. *Am J Occup Ther;* 1990;44 (11):971–976.

Braun BG, Gray, GT: Report on the 1985 questionnaire on multiple personality disorder, in Braun BG (ed): *Proceedings of the Third International Conference on Multiple Personality/Dissociative States.* Chicago, Rush University, 1986; 111.

Braun BG, Sachs RG: The development of multiple personality disorder: Predisposing, precipitating, and perpetuating factors, in Kluft RP (ed): *Childhood Antecedents of Multiple Personality.* Washington, DC: American Psychiatric Press, 1985; 37–64.

Coons PM: Treatment programs in 20 patients with multiple personality disorder. *J Nerv Ment Dis;* 1986, 174(12):715–721.

Coons PM, Sterne AL: Initial and follow-up psychological testing on a group of patients with multiple personality disorder. *Psychol Rep;* 1986, 58: 43–49.

Curtain SL: Recognizing multiple personality disorder. *J Psychosoc Nurs Ment Health Ser;* 1993, 31(2):29–35.

Decher HS: The lure of non-materialism in materials Europe, in Quen J (ed): *Split minds/Split Brains.* New York: New York University Press; 1986; 31–62.

Diagnostic and Statistical Manual of Mental Disorders, 4th ed. Washington, DC: American Psychiatric Association: 1994.

Fike ML: Considerations and techniques in the treatment of persons with multiple personality disorder. *Am J Occup Ther;* 1990, 44(11):999–1007.

Kluft RP: Treatment of multiple personality disorder: A study of 33 cases. *Psychiatr Clin North Am;* 1984a, 7: 9–29.

Kluft RP: Aspects of the treatment of multiple personality disorder. *Psychiatr Ann;* 1984b, 14: 51–55.

Kluft RP: Multiple personality in childhood. *Psychiatr Clin North Am;* 1984c, 7: 121–134.

Kluft RP: The natural history of multiple personality disorder, in Kluft RP (ed): *The Childhood Antecedents of Multiple Personality.* Washington, DC: American Psychiatric Press. 1985a, (pp.45–67).

Kluft RP: Childhood multiple personality disorder: Predictors, clinical findings, and treatment results, in Kluft RP (ed); *The Childhood Antecedents of Multiple Personality.* Washington, DC: American Psychiatric Press. 1985b, (pp167–196).

Kluft RP: Hospital treatment of multiple personality disorder: An overview. *Psychiatr Clin North Am;* 1991a, 14(3):695–719.

Kluft RP: Multiple personality disorder, in Tasman A (ed): *American Psychiatric Press Annual Review of Psychiatry, vol. 10.* Washington DC: American Psychiatric Press, 1991b, (pp. 161–188).

Kluft RP: Multiple personality disorder: A contemporary perspective. *Harvard Ment Healt Letter;* 1993, 10(4):5–7.

La Bruzza AL: *Using DSM-IV.* Northvale, NJ: Jason Aronson, 1994.

Lowenstein RJ: An office mental status examination for complex chronic dissociative symptoms and multiple personality disorder. *Psychiatr Clin North Am;* 1991, 14: 567–604.

Mackay S & Purcell SD: Somataform and dissociative disorders. In Goldman H (ed), *Guide to General Psychiatry,* Stamford, CT: Appleton and Lange, 1995.

Prince M: *The Dissociation of Personality.* New York: Longman, 1906.

Putnam FW: The treatment of multiple personality: State of the art, in Braun BG (ed): *The Treatment of Multiple Personality Disorder.* Washington, DC: American Psychiatric Press, 1986a, (pp. 49–67).

Putnam FW: The scientific investigation of multiple personality disorder. In Quen, JM (ed): *Split Minds/Split Brains.* New York: New York University Press, 1986b, (pp109–217).

Putnam FW: *Diagnoses and Treatment of Multiple Personality Disorder.* New York: Guilford Press, 1989.

Putnam FW: Recent research on multiple personality disorder. *Psychiatr Clin North Amer;* (1991), 14(3):489–502.

Putnam FW: Diagnosis and clinical phenomenology of multiple personality disorder: A North American perspective. *Dissociation: Progr in the Dissoc Disorders; 1993, 6* (2–3): 80–86.

Putnam FW, Post RM: *Multiple Personality Disorder: An Analysis and Review of the Syndrome.* Unpublished manuscript, 1988.

Putnam FW, Guroff JJ, Silbermann EK et al: The clinical phenomenology of multiple personality disorder: 100 recent cases. *J Clin Psychiatry;* 1986, 47: 285–293.

Ross CA: *Multiple Personality Disorder: Diagnosis, Clinical Features, and Treatment.* New York: John Wiley and Sons, 1989.

Ross CA, Heber, S, Norton et al: The dissociative disorders interview schedule: A structured interview. *Dissociation;* 1989, 2: 169–189.

Ross CA, Norton GR, Wozney K: Multiple personality disorder: and analysis of 236 cases. *Can J Psychiatry;* 1989, 34(5):413–418.

Saks, ER: Does multiple personality disorder exist? The beliefs, the data, and the law. *Int J Law Psychiatry;* 1994, 17(1):43–78.

Saks, ER: The criminal responsibility of people with multiple personality disorder. Special issue: research in mental health and law. *Psychiatr Quarterly;* 1995, 66(2): 119–131.

Varma VK, Bouri M, Wig NN: Multiple personality in India: comparisons with hysterical possession state. *Am J Psychotherapy;* 1981, 35:113–120.

2

Level 2

Transitional and Altered Self-Regulatory Patterns

Level 2 of the stress–crisis continuum reflects two types of stress: stress that occurs during life transitions and passages, and over which a patient may or may not have substantial control; and stress due to alterations in self-regulatory patterns.

Examples of disruptive life events that result in stress typical of Level 2 include birth, premature birth, or birth injury; childhood learning problems; pregnancy during adolescence; parenthood or infertility; the legal issues of divorce and child custody; grief, work disruption, or chronic illness in adulthood; and forced retirement in elderhood. The etiology is the unexpected stress from a normative experience. Patient response to the stress may be anxiety, depression, or loss of cognitive coping behaviors.

The second type of Level 2 stress involves disruption of patterns that are normally self-regulated. Dysregulation may be in sleeping, eating, mood, emotion, sex, or thinking. The etiology of altered self-regulatory patterns may be biochemical, familial, or interpersonal stress.

Several interventions may address Level 2 stress. The primary task of a psychiatric nurse is to educate the patient about the changes that did or will occur in the patient's life, and to explore the psychodynamic implications of these changes during individual sessions of limited duration. In addition, support is provided. Anticipatory guidance will help an individual plan an adaptive coping response to problems encountered during transitional events. Crisis intervention techniques may be used if disruption of self-regulatory patterns occur without anticipatory information having been given.

A group approach may also be taken in intervention. Self-help groups specific to transitional issues are Parents Without Partners; Parents of Children with Chronic Illness; pre-retirement groups; and Lamaze childbirth groups. Altered self-regulatory patterns may be addressed by referring individuals to clinics specializing in eating, sleep, or pain disorders.

Conditions representative of transitional or altered self-regulatory patterns are discussed in the following eight chapters:

- *Loss, Grief, and Bereavement*
- *Childhood Disorders*
- *Issues in Adolescent Mental Health*
- *Delirium, Dementia, and Aging*
- *Mood Disorders*
- *Sexual Issues, Disorders, and Deviations*
- *Eating Disorders*
- *Sleep Disorders*

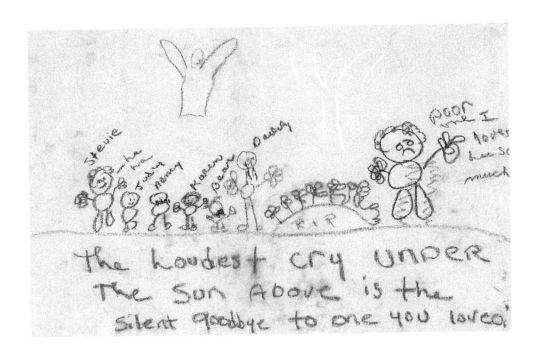

The loudest cry under the sun above is the silent goodbye to one you loved.

Grief fills the room up of my absent child,
Lies in his bed, walks up and down with me,
Puts on his pretty looks, repeats his words,
Remembers me of all his gracious parts,
Stuffs out his vacant garments with his form.

King John
William Shakespeare (1564–1616)

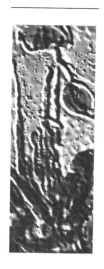

16

Loss, Grief, and Bereavement

Mary Pickett

The concept of transition is prominent in the literature describing family-centered care designed to help people to cope with changes associated with loss. Research findings support the concept that transitions require major reorganization of each individual's psychological perspective (Cowan, 1991). Previously held assumptions about how the world works may no longer apply after a significant loss experience (Parkes, 1971). The need for adaptive behavior in response to a transition offers the opportunity to stimulate developmental growth or dysfunction (Cowan, 1991). A review of the nursing literature supports the belief that the character and consequences of transitions are influenced by meanings, expectations, level of knowledge and skill, environment, level of planning, and emotional and physical well-being (Schumacher and Meleis, 1994). Psychological distress is commonly linked to life events that are associated with loss or expected loss. Serious illness, divorce, change in residence, retirement, and the death of a loved one are examples of loss experiences that precipitate grief responses and bereavement.

The bereavement process is not linear; rather, there are periods of overlap and regression. Bereavement may result in psychological growth, no substantial change, or an adverse change in health or functioning. It is important to *recognize that each bereaved individual is unique and that the course of bereavement is variable. Table 16-1 summarizes selected 20th century views of grief.*

Professional nurses can enhance their assessment skills, communication abilities, and interventions to create supportive environments for bereaved individuals. Interventions may be developed and refined in nursing practice. Nurses may expand their knowledge of bereavement care by participating in independent study, attending conferences focused on loss and grief, communicating with local community hospice organizations, and interacting with professionals who can provide information about their own experiences in caring for bereaved individuals and families.

Nurses who frequently encounter bereaved individuals need to periodically conduct an assessment of their own stress levels and resources. It is important for nurses to build and maintain their resources so that they can meet the challenges of caring for terminally ill persons and provide therapeutic interventions for bereaved individuals and families.

■ THE VOCABULARY OF LOSS, GRIEF, AND BEREAVEMENT

Loss is a universal experience repeatedly encountered throughout life. Any loss results in deprivation, either tangible or symbolic. A loved one's death is usually experienced as a significant loss event. The degree of importance associated with the loss will vary with the meaning the individual attaches to the experience.

Grief is the process of psychological, social, and somatic reactions to loss, and is considered a normal reaction. Grief reactions or symptoms might include anger, guilt, anxiety, sorrow, depression, relief, and sadness (Worden, 1991). The intensity of the symptoms varies among individuals, and is influenced by the type of loss, the situation surrounding the loss, personality factors of the bereaved, concurrent stressors, the availability of social support, and the strength of attachment to the deceased (Parkes and Weiss, 1983).

Disenfranchised grief is defined as "the grief that persons experience when they incur a loss that is not or cannot be openly acknowledged, publicly mourned, or socially supported" (Doka, 1989, p. 4). This construct recognizes that societal norms attempt to specify who, when, where, how, how long, and for whom people should grieve. Examples of disenfranchised grief include significant losses related to perinatal death, abortion, divorce, adoption, the death of pets, and extramarital or non-kin relationships.

Bereavement may be viewed as a state of loss of a significant other through death. *Mourning* represents the culturally defined rituals and behaviors that are usually performed after a death.

Dying refers to a process that may last from a few hours to days, depending on the cause. The length of the dying process can be rapid in the case of sudden traumatic injury, or can persist over months, as in the

TABLE 16–1. SELECTED VIEWS OF GRIEF: 20TH TO 21ST CENTURY

Theorist	View of Grief
Freud, S. (1917)	Psychoanalytic View—Depression Model of Grief

Psychoanalytic views of mourning were described in case studies of individuals who had experienced major loss events. Descriptions of normal grief responses and pathological expressions of grief were offered in an attempt to differentiate mourning, anxiety, and pain resulting from loss. Freud documented expressions of grief in the classic paper *Mourning and Melancholia* (1917/1959) that included anniversary reactions, feelings of guilt and responsibility for the death in an ambivalent relationship, and an explanation of "decathexis," the process of detaching and modifying emotional bonds so that new relationships can develop.

Deutsch, H. (1937)	Psychoanalytic View—Absent Grief Response

Absence of grief response in bereaved individuals was recognized as a form of pathologic grief. Case studies supported this hypothesis through descriptions of how bereaved individuals expressed their grief in other ways (eg. neurotic symptoms or narcissistic schizoid character traits).

Lindemann, E. (1944)	Acute Grief Syndrome

A pattern of psychological and somatic symptoms of acute grief was developed through clinical observations and interviews with bereaved persons. The grief syndrome was characterized by preoccupation with thoughts of the deceased, feelings of hostility and guilt, loss of usual patterns of behavior, and somatic symptoms. The constellation of somatic symptoms associated with grief included: sighing, shortness of breath, tightness in the throat, lack of strength, exhaustion, and gastric distress. The term 'anticipatory grief' was proposed as the experience of grief in anticipation of a loss. Lindemann conceptualized three tasks of grief: emancipation from bondage to the deceased; readjustment to the environment without the deceased loved one; and formation of new relationships. Abnormal patterns of grief were described as 'distorted or delayed' grief reactions and were viewed as having potential to influence physical and mental health.

Pollock, G.H. (1961)	Ego-Adaptive View

The mourning process was described as an ego-adaptive process that attempts to maintain the internal psychic equilibrium. A revised view of mourning was posited to include the theory of adaptation, the concepts of homeostasis, and Darwin's phylogenetic evolution. Responses during the acute stage of grief were conceptualized as shock, acute regression, and immobilization. Hyperactivity, deep despair, sorrow, anxiety, energy impoverishment, and intense psychic pain were also described as grief responses. Integration of the loss experience into reality was thought to be facilitated by adaptive mechanisms in the stage of chronic grief.

Caplan, G. (1961)	Crisis Theory View

Initially, bereavement was viewed as a life event that had the potential to initiate a "crisis" that could be resolved in a relatively short span of time (4 to 8 weeks). Crisis theory suggested a more inclusive view of the balance between the person's available resources and stressors. A crisis was viewed as a pivotal time when an individual had an increased desire for help, and could be more readily influenced by others.

Engel, G.L. (1961, 1964)	Biochemical/Physiological View

A medical model approach advanced that grief was a multidimensional phenomenon with biochemical, physiological, and psychological aspects. Engel suggested a theory of grief that included the following stages: shock and disbelief; developing awareness; restitution; and resolution. Successful mourning was signalled by the bereaved individual's 'ability to remember comfortably and realistically both the pleasures and disappointments of the lost relationship' (1962, p. 279). Engel identified predictors of difficult mourning: individuals who want to cry but are unable to, identification with the negative traits of the deceased, and an exaggerated need to fulfill the wishes of the deceased.

Parkes, C.M. (1964, 1972)	Life-Transition View

Grief is viewed as a process that requires bereaved individuals to change their relationship with the deceased. Parkes' systematic observations of individuals' adjustment after spousal loss contributed to the description of grief as a major life transition. The phases of grief that are included in this life transition view are: numbness, yearning and protest, disorganization, and reorganization. Antecedent and concurrent variables were tested for their ability to predict mental and physical health outcomes of bereaved individuals. A profile of high risk factors for bereavement recovery included: low socioeconomic status, concurrent multiple losses, sudden unexpected loss, relationship characterized by ambivalence, and early severe distress.

Bowlby, J. (1969, 1980)	Attachment Theory View

Attachment theory was developed on extensive clinical observations of adults and children in scientific and medical settings. Attachment was viewed as a basic biological mechanism that protects the survival of the individual and the species. Bowlby's theory (1981) integrates concepts from psychoanalytic theory and ethology. Adult response to loss was described as a four phase process that included: numbing; the urge to recover the lost object (yearning and searching); disorganization and despair; and reorganization. Bowlby described the state of 'chronic mourning' as unusually intense, prolonged emotional responses that include anger and self-reproach, and sorrow is conspicuously absent.

Krupp, G. (1972)	Intrapsychic/Ecological View

In a paper that describes intrapsychic maladaptive reactions to grief, Krupp discussed family systems dynamics and how unresolved mourning can characterize an entire family. Grief reactions of an individual that permeate all members of a family unit require both individual and family level intervention. There is also reference to societal influences on grief resolution, such as the smaller circle of close relationships, and fewer opportunities to express and resolve intense emotions characterizing life in the later part of the 20th century.

Bugen, L. (1977)	Human Grief Model

This conceptualization of grief posits that the intensity and duration of grief is best predicted by the magnitude of closeness within the relationship (central or peripheral) and the degree to which survivors perceive that the death was preventable. Within this view, intense bereavement response would be anticipated in a mourner who feels responsible for the loved one's death.

continued

TABLE 16–1. SELECTED VIEWS OF GRIEF: 20TH TO 21ST CENTURY—CONTINUED

Theorist	View of Grief
Raphael, B. (1983)	Life-span Development View

In a review of bereavement literature, Raphael summarized the forms of human grief resulting from lost relationships across the lifespan. Implications for providing comfort, consolation, and facilitating recovery for the bereaved are offered in the comprehensive work entitled: *The Anatomy of Bereavement.*

Martocchio, B. (1985)	Theory of Grieving

According to Martocchio's framework, grief is defined as the process of moving through the pain of loss. The process of grief is characterized by complex thoughts and emotions, and is a time for healing, adaptation and growth for the bereaved. Martocchio, a nurse researcher, described clusters of reactions that are not bound in time, and may overlap. The clusters that form the framework include: shock and disbelief; yearning and protest; anguish, disorganization, and despair; identification in bereavement; and reorganization and restitution. The time line for grief resolution defined by Martocchio is variable. Periods of time that grief resolution may occur are defined as ranging from shorter to much longer than one year. Martocchio asserted that loss reactions may last a life time. Anniversaries and holidays may be times that are particularly difficult for survivors as they recall memories of the deceased loved one. The goal of successful grief work, according to this framework, is to be able to remember the loved one without major emotional pain and to reinvest emotional energy in living.

Stroebe, W. and Stroebe, M.S. (1987)	Deficit Model of Partner Loss

This framework applies the general psychological stress model to the experience of conjugal loss. Widowhood results in situational demands and loss of coping resources previously available in the conjugal relationship such as instrumental support, validational support, and emotional support. The loss is thought to have a negative impact on the surviving partner's definition of self and social identity.

Sanders, C. (1989)	Integrative Theory of Bereavement

This perspective includes both biological and psychological factors. An individual's psychological health and successful use of coping strategies in the past will influence the ability to cope with the loss of the loved one. External factors such as availability of social support systems, the circumstances surrounding the death, the relationship to the deceased, socioeconomic status, and concurrent stressors influence bereavement patterns. Internal mediators included in this theory are: age, gender, personality, health, feelings about relationship with deceased loved one. There is wide variation in the ways people grieve and in the time required to get through the phases of the grief process. The phases of the bereavement are: shock, awareness of loss, conservation-withdrawal, healing, and renewal.

case of a chronic illness such as cancer. Intervals of remission and relapse during terminal illness are difficult transitions for patients, family members, and professional care-givers.

Anticipatory grief refers to the anticipation of a future loss, and includes many of the symptoms and processes of grief following a loss; it may be experienced by the dying person as well as the family and friends of the terminally ill. Anticipatory grief is characterized as a multi-dimensional process that includes psychosocial and somatic reactions to predicted future loss. Lindemann (1944) introduced the term "anticipatory grief" to distinguish grief reactions that result from expected loss in contrast to those that result from sudden, traumatic events. Lebow (1976, p. 459) outlined the multiple dimensions of anticipatory grief as a "total set of cognitive, affective, cultural, and social reactions to expected death." Fulton and Fulton (1971) identified the following aspects of anticipatory grief: depression, intensified concern for the terminally ill individual, rehearsal of the impending death, and attempts to adjust to the death.

Dimensions of time and certainty have been included in discussions about the construct of anticipatory grief. Neale (1974) combined the dimensions of time and certainty, and suggested four perspectives on viewing one's own future death: near and certain, near

and uncertain, distant and certain, and distant and uncertain. Neale (1974) postulated that ways of viewing death can play a significant role in modifying responses to the actual event.

Death may be defined across four dimensions of life: social, psychological, biological, and physiological (Sudnow, 1967). *Social death* is the symbolic death of a patient because of life-style changes brought about by illness. Decreased functional capacity related to illness may interfere with usual patterns of work and recreation, resulting in limited opportunities for social contact. *Psychological death* refers to the withdrawal of certain aspects of a dying person's personality. Causes of psychological death include loss of autonomy; biochemical changes precipitated by disease and medication; grief reactions to anticipated future losses; and changes in relationships related to declines in functional or cognitive abilities. *Biological death* occurs when consciousness and awareness no longer exist. Artificial life-support systems may sustain organ function; however, the self-sustaining mind–body whole of the person is no longer present. *Physiological death* occurs when there is cessation of all vital organs.

Chronic mourning is an unusually intense, prolonged emotional response to loss that is accompanied by anger, self-reproach, and the absence of sorrow (Bowlby, 1980, pp. 137–138). Depression is the principal symptom, and is often concurrent with anxiety, agoraphobia, hypochondria, or alcoholism.

Complicated mourning is some compromise, distortion, or failure to successfully engage in the complete process of mourning (Rando, 1993). In all forms of complicated mourning, the bereaved individual attempts to deny, repress, or avoid aspects of the loss, and to hold onto and avoid relinquishing the lost loved one.

■ COMPLICATED GRIEF AND LOSS REACTIONS

Persons who have experienced multiple deaths of significant others within a relatively short period have an increased risk of experiencing **complicated grief and mourning.** Parkes and Weiss (1983) identified a profile of families at risk for problems after the death of significant others. The high risk factors associated with complicated grief that they reported include:

- Low socioeconomic status
- Poor health status
- Sudden death or a short period of illness
- Perceived lack of available social support
- Lack of support from one's religious belief system
- Lack of a supportive family
- History of psychiatric illness
- Multiple concurrent losses
- Dysfunctional family relationships
- Geographic distance from extended family
- Guilt within family relationships
- High level of dependency among survivors
- Ambivalent relationships within family

PATHOLOGIC GRIEF

Efforts to establish consensus criteria for diagnosing pathologic grief led to the concept of three variants of **pathologic grief:** (1) delayed or absent grief; (2) inhibited grief; and (3) chronic grief (Raphael, 1989). The criteria for pathologic grief are based on unusually severe or prolonged manifestations of grief, or conversely, on inhibited manifestations of normal grief. Jacobs (1993) summarized the variants of pathologic grief in the following descriptions: *Delayed grief* is suspected if the typical manifestations of separation and progressive evolution of grief are delayed for more than 2 weeks after a loss. The prolonged absence of grief is termed *absent grief*. The diagnosis of *inhibited grief* refers to diminishment of typical responses of grief under circumstances in which one would expect these manifestations. *Chronic grief* is diagnosed when the intensity of separation anxiety does not diminish during the first year of bereavement.

■ EPIDEMIOLOGY

Psychiatric complications of bereavement are among the more common disorders encountered in outpatient psychiatric settings and psychiatric consultation services. Pathologic grief, major depressions, anxiety disorders, post-traumatic stress disorder (PTSD), and substance abuse are complications of bereavement that require professional intervention. Osterweis et al. (1984) noted that more than 800,000 men and women in the United States experience the loss of a spouse annually. This number does not take into account bereaved parents, siblings, and children who also experience grief responses after the loss of loved ones. Approximately 2 million deaths occur annually in the United States, with each death resulting in from 8 to 10 bereaved family members (Hocker, 1989; Redmond, 1989). A total of 16- to 20-million newly bereaved individuals in the United States can be estimated from annual mortality data (Rando, 1993). Raphael (1983, p. 64) estimates that as many as one in three bereavements result in pathological patterns of grief. Rando (1993, p. 5) suggests that if Raphael's statistic is applied, there is the potential for 5 to 6 million new cases of pathologic grief each year.

A recent review by Jacobs (1993, pp. 41–42) of epidemiological studies of clinical complications of bereavement suggested that bereavement is an important cause of depressive complications. Jacobs (1993, pp. 42–45) also reviewed clinical bereavement outcome studies published between 1968 and 1992 and found the following estimates of the occurrence of complications of grief among adults: pathologic grief - 14 to 34%; major depression - 4 to 31% panic disorder 6 to 13%; and generalized anxiety disorder - 39%. Jacobs (1993, p. 45) concluded from his extensive review that estimates of bereavement complications tend to center around 20%, which is the crude rate of complications of acute bereavement cited by many clinicians. This 20% rate of complications during the first year of bereavement is a substantial figure when one considers that more than 800,000 spouses are widowed each year in the United States. Furthermore, this number does not estimate the numbers of other bereaved individuals who are affected by such a loss, and who may develop bereavement complications.

■ DIVERSITY AND SOCIO-CULTURAL ISSUES

Personal values and beliefs, socioeconomic status and cultural background, and religious or existential belief systems are among the factors that influence bereaved individuals' grief processes (Berger et al., 1989; Johnson and McGee, 1991). Religious and cultural beliefs in an afterlife influence perceptions surrounding dying and death, and may even influence utilization patterns for psychosocial help. For example, survivors of victims of suicide who are members of religions that exclude suicide victims from customary funeral rites and social support are very vulnerable to high levels of distress. Bereaved family members who usually find comfort and hope in the teachings of their religious affiliation may experience a high level of distress because they fear that their loved one will not be at peace in the afterlife. Bereaved survivors of suicide victims may turn to individual or group counseling for social support or to resolve conflicts.

Secularization of the American culture has diminished the former role of religious organizations in supporting the bereaved. Worden (1982) has suggested that changes in American culture have contributed to the fact that more people are turning to mental-health professionals to assist them with grief. Increasing mobility has created an environment in which cohesiveness among inter-generational families and close relationships with neighbors are rare. The sense of community support that was prevalent in the first half of the 20th century has diminished considerably.

SPIRITUALITY

Nurses have an obligation to respect individuals' belief systems, and to have a non-judgmental perspective if patients' spiritual philosophies are different from their own. A brief spiritual-assessment interview can provide more information about how an individual's or family's spiritual-belief system influences the process of grief after the loss of a loved one. Religious traditions, for example, may require mourners to perform memorial rituals or prayers for the deceased on designated days of the year. Some religious traditions practiced by Americans of Chinese descent for honoring deceased ancestors include prayers and ritual offerings at an altar in the home. In addition, religious traditions may guide thinking about loss, dying, an afterlife, and the expression of grief. Questions (Burkhardt and Nagai-Jacobsen, 1985) that might be helpful include:

- What gives meaning to your life?
- Is religion or God significant to you?
- What is your source of strength or hope?
- What helps you the most when you feel afraid or need special help?
- Are there any spiritual practices that help you (prayer, meditation)?
- Is there someone (clergy, church members, etc.) that I could contact for you who could assist you with your spiritual practices?

Nurses need to be aware of their own spiritual beliefs in order to assist bereaved individuals with this aspect of human life. The following points, based on Burkhardt and Nagai-Jacobson's (1985) work, help the nurse in preparing to facilitate the spiritual dimension:

- Know yourself as a spiritual being.
- Understand that spirituality is not limited to definitions of God or Ultimate Being.
- Encourage and share in reminiscing; experience the present moment whatever joy, pain, or grief it may hold.
- Recognize the importance of *"being present with"* as clients describe the meaning or pain in their lives.
- Know that ambiguities, struggles, and searching are aspects of spirituality that may remain as unanswered questions.
- Recognize that each individual is the "expert" about his or her own life journey. Nurses can assist individuals through receptive listening.

CULTURAL PRACTICES

Cultural practices also guide thinking, decisions, and actions in a patterned way. Members of cultural groups may have certain expectations of newly bereaved community members with respect to participation in festivities and the formation of new attachments. Mourning traditions restrict the style and color of clothing of mourners for a defined period after a loved one's death. Widows of Mediterranean descent may wear conservative black clothing for a full year or even a lifetime after the death of a spouse.

It is inappropriate, however, to make assumptions about patients and their families solely on the basis of awareness of their cultural heritage. It is important for nurses to assess families' cultural backgrounds in order to plan appropriate interventions for grief. Assessments of family roles, usual life-style, developmental level, authority patterns, and resources within the family network enable the nurse to identify strengths and needs within the family system. The following questions (Tripp-Reimer and Brink, 1985) will guide the nurse to gain a more complete understanding of families' world views.

- What roles did the deceased person relinquish?
- Who are the people affected by the loss of this person?
- What are the expectations of the family members?
- What are the occupational patterns?
- What adaptations need to be made?
- Who are the deceased's close friends and family?

- What are the family's economic resources?
- Are there any other concurrent stressors?
- What child-rearing activities exist?
- Are there other caregiving responsibilities?
- Who will participate in decision making?
- What is the level of participation in religion?
- Does the spiritual tradition provide hope?

GROUP PRACTICES

The expression of loss and grief takes a variety of forms among members of diverse cultures. Cultural and sub-cultural norms influence the expression of grief. It is critical that nurses recognize, understand, and respect each family's culture-specific patterns of behavior in loss situations. These practices and beliefs may, however, vary widely among members of a group. Brief summaries of selected religious and cultural traditions are provided below to demonstrate the broad range of patterns and expectations across different cultural groups.

Orthodox Jews participate in highly structured mourning rituals that prescribe customs for a period of one year after the death of a family member. Jewish customs are highly supportive of the bereaved, and are consistent with the psychological phases of a healthy grief trajectory (Pollock, 1972). Full participation of the bereaved is expected during the specific mourning periods, and a code of behaviors specified in the Torah guides the bereaved and other members of the community. During *Shiva*, the period of 7 days of mourning following the burial of the deceased, community members go to the home of the bereaved family to verbally express their sorrow and concern, and to provide comfort to and assist the family with household duties, such as food preparation. *Shiloshem* extends through 30 days after the burial and signals the end of ritual mourning and return to a more active involvement in work and social life. The *unveiling* of the deceased persons' headstone is held at the end of Sheloshim, during a commemorative service. The deceased is remembered by survivors on anniversaries and certain holidays throughout the year. Sadness among survivors is expected on these anniversaries, but excessive grief is not viewed favorably within the community (Goldberg, 1981).

Native Americans represent a broad diversity of cultures encompassing more than 500 federally recognized tribal entities. The greatest concentration of the Native American population is located in Oklahoma, Arizona, and California, with over 2,000 native languages represented in these states. Most Native Americans value self-reliance, but there is a tradition of shared decision-making among extended family members. Many Native Americans are death-accepting and view life and death in circular fashion. Children are

taught, through ceremonies and stories, that death is a part of life. Dying and death are usually accepted in a stoic manner. *Navajo Indians* have traditional mourning norms that limit the expression of mourning to a period of 4 days, and set expectations for members of the bereaved family to resume full participation in work and social life thereafter. This abbreviated mourning period is in sharp contrast to the Western trajectory of mourning, which may last more than a year. Navajos express fear of death and of the ghost of the deceased person (Miller and Schoenfeld, 1973).

Many *African-Americans* believe in immortality, and observe funeral rites characterized as celebrations of life. There are strong multigenerational ties among members of extended African-American families. Research has found that non-verbal patterns of communication are emphasized in African-American culture. Therefore, actions in response to immediate situations are more highly valued than discussions of the future. Open expressions of feelings are valued. African-Americans may perceive little control over their own lives as a consequence of many years of living with oppression imposed by the dominant culture. Death has been more visible to Americans of African descent than to European Americans; violent deaths among young African-American men are common in urban centers. During mourning, members of the deceased's extended family, friends, and church members openly demonstrate expressions of support for the bereaved family members. For many African-Americans death is perceived to be a reunification with those who have died in the past, and passage to a better life.

Americans of European descent comprise the dominant American culture and represent many unique sub-groups. Expressions of sadness and grief within this culture are learned within the family setting, and the demonstration of emotions varies widely among this group of Americans. Bereaved family members may display stoicism. Indeed, Western culture has become characterized as a death-denying culture. Death is less visible in this culture because of a decline in multi-generational co-habitation. Many Americans of European heritage believe in immortality, usually put a high value on family closeness, and demonstrate variations in spiritual beliefs and traditions across specific cultural sub-groups.

Hispanic Americans are represented by diverse cultures, including the Mexican-American, Latino, Spanish-American, and Chicano cultures. Each of these sub-groups may differ in traditional beliefs and practices in the care of the dying. Death is a family event and children are full participants in the rituals and customs surrounding death. Hispanic-Americans have a long tradition of a death-accepting culture that can be traced to Spain and Mexico. Frequently, Hispanic-Americans' religiosity is non-institutional, tending to be home-centered rather than church-centered. Symbols and rituals are very important among many Hispanic-Americans. These symbols provide comfort to the dying person and family members. Open expressions of grief among Hispanic women are expected, but are uncommon among Hispanic men.

Asian Americans are represented by many subgroups including Chinese, Japanese, Koreans, Filipinos, Cambodians, Hmong, Laotians, and Vietnamese. Their beliefs and values are diverse. As a group, however, Asian-Americans share a holistic conception of health and illness in which physical and mental functioning are intimately linked. Many Asian-Americans believe in both Eastern and Western medicine. They revere past generations of ancestors. Ritual ceremonies that honor dead ancestors may be incorporated into the care of the dying. Traditional Asian families play a key role in decision making about medical care. Individuals who follow traditional Asian cultural patterns relinquish their right to autonomous decision making.

■ NURSING ASSESSMENT OF BEREAVED PERSONS

Feelings of anxiety, sadness, loneliness, spiritual distress, depression, and guilt have been reported by bereaved persons. It is not uncommon for bereaved persons to display flattened or inhibited affect during the grief reaction. The timing of these feelings, however, may not coincide among family members. This presents a complex situation for nursing assessment, in that family members may need different types of support at different times. Bereaved individuals may experience any combination of somatic, psychological, and cognitive responses during the course of normal grief.

Somatic responses in grief may include:

- Appetite disturbance (loss or gain of weight)
- Gastrointestinal disturbances (diarrhea)
- Sleep disturbance (inability to sleep, interrupted sleep)
- Crying and tearfulness
- A tendency to sigh
- Lack of strength
- Physical exhaustion
- Feelings of emptiness and heaviness
- Feelings of "something caught in the throat"
- Heart palpitations
- Nervousness and tension
- Loss of sexuality or hypersexuality
- Lack of energy and psychomotor retardation
- Restlessness and searching for something to do
- Shortness of breath
- Dizziness
- Feelings of numbness
- Headache

Psychologic and cognitive responses in grief include:

- Disbelief
- Sadness
- Sorrow
- Depression
- Anxiety
- Irritability
- Self-blame
- Guilt
- Anger
- Fear
- Anxiety
- Relief
- Flattened or inhibited affect
- Hallucinations
- Confusion
- Difficulty concentrating
- Impaired memory
- Slow, disordered thought processes
- Restlessness and inability to sit still
- Inability to initiate and maintain organized patterns of activity
- Withdrawal from social interaction
- Preoccupation with thoughts of the deceased
- Dreaming about the deceased loved one
- Searching for the deceased in familiar places
- Learning to live without the deceased loved one
- Experience of loneliness
- Anniversary reactions occur on dates throughout the year (i.e., birthdays, wedding anniversary, holidays, etc.)

RANDO'S SCHEMA OF GRIEF AND MOURNING

This schema is a framework meant to guide the assessment of bereaved individuals over time. Rando (1993) has proposed that the bereaved individual experiences six major mourning processes (see Table 16–2: Rando's Six "R" Processes of Mourning). Those common responses to major loss are described by Rando (1984) over three phases or time periods: avoidance, confrontation, and accommodation. The phases do not occur separately from one another, but rather the mourner will probably move back and forth between phases. The unique characteristics of the bereaved individual and the particular circumstances associated with the loss will contribute to the progression of movement between the phases of grief.

Avoidance

During the avoidance phase of mourning, the news of the death of the significant other is received, and there is a desire to avoid acknowledging the death. Emotional numbness, confusion, bewilderment, and disorganized

TABLE 16-2. RANDO'S SIX "R" PROCESSES OF MOURNING

Avoidance phase
1. Recognize the loss
   - Acknowledge the death
   - Understand the death

Confrontation phase
2. React to the separation
   - Experience the pain
   - Feel, identify, accept, and give some form of expression to all of the psychological reactions to the loss
   - Identify and mourn secondary losses
3. Recollect and reexperience the deceased and the relationship
   - Review and remember the relationship realistically
   - Revive and re-experience the feelings in the relationship
4. Relinquish the old attachments to the deceased and the old assumptive world

Accommodation phase
5. Readjust to move adaptively into the new world without forgetting the old
   - Revise the assumptive world
   - Develop a new relationship with the deceased
   - Adopt new ways of being in the world
   - Form a new identity
6. Reinvest personal energies

Printed with permission from: Rando, T.A. (1993). *Treatment of Complicated Grief.* Champaign, IL: Research Press, p. 45.

thought, emotion or behavior are common during this phase (Rando, 1993).

Confrontation

The confrontation phase is a painful time when the bereaved individual confronts the reality of the loss, and experiences intense biopsychosocial and behavioral reactions to separation from the significant other.

Accommodation

The accommodation phase of mourning (Rando, 1993), formerly called the re-establishment phase (Rando, 1984), is characterized by a gradual decline of the symptoms of acute grief, and re-entry into everyday life. The bereaved individual is able to recognize the loss in a way that does not preclude healthy, life-affirming living (Rando, 1993).

NORMAL GRIEF RESPONSES

Bereavement is listed as a category in *DSM IV* when the focus of clinical attention is a reaction to the death of a loved one. Bereaved individuals typically experience symptoms characteristic of a major depressive episode (e.g., sadness, insomnia, poor appetite, weight loss).

Professional help may be sought to relieve symptoms associated with "normal" bereavement, such as loss of appetite or insomnia. It is important to differentiate sadness from reactive depression; depression should be treated.

COMPLICATED GRIEF

The assessment of depression in bereaved individuals is more complex because some symptoms of grief and depression overlap. Depression is a distressing illness characterized by dysphoric mood, with a loss of interest in all or many of one's usual activities. The symptom profile of depression includes poor appetite or weight loss, sleep disturbance, fatigue, psychomotor agitation or retardation, decreased ability to concentrate, feelings of guilt or reproach, and recurrent thoughts of suicide. Persistent feelings of low self-esteem, unworthiness, and a reduced capacity for pleasure and enjoyment may signal depression in bereaved persons. Because bereaved persons who experience unrelieved symptoms of depression may verbalize a desire to commit suicide, discussion of suicide should not be avoided. The diagnosis of major depressive disorder in bereaved individuals is generally not made unless the appropriate symptoms persist for 2 months after a loss. The following symptoms help to identify a major depressive episode:

- Guilt about issues other than actions taken by the survivor at the time of the deceased person's death.
- Thoughts of death other than feelings that the survivor would be better off dead or should have died with the deceased person.
- A morbid preoccupation with worthlessness.
- Marked psychomotor retardation.
- Prolonged and marked functional impairment.
- Hallucinating experiences other than thinking that one hears the voice of or transiently sees the image of the deceased person. (*DSM IV*, pp. 684–685).

Parkes (1988) suggested that four salient characteristics of life-change events were commonly associated with the onset of mental illness. A life-change event that happened rapidly, was perceived as negative, had lasting implications, and required a major revision in assumptions about the world would be defined as a situation that might precede disruptions in mental health. Empirical study has identified variables that may enhance or impede adaptation to circumstances following life-change events. These variables include the type and magnitude of the life-change event; the degree of warning of its occurrence; the affected individual's previous personality, coping styles, and past life experiences; and the availability of social support. *Assessment* of these variables is important when planning intervention. Empirical studies indicate that bereaved persons report decreased physical and mental symptoms and an increased quality of life if appropriate intervention is available at the right time (Mor, 1987; Parkes, 1981; Raphael, 1977).

■ ANTICIPATORY GRIEF REACTIONS OF TERMINALLY ILL INDIVIDUALS

Individuals who anticipate dying may engage in activities that will keep their memory alive for family members and friends. Writing journals and letters, recording shared times on videotape, recording personal messages on audiotape, and distributing photographs and personal possessions to loved ones are meaningful ways of completing personal business. Dying individuals may convey preferences about types of medical care and the procedures to be used, and make decisions related to estate planning, funeral arrangements, and choice of a location in which to die.

Active listening and being present with the terminally ill patient facilitate an environment in which the patient defines the context and meaning of his or her own life (Herth, 1990; Jones, 1993). Abandonment and isolation, uncontrollable pain, and devaluation of personhood were identified by terminally ill persons as factors that interfered with their hope (Herth, 1990). There exists no universal definition of hope with which to capture the meaning of this construct for all people. Personal values, beliefs, experiences, and resources influence the meaning of hope for each individual. Clinicians and researchers observe that maintenance of hope is instrumental in the coping processes of chronically ill persons (Herth, 1989; Scanlon, 1989; Weisman, 1979). Herth's (1990) findings about the meaning of hope and hope-fostering strategies in a convenience sample of adults (n = 30) enrolled in hospice programs contribute to an understanding of hope within the context of terminal care. The patients were aware that their life expectancies were projected to be 6 months or less. Herth interpreted their descriptions of hope as being a dynamic and complex phenomenon that involves thoughts, feelings, and actions that provide a new awareness of what is possible in life; an ability to "put pieces of life into a (new) pattern"; and an ability to "face the shortness of life constructively" (Herth, 1990, p. 1256). Herth identified hope-fostering strategies from patient interviews and sorted them into the seven categories of interpersonal connectedness; attainable aims; spiritual base; personal attributes; light-heartedness; up-lifting memories; and affirmation

of worth. These categories of hope-fostering strategies provide direction for the support of terminally ill individuals.

A critical element of hope is the presence of a caring relationship during terminal illness. Interpersonal relationships may change when awareness of a shortened lifespan becomes part of an individual's life experience. Nurses can influence internal and external conditions that foster caring relationships by providing the patient, family, and friends with physical and emotional support, information about hope and dying, encouragement to create an environment of closeness, and a sense of belonging (Herth, 1990). Dufault and Martocchio (1985) advanced a multi-dimensional model of hope, based on information obtained through interviews and observations of elderly persons with cancer. Nursing strategies are focused on creating an environment that offers patients opportunities to express their hopes by communicating thoughts and feelings; maintaining significant relationships; and reflecting on continuity between past, present, and future hopes (Dufault and Martocchio, 1985).

■ ANTICIPATORY GRIEF REACTIONS OF FAMILY MEMBERS

Anticipatory grief reactions are commonly associated with the physical decline of the patient with advanced cancer (Northouse, 1984; Parkes and Weiss, 1983; Rando, 1984; Sanders, 1982–83). The emotional resources of the patient's family members are challenged by the stress associated with feelings of loss as they anticipate separation from their loved one. Although each family member has a subjective experience of loss, the family experiences dynamic shifts in expected roles and responsibilities in relation to the new demands imposed by the patient's illness (Lewis, 1983). Care of a dying person in the home setting may strain the physical, psychosocial, and financial resources of a family. Major changes in a family's life-style patterns may be required in order to accommodate the demands of caring for a terminally ill family member. Unresolved conflict and difficulties in relationships and communication patterns among family members may worsen with the stress of the patient's terminal illness. Family members need to know that the disequilibrium within the family is not unexpected, and that problem-solving approaches may prevent or defuse some family tensions. Lewis (1993) emphasizes the importance of maintaining "non-illness-related aspects of family life" so that the family continues to live as a family. Additional help and respite care may be needed for families to participate in the non-illness-related aspects of their lives.

■ CHILDREN'S NEEDS

Children require special consideration when they reside in a household with a seriously ill family member. In the past, children were often sheltered from the truth about the gravity of a close relative's illness by parents and professionals. Siegel et al. (1992) emphasize that children are sensitive to changes in family dynamics and may experience distress associated with loss and separation related to hospitalizations, increasing limitations in both parents' physical and emotional availability and role functioning, changes in family routines, a shift in the family's emotional climate, and a decrease in financial resources as efforts are directed toward providing care for an ill family member. Siegel et al. (1992) found that depressive symptomatology and anxiety were significantly greater in children (n = 62) with a terminally ill parent than in a comparison sample of children in the community. They also identified diminished self-esteem and deficits in social competence in children with a terminally ill parent. Further complications may be expected from these children's decreased participation in social activities and poor school performance.

Christ et al. (1993) and her colleagues examined the impact of parental terminal cancer on children 7 to 16 years of age. Common concerns of these children reported during interviews included fears related to symptoms of the cancer and the side effects of treatment (i.e., weight loss, hair loss, vomiting, weakness, etc.); fear of the parent's future death; anxiety or panic related to uncertainty about and rapid changes in the parent's status; guilt about the cause of the parent's illness; and concern that the healthy parent might also be vulnerable to illness. Clinical observations indicate that children experience greater stress during the terminal stage of cancer than after a parent's death from the disease (Christ et al., 1993). Nurses need to determine whether there are children in a dying patient's family, and to identify the family member who has major responsibility for their care. Appropriate referrals may have to be made in order to support families during this stressful time, and age-specific needs may require special guidance from professionals skilled in family relations.

Professionals who feel comfortable talking about issues surrounding terminal illness may offer guidance to parents dealing with overwhelming changes brought on by such illness in the family (Schonfeld, 1993). Bourne and Meier (1988) have developed a booklet for children (pre-school to 10 years old) that sensitively addresses the topic of advanced illness. Parents should be encouraged to read this booklet with their children so as to facilitate an open discussion about existing and expected changes caused by advanced illness in a family member. Parents also need to be aware of the differences between children's and adults' grief reactions. Children's questions and reactions related to the loss of a loved one may seem insensitive, but these responses are usually consistent with a child's social, emotional, and cognitive development. Nurses should encourage honest discussion of terminal illness among adults and children within the family setting. Children's fantasies about death will decrease if information is presented at the appropriate cognitive level. Older family members should be encouraged to discuss their true feelings openly with the family's children if this is a cultural norm. Lies and distortions of truth should be avoided. In certain cultures, open expression of grief establishes a model for children that may be fostered within the family culture. Families that follow a cultural or religious tradition should be encouraged to share with their children its values, beliefs, and rituals related to death. Children need assurance that family integrity, the home, and love will continue despite the sadness related to illness and death.

■ COPING STRATEGIES

It is not uncommon for family members who provide care for a terminally ill member to experience loss and anticipatory grief while doing this. Nursing interventions should be directed toward assisting these caregivers in using coping strategies for managing their feelings of loss and grief.

Hull (1992) reported coping strategies used by 14 family caregivers providing hospice home care. The most frequently reported coping strategy in this study was taking time away from care-giving responsibilities, such as a few hours of uninterrupted respite at home or outside the home to pursue hobbies or contact friends. The strategy of downward comparison, in which family care-givers believed that their own situation was not as bad as someone else's, enabled some of them to continue their responsibilities. A cognitive re-formulation process was another strategy used by some family caregivers to minimize the negative aspects of their situation and transform them into meaningful opportunities.

Family care-givers also reported using avoidance in order to direct their energy away from their lack of control over the impending death of a loved one, and to actively expend their efforts toward aspects of care that were within their control. Family care-givers also reported "taking one day at a time" to cope with the uncertainty of their situations, and used attitudes of acceptance and rationalization to cope with changes brought about by cognitive disorientation in a loved one. Social-support networks were identified as a major factor in coping with the stresses associated with caring for a dying family member at home (Hull, 1992).

Warner (1992) suggests that providing information about coping strategies will enhance the effectiveness of family members who provide home care to a seriously ill relative, and will improve their own quality of life. Health professionals can offer anticipatory guidance about expected future events in an effort to decrease uncertainty and increase the care-givers' feelings of control and competence. These professionals can review decision-making and assertiveness skills with family care-givers in order to help them make the best use of available resources during these stressful times. Specific stress-management techniques (i.e., progressive relaxation, imagery), distraction techniques (i.e., music, reminiscing, reviewing photo albums), and time-management techniques are all hold the potential to enhance care-givers' lives (Warner, 1992).

Care-givers to persons with AIDS (PWAs) encounter very complex situations because many of their patients are young and face an abbreviated lifespan. AIDS patients' care-givers who are immersed in the gay community are also constantly aware of the deaths of friends and associates. Brown and Powell-Cope (1993) identified central themes of "facing loss" and "transformed time" in a qualitative study of 53 care-givers to persons with AIDS. The care-givers faced multiple losses, including the loss of interpersonal relationships, future dreams, personal freedom, and their previous life-styles. In order to cope with anticipatory grief, the care-givers in this study reported "taking one day at a time," "living fully in the moment," and "actualizing future dreams" (Brown and Powell-Cope, 1993).

Herth (1993) reported that family care-givers to terminally ill persons identified the following strategies as fostering hope: sustaining supportive relationships; using cognitive reframing (e.g., positive self-talk, praying/meditating); changing their perception of space or focus of time (e.g., taking one day at a time); defining attainable goals; engaging in spiritual practices (e.g., listening to music, reading inspirational books); and balancing available internal energy with external demands (e.g., priority setting and using available resources). Information about these approaches may be offered to increase the range of strategies that family care-givers can use as they face the demands of terminal care for a loved one.

■ SUPPORT SERVICES

Many households in America are headed by adults who work full-time or part-time outside the home. The im-

pact on financial income, roles, and work patterns of caring for a terminally ill family member at home is evident when families decide to do this. The Federal Family and Medical Leave Act (1993) offers working family members unpaid leave from the workplace to care for a seriously ill family member, with continuation of benefits (health insurance, retirement contribution, etc.) for a maximum period of 12 weeks per 12-month period.

Literature about the care-giver's burden, stress, and coping indicates a need for interventions designed to support family members in providing terminal care in the home setting (Decker and Young, 1991; Dobratz, 1990; Ekberg, Griffith, and Foxall, 1986; Gaynor, 1990; Lev, 1991; Masters and Shontz, 1989; Oberst, Thomas, and Ward, 1990; Reimer, Davies, and Martens, 1991; Robinson, 1990; Wingate and Lackey, 1989). Lewis (1990) identified support services needed by families facing the challenges associated with breast cancer. She identified the following support services as being needed across the trajectory of the illness: information about diagnosis, treatment, and illness course; anticipatory guidance; dealing with school-age children; cognitive and emotional processing (the meaning of the illness for all family members); and access to problem-focused services (physical and psychological care) (Lewis, 1990).

■ NORMAL GRIEF

No single therapeutic approach is effective in all bereavement situations, because an individual's grief response is influenced by multiple psychological, sociocultural, and developmental factors. A broad knowledge of therapeutic approaches is advantageous. The nurse plays a critical role in selecting interventions that are best suited to the particular needs of the bereaved individual. Worden (1991) identified tasks of mourning that guide survivors in adapting to life after the death of a loved one. He found that the mourning process is complete when the following tasks have been accomplished:

- Accepting the reality of the loss.
- Working through the pain of grief.
- Adjusting to the world without the loved one.
- Re-investing emotional energy in a new relationship.

A review of simple measures for maintaining personal emotional and physical well-being may open lines of communication with bereaved individuals. Addressing common emotional concerns (e.g., uncertainty, anxiety, fear, loss), encouraging health-promoting behaviors (e.g., exercise, balanced nutrition, contact with friends and family network, avoidance of alcohol and drugs), and presenting stress-management strategies (e.g., relaxation techniques, giving oneself permission for "time out") may prevent health problems associated with bereavement.

COMPLICATED GRIEF

Physiological, behavioral, and social origins of complications of grief, along with suggested strategies for treating these complications, are summarized in Table 16–3. Table 16–4 lists the goals of pharmacologic, psychotherapeutic, and mutual-support-group strategies for managing complications of bereavement. In a review of therapeutic approaches to grief, Barbato and Irwin (1992) emphasize the importance of the patient's focusing on his or her feelings during the initial stages of grief therapy in order to accept the loss as a reality and work through the pain of grief. Some bereaved individuals successfully avoid feelings and thoughts about the loss.

INTERVENTIONS

Interventions that facilitate the expression of emotional pain and simultaneously normalize the grief experience are most helpful to grieving individuals. Patient-centered and gestalt therapies are used to guide bereaved individuals toward expressing their feelings. If an individual's grieving is sustained, referral for bereavement counseling may be necessary.

Family intervention is indicated for surviving family members in order to avert marital dysfunction, family dysfunction, and poor school performance by children. The value of family therapy for bereaved children has been reported by Black (1979). Strategies that strengthen family interaction, communication, cooperation, and social and emotional involvement are described in the literature (Giacquinta [nee Stewart], 1977, 1989, 1990; Stewart, 1994).

CLIENT-CENTERED THERAPY

Patient-centered counseling facilitates the expression of feelings. Such counseling relies on building a trusting relationship in which acceptance, empathy, genuineness, openness, and unconditional positive regard create a climate in which the bereaved individual can express his or her feelings and become more conscious of the experience of grief. Non-directive techniques, such as reflection, enable the therapist to act as a "mirror" to the patient's feelings, thereby heightening

TABLE 16–3. ORIGINS AND TREATMENT STRATEGIES FOR COMPLICATIONS OF BEREAVEMENT

Origins	Recovery	Treatment
Physiological		
Stress/arousal (corticotropin-releasing hormone, locus coeruleus, norepinephrine)	Homeostasis	Possibly alprazolam Stress management
Norepinephrine dysregulation	Homeostasis Substitution (remarriage) Self-care	Antidepressant drugs Cognitive and interpersonal psychotherapy Mutual supports
Behavioral		
Learned helplessness	Effective coping	Antidepressant drugs Cognitive and interpersonal psychotherapy Psychoeducation Mutual supports
Insecure attachments	Substitution Growth Grief work	Brief, dynamic psychotherapy
Poor health practices	Healthy life-style	Health education Psychoeducation
Social		
Social isolation/loss of care	New interests New friends	Social services Mutual supports
Decline in socio-economic status	Work Recognition	Social services Mutual supports
Psychosocial transitions	Effective coping New identity New assumptions about the world Future orientation	Psychoeducation Brief, dynamic psychotherapy Mutual supports

awareness of painful feelings the patient has avoided in an attempt to blunt the pain.

GESTALT THERAPY

Gestalt therapy guides the bereaved individual to "relive" the loss of a loved one as fully as possible. Past experiences are dealt with in their immediate present context. This can help individuals who have delayed dealing with grief.

Gestalt therapy directs patient's to gain a greater awareness of their grief through awareness of their non-verbal expressions. In the "empty chair technique," the client is directed to have a dialogue with the deceased. The patient is asked to sit in the "deceased's" chair and

TABLE 16–4. GOALS OF TREATING PSYCHIATRIC COMPLICATIONS OF BEREAVEMENT

Modality	Goals
Psychotropic drugs	Treat major depressions and anxiety disorders
	Alleviate symptoms that are subjectively overwhelming or that interfere with functioning
	Facilitate the natural healing of grief
Psychotherapy	Counter demoralization
	Provide psychoeducation
	Solve problems
	Clarify interpersonal problems
	Elucidate maladaptive relationship patterns
	Clarify pessimistic cognitive schemas
	Desensitize the phobic avoidance
Mutual-support groups	Provide membership and friendship
	Exchange information about grief, coping, and community resources
	Offer a milieu for practicing social skills
	Empower through publicity and advocacy
	Promote self-esteem

Reprinted with permission from: Jacobs, S. (1993). *Pathologic Grief Maladaptation to Loss*, Washington, DC: American Psychiatric Press, p. 238.

participate in the dialogue. This dialogue enables the patient to experience his or her feelings and gain insight into thoughts they may have projected onto the deceased. This technique is also helpful for bereaved individuals who were unable to say a last good-bye to a deceased person.

COGNITIVE AND BEHAVIORAL THERAPIES

Barbato and Irwin (1992) suggested that cognitive and behavioral therapies may be effective for patients experiencing prolonged or exaggerated grief responses. Cognitive therapies, such as rational-emotive therapy (RET) and transactional analysis (TA), are directed toward teaching patients to think rationally. The underlying basis of these therapies is that the negative event is not the problem, but rather how the client thinks about the event. Techniques of rational-emotive therapy (RET) are directed toward helping patients become aware of the irrationality of beliefs about a loss, and to then substitute negative thoughts with positive statements. Transactional analysis (TA) directs the patient to recognize destructive thought patterns and encourages constructive behavior. TA techniques may be particularly useful in bereaved patients who have low self esteem or were very dependent on the deceased (Barbato and Irwin, 1992).

Behavioral interventions for bereaved patients would be directed to the specific behaviors that are im-

peding grief resolution. Counseling bereaved patients to become more self-sufficient by learning new skills and acquiring increased confidence in new areas may be done by coaching and assertiveness-training strategies. Some physical symptoms of grief may be effectively resolved through a problem-solving approach that includes a process of problem identification, goal setting, and learning new skills. Gastrointestinal symptoms associated with grieving may be effectively resolved by eating small, frequent meals. Behavioral techniques are helpful strategies for patients with an excessive intake of alcohol, caffeine, or nicotine. Healthy changes in physical status can also be achieved through behavioral interventions directed at physical exercise, sexual contact, and stress reduction.

HOSPICE BEREAVEMENT SERVICES

Hospices are health-care services designed to meet the needs of patients and their families during the last 6 months of life. The goals of hospice care are to support physical, emotional, social, and spiritual aspects of life until the end of life; to preserve human dignity, maintain comfort, and provide the dying individual with autonomy and the power to make decisions; and to assist family members and friends to cope with the reality of terminal illness. The availability of hospice services varies across the United States; rural areas are underserved. Many hospice-care programs provide a bereavement home visit for surviving family members and ongoing bereavement support-group meetings.

GROUP BEREAVEMENT COUNSELING

Mutual support groups for bereaved individuals are offered through community and hospital-based hospices, mental-health agencies, and religious organizations. Their goal is to provide a social organization that is directed to meet the needs of the bereaved and a forum for valuable information and social support. Both formal and informal aspects of mutual-support groups provide opportunities for bereaved individuals to learn about grief, how others cope with it, and available community resources for helping with this (Jacobs, 1993). Mutual-support groups also provide opportunities for bereaved individuals to decrease their social isolation, validate their feelings, and experience reality checking. Not all individuals and families choose to accept available bereavement support from community agencies.

Bereaved individuals often experience high levels of anxiety and confront altered expectations about the future. Research has demonstrated that "widow-to-widow" or "parent-to-parent" groups provide a forum for individuals facing similar losses (Silverman, 1987; Segal, Fletcher, and Meekison, 1986). Mutual-support groups for bereaved persons provide key elements of support, including person-to-person exchange based on identification and reciprocity; access to a body of information; opportunity to share coping techniques and increase one's sense of personal worth; and a forum for advocacy, change, feedback on performance, and "reality checking" with peers. Within these groups, bereaved members act as role models for newly bereaved individuals (Osterweis, Solomon, and Green, 1984). Information about selected survivor support groups is presented here for future referral.

ASSISTANCE FROM ORGANIZATIONS

The American Association of Retired Persons provides information about local support groups for widowed persons at the telephone number 1-202-872-4700. The death of a spouse is considered one of the greatest loss events of a lifetime, and adjustment to living without a spouse is very difficult. Mutual assistance groups help widowed persons in a social setting.

The Compassionate Friends, Inc. is a national organization that has more than 600 local chapters in the United States. Bereaved parents, siblings, and grandparents who have lost a child at any age may join its local group support meetings. Parents whose children have died demonstrate the range of grief reactions and may experience intense survivor guilt responses. Parents' grief symptoms are usually severe and long-lasting. Parents may feel that they failed to protect their child. Many will require assistance in identifying irrational beliefs and expectations that intensify their feelings of guilt. Individual counseling or group support settings may be beneficial for this.

The National Sudden Infant Death Syndrome (SIDS) Foundation offers education and support to parents who have suffered the loss of an infant through SIDS.

Unite, Inc. is a supportive organization for parents who have experienced miscarriage, stillbirth, or infant death. It provides telephone support service, educational programs, and parent-to-parent discussions.

Resolve Through Sharing Bereavement Services (RTS), located in La Crosse, Wisconsin, also provides information and supportive services nationwide to parents who have experienced miscarriage, stillbirth, or infant death. Grief-training sessions are also available for professionals who interact with bereaved parents.

The American Association of Suicidology, based in Denver, Colorado, provides information about local support groups for persons who have lost a loved one as a result of suicide. Suicide poses difficult problems of grief resolution for many survivors. Western culture has traditionally perceived suicide as sinful, criminal, or a weakness in character. In contrast, other cultures view suicide as a rational choice or even an honorable act. Survivors of suicide should be offered information about available grief-counseling services. These survivors may blame themselves for failing to prevent the suicide. They may also need to work through feelings of anger and abandonment. Suicide that was consciously chosen to end debilitating illness may offer survivors an explanation for the act, and thereby assist them. On the other hand, recovery from loss may be slowed when survivors of suicide experience social stigmatization.

National clearinghouses for victim information include: Parents of Murdered Children, Inc., at 1-513-721-5683; the National Victim Center, at 1-703-276-2880; and the National Organization for Victim Assistance, at 1-202-232-6682. When someone dies suddenly and violently, survivors may experience intense grief reactions as well as anger and rage. Information and support resource networks have been established across the United States to meet the needs of family members and friends of murder victims. Referrals to local and national agencies that provide information and guidance about criminal justice, crime victims' compensation, court accompaniment, and bereavement services are important in establishing ongoing support for grieving survivors of violent death.

PHARMACOLOGIC INTERVENTIONS

Clinical experience and results from a limited number of empirical studies indicate that the course of normal manifestations of grief, such as separation distress, is independent of the course of depressive symptoms (Jacobs, 1993). The goals of using psychotropic drugs to treat complications of bereavement are to treat major depressions and anxiety disorders; alleviate symptoms that are subjectively overwhelming or that interfere with functioning; and facilitate the natural resolution of grief (Jacobs, 1993). Intervention that integrates psychotherapeutic, pharmacologic, and mutual-support-group strategies is a comprehensive approach to complications of bereavement. Chapter 40 reviews pharmacotherapy.

■ LEGAL/ETHICAL IMPLICATIONS

The constitutional right of individuals to engage in decision-making about medical interventions at end-of-life is now protected through federal legislation. The Patient Self-Determination Act (PSDA) of 1990 requires all Medicare- and Medicaid-funded health-care facilities to advise patients of their legal rights to refuse or accept medical treatment. Patients may prospectively determine and record their choices about end-of-life treatment through living wills and the assignment of a durable power of attorney for health care (Dimond, 1992; 1994).

THE LIVING WILL

The living will promotes the right of self-determination by preventing unwanted heroic medical interventions. The living-will statute offers competent individuals a mechanism by which to document the medical interventions that they do and do not want in case they become mentally incompetent and require medical technology to keep them alive.

DURABLE POWER OF ATTORNEY

A durable power-of-attorney document provides a means for control of the process and content of decision-making about medical interventions in case of an individual's mental incapacity by naming an authorized other person to make decisions consistent with the declarant's specific instructions as stated in this document.

Business affairs must be concluded after the death of an individual. It is not uncommon for bereaved survivors to engage in family conflicts while business affairs are being settled. All debts, taxes, funeral and administrative expenses must be paid, and the property owned by the deceased at the time of death must be distributed to others. The management, administration, and transfer functions necessary for this are accomplished through the probate process under the supervision of a court (Scheible, 1988).

WILLS

Individuals are free to distribute their property to anyone they wish according to the terms stated in a formal will. Wills are guided by statutory formalities that vary from one state to another. A formal will must be signed by at least two witnesses who stand to gain nothing as a result of the will. A will that does not comply with the statutory formalities has no legal effect, and the decedent's property will be transferred under the laws of intestacy. A person dying without a valid will is regarded as having died intestate. Intestacy statutes are drafted and enacted by state legislators. Although the details of these statutes vary from state to state, a surviving spouse and children are generally the preferred heirs.

WILL SUBSTITUTES

To avoid the expense and time of the probate process, individuals may chose to transfer their property to their heirs while they are still alive. State regulations guide this transfer process.

O AN OVERVIEW

- Bereavement may result in psychological growth, no substantial change, or an adverse change in health or functioning.

- Psychiatric complications of bereavement are among the more common disorders encountered in outpatient psychiatric settings and psychiatric consultation services.

- Secularization of American culture has diminished the role of religious organizations in supporting the bereaved.

- Mourning practices differ among various cultural groups, such as Orthodox Jews, Native Americans, African-Americans, persons of European descent, Hispanic-Americans, and Asian Americans.

- Rando's Assessment Guide is a framework for evaluating a bereaved individual in terms of three stages: avoidance, confrontation, and accommodation.

- Sadness and reactive depression must be differentiated in a bereaved individual, since depression should be treated.

- Anticipatory grief reactions are experienced by terminally ill patients and their family members.

- No single therapeutic approach is effective in all bereavement situations because an individual's grief response is influenced by multiple psychological, sociocultural, and developmental factors.

- Therapies for complicated grief include family-centered, Gestalt, cognitive (rational-emotive therapy and transactional analysis), and behavioral therapy.

- Many national organizations provide support and other social services to persons experiencing grief.

TD TERMS TO DEFINE

- anticipatory grief
- bereavement
- chronic mourning
- complicated grief and loss reactions
- complicated mourning
- death
- delayed grief
- disenfranchised grief

- dying
- grief
- loss
- mourning
- pathologic grief

Q STUDY QUESTIONS

Short Essay Responses

1. Select a cultural group that is unfamiliar to you. Search the literature about the beliefs and traditions of the group's culture and interview someone from the group about a loss experience. Plan a supportive bereavement intervention that incorporates what you have learned about the cultural group.

2. Describe supportive interventions that you can offer to family members who are experiencing anticipatory grief during the terminal illness of a beloved family member.

3. Differentiate characteristics of normal grief from those of pathologic grief. Describe how you would discuss this information with an individual who is newly bereaved.

Multiple Choice Questions

4. Identification of depression in bereaved individuals is complex because
   a. cognitive functioning in bereaved persons remains unchanged.
   b. symptoms of grief overlap with symptoms of depression.
   c. bereaved individuals may not openly disclose feelings.
   d. poor appetite and weight loss are usually absent in bereaved persons.

5. Family members caring for a terminally ill member need to know that
   a. unresolved family conflicts and relationship difficulties may exacerbate.
   b. a similar pattern of grief reaction will be shared by all family members.

   c. nonillness-related aspects of family life should be delayed until after the death.
   d. communication of feelings about expected loss is not recommended.

6. Which of the following is NOT a coping strategy used by family caregivers of terminally ill loved ones?
   a. Taking action to make loved one comfortable
   b. Use of distraction, such as reading and music
   c. Time management strategies
   d. Developing new interests

7. Anticipatory grief is a concept that
   a. applies only to terminally ill individuals.
   b. applies only to family members of terminally ill individuals.
   c. includes many symptoms of grief following a loss.
   d. applies to sudden traumatic loss situations.

8. The intensity of grief symptoms is NOT influenced by
   a. information about local sources of mutual support groups for survivors.
   b. concurrent stressors.
   c. strength of attachment to the deceased.
   d. circumstances surrounding the loss.

9. All of the following drugs might be used to treat bereavement complications EXCEPT
   a. monoamine oxidase inhibitors (MAOIs).
   b. antihistamines.
   c. antidepressants.
   d. benzodiazepines.

■ REFERENCES

Diagnostic and Statistical Manual of Mental Disorders, ed 4. Washington, DC, *American Psychiatric Association, 1994.*

Barbato A, Irwin HJ: Major therapeutic systems and the bereaved client. *Aust Psychol* 1992; 27(1):22–27.

Black D: The bereaved child. *J Child Psychol Psychiatry* 1979; 19:287–292.

Berger A, Badham P, Kutscher A, Berger J, Perry M, Beloff J (eds): *Perspectives on Death and Dying: Cross-cultural and Multidisciplinary Views.* Philadelphia, The Charles Press, 1989.

Bourne V, Meier J: What is happening? A booklet to be read to young children experiencing the terminal illness of a loved one. *Oncol Nurs Forum* 1988; 15(4):489–493.

Bowlby J: *Attachment and Loss: vol. 1. Attachment.* New York, Basic Books, 1969.

Bowlby J: *Attachment and Loss: Vol. 3. Loss, sadness, and Depression.* New York, Basic Books, 1980.

Brown MA, Powell-Cope G: Themes of loss and dying in caring for a family member with AIDS. *Res Nurs Health* 1993; 16:179–191.

Bugen L: Human grief: A model for prediction and intervention. *Am J Orthopsychiatry* 1977; 47(2):197–206.

Burkhardt M, Nagai-Jacobson MG: Dealing with spiritual concerns of clients in the community. *J Commun Health Nurs* 1985; 2(4):191–198.

Caplan G: *An Approach to Community Mental Health.* New York, Basic Books, 1961.

Christ GH, Siegel K, Freund B, Langosch D, Henderson S, Sperber D, Weinstein L: Impact of parental terminal cancer on latency-age children. *Am J Orthopsychiatry* 1993; 63(3):417–425.

Cowan PA: Individual and family life transitions: A propoal for a new definition, in Cowan PA, Hetherington M (eds): *Family Transitions.* Hillsdale, NJ, Lawrence Erlbaum Associates, 1991, pp. 3–30.

Decker S, Young E: Self-perceived needs of primary caregivers of home-hospice clients. *J Commun Health Nurs* 1991; 8(3):147–154.

Deutsch H: Absence of grief. *Psychoanal Q* 1937; 6:12–22.

Dimond EP: The oncology nurse's role in patient advance directives. *Oncol Nurs Forum* 1992; 19(6):891–896.

Dimond EP: Two years of the patient self-determination act. *Oncol Nurs Patient Treatment Support* 1994; 1(2):1–14.

Dobratz MC: Hospice nursing: Present perspectives and future directives. *Cancer Nurs* 1990; 13(2):116–122.

Doka KJ: *Disenfranchised Grief: Recognizing Hidden Sorrow.* Lexington, MA, DC Heath and Company, 1989.

Dufault K, Martocchio B: Hope: its spheres and dimensions. *Nurs Clin North Am* 1985; 20(2):379–391.

Ekberg J, Griffith N, Foxall M: Spouse burnout syndrome. *J Adv Nurs* 1986; 11:161–165.

Engel GL: Is grief a disease? A challenge for medical research. *Psychosom Med* 1961; 23:18–22.

Engel GL: *Psychological Development in Health and Disease.* Philadelphia, WB Saunders, 1962.

Engel GL: Grief and grieving. *Am J Nurs* 1964; 64:93–98.

Federal Family and Medical Leave Act. Public Law 103-3, 107 STAT.6, (U.S.C. 2101 ct. SEq.) (1993). United States.

Freud S: Mourning and melancholia, in Riviere J (Trans). *Collected papers,* vol 4. (Original work published in 1917). New York: Basic Books, 1959, pp. 152–170.

Fulton R, Fulton J: A psychosocial aspect of terminal care: Anticipatory grief. *Omega* 1971; 2:91–99.

Gaynor S: The long haul: The effects of home care on caregivers. *Image* 1990; 22(4):208–212.

Giacquinta (nee Stewart) B: Helping families face the crisis of cancer. *Am J Nurs* 1977; 77:1585–1588.

Giacquinta (nee Stewart) B: Researching the effects of AIDS on families. *Am J Hospice Care,* 1989; 6(3):31–36.

Giacquinta (nee Stewart) B: Psychosocial case report: Attachment responses in a family affected by AIDS. *AIDS Patient Care* 1990; 4(2):19–22.

Goldberg HS: Funeral and bereavement rituals of the Kota Indians and Orthodox Jews. *Omega* 1981; 12:117–128.

Herth K: The relationship between level of hope and level of coping response and other variables in patients with cancer. *Oncol Nurs Forum* 1989; 16(1):67–72.

Herth K: Fostering hope in terminally-ill people. *J Adv Nurs* 1990; 15:1250–1259.

Herth K: Hope in the family caregiver of terminally ill people. *J Adv Nurs* 1993; 8:538–548.

Hocker W: President's perspective. *Director,* 1989; 60(7):5,8.

Hull M: Coping strategies of family caregivers in hospice homecare. *Oncol Nurs Forum* 1992; 19(8):1179–1187.

Jacobs S: *Pathologic Grief—Maladaptation to Loss.* Washington, DC, American Psychiatric Press, 1993.

Jacobs SC, Hansen FF, Kasl SV, Ostfeid A, Berkman L, Kim K: Anxiety disorders during acute bereavement: risk and risk factors. *J Clin Psychiatry* 1990; 51:269–274.

Jacobs SC, Nelson JC, Zisook S: Treating depressions of bereavement with antidepressants: a pilot study. *Psychiatr Clin North Am* 1987; 10:501–510.

Johnson C, McGee M: *How Different Religions View Death and Afterlife.* Philadelphia, PA, The Charles Press, 1991.

Jones SA: Personal unity in dying: Alternative conceptions of the meaning of health. *J Adv Nurs* 1993; 18:98–94.

Krupp G: Maladaptive reactions to the death of a family member. *Soc Casework* 1972; 53:425–434.

Lebow GH: Facilitating adaptation in anticipatory mourning. *Soc Casework* 1976; 57:458–465.

Lev E: Dealing with loss: Concerns of patients and families in a hospice setting. *Clin Nurse Specialist* 1991; 5(2):87–93.

Lewis FM: Psychosocial transitions and the family's work in adjusting to cancer. *Semin Oncol Nurs* 1993; 9(2):127–129.

Lewis FM: Strengthening family supports: Cancer and the family. *CA* 1990; 65:158–165.

Lewis FM: Family level services for the cancer patient: Critical distinctions, fallacies, and assessment. *Cancer Nurs* 1983; 6:193–200.

Lindemann E: Symptomatology and management of acute grief. *Am J Psychiatry* 1944; 101:141–148.

Masters M, Shontz F: Identification of problems and strengths of the hospice client by clients, caregivers, and nurses. *Cancer Nurs* 1989; 12(40:226–235.

Martocchio B: Grief and bereavement: healing through hurt. *Nurs Clin North Am* 1985; 20(2):327–341.

Miller SI, Schoenfeld L: Grief in the Navajo: Psychodynamics and culture. *Int J Soc Psychiatry* 1973; 19:187–191.

Mor V: *Hospice Care Systems: Structure, Process, Costs and Outcome.* New York, Springer, 1987.

Neale RE: Initiatory grief, in Schoenberg B, Carr AC, Kutscher AH, Peretz D, Goldberg I (eds): *Anticipatory Grief* New York, Columbia University Press, 1974, pp. 333–342.

Northouse L: The impact of cancer on the family: an overview. *Int J Psychiatry Med* 1984; 14:215–243.

Oberst M, Thomas S, Ward S: Caregiving demands and appraisal of stress among family caregivers. *Cancer Nurs* 1990; 12(4):209–215.

Osterweis M, Solomon F, Green M, (eds): *Bereavement: Reactions, Consequences, and Care.* Washington, DC, National Academy Press, 1984.

Parkes CM: Effects of bereavement on physical and mental health—A study of the medical records of widows. *BMJ* 1964; 2:274–279.

Parkes CM: Psycho-social transitions: A field for study. *Soc Sci Med,* 1971; 5:101–115.

Parkes CM: *Bereavement: Studies of Grief in Adult Life.* New York, International Universities Press, 1972.

Parkes CM: Evaluation of bereavement service. *J Prev Psychiatry* 1981; 1:179.

Parkes CM: Bereavement as a psychosocial transition: Processes of adaptation to change. *J Soc Iss* 1988; 44(3):53–65.

Parkes CM, Weiss RS: *Recovery from Bereavement.* New York, Basic Books, 1983.

Pasternak RE, Reynolds CF, Schlernitzauer M, Hoch, CC, Buysse, DJ, Houck PR, Perel JM: Acute open-trial nortriptyline therapy of bereavement-related depression in late life. *J Clin Psychiatry* 1991; 52:307–310.

Pollock GH: Mourning and adaptation. *Int J Psychoanal* 1961; 42:341.

Pollock G: On mourning and anniversaries: The relationship of culturally constituted defense systems to intra-psychic adaptive processes. *Isr Ann Psychiatry* 1972; 10:9–40.

Rando TA: *Grief, Dying, and Death: Clinical Interventions for Caregivers.* Champaign, IL, Research Press Company, 1984.

Rando TA: *Treatment of Complicated Mourning.* Champaign, IL, Research Press, 1993.

Raphael B: Preventive intervention with the recently bereaved. *Arch Gen Psychiatry* 1977; 34:1450.

Raphael B: *The anatomy of bereavement: A handbook for the caring professions.* London: Hemisphere, 1983.

Raphael B, Middleton W, Dunne M, Martinek N, Smith S: Normal and pathological grief: The need for diagnostic criteria. Manuscript submitted for publication, 1990.

Redmond L: *Surviving: When Someone You Love was Murdered.*

Clearwater, FL, Psychological Consultation and Education Services, 1989.

Reimer J, Davies G, Martens N: Palliative care: The nurse's role in helping families through the transition of 'fading away'. *Cancer Nurs* 1991; 14(6):321–327.

Robinson K: Predictors of burden among wife caregivers. *Schol Inq Nurs Pract Int J* 1990; 4(3):189–203.

Sanders CM: Effects of sudden vs. chronic illness death on bereavement outcome. *Omega* 1982–1983; 13:227–241.

Sanders C: *Grief: The Mourning After.* New York, John Wiley & Sons, 1989.

Scanlon C: Creating a vision of hope: The challenge of palliative care. *Oncol Nurs Forum,* 1989; 16(4):491–496.

Scheible SS: Death and the law, in Wass H, Berardo FM, Neimeyer RA (eds): *Dying: Facing the Facts.* Washington, Hemisphere Publishing Corporation, 1988, pp. 301–319.

Schonfeld DJ: Talking with children about death. *J Pediatr Health Care* 1993; 7:269–274.

Schumacher KL, Meleis AI: Transitions: A central concept in nursing. *Image* 1994; 26(2):119–127.

Segal S, Fletcher M, Meekison WG: Survey of bereaved parents. *Can Med Assoc J* 1986; 134(1):38–42.

Siegel K, Mesagno FP, Karus D, Christ G, Banks K, Moynihan R: Psychosocial adjustment of children with a terminally ill parent. *J Am Acad Child Adolesc Psychiatry* 1992; 31(2):327–333.

Silverman P: In search of new selves: Accommodating to widowhood, in Bond LA, Wagner BM (eds): *Families in Transition: Primary Prevention Programs that Work.* Beverly Hills, CA, Sage, 1987.

Stewart BM: End-of-life family decision-making from disclosure of HIV through bereavement. *Schol Inq Nurs Pract* 1994; 8(4):321–352.

Strobe W, Strobe MS: *Bereavement and Health: the Psychological and Physical Consequences of Partner Loss.* New York, Cambridge University Press, 1987.

Sudnow D: *Passing On: The Social Organization of Dying.* Englewood Cliffs, NJ, Prentice-Hall, 1967.

Tripp-Reimer T, Brink P: Culture brokerage, in Bulechek G, McCloskey J, (eds): *Nursing Interventions Treatments for Nursing Diagnoses.* Philadelphia, WB Saunders, 1985.

Warner JE: Involvement of families in pain control of terminally ill patients. *Hospice J* 1992; 8(1–2):155–170.

Weisman A: *Coping with Cancer.* New York, McGraw Hill, 1979.

Wingate A, Lackey N: A description of needs of non-institutionalized cancer patients and their primary caregivers. *Cancer Nurs* 1989; 12(4):216–225.

Worden JW: *Grief Counseling and Grief Therapy,* ed. 2. New York, Springer Publishing Company, 1991.

Worden JW: *Grief Counseling and Grief Therapy,* ed. 1. New York, Springer Publishing Company, 1982.

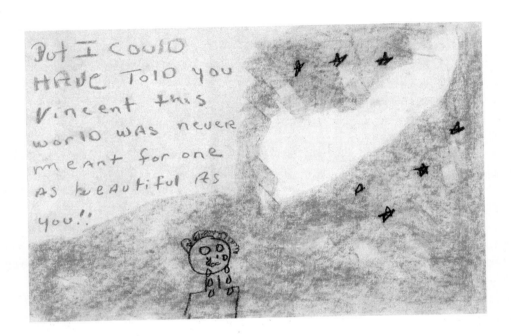

The child's sob in the silence curses deeper
Than the strong man in his wrath.

Elizabeth Barrett Browning (1806–1861)
The Cry of the Children

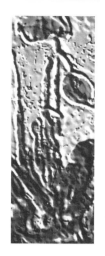

17

Childhood Disorders

Maureen P. McCausland / Laureen M. Burgess

The first children to receive psychiatric attention in America were troubled adolescents. In the 1890s the courts became concerned about such problematic teenagers and established the first juvenile court. In 1909, psychologist William Healy, in association with the Cook County Juvenile Court of Chicago, started a behavior clinic for the study of delinquents. It is from this development of what later became known as the Institute for Juvenile Research that the child guidance movement began. Healy's study of delinquency concluded that pathological behavior was the product of multiple factors, including the family (Healy, 1934). Neurological deficit, heredity, and organ impairment were deemphasized as causes of juvenile delinquency.

The field of child psychiatry was greatly influenced by the psychoanalytic school of thought. Sigmund Freud (1963) emphasized the crucial nature of childhood experience in adult mental health. Two European psychoanalysts, Anna Freud and Melanie Klein, influenced the development of child psychiatry in the 1920s. Anna Freud (1965) used play to communicate with children and to foster their understanding. Klein (1932) pioneered the use of play therapy with children in a way that was similar to the use of free association with adults. She regarded the child's play as a symbolic representation of unconscious content, and interpreted it as such directly to the child.

Jean Piaget (Ginsburg and Opper, 1979), a Swiss psychologist, studied the development of the child's perceptual and sensorimotor systems. The behaviorists Pavlov, Watson, and Skinner contributed the concept of stimulus-response, which has been used to modify troubled behavior in children (Levenson and Pope, 1995).

Historically, educators have presented the idea that children require learning as well as caring if they are to fully develop their potential. Binet and Binet (1916) and Catell (1980) were pioneers in the field of measuring intelligence in children.

Child-guidance clinics were established in the 1920s and 1930s in the United States, with services for children who were not delinquents. A multidisciplinary treatment team was introduced. Child psychiatrists, social workers, psychologists, educators, and criminal-justice professionals worked together to diagnose and treat the child, the family, and their environment. Today, children's services are provided by multidisciplinary teams in a variety of hospital and community settings.

The concepts of health and disease in children are different from those applicable to adults, and depend on the child's capacities at a particular stage of development, the current nature of family-transactional operations, and other factors. In assessing the child or adolescent psychiatric patient, the parameters of normal growth and development (Chapter 7) provide an initial framework. The nurse, however, must remember that among children and adolescents, the "normal" growth and developmental patterns vary from one individual to another.

PSYCHIATRIC DISORDERS ASSOCIATED WITH CHILDHOOD

Mental illness in children has a complex, multifactorial etiology. It cannot be stressed enough that emotional disorders among children usually have more than one etiologic component, including:

- Genetic background and family history of mental illness.
- Faulty training and faulty life experiences.
- Surface conflicts between children and parents that arise from such adjustment tasks as relations among siblings, school, and social and sexual development.
- Deeper conflicts within the child (the so-called neuroses).
- A difficulty associated with physical handicaps and disorders.
- Difficulties associated with severe mental disorders, such as psychoses.

The first category may have a role in the others; it is estimated that 80% of emotional problems in children are related to the second and third categories; 10% to the fourth category; and 10% to the fifth and sixth categories. Any combination of the above factors may contribute to a psychiatric disturbance arising in a child at any phase of its development.

ATTENTION DEFICIT–HYPERACTIVITY DISORDER

Children with attention deficit hyperactivity disorder are described as restless, inattentive, distractible, impulsive, and fidgety *(DSM-IV)*. They may be classified as having one of three subtypes of ADHD: attention deficit only; hyperactivity; or both, which is the most common form of the disorder. Previously, it was erroneously thought that children with ADHD had a brain dysfunction.

EPIDEMIOLOGY

Attention deficit hyperactivity disorder (ADHD) is generally more common in boys than in girls, at least when studied in the clinical setting. No real data exist about the prevalence of ADHD in boys in the general population or school setting. It has been estimated, however, that this disorder is more common in boys than girls, can be found in all socioeconomic groups, and has a prevalence of around 3–5% in school aged children (Huberman, 1995).

ETIOLOGICAL FACTORS AND FAMILY PATTERNS

Among children with ADHD, higher rates of the disorder have been shown in the immediate family. It has also been suggested that neurotransmitter abnormalities exist in ADHD, but this is not fully documented. Delayed or abnormal maturation of the frontal lobes of the brain may also cause this disorder. Other suggested causative factors include complications of pregnancy, maternal smoking or use of alcohol, long labor, malnutrition in infancy, lead poisoning, and phenylketonuria.

AGE OF ONSET AND COURSE

Attention deficit hyperactivity disorder manifests itself no later than age of 7 years. If "ADHD-like" symptoms develop after that, they are most likely from another disorder, possibly an adjustment disorder. Symptoms of ADHD must persist for at least 6 months and be extreme for the child's age and intelligence in order for the condition to be formally diagnosed. The symptoms do not have to be present all the time, but must be exhibited often.

IMPAIRMENT AND COMPLICATIONS

Possible symptoms of ADHD include restlessness, distractibility, difficulty in staying seated, difficulty in waiting in lines, impulsive speech, difficulty in following instructions, a short attention span, seeming inability to listen, forgetfulness, difficulty in organizing oneself, losing things, and making careless mistakes. The symptoms of ADHD generally occur in different situations, and often vary from one time to another.

The child with ADHD does not complete tasks and has difficulty organizing and completing work. The work is often messy and done carelessly and impulsively. Performance at school is usually impaired. The group-learning situation in the classroom tends to exaggerate the attentional difficulties of children with this disorder.

Most children in whom ADHD is diagnosed have experienced difficulties with learning, achievement, and finishing school work by the time they are identified as having this disorder. Further effects of ADHD are depression and low self-esteem. Many affected children have problems forming friendships, since they often appear to be "bossy," loud, and uncooperative in social situations.

NURSING ASSESSMENT AND NURSING DIAGNOSES

Multiple sources of data should be used to assess whether a child has ADHD. Teacher and parent evaluations, should be done using standardized tests such as

TABLE 17-1. ASSESSMENT TESTS AND SCALES FOR CHILDREN

Intelligence Tests

Bayley Scales of Infant Development (2nd) for 1 month-3½ years
Wechsler Preschool and Primary Scale of Intelligence-revised (WPPSI-R) for 4-6 years
Wechsler Intelligence Scale for Children-III (WISC-III)
Stanford-Binet for 2 years-adult
Leiter International Performance Scale for 2-13 years (does not require verbal language)
Peabody Picture Vocabulary Test-revised (PPVT-R) for 4-adult (only measures receptive vocabulary)
Raven's Coloured Progressive Matrices-for 5-11 years (test of non-verbal reasoning)

Neuropsychological Tests

Visual-Motor Integration assessed by copying figures, Bender Visual Motor Gestalt, Beery Visual Motor Integration
Batteries of tests for the detection of suspected brain damage:
Reiton-Indiana test battery, Halstead-Reiton test battery, Luria-Nebraska neuropsychologic battery

Academic Achievement Tests

Tests for reading, math, spelling and written language achievement such as:
Woodcock-Johnson, Wide Range Achievement (WRAT), Stanford Achievement Test, Wechsler Individual Achievement Test (WIAT)

Personality Assessment

Children's Apperception Test (CAT)
Rorschach inkblots
Sentence completion
Draw-a-person (DAP)
Personality Inventory for Children (PIC)

Adaptation

Vineland Adaptive Behavior Scales
(Questionnaires to assess daily living skills, communication and socialization)

Child Behavior Checklist (CBCL)

Parent report form which asks about the child's usual activities and relationships, and has a 113 item symptom checklist (Achenbach and Edlebroch, 1983)

Conner's Parent Questionnaire/Conner's Teacher Rating Scale

Short rating scale inquiring about presence and severity of symptoms of Attention Deficit Hyperactivity Disorder. Although not diagnostic, it can be used in assessment, and to follow effectiveness of treatment

Denver Developmental Screening Test

Used frequently by pediatricians, this test includes simple ways to test a 1 month to 5 year old child's development in language, gross motor, fine motor and personal-social areas. Requires special items (wooden blocks, specific pictures, etc.)

the Child Behavior Checklist (Auchenbach and Edlebroch, 1983). Psychological testing is useful for evaluating the child's intelligence quotient (IQ) and identifying any accompanying specific developmental disorders. Tests useful in assessments of children are listed in Table 17–1 (Huberman, 1995).

■ PERVASIVE DEVELOPMENTAL DISORDERS

Pervasive developmental disorders are characterized by very early distortions, based on the child's chronological and mental ages, in three areas of development: social interaction; behavioral patterns; and communication, including attention, perception, and reality testing. Of the pervasive developmental disorders, this section focuses on **autism.** Children with autism often appear physically normal and come from loving families, but behave in peculiar and disturbing ways.

EPIDEMIOLOGY

Autistic disorders occur in 4 children out of 10,000, with boys being more likely to be affected than girls, in a ratio of 3 or 4 to 1. Other pervasive development disorders occur at a rate of 10 to 20 cases per 10,000 children (Dulcan, 1994).

ETIOLOGIC FACTORS AND FAMILY PATTERNS

In the past, it was believed that autism was rooted in poor parenting; much blame was placed on a cold, unemotional mother figure. Today it is believed that autism has only biological causes. It seems more common in children with certain chromosomal abnormalities, such as Fragile X syndrome. Some cases of autism stem from maternal infections during pregnancy (rubella) or trauma to the developing central nervous system. A genetic link is found in cases in which the family history includes autism, dyslexia, lung disorders, and mental retardation. Families with one autistic child are at somewhat greater risk of having another child born with this disorder. Children born with autism may be mentally retarded, and develop seizures in later childhood (Dulcan, 1994).

AGE OF ONSET AND COURSE

Autism is typically first seen in infancy or early childhood, although some autistic children may appear normal until age 2 or 3 and then show autistic behavior more vividly at the point at which their communication and social-interaction skills are expected to become more advanced.

E CASE EXAMPLE

▶ ATTENTION DEFICIT HYPERACTIVITY DISORDER

Andy was an 11-year-old white male who had exhibited problems since age 6. Problems his mother reported were constant fidgeting, inattention, impulsivity, and difficulty in following direction. When playing with other children, he often interrupted and was bossy. Other children teased him. The teacher reported that he had difficulty in concentrating and staying on a task, failed to complete assignments, and was over-active. He was performing below his grade level despite being of average intelligence. Andy had lived with his biological parents until he was 2 years of age, when they divorced. He then lived with his mother for 6 months and subsequently moved in with his father when his mother had financial difficulties. Both Andy and his mother report that his father was physically abusive. He returned to his mother at age 6 and has remained with her. His mother had several male friends live with her in the household during this time, and married one of them 6 months ago. Andy gets along with his stepfather.

Andy frequently over-reacts to requests asked by his parents, teachers, and peers. He has been increasingly aggressive. On the day of his admission to the child/adolescent inpatient program, he became angry at his teacher and overturned his desk. For approximately 2 weeks he has been making statements and writing notes about wishing he were dead. He has been on methylphenidate (Ritalin) 10 mg TID for 2 years.

▶ NURSING DIAGNOSES FOR ANDY:

- Risk for violence: self-directed or directed at others.
- Ineffective individual coping.
- Impaired social interactions.
- Disturbance in self-esteem.
- Ineffective family coping.

This case was contributed by Roberta M. Kepner.

▶ NURSING INTERVENTION

- Keep patient safe
  Provide safety with 30-minute checks; gradually increase checking intervals as teaching increases.
  Educate patient about safe and unsafe behavior in brief teaching sessions and by discussing his behavior with him.
  Hold patient accountable to rules and structure of milieu; for example, have him remain in open, visible area for nurses to observe; impose consequence as soon as possible following undesired behavior.
- Physical care
  Observe patient's behavior in milieu and record.
  Obtain baseline height, weight, blood pressure, heart rate.
  Parent education
  Using patient-teaching materials, help parents to understand ADHD.
  Engage parents to visit by seeking them out and asking how they perceive patient's progress. Inquire if parents are interested in attending parent-support group; provide information.
- Discussion in team meeting about patient assignment to group.
  Group therapy—relationships in group will mimic family and peer relationships.
  Problem-solving—patient is taught a systematic way to solve problems.
  Anger control—patient is taught to recognize physical and emotional signs of anger in self; coping skills; anger management; and relaxation techniques.
  Social skills—patient is taught good communication skills, eye contact, sharing, and cooperation
- Communicate with school personnel. Share strategies for classroom management with school personnel.

IMPAIRMENT AND COMPLICATIONS

As the autistic child develops, several abnormal behaviors become evident. The child often has an aversion or indifference to being held or hugged; will not engage in imaginative or social play; often clings to an inanimate object; exhibits delayed or abnormal language and speech abilities; and shows hand-flapping and head-banging tics.

NURSING ASSESSMENT AND NURSING DIAGNOSES

Children with autism generally exhibit more bizarre or uneven behaviors than those who are mentally retarded. Differentiating between schizophrenia and autism can be difficult in the very young or in nonverbal children. A thorough developmental history and medical examination are needed to show that autism actually exists, and that a child's behavior is not due to sensory deficits, metabolic disorders, or degenerative diseases.

■ MENTAL RETARDATION

The DSM-IV outlines **mental retardation** as significantly subaverage intellectual functioning, with onset before age 18, accompanied by impairment in at least two of the following areas: communication, self-

E CASE EXAMPLE

▶ ATTENTION DEFICIT HYPERACTIVITY DISORDER

Julie B. is an 8-year-old child who has been living with her natural father and step-mother for the past 2 months. Before that, and after her parents separation and divorce 5 years ago, she had lived with her maternal grandmother in a southern state. Julie's mother had custody of her, but shortly after the separation the mother moved, leaving Julie with her grandmother. Julie's mother has since remarried and has another child. Her contacts with Julie have been sporadic, and she made no attempt to regain custody until Julie's father filed for custody of the child.

Julie's father was transferred to the mid-west shortly after his separation from her mother, but remained in constant contact with Julie through weekly phone calls and bi-monthly visits. Prior to his recent attempt to gain custody, his relationship with the maternal grandmother was cordial, although his relationship with Julie's mother was strained. After the court battle, which resulted in Julie's father obtaining custody, the relationships of Julie's father with her mother and grandmother have been very poor.

For several years, Julie had exhibited problem behaviors at school and at home. At school, she demanded excessive teacher attention, left her seat unexcused, disturbed others, was inattentive to instruction, was restless and overactive, had a short attention span, and was passively uncooperative. She also had difficulty relating to peers, was unaccepted by them, and had few friends. At home she frequently threw temper tantrums and was openly defiant and argumentative. She also had difficulty sleeping, and sometimes reverted to regressive behavior, such as thumb sucking when upset. Developmentally she had reached all of the childhood milestones at about the normal time. Nine months ago, at her father's insistence, Julie was seen by her pediatrician and was referred to a neuropsychologist for testing. She was diagnosed as having attention deficit—hyperactivity disorder and was begun on therapy with methylphenidate and enrolled in a behavior-modification program. Her behavior at home improved, and her behavior in school improved somewhat, as measured by the Child Behavior Checklist (Achenbach & Edelbrock, 1978).

Julie's father and stepmother sought counseling because of her continued disruptive behavior at home, which became worse before and after visits with her mother and grandmother. Moreover, although she seemed to be functioning adequately in school, her peer relationships remained poor. A nursing assessment was done with the family by helping them to construct a family genogram. The goal was to assist the family to see its relationships while making the child the focus of these. The assessment revealed that Julie was the focus of all anxiety in the extended family system. It would be essential for the relationships between Julie's father, mother, and grandmother to improve before Julie's symptoms decreased and she was able to make a smooth transition between the three homes.

▶ NURSING DIAGNOSIS: INEFFECTIVE FAMILY COPING: COMPROMISED

One therapeutic goal in Julie's case was to coach her father toward improving his relationships with Julie's mother and grandmother. Although this was a difficult task, it was essential to remove Julie as the focus of these family triangles. Julie's behavior would be a good barometer for the effect of her father's efforts. Outcome criteria were:

- Julie would experience less distress surrounding visits with her mother and grandmother, as evidenced by an absence of temper tantrums, by achieving the goals on her behavior chart in 80% of instances, by a lack of insomnia, and by an absence of thumb sucking before and after her visits.
- Julie's behavior at home would improve according to these same criteria;
- Julie's performance at school would continue to be good, as evidenced by daily reports from her teachers, functioning at her appropriate grade level, and satisfactory behavior on her report card.
- Julie's peer relationships would improve, with the formation of at least one peer relationship in the following 3 months.

Once the immediate problem of Julie's behavior was resolved, her father and stepmother would need to decide whether they wanted to continue their work with their family of origin.

Case contributed by Carole S. Burdge

---

care, home living, social skills, community use, self-direction, health and safety, functional academics, leisure, and work. Along with these deficits in adaptive functioning, the affected individual's IQ is 70 or less.

Some children may test in the retarded range without being clinically mentally retarded. This often includes children who are severely neglected and may suffer from specific developmental disorders. Other children may be diagnosed as having other disorders, such as ADHD, when in fact they are mentally retarded. The incidence of emotional disorders in mentally retarded individuals is also very high

(i.e., from three to five times that in the general population).

Four degrees of severity of mental retardation exist, ranging from mild to profound (DSM-IV, 1994).

	IQ	Proportion of Retarded Population
Mild	50–55 to 70	85%
Moderate	35–40 to 50–55	10%
Severe	20–25 to 35–40	3–4%
Profound	Below 20–25	1–2%'

E CASE EXAMPLE

▶ AUTISM

James, 4-years-old, is brought for evaluation because of delayed language development. Unlike his older brother, who spoke full narratives when he was 4, James speaks only a few isolated words spontaneously. His mother reports that at times he repeats sentences from commercial jingles he hears on television. He is withdrawn and won't play with his brother or other children. Instead, he amuses himself in playing with crayons, often lining them up in long rows but rarely coloring with them. He loves puzzles and can complete complicated ones that baffle his sibling. He sometimes has temper tantrums, which appear to be caused by his mother's attempts to rearrange items in the home. After describing her son's problems, she says sadly, "I think I've known some-thing was wrong from the beginning. He isn't like other children. He doesn't care about people."

Nursing problems of such children are complex and require many levels of intervention. Emphasis on supporting ego development is central to care, with the child encouraged to engage in appropriate behavior, decrease clinging, and reduce anxiety. Reducing sensory stimulation and establishing daily routines may help. The most effective treatment for autism is a specialized educational program that combines development in social, language, and behavioral skills. This type of program can begin as early as age 2, and such early intervention is known to be vital to helping the child avoid institutionalization.

EPIDEMIOLOGY

In the United States, approximately 1 to 3% of the population is mentally retarded. In 1983 there were 6-million mentally retarded persons, which is twice the combined total of those who suffer from blindness, poliomyelitis, cerebral palsy, and rheumatic heart disease. Males predominate over females in a ratio of 1.5 to 1 (Flohr & Phillips, 1995).

ETIOLOGIC FACTORS AND FAMILY PATTERNS

In the case of mild retardation, the genetic endowment of the parents may already be poor for intellectual competence, or psychosocial influences such as poverty and deficient external stimulation may be factors. Moderate to profound mental retardation is generally linked to genetic abnormalities or metabolic, traumatic, and toxic injury. The most frequent genetic disorder causing mental retardation is Down's syndrome. This syndrome produces physical characteristics that allow it to be easily diagnosable at birth, but the future intellectual and social functioning of the affected individual cannot be predicted with certainty at that time. Children born with Down's syndrome can have an IQ ranging from 0 to 100, with the mean at the high end of the moderately retarded range.

AGE OF ONSET AND COURSE

The diagnosis of mental retardation is made if an individual meets the description listed above before the age of 18. For the vast majority of such persons—the mildly

E CASE EXAMPLE

▶ MENTAL RETARDATION

Tommy, a well-adjusted 10-year-old boy, was noted by his teacher to be a slow learner. She asked for an evaluation of him and consultation with the school psychologist. Testing indicated that Tommy had an IQ in the range of 63 to 69. His teacher continued to give him individually paced instruction in her class. A similar approach, with individual tutoring as needed, was followed when he reached high school. The boy enjoyed participation on the track team and was accepted by his peers. His family encouraged his interest in fishing, and at age 16 he began to learn about commercial fishing at a local firm. When he was subsequently hired by the firm, he told his family, "I may never make it to manager, but I'll always make a decent living." He later married and had two children.

The existence of special-education programs has been critical to allowing many mentally retarded individuals to function in society. Specialized infant and toddler stimulation programs can reduce the degree of deficits experienced by the child. Today, only children who are severely retarded, with additional medical disorders or severe behavioral problems, are institutionalized.

retarded—difficulties begin during the school years. During this period, the mentally retarded child reaches the age at which the ability to function independently becomes important yet may not be possible.

Several misconceptions exist about the limitations produced by mental retardation. For example, many people believe that all mentally retarded individuals are alike, and that their problems cannot be alleviated. The case example illustrates that not all mentally retarded individuals are limited to functioning "outside of society," but can instead lead essentially "normal," highly functional lives.

■ SPECIFIC DEVELOPMENTAL DISORDERS (SDD)

Children with **specific developmental disorders** show a developmental delay that leads to functional impairments. The delay must not be attributable to a physical disorder, pervasive developmental disorder, mental retardation, or inadequate educational opportunity. Specific developmental disorders are generally centered around reading, arithmetic, language, or verbal articulation (DSM-IV).

ETIOLOGICAL FACTORS

Genetic factors are suggested as playing a role in specific developmental disorders, since members of certain families exhibit a prevalence of these disorders. The disorders are presumed to relate to delayed or abnormal maturation of areas within cerebral cortex. Their etiology is complex, and it is not clear whether their cause is biologic or nonbiologic.

AGE OF ONSET AND COURSE

No information is available about the age of onset of specific developmental disorders. Generally, they are first seen when a child reaches school age and shows developmental delays. Children do not outgrow these disorders; if they are not treated, they may experience difficulties into adulthood.

IMPAIRMENT AND COMPLICATIONS

It is common for a child to have more than one specific developmental disorder. Secondary symptoms are behavioral problems, low self-esteem, and demoralization, which can be dramatically reduced by the early diagnosis and treatment of these disorders.

NURSING ASSESSMENTS AND NURSING DIAGNOSIS

The diagnostic tools for identifying specific developmental disorders include IQ tests; academic achievement tests; language, speech, and motor-function tests; neurological examinations; and school attendance and performance reports. Visual and hearing tests are also necessary to rule out impairments of these systems as the cause of a disorder.

RECOMMENDED TREATMENT

The care of patients with specific developmental disorders is often provided by a specialized, multidisciplinary team. Nurses provide the support necessary for patients to cope with their disability. The emphasis is on the exploration of feelings; structuring of situations so that the patient can gain mastery of them; and promoting peer relationships. Other techniques useful in treating specific developmental disorders incorporate behavior modification to help the child practice and learn skills that have been difficult; special education classes; and physical, language, and/or occupational therapy.

■ CONDUCT DISORDERS

Children with **conduct disorders** (CD) have a repetitive and persistent pattern of disruptive, willfully disobedient behavior. This pattern involves a violation of basic age-appropriate norms and social rules. A significant minority of children with conduct disorders become substance abusers or develop antisocial personality disorders (DSM-IV).

EPIDEMIOLOGY

From 3 to 7% of children have conduct disorders. Such disorders, more common in boys than in girls, have become the most common reasons for referrals to child psychiatric clinics and hospitals (Huberman, 1995).

ETIOLOGICAL FACTORS AND FAMILY PATTERNS

No known single cause and no particular combination of factors are present in every case of conduct disorder. Oppositional defiant disorder and attention deficit–hyperactivity disorder often precede conduct disorders. Conduct disorders may also result from mania, depression, or psychosis. Some combination of the following factors generally leads to a conduct disorder (Dulcan, 1994).

- Temperament; child's adaptability, high-activity level, intense reactivity.
- Parental attention to problem behavior rather than good behavior; lack of adequate discipline, instead discipline is ineffective, inconsistent, too lax, or too punitive.
- Poor peer-group identification; the individual belongs to a delinquent group of children.

- Genetic predisposition.
- Modeling of parent's negative behavior.
- Poverty.
- Parental marital problems.
- Placement outside the home at an early age.
- Low IQ

AGE OF ONSET AND COURSE

Conduct disorder is usually diagnosed in school-age children. Younger children diagnosed as having this disorder are often aggressive boys with a poor prognosis. Rule-violating behavior is graded on a continuum; and is determined according to certain acts performed by the child at certain ages. These acts may include stealing, lying, drug use, running away, low achievement in school, truancy, fire-setting, vandalism, cruelty to animals, bullying, forcing sexual activities on others, and physical aggression. For a child to be diagnosed as having a conduct disorder, three or more of the foregoing criteria must have been present in the previous 12 months, with at least one criterion having been met in the previous 6 months (DSM-IV). Not all children who exhibit these behaviors named above have conduct disorder. A single such act may be seen as a childhood adjustment disorder, and several such acts could be diagnosed as an adjustment disorder with disturbance of conduct.

IMPAIRMENT AND COMPLICATIONS

Many children with conduct disorders seem to lack appropriate feelings of remorse, guilt, empathy, and responsibility for their behavior. They may also exhibit tantrums, cheating, low frustration levels, irritability, provocativeness, and an inability to delay gratification. Sexual precociousness and promiscuous sexual activity are often seen. Poor social skill with peers and adults is also common.

NURSING ASSESSMENT AND NURSING DIAGNOSIS

Assessment interviews with children who may have a conduct disorder can be difficult, since they often attempt to deceive people, show a false bravado and tough exterior, and are unwilling to let go of their defenses. The case example below describes assessment and treatment techniques for a child with a conduct disorder.

Treatment of a child with CD needs to be multifaceted, with first consideration given to diagnosing associated, potentially treatable conditions, both common (depression) and less common (seizure disorders). Educational intervention for learning disabilities and out-of-home placement for children in abusive or negligent environments are important.

It must be emphasized that the case of the child with a conduct disorder requires consistency on the part of both primary-care providers and limit-setting for impulsive, egocentric, or aggressive behavior. Feelings evoked in the care staff by such patients often include anger, fear, and frustration. The staff must have an opportunity to identify and express such reactions in supervision in order to prevent them from acting out their feelings with the patient. Therapeutically, it is essential that patients feel and believe that the care staff can limit their inappropriate behavior.

E CASE EXAMPLE

▶ CONDUCT DISORDER

Sam, who is 11 years old, is admitted to an inpatient child psychiatry unit for behavioral changes that have begun within the past 6 months. He has been oppositional and defiant at home; he has poor impulse control; vandalizes property; and is difficult to engage in cooperative play and social interaction with his peers. He frequently becomes physically aggressive. During the assessment process, he repeatedly answers questions by saying "I don't know" or "I don't care." Sam's mother accompanies him to the interview and states that Sam has no history of psychiatric problems and no medical problems; that his school grades are Bs and Cs; that he is developmentally on target for his age; and that a traumatic event in his life is a parental divorce, leaving his mother to raise seven children on her own. Sam tends to be a loner with only a few friends. He typically prefers to play with his siblings.

Sam is diagnosed as having conduct disorder. He shows a potential for violence, poor peer relationships, poor role identity, and underlying anger. He begins treatment in several different programs:

- Group therapy, to help him role play and express feelings appropriately.
- Group play therapy, to assess his ability to engage in cooperative and creative play with peers and to promote sharing and the ability to follow group activities
- Creative Art therapy, to encourage his expression of emotions and ideas through art, music, or movement.

One-to-one play therapy with the psychiatrist and medication therapy were also instituted. Goals for Sam were established to help him function more appropriately with others, and an evaluation system was set up to monitor his progress.

■ SEPARATION ANXIETY DISORDER

Separation anxiety disorder involves excessive anxiety about separation from parents, other attachment figures, the home, or other familiar surroundings. When separation occurs, the child with separation anxiety disorder often panics and shows a reaction that is beyond what is expected for the child's developmental level. All children experience some sort of developmentally expected separation anxiety during infancy, which may continue through the ages of 4 or 5. Separation anxiety disorder is the persistence or return of fears of separation after a child would be expected to have outgrown them (Diagnostic and Statistical Manual, Fourth Edition, 1994).

EPIDEMIOLOGY

From 2 to 15% of children have anxiety disorders, with separation anxiety disorder being the most common such disorder. This condition is one of the few childhood disorders that is more prevalent in girls than in boys (Huberman, 1995).

ETIOLOGICAL FACTORS AND FAMILY PATTERNS

A strong familial link exists between separation anxiety disorder and other anxiety disorders. Families of children with separation anxiety disorder also have increased rates of panic disorder, agoraphobia, depression, and alcoholism.

AGE OF ONSET AND COURSE

The onset of separation anxiety disorder occurs before the age of 18, and its early onset occurs before the age of 6. The disturbance must last for at least 4 weeks to be classified as a true separation anxiety disorder. The prognosis is better when the disorder appears in a younger child, and worsens as the child gets older.

IMPAIRMENT AND COMPLICATIONS

A child with separation anxiety disorder may be reluctant to go to school, fear being alone, have difficulty sleeping alone, have separation nightmares, and even develop physical symptoms when faced with an impending separation from an attachment figure. Other disorders commonly present with separation anxiety disorder are depression and other anxiety disorders.

As seen in this case, intervention with children suffering from separation anxiety disorder is aimed at reducing the level of the child's anxiety. Progress with treatment cannot be attained while the child is experiencing severe anxiety. First, basic trust must be established with a minimum number of care-givers. The growing perception that the attachment figure always returns is a major step for the child. Sometimes a staff member stays with the child until he or she falls asleep. Play therapy and stories such as "Hansel and Gretel" provide an opportunity for the symbolic expression of fears and mastery over the child's situation.

■ OPPOSITIONAL DEFIANT DISORDER (ODD)

Oppositional defiant disorder (ODD) is a relatively new diagnostic category characterized by the behavioral traits of milder forms of conduct disorder. The behavior of children with oppositional defiant disorder is not as extreme as that of conduct disorder and does not appear to violate the rights of others to the same extent. Largely, the child with oppositional defiant disorder exhibits behavior that is in opposition to authority figures.

EPIDEMIOLOGY

From 6 to 10% of young persons have oppositional defiant disorder; males with the disorder outnumber females in a ratio of 2 or 3 to 1. The disorder is quite common in psychiatric clinical settings. (Dulcan, 1994; Huberman, 1995).

ETIOLOGICAL FACTORS AND FAMILY PATTERNS

Oppositional defiant disorder may be linked to an inherited quality of temperament. Children may imitate parental behavior resembling that seen in the disorder, and parents may fail to reward good behavior and set clear, consistent limits.

AGE OF ONSET AND COURSE

No age of onset has been identified for oppositional defiant disorder, although negative behavior and tantrums are normal for children under the age of 3. However, the same behavior exhibited after this age can be an indicator of the disorder. Children who show behavior resembling that of oppositional defiant disorder but only when in school may have a specific developmental disorder or mental retardation.

IMPAIRMENT AND COMPLICATIONS

Children with oppositional defiant disorder display chronic stubbornness, negativism, provocativeness, hostility, and defiance. They are difficult to manage in the home, but can also be a problem in school and with peers. They tend to resist compliance at all costs, even

E CASE EXAMPLE

▶ SEPARATION ANXIETY

Sierra is an attractive, healthy, 30-month-old child who presents at a child health clinic for a routine examination. As she and her mother approach the examination room, Sierra begins to cry, then to sob uncontrollably, and throws herself to the floor. She refuses to have blood drawn from her or to be seen by the physician. Her mother complains that Sierra has been terrified of doctors and nurses since a recent hospitalization. The clinic staff try to comfort her, and when this fails reschedule Sierra's visit for another day. Her mother is asked to bring Sierra to the clinic office later that same day to talk with the nurse.

A month before her visit, Sierra was hospitalized for pneumonia and dehydration. She remained in the hospital for 3 days and was treated with intravenous fluids and antibiotics. While hospitalized, she was very quiet and withdrawn. Her mother, a single parent, works during the day and was not able to spend much time with her in the hospital. Since returning home Sierra has had problems sleeping and eating, and clings to her mother. She lives alone with her mother and before her hospitalization had been attending a day care center while her mother worked.

▶ NURSING ASSESSMENT

During the assessment interview, the nurse met with Sierra's mother. The nurse asked about Sierra's recent hospital experience, previous illnesses or hospitalizations, family interactions, coping patterns, past experiences with separation from her mother, and other questions that would provide information about Sierra's level of functioning and her recent anxieties. The nurse also interviewed Sierra, but was unable to obtain additional information from her. Sierra was quiet and attentive, but would say no more than a few words to the nurse.

▶ NURSING DIAGNOSIS

Anxiety related to Sierra's recent hospitalization.

▶ RECOMMENDED TREATMENT

The nurse suggested structured play therapy sessions that would provide Sierra with an opportunity to act out her anxieties and fears in a safe, developmentally appropriate way. After explaining the purpose of the therapy to the child and her mother, the nurse scheduled the first of six play therapy sessions.

The child was seen twice each week. The sessions were held in a clinic conference room, with a doll family, stuffed animals, a doctor's kit, toy stethoscopes, an old tympanic thermometer, band aids, and other hospital-related materials. Because Sierra was hesitant to leave her mother, the conference-room door was left open and her mother seated directly outside the room. The nurse told Sierra that she could play with anything in the room. Sierra walked around the room for several minutes before choosing to play with a stuffed animal. During the second session Sierra cautiously approached the various medically related items with her "favorite" stuffed animal in hand. During the remaining sessions Sierra "examined" her stuffed animal, took its temperature, gave it injections, and bandaged it repeatedly. She talked to the stuffed animal and treated it like a patient.

During the play therapy sessions the nurse quietly observed Sierra, answered questions the child raised, reflected back feelings that the child expressed, and occasionally became the "patient." Sierra's mother remained closeby, but the conference room door was closed by the third session. By the sixth session the child lost interest in playing doctor and was looking for other toys. The child's mother reported that Sierra's behavior had returned to normal and that she had returned to day care.

Play therapy has become one of the most popular clinical modalities for therapists working with children. Providing a child with a safe, accepting, and friendly environment encourages the child to communicate his or her feeling, wishes, fears, and fantasies through the natural act of play. Current research suggests that play therapy will realize more of its promise as it expands its focus to include the family context.

This case was contributed by Kathryn Balcziunas.

---

when cooperation would be in their best interest. They often have attention deficit-hyperactivity disorder, with other traits including frequent loss of temper, argumentativeness, vindictiveness, and blaming.

NURSING ASSESSMENT AND NURSING DIAGNOSIS

Oppositional defiant disorder is difficult to assess if the child is calm, relaxed, and not in the presence of familiar people. If demands are made on the child and the family is present, the behavior characteristic of the disorder will manifest itself.

Treatment requires patience and continual acceptance of the child regardless of the negative behavior it displays. Structuring a corrective life experience through behavior modification has proven useful. Parents, and possibly teachers, should be taught methods for reinforcing good behavior and helping the child to find appropriate alternatives to negative behavior.

■ PHOBIAS

A phobia is a specific, persistent fear that is disproportionate, to the danger that activates it. In children, this fear leads to difficulty in functioning at school or in social situations. Phobias persist because avoiding the feared object reduces the child's anxiety.

EPIDEMIOLOGY

Girls report phobias more often than do boys. It is not certain whether this is due to boys' role-related resistance to reporting fears.

AGE OF ONSET AND COURSE

Fears in children vary according to their age, and are usually quite normal. The diagnosis of phobia largely depends on how the child responds to a fear rather than to the object of the fear. Infants tend to fear loud noises and the loss of physical support. Toddlers (age 1 to 3) are afraid of storms, the dark, separation from parents, and some animals. Three- to 5-year-olds experience fears similar to those of toddlers, but are also afraid of monsters. School-age children are concerned about bodily injury, being punished or kidnaped, getting sent to the principal's office, and academic or social failure.

NURSING INTERVENTION

Nursing interventions for childhood phobias are directed at decreasing fear and anxiety. The appropriate interventions are selected through team discussions in which mental-health practitioners identify a consistent approach to the child.

■ ENURESIS

Enuresis is repeated, involuntary urination into the bed or clothing after the age of 5 years.

EPIDEMIOLOGY

Urinary control is generally achieved between 2 and 3 years of age. By age 4, most children are continent throughout the day. Nocturnal continence is more difficult to achieve and is more of a problem to achieve than daytime continence. Boys are slower to reach continence than girls. Among 5-year-olds, 14% of girls and boys wet their beds once a month. Ten percent of first graders are nocturnally enuretic. At age 14, 1% of boys and 0.5% of girls remain enuretic. The rate of spontaneous remission of nocturnal enuresis is high (Dulcan, 1994).

ETIOLOGICAL FACTORS AND FAMILY PATTERNS

Enuresis has been linked to family genetics, psychological disorders, and physiological problems. Seventy-five percent of enuretic young persons have a parent with a history of enuresis or a family history of this problem. Some of the childhood factors related to enuresis are: attention deficit-hyperactivity disorder, oppositional defiant disorder, abuse, witnessing domestic violence, and adjustment disorder. Physiological links are delayed maturation of bladder control mechanisms, a small bladder, and constipation. Improper toilet-training techniques can also increase the rate of enuresis.

AGE OF ONSET AND COURSE

True enuresis occurs when a child reaches the age of 5 and experiences incontinence twice a week for 3 consecutive months, or exhibits a sudden, marked impairment of bladder control.

IMPAIRMENT AND COMPLICATIONS

Enuresis may result in significant family conflict, with the child being ashamed, teased by peers, and having low self-esteem.

NURSING ASSESSMENT AND NURSING DIAGNOSIS

As noted earlier, enuresis has psychological, physical, and physiological roots. When the diagnosis is made, treatment will depend on the information gathered from examination of the child. The clinician must differentiate enuresis caused by such medical factors as urethritis caused by a bubble bath from enuresis caused by urinary tract infection, diabetes, seizure disorder, and genitourinary malformation.

RECOMMENDED TREATMENT

Treatment of enuresis requires patience and support. The family environment must be flexible enough to allow the child to assume some control over the condition (allowing the child to change his or her own sheets), and must never involve ridicule of the child. A system of rewards should be attempted. Also, medications may help in treating the disorder, although it usually returns when they are discontinued.

■ ENCOPRESIS

Encopresis is the involuntary pattern of passing feces into clothing or in other inappropriate places (closet, floor) after age 4.

EPIDEMIOLOGY

Bowel control is usually reached between 30 months and 4 years of age. Encopresis affects 1.5% of children after age 5, and this percentage decreases as age increases. The condition is more frequent in boys than in girls in a ratio of 6 to 1. One-fourth of encropretic children are also enuretic (Dulcan, 1994).

ETIOLOGICAL FACTORS AND FAMILY PATTERNS

In most cases of encopresis, subtle colon or sphincter abnormalities exist. Fifteen percent of encopretic children have fathers who were also encopretic as children. Chronic, severe constipation may also lead to encopresis. This occurs when some factor, such as a painful anal fissure, anal rash, diet, punitive toilet training, or unresolved fear of the toilet triggers constipation. This may result in suppression of the urge to defecate, and can lead to anal blockage. Eventually, feces will involuntarily leak around the blockage. The affected child often becomes habituated to the smell of his or her feces and is unaware of having soiled.

Encopresis can also be secondary to sexual abuse, oppositional defiant disorder, attention deficit-hyperactivity disorder, conduct disorder, phobias, or adjustment disorder. Temporary encopresis can arise from such stressors as hospitalization or parental divorce.

AGE OF ONSET AND COURSE

After the age of 4, encopresis is defined as involuntary defecation at least once a month for 3 successive months. The affected child rarely passes feces during sleep. Older children are less responsive to treatment for this disorder.

IMPAIRMENT AND COMPLICATIONS

Encopretic children suffer from peer rejection and school and family problems. Some medical causes for this disorder include hypothyroidism, lactase deficiency, and anal fissures.

NURSING ASSESSMENT AND NURSING DIAGNOSIS

A complete medical, psychological, and toilet training history must be taken. The nurse must help the child to explore his or her feelings about the soiling behavior. One goal is to help the child learn to clean up after each episode of soiling. Before the nurse can intervene therapeutically, he or she must understand his or her own feelings and attitudes toward fecal soiling. Avoidance of a punitive response by parents can improve the child's recovery as well as bolster the child's self-esteem.

■ MOOD DISORDERS

A childhood **mood disorder** can be serious, long-lasting, and recurrent. Such disorders encompass depression and bipolar (manic) disorders, and generally involve varying levels of depression, elation, or irritability. For children, irritability is more prevalent than depression, and the inability to gain weight is more common than weight loss.

EPIDEMIOLOGY

An increase in the frequency of childhood mood disorders, with the age of onset decreasing for bipolar disorders, has been seen in the past decade. Two percent of children experience major depression. Prior to puberty, depression is more common in boys than in girls, and mania is rare in both genders (Dulcan, 1994).

ETIOLOGICAL FACTORS AND FAMILY PATTERNS

Strong familial genetic links exist for mood disorders, especially with bipolar disorder.

AGE OF ONSET AND COURSE

A mood disorder can occur at any age. It is difficult to diagnose in very young children who can't communicate thoughts and feelings.

IMPAIRMENT AND COMPLICATIONS

Behaviors of depressed children vary according to their age-appropriate developmental level. Mood disorders may lead to poor school performance, a decreased desire to interact with other children, complaints of boredom, sleep problems, stomachaches and headaches, separation anxiety, and impaired concentration.

Major depression in children can be an indicator of a bipolar disorder, especially when there is a family history of this disorder. Mood disorders can be confused with conduct disorder, attention deficit-hyperactivity disorder, and anxiety disorders.

NURSING ASSESSMENT AND NURSING DIAGNOSIS

Observing and interviewing a child are ways of assessing whether it is depressed. When interviewing a child, the clinician must use age-appropriate language to which the child can relate. Evaluating for suicidality is also very important, and posing this question to a child does not increase the likelihood of self-destructive behavior.

RECOMMENDED TREATMENT

Treatment for childhood mood disorders involves supportive individual and family therapy and, for some children, medication after therapy has begun, although the efficacy of antidepressants in children is less clear than in adults.

■ RUMINATION DISORDER OF INFANCY

Rumination disorder, also known as "failure to thrive," is the repeated, voluntary regurgitation and rechewing of food with weight loss or failure to gain weight. Affected children appears to do this in order to release tension or as a source of pleasure.

EPIDEMIOLOGY

Rumination disorder is more prevalent in males than in female children by a ratio of 5 to 1 (Dulcan, 1994).

ETIOLOGICAL FACTORS AND FAMILY PATTERNS

One-third of infants with rumination disorder come from mothers who have experienced obstetrical complications. One fourth of these infants have developmental delays related to mental retardation or pervasive developmental disorder. Rumination disorder has also been linked to poor infant care in the form of neglect or harsh handling. Maternal depression is often the cause of this poor parenting.

AGE OF ONSET AND COURSE

Rumination disorder occurs in infants aged of 3 months to 1 year, and in persons with moderate to severe mental retardation.

IMPAIRMENT AND COMPLICATIONS

When not ruminating, the child with rumination disorder may be withdrawn and apathetic, irritable, and fussy, or may appear normal. The condition can also be the result of some medical disorders, such as congenital malformations, gastrointestinal infections, or a hyperactive gag reflex.

NURSING ASSESSMENT NURSING DIAGNOSIS, RECOMMENDED TREATMENT

Hospitalization is usually required for the evaluation of children with rumination disorder, which includes medical testing, parental interviews, and observation. Supportive therapy is important for parents, along with teaching them positive ways in which to feed and interact with an affected infant. Some cases of rumination disorder may be so severe—and potentially life threatening—that the infant needs to be hospitalized for treatment.

AN OVERVIEW

- Emotional disorders among children usually have more than one etiologic factor, including genetic background or family history; surface conflicts between children and parents that arise from adjustment tasks; deeper conflicts within the child (so-called neuroses); or difficulty associated with a physical handicap or disorder, or with a mental disorder (psychosis).

- Children with attention deficit–hyperactivity disorder (ADHD) may be classified as having one of three subtypes of this disorder: attention deficit only; hyperactivity; or both, which is most common.

- ADHD begins no later than age 7; if similar symptoms develop after that age, they are most likely caused by another disorder. Symptoms of ADHD must be frequently in evidence and must persist for at least 6 months, although they need not be present all the time.

- Pervasive development disorder (PDD) is characterized by very early distortions in the development of social interaction, behavioral patterns, or communication.

- Autism, a pervasive development disorder, is first seen in infancy or early childhood, although some autistic children may appear normal until 2 or 3 years of age, when their communication and social-interaction skills are expected to move to a higher level but do not.

- Contrary to earlier beliefs, autism is thought to have only a biological origin; its causes include certain chromosomal abnormalities, maternal infection during pregnancy, trauma to the developing central nervous system, or genetic abnormalities.

- Autistic children often have an aversion or indifference to being held or hugged; they will not engage in imaginative or social play, often cling to an inanimate object, exhibit delayed or abnormal language and speech abilities, and show hand-flapping and head-banging tics.

- Mental retardation is defined as "significantly subaverage intellectual functioning originating during the developmental period, accompanied by impairment in at least two areas: communication, self-care, home living, social skills, community use, self-direction, health and safety, functional academics, leisure and work." Along with these deficits in adaptive functioning, the IQ is 70 or less.

- Mental retardation may be mild, moderate, severe, or profound.

- Some specific developmental disorders centered around reading, arithmetic, language, or verbal articulation can lead to functional impairment.

- Children with conduct disorders (CD) have a repetitive, persistent pattern of disruptive, willfully disobedient behavior. Not all children who exhibit such behavior have CD: a single disruptive act may be seen as representing childhood adjustment disorder, and several such acts as representing adjustment disorder with disturbance of conduct.

- Separation anxiety disorder involves excessive anxiety, often to the level of panic, concerning separation from parents or another attachment figure, from home, or from other familiar surroundings. Although anxiety is developmentally appropriate in children, children older than 5 years who persistently exhibit excessive anxiety may be diagnosed as having separation anxiety disorder.

- Children with oppositional defiant disorder (ODD), a relatively new diagnostic category, exhibit behavior that is less extreme than that seen in conduct disorder; their behavior does not appear to violate the rights of others, as does the behavior of children with conduct disorder.

- A phobia is a specific, persistent fear that is out of proportion to the danger that triggers it. It leads to difficulty in functioning at school or in social situations.

- Enuresis, which is repeated, involuntary urination into bed or into clothing after a child reaches 5 years of age, has psychological, physical, and physiological roots. It may precipitate significant family conflict, shame in the child, peer teasing, and low self-esteem.

- In encopresis, which is the involuntary pattern of defecating into clothing or in other inappropriate places after age 4, a subtle colon or sphincter abnormality exists. Encopresis may also be secondary to sexual abuse, oppositional defiant disorder, attention deficit hyperactivity disorder, conduct disorder, phobias, or adjustment disorder; temporary encopresis can arise from such stressors as hospitalization or parental divorce.

- A childhood mood disorder generally involves varying degrees of depression, elation, or irritability; irritability is more prevalent than depression, and the inability to gain weight is experienced rather than weight loss.

- Rumination disorder in infancy (failure to thrive) is the repeated voluntary regurgitation and re-chewing of food with weight loss or failure to gain weight. The action appears to release tension and to be a source of pleasure.

TD TERMS TO DEFINE

- attention deficit hyperactivity disorder (ADHD)
- autism
- conduct disorder (CD)
- encopresis
- enuresis
- mental retardation
- mood disorders
- oppositional defiant disorder (ODD)
- phobia
- pervasive developmental disorders (PDD)
- rumination disorder
- separation anxiety disorder
- specific developmental disorders

Q STUDY QUESTIONS

1. What is the advantage of using a developmental framework to assess a child or adolescent psychiatric patient?

2. What nursing interventions are appropriate to use with a 9-year-old male with a socialized, nonaggressive conduct disorder?

3. Which of the following statements describes attention deficit hyperactivity disorder?
    a. It appears when the child is not older than 5 years.
    b. Symptoms are present for at least 6 months.
    c. Symptoms are extreme for the child's age and intelligence.
    d. Symptoms violate the basic age-appropriate norms and rules of society.
    e. The child is often restless, inattentive, distractible, impulsive and fidgety.

4. T F Separation anxiety disorder involves any level of anxiety experienced by the child when separated from its parents, another attachment figure, home, or other familiar surroundings.

5. Discuss treatment for an enuretic child and what you would teach the parents about helping the child overcome this disorder.

6. A toddler is afraid of storms. To determine whether he is suffering from a phobia, what additional information would you need?

7. How is oppositional defiant disorder different from conduct disorder? How is oppositional defiant disorder different from specific developmental disorder?

8. What behavior would you expect of a child with conduct disorder?

9. What childhood disorder is also known as a "failure to thrive"?

10. A mother tells you that her 6-year-old son has begun soiling himself while at school. She asks your advice. What would you recommend?

11. Why is the technique of limit setting especially important in child-psychiatric nursing?

■ REFERENCES

Achenbach T, and Edelbrock C: The classification of child psychopathology: A review and analysis of empirical effects. *Psychological Bulletin*, 85, 1983, 1275–1285.

Standards of Psychiatric and Mental Health Nursing Practice. Kansas City, American Nurses' Association, 1994.

Diagnostic and Statistical Manual of Mental Disorders, ed 4 Washington, DC, American Psychiatric Association, 1994.

Binet A, Binet S: *The Development of Intelligence in Children.* Baltimore, Williams & Wilkins, 1916.

Catell J: Mental tests and measurements. Mind 1980; 15:373.

Dulcan MK: Psychiatric disorders of childhood and adolescence, in Stoudemire A (ed): *Clinical Psychiatry for Medical Students,* ed 2 Philadelphia, JB Lippincott, 1994.

Erikson E: Growth and crises of the healthy personality, in *Identity and the Life Cycle: Psychological Issues,* E. Erikson (ed.) (Monograph No. 1). New York, International Universities Press, 1959.

Flohr LM & Phillips I. Mental retardation, LM Goldman HH (ed). Review of General Psychiatry, 4th ed, Stamford, CT, Appleton & Lange, 1995.

Freud A: *Sexual Enlightenment of Children.* New York, Macmillan, 1963.

Freud A: *The Psychoanalytic Treatment of Children.* New York, International Universities Press, 1965.

Ginsburg H, Opper S: *Piaget's Theory of Intellectual Development,* ed. 2. Englewood Cliffs, NJ, Prentice-Hall, 1979.

Healy W: *Twenty-Five Years of Child Guidance.* Chicago, Institute for Juvenile Research, 1934.

Helmer L, Lalibert M: Assessment groups for preschool children: A preventive program. *Arch Psychiatr Nurs,* 1987; 1:334–340.

Huberman R: Childhood mental disorders and child psychiatry, in Goldman HH (ed): *Review of General Psychiatry,* ed 4. Stamford, CT, Appleton and Lange, 1995.

Klein M: *The Psychoanalysis of Children.* London, Hogarth Press, 1932.

Last C, Hersen M, Kazdin A, Francis G, Grubb A: Psychiatric illness in the mothers of anxious children. *Am J Psychiatry* 1987; 144:1580–1583.

Levitan S, Belous R: *What's Happening to the American Family?* Baltimore, Johns Hopkins University Press, 1981, p. 29.

National Center on Child Abuse and Neglect: Child Sexual Abuse: Incest, Assault and Sexual Exploration. Department of Health and Human Services Publication No. (OHDS) 81-30166. Washington, DC, US Government Printing Office, 1981.

Simmons JE: *Psychiatric Examination of Children,* ed 4. Philadelphia, Lea and Febiger, 1987.

Wiener JM (ed): *Textbook of Child and Adolescent Psychiatry.* Washington, DC, American Psychiatric Press, 1991.

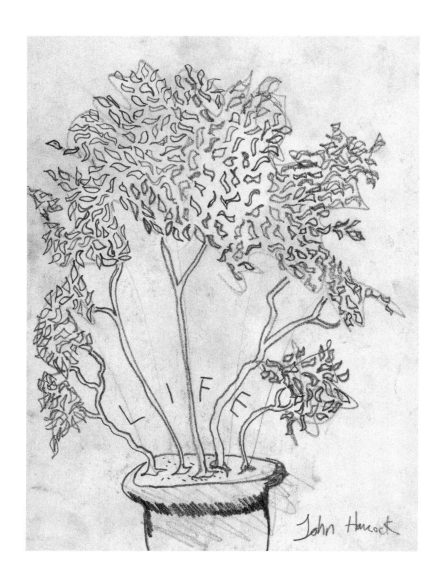

Endure that toil of growing up;
The ignominy of boyhood; the distress
Of boyhood changing into man.

William Butler Yeats (1865–1939)
A Dialogue of Self and Soul II, st.1

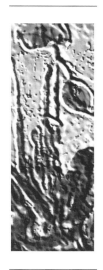

18
Issues in Adolescent Mental Health

Wanda K. Mohr

The word adolescence evokes a variety of reactions among different people. Many remember adolescence fondly as a carefree time spent "hanging out" with friends, dating, and talking at length on the telephone about nothing in particular. Others remember it as a time of intense conflict with parents, grinding peer pressure, and confusion. As diverse as the recollections of those who have passed through it are the misconceptions and myths that have been perpetuated about the adolescent experience. Because of these persistent misconceptions and myths, nurses who work with adolescents need to be aware of recent studies that resist the pull of theoretical sacred cows and ethnocentric assumptions.

This chapter provides an overview of current approaches to adolescent mental health. Opening with definitions of "normal" adolescence and adolescent development, the chapter next considers high-risk and deviant behaviors and the typical health-related issues of adolescence. It also surveys common mental-health problems and treatments, as well as strategies for nursing care of the adolescent.

■ THEORIES OF ADOLESCENT DEVELOPMENT

Theories are neither true nor false, although their implications may be. Theories are useful in nursing practice because they facilitate gathering relevant information; they are a working framework that focuses the nurse. Theories may be viewed as compasses for decision-making, in that they guide a nurse's interpretations and evaluations about what is appropriate patient behavior, environment, and development. Note that theories are compasses, not maps to be exhaustively followed.

Although some scholars have argued that biological influences are the prime determinants of adolescent development (Gesell *et al.,* 1956) and others have concentrated on moral development (Kohlberg, 1969), personality theorists have dominated adolescent psychology. Historically, several theories of **personality development** have been relevant to the study and treatment of adolescents:

- psychoanalytic theory (Sigmund Freud)
- interpersonal theory (Harry Stack Sullivan)
- psychosocial development theory (Eric Erikson)
- cognitive development theory (Jean Piaget)

Stated briefly, each of these theories identifies behaviors with different developmental stages through which the individual is presumed to pass. These stages, which are associated with age, provide a basis to evaluate the appropriateness of certain behaviors. The value of these theories is their insistence that developmental events taking place in the present are systematically linked to past events, and that development is a consistent process.

More recent approaches to adolescent psychology and psychiatry have been accompanied by significant developments in psychobiology and behavioral biology. The systematic investigation of genetic determinants of behavior, at a time when the traditional American emphasis on environmental factors is less pronounced, has led to broader and deeper knowledge of the way in which biological factors influence and are influenced by behavior. Promising research findings have addressed such complex human behaviors as aggression, altruism, and cooperation and their relationship to various environmental contingencies: the presence or absence of a second parent, the impact of divorce, the child-rearing styles of a family, and the presence of violence in the environment. These studies suggest that biology will have a greater role in approaches to personality development and adolescent mental health than it has had in the past.

■ STAGES OF ADOLESCENCE

Adolescence is a period distinct from childhood or adulthood, one marked by ever-changing influences and conditions that make it increasingly difficult for intergenerational understanding to take place. Many people think of adolescence as being defined only by physiological changes. For many years, the child's entry into puberty was the most widely accepted indicator of the beginning of adolescence. Eliott and Feldman (1990), however, argue that in addition to biological factors, social factors—such as starting high school or obtaining a driver's license—define this transition.

During adolescence, certain tasks must be completed: becoming physically and sexually mature, acquiring skills to carry out adult roles, and gaining increased autonomy from parents. At the same time adolescents need to establish and realign their social interconnections with their peers (Nicholi, 1988).

EARLY ADOLESCENCE AND PUBERTY

Adolescence is commonly subdivided into early, middle, and late stages (Elliot and Feldman, 1990; Nicholi, 1988). **Early adolescence** (ages 10 to 14) typically encompasses the physical and social changes that occur with puberty, as maturation begins and social interactions become increasingly centered on members of the opposite sex. Early adolescence, sometimes known as preadolescence or prepubescence, is the period lasting up to 2 years before **puberty,** during which certain physical changes occur (Nicholi, 1988). Most girls have a growth spurt at about 9 ½ years of age and most boys, on the average, 2 years later.

Preparatory changes in girls that occur before the onset of puberty are an increase in estrogen levels and the appearance of specific feminine characteristics. Breasts begin to develop, areolae and nipples increase in size and pigmentation, the pelvis widens, and layers of subcutaneous fat alter the contours of the body. Girls also begin to grow pubic and then axillary hair at this time.

In boys, physical changes begin about one year after the testes begin to secrete testosterone. Boys' shoulders broaden, their genitals enlarge slightly, and their voices begin to deepen as the larynx increases in size. They gradually begin to grow pubic, axillary, facial, and chest hair, in that order.

The beginning of the menstrual flow (menarche) and the manifestation of seminal emissions (spermarche) denote the onset of puberty in girls and boys, respectively (Brooks-Gunn, 1989). Boys and girls experience pubertal events differently, and the meaning of these events varies according to gender.

Girls report ambivalent reactions to menarche. Those who menstruate early, as well as those who are unprepared for the event, report more negative experiences than those who have been prepared (Grief and Ulman, 1982). Girls will seek information and discuss menarche and other pubertal changes with their peers and mothers, but almost never with their fathers or other males (Brooks-Gunn and Ruble, 1982).

Very little is known about the meaning of spermarche, although it might seem to be as critical an event for boys as menarche is for girls. Boys are reluctant to discuss spermarche with parents or peers. What little study has been done indicates that boys' emotional reactions to spermarche are not very intense, but that the event is slightly frightening, which is much the same reaction that girls have to menarche (Gaddis and Brooks-Gunn, 1985).

For many adolescents this can be a confusing time, in that the effects of maturational timing are different for different individuals. Significant differences in pubertal maturation with respect to one's peers are associated with potentially negative consequences for both girls and boys. For example, girls who mature earlier than their peers and boys who mature later are proposed to be at greater risk for emotional and adjustment problems than their peers (Brooks-Gunn *et al.*, 1985).

Beginning in early adolescence, the peer group becomes increasingly significant as a socializing body, and although the effect of the family is reduced, it is not eliminated (Baumrind, 1985). Adolescents may conform to peer standards up to a point in order to attain status and identity within the peer group. Therefore, although the influence of friends predicts adolescents' initiation to alcohol and marijuana, the primary influence on their long-range educational aspirations and occupational plans appears to remain with the parents. Social cliques tend to discourage academic strivings. As the importance of parental approval wanes with the increasing importance of peer approval, high achievers can be faced with a dilemma.

MIDDLE ADOLESCENCE

Pubertal processes may also extend into **middle adolescence** (Brooks-Gunn, 1988). Middle adolescence is said to range from ages 14 to 15 to ages 15 to 17 (Nicholi, 1988), and is described as a time of increasing independence. For some individuals it may mark the end of adolescence, if they complete their tenure at school or otherwise become emancipated. During middle adolescence, individuals must come to terms with their newly maturing bodies and their sexual identity. Sexual impulses that emerged in early puberty remain high during this phase (Nicholi, 1988). Although gender roles exist before puberty, they intensify during this time; the reasons for this are not known, but may involve a combination of pronounced reproductive differences, peer influences, parental expectations, and cultural messages (Hill and Lynch, 1983). Teens' relationships with their peers take on special significance in these years, as the initial effort to separate from parents takes place (Harter, 1986; Damon and Hart, 1988).

LATE ADOLESCENCE

Late adolescence is an indefinite period from age 18 to the mid 20s. The variance in the age range during which it occurs is a function of individual factors, such as educational goals, that delay adolescents' entry into adult roles. For many individuals late adolescence begins upon high-school graduation. Their task in this phase is to define who they are and what their future direction will be.

■ ADOLESCENT HEALTH ISSUES

Today's adolescent experience cannot be compared with that of 10 years ago. For parents and other adults who may legitimately attempt to comprehend a child's life by remembering their own, this is perhaps the most difficult concept to understand.

The consensus in the 1970s was that young people were victims of social forces beyond their control, such as a breakdown in tradition or a reduced material standard of living, and that problematic youthful behavior was a function of these forces. The 1980s saw a re-labeling of problems as risk-taking behavior. This re-labeling shifted the locus of responsibility away from social forces and implied that young people are the victims of problems that they themselves create. Like other facile explanations for behavior, however, both of these interpretations have been challenged.

Adolescents frequently lament that they feel like outsiders. This is not necessarily idle discontent or whining. According to Baumrind (1987), adolescents are, from a sociological perspective, indeed outsiders in modern Western societies. Adolescent dependency on peer relationships and other non-family influences over the past 25 years has increased while the influence of parents has waned correspondingly. In addition, adolescent well-being has declined and problem behaviors have increased, as illustrated by rising rates of academic failure, delinquency, suicide, and sexual license. Although causality is difficult to trace, efforts to explain this decline continue. Many professionals in the field of adolescent psychology (Uhlenberg and Eggebeen,

1986; Baumrind, 1987; Nicholi, 1988) strongly suggest that parental influence has decreased primarily because parents have chosen to withdraw from the lives of their youngsters. They argue that emotional withdrawal, irrespective of the makeup of the family unit, creates an emptiness in the life of the child and lays the groundwork for feelings of abandonment and alienation.

The health status of adolescents has declined over the past several decades (Wilson and Joffe, 1995). In contrast to health problems in children and adults, morbidity and mortality among adolescents are attributed primarily to social, environmental, and behavioral determinants rather than to biomedical factors. Mortality rates in adolescent females are half those in adolescent males, and life expectancy is lowest among African-American males (Wetzel, 1987). Since 1984, adolescent health problems have changed not qualitatively but quantitatively, with violence continuing to pose the greatest health risk for young people. The major declines in health status can also be linked to substance abuse, accidental injuries, and the consequences of unprotected sexual activity, which results in teen pregnancies and sexually transmitted diseases, including human immunodeficiency virus (HIV) and acquired immune deficiency syndrome (AIDS).

SUBSTANCE ABUSE

In their Monitoring the Future study, researchers at the University of Michigan found an unprecedented increase during the past two decades in the abuse of alcohol and drugs by adolescents (Johnston, O'Malley, and Bachman, 1994). Marijuana use among 8th graders has more than doubled since 1991, and after a brief decline during the 1980s, drug use has increased overall among all teenagers. Alcohol consumption was reported by 92% of a national sample of high-school seniors, and daily cigarette smoking is reported by 18% of all high-school seniors. Drug and alcohol abuse and addiction present a variety of clinical pictures, which are extensively discussed in the Diagnostic and Statistical Manual of Mental Disorders, Fourth Edition (*DSM IV,* 1994).

Studies show that the drug experience both affects and is affected by the developmental phase of the adolescent user. Baumrind (1985) makes a strong case against "recreational" and chronic early-adolescent drug use, which may either activate difficulties or intensify and exacerbate pre-existing problems. These negative consequences include impairment of attention and memory, a developmental lag in the cognitive, moral, and psychosocial domains, and an **amotivational syndrome** (pattern of apathy). In addition, drug and alcohol use and the resulting negative reactions of the family and other social groups can lead to the development of negative identity, social alienation, and estrangement at a time when adolescents need social support (Stanton and Todd, 1982).

ACCIDENTS

More than half of all deaths among young people aged 10 to 19 are due to accidents, and most of these involve motor vehicles. (Pipkin *et al.,* 1989). Risky driving habits such as speeding, tailgating, and driving under the influence of alcohol or other drugs is a more significant cause of accidents than lack of driving experience (Insurance Institute for Highway Safety, 1984). In over half the motor vehicle fatalities involving an adolescent driver, he or she has a blood alcohol level above 0.10% (Center for Disease Control, 1983a; 1983b; Insurance Institute for Highway Safety, 1984), or two times the legal limit for being "under the influence" in some states. Studies also show high rates of intoxication among samples of adolescents who die as pedestrians or while using recreational vehicles. (Pipkin *et al.,* 1989). The most common non-fatal injuries resulting from vehicular accidents account for the largest number of hospital days among adolescents between the ages of 12 and 17; most involve the use of alcohol (Millstein and Irwin, 1988).

SEXUAL ACTIVITY

By the age of 19, more than 77% of males and more than 62% of females have engaged in sexual intercourse (Hofferth and Hayes, 1987). The main problems associated with teen-age sexual behavior are sexually transmitted disease (STD) and pregnancy. STD rates are higher among adolescents than among any other group, with 25% of sexually active adolescents becoming infected during their high-school careers. For unknown reasons, STD rates are significantly higher among black than among white teen-agers (Shaffer et al., 1984). Risk factors for STD include multiple partners and failure to use condoms (Bell and Holmes, 1984).

Studies (Zelnick and Shah, 1983; Morrison, 1985) have found that most adolescents do not use contraception in their first sexual encounter, and that only 29% of sexually active teenagers use contraception of some kind on a consistent basis. As a result, at least one million adolescents become pregnant in the United States every year, many within 6 months of their initiation into sexual activity. Approximately 50% of these teen-agers give birth. (Zelnick and Shah, 1983).

FADS

Several recent fads among adolescents have the potential to cause injury or illness. One is known as **body marking,** which includes body piercing, scarring, and tattooing. No research is currently available about the meaning of body marking to adolescents, but its purpose seems to be to provide information about group membership and to make statements about individuality, rank, social status, and a particular set of values (Hambly, 1975). Tattooing creates patterns or pictures by introducing pigments through puncture marks in the skin. Ornamental scarring, also known as "cicatrization," is the induction of an injury that results in the formation and contraction of fibrous scar tissue. This is done by cutting or burning, with irritants often rubbed into the resulting wounds in order to raise weals or keloids (Strathern and Strathern, 1971). Body piercing ranges from multiple ear piercing to the piercing of other body parts, including nipples, labia, eyelids, tongues, and noses. No data exist on the rates of injury or infection resulting from these particular marking activities, but it seems reasonable to speculate that adolescents may potentially become systemically or locally infected through the use of unsterile instruments or the presence of unhygienic conditions.

Another fad that has become commonplace is moshing (slam-dancing), described by young people as a kind of chaotic dance. Moshing includes body surfing, hurling oneself into a crowd of spectators, and stage diving. Again, little research has been done into the significance or meaning of these particular behaviors, but their potential for severe injury is a significant concern.

■ ADOLESCENT MENTAL HEALTH

Clinicians have expressed the need for comprehensive epidemiologic research on adolescents and mental health; however, only limited populations, such as groups of undergraduate college students, have been studied (Nicholi, 1988). What the literature indicates is an apparent peak in the incidence of mental disorders during the adolescent years that covers the entire range of the psychopathology experienced by adults (Nicholi, 1988). Other reports on adolescent mental-illness rates, such as those represented by hospital admissions, have been flawed in the past decade. Researchers have noted that part of this may have been due to a rash of over-diagnosing related to the unrestrained proliferation of for-profit psychiatric hospitals and the unregulated state of the mental-health "industry," as well as reimbursement practices that led to diagnostic manipulation and the unnecessary hospitalization of adolescents (Schwartz et al., 1984; 1989; Weithorn, 1988; Mohr, 1994). Moreover, confusion surrounds the pathology of adolescence, and diagnostic errors of commission and omission are often made by the most experienced and

honest of clinicians. One reason for the confusion is that it is difficult to distinguish among normal adolescent turmoil, turmoil due to family dysfunction, and incipient mental problems.

Overall rates of mental illness among adolescents do not differ by sex. However, the frequencies within categories of diagnosis are different for males and females, with females more often given the diagnosis of depression and males the diagnosis of conduct disorder (Institute of Medicine, 1989).

ADJUSTMENT DISORDER

The most frequent and least reliable diagnostic category given to adolescents is **adjustment disorder** (Nicholi, 1988). As described in *DSM-IV*, adjustment disorder is a pathological reaction to an identified internal or external stressor. Such stressors can range from physical illness to divorce (Enzer and Cunningham, 1991). Among adolescents, adjustment disorder persists for up to 6 months and impairs social functioning. The symptoms vary with the developmental phase, previous patterns of coping, and the familial/environmental circumstances of the affected individual (Newcorn and Strain, 1992). *DSM-IV* describes several subtypes, in which adjustment disorder is linked with one of several specific factors: academic inhibition, anxiety, physical complaints, conduct disturbance, depression, or social withdrawal. Some symptoms include defiance, aggression, drug and alcohol use, and outbursts of rage.

EATING DISORDERS

Eating disorders represent another psychological disorder that appears in the teenage years. Eating disorders among young women were reported in the medical literature as early as the 17th century (Herzog, 1988). These disorders typically refer to the syndromes of anorexia nervosa and bulimia nervosa. Anorexia nervosa and bulimia may co-exist or one may manifest itself after the appearance or resolution of the other. In the two decades from 1965 to 1985, the incidence of anorexia nervosa doubled. The syndrome is estimated to occur in 0.5% of females from aged 12 to 18 years (Kennedy and Garfinkel 1985). Reports on the incidence of bulimia indicate that this condition is more widespread and increasing in prevalence. At least 5 to 18% of young women in high school are afflicted with the disorder (Herzog et al., 1985). There is some dispute about whether eating disorders are increasing in number or whether they are simply being acknowledged, recognized, or diagnosed more extensively. Although these disorders are common in females, bulimia can also occur in males. Socio-cultural factors, in the form of a high value for thinness, have been strongly implicated in the genesis of eating disorders.

Anorexia nervosa most often begins in the female adolescent as early as 12 years of age, with the affected individual perceiving herself as overweight whether or not this perception is reality based, and even when others tell her she is not. She achieves rapid and extreme weight loss by drastically restricting her caloric intake, purging herself through vomiting, fasting, the use of laxatives or diuretics, and excessive physical activity. Because of complications related to starvation, anorexia nervosa is accompanied by the highest reported morbidity and mortality rates among all psychiatric illnesses. Physical problems related to anorexia nervosa involve all body systems, and its manifestations include osteoporosis, cardiac arrhythmias, renal failure, endocrine imbalances, anemias, and amenorrhea. The condition is associated with a mortality rate of 10 to 15% (Herzog and Copeland, 1985). Three of the hallmarks of anorexia nervosa are secretiveness, massive denial that a problem exists, and resistance to psychotherapy or any treatment that will cause a gain in weight (Halmi, 1983).

Bulimia occurs more typically in later adolescence, usually between the ages of 17 and 25, in young women who have tried a variety of diets with little success. These young women are concerned with weight control. Either through talking with friends or by accident, they discover that laxative abuse and vomiting can be a way of weight management. They then begin to follow a pattern of "bingeing," or eating large amounts of (usually high-calorie, starchy) food, followed by self-induced vomiting, diuretic or laxative use, vigorous exercise, or fasting (Herzog, 1982). Bulimia often produces dental-enamel erosion, electrolyte imbalances, and esophagitis, but does not cause amennorhia or severe weight loss (Halmi, 1983).

Among the weight-related problems affecting the mental health of young people is obesity. Obesity occurs in approximately 15% of adolescents (Peck and Ulrich, 1985). By conventional agreement, obesity is said to exist when an individual's body weight exceeds the recommended levels (which are now under revision) by at least 20%. Females are more likely to be obese than males, and obesity is more frequent in children of lower socio-economic status and in ethnic minority groups. The results of research on causes of obesity in the population as a whole are inconclusive, but the most common cause of obesity in adolescents is chronic overeating. Given the emphasis and desirability of slenderness in the American body ideal, adolescents who are obese or overweight often suffer from depression and low self-esteem. Diminished self-esteem presents a special risk to young adolescents. This is because pubertal changes bring dramatic discontinuities in body image,

and youngsters may feel less physically attractive when their awareness of self and others is developing. Coupled with social pressures that support what Naomi Wolf (1991) calls the "ideology of semi-starvation," overweight teenagers may become vulnerable to cognitive and emotional disturbances or maladaptive behaviors such as those discussed under eating disorders.

DEPRESSION

Depression in adolescence may be a temporary, situational reaction or a chronic condition with all of the crippling symptoms of adult depression. The incidence of depression in adolescents is difficult to determine because of variations in its definition and measurement (Brage, 1995). Various researchers estimate that 5 to 7% of high-school students experience severe depression, and that 21 to 27% experience moderate depression (Terri, 1982; Worchel et al., 1987). Depression is a debilitating affective state characterized in *DSM-IV* as consisting of a dysphoric mood or loss of interest or pleasure in usual activities. It is marked by persistent symptoms such as hopelessness, irritability, or "feeling blue or sad" (*DSM-IV*, 1994).

The clinical picture of depression in adolescents may differ somewhat from that in adults. These differences may reflect the stage of development at which the depression is manifested. Symptoms may include poor academic performance, restlessness, listlessness, and aggressive or sexual acting-out behavior (Nielsen, 1983). In addition, the adolescent may appear bored or engage in other high-risk behaviors, such careless driving of vehicles or alcohol and drug use (Nicholi, 1988). Adolescent depression has not been taken as seriously as it should be. Nevertheless, the alarming statistics on adolescent suicide show that depression can be a grave, life-threatening condition that merits careful consideration.

SUICIDE

Suicide accounts for 6% of deaths in the 10- to 14-year age group. Between the ages of 15 and 19 it accounts for 12% of deaths. It is the second leading cause of death among white adolescents and the fifth leading cause of death among black teen-agers (U.S. Dept of Health and Human Services, 1991). Adolescents who commit suicide have usually made previous attempts, and for many of them, other major clinical factors increase the likelihood of suicidal behavior. These factors include the presence of a major psychiatric disorder and a family history of suicide or psychiatric illness (Holinger et al., 1994). Suicidal behavior is associated with a history of bipolar disorder, schizophrenia, character disorders, substance abuse, depression and learning disorders. Among vulnerable youth, common stressors, such as family conflicts, rejection by peers, or romantic involvement may be sufficient to trigger a suicidal gesture or attempt. (Brent et al., 1988).

As many as 30% of adolescents who commit suicide are abusers of drugs and alcohol. Adolescents who use drugs and alcohol are three times more likely to attempt suicide than those who do not, and studies show that suicidal ideation increases dramatically after drug or alcohol use begins (Berman, 1991). Retrospective studies (Hilliard et al., 1987; Berman, 1991) also note that conduct disorder occurs at a particularly high rate in adolescent boys who complete suicide. Other traits considered common risk factors for suicide are poor mood regulation, intense rage, impulsive behavior, and limited tolerance for frustration.

Researchers (Schaffer et al., 1988) have concluded that many common approaches to suicide prevention that have been touted by the media are ineffective. School-based programs are not cost effective, there is no evidence that they have any impact, and their effect on students who are not considering suicide is unknown. Telephone hotlines and other crisis-intervention services do reduce suicide attempts among white women, who are the most frequent callers, but studies also show that callers do not usually take the advice given on hot lines.

OPPOSITIONAL DISORDER

Oppositional disorder is a controversial diagnostic category that includes persistent disobedience, negativism, and provocative opposition to authority figures, rule violation, argumentativeness, provocative behavior, and stubbornness (*DSM-IV*, 1994). The presence of oppositional behavior in adolescents is not necessarily diagnostic of the disorder, as much oppositional behavior is normative and adaptive during maturation. Data on the incidence of oppositional disorder are questionable, since it was a diagnostic label commonly applied to adolescents during the years of greatest psychiatric hospital misuse during the late 1980s (Mohr, 1994; Schwartz, 1989; Schwartz et al., 1984). Oppositional behavior can be caused by situational crises, and is also seen in depressed teens. Oppositional disorder is diagnosed more often in male adolescents, and the long-term prognosis is considered poor when it occurs as a long-standing pattern of behavior (Doke and Flippo, 1982).

CONDUCT DISORDER

The diagnostic category of **conduct disorder** accounts for 10 to 15% of referrals of children to psychiatric treatment centers. Although adjustment dis-

order is the most commonly made diagnosis in adolescents, conduct disorder is the most common psychiatric diagnostic category in referrals to child mental-health services (Sholevar, 1995). The diagnosis of conduct disorder is made more commonly in male children, especially those who come from lower socio-economic backgrounds and environments in which harsh punishment and domestic violence are frequent. As with adjustment disorder and oppositional disorder, conduct disorder is a diagnosis that provokes controversy because of its non-specificity, including difficulty in differentiating its symptoms from those of attention deficit disorder. Two subtypes of conduct disorder are recognized in the *DSM-IV*: the aggressive type, in which the adolescent is asocial and isolated, and the group type, which involves the organized group pathology of gangs and involves a number of individuals who share similar problems and mind sets.

Conduct disorder is characterized by academic problems, overt or covert hostility, disobedience, physical and verbal aggressiveness, quarrelsomeness, vengefulness, and destructiveness (*DSM-IV*, 1994). Lying, solitary stealing, and temper tantrums are other common behaviors in adolescents diagnosed as having conduct disorder. Moreover, a powerful association exists between early-onset conduct disorder and later substance abuse in adolescents (Hesselbrock, 1986). Teenagers with conduct disorder often tend to be sexually uninhibited and inclined toward sexual aggressiveness, and some may engage in fire-setting, vandalism, and even homicidal acts. Fire-setting is considered a very serious symptom by most clinicians, and is associated with poor future social adjustment (Rapoport and Ismond, 1984). Other terms that have been applied to such behavior in adolescents include antisocial behavior, delinquency, and externalizing behavior (Sholevar and Sholevar, 1995).

Some of the factors implicated in the etiology of conduct disorder are deficits in parental skills, parental alcoholism, sociological factors that affect psychosocial and economic status, school and neighborhood environments, social immaturity (undersocialization), and aggressive personality traits that may have a biological component (Sholevar and Sholevar, 1995; Shaw and Campo-Bowen, 1995). Many clinicians agree that treatment for conduct disorder is likely to be ineffective, and the syndrome is strongly associated with psychopathology and criminal behavior in adulthood, with 50% of affected youths going on to exhibit antisocial personality disorder. In general, the less aggression adolescents exhibit, the better their prognosis for future social adjustment (Shaw and Campo-Bowen, 1995; Rapoport and Ismond, 1984; Robins, 1978).

SCHIZOPHRENIA

Schizophrenia most often appears for the first time between the ages of 15 and 25. It becomes a family problem as it disrupts the family of the affected individual. The syndrome presents itself slowly and is often difficult to diagnose, since it may be mistaken for another, less pernicious condition such as oppositional disorder, or may even be considered "moody adolescence" that the child will outgrow. Moreover, professionals are reluctant to make the diagnosis of schizophrenia in a young person. One reason for this is that it may become a label that will haunt the affected individual for life. However, this misguided altruism has sometimes delayed crucial treatment that could have reduced the suffering of the patient and his or her family. Vine (1982) found that nearly 70% of parents of schizophrenic individuals had not learned the serious nature of the diagnosis until more than 2 years after the appearance of the first psychotic symptoms.

Schizophrenia particularly presents major problems for the family of the afflicted individual, for a number of different reasons, not the least of which is having to cope with the knowledge that the family may have to relinquish many of its hopes for their child (Vine, 1982). The families of adolescents diagnosed as having schizophrenia often feel isolated and embarrassed, blaming themselves on the one hand and wondering about the extent to which the schizophrenic symptoms are under the adolescent's control. They are often torn by dilemmas presented by the time and cost of treatment to the detriment of other children in the family. They may also become extremely overprotective of the patient, in much the same way as parents of children with other chronic debilitating diseases (Anderson et al., 1986).

Hope for victims of schizophrenia has grown with recent research showing that the disease is not a degenerative disorder that becomes more serious with age. The symptoms rarely worsen after the first 2 years, and the drug dose required for treatment of the disease usually decreases (Pardes et al., 1989). A review of 22 studies conducted over several decades has shown that early treatment of schizophrenia with antipsychotic drugs not only cuts short the acute psychotic episode but improves the long-term outcome. Wyatt (1991) found that patients who began taking drugs at an early stage of their illness relapsed less quickly, spent less time in mental hospitals, and were more capable of working even if they did not receive preventive maintenance therapy.

DEVIANCE AND DELINQUENT BEHAVIOR

One of the most troublesome and extensive problems in adolescence is delinquent behavior, such as the destruction of property, violence, and other behavior that infringes the rights of others and violates society's rules. Delinquent behavior ranges from truancy and incorrigibility to serious criminal offenses; not surprisingly, it is also highly correlated with youthful drug and alcohol abuse (Rapoport and Ismond, 1984).

Explanations of adolescent deviance generally focus on social and community factors that influence opportunities as well as biogenetic susceptibilities, personality and character traits, parental inadequacies, and vulnerability to peer influence McCord (1988). Traditional theories are unsatisfactory in explaining adolescent deviance, and some, such as the biogenic and trait theories, are difficult to establish empirically. However, deviance theorists consistently point to the negative consequences of premature adolescent emancipation from parental control. It therefore seems safe to say that postponing adolescent emancipation as long as possible may be one prescription for preventing deviant behavior.

With respect to other treatment or prevention modalities for deviance and delinquency, imprisonment fails to deter crime, and diversion programs are ineffective (Wolfgang et al., 1972; Hawkins et al., 1987; McCord, 1988). Job programs and counseling used as preventive techniques have also failed to live up to their promise, with most counseling programs having been found ineffective and often harmful (Cass and Thomas, 1979; McCord, 1981).

Violence

Victimization of children and adolescents in the form of assault or sexual abuse has been recognized as a national problem chiefly through the intense focus of the news media. In 1991 the Surgeon General of the Public Health Service (Novello, 1991) wrote that violence in all forms was a greater killer of children in the United States than were diseases. The data on the prevalence of sexual and physical abuse are incomplete and such events are probably underreported, but are thought to be increasing significantly. A recent study of 10- to 16-year-olds indicated that 25% had experienced an assault or sexual abuse in the previous year (Finkelhor and Dziuba-Leatherman, 1994) Among 12- to 15-year-olds the rate in 1995 was three times greater than the rate reported in 1991 by the National Crime Survey (Wilson and Joffe, 1995; National Crime Survey, 1992). Homicide is the leading cause of death among young black males, particularly those living in impoverished, high-density urban areas (Bureau of Justice Statistics, 1992). It accounts for 33% of deaths in the 15- to 19-year age group. Homicides most often occur during altercations between young men, and usually involve lethal weapons (Huizinga and Elliott, 1990).

Exposure to violence is a serious problem for young children and adolescents. Children and adolescents who have witnessed the killing of a parent, sexual assault of a parent, suicide attempts by a parent, gang warfare, sniper attacks, or any other form of environmental violence evolve thoughts and fantasies that frequently provoke enduring anger or self-blame (Pynoos and Eth, 1984). They can also develop post-traumatic stress disorder (Chapter 14), which can consist of intrusive traumatic images during which they re-experience the violent scenes. Because of the persistent arousal it engenders, this may seriously affect their cognitive emotional and interpersonal development and later emerge behaviorally in the form of violence and other kinds of impulsive acting out.

Running Away

Up to 2 million young people in the United States run away from home each year, and another 500,000 have no home. Studies (Shane, 1989) indicate than less than 30% of children are true runaways, which is to say that they are absent from the family home without the approval of their parents. Sixty percent are thrown out ("throwaway kids"), agree to leave their families, or are removed by authorities. Before they run away, most such children live with their biological mothers, and about 40% live in two-parent families. Almost 50% report physical or emotional abuse at home and 10% report sexual abuse. Other family problems include serious conflict, drug or alcohol abuse, violence, and poor physical or mental health. Shane (1989) argues that this high level of severe domestic dysfunction keeps most runaway and homeless adolescents from returning to their families.

Cults and Adolescents

Recently, attention has been focused on adolescent involvement in cult activity. This may include involvement in occult practices or religious cults. It is difficult to understand how some cult leaders of recent notoriety, such as Charles Manson, David Koresh, or Jim Jones, could have attracted and held their devoted followers and induced them to commit acts they might otherwise never have thought of committing, including theft and murder. Yet history is full of examples of blind devotion to charismatic cult leaders. Social psychologists (Mixon, 1989) believe that cults flourish in times of violence, social disorganization, and great uncertainty. They offer their adherents security and absolute truth. Galanter (1989) writes that adolescents who become involved in cults are often socially alienated and estranged from their families. They come from families that show a high degree of tolerance for deviant behavior, and

whose members have unresolved and unspoken conflicts from which they distance themselves.

Adolescents who join cults generally have low self-esteem and poor social skills. Identification with and loyalty to a cause or leader gives their lives meaning. Unless it is a gang, the cult may stand for noble values. Once they become involved in the cult, adolescents become subject to powerful pressures from other group members, and may do whatever they have to do to prove their absolute commitment to the leader. This may include sleep deprivation, fasting and starvation, degrading sexual activity at the behest of the leader, organized begging, and other ritualistic or personally demeaning behavior and criminal activity (Galanter, 1989).

■ APPROACHES TO TREATMENT

Adolescents with psychological disorders are seen and treated in a variety of settings, including residential treatment schools for long-term therapy, hospitals for acute psychiatric emergencies, day hospitals and clinics, and community health centers. Nurses will normally be the first professionals that children encounter when they are admitted for hospital treatment, and among the first whom they encounter in outpatient settings. Working with adolescents can be both intensely rewarding and intensely frustrating. Nurses must be aware of their feelings and reactions toward belligerent, impulsive and frequently obnoxious adolescent behavior, and acknowledge personal fear while keeping it under control. Because being on the receiving end of a barrage of abusive language can be frightening, some nurses may find themselves wanting to retaliate or becoming impatient with an adolescent patient, particularly under situations of time pressure. Nurses with unresolved issues within their own histories may project their insecurities or over-react in ways that do not benefit the adolescent or the nurse. This is particularly true on busy adolescent units or in busy psychiatric emergency rooms when tasks, noise, and general mayhem can threaten to overwhelm the most confident nurses with doubts about their competence. In order to avoid being caught off guard when working with adolescents, it is important that nurses practice effective stress management with respect to their own day-to-day reactions. It is also of great importance in communicating with adolescent children that nurses carefully examine their own memories and experiences, and the emotional sediment that these may have left in them.

Occasionally the adolescent experiences so much psychic pain that it makes them agreeable to intervention and treatment. Most adolescents, in this author's experience, come to treatment manifesting obvious distrust and hostility. They are likely to be crude and rude, and if their parents are present, they will often act in a way that maximally embarrasses and provokes the parents. They may also attempt to antagonize and humiliate the nurse. The nurse should anticipate this situation and try to be as good-humored and calm as possible. Respect and understanding are essential elements in communicating with adolescent patients, just as they are in any other meaningful human encounter. Using jargon or adolescent street talk, however, is usually not beneficial, and is most often interpreted by the adolescent as patronizing and artificial (Youniss and Smollar, 1985). Adolescents are like anyone else in that they want to be accepted, approved, and understood. They respond to firmness, honesty, genuine affection, and consistent behavior on the part of authority figures. Although this may seem like nothing more than common sense, it has been this author's experience over the years that attaining and maintaining such an attitude in residential or in-patient settings is exceedingly difficult. In particular, consistency of behavior, mutual respect, and team cohesiveness on the part of staff members are elements that are frequently problematic and difficult to achieve.

Because adolescents value their independence and sense of control, it is crucial that nurses communicate directly with them as much as possible, rather than doing so through intermediaries. The adolescent, like any patient, has the rights and privileges accorded to all human beings. Because trust and honesty are crucial, nurses must thoroughly explain confidentiality and clearly delineate the issues it entails and excludes.

Adolescents with a history of violent, impulsive behavior pose a special challenge to nursing-staff members. Warning signs of potentially explosive behavioral episodes include a loud strident voice, tense posture, fist clenching, or inability to sit still. Nurses should be particularly careful when assessing adolescents who show no remorse or discomfort when discussing their violent acts. In an initial contact with a potentially violent adolescent, the nurse and patient should not be alone. From the beginning, the nurse must calmly state (without issuing hostile directives or ultimatums) that violent behavior will not be tolerated. Nurses should speak slowly and clearly, and listen to uncritically to the potentially violent adolescent patient. Offering a soft drink or snack can sometimes help to reduce the patient's agitation; speaking softly can be helpful when an adolescent patient is particularly belligerent (Howells and Hollin, 1989).

In addition to dealing with the impulsivity and acting-out behavior of adolescents, the nurse must also remember that regardless of the structure or setting, there may be many obstacles to treatment if the latter is involuntary. This is simply because no human being takes pleasure in being incarcerated, nor do they relish the perception of being forced to do the will of others. Part of the difficulty in involuntary treatment is that it heightens the disparity in power between the adolescent patient and staff member, and exacerbates already existing conflicts over authority. Involuntarily committed adolescents may be hostile, guarded, and suspicious, or deceptively placating and submissive. Nurses and other staff members may sometimes lose hope for the adolescent patient's future, come to fear the patient, or have sadistic fantasies about the patient. All of this makes it difficult to maintain a consistent and therapeutic attitude. To develop a meaningful and mutually respectful relationship with a reluctant adolescent, nurses must keep these difficulties in mind and concentrate on helping the patient, emphasizing and re-emphasizing both verbally and by their actions that their obligation is primarily to the adolescent and his or her welfare.

■ NURSING CARE OF THE ADOLESCENT

The nursing process is carried out for adolescents as it is for any other patient. Of particular importance is the nurse's awareness of the developmental needs and key issues unique to adolescents, such as those related to puberty. Efforts must be made to create a comfortable climate in which to talk about these issues.

ASSESSMENT

Assessment is a means of gathering information, and in work with adolescents should include all of the elements that are important to know about any client. In addition, because the epidemic of new and deadly STDs is today a high-risk consequence of sexual activity, the nurse should gather information about the adolescent patient's sexuality and sexual behavior, sexual identity, and need for knowledge about sexual issues. Most experts in adolescent psychology suggest that both the adolescent and parent figures should be interviewed, and also argue that it is useful to express an awareness of multiple points of view about sexuality and that the professional is willing to listen to all of them (Miller, 1983).

DIAGNOSIS

The diagnosis portion of the nursing process in working with adolescent patients involves analysis of the data gathered during the assessment portion of the interview process, which becomes the basis for the planning of care. Diagnoses are labels that identify certain real and potential problems in a patient. Although diagnosis is a useful procedure, nurses should keep in mind that the labels it yields are often negative and liability oriented, and say nothing about a patient's assets or strengths.

PLANNING

Planning for intervention should be determined by the priority of the patient's problems, with safety issues being of paramount importance. It should include working with the patient's assets and strengths as well as the patient's liabilities. Planning is always goal-directed and based on desired outcome objectives that can be measured. It includes discharge planning for hospitalized patients as well as the development of strategies for in-patient and out-patient care. Planning for care with adolescents should be a collaborative process, with the patient being allowed to maintain some sense of control over his or her circumstances. Although limits should be set on impulsive acting-out or abusive behaviors, adolescents will be much more inclined to adhere to treatment regimens and participate in their care if power struggles with staff members are avoided.

Some sense of autonomy and self-direction can be instilled by simply presenting the adolescent patient with a forced choice, such as by having the patient decide whether to take showers in the morning or evening. Because adolescent problems take place within a family context, the patient's family should be included in planning. Planning in psychiatric settings should always involve a multidisciplinary team consisting of a group of psychiatric specialists, subspecialists, and other behaviorally oriented professionals. The concept underlying the multidisciplinary approach is the belief that because health care is provided in complex institutions, by multiple skilled personnel, a collaborative approach to patient care will reduce fragmentation and offer a more holistic approach to such care (Brown, 1982).

INTERVENTION

Interventions are processes concerned with assisting individuals to achieve their goals or to function more effectively. The purpose of intervention can be remedial (resolving an existing problem), prevention (developing skills and programs to prevent a specific problem), or developmental (with the goal of educating or increasing a patient's functioning or coping). Counseling and psychotherapy are remedial, preventive, and developmental interventions employed in psychiatric settings. The other treatment modality for adolescents experiencing mental-health problems is medication targeted at individual symptoms.

Although the staff nurse does not practice classical psychotherapy, Peplau (1969) has argued that it is essential for staff nurses who work in psychiatric settings to have a general knowledge of basic counseling techniques. Peplau has written extensively about the phases of relationship development and the basic principles of counseling techniques. Because it is the ethical responsibility of nurses (ANA, 1985) to acquire the skills that have been shown to be effective in psychiatric settings, nurses considering work in this environment are strongly encouraged to become acquainted with Peplau's work before entering such practice.

It is uncommon for any single form of therapy to be the correct one for a particular disorder. Although opinions differ about therapy for adolescents, several general conclusions are agreed upon. These include flexibility of approach, focusing on the patient's existing functioning in a directive and direct manner as opposed to interpretation and analysis (Miller, 1983; Shaffer et al., 1988).

Family therapy has recently begun to play an important part in the treatment of adolescent problems. Therapists have realized that adolescent turmoil and other symptoms may often directly reflect disturbed family functioning. Gadpaille (1985, p. 1809) argues that "in the best of all possible worlds, family therapy would be the one modality employed . . . in the treatment of all disturbed adolescents who are still actively involved with their parents." Group therapy has been found effective in some cases. However, because of adolescents' fragile self-images, the selection of patients for adolescent group therapy must be done carefully. This is because group therapy, rather than helping, may confirm adolescents' worst fears about themselves. Groups seem to be most effective for adolescents whose problems manifest themselves primarily in interpersonal difficulties and who show a pattern of withdrawal and isolation, or who become involved in gangs that are bound together by destructive behavior (Miller, 1983).

EVALUATION

The evaluation portion of the nursing process entails determining whether there is agreement by the patient, nurse, and treatment team about the outcomes of the interventions to be used. The evaluation does not have to be restricted to outcomes only, but should properly include an evaluation of the processes for implementing the program of care. Attention to the implementation and care process is as important as attention to outcomes, and can help in future planning and in fine-tuning interventions, as well as in establishing links between qualitatively different interventions and behavioral outcomes.

E CASE EXAMPLE

▶ NURSING CARE PLAN AND INTERACTION SAMPLE FOR AN ADOLESCENT WITH CONDUCT DISORDER

Background: Jason is a 16-year-old who is admitted to an inpatient psychiatric facility following a period during which he had increasingly serious problems in school. He had been truant, his grades were failing, he was provocative toward his peers, and belligerent with his teachers. He fancied himself to be the "class clown." On the day preceding his admission, Jason had played a "practical joke" that consisted of his setting fire to the tail of a cat and letting the animal loose in his English class. He was suspended from school and his parents were contacted. His admission to the hospital was precipitated by his having attacked his father at home. His father, who has a history of alcohol abuse, has been known when provoked to be physically abusive toward Jason and his mother, and became enraged when he found out that Jason had been suspended from school. When he came home in the evening the father began to punch Jason with his fists and Jason had tried to stab him with a kitchen knife. The police were called and Jason is admitted to the inpatient facility as a danger to others. At the point of this interaction, Jason is already beginning to make plans for his discharge, and he was no longer considered a danger to others. The treatment team has been making plans with Jason for his re-integration into his community. Jason has been asked to take specific steps to facilitate this integration, but has been somewhat resistant about them.

Nursing diagnosis: Jason is diagnosed as having a disturbance in role performance related to failure at life events, as evidenced by his poor academic performance, suspension from school, and not taking responsibility for himself.

Outcome criteria: The outcome criteria in Jason's case call for him to realistically identify and evaluate what can be actively influenced by his own actions. He develops a plan to cope with his age-appropriate roles. Possible interventions: assist Jason in understanding his poor academic performance; encourage his participation in a plan for his return to school; explore his lack of action, and stress the need for his self-direction and accountability.

Examples of interaction related to Jason's case are as follows:

Nurse: So, how have things been going? (Open question.)

Jason: Well, I thought real hard about how to get back into the swing of school again. Nothing really came to mind.

Nurse: So you've been thinking real hard. What specific thoughts have you had along those lines?

Jason: Oh, lots, I've been pretty busy here, what with groups and all (vague, changes the subject, gives excuses).

Nurse: Yes, it can get pretty busy. So tell me about some of the thoughts that you say you've had. (Directive.)

Jason: Well, I was thinking I might call one of my buddies to get caught up with what I missed. You know I missed a lot when I got suspended and I'm really gonna be behind. It's gonna be a drag. I'm not even sure whether anyone would come and bring the work here to the nuthouse.

Nurse: Which buddy?

Jason: Maybe Joe, but he probably wouldn't.

Nurse: Have you asked him or contacted him to ask him if he would mind?

Jason: Well, no.

Nurse: So although you say that you want to get back to your regular routine, you really haven't moved to do anything, like calling some of your friends about getting transitioned back to school? (Interpreting, confronting, and paraphrasing.)

Jason: Well, no I guess not.

Nurse: There, it sounds as if you're beginning to take some responsibility for not moving on the issue of school.

Jason: Well, yeah. But . . . ,

Nurse: But what?

Jason: Well I don't really like to look at it as me not moving. But I guess it is.

Nurse: So let's start by discussing who you could call who might be able to help you out with the school assignments and bring you up to date on what's been going on while you've been away.

■ NURSING RESEARCH AND ADOLESCENCE

The period of adolescence has been extensively, although often inadequately, researched. Studies of this period been flawed in many respects, most especially in terms of sampling. The inattention to girls has been noted as a significant shortcoming in the study of the adolescent experience (Gilligan, 1987), and minority youth have been significantly underrepresented (Elliot and Feldman, 1990). These problems are being addressed by current research efforts.

Nurses who work with hospitalized adolescents are conducting research that significantly contributes to the quality of care these patients receive. One such study (Peterson et al., 1994) instituted a new behavioral-milieu program that included two components. One component was a positive behavioral point system in which patients earned up to 100 points in a 24-hour period for certain positive behaviors on a psychiatric unit, at meals, in school, in family meetings, and in group therapy. The entire staff was expected to be consistent in the allocation of points. The second aspect was the implementation of 15 nurse-led groups. These groups provided a forum for teaching and assessing adolescents, and included a self-esteem group, drug abuse group, and boys' and girls' issues group. The groups dealt with social skills, communication skills, critical thinking, and other issues that were relevant to adolescent populations and focused on promoting each adolescent's sense of responsibility. The outcomes of this study included decreased use of mechanical restraints for 56% of the patients in the first 3 months of implementation, and for 82% in the second 3 months. This study is important in that it can assist nurses in implementing changes on their own hospital units that promote more adaptive and less restrictive ways of dealing with maladaptive or aggressive behavior.

A second study illustrates the increasing sensitivity among nurse-researchers to the issue of under-represented groups in adolescent health research. Dashiff et al. (1995) conducted a study to see whether African-American and white fifth-grade girls had different attitudes about menarche and menstruation. Administering a questionnaire to 55 premenarcheal girls, they found no difference between black or white girls in their attitudes toward this life change. The authors concluded that the instrument was not culturally sensitive enough to use as a way of assessing the efficacy of future interventions with different populations. The importance of this article lies in its underscoring the issue of cultural sensitivity when considering intervention research in a health-care environment that involves diverse and heterogeneous populations.

O AN OVERVIEW

- Adolescence is a period of development characterized by a number of tasks and shifts in learning. It is determined by chronological age, a variety of physical, sexual, and emotional factors, and contextual factors such as historico-socio-cultural influences.

- A number of theories and models attempt to explain the adolescent experience; some models are more useful than others. They are a short-hand for characterizing the resolution of adolescent task attainment.

- Adolescent issues that can disrupt resolution of this period of development include sexual activities, social roles, peer influences, family dynamics, body image, and dependence-in-dependence negotiations.

- Adolescents may engage in several high-risk behaviors: substance abuse, unprotected sexual activity, behaviors that are related to accidental injury, body marking, and moshing.

- Adolescents may experience various maladaptive disorders: adjustment disorders, conduct disorders and violence, depression, suicidal behavior, eating disorders, oppositional-defiant disorder, schizophrenia, and delinquent behavior.

- Strategies for working with disturbed adolescents include group, individual, milieu and family therapies, psychopharmacology, communications skills, and behavior modification.

TD TERMS TO DEFINE

- personality theory
- early adolescence
- puberty
- middle adolescence
- late adolescence
- amotivational syndrome
- body marking
- adjustment disorder
- eating disorders
- depression
- oppositional disorder
- conduct disorder
- delinquent behavior

Q STUDY QUESTIONS

1. Discuss adolescence as a developmental process and differentiate the concept of process from the idea of developmental stages.

2. Identify some ways in which research on the adolescent experience can be more inclusive of the ways in which various under-represented youth groups perceive it.

3. Thinking back on your own adolescent experience, identify one adolescent conflict that might affect your role as a nurse on an adolescent psychiatric unit or in an adolescent psychiatric clinic. Discuss ways in which your own value system might influence your care of an adolescent (e.g., if you have a negative reaction toward obesity). How would you deal with your own issues and engage in the process of values clarification?

4. Identify the ways in which males and females experience puberty differently.

5. In communicating with and assessing adolescents, what factors must be taken into account that differ from those in the care of adult patients?

6. Discuss the various factors that can negatively affect "normal" adolescent health.

7. Discuss the variables that can result in adolescent psychiatric disorders.

8. A young man of age 13 is admitted to your unit after having stabbed to death his girlfriend in a jealous rage. Discuss your plan of care for this patient.

9. Read one book of fiction about an adolescent experience. This can be one involving a psychiatric illness or a "normal" experience. What are the conflicts as narrated by the author? Knowing what you know about the adolescent experience, do these conflicts ring true to you? Why or why not? If this novel involves a psychiatric situation, construct a plan of care for this adolescent.

10. Discuss the role of the family and family dynamics in adolescent mental health care. Why is it crucial to have family involvement in the care of the adolescent patient?

■ REFERENCES

Standards of Psychiatric Mental Health Nursing. Kansas City, American Nurses' Association, 1982.

Code Book with Interpretive Statements. Kansas City, American Nurses' Association, 1985.

Diagnostic and Statistical Manual of Mental Disorders ed. IV. Washington, DC, American Psychiatric Association, 1994.

Anderson CM, DJ, Hogarty GE *Schizophrenia and the family.* New York, Guilford Press, 1986.

Baumrind D: Familial antecedents of adolescent drug use: A developmental perspective, in Jones CL, Battjes RJ (eds): *Etiology of Adolescent Drug Abuse: Implications for Prevention.* NIDA Research Monograph No. 56. Rockville, MD, National Institute on Drug Abuse, 1985.

Baumrind D: (1987) A developmental perspective on adolescent risk taking in contemporary America, in Irwin C (ed): *Adolescent Social Behavior and Health* Cambridge, MA, Cambride University Press, pp. 93–125.

Bell TA, Holmes KK: Age-specific risks of syphilis, gonorrhea and hospitalized pelvic inflammatory disease in sexually experienced U.S. women. *Sex Transm Dis* 1984; 11:291–295.

Berman AL: *Adolescent Suicide: Assessment and Intervention.* Washington, DC, American Psychological Association, 1991.

Brage D: Adolescent depression: A review of the literature. *Archi Psychiatr Nurs* 1995; 9(1):45–55.

Brent D, Perper J, Goldstein C, Kolko D, Allen M, Allman C, Zelenak J: Risk factors for adolescent suicide: A comparison of adolescent suicide victims with suicidal pts. *Arch Gen Psychiatry* 1988; 45:581–588.

Brooks-Gunn J, Ruble DN: The development of menstrual related beliefs and behaviors during early adolescence. Child Dev 1982; 53:1567–1577.

Brooks-Gunn J, Petersen AC, Eichorn D: The study of maturational timing effects in adolescence. *J Youth Adolesc,* 1985; 14 pp. 3, 4.

Brooks Gunn J: Transition to early adolescence, in Gunnar M., Collins WA. (eds): *Development During Transition to Adolescence: Minnesota Symposia on Child Psychology,* vol 21. Hillsdale, NJ, Lawrence Erlebaum, 1988, pp. 189–208.

Brooks-Gunn J: Pubertal processes and the early adolescent transition. In W. Damon Ed. *Child development today and tomorrow.* San Francisco; Jossey-Bass, 1989; pp. 155–176.

Brooks-Gunn J, Reiter EO: The role of pubertal processes. 16–54 *At the Threshold* Cambridge, MA, Harvard University Press, 1990.

Brown TM: A historical view of health care teams, in Agich GJ (ed): *Responsibility in Health Care.* Boston, D. Reidel, 1982.

Bureau of Justice Statistics National Crime Survey. Washington, DC, U.S. Department of Justice, 1992.

Cass LK, Thomas CB: Childhood pathology and later adjustment, in Rossi PH, Berk RA, Lenihan KJ (eds): *Money Work and Crime.* New York, Academic Press, 1980.

Centers for Disease Control: Patterns of alcohol use among teenage drivers in fatal motor vehicle accidents: US, 1977–81 *Morbid Mort Wk Rep* 1983a; 32:344–347.

Centers for Disease Control: Alcohol as a risk factor for injuries: *US Morbid Mortal Wkly Rep* 1983b; 32:61–62.

Damon W, Hart D: *Self-Understanding in Childhood and Adolescence.* New York, Cambridge University Press, 1988.

Dashiff CJ, Buchanan LA: Menstrual attitudes among black and white premenarcheal girls. *J Child Adolesc Psychiatr Nurs* 1995; 8(3):5–14.

Doke LA, Flippo JR: Aggressive and oppositional behavior, in Ollendick T., (ed): *Handbook of Child Psychopathology* New York, Plenum Publishing, 1982, p. 222.

Elliott GR, Feldman SS: Capturing the adolescent experience 1–15, in Elliot GR, Feldman SS (eds): *At the Threshold.* Cambridge, MA, Harvard University Press, 1990.

Enzer NB, Cunningham SD: Adjustment and reactive disorders, in Wiener JM (ed): *Textbook of Child and Adolescent Psychiatry.* Washington, DC, American Psychiatric Press, 1991.

Finkelhor D, Dziuba-Leatherman J: Children as victims of violence: a national survey. *Pediatrics* 1994; 94:413–420.

Gaddis A, Brooks-Gunn J: The male experience of pubertal change. *J Youth Adolesc* 1985; 14(1):61–69.

Gadpaille WJ: Psychiatric treatment of the adolescent, in Kaplan HI, Sadock BJ (eds): *Comprehensive Textbook of Psychiatry*, vol 4. Baltimore, Williams & Wilkins, 1985, pp. 1805–1812.

Galanter M: *Cults and New Religious Movements*. Washington DC, American Psychiatric Press, 1989.

Gessell A, Ames L: *Youth: The Years from Ten to Sixteen*. New York, Harper & Row, 1956.

Gilligan C: Adolescent development reconsidered, in Irwin C (ed): *Adolescent Social Behavior and Health*. San Francisco, Jossey-Bass, 1987 pp. 63–92.

Grief EB, Ulman KJ: The psychological impact of menarche on early adolescent females: A review of the literature. *Child Dev* 1982; 53:1413–1430.

Halmi KA: The state of research in anorexia nervosa and bulimia, in Guze S, Roth M (eds): *Psychiatric Development, Advances and Prospects in Research and Clinical Practice*. New York, Oxford University Press, 1983, pp. 247–60.

Hambly WD: *The History of Tatooing and Its Significance*. New York, Basic Books, 1975.

Harter S: Cognitive-developmental processes in the integration of concepts about emotion and the self. *Soc Cogn* 1986; 4:119–151.

Hawkins JD, Lishner DM, Jenson JM, Catalano RF: Delinquents and drugs: What the evidence suggests about prevention and tx. programming, in Brown BS, Mills AR (eds): *Youth at High Risk for Substance Abuse*. Rockville, MD, National Institute on Drug Abuse, 1987.

Herzog DB: Bulimia: the secretive syndrome. *Psychosomatics 1982; 23:481–487.*

Herzog DB, Pepose M, Norman DK, Rigotti NA: Eating disorders and social maladjustment in female medical students. *J Nerv Ment Dis* 1985; 173:734–737.

Herzog DB, Copeland PM: Eating disorders. *N Engl J Med* 1985; 313:295–303.

Herzog DB: Eating disorders, in Nicholi AM (ed): *The New Harvard Guide to Psychiatry*. Cambridge, MA, Harvard University Press, 1988, pp. 434–445.

Hesselbrock N: Childhood behavior problems and adult antisocial disorder in alcoholism, in Meyer RE (ed): *Psychopathology and Addictive Disorders*. New York, Guilford Press, 1986, pp. 307–324.

Hill JP, Lynch ME: The intensification of gender related role expectations during early adolescence, in Brooks-Gunn J., Peterson AC (eds): *Girls at Puberty: Biological and Psychosocial Perspectives*. New York, Plenum Publishing, 1983, pp. 201–228.

Hilliard JR, Slomowitz M, Levi LS: A retrospective study of adolescent visits to a general hospital psychiatric emergency service. *Am J Psychiatry* 1987; 145:1416–1419.

Hofferth SL, Hayes CD: *Risking the Future: Adolescent Sexuality, Pregnancy and Childbearing,* vol 2 Washington, DC, National Research Council, National Academy Press, 1987.

Holinger PC, Offer D, Barter JT, Bell CC: *Suicide and Homicide Among Adolescents*. New York, Guilford Press, 1994.

Howells K, Hollin CR: *Clinical Approaches to Violence*. New York, John Wiley & Sons, 1989.

Huizinga D, Elliott DS: Juvenile offenders: Prevalence, offender, incidence and arrest rates by race. *Crime Delinq* 33:206–223, 1990.

Insurance Institute for Highway Safety. *1984 Status report* 19(7), Washington DC 1–11, 1984.

Institute of Medicine, Division of Mental Health and Behavioral Medicine: *Research on Children and Adolescents with Mental, Behavioral and Developmental Disorders: Mobilizing a National Initiative*. Washington, DC, National Academy Press, 1989.

Johnston LS, O'Malley PM, Bachman JG: *National Survey results on drug use from the monitoring the future study 1975–1993*. Publication No. 94–3809. Rockville, MD, National Institute on Drug Abuse, 1994.

Justice B: Evidence fails to support more punishment as a remedy for childhood violence. *Psychol Rep* 1991; 69:1193–1194.

Kennedy S, Garfinkel PE: Anorexia nervosa, in Francis AJ, Hales RE (eds): *American Psychiatric Association Annual Review*. Washington, DC, American Psychiatric Press, 1985.

Kohlberg L: Stage and sequence: The cognitive-developmental approach to socialization, in Goslin DA (ed): *Handbook of Socialization Theory and Research* Chicago, Rand McNally, 1969, pp. 347–480.

McCord J: Consideration of some effects of a counseling program, in Martin WE, Sechrest LB, Redner R (eds): *New Directions in the Rehabilitation of Criminal Offenders*. Washington, DC, National Academy of Sciences, 1981, pp. 394–405.

McCord J: Deterrence and the light touch of the law, in Farrington DP, Gunn J. (eds): *Reactions to crime: The public, the Police Courts and Prisons*. London, Wiley, 1988, pp. 73–85.

Millstein SG, Irwin CE: Accident related behaviors in adol: A biopsychosocial view. *Alcohol, Drugs Driving* 1988; 4(1):21–29.

Miller D: *The Age Between: Adolescence and Therapy*. New York, Jason Aronson, 1983.

Mixon D: *Obedience and Civilization: Authorized Crime and the Normality of Evil*. Winchester, MA, Pluto Press, 1989.

Miller D: *The Age Between: Adolescence and Therapy*. New York, Jason Aronson, 1983.

Mohr WK: The private psychiatric hospital scandal: A critical social approach. *Arch Psychiatr Nurs* 1994; 8(1):3–8.

Morrison DM: Adolescent contraceptive behavior: A review. *Psychol Bull* 1985; 98(3):538–568.

Newcorn JH, Strain J: Adjustment disorder in children and adolescents. *J Am Acad Child Adolesc Psychiatry* 1992; 31(3):318–327.

Nicholi AM: The adolescent, in Nicholi AM (ed): *The New Harvard Guide to Psychiatry*. Cambridge MA, The Belknap Press of Harvard University Press, 1988.

Nielsen G: *Borderline and Acting Out Adolescents*. New York, Human Services Press, 1983.

Novello AC: Violence is a greater killer of children than disease. *Pub Health Rep* 1991; 106(3):231–232.

Pardes H, Kaufmann C, Pincus HA, West A: Genetics and psychiatry: past discoveries, current dilemmas and future directions. *Am J Psychiatry* 1989; 146:435–443.

Peck EB, Ullrich HD: *Children and Weight: A Changing Perspective*. Berkeley; CA, Nutrition Communications Associates, 1985.

Peplau H: *Basic Principles of Patient Counseling*, 2nd ed. Philadelphia, Smith Kline and French Laboratories, 1969.

Petersen AC: The nature of biological-psycholsocial interactions: The sample case of early adolescence, In Lerner RM, Foch TT (eds): *Biological-Psychosocial Interactions in Early Adolescence: A Life-Span Perspective*. Hillsdale, NJ, Lawrence Erlbaum, 1987, pp. 35–61.

Peterson EJ, Gray KA, Weinstein SR: A look at adolescent treatment in a time of change. *J Child Adolesc Psychiatr Nurs,* 1994; 7(2):5–15.

Pipkin NL, Walker LG, Thomason MH: Alcohol and vehicular injuries in adolescents. *J Adolesc Health Care* 1989; 10:119–121.

Pynoos RS, Eth S: Child as criminal witness to homicide. *J Soc Iss* 1984; 40:87–108.

Rapoport JL, Ismond DR: *DSM III Training Guide for Diagnosis of Childhood Disorders.* New York, Brunner-Mazel, 1984.

Robins LN: Sturdy childhood predictors of adult antisocial behavior: replications from longitudinal studies. *Psychol Med* 1978; 8:611–622.

Robins LN, Tipp J, McEvoy L: Antisocial personality, in Robins LN, Regier D (eds): *Psychiatric Disorders in America,* New York, The Free Press, 1991.

Rutter M, Graham P, Chadwick OFD, Yule W: Adolescent turmoil: fact or fiction? *J Child Psychol Psychiatry,* 1976; 17:35–56.

Shaffer D, Blain B, Beck A, Dole P, Irwin CE, Sweet R, Schachter JB. *Chlamydia trachomatis:* Important relationships to race, contraceptive use, lower genital tract infection and Papanicolaou smears. *J Pediatr* 1984; 104:141–146.

Shaffer D, Garland A, Gould M, Fisher P, Trautman P: Preventing teenage suicide: a critical review. *J Am Acad Child Adolesc Psychiatry* 1988; 27:675–687.

Shane PG: Changing patterns among homeless and runaway youth. *Am J Orthopsychiatry* 1989; 59(4):208–214.

Shaw JA, Campo-Bowen A: Aggression, in Sholevar GP (ed): *Conduct Disorder in Children and Adolescents,* Washington, DC; American Psychiatric Press, 1995, pp. 45–59.

Sholevar GP: *Conduct Disorders in Children and Adolescents.* Washington, DC, American Psychiatric Press, 1995.

Sholevar GP, Sholevar EH: Overview, in Sholevar GP (ed): *Conduct Disorders in Children and Adolescents,* Washington, DC; American Psychiatric Press, 1995, pp. 3–27.

Schwartz IM, Jackson-Beeck M, Anderson R: The "hidden system of juvenile control. *Crime Delinq* 1984; 30(3):371–385.

Schwartz IM: Hospitalization of adolescents for psychiatric and substance abuse treatment. *J Adolesc Health Care* 1989; 10(6):1–6.

Stanton MD, Todd TC: *The Family Therapy of Drug Abuse and Addiction.* New York, Guilford Press, 1982.

Steinberg L: Single parents, step parents and the susceptibility of adolescents to antisocial peer pressure. *Child Dev* 1987; 58:269–275.

Stratern A, Strathern M: *Self Decoration in Mount Hagen.* London, Lippincott, 1971.

Strunkard AJ, Stellar E: *Eating and its Disorders.* New York, Raven Press, 1983.

Teri L: Depression in adolescence: Its relationship to assertion and various aspects of self-image. *J Clin Child Psychol* 1982; 13:475–487.

Uhlenberg P, Eggebeen D: The declining well-being of American adolescents. *Public Interest* 1986; 82:25–38.

U.S. Department of Health and Human Services: *Healthy People 2000: National Health Promotion and Disease Prevention Objectives.* Washington, DC, U.S. Public Health Service, 1991.

Vine P: *Families in Pain: Children, Siblings, Spouses and Parents of the Mentally Ill Speak Out.* New York, Pantheon, 1982.

Vygotsky LS: *Mind in Society* Cambridge, MA; Harvard University Press, 1978.

Weithorn LA: Mental hospitalization of troublesome youth: An analysis of skyrocketing admission rates. *Stanford Law Rev* 1988; 40:753, 773–838.

Wetzel J: *American Youth: A Statistical Snapshot.* Washington, DC, William T. Grant Foundation Commission on Work, Family, and Citizenship, 1987.

Wilson MD, Joffe A: Adolescent medicine. JAMA 1995; 273(21):1657–1659.

Wolf N: *The Beauty Myth: How Images of Beauty are Used Against Women.* New York, William Morrow & Co., 1991.

Wolfgang ME, Figlio RM, Sellin T: *Delinquency in a Birth Cohort.* Chicago, University of Chicago Press, 1972.

Worchel F, Nolan B, Wilson V: New perspectives on child and adolescent depression. *J School Psychol* 1987; 25:411–414.

Wyatt RJ: Neuroleptics and the natural course of schizophrenia. *Schizophr Bull* 1991; 7(2):325–351.

Youniss J, Smollar J: *Adolescents' Relations with Mothers, Fathers, and Friends.* Chicago, University of Chicago Press, 1985.

Zelnick M, Shah FK: First intercourse among young Americans. *Fam Plan Perspect* 1983; 15:64–72.

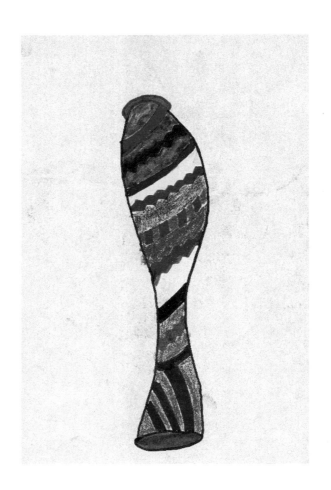

"Thank God for the way I am."

Elsie Immerman,
a 94-year-old woman

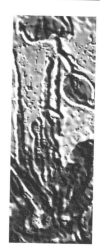

19

Aging and Mental Health

Sandra L. Rosen

Americans are growing older. Since the turn of the century, the number of people aged 65 years and older in the United States has increased tenfold (National Institute on Aging [NIA], 1991). In the span of one decade, between 1980 and 1990, the number of people over age 85 grew by 38%, while the 65- to 84- and under-65 age groups grew by only 20% and 8%, respectively, (NIA, 1991). These statistics indicate that the fastest-growing segment of the older population is the "very old." Almost 7-million people were at least 80 years of age in 1990, approximately 3 million of them were at least 85 years old, and almost 1 million at least 90 years of age (NIA, 1991); 36,000 had reached or surpassed the century mark (NIA, 1991). As of 1990, the life expectancy at birth was 75 years, and the odds of reaching age 65 were 80% (NIA, 1991). Burnside (1990) has projected annual percentage growth rates for the United States population through the year 2020, with an emphasis on increases in the number of older adults (Figure 19-1).

Statistics reveal that approximately 12.5% of Americans are over 65 (NIA, 1991). The stereotyped image American society has of its older adults represents them as frail and heavily dependent on others. However, this portrait is far from accurate. For instance, less than 5% of those aged 65 to 69 require assistance with bathing (Blazer, 1990), and more than 70% of those aged 85 and up can bathe independently (Blazer, 1990). Most elders in the United States have at least one chronic medical problem; yet the majority do not suffer disabling functional impairment. Since the aging process is not necessarily a pathway to dysfunction and dependency, most older adults live in the community, with only 5% residing in institutions, such as nursing homes (Blazer, 1990). Many elders lead active lives, and some, such as marathon runners, are more active than most people half their age.

Almost no age group is immune from emotional problems. Toddlers, school-aged children, adolescents, young adults, and middle-aged people seek psychiatric help. The elderly are no exception. Since the older adult population is both large and fast growing, and since most elderly persons reside in the community, nurses may encounter them in a wide variety of settings, such as acute-care hospitals, personal-care homes, adult day-care centers, psychiatric hospitals, out-patient clinics, geriatric-evaluation clinics, community mental-health centers, primary-care physician's offices, and even on the streets. Of the patients enrolled with home health-care agencies, 45 to 65% are over age 65; 50 to 70% have behavioral, emotional, social, and mental disorders (Harper, 1990).

This chapter examines mental health in the older adult. Following an overview of the aging process, typical changes of later life, and nursing assessment of the geriatric patient, detailed attention is given to three disorders commonly seen in old age: depression, delirium, and dementia, including Alzheimer's disease. The chapter concludes with a discussion of the role of families as care-givers for the elderly.

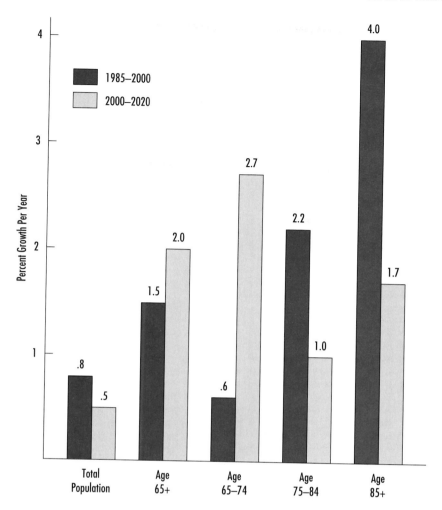

Figure19–1. Projected annual percentage growth for United States Population.

From Burnside I: Reminiscence: An independent nursing intervention for the elderly. *Issues Ment Health Nurs.* 1990; 11:36.

■ THE FINAL STAGE OF PSYCHOSOCIAL DEVELOPMENT

Erik Erikson (1950) developed a paradigm of psychosocial development that he called the Eight Stages of Man. His theory is based on the process of socialization, with heavy emphasis on the influence of parents, significant other persons, and the environment on this process. Erikson perceived development as a continuous struggle for emotional–social equilibrium. For each of the eight stages of development in his theory, there is a dominant psychosocial crisis and a specific task to be accomplished. Through such task accomplishment, the individual is said to have resolved the conflict of the stage, thereby attaining emotional–social equilibrium.

The final stage in Erikson's framework is the achievement of **ego integrity** as opposed to **despair.** During this final stage, older adults review their lives for meaning, purpose, and a sense of worth. They are sharply aware that their past, including mistakes, perceived failures, poor decisions, and omissions, cannot be changed, and they experience either acceptance or regret. If elders feel reasonably pleased with the way they have lived and what they have accomplished, the developmental task has been successfully accomplished, and ego integrity is achieved. If instead they face many regrets, despair and resentment may ensue. Of course, such despair may lead to depression. It is important to recognize that individuals differ in their readiness for death. Some elders may indicate goals, realistic or unrealistic, that they still hope to achieve.

■ CHANGES OF LATE LIFE

Americans have formed several misconceptions about the aging process, which in turn contribute to unpleasant myths and stereotypes. For example, older adults are sometimes described as crotchety, cranky old people. However, since a person's basic personality style is established during early adulthood and remains the same thereafter (Blazer, 1990), the truth is that drastic personality changes are not occurring in the elderly. What may happen is a strengthening of the established personality, which becomes more evident to others. Perhaps the major misconception about this cohort involves senility and the incorrect perception that confusion is a normal part of aging. On the contrary, confusion is definitely not a part of the normal aging process.

A few changes in mental function are likely to occur as people age. Occasional forgetfulness, especially of the recent past, and an increase in the time needed for processing information are not danger signs. Likewise, the older adult may take longer to respond to questions and requests and to process multiple stimuli (Blazer, 1990). Another change affecting members of this cohort is the likelihood of shorter sleeping periods; many older adults complain of insomnia.

Hearing difficulty is both the most common and the most disabling sensory problem of aging (Blazer, 1990); a decrease in both pitch discrimination and hearing acuity may occur. As for visual changes, acuity, accommodation, and adaptation to darkness all may decrease, whereas sensitivity to glare increases. Of visual problems, presbyopia is common, but cataracts and glaucoma are more serious (Blazer, 1990). Normal changes need to be assessed to ensure early intervention, such as providing a hearing aid or eyeglasses, and appropriate communication with elders.

■ STRESSES AND LOSSES OF OLDER ADULTHOOD

At a time when older adults are looking back on their lives, they most likely are also forced to deal with present losses. Often these losses are multiple and may include the deaths of family members and friends. Although the death of a spouse is a devastating loss, a living but ailing spouse adds extra stress. Other potential losses include decreased income and financial status, and declining health and physical capabilities. Loss of independence may be particularly disturbing to the older adult. Furthermore, today's high rate of crime and violence may be especially frightening to members of this cohort, whom others, and they themselves, see as vulnerable.

A study of 1,415 elderly people found that the frequency of loneliness increased with older age (Bowling, Farquar, and Browne, 1991). Another source of stress is relocation, which can occur in a variety of configurations, including a move from a house to an apartment, from one's own home to the home of relatives, or from a community residence to a nursing home. A variety of losses often accompany relocation, such as giving up belongings and possessions, decreased privacy, and decreased independence. Elders feel a greater sense of control when residing in a familiar environment; this is true even when the environment appears objectively detrimental to the quality of life (Silverstone and Horowitz, 1992). Likewise, elderly persons may feel a loss of control when well-meaning relatives make decisions about relocating them without taking into consideration their choices and preferences.

Retirement is usually viewed as another loss, with changes in role, time structure, and financial status. However, Bosse and colleagues (1991) studied 1,516 men, 45% of whom were retired. Participants completed an Elders Life Stress Inventory (Aldwin, 1990), which focuses on 31 possible events. In this sample, the three stressful events most frequently cited were deterioration of memory, the death of a friend, and major deterioration in the health or behavior of a family member. The three most stressful events by ranking were the death of the spouse, the death of a son or daughter, and the institutionalization of a spouse. Respondents who had retired within the prior year rated their own and their spouse's retirement as the least stressful of 31 events. In fact, retirement was found stressful by only 30%. The investigators found retirement more likely to be stressful when accompanied by negative implications, such as forced, unexpected, or involuntarily separation from employment (due to health, plant closings, etc.); health problems after retirement; or financial decline. Retirement planning should always be considered a worthwhile intervention, best undertaken during middle- to late-middle-age. Components of this anticipatory work include areas such as finances, post-retirement activities, living arrangements, role changes, health-care needs, and legal affairs.

■ THE GERIATRIC ASSESSMENT

The psychological assessment of the older adult patient is much like that of younger individuals. Table 19–1 provides a quick reference for components of the geriatric assessment. To begin, the nurse should determine the chief complaint or reason for referral—in other words, the reason for the interview. Demographics including sex, age, culture, and living arrangements should be explored. A thorough medical and psychiatric history is important, as well as a current evaluation of overall medical health. A physical examination with a complete review of the patient's systems is necessary. Likewise, all

TABLE 19–1. THE GERIATRIC ASSESSMENT

Chief complaint/reason for interview

Demographical information

Medical and psychiatric histories

Current overall medical health

Physical examination and laboratory tests

Medication inventory and compliance

Drug and alcohol use

Mental status examination

Stressors and coping style

Nature of support system

Functional status

Cultural and spiritual assessments

Tests/screening tools as needed

Patient concerns and goals

cranial nerves should be checked. Studies such as a complete blood count, blood chemistry analyses, thyroid function tests, vitamin levels, urinalysis, a urine drug screen, a chest X-ray, an electrocardiogram (ECG), and electroencephalogram (EEG) may be indicated to rule out physical disturbances such as electrolyte imbalances, vitamin deficiencies, anemia, dehydration, or systemic infections. Symptoms of physical disturbances may mimic symptoms of emotional problems. While most older adults are neither seriously ill nor have significant functional disability, the presence of physical illness in later life does increase the risk of emotional problems, especially if the physical problems are multiple (Blazer 1990). Moreover, physical problems can lead to social stigma and isolation, economic difficulties, and functional impairments. An inventory of all the patient's medications, the patient's knowledge about them, and the extent of compliance with treatment needs to be completed. Drug and alcohol use should be assessed regardless of a patient's age.

Assessment of mental status should include the following elements:

- General appearance
- Reaction to interview
- Level of consciousness
- Orientation
- Consistency and appropriateness of behaviors
- Mood and affect
- Thought content
- Judgment and insight
- Recall and memory
- Intellectual function
- Comprehension
- Concentration and attention

Buckwalter and Stolley (1991) identify warning signs of mental illness in the older adult:

- Significant personality changes
- Confused thinking
- Strange or grandiose ideas
- Prolonged and severe depression
- Apathy
- Extreme mood changes
- Severe anxiety
- Extreme fear
- Suspiciousness
- Blame of others
- Withdrawal
- Isolation
- Denial
- Suicidal ideation
- Suicide talk
- Exaggerated anger
- Psychosis
- Drug and alcohol abuse
- Inability to cope with daily life

These are not unlike warning signs of mental illness in any population.

Assessment of the patient's support system, including kin, friends, neighbors, organizations (church, clubs, self-help groups), and professionals (health-care providers), is important Does the patient have a confidant, someone with whom he or she feels safe in sharing concerns and problems? Social support and/or an intimate confidant may act as a "buffer" mediating the influence of stressful life events (Kurlowicz, 1993). How does the patient describe the quality and quantity of his or her social interactions? What is the patient's perception of his or her social activity and the availability of support? With an effective social network in place, there are opportunities for improved self-esteem, positive feedback and approval, acceptance, love, and support.

Functional status must be explored, especially basic self-care needs. Is the patient toileting, bathing, grooming, dressing, and feeding him- or herself independently? Is the patient able to shop, carry groceries, cook, and wash dishes independently? What about light housekeeping tasks? What about heavier tasks, such as vacuuming, washing the floors, and shoveling snow? Can the patient manage his or her own finances? If assistance is needed with any of these functions, is the patient receiving it? Mobility is critically important but may be affected by arthritis, reductions in orthostatic blood pressure, and an unsteady gait. Are there stairs in the home, and if so, is the elder able to handle them? What transportation is available to the older adult? Is the neighborhood a generally safe one? How often does the patient get out of the home? Does the patient work? If so, how much and doing what? Is the patient satisfied with his or her job/retirement? Does the patient do any volunteer work? Is he or she having sleep difficulties? Does the patient report any sexual concerns? Very important is determining the patient's access to health care. Does the older adult describe any burdens, and what is his or her knowledge of available resources? What is a typical day like for this older adult? A typical night?

Cultural and spiritual assessments should be included, as people often find security in their beliefs, values, and customs. Moreover, customs and beliefs affect attitudes toward health, illness, aging, death, health-care providers, gender-role differences, and family roles. A patient's cultural background and value system influence reported symptoms. For example, culture often affects pain reactions, and depressive-type symptoms may not be revealed without some gentle probing by the interviewer. The American Psychiatric Association (*DSM-IV,* 1994, p. 324) acknowledges the impact of culture on emotional function; the organization states the following about symptoms of depression: "Complaints of 'nerves' and headaches (in Latino and Mediterranean cultures), of weakness, tiredness, or 'imbalance' (in Chinese and Asian cultures), of problems of the 'heart' (in Middle Eastern cultures), or of being 'heartbroken' (among Hopi) may express the depressive experience." Some older adults and their families may be wary of the health-care system because of previous experiences with discrimination. Assessing the role of religion in the patient's life is significant, because religious beliefs influence attitudes and practices. Furthermore, religious persons and organizations may be part of the elder's support system. Noting the patient's socio-economic status and educational background is important for similar reasons.

Asking the patient about any concerns he or she may have is vital and ideally leads to preventive measures and anticipatory guidance. Common themes for older adults include somatic concerns, losses (including loss of control), review of life, and death (Blazer, 1990). Themes that recur among elderly patients who are "alone" are mortality, personal regrets, the need for forgiveness, and expressions of love for dead and living family members and friends (Genevay, 1992). It is noteworthy that 30% of persons aged 75 or older report concerns about emotional problems or social support (Wasson and Jeste, 1993). The patient's goals and ideas need to be assessed and seriously considered. Helping the patient to set realistic goals is an important nursing function. As with any patient, mutual definition of treatment goals and intervention modalities is optimumal with the elderly patient.

TESTS AND SCREENING TOOLS

Psychiatric nurses have many screening tools to aid their assessments. One benefit of using such tools is that patient status is evaluated on an objective level, so that reports from different nurses and shifts are comparable. Likewise, progress and decline are easier to detect by simply re-testing and comparing the results. Some screening tools have been developed for all patients regardless of age, and others are designed specifically for older adults. Moreover, there are tools to measure different aspects of a person's well-being. Table 19–2 provides a modest list of screening tools, tests, and scales.

OPTIMAL APPROACHES TO INTERVIEWING AND TESTING

Building rapport and a trusting therapeutic relationship is important in helping the older patient to feel at ease and able to discuss concerns openly and honestly. If the assessment is the first meeting between the patient and the psychiatric nurse, the time for building rapport will be limited. However, the nurse can assist the patient to feel comfortable and safe and can get accurate testing results in a number of ways. Late morning may be the time of optimum cognitive functioning, prior to afternoon fatigue, but this can vary among individuals. On the other hand, it may be better to test a patient's functioning at a variety of times if there is some question about cognitive ability. A quiet, un-busy location is needed for testing, since sensory overload can contribute to anxiety as well as interfere with memory and learning. After introducing her- or himself, the nurse should explain the purpose and length of the interview and screening tests. Before beginning, it is important that the older adult be wearing any sensory aids prescribed to reduce the impact of sensory deficits. The nurse should speak clearly, avoiding both medical terminology and slang. When the patient's hearing is decreased, it is especially important to look at the patient while speaking. When asking questions or giving directions to perform an action, it is crucial not to assume that the patient does not know the answer, cannot remember, or is confused, since the older adult's reaction time to verbal requests and questions may be normally slowed. Likewise, the older adult is not to be rushed; instead, the nurse should demonstrate patience and comfort with silence. Demonstrating a non-judgmental attitude is equally important to minimize test anxiety. Of course, assessing a patient's understanding of questions and requests is necessary. Clarification would then be provided as needed.

Slight changes in testing procedure may lead to increased comfort and more valid results with elderly patients. For instance, when a screening tool is lengthy or emotionally or physically taxing, a fatigued patient may benefit from rest periods. However, it is imperative to first check whether such changes are permissible for the tool. A patient's position may make a difference, such as lying in bed, sitting up in a chair, or being allowed to have stretch periods to prevent joint stiffness

TABLE 19–2. LIST OF TESTS/SCREENING TOOLS

Test/Scale	Author(s)	Year	Measures
ADL's/Functioning:			
CADET	Rameizl	1983	Self-care
Geriatric Functional Rating Scale	Grauer and Birnbom	1975	Functioning, to determine need for institutional care
Index of Independence in Activities of Daily Living	Katz, Ford, Inoskowitz, Jackson, and Jaffe	1963	Asks about behaviors most people encounter daily
Instrumental Activities of Daily Living Scale	Lawton and Brody	1969	Self-maintaining and instrumental activities of daily living
OARS Instrument	Duke Univ. Ctr. for the Study of Aging and Human Develop.	1978	Functional ability
Townsend's Activities of Daily Living Scale	Townsend	1979	Functional status
Depression:			
Beck Depression Inventory (BDI)	Beck	1961	Depression
The Geriatric Depression Scale	Yesavage Brink, Rose, Lum, Huang, Adey, and Leiter	1983	Depression
Zung Self-Rating Depression Inventory (SDS)	Zung	1965	Depression
Dementia:			
Blessed Dementia Rating Scale	Blessed, Tomlinson and Roth	1968	Dementia
A Dementia Rating Scale	Lawson, Rodenberg and Dykes	1977	Dementia
FROMAJE	Libow	1981	Dementia, depression
Mental Status/Cognition:			
Assessment of Confusion	Vermeersch	1986	Presence/severity of acute confusion in
Confusion Rating Scale	Williams, Ward, Campbell	1988	Subtle manifestations and rapid changes of acute confusion
The face-hand test (FHT)	Fink, Green and Bender	1952	Adjunct in assessment of organic mental disorders, to distinguish patients with brain damage from those who are psychotic without an organic cause
Mental Status Questionnaire (MSQ)	Kahn	1960	Severity of brain syndrome, a gross measure of mental status and cognitive function changes
The Mental Status Questionnaire for Evaluation of Brain Dysfunction in the Aged	Kahn	1971	Mental status
Mini-Mental Status Examination	Folstein and McHugh	1975	Cognitive function
Nurses' Observation Scale for Inpatient Evaluation (NOISE)	Honigfeld and Hendricks	1981	Patient behaviors, incl. factors of social competence and interest, cooperation, and psychotic depression
Sandoz Clinical Assessment-Geriatric (SCAG)	Shader, Harmatz, and Salzman	1974	Mental status, mood, motivation, social ability, fatigue, and anxiety
Short Portable Mental Status Questionnaire (SPMSQ)	Also, Duke University	1978	Mental status: intact to severe impairment
Others:			
Delighted-Terrible Faces Scale	Andrew and Withey	1976	Current and overall life satisfaction
Elders Life Stress Inventory (ELSI)	Aldwin	1990	Stress of events of past year
General Health Questionnaire (GHQ)	Goldberg and Williams	1988	Psychiatric morbidity
Neugarten's Life Satisfaction Scale Index A	Neugarten, Havighurst, and Tobin	1961	Current and overall life satisfaction
PACE II	U.S. Dept. of Health, Educ. and Welfare	1978	Physical health of nursing home patients
Social Network Scale	Hirsch	1980	Network size and type
	Stokes	1983	

in elders susceptible to this. Moreover, one patient may prefer a hard, wooden chair and another a soft, cushiony chair.

■ MENTAL ILLNESS IN OLDER ADULTS

Careful assessment of the elderly patient may reveal signs and symptoms of an emotional disorder or mental illness. Among the conditions typically encountered in this age group are depression, delirium, and dementia. It is important to understand the clinical manifestations, risk factors, and etiology characteristic of each, as well as the appropriate treatment regimens.

DEPRESSION

Depression is not only the most prevalent emotional disorder plaguing older Americans it is also believed by some to have the most disturbing symptoms (Keane and Sells, 1990). According to an epidemiologic catchment-area study (National Institutes of Health [NIH] Consensus Development Panel on Depression in Late Life, 1992), depressive symptoms occurred in approximately 15% of the studied community's residents who were over age 65. The rates of major or minor depression in older adults range from 5% in primary-care clinics to 15 to 25% in nursing homes. Moreover, 13% of nursing-home residents will develop a new episode of major depression within any 1-year period (NIH Consensus Development Panel on Depression in Late Life, 1992).

Underdetection

Although depression is the most treatable mental disorder in later life (Keane and Sells, 1990), it is often undetected. By one estimate, only about 10% of the elderly who are in need of psychiatric treatment ever receive it (NIH Consensus Development Panel on Depression in Late Life, 1992, p. 1020). The consequences of such underdetection are tragic. In addition to suffering and mental anguish, the elderly population experiences devastatingly high suicide rates. The American Psychiatric Association (1994) notes that not only do up to 15% of persons with severe major depressive disorder commit suicide, but that the death rate increases fourfold for those with major depressive disorder who are over 55 years old. Reducing this high percentage of suicide fatalities is possible, especially since most elders contemplate suicide for 1 to 2 months before making the attempt (Frierson, 1991). According to recent data more than 75% of elderly suicide victims visited their primary care physician within the month prior to suicide (NIH Consensus Development Panel on Depres-

sion in Late Life, 1992), and 33% to 50% did so within the prior week (Frierson, 1991). However, far too many of these adults at risk are not receiving life-saving intervention.

The National Institutes of Health Consensus Development Panel on Depression in Late Life (1992) identified several reasons for underdetection of mental disorders in the elderly. Frequently, depression is unnoticed in the older adult who has many physical problems. Furthermore, a depressed mood may be a less prominent symptom in this age group than loss of appetite, sleeplessness, anergia, decreased interest in and enjoyment of activities, and somatic symptoms. Health-care professionals all too often conclude that depression is a normal consequence of the circumstances of old age, such as physical illness, economic difficulties, and social problems. Likewise, the symptoms experienced by an older person may be noticed but then incorrectly labeled as part of the usual aging process. A compounding problem is that older adults often do not see themselves as depressed or will not admit experiencing depression, possibly because of the belief that there is no hope for help, or for reasons of fear of stigma.

Other investigators suggest that the diagnostic criteria for psychiatric disorders may not be "age-fair." Consequently, a high number of symptoms may be reported in an older person but no actual disorder diagnosed. Without a diagnosis, treatment is not offered (George, 1990).

Clinical Manifestations

The depressed older adult may experience loss of appetite, disturbed sleep, decreased energy and enjoyment, and a range of physical symptoms. These manifestations may be more evident than a depressed mood *per se* (NIH Consensus Development Panel on Depression in Late Life, 1992).

Careful and thorough screening for depression is emphatically needed with the older adult population. Interviews with not only the older adult but also family members and care-givers are frequently indicated. Another way to enhance detection is to utilize sound screening tools (see Table 19–2) in conjunction with the nursing interview. For example, Keane and Sells (1990) investigated the reliability of the Beck Depression Inventory (BDI) and Zung Self-Rating Depression Inventory (SDS) as indicators of depression in the elderly. They found both to be adequately reliable as clinical screening instruments with an elderly population. However, they noted that the SDS may result in a higher number of false positives, diagnoses, and for this reason the BDI might be a preferable screening instrument (Keane and Sells, 1990, p. 24). The Geriatric Depres-

TABLE 19–3. DIAGNOSTIC CRITERIA FOR DEPRESSION

Criteria for Major Depressive Episode

- Five (or more) of the following symptoms have been noted over a 2-week period and represent a change from previous functioning; at least one of the symptoms is either (1) depressed mood or (2) loss of interest or pleasure. The symptoms are not due to a medical condition, use of a substance, or bereavement.
  1. Depressed mood most of every day, as indicated by either subjective report (e.g., feels sad or empty) or observation made by others (e.g., appears tearful).
  2. Markedly diminished interest or pleasure in all, or almost all, activities most of the day.
  3. Significant weight loss when not dieting or weight gain (e.g., a change of more than 5% of body weight in a month), or decrease or increase in appetite.
  4. Insomnia or hypersomnia nearly every day
  5. Psychomotor agitation or retardation
  6. Fatigue or loss of energy
  7. Feelings of worthlessness or excessive or inappropriate guilt (which may be delusional, not merely self-reproach or guilt about being sick)
  8. Diminished ability to think or concentrate, or indecisiveness.
  9. Recurrent thoughts of death (not just fear of dying), recurrent suicidal ideation without a specific plan, or a suicide attempt or a specific plan for committing suicide.

(*Diagnostic and Statistical Manual of Mental Disorders*, ed. 4, Washington, DC, American Psychiatric Association, 1994. p. 327)

sion Scale may be a good choice, since it emphasizes psychosocial symptoms instead of vegetative ones. The diagnostic criteria for major depression are listed in Table 19–3, and the criteria for adjustment disorder with depressed mood in Table 19–4.

Risk Factors

According to the NIH Consensus Panel, the major social and demographic risk factors for depression in the elderly are basically the same as those for younger adults: females, unmarried persons (especially widowed) individuals, and those experiencing stressful life events and lacking a supportive social network are most at risk. A host of disturbances associated with late-life depression have been identified, including neurotransmitter imbal-

ance, structural brain changes, dysregulation of endocrine function, physical illness, cognitive distortions, mourning, sleep-wake cycle disturbances, unsuccessful developmental task accomplishment, stressful life events, chronic social stress, and extreme social isolation (Leuchter (1991) and Blazer (1990). It is important to reiterate that there is a connection between physical illness and depression. According to Kurlowicz (1993), a strong relationship exists between depression and physical illness or disability at all ages. The *DSM IV* (1994) noted that up to 25% of people with certain medical conditions, such as diabetes, myocardial infarction, carcinomas, and stroke, may develop a major depressive disorder. Moreover, from 4 to 8% of older adults have significant depressive symptoms secondary to an adjustment disorder related to physical illness (Blazer, 1990). Bowling and Browne (1991) conducted a study of elders aged 85 and older living in inner London. They were looking at life satisfaction and found that health status (measured by functional ability and number of health problems) was a more powerful predictor of overall life satisfaction than social-network variables (i.e., number of friends and relatives).

As previously discussed, loss is a stressful life event for older adults. Bereavement, for example, "too often leads to the feeling that all life is loss, that nothing good does or can occur" (Zerhusen, Boyle, and Wilson, 1991, p. 17). Since old age is, as Erikson noted, a time to review one's life, such negative thoughts may lead to depressive emotions (Zerhusen, et al., 1991).

Depression Versus Bereavement

A loss occurs when someone or something is missing or no longer possessed. Approximately 800,000 people are

TABLE 19–4. DIAGNOSTIC CRITERIA FOR ADJUSTMENT DISORDER

Diagnostic Criteria for Adjustment Disorders

- The development of emotional or behavioral symptoms in response to an identifiable stressor(s) occurring within 3 months of the onset of the stressor(s).
- These symptoms or behaviors are clinically significant as evidenced by either of the following:
  1. Marked distress that is in excess of what would be expected from exposure to the stressor
  2. Significant impairment in social or occupational (academic) functioning
- The symptoms do not represent Bereavement.
- Once the stressor is eliminated, the symptoms do not persist for more than an additional 6 months.
- May be acute or chronic.

Diagnostic and Statistical Manual of Mental Disorders, ed. 4. Washington, DC, American Psychiatric Association, 1994, pp. 626–627.

widowed each year, most of them older adults (NIH Consensus Development Panel on Depression in Late Life, 1992).

Although such a loss may lead to depression, bereavement and depression are not identical. A few symptoms of normal bereavement resemble depressive symptoms. Like an older person who is depressed, one who is bereaved may voice more somatic complaints and make more physician visits. Normal symptoms of the grieving process include decreased interest in usual activities, reduced energy, sleeping difficulties, crying, decreased concentration, tightness in the throat, shortness of breath, sighing, a decreased appetite, preoccupation with the image of the deceased, irritability, and hostility (Blazer, 1990). Expressions of guilt concerning things done or not done at the time of the loved one's death are not abnormal; such guilt is specific instead of global. The bereaved older adult still sees him- or herself as a good person; there is no morbid preoccupation with worthlessness (Blazer, 1990). While the bereaved older adult may think that he or she would be better off dead, there is no suicidal ideation.

Generally, treatment of the bereaved is supportive in nature. Medications must not be used to sedate or numb the grief-stricken patient. The availability of one nurse with whom the patient can talk is important. This nurse might choose to begin by educating the older adult about the grieving process. Encouraging the patient to talk of the relationship, death, and resulting feelings is a significant aspect of **grief** work. Referrals to support groups, such as widow-to-widow programs, may also be indicated. Sometimes, more extensive referrals may be necessary. A man who has not cooked or cleaned may need housekeeping help or a meal program after losing his wife. Likewise, a woman who has not been a part of financial planning may require assistance with bills and budgeting if her husband dies.

Suicide Risk

At highest risk for suicide are elderly white males (NIH Consensus Development Panel on Depression in Late Life, 1992). According to Frierson (1991), suicide rates for these men increase with every decade after age 60. Although there are many suicide attempts in younger age groups, completed suicides among older adults are likely related to the use of more lethal methods. Frierson (1991) conducted a chart review study of 95 patients who were evaluated by a psychiatric consultation service following an unsuccessful suicide attempt. The patients ranged in age from 60 to 90. He found the top three precipitants to be ill health, loneliness, and bereavement. He also found that characteristics of these survivors included premeditation, a greater tendency

(than younger attempters) toward firearm use and wounds to the head, male sex, co-existing medical problems, a serious intent to commit suicide that increased by decade, solitary living arrangements, presence of a serious psychiatric condition or history, and ill health identified as a major precipitant to suicidality (Frierson, 1991, p. 144).

In another study, of a group of 60 completed suicides committed by elders 65 years or older, 18 had given reasons for their suicide (Loebel et al., 1991). The most common reason was fear of nursing-home placement (44.4%); second was pain (22.2%); third was a tie between interpersonal difficulties and incapacity (each 11.1%); and last was a tie between finances and remorse (each 5.6%). Although the study sample was small, and the number of subjects providing specific suicide reasons was only 18, the results are still noteworthy. Prevention of suicide is more likely when reasons for attempting it can be identified and dealt with. For instance, anticipatory work can be undertaken with likely nursing-home candidates. Pain management is crucial in any population, but unfortunately, since the aged population verbalizes many physical complaints, cries of pain from older persons are not taken as seriously as they should be.

Etiology

The many theories about mental illness derive from biologic, psychodynamic, sociocultural, and behavioral frameworks. One theory of depression is that an imbalance of the neurotransmitters norepinephrine and serotonin in the brain causes depression (Blazer, 1990). Some theorists are paying specific attention to the site where these neurotransmitters attach to the postsynaptic neuron. A quantity of evidence exists that these receptors are "down-regulated" in depressed people (Blazer, 1990).

Clinical Management

"Talking" Therapies. The NIH Consensus Development Panel on Depression in Late Life (1992) listed the following goals of treatment: decrease symptoms, decrease risk of relapse, increase quality of life, increase medical health, and decrease health-care costs and mortality. A variety of noninvasive techniques can be used to treat the depressed older adult patient. Koenig and Breitner (1990, p. 29) suggest that "because some symptoms of depression are situational, counseling and supportive care should be offered, regardless of whether antidepressants are prescribed." Blazer (1990, p. 65) warns that antidepressants "are of little benefit in treating adjustment disorders and actually may complicate the

physical problem." Therefore, "talking therapy" may be particularly appropriate for a patient with an adjustment disorder with a depressed mood related to difficulty in adjusting to a medical illness. Use of empathy helps to encourage the expression of feelings. Relaxation therapy may also be beneficial for the depressed anxious patient. Examples include progressive muscle relaxation, rhythmic breathing exercises, and/or guided imagery. Expanding the elder's support system or working to motivate the one already in place is sometimes necessary.

Of course, even those professionals who provide "talking therapy" may employ a number of different modalities (psychoanalytical, supportive, cognitive, behavioral, systems, etc.). However, certain techniques are strikingly appropriate with elderly patients. Life review and reminiscing are two examples of approaches to use with this cohort. Each gives the patient a chance to reorganize and resolve issues. When these techniques are being used, patients may be asked to write brief autobiographies or to verbally share experiences relating to a specific historical or personal event or to a particular personal relationship.

Zerhusen, Boyle, and Wilson (1991) conducted a study comparing cognitive therapy and music therapy to treat depression in men and women aged 70 to 82. Such cognitive therapy techniques as graded task assignments and cognitive rehearsal (both designed by Aaron Beck, 1979) were used, and BDI scores before and after intervention were compared. If met, it was held that the goals of cognitive therapy—"to replace the faulty and negative perceptions with more valid and positive ones" (p. 21)—would decrease depression. Cognitive therapy was found to be an effective modality in this study. However, more studies focusing on effects of noninvasive therapies with older adults are needed. Identification of the approaches that work best with different diagnoses is greatly needed. A general nursing-care plan for older adults with depression is presented in Table 19–5.

TABLE 19–5. NURSING CARE PLAN: DEPRESSION

Providing an Accepting, Comforting Atmosphere	Problem-Solving
Establish rapport	Include family therapy when indicated
Display empathy	
Encourage expression of feelings	Teach relaxation techniques to decrease anxiety
Allow time for responses, show patience	Assist with utilization of constructive problem solving process
	Assist with structuring of daily activity
	Assist with realistic goal formation
	Deemphasize importance of unrealistic goals

Maintaining Safety	Increasing Self-Esteem
Assess suicidality carefully and repeatedly	Assist to reduce negative thoughts via examination of perceptions/conclusions
Hospitalize when necessary	Limit negative self-criticism
Provide close supervision as needed	Stimulate participation in activities/hobbies
Assess and maintain physiological status	Encourage exercise, adjusted to health level
Assure that self-care needs are met	Encourage independence
Encourage appropriate expression of anger	Provide positive feedback
	Encourage socialization
	Assist with life review

Medication. In accordance with the theory that maintains that depression is due to a deficiency of certain neurotransmitters in the brain, many of the antidepressant drugs act to increase the concentration of chemical messengers in the synaptic clefts. In other words, these drugs increase the amounts of neurotransmitters such as norepinephrine and serotonin between nerve cells in the brain. For example, tricyclic antidepressants work specifically by blocking the re-uptake of neurotransmitters that are excreted from one end of a nerve cell at the synapse (Blazer, 1990).

Antidepressants may be used with the older depressed population. However, because of changes in pharmacokinetics in this group, the judicious use of any medication is imperative, owing to the potential for adverse side effects. Table 19–6 provides a list of common side effects of this category of drugs. For instance, **tricyclic antidepressants** may increase the risk of cardiac-rhythm irregularities, cause a decrease in blood pressure, increase urinary hesitancy and retention, and interact with many medications used for physical ailments (Blazer, 1990). Koenig and Breitner (1990) recommend that when tricyclic drugs are given to older hospitalized patients, a preliminary electrocardiogram should be done, as well as another one week after initiation of therapy. They go on to suggest checking the patient's orthostatic blood pressure before treatment begins, on the morning after the first dose, and again whenever dosage changes are instituted. Moreover, they reiterate the need for checking the blood levels of psychiatric medications. According to the NIH (NIH Consensus Development Panel on Depression in Late Life, 1992), the most commonly used antidepressants with older adults are the secondary amine tricyclic drugs

TABLE 19–6. ANTIDEPRESSANTS: SIDE EFFECTS PROFILE

Tricyclics

Anticholinergic effects:	Other effects:
Dry mouth	Lightheadedness
Blurred vision	Dizziness
Tachycardia	Sedation
Urinary hesitancy/retention	Photosensitivity
Constipation	Headache
Nausea	EPRs
Vomiting	Hypotension
	Cardiac rhythm disturbances

MAO-I's

Restlessness, jitteriness, hyperactivity

Insomnia

Fatigue

Weakness

Dizziness

GI disturbances, i.e., anorexia, nausea, diarrhea, abdominal cramping

Headache

Dry mouth

Blurred vision

Orthostatic hypotension

Cardiac rate and rhythm changes

Risk of hypertensive crisis

TABLE 19–7. CONTRAINDICATIONS TO USE OF ANTIDEPRESSANT MEDICATIONS IN OLDER PATIENTS WITH PHYSICAL ILLNESS

Relative contraindications

Symptoms of urinary obstruction
  benign prostatic hypertrophy
  urinary retention due to outlet obstruction

Delirium

Marked sedation or agitation

Use of multiple drugs with anticholinergic side effects
  antipsychotics   antiparkinsonian agents
  antihistamines
  atropine-containing drugs

Use of other drugs with the potential for serious interactions with tricyclics
  guanethidine, methyldopa, clonidine
  anti-arrhythmics, such as quinidine or pronestyl

Orthostatic hypotension

Severe hypertension

Moderate to severe congestive heart failure

Unstable angina

Conduction disturbances
  any combination of two of the following:
    first-degree heart block
    left anterior hemiblock
    left or right bundle-branch block

Poorly controlled seizures

History of allergy to a tricyclic antidepressant

Absolute contraindications

Recent myocardial infarction (within six weeks)

Acute ischemia on electrocardiogram

Acute angle closure glaucoma (rare)

Second- or third-degree heart block

New bundle-branch block following initiation of tricyclic treatment

Increased ventricular arrhythmias following initiation of tricyclic treatment

Reprinted from Koenig HG, Breitner JCS: Use of antidepressants in medically ill older patients. *Psychosomatics* 1990; 31: p. 24.

nortriptyline and desipramine, which have a more favorable side effect profile. The NIH warns that the use of the tertiary tricyclics amitriptyline and imipramine may produce such side effects as orthostatic hypotension, anticholinergic effects, cardiovascular consequences, and sedation. Table 19–7 presents a list of relative and absolute contraindications to the use of antidepressant medications in older patients with physical illness, as identified by Koenig and Breitner (1990).

The **monoamine oxidase inhibitors** (MAOI) are safe and effective in treating depression in the older adult, but are infrequently prescribed. Jeste and Krull (1991) suggested that this may be related to fears about the dietary and medication restrictions, hypotension, and insomnia. Several newer drugs are available in the fight against depression, such as trazadone, bupropion, and fluoxetine. These may be good choices for the older age group because they produce fewer anticholinergic and cardiovascular side effects (NIH Consensus Development Panel on Depression in Late Life, 1992), making them especially good choices for depressed patients with cognitive impairment (Koenig and Breitner, 1990).

In addition to side-effect profiles, the patient's medical status, previous response, symptom patterns, lifestyle, level of functioning, and knowledge base should be considered when selecting a drug. Once an antidepressant is chosen, conservative dosing is the key to safety, especially with older physically ill patients. Dosing should begin at a low level and be increased gradually. It is important for the treatment team to recognize that a significant antidepressant response frequently occurs later in older than in younger patients, often requiring at least 6 to 12 weeks before it appears (NIH Consensus Development Panel on Depression in

Late Life, 1992). Furthermore, since up to 40% of older patients will continue to experience depression over time, it is best to continue treatment for 6 months after the first episode of major depression and for at least 12 months if the episode is the second or third (NIH Consensus Development Panel on Depression in Late Life, 1992). The NIH (NIH Consensus Development Panel on Depression in Late Life, 1992) explains that about 80% of elderly patients who are maintained on antidepressant drug doses that produce a remission of the acute episode will remain in remission over an extended follow-up period.

Compliance is often a problem with older adults. An estimated 70% of such patients fail to take between 25% and 50% of their medication (NIH Consensus Development Panel on Depression in Late Life, 1992). Therefore, a thorough assessment, effective teaching

about medication, and a return demonstration are all key components to successful drug therapy. Facets of the assessment include previous and current medication compliance, perceptions of antidepressant treatment, the condition of the patient's memory, motivation, opportunities and financial means for obtaining prescribed medications, and availability of any needed assistance. If the patient has been non-compliant with medications, the reasons for this must not be overlooked. Careful planning and continued monitoring can help minimize the risk of non-compliance.

Electroconvulsive Therapy. **Electroconvulsive therapy** (ECT) may be the treatment of choice for the older depressed patient when delusions, catatonia, or life-threatening behaviors (i.e., refusal to eat) are also present. For pa-

E CASE EXAMPLE

▶ DEPRESSION

Terry Hampton is a 65-year-old widowed white female who has been living alone since the death of her husband from a myocardial infarction 4 years ago. Terry gets up each morning and attends to her grooming needs independently. Yet she then stays home all day watching television or listening to the radio while sitting next to her dog. Her medical history reveals that she has had insulin-dependent diabetes mellitus (IDDM) since age 30, had an occipital stroke 1½ years ago, has hypertension, arthritis, and slight dyspnea on exertion, and had early cataracts. Terry uses a cane to walk, and moves very slowly. She wears glasses but still complains of not being able to see. Her hearing is intact. She does her own finger sticks for blood glucose testing—three times on Monday, and each morning from Tuesday through Sunday. She reports that her glucose levels are usually in the low 100s, with an occasional spike related to an ice-cream indulgence. She admits that when she was younger she did not follow her diabetic diet because of a fancy for sweets, but adds that recently she has been more careful. Her insulin coverage is 40 units (70 NPH, 30 Reg) every morning. A visiting nurse goes to her home once a week to prepare seven syringes of insulin, after which Terry administers one to herself each morning. She feels that "they" have taken away her ability to draw up her own insulin. However, she also verbalizes understanding of why she is not "allowed" to do it herself, acknowledging her poor eyesight and the risk of making an error that could put her health, and even her life, in jeopardy. Her other medications are Procardia, 10 mg P.O. b.i.d., calcium 500 mg P.O. b.i.d., and aspirin 500 g P.O. b.i.d.

At one time Terry was quite active. She spent most of her life working at a local factory, but retired 5 years ago when she broke her leg. In her leisure time, she used to especially enjoy dancing with her husband. However, she currently ambulates slowly, with a cane, and leads a very inactive life, choosing to isolate herself. Both of Terry's

parents are deceased, as is also her sister, who died at age 35 from diabetes.

Terry has no children. The only family she has are her sister-in-law Marie and Marie's husband. Marie calls Terry daily, but they do not actually get together because Terry does not consider herself worthy enough for Marie to take time out of "her own busy life." She states that she has no friends because they have all either died or moved away. She insists that she is not good at starting conversations with people or making friends.

Terry has been referred to a partial hospitalization program. A psychiatric nurse admits her and completes a nursing assessment. Terry is awake, alert, and oriented to person, place, time, and situation, but also anxious, depressed, and withdrawn. She sits looking down at her hands in her lap, which she wrings intermittently during the interview. Her speech is soft and slow. Her immediate recall is intact, but she is uncooperative with testing of recent and remote memory. Both her concentration and insight are poor. She denies thoughts or past actions of harming herself or others, and is able to contract for safety. She reports sleeping from 9 P.M. to 9 A.M., which she labels "too much." No evidence of psychosis is noted.

An initial treatment plan is devised to address Terry's depression. Her social isolation, anxiety, physical problems, and low self-esteem are key objects of the plan. She is started on sertraline (Zoloft) 50 mg P.O. q.d. Terry is scheduled to attend a day program from 9:30 A.M. to 3:00 P.M. Monday, Wednesday, and Friday. It will include health education, group therapy, relaxation group, art psychotherapy, communication/social skills, assertiveness training, and a reminiscence group. The nurse will review Terry's diabetic diet with her and make suggestions for easier compliance, such as eating sugarless ice cream. In addition, an appointment is made for an eye exam because Terry has not had an examination in more than a year.

tients who are suicidal and for whom no other treatment has been effective, ECT may be life-saving. Jeste and Krull (1991) cite ECT as good for depression with dementia. A study by the National Institutes of Mental Health (NIMH) showed that patients over 61 years of age are the largest group receiving ECT, and that its short-term efficacy is strong (NIH Consensus Development Panel on Depression in Late Life, 1992). ECT may be safer than antidepressant drugs for these patients. However, there is fear and stigma about such treatment, partly related to its depiction in old movies, and an increased risk for post-ECT confusion has been identified in the older age group (NIH Consensus Development Panel on Depression in Late Life, 1992). Memory difficulties may be reduced by performing ECT unilaterally,

by inducing a seizure only in the nondominant hemisphere of the brain: the hemisphere less associated with memory (Blazer, 1990). Six to ten treatments are usually required, but Blazer (1990, p. 83) declares that "in most cases, improvement is evident after one treatment." The exact reason why ECT works has not been firmly concluded; the seizure may re-set the nerve-cell receptors for the chemical messengers in the brain (Blazer, 1990).

■ DELIRIUM

Delirium and dementia are two major mental conditions in the elderly. **Delirium** is a syndrome that goes by

E CASE EXAMPLE

▶ DEPRESSION

Jane Smith, age 66, lives alone. One year ago, her husband Tom died of a myocardial infarction, just 2 weeks after they celebrated their 40th wedding anniversary. They had raised two sons. One is married and lives with his wife and their two children just around the corner from Jane. The younger son married and had one child before being killed in an automobile accident 5 years ago. His wife and child survived the crash without any permanent injury and live 1½ hours from Jane. Jane's health has been fairly good. She takes propranolol for hypertension, but no other prescription medications. Aspirin had been helpful in relieving her arthritis pain in the past, but since her arthritis began to seriously flare up 3 weeks ago, aspirin no longer reduces the pain and swelling.

At a family barbecue yesterday, Jane broke out in tears, stating that she could not go on "like this." She wept about "everyone" leaving her when referring to her late husband and son. She went on to say that she was no good anymore because her arthritis pain kept her from baking cookies for her grandchildren. She cried for nearly 30 minutes despite hugs and positive remarks from her son and both daughters-in-law. It was not until one of her grandchildren climbed on her lap and said, "Grandma, please don't cry" that she dried her tears. She then worked to brighten her spirits for the "sake of the children."

Today, Jane's son calls the local mental-health center from concern for his mother. He would like to bring his mother in "so she has someone to talk to." He states, "I'm afraid for mom. She's so sad and depressed all the time lately, and none of us knows how to help her. We try to comfort her, to tell her how much she means to us, but it doesn't help." The mental-health nurse asks if he has talked with his mother about bringing her to the center. He quickly responds that he has in fact discussed this with his mother, and that she told him, "whatever you want . . . I don't care." An appointment is made for later the same day.

Once Jane and her son arrive at the mental health center, an intake assessment is performed. Jane is awake, alert, oriented, and cooperative with the intake process.

Her physical health is good except for arthritis pain in her hands, back, and knees, which she rates as 9 to 9.5 on a 0- to 10-point (10 representing the worst pain imaginable) pain scale. Her thought processes are clear and goal directed; there is no evidence of psychosis. Jane has no prior psychiatric history. She and her son each describe the good relations she had with her husband during their marriage, and the strong ties she still has with her family. She has one close friend, from college. Jane is a retired home-economics teacher. She "makes" herself perform activities of daily living and basic housekeeping chores despite her arthritis, but the pain keeps her from doing the "extra things" she enjoys—baking and knitting. Although Jane reports a decreased appetite, thus far she has not lost any weight. She also reports difficulty in going to sleep and staying asleep as a result of her arthritis pain. During the intake interview she repeatedly makes comments indicative of feelings of worthlessness. She denies suicidal ideation, firmly stating that she would never harm herself because she believes that whether she lives or dies is not to be in her hands. She describes herself as a "Catholic Church-goer but not overly religious." Jane agrees to come bi-weekly to the center to talk with someone about the things bothering her, although she voices doubt that this will help. She agrees to try a different medication for her arthritis, but refuses even to discuss the possibility of taking an antidepressant. She is prescribed naproxen sodium, 250 mg P.O. b.i.d. to take in place of aspirin.

As he drives Jane home from her seventh appointment, Jane's son asks her how she is doing. She responds that her arthritis is still present but "much, much better" with the naproxen. Knitting is still not possible. Jane affirms that she likes going to the center to meet with her "nurse" (a master's-prepared clinical nurse specialist), because she now has someone to talk to about "everything" without "bothering" her family. Jane's son tries to reassure his mother that she is not a bother, but she shushes him, instructing him to drive faster because she wants to bake a batch of cookies for him to take to his children.

many names, including but not limited to acute confusional state, pseudosenility, toxic confusional state, and toxic delirious reaction (see Table 19–9). The implication is that delirium is a temporary illness from which a person will return to normal functioning. Unfortunately, as with depression, delirium in an older adult is often unidentified. This can lead to various complications and even result in death.

CLINICAL MANIFESTATIONS

Delirium may be manifested in any combination of several signs and symptoms. These include changes in cognition, such as difficulties with memory, concentration, focusing, registration, and directed thinking, which may arise and tend to fluctuate throughout the day in an unpredictable manner. Likewise, problems with attention fluctuate in a non-regular way. Orientation may be disturbed, especially in terms of the patient's time sphere. Psychomotor behavior may either be increased, retarded, or both (the hyperactive, hypoactive, and mixed variants, respectively). The characteristics of hyperactive and hypoactive variants of delirium are listed in Table 19–10. The hypoactive and mixed variants are the most common forms in older adults. According to Lipowski (1989, p. 579), a patient with the hypoactive variant of delirium "appears lethargic and drowsy, responds to questions slowly, initiates hardly any action, and is apt to be overlooked or misdiagnosed as depressed." When increased motor behaviors exist, agitation and wandering can become stressful management problems for nurses. The patient may also experience psychotic thoughts, including hallucinations and delusions. The delusional patient may present as irritable, restless, and fearful. A delirious patient may engage in inappropriate communication (i.e., using nonsensical words, yelling, swearing, or keeping an unusual si-

lence), inappropriate maneuvers (i.e., pulling out intravenous lines or catheters), impulsive actions, and/or unsocial behavior (i.e., combativeness). Furthermore, illusions may occur. Also important to note is that general physical and neurologic changes such as dysphasia, tremor, asterixis, coordination problems, urinary incontinence, and focal neurologic signs, as well as clues to autonomic nervous system dysfunction, are more common with older than with younger adults who suffer from delirium (Liston, 1981).

Delirium is not a neat and tidy syndrome for which doctors and nurses can simply check-off a list of signs and symptoms to arrive at a diagnosis. The variability in signs and symptoms may account in part for the problem of underdetection of this condition. The diagnostic criteria for delirium are listed in Table 19–11.

PATHOGENESIS

There are four basic theories of delirium. These hold that it is due to: (1) A generalized cerebral insufficiency re-

TABLE 19–10. CHARACTERISTICS OF HYPERACTIVE VERSUS HYPOACTIVE VARIANTS OF DELIRIUM

Hyperactive	Hypoactive
Increased psychomotor activity	Decreased psychomotor activity
Mixed fast and slow frequencies on EEG excitability, hyperarousal of autonomic system	Diffuse slowing on EEG
Agitated, belligerent, restless	Decreased alertness, arousal, excitability
Pressured speech, loud	Lethargic, drowsy, quiet, calm
Psychotic tendencies	Responds slowly to questions

Reprinted with permission from Rosen SL: Managing delirious older adults in the hospital; *Med Surg Nurs*, 1994; 3: 181–189.

TABLE 19–9. ALTERNATIVE NAMES USED TO LABEL DELIRIUM

Acute brain failure	Clouded states	Subacute befuddlement
Acute brain syndrome	Exogenous psychosis	
Acute cerebral insufficiency	ICU Psychosis	Sundown syndrome
Acute confusional state	Metabolic encephalopathy	Toxic confusional state
Acute organic psychosis	Pseudosenility	
Acute organic reaction	Post cardiotomy delirium	Toxic delirious reaction
Acute organic syndrome	Rapid-onset confusion	
Acute psycho-organic syndrome	Reversible brain syndrome	Toxic encephalopathy
	Reversible dementia	Toxic psychosis
Cerebral insufficiency syndrome	Reversible toxic psychosis	Transient impairment

Reprinted with permission from Rosen SL: Managing delirious older adults in the hospital; *Med Surg Nurs*, 1994; 3: 181–189.

TABLE 19–11. DIAGNOSTIC CRITERIA FOR DELIRIUM DUE TO MEDICAL CONDITION

- Disturbance of consciousness (i.e., reduced clarity of awareness of the environment) with reduced ability to focus, sustain, or shift attention.
- A change in cognition (such as memory deficit, disorientation, language disturbance) or the development of a perceptual disturbance that is not better accounted for by a preexisting, established, or evolving dementia.
- The disturbance develops over a short period of time (usually hours to days) and tends to fluctuate during the course of the day.
- There is evidence from the history, physical examination, or laboratory findings that the disturbance is caused by the direct physiological consequences of a general medical condition.

(*Diagnostic and Statistical Manual of Mental Disorders* ed. 4. by Washington, DC, American Psychiatric Association, 1994, p. 129.)

lated to a decrease in the mechanisms for cerebral oxidation. (2) Changes in neurochemical mechanism with a decrease in acetycholine synthesis. (3) A reaction to acute stress with an accompanying increase in levels of plasma cortisol. (4) Acute lesions of the brain, especially of the right hemisphere. (Wanich, personal communication).

RISK FACTORS

Just as the older adult population is composed of more women than men, so too are there more female elders with delirium (*DSM-IV*, 1994). Substance abuse, polypharmacy, surgery, structural brain pathology, chronic illness, impaired vision, sleep deprivation, advanced age, social isolation, unfamiliar environment, and weakened psychological defenses are among the factors that predispose older adult patients to this condition (Liston 1984). Studies of older adult patients with hip fractures, conducted in 1979 and 1985, found the following risk factors for the development of delirium during hospitalization: confusion on admission, loss of mobility, elimination difficulties, and use of narcotics and tranquilizers (Williams, cited in Stanley, 1991). Polypharmacy and altered pharmacokinetics are contributing factors. Table 19–12 is a list of medications that can cause delirium. It is easy to recognize that any older adult is likely to have one or several factors predisposing to delirium.

ETIOLOGY

The list of causes of delirium is even more extensive than the list of syndrome characteristics or of risk factors. Foreman's research (1986, 1989, 1990) divides the causes of delirium into three large categories: physiological, psychological, and environmental. Physiological components include primary cerebral disease stemming from vascular insufficiency, infection of the central nervous system, trauma, or tumors; or entracranial diseases such as cardiovascular diseases (i.e., congestive heart failure, arrhythmias), pulmonary abnormalities (i.e., pneumonia), systemic infections (i.e., pyelonephritis), metabolic disturbances (i.e., acidosis, alkalosis, renal failure), drug intoxications (i.e., misuse of over-the-counter or prescribed medications), endocrine problems (i.e., diabetes), malnutrition and anemia, and disruptions in temperature regulation. Medications at dosages given to younger patients can be detrimental in older patients as the result of changes in **pharmacokinetics.** Additionally, drug withdrawal (i.e., alcohol, barbiturates, chloral hydrate, diazepam) can cause delirium. Psychological factors causing delirium include anxiety, depression, fatigue, pain, and grief. Environmental factors include unfamiliar surroundings, sensory overload or deprivation, and sleep deprivation.

UNDERDETECTION AND ITS IMPLICATIONS

Although prevalence rates of delirium vary, the numbers are disturbing. According to the *DSM IV*, about 10% of patients over age 65 and hospitalized with a medical condition have delirium on admission, and another 10 to 15% of such patients may develop delirium during their hospital stay (1994). Foreman's 1989 study of 71 non-surgical patients over the age of 60 found a 38% incidence of confusion within 6 days after admission. Even more troublesome is Foreman's observation that of all older hospitalized adults, up to 80% may develop acute confusion; nevertheless, as many as 7 in 10 patients who become delirious while hospitalized are never identified as delirious by nurses or physicians (Foreman, 1990).

What accounts for such drastic underidentification of delirium in older adult patients? In her discussion of delirious older adults in the intensive care unit (ICU), Stanley (1991, p. 63) asks whether there is "an attitude among nurses that some degree of disorientation is expected in the elderly and that these aspects of care [assessments of cognitive function] are not as critical as the physiologic aspects of care." Most likely, the primary reason for most missed diagnoses of delirium is the myth that older persons become confused as part of the normal aging process. Furthermore, the staff may hold the prejudiced view that therapy will be useless, since the confusion is seen as resulting from "the normal aging process." Other potential reasons for the nondetection of delirium include the high incidence of hypoactive and mixed variants (as described above) and the variety of names given to the syndrome.

Other barriers to detection of delirium in the older adult population are identified by Kurlowicz. (1993) One is that nurses fear insulting patients. Others

TABLE 19–12. TYPES OF MEDICATIONS WITH THE POTENTIAL FOR CAUSING DELIRIUM

Analgesics	Antiinflammatory agents	Coronary vasodilators
Anesthetics	Antinauseants	
Antiarrhythmics	Antineoplastics	Decongestion
Anticholinergics	Antiparkinsonism agents	Diuretics
Anticonvulsants	Antispasmodics	Expectorants
Antidiabetic agents	Antipsychotics	Hypnotics
Antidiarrheals	Antituberculosis agents	Muscle relaxants
Antihistamines	Antitussives	Sedatives
Antihypertensives	Cardiac/digitalis glycosides	

Reprinted with permission from Rosen SL: Managing delirious older adults in the hospital; *Med Surg Nurs*, 1994; 3: 181–189.

are that nurses do not perform comprehensive examinations, and gaps in communication occur, with nurses not informing physicians of changes in a patient's state of consciousness. Moreover, Kurlowicz recognizes the unfortunate reality that "in general, ageism prevailing in society gives mental health needs of elders a low priority." This ageism influences the care provided in all settings (Kurlowicz, personal communication, May 10, 1993).

The missed diagnosis of delirium leads to enormous implications. For example, delirious patients often require longer hospital stays, resulting in inflated hospital costs. In fact, Foreman (1990, p. 136) has said that "if the length of stay of each acutely confused elderly hospitalized patient could be reduced by just one day, the savings to Medicare would total $1 to 2 billion each year." The personal "cost" of underdetection of delirium is preventable death. Delirium in older adults should be considered a medical emergency (Davies, 1991), and should therefore receive immediate attention. According to Liston (1984, p. 116), recovery from delirium "is inversely related to age and to the duration of the syndrome." Even mild confusion can lead to injuries. Patients with the hyperactive variant are especially at risk for falls, fractures, head injury, and even cardiovascular collapse (Liston, 1984). Additionally, complications may be exacerbated if the patient fails to comply with or resists necessary medical treatment. If delirium is not identified, then the underlying problem is not treated and may become fatal. Likewise, delirium can progress to chronic organic brain impairment and then death. Progression to death may occur quickly in older adults who are also suffering from uncorrected dehydration and malnourishment (Liston, 1982). Liston (1984) notes that from 15% to 30% of older adult patients with delirium progress to stupor, coma, and death.

When hospitalized or placed in some other kind of facility such as a nursing home, patients require a comprehensive assessment of their physiological and cognitive status at the time of admission; frequent reevaluations cannot be overemphasized for the early detection of problems. Marr (1992, p. 31) recognizes that "nurses will have a key part to play in the assessment of acute confusional state as they are able to provide a 24-hour account of the patient in various situations in or out of the ward." Foreman (1990) suggests using the **Mini-Mental Status Examination** along with a behavioral scale for assessment. Such screening tools are best administered at different times of the day. The patient's mood should also be considered. The speed, mode, onset, and duration of actions need to be included in the assessment process to assist with accurate diagnosis. Additionally, screening for sensory/perceptual disturbances is important in order to avoid incorrect diagnosis. Direct questions should be asked to assess the

presence of psychotic features (i.e., hallucinations). Prompt diagnosis is more likely when nurses consider questions such as the following:

- Is the patient demonstrating attention difficulties?
- Is the patient disoriented?
- Is the patient experiencing a decreased level of consciousness?
- Is the patient having difficulty remembering?
- Is the patient engaging in inappropriate behavior, such as pulling out tubes?
- Is the patient climbing out of bed when he or she understands that this is not supposed to be done?
- Is the patient more withdrawn or quiet than usual?
- Is the patient suffering from a drastic change in the sleep-wake cycle?
- Is the patient physically agitated or even combative?
- Is the patient speaking incoherently or with nonsensical words?
- Is there evidence of psychotic symptoms?

CLINICAL MANAGEMENT

The first line of care for a delirious patient is determining the underlying cause of the confusion and treating it aggressively. However, the management of such patients goes beyond this to encompass five areas: physiology, environment, communication, protection, and medication.

Physiological Support

The list of potential physiological causes of delirium is long, and interventions that improve the patient's physiological status become very important in caring for a delirious older adult. Stanley (1991, p. 65) notes that an elderly patient has less tolerance for abnormalities in physiologic functioning than does a young patient. Significant attention must be paid to maintenance of hydration, nutrition, and electrolyte balance. Furthermore, such conditions as hypoglycemia and ketoacidosis must be dealt with immediately. Careful, precise monitoring of fluid intake and output, along with assessments of skin turgor, quality of salivation, and moistness of mucous membranes is imperative. Additionally, laboratory results should receive more than a quick perusing.

Older patients may have difficulty adjusting to hospital mealtimes and/or foods, which can negatively affect their nutritional status (Patrick, 1967). An example of a simple but helpful intervention is to allow the patient as much choice as possible with food selection. Assisting patients to easily meet elimination needs should also be a priority. Both the call bell and a urinal/bedpan should be placed within the patient's reach. Additionally, a nurse must promptly answer a request for assistance with toileting.

With delirium, the sleep-wake cycle is often impaired; at times a reversal of the usual diurnal rhythm even occurs (Liston, 1984). As a result, according to Lipowski, (1989, p. 579), "at night sleep is, as a rule, shortened and fragmented." Disruptions in usual sleep and activity patterns should be kept to a minimum. Liston (1982) notes that older adults with nocturnal exacerbations of delirium may endure more complications. Sleep-enhancing measures implemented in the evening (i.e., relaxation exercises, warm milk, and/or soft music) may be helpful. Frequent interruptions of the patient's sleep, such as for the recording of routine vital signs, may cause more harm than good, and need to be re-evaluated (Stanley, 1991). Grouping night treatments is one method to limit disruptions. Allowing for and encouraging activity that is appropriate and tolerated should also be an aim; enlisting a physical therapist or occupational therapist to become an active member of the patient's care team leads to high-quality, holistic care.

Environment

The best environment for the patient with delirium is one that is familiar, provides many orienting clues, maintains an appropriate balance of sensory stimulation, and is secure. When the older adult is hospitalized or placed in a nursing home, the nursing staff is in a good position to promote these measures.

An older adult may become confused in a confusing environment. Measures to make the environment more familiar may include decorating the room with the patient's favorite pictures, having his or her favorite books and objects in sight, and encouraging the family to bring in the patient's own quilt or bedspread from home (Davidhizar and Cosgray, 1990). McBride (1992) cautions that staff members sometimes pull curtains around the patient's bed to help block out external noise, but in so doing also block out familiar objects. Moreover, a patient who cannot locate a desired object may become anxious and insecure, which may then lead to confusion (Patrick, 1967). Room changes should be kept to a minimum.

Encouraging family and friends to visit is also helpful to the patient in the unfamiliar hospital environment or the patient beginning nursing-home adjustment. However, it is important for a nurse to educate visitors about their loved one's status prior to their entering the patient's room. For example, each visitor should understand that he or she may need to answer the same questions and provide the same explanations repeatedly. Patrick (1967, p. 2537) makes a good point that "sitting in silence across the room from the patient will be of little help"; instead, "the family member should sit near enough to the bed to be able to touch the patient frequently to let him know he is not alone." Even though a delirious patient may not recognize friends or family, having them around may make the environment more familiar. In fact, "a familiar person can provide reality feedback, comfort, and a sense of continuity with the patient's life before hospitalization" (Davies, 1991, p. 485). Moreover, family and friends can be instructed on reminiscence therapy and encouraged to utilize this technique with their loved one. Simply focusing conversation on a "familiar" topic, such as children, pets, or hobbies, may prove beneficial. Altering hospital rules to allow for overnight visitors should be considered.

Improved orientation can result from simply manipulating the environment to make it more familiar to the patient. A large clock and a calendar (with year) in view are helpful in keeping the patient oriented to time. However, the dates of the calendar need to be marked off daily if it is to do any good. Moreover, it is important to mark the calendar at approximately the same time every day (i.e., at breakfast time or with the evening snack) while verbally telling the patient the date. If the patient has a wristwatch, he or she should be encouraged to wear it. A window in the patient's room through which he or she can look out can provide clues about the season and time of day (Davidhizar and Cosgray, 1990).

The confused older patient should not be supported in his or her disorientation (Patrick, 1967, p. 2538). Instead, the nurse should attempt to orient the patient to reality. If the patient begins to argue about reality, the nurse need not get into an argument. However, the nurse may try to discover the emotion behind the patient's non-reality-based statements (i.e., fear), change the subject, or attempt to engage the patient in a diversional activity. Staff should reinforce the patient's reality-based behaviors.

Controlling the amount and quality of stimulation to which the delirious older patient is exposed is important in management of this syndrome. Both sensory overload and sensory deprivation can result in increased confusion. Additionally, perceptual problems can add to morbidity. Visual and hearing assessments should be done on all older adult patients. Any deficiencies noted need to be corrected, if possible, to decrease the risk of the patient's misperceiving sights and sounds, and to improve the quality of the patient's life. The patient who has an assistive device, such as dentures, glasses, or a hearing aid, should wear it. When not in use, any prosthesis should be kept in a place within the patient's reach.

Darkness contributes to confusion in elderly delirious patients. In older adults, the size of the pupil is reduced, which makes it more difficult to adjust to changes in light (Patrick, 1967). Moreover, visual acuity is not as good. Therefore, leaving a light on in the older adult's room during the night may be helpful. Furthermore, a patient who is confused at night may benefit from being given his or her eyeglasses so as to make better sense of the environment. Lighting, Davies cautions, "should be soft and diffuse to avoid sharp contrasts and shadows that can be misperceived" (1991, p. 486).

There are many opportunities for sensory overload in the hospital setting. To prevent overstimulation, the delirious older adult patient should be given a private room. Placing a confused older patient in a room across from the nursing station for closer observation must be analyzed critically, since the nursing station is often the center of activity. Staff conversations, ringing telephones, visitors asking questions, and a buzzing intercom system may subject a patient placed near such activity to sensory overload. This is especially a risk if the patient has perceptual disturbances. Likewise, conversation immediately outside the patient's room may contribute to overload and should be avoided (Stanley, 1991). Stanley suggests that "a useful exercise to raise the nursing staff's awareness of the amount of noise in a unit is to have each nurse spend approximately 4 hours in a bed, with wrist restraints in place" (1991, p. 66).

Sensory overload may be avoided by providing the patient with clear, understandable explanations of machine equipment (e.g., the beeps of monitors), as well as setting monitor alarm limits so as to reduce unnecessary soundings. Ideally, the patient should have rest periods between appointments with different health-care providers. This has an added advantage of spaced-out contacts to decrease social isolation. If, however, more than one staff member is with the patient, they ought to be careful to speak one at a time.

Sensory deprivation can also lead to confusion. Visits from family and friends should be encouraged. Interpersonal communication prompted by staff members is also important. When human contact is minimal, the patient may watch television or listen to the radio for "companionship."

Communication

The nurse has a key role in promoting the patient's comfort and self-esteem, providing support and reassurance, and encouraging independence. It is important that continuity of staff be maintained for the confused patient as much as possible, since this helps with accurate detection of even minute changes in patient status, and also helps the patient's familiarity with the environment. In considering communication, both content and process require attention.

The patient should be addressed by name as a reminder of his/her name and for the personal effect. More importantly, nurses should always introduce themselves and not simply assume that they will be remembered from the last contact. Wearing a large name tag can serve as an additional orienting clue (Stanley, 1991). Attaining the patient's attention is important before beginning a conversation or providing direction. Methods for gaining and maintaining attention include the use of touch, eye contact, and name repetition, and also standing in front of the patient (Hahn, 1980). Additionally, since the patient may be helped by reading lips, the nurse should look at the patient while speaking. C. Wanich identifies arm's length as a good distance for communication with the delirious older adult patient (personal communication, March 3, 1993).

The nurse should speak clearly and distinctly. The pace must not be rushed and pressured, but should be slow and relaxed. Although the nurse should avoid shouting, the voice must be audible over background noises. Short and simple sentences are best. The nurse should assess the patient's understanding and repeat what is she said when necessary. Instructions should be given in concrete, specific terms and only one at a time (Hahn, 1980). Furthermore, any procedure needs to be explained to the patient before it is initiated. It is demeaning, however, to talk to an older adult patient in childish tones.

The delirious patient is likely to be anxious. To reduce this uncomfortable emotion, the nurse should make time to listen to the patient's concerns. The nurse can provide reassurance and support through verbalizations and gestures. During daily activities of physical care, such as bathing and repositioning, the nurse can use touch to convey a sense of warmth and caring. Additionally, promotion of physical comfort and relief of pain can serve to reduce anxiety. The nurse should encourage independence and allow the patient as much control as he or she can handle. Moreover, providing the patient with opportunities for activity—both safe physical mobility and stimulating mental activity—can decrease anxiety. Teaching the patient relaxation techniques may be of additional benefit, as may playing the patient's favorite music. Asking the patient such questions as "'What brought you to the hospital?' or 'What has happened to you since you were admitted'" provide an opportunity to assess intellectual ability. However, beyond that, such questions convey interest and offer "the patient a chance to recount the events that have occurred, thus giving meaning to the events and the individual" (Stanley, 1991, p. 65). Debriefing is another extremely important nursing function, especially since partial or total amnesia about the whole experience usually occurs after the delirium resolves (Lipowski, 1989.)

Protection

Older adult patients with the hyperactive variant of delirium may be at an increased risk of injury during states of extreme confusion. Patients may unintentionally engage in self-injurious behaviors such as pulling at intravenous and catheter tubing, ripping off dressings, or trying to climb out of bed when not strong enough to walk. Furthermore, in a search for the familiar, the confused patient may wander out of his or her room and off the unit. Nurses often worry about the risk of falls. In contrast, the patient may become agitated and combative, risking injury to the staff. All of these risks represent real concerns that warrant intervention.

Because of the risk in the older adult population for falls and injuries, the patient is too often restrained physically or chemically (i.e., with major tranquilizers), which leads to increased confusion and greater injuries (in discussion of ICU, Stanley, 1991). Strumpf, Evans, and Schwartz (1990) estimate that more than 500,000 people are physically restrained in beds or chairs each day in America's hospitals and nursing homes; they note further that "restraints seldom eliminate falls or the risk of injury" (Evans, Strumpf, and Williams, 1991, p. 86). A plethora of problems result from the use of physical restraints. For example, fighting against the restraints can cause skin damage, and tightness or restriction predispose to problems of elimination, pneumonia, or other complications of immobility (Patrick, 1967). Accidental strangulation has even been reported (Evans et al., 1991). Additionally, a patient may feel that he or she is being punished and may consequentially suffer emotionally. Loss of self-image, increased psychologic dependency, increased confusion, and withdrawal are also observed (Evans et al., 1991, p. 88). As for actual behavioral changes, restraint of frightened delirious patients can increase panic and fear and produce increasingly angry, belligerent, agitated, or combative behavior (Evans, et al., 1991, p. 88).

When a patient seems at great risk for injury and is determined to be uncontrollable and in need of **physical restraint** for protection of him- or herself or others, it is important to first rule out other, less restrictive measures. Restraints must be used only when less restrictive measures have been exhausted or have been deemed inappropriate for the particular patient by the health-care team. If indeed the patient is restrained, the restraints should be removed as soon as indicated. This requires frequent reassessments by the nursing staff and close communication with the medical staff. Debriefing with the patient should be done.

If restraints are to be used as a last resort, staff members must be aware of the mechanisms that can be attempted first to ensure safety. Frequent observation of the patient is a priority. Reassurance should be provided during these contacts. Even though a room by the nursing station may cause additional problems due to potential for sensory overload, the risk-benefit ratio should be critically evaluated. The patient may be placed on a low bed, or even on only a mattress on the floor in order to prevent him or her from falling out of bed. The room should be uncluttered, and harmful objects should be removed. Close observation provided by family, friends, or staff members can diminish the need for restraints. The head nurse can be helpful in providing coverage on the unit when a delirious patient requires much time spent under surveillance. A private duty nurse hired by the family is yet another option.

The worry of a patient wandering away is a reason for the overuse of restraints. Here again there are other, less restrictive measures to be tried. Davidhizar and Cosgray (1990, p. 281) write of utilizing "definite spatial limits," such as setting up "waist-high fences that don't obstruct the person's view of the environment but offer a sense of security and protection." Pace and Emerich (1990) write about a system that was implemented successfully on a rehabilitation unit, in which each patient was rated on cognition, communication, and mobility. The patient was then classified in terms of how much supervision he or she required, and was given a wristband to wear that was color-coded to identify the patient's supervision level. The system was shared with other hospital employees and also explained to visitors through posted signs. The signs included what to do if a wandering patient was spotted. Davidhizar and Cosgray conclude that "not only did (this system) help to prevent injuries to these patients, but it also encouraged our staff, families, and visitors, to work together" (p. 64).

A few last words about restraint use will hopefully further illustrate the significance of this issue. Mattice and Mitchell (1990. p. 16) write about an elderly man who had been labeled "severely demented because he repeatedly yelled out nonsense words." This man "had been restrained in a darkened room most of the time with little human contact." One day a nurse asked him why he yelled so much. Said the patient, 'It is the only way I know I am still alive.'" It is essential to remember that all behavior does have meaning!

Medication

Medications can be a predisposing factor and/or cause of delirium in older adults. Yet medications are also often used in treating medical, surgical, and psychiatric problems. Therefore, care must be taken in determining what medication to use, how much, and when. Sullivan and colleagues (1991, p. 827) suggest that "the nurse should assess all standing and prn medications with the medical team every day." Certain categories of drugs, such as phenothiazines, should be avoided because of their propensity for increasing confusion in response to anticholinergic effects. For psychotic components of delirium, medication should be used in an amount that will eliminate psychotic features without sedating the patient. The butyrophenones, especially haloperidol, are suggested (Liston, 1984). Careful monitoring for side-effects is imperative. In general, barbituates, sedatives, and hypnotics should be avoided (Stan-

ley, 1991). Instead, since elderly delirious patients may suffer from severe sleep disturbances, a benzodiazepine with a short half-life (i.e., temazepam) may be prescribed (Liston, 1984). Davies (1991) cautions that a starting dose of any such medication recommended should be only one-third of the usual adult dose.

■ VASCULAR DEMENTIA

Vascular **dementia** (also called multi-infarct dementia) is second to Alzheimer's disease as the most common cause of dementia. It is caused by tiny strokes. While

E CASE EXAMPLE

▶ DELIRIUM

Mike Henley is a 70-year-old married white man admitted to a hospital cardiac unit for congestive heart failure. A physical history and examination reveal that he has: insulin-dependent diabetes mellitus (IDDM) a coronary artery bypass graft performed 6 years ago, and much shortness of breath when anxious. He is farsighted and wears bifocal lenses; he also experiences difficulty in hearing, but does not have a hearing aid. On admission his medication profile is as follows: capoten 50mg P.O. t.i.d., digoxin 0.125mg P.O.q.d., furosemide 40mg P.O.b.i.d., K-Lor 20 meq P.O.q.d., coumadin 5mg P.O.q.d., and insulin 24 units (70 NPH, 30 Reg) s.q. q.d. He verbalizes knowledge of his medications and reports being compliant with their prescribed use. Mike denies substance abuse or a psychiatric history.

For the first 3 days of his hospitalization, Mike is cooperative with treatment and pleasant during interactions. He is appropriately concerned about his status, while also able to engage in diversional activity and talk about his feelings. He remains awake much of the third night. Then, on the next day, he sleeps a lot. Additionally, the nurses have noticed other drastic and sudden changes in his behavior. For example, he is sometimes alert, but at other times not. Most notable is how much Mike's concentration and attention have decreased. Other changes include slight memory problems, slowed speech and psychomotor behavior, slow responses to questions and directions, and lethargy. He is oriented to person and place, but gets confused with time. This depressed and withdrawn patient is very different from the "admitted Mike." His primary nurse mentions her observations to Mike's physician, but the doctor and staff assume that these problems reflect a normal reaction to having a life-threatening illness. However, when Mike begins to experience illusions, his wife asks, "Is my husband getting Alzheimer's?"

The staff discuss Mike's status during a meeting later that afternoon. One member again speculates that the changes the staff are seeing are a part of aging and a nor-

mal response to such overwhelming circumstances. Another is concerned that Mike does in fact have beginning Alzheimer's disease. Then, one nurse speaks up loudly that the patient may be delirious—with the hypoactive variant of that condition. She educates the staff about delirium in the elderly, including what it is, its risk factors, signs, and symptoms, and its consequences if untreated. They listen with interest and verbalize agreement that Mike is certainly at risk for delirium (i.e., advanced age, unfamiliar environment, congestive heart failure, diabetes, weakened psychological defenses, decreased hearing, and certain medications [antiarrhythmic, antidiabetic, antihypertensive, cardiac glycoside, diuretic]). A decision is made to call Mike's physician immediately with the staff members' concerns.

Mike's physician is receptive to the call, and a team conference is immediately held. An active discussion ensues, resulting in several agreed upon initial interventions and goals:

- All staff will participate in educating Mrs. Henley and providing frequent updates about her husband's status.
- Mike's primary nurse will ask Mrs. Henley to bring in some items from home to make Mike's hospital room more familiar.
- The nurses will spend time with Mr. Henley each day, trying to engage him in activity—for example, a game of checkers.
- Mike's physician will order comprehensive blood studies.
- Nursing staff will chart Mr. Henley's intake and output strictly.
- The staff will maintain proper nutrition and hydration.
- Mr. Henley's bifocals will remain in his reach; he will be encouraged to wear them.
- Mr. Henley will be evaluated and fitted for a hearing aid.
- A medication specialist will be consulted.

these tiny strokes are often individually unrecognizable, their summation eventually destroys enough brain tissue to impair memory and other intellectual functions (Davidhizar and Cosgray, 1990). Hypertension is associated with this kind of dementia (Blazer, 1990). Unlike Alzheimer's disease, whose course is progressive, multi-infarct dementia has a stepwise course, producing "patchy" deficits (Blazer, 1990). For example, the patient may be agitated and severely depressed, but suffer only from minimal memory loss. Usually with multi-infarct dementia, neurological symptoms are evident, such as increased deep-tendon reflexes, unilateral weakness, gait difficulty, pseudobulbar palsy, and an extensor plantar response (*DSM-IV*, 1994). Table 19–13 for a lists the diagnostic criteria for multi-infarct dementia. Diagnosis is aided by laboratory evidence of vascular disease (*DSM-IV*, 1994). Computed tomography (CT) and magnetic resonance imaging (MRI) usually reveal multiple vascular lesions in both the white and grey matter of the cerebral cortex and subcortical structures (*DSM-IV*, 1994). These tests may also demonstrate evidence of old infarctions, such as focal atrophy.

■ DEMENTIA OF THE ALZHEIMER'S TYPE

Dementia of the Alzheimer's type (frequently referred to simply as Alzheimer's disease), is named for the German neurologist, Alois Alzheimer, who in 1906 first described the neurofibrilary tangles characteristic of the disease. Alzheimer's disease is the most common form of dementia (National Institutes of Health [NIH], 1991). In fact, 50% or more of older adults with severe

intellectual impairment suffer from Alzheimer's disease (NIH, 1991). The prevalence rates are 2 to 4% for those over 65 years of age and 20% or more for those over 85 years old (*DSM-IV*, 1994). The disease causes intellectual impairment in 4 million American adults (Kuhlman *et al.*, 1991). Furthermore, it is the fifth leading cause of total disability in the United States, and the fourth leading cause of death for adult Americans (Kuhlman *et al.*, 1991, p. 331).

CLINICAL MANIFESTATIONS

Although a CT scan or MRI may reveal cerebral atrophy, focal brain lesions, hydrocephalus, or periventricular ischemic brain injury (*DSM-IV*, 1994), a definitive diagnosis of Alzheimer's disease is not possible during life (Abraham and Neundorfer, 1990). Therefore, clinical symptoms can only point to possible or probable Alzheimer's disease. The criteria for such a diagnosis are listed in Table 19–14, and distinguishing characteristics between delirium and dementia are given in Table 19–15. A number of scales are available to aid with patient assessment, such as the Global Deterioration Scale, the Clinical Dementia Rating, and the Alzheimer's Disease Assessment Scale (Abraham and Neundorfer, 1990). Tragically, the symptoms of the disease, which may appear to be mild at an early stage, are progressive. Thus, the patient may initially present as somewhat for-

---

TABLE 19–13. DIAGNOSTIC CRITERIA FOR VASCULAR DEMENTIA

- The development of multiple cognitive deficits manifested by both
- Memory impairment (impaired ability to learn new information or tore call previously learned information)
- One (or more) of the following cognitive disturbances:
  - (a) Aphasia (language disturbance)
  - (b) Apraxia (impaired ability to carry out motor activities despite intact motor function)
  - (c) Agnosia (failure to recognize or identify objects despite intact sensory function)
  - (d) Disturbance in executive functioning (i.e., planning, organizing, sequencing, abstracting)
- Significant impairment in social or occupational functioning and a decline from a previous level of functioning.
- Focal neurological signs and symptoms (e.g., exaggeration of deep tendon reflexes, extensor plantar response, pseudobulbar palsy, gait abnormalities, weakness of an extremity) or laboratory evidence indicative of cerebrovascular disease.

Diagnostic and Statistical Manual of Mental Disorders ed. 4. Washington, DC, American Psychiatric Association, 1994, p. 146.

TABLE 19–14. DIAGNOSTIC CRITERIA FOR DEMENTIA OF THE ALZHEIMER'S TYPE

- The development of multiple cognitive deficits manifested by both
- Memory impairment (impaired ability to learn new information or to recall previously learned information)
- One (or more) of the following cognitive disturbances:
  - (a) Aphasia (language disturbance)
  - (b) Apraxia (impaired ability to carry out motor activities despite intact motor function)
  - (c) Agnosia (failure to recognize or identify objects despite intact sensory function)
  - (d) Disturbance in executive functioning (i.e., planning, organizing, sequencing, abstracting)
- The cognitive deficits cause significant impairment in social or occupational functioning and represent a significant decline from a previous level of functioning.
- The symptoms have a gradual onset and continuing cognitive decline.
- The symptoms are not due to
  - Other central nervous system conditions
  - Systemic conditions that are known to cause dementia (e.g., hypothyroidism, vitamin B$_{12}$ or folic acid deficiency, niacin deficiency, hypercalcemia, neurosyphilis, HIV infection)
  - Substance-induced conditions

Diagnostic and Statistical Manual of Mental Disorders (4th ed.) Washington, DC, American Psychiatric Association, 1994, pp. 142–143.

TABLE 19–15. DISTINGUISHING CHARACTERISTICS OF DELIRIUM VERSUS DEMENTIA

Characteristic	Delirium	Dementia
Age of onset	Any	Usually >65, highest >85
Onset	Sudden, usually over a period of hours to days	Gradual
	Frequently during the night	
Duration	Brief, days to months	Long term, months to years
Course	Tends to fluctuate, often worse at night	Relatively stable decline
Consciousness	Clouded	Usually normal
Alertness	Tends to fluctuate	Usually normal
Cognition	Periods of lucidity	Consistent loss
Memory	Recent impaired	Recent and remote impaired
Attention	Ability to maintain or shift always impaired	Usually normal
Affect	Intermittent fear, anxiety or puzzlement	Flat or indifferent
Judgment/Insight	Good during periods of lucidity	Poor
Sleep-wake cycle	Disrupted sometimes with a complete reversal	Sleep fragmented

getful. As the patient's memory deteriorates, however, the patient may become suspicious of others, even accusing them of stealing or hiding his or her belongings. Other symptoms of dementia include decreased judgment and attention, inappropriate behavior, labile affect, language disturbance, altered motor skills, and restlessness. Usually, patients with Alzheimer's disease will show a decline of 3 or 4 points annually (a perfect score is 30) on the Mini-Mental Status examination (*DSM IV,* 1994). Cooper and colleagues (1991) found that among 677 subjects with probable Alzheimer's disease, the overall prevalence of psychotic symptoms was 31%. The two most common forms of psychosis in demented patients are: (1) non-elaborate persecutory delusions; and (2) simple auditory or visual hallucinations (Jeste and Krull, 1991). Approximately 85% of demented patients will develop agitation (Jeste and Krull, 1991). According to the APA, the average duration of Alzheimer's disease is 8 to 10 years from the development of symptoms to death (1994).

ETIOLOGY

Specifically, what occurs with Alzheimer's disease is an accumulation of abnormal fibers in the proteins of the nerve cells in the cerebral cortex of the brain. Blazer (1990) notes that although an excessive amount of aluminum is found in these damaged nerve cells, exposure to aluminum in the environment is not now considered a risk factor for Alzheimer's disease. Another contributor to the disease process is the degeneration of groups of nerve endings in the cortex, producing lesions referred to as plaques, which in turn

disrupts the passage of electrochemical signals between nerve cells (NIH, 1991). Thus, the two major causes of Alzheimer's disease are neurofibrilary tangles and plaques. However, Kuhlman and his colleagues (1991) summarize additional possible causes suggested by others, including a genetic predisposition (autosomal dominant trait), decreased levels of choline acetyltransferase and other neurotransmitters, and decreased oxygen as the result of sleep apnea. They also mention environmental toxins, infectious agents, dietary habits, and immune system deficits as contributing factors to Alzheimer's disease. These possibilities, however, require further investigation: For example, acetyocholine is important to memory, and it is decreased in Alzheimer's disease patients, but is the reduction cause or result?

CLINICAL MANAGEMENT

When a demented patient is hospitalized or admitted to a nursing home, many of the interventions performed by nurses will resemble those used in working with a delirious patient (discussed earlier in the chapter). Table 19–16 provides a general dementia nursing-care plan. **Reminiscence therapy** may be particularly appropriate with this population. In fact, a nursing director in a Canadian nursing home constructed for each patient a metal ring of cards that contained cues such as "He was a boxer when he was in his 20s," or "He served in World War I in France," or "She once sang in the opera" (Burnside, 1990, p. 40). These cue cards promoted the use of reminiscence techniques by the nursing staff.

TABLE 19–16. NURSING CARE PLAN: DEMENTIA

Demonstrating effective communication
Speak slowly and calmly
Use simple words and sentence structure
Ask only one question at a time
Repeat questions/statements exactly when repetition is needed

Maintaining safety
Be firm but gentle with an agitated patient
Determine the agenda/feelings behind inappropriate behaviors and wandering
Always, use least restrictive means
Provide diversional activity as needed
Be careful not to put unnecessary restraints on independence

Educating patients and family
Describe the usual progression of disease
Inform the patient of his condition/progress when patient is lucid
Teach the family orienting and reminiscing techniques: use role-play
Provide written instructions
Suggest further reading materials
Refer to community resources as needed

EDUCATING LOVED ONES

It is important for family members and close friends to understand the disease process in Alzheimer's disease along with patient management. This education is essential if these persons are also serving as primary care-givers but is an important nursing responsibility when working with dementia patients regardless. Since safety is always a priority, steps should be taken to maintain safety for the older adult patient and others. Removing potentially hazardous materials, such as cigarette lighters, matches, poisons, and medications, minimizes risks. Likewise, placing gates at stairwells, installing door and window alarms, and applying identification bracelets may be indicated to keep wandering, demented adults safe. Having a well-lit, clutter-free environment decreases the risk of falls. Signs and labels (e.g., "bathroom") may be helpful, but the demented patient's ability to read and comprehend must be repeatedly checked. Signs do not have to involve written words; a creative care-giver may choose to draw a picture of a toilet!

Since patients with dementia are likely to require assistance with personal care at some point, family members should be provided with "tips." It may, for example, be best to store inappropriate clothing including items out of season, ill-fitting, or soiled/torn, beyond the reach of the patient. Buying articles that are easy to put on, adjust, and remove is preferable. Verbal prompts during dressing may be necessary. Scheduling regular bathroom visits, including visits during the night, can help with the problem of urinary incontinence. Providing the older adult with a task, such as folding laundered linens, serves more than one purpose: Not only is the elder kept busy, but the completion of a "job" provides him or her with a sense of worth and accomplishment.

Care-givers working with Alzheimer's disease patients may request direction in finding financial assistance, legal aid, support groups, and/or good educational materials and books about Alzheimer's disease. Also, the family may be interested in therapeutic day care settings for their own respite. Abraham and Neundorfer (1990, p. 119) describe the goals of such places as "to provide socialization, rehabilitation, training, and health and supportive services in a controlled environment that supports maximum functioning of the patient." The nurse who understands the benefits of interdisciplinary planning may ask a social worker to talk with the family about day care and other options for help.

MEDICATION

There is currently no cure for Alzheimer's disease. Moreover, Jeste and Krull (1991) warn that several of the common symptoms of dementia are not usually amenable to management with **neuroleptic drugs.** Such symptoms include cognitive deficits, wandering, pacing, and non-aggressive verbalizations. Gomez and Gomez (1990, p. 7) agree, warning that "in the absence of a true psychosis, neuroleptics should not be used." However, psychosis and other symptoms of Alzheimer's disease, such as excitement and hostility, may be decreased by neuroleptic drugs (Jeste and Krull, 1991). Gomez and Gomez (1990) have written an article about neuroleptic-drug use in this population, which includes data on side effects, interactions, and contraindications, as well as case examples.

Higher blood levels of neuroleptic drugs occur in older adult patients in relation to altered absorption, metabolism, distribution, and elimination (Gomez and Gomez, 1990). In fact, Jeste and Krull (1991) remind practitioners that demented patients should receive only one-fourth to one-third of the usual adult doses of neuroleptic drugs, be subject only to gradual increases in their dosage, and be monitored closely for side effects. Gomez and Gomez (1990) suggest that antipsychotic agents be avoided in hypertensive patients taking guanethidine, since these neuroleptic drugs can increase the hypotensive effect of the guanethidine and cause severe hypotension. They also warn that since the low-potency, high-dose antipsychotics drugs such as thorazine and mellaril are generally not only more sedating but also cardiotoxic, they should not be given to patients with cardiac problems (Gomez and Gomez, 1990). Medications that have a sedating effect should be used with caution because of the risk of falls and fractures. On the other hand, medication choice requires a balance of benefits and risks; for instance, a slightly sedating drug may be best for an agitated, restless, demented patient.

Nurses must carefully and repeatedly assess patients receiving neuroleptic drugs for any signs of extrapyramidal reactions (EPRs) and neuroleptic malignant syndrome (NMS). Unfortunately, the estimated prevalence of tardive dyskinesia (TD) in demented elderly patients treated with neuroleptic drugs is 50% (Jeste & Krull, 1991). Risk factors for developing tardive dyskinesia include brain damage, a history of mood disorder, early extrapyramidal reactions, and intermittent use of neuroleptic drugs (Jeste and Krull, 1991). According to Addonizio (1991) symptoms of neuroleptic malignant syndrome are sometimes mistakenly attributed to other ailments of aging or to medical problems. Such error can lead to tragic consequences, since fatality in older adults with this syndrome is greater than in young adults (Addonizio, 1991). Therefore, it is again evident that as with depression and delirium, stereotypes of aging can lead to missed diagnosis and death.

As already mentioned, acetylcholine is a neurotransmitter important to memory and also deficient in Alzheimer's disease patients. Cholinesterase is an enzyme involved in the breakdown of acetylcholine, and an agent that antagonizes cholinesterase will therefore increase the concentration of acetylcholine in the brain and nervous system. The drug physostigamine is such an agent. Some studies show it to be effective at improving the memory of patients with mild to moderate Alzheimer's disease for at least a few weeks or months (Blazer, 1990). However, more studies are needed.

■ WORKING WITH FAMILIES

A family is a system with interrelated members, each influenced by and influencing the others. A family genogram including the identification of family roles is often helpful to the health-care provider who takes the time to construct one. In constructing the genogram the older patient is asked about the nature of contacts with family members. Often, also evaluating the family alone, without the elder, will reveal significant issues. All weighty stressors in the family system are to be noted.

Long-term care of older adults is largely maintained within the family system. An obvious benefit of this is that the family probably knows the older adult

best, including knowledge of his or her lifetime experiences, personal goals, values, and fears. Family members may respond in different ways to an ill loved one, depending on the level of coping achieved. Various responses may include denial, overinvolvement, anger, or guilt. A family member's response pattern will often change as time goes on, in relation to changes in the elder's status, changes in coping techniques used, and/or changes in the extent and types of support available and provided. Each response style correlates with specific nursing interventions aimed at bringing the caregiver closer to acceptance. Typically, the family in denial needs gentle but firm confrontation, along with education. The overinvolved may require family sessions with the elder to learn the latter's feelings about not being allowed to do things for him- or herself. Consequences of such overinvolvement need to be discussed. Listening to the family ventilate about burdens of care-giving may be much of what is required. Referrals for assistance may then also be made. When a member is feeling guilty, it may be due to dilemmas about nursing home placement. Again, listening, educating, and providing general support are indicated once the nature of the guilt is determined. However, guilt related to abuse or neglect requires special intervention to protect the older adult patient.

Autonomy refers to independence, or self-determination. When issues relating to autonomy in the older population are considered, two opposite risks are apparent. First, the family may do too little for the older adult, leaving the latter vulnerable to various negative consequences, including injury and disease. On the other hand, family members may do too much, potentially contributing to feelings of uselessness in the elder. Horowitz, Silverstone, and Reinhardt (1991) studied visually impaired older adults being cared for by family members. The results showed that families tend not to hinder autonomy by providing too little or too much assistance with functional tasks. The older adults were more likely than care-givers to report exceptions, all of which, in the study, involved receiving too little help in a particular task. Another part of the same study focused on attitudes toward autonomy rather than on actual behaviors. Assessments were made using reactions to vignettes of hypothetical family situations depicting conflicts relating to autonomy. Interestingly, the care-givers were more sensitive to autonomy, while the older adults studied were more concerned with the health and safety of older adults in the vignettes than with compromised autonomy. The majority of both older adults and care-givers in the study believed that elders generally have freedom of choice in their lives. They see the major barriers to autonomy as the intrinsic conditions of aging—its physical and mental disabilities. This study's results seem positive, but the elders were all visually impaired or blind, not mentally impaired. Since mental illness is obviously different, a study similar to the one conducted by Horowitz and his colleagues but involving emotionally disturbed adults is much needed.

Nowadays, care-giving functions may be performed by a spouse, child, grandchild, or another person. In fact, Silverstone and Horowitz (1992) call attention to the statistic that 75% of community-dwelling, frail older adults get all their support from family members and friends. Genevay (1992, p. 62) states "that older adult children may now spend more of their lives taking care of elderly parents than they did raising children." Moreover, the majority of potential care-givers are adult children aged 45 to 64; 17% of 45- to 54-year-olds have a disabled parent (Cantor, 1992). With many four-generational families existing, in some systems the old are taking care of the very old; and in the future, this

may occur with even greater frequency. Keeping all of this in mind, it is easy to understand why psychoeducation provided to the elderly patient and to family members and other care-givers is so significant. Education about the aging process is needed so that family care-givers will know how to differentiate normal from abnormal in order to detect even minor changes and problems in an elderly relative at an early point. The specifics of any disease processes affecting the particular older adult, and treatments for them, should be covered. Furthermore, discussion of potential behavior problems and of ways to handle them safely must not be overlooked. Family members and care-givers may not be comfortable with setting limits. For example, a woman whose father was a strict disciplinarian while she was growing up might find it difficult to set limits with her aging, demented father. Such discomfort with this role reversal can be explored. Culture too may affect

E CASE EXAMPLE

▶ DEMENTIA

Sarah, age 47, brings her 75-year-old mother, Alice, to a community hospital, asking to have her admitted to the psychiatric unit. Greatly distressed, Sarah quickly starts by recounting that after her father died 7 years ago, her mother had moved in with herself, her husband, and their three teenagers. The move occurred solely for financial reasons. Sarah states that her mother has been in excellent physical health. Furthermore, says Sarah, although her mother had certainly grieved for the death of her husband, she has remained active with her Bridge group and church, and had seemed to be handling it all fairly well. Sarah goes on to describe that a year ago she began to notice her mother becoming slightly forgetful, such as, with names. She states that initially, Alice herself had also been aware of this and was frustrated by it. Both the mother and daughter figured that the change was "part of aging." As the year passed, however, Alice's memory difficulties worsened, although she no longer seems concerned about her failing memory. The problem has become so severe that Alice often cannot remember where she has put her belongings and clothing. Things began to reach a "crisis level" when Alice accused Sarah's husband of stealing her earrings. Likewise, an incident occurred a week ago in which Alice accused her grandson of taking her girdle, which resulted in a long and loud argument at the Sunday dinner table. Alice also gets confused and talks of her late husband as if he were alive. She talks of needing to buy groceries to make him dinner; neighbors have twice found her wandering down the street (most recently, the night before she came to the hospital). Fortunately, neighbors called Sarah, and both times she was able to re-direct her mother into the car and take her home. However, she is extremely worried about her mother's status and safety.

Alice is admitted. More data are collected from the patient and her family, and a full medical work-up is performed, including physical, neurological, and psychiatric examinations. There is no impairment of Alice's cranial nerve function, and her sensory functions are intact. The laboratory work done for her includes a complete blood count, blood chemistries, thyroid function tests, vitamin level assays (B_{12} and folic acid), urinalysis, lumbar puncture, chest X-ray, and electrocardiogram. None of the test results indicate a specific central nervous system disease or systemic condition. An electroencephalogram shows general slowing of brain waves. A computed axial tomography scan and MRI reveal atrophy of the cortex of the brain. Also notable from the assessment is that Alice has difficulty remembering the names of objects, although she is able to describe their functions. For example, she knows "it is how you talk with other people over lines," but not "telephone." Moreover, she is also unable to classify similar objects, such as recognizing that both apples and oranges are fruits. During the face-hand test, Alice reports her cheek being touched but not her hand. Throughout all the testing, Alice seems indifferent to what is happening to her.

As other diagnoses are ruled out, it becomes increasingly probable that Alice is suffering from dementia of the Alzheimer's Type. A family meeting is held. To begin, the nurse provides the family with information, both verbal and written, about Alzheimer's disease, and gives them opportunities to ask questions. Alternatives for care are discussed, and each family member discusses his or her feelings about Alice's status and about how it affects them. A decision is made to place Alice in the same nursing home in which Sarah's grandmother had once been placed for debilitating medical illnesses (she died at age 90, 10 years ago). Alice at this point does not seem to understand what is going on, but is happy to be going to the home where her mother once lived.

the care-giving experience; and discussion about care-taking patterns, beliefs, and practices may therefore also be significant.

Care-givers often find their loved one's incontinence, memory problems, accusations, or other disturbances stressful. Stress needs to be handled effectively and safely. Care-giving sometimes becomes a burden, which is defined by Gregory, Peters, and Cameron (1990, p. 21) as "the perceived negative consequences that result from providing care." As a result of care-taking duties, family members may experience fatigue, anger, depression, conflict, and other stress-related symptoms. They may also have less time for themselves and for friends, and experience a decrease in life satisfaction (Blazer, 1990). In fact, care-givers report as much as a threefold greater number of stress-related symptoms than do comparison groups (Blazer, 1990, p. 225). They also report a decrease in life satisfaction (Blazer, 1990). Ideally, education, anticipatory guidance, and strengthening the support system will thwart some of these problems. By understanding an elderly relative's disease process, care-givers may be more tolerant to such annoyances as repetitive questioning by person's with Alzheimer's disease. They may be better able to stay calm and figure out the relative's emotions and agenda behind wandering. Problems do occur and should be discussed. Assistance with constructive problem-solving and with developing and utilizing effective coping techniques should be included. Referring families to support groups and other community resources is often an important step.

Tragically, there are situations in which the care-giving burden leads to abuse of the elderly. Research suggests that such abuse affects 3 to 5% of persons over age 60 (Nemeth, 1994). Another statistic indicates that there are approximately 1.5 million cases of elder abuse in domestic settings annually, but that only one in eight cases comes to the attention of state elder-abuse reporting systems (Quirk, 1991). Immediate, intensive intervention is indicated for these dysfunctional families. Vitaliano, Young, and Russo (1991) reviewed and critiqued measures that have been used among care-givers of demented individuals.

■ PREVENTING ILLNESS

The population of older adults is vast, and more of the very old are surviving. Stereotypes and myths about older age can negatively affect the last years and days of life. Therefore, society's members must begin to look at the realities of later life. A misunderstood and sometimes neglected cohort, older adults too often do not

receive enough attention, proper diagnosis, or necessary treatment.

Maintaining good health in this population presents unique problems. The primary nursing prevention of health promotion and illness prevention must be on the forefront of health-care goals. Much can be accomplished through well-planned educational programs. Detection and reduction, if not elimination, of risk factors should be a priority. Examples of health-promoting activities include preserving independence and encouraging exercise (a pre-exercise physical examination and repeated checks are musts).

Secondary prevention, screening, and early detection of problems are essential to limit disability and disturbances that compound existing illnesses. Unfortunately, a patient may be plagued by more than one of the three "D's" (depression, delirium, dementia). For instance, he or she may have depression and dementia, or a delirium superimposed on Alzheimer's disease. Therefore, thorough assessments and treatments are crucial. In the United Kingdom, general practitioners must offer patients aged 75 and older a home visit to satisfy the enhanced annual capitation fee for patients in this age group. The home visit includes assessments of mobility, functioning, mental status, hearing, and continence (Freer, 1990). Another component of this home visit is a medication review (Freer, 1990). Thus, the special importance of providing health-care services to the elderly is the message sent to British practitioners. Studies of the effects of the British system would be interesting. In the United States, The Omnibus Budget Reconciliation Act of 1987 (Public Law 100-203) mandates pre-admission screening of all nursing home applicants for both mental illness and mental retardation (Harper, 1990). It also mandates 75 hours of training for nurse's aides (Harper, 1990). However, greater community outreach is needed in the United States. The third and final aspect of health care is tertiary prevention, which focuses on rehabilitation and limiting disability.

Ideally, each older adult will look back on his or her life and be satisfied with the review, and will also find his or her last days of life enjoyable and equally satisfying. The second objective of the Older Americans Act of 1965 is to give elders the opportunity for "the best possible physical and mental health which science can make available and without regard to economic status" (McConnell and Beitler, 1991, p. 10). Unfortunately, as George (1990) notes, a psychiatric disorder affects about 8 to 13% of persons aged 65 and older at any given time. Psychiatric nurses are vital to the emotional health of members of this cohort. Nurses can influence this final stage of life by educating society and by demanding comprehensive, high-quality care for elders.

O AN OVERVIEW

- Stereotypes and myths about older age can have a negative impact on individuals in the last years and days of life.

- Too often, older adults do not receive enough attention, proper diagnosis, or necessary treatment.

- Primary prevention—the promotion of health (e.g., preserving independence, encouraging exercise)—and illness prevention should be foremost among health-care goals for the elderly.

- Detecting and reducing risk factors among the aging population is a nursing priority.

- Secondary prevention—screening and the early detection of problems—is essential to limiting disability and disturbances that compound the patient's illness.

- Thorough assessment of an aging individual is crucial to detect depression, delirium, or dementia, or the concurrent presence of more than one of these conditions.

- The Omnibus Budget Reconciliation Act (OBRA) of 1987 mandates that before nursing-home applicants are admitted for care, they be screened for mental illness and mental retardation.

- Tertiary prevention focuses on rehabilitation and limiting disability.

- In the United States, psychiatric disorders affect from 8 to 13% of persons 65 years of age and older.

TD TERMS TO DEFINE

- autonomy
- delirium
- dementia
- depression
- ego integrity versus despair
- electroconvulsive therapy (ECT)
- grief
- incompetency
- informed consent
- loss
- mental status examination
- monoamine oxidase inhibitors (MAOIs)
- neuroleptic drugs
- pharmacodynamics
- pharmacokinetics
- physical restraint
- polypharmacy
- presbyopia
- reality orientation
- reminiscence therapy
- respite care
- senility
- sundowning
- tricyclic antidepressants

Q STUDY QUESTIONS

1. Considering past and present statistics, and future projections, in the next 25 years the population of elderly will most likely
   a. continue to increase.
   b. decrease.
   c. stay relatively stable.

2. According to Erik Erikson, old age is primarily a time to
   a. guide and teach the new generation, termed *generativity.*
   b. review one's life to find meaning.
   c. both a and b.
   d. re-invest trust in new people as losses occur, which he termed *trust vs. mistrust.*

3. Expected late-life alterations may include
   a. occasional forgetfulness of recent memories, presbyopia, a need for more time to respond to questions and requests.
   b. occasional forgetfulness of recent memories, changes in personality style.
   c. occasional forgetting of one's own name, presbyopia, a need for more time to respond to questions and requests.
   d. a decrease in pitch discrimination (hearing), myopia, longer sleeping periods.
   e. occasional confusion, reversal of the sleep-wake cycle, presbyopia.

4. When performing a geriatric assessment, the nurse recognizes that

   a. questioning the patient about current use of illegal drugs and alcohol is unnecessary.
   b. interviewing a family member is often helpful.
   c. interviewing a family member steps over family boundaries and goes against the principles of establishing a therapeutic relationship with the patient.
   d. a thorough physical history and work-up are important, even when the chief complaint/reason for referral seems clearly psychiatric.
   e. both b and d
   f. a, c, and d

5. For optimum communication, the nurse knows it is best to

   a. speak very loudly.
   b. repeat questions and statements that are not heard in different ways, so that the patient has the best chance for understanding.
   c. assess the patient's understanding of requests and directions.
   d. interview quickly because the patient will need time to rest after the exhausting interview.

6. Depression in the older adult is

   a. common only among those who reside in nursing homes.
   b. an expected reaction to the potential multiple losses of old age, such as deaths, retirement, relocation, and decreased financial income.
   c. often undetected by health-care professionals.
   d. not likely to respond successfully to treatment.

7. Among the following symptoms reported by a grieving older adult, which should concern the nurse the most?

   a. Occasional shortness of breath
   b. Thoughts of being better off dead
   c. Guilt about what was not done at the time of a loved one's death
   d. A morbid preoccupation with worthlessness

8. Concerning suicide, the nurse recognizes that

   a. elderly white males are at highest risk for suicide.
   b. widowed females are at highest risk for suicide.
   c. older adult suicide is more preventable, as up to 50% of elderly suicide victims visit their primary-care physicians within the week prior to suicide.
   d. both a and c
   e. both b and c

9. Recent studies show that the single most successful method to treat depression in older adults is

   a. the "talking therapies," especially supportive counseling and grief work.
   b. medication, because talking therapy is often too exhausting for depressed elders.
   c. electroconvulsive therapy (ECT), because it is the most short-term therapy (6 to 10 treatments are usually required).
   d. unknown, as there is not one ultimate treatment method.

10. The two most common antidepressants used for older adults are

    a. nortriptyline and fluoxetine.
    b. nortriptyline and desipramine.
    c. desipramine and nardil.
    d. desipramine and fluoxetine.

11. A patient prescribed a tricyclic antidepressant drug is at risk for which one of the following side effects?

    a. Photosensitivity
    b. Extrapyrimidal reactions (EPR's)
    c. Hypertensive crisis
    d. a and c
    e. b and c
    f. a and b

12. A patient with delirium may exhibit which of the following symptoms?

    a. Memory problems
    b. Restless behavior, such as agitation, wandering, and pulling at intravenous tubing
    c. Disorientation
    d. Lethargic appearance, and quiet, withdrawn behavior
    e. All of the above
    f. a, b, and c

13. Undiagnosed and untreated delirium may lead to

    a. falls and fractures.
    b. long hospital stays.
    c. death.
    d. all of the above.
    e. none of the above.

14. With a delirious patient it is important to

    a. limit fluid intake.
    b. take vital signs every 4 hours, including throughout the night
    c. recognize that restraining agitated patients may only increase their agitation and risk of injury
    d. administer phenothiazines.
    e. both c and d.

15. Vascular dementia is caused by tiny strokes and is
    a. the most common form of dementia.
    b. destructive of brain tissue, which leads to dementia.
    c. temporary and reversible.
    d. progressive, similar to Alzheimer's disease.

16. The percentage of older adults with severe intellectual impairment who probably have Alzheimer's disease is approximately
    a. 5–10%
    b. 25%
    c. 33%
    d. >50%

17. Which of the following statements is true of Alzheimer's Disease?
    a. Its two major causes are plaques and neurofibrillary tangles.
    b. It is reversible if detected early.
    c. It can be diagnosed only by performing both an MRI and CT scan.
    d. Its course can be halted and reversed among a small number of patients with the administration of physostigamine.

18. Working from a systems framework, the psychiatric nurse caring for a demented patient will
    a. prefer to maintain the older adult in the family home throughout the disease process.
    b. interview the patient only with the family present.
    c. assess how the patient's condition is impacting other family members.
    d. All of the above.

19. Which of the following measures would be best for decreasing stress in a caregiver?
    a. Encouraging occasional respite care
    b. Providing education
    c. Insisting that the family place the elder in a nursing home.
    d. a and b

20. Jack, a 71-year-old, divorced (for 15 years) white male, recently moved in with his daughter Ann, her husband, and their two young children, due to the high rent of his apartment, which was an hour's drive from Ann's home. Ann is concerned because at times her father seems confused and unable to concentrate or remember recently learned information. At other times he is lucid, clear, and oriented. His only prescribed medication has been an antihypertensive. Which of the following descriptions of Jack's condition is most probably accurate?
    a. Jack is suffering from delirium. This diagnosis is based on the following: He is in a new environment (risk factor) and is taking an antihypertensive drug (a contributing risk factor). His confusion and inability to remember new information or concentrate are intermittent.
    b. Jack is suffering from vascular dementia, a dementia that has been linked to hypertension.
    c. Jack is depressed because of his decreased financial independence, loss of apartment, and loss of friends.
    d. Jack may be suffering from a depression, delirium, or dementia, or a combination of these. More data are needed.

■ REFERENCES

Abraham IL, Neundorfer MM: Alzheimer's: A decade of progress, a future of nursing challenges. *Geriatr Nurs* 1990; 11:116–119.

Addonizio G: NMS in the elderly—An under-recognized problem. *Int J Geriatr Psychiatry* 1991; 6:547–548.

Aldwin C: The Elders Life Stress Inventory (ELSI): Egocentric and nonegocentric stress, in Stephens MAP, Hobfoll SE, Crowther JH, Tennenbaum DL (eds): *Stress and Coping in Late Life Families* New York, Hemisphere, pp. 49–69.

Diagnostic and Statistical Manual of Mental Disorders ed 4, Washington, DC, American Psychiatric Association, 1994.

Beck AT, Rush AJ, Shaw BF, Emergy G: *Cognitive Therapy of Depression.* New York, Guilford, 1979.

Blazer D: *Emotional Problems in Later Life: Intervention Strategies of Professional Caregivers.* New York, Springer, 1990.

Bosse R, Aldwin CM, Levenson MR, Workman-Daniels K: How stressful is retirement? Findings from the normative aging study. *J Gerontol* 1991; 46:9–14.

Bowling A, Browne P: Social support and emotional well-being among the olders old living in London. *J Gerontol* 1991; 46:20–32.

Bowling A, Farguhar M, Browne P: Life satisfaction and associations with social network and support variables in three samples of elderly people. *Int J Geriatr Psychiatry* 1991; 6:549–566.

Buckwalter KC, Stolley J: Managing mentally ill elders at home. *Geriatr Nurs* 1991; 12:136–140.

Burnside I: Reminiscence: An independent nursing intervention for the elderly. *Issues Ment Health Nurs* 1990;11:33–48.

Cantor MH: Families and caregiving in an aging society. *Generations* 1992; (Summer):67–70.

Cooper JK, Mungas D, Verma M, Weiler PG: Psychotic symptoms in Alzheimer's Disease. *Int J Geriatr Psychiatry* 1991; 6:721–726.

Davidhizar R, Cosgray R: Helping the wanderer. *Geriatr Nurs* 1990; 11:280–281.

Davies HD: Dementia and delirium, in Chenitz, WC, Stone JT, Salisbury SA (eds): *Clinical Gerontological Nursing* Philadelphia, WB Saunders, 1991, pp. 455–489.

Erikson E: *Childhood and society.* New York, WW Norton, 1950.

Evans LK, Strumpf NE, Williams CC: Redefining a standard of care for frail older people: Alternatives to routine physical restraint, in Katz PR, Kane RL, Mezey MD (eds): *Advances in Long Term Care.* New York, Springer, pp. 81–108.

Folstein MF, McHugh PR: "Mini-Mental State": A practical method for grading the cognitive state of patients for the clinician. *J Psychiatr Res* 1975; 12:189–198.

Foreman MD: Acute confusional states in hospitalized elderly: A research dilemma. *Nurs Res* 1986; 35:34–38.

Foreman MD: Confusion in the hospitalized elderly: Incidence, onset, and associated factors. *Res Nurs Health* 1989; 12:26–29.

Foreman MD: Complexities of acute confusion. *Geriatr Nurs* 1990; 11:136–139.

Freer BB: Screening the elderly. *BMJ* 1990; 300:1447–1448.

Frierson RI: Suicide attempts by the old and the very old. *Arch Intern Med* 1991; 151:141–144.

Genevay B: 'Creating' families: Older people alone: What is the role of service providers? *Generations* 1992; (Summer,):61–64.

George LK: Gender, age, and psychiatric disorders. *Generations* 1990; (Summer):22–27.

Gomez GE, Gomez EA: The special concerns of neuroleptic use in the elderly. *J Psychosoc Nurs* 1990; 28:7–14.

Gregory DM, Peters N, Cameron CF: Elderly male spouses as caregivers: Toward an understanding of their experience. *J Gerontol Nurs* 1990; 16:20–24.

Hahn K: Using 24-hour reality orientation. *J Gerontol Nurs* 1980; 6:130–135.

Harper MS: Psychogeriatric Nursing. *Counc Gerontol Nurs* 1990; 7:1, 3–6.

Horowitz A, Silverstone BM, Reinhardt JP: A conceptual and empirical exploration of personal autonomy issues within family caregiving relationships. *Gerontologist* 1991; 31:23–31.

Jeste DV, Krull AJ: Behavioral problems associated with dementia: Diagnosis and treatment. *Geriatrics* 1991; 46:28–34.

Keane SM, Sells S: Recognizing depression in the elderly. *J Gerontol Nurs* 1990; 16:21–25.

Koenig HG, Breitner JCS: Use of antidepressants in medically ill older patients. *Psychosomatics* 1990; 31:22–32.

Kuhlman GJ, Wilson HS, Hutchinson SA, Wallhagen M: Alzheimer's Disease and family caregiving: Critical synthesis of the literature and research agenda. *Nurs Res* 1991; 40:331–337.

Kurlowicz LH: Social factors and depression in late life. *Arch Psychiatr Nurs* 1993; 7:30–36.

Leuchter AF: Brain structural and functional correlates of late life depression [Abstract]. *National Consensus Development Conference Diagnosis and Treatment of Depression in Late Life.* National Institutes of Health, Bethesda, MD, November 4–6, 1991.

Lipowski ZJ: Delirium in the elderly patient. *T N Engl J Med* 1989; 320:578–582.

Liston EH: Delirium in the aged. *T Psychiatr Clin North Am* 1982; 5:49–66.Liston EH: Diagnosis and management of delirium in the elderly patient. *Psychiatr Ann* 1984; 14:109–118.

Loebel JP, Loebel JS, Dager SR, Centerwall BS, Reay DT: Anticipation of nursing home placement may be a precipitant of suicide among the elderly. *J Am Geriatr Soc* 1991; 39:407–408.

Marr J: Acute confusion. *Nurs Times* 1992; 88:31–32.

Mattice M, Mitchell GJ: Caring for confused elders. *T Can Nurse* 1990; 88:16–18.

Matzo M: Confusion in older adults: Assessment and differential diagnosis. *Nurse Practi* 1990; 15:32–46.

McBride S: Confusion in the elderly hospitalized patient. *Can Nurse* 1992; 88:35–36.

McConnell S, Beitler D: The older americans act after 25 years: An overview. *Generations* 1991; (Summer/Fall):5–10.

National Institute on Aging: *Profiles of America's Elderly: Growth of America's Elderly in the 1980's.* Washington, DC, U.S. Government Printing Office, 1991.

National Institutes of Health. *Alzheimer's disease Q & A* (NIH Publication No. 91-1646). Washington, DC, U. S. Government Printing Office, 1991.

National Institutes of Health Consensus Development Panel on Depression in Late Life. Diagnosis and treatment of depression in late life. *JAMA* 1992; 268:1018–1024.

Nemeth M: Amazing greys. *MacLean's,* January 10, 1994, pp. 26–29.

Pace K, Emerich M: Keeping track of confused patients. *Nursing 90,* 1990; 20:64.

Patrick ML: Care of the confused elderly patient. *Am J Nurs* 1967; 67:2536–2539.

Quirk DA: From the executive director of NASUA: An agenda for the nineties and beyond. *Generations* 1991; (Summer/Fall,):23–26.

Ray T, Baretich M: Factors affecting the incidence of patient falls in hospitals. *Med Care* 1987; 25:185–194.

Rosen SL: Managing delirious older adults in the hospital. *MEDSURG Nurs* 1994; 3:181–189.

Silverstone BM, Horowitz A: Aging in place: The role of families. *Generations* 1992; (Spring):27–30.

Stanley M: Ensuring a safe ICU stay for your confused elderly patient. *Dimens Crit Care Nurs* 1991; 10:62–67.

Strumpf NE, Evans LK, Schwartz D: Restraint-free care: From dream to reality. *Geriatr Nurs* 1990; 3:122–124.

Sullivan EM, Wanich CK, Kurlowicz LH: Nursing assessment, management of delirium in the elderly. *AORN J* 1991; 53:820–828.

Vitaliano PP, Young HM, Russo J: Burden: A review of measures used among caregivers of individuals with dementia. *Gerontologist,* 1991; 31:67–75.

Wasson J, Jette AM: Partnerships between physicians and older adults. *Generations* 1993; (Fall):41–44.

Williams MA, Holloway JR, Winn MC, Wolanin MO, Lawler ML, Westwick CR, Chin MH: Nursing activities and acute confusional states in elderly hip fractured patients. *Nurs Res* 1979; 28:25–35.

Zerhusen JD, Boyle K, Wilson W: Out of the darkness: Group cognitive therapy for depressed elderly. *J Psychosoc Nurs* 1991; 29:16–21.

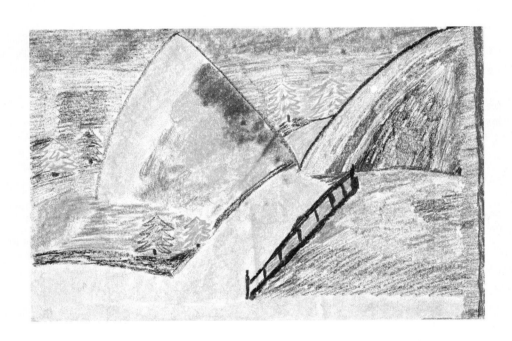

Those who have become eminent in philosophy, politics, poetry, and the arts have all had tendencies toward melancholia.

Aristotle (4th Century B.C.)

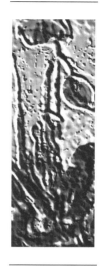

20
Mood Disorders

Ann Wolbert Burgess / Laureen M. Burgess

Mood, a prolonged emotion that colors the whole of psychological life, generally involves either elation or depression. One's mood is the persisting affective lens through which one views the world.

The mood disorders, a heterogeneous mix of psychiatric conditions, generally involve varying levels of depression, euphoria, and irritability. An altered mood, however, does not indicate a mood disorder. Such a diagnosis comes from a careful analysis of signs and symptoms that occur over a specified period of time and present at a certain level of disability.

The term depression stems principally from attempts of the 19th century psychiatrist Emil Kraeplin to introduce a term that would have greater diagnostic specificity than the classic term melancholia.

Currently, mood disorders are not completely understood by the psychiatric community. Their etiologies are uncertain, and researchers speculate that varying combinations of stress, the personality, central nervous system changes, and other factors contribute to one's behavioral state at any given time.

■ THE OVERALL PICTURE

Mood disorders are often either misdiagnosed or under-diagnosed in primary care settings. It is estimated that as many as one-third to one-half of individuals who suffer from a major depressive disorder are misdiagnosed by nonpsychiatric clinicians. This may be due to the social stigma associated with a mood disorder, to the patient's unwillingness to report symptoms or even recognize them, or to clinicians being unfamiliar with the signs and symptoms of a mood disorder. Clinicians also tend to have a low index of suspicion for such disorders. Often, diagnosing depression in the elderly is difficult because many of its symptoms are similar to dementia and other common geriatric medical conditions.

The societal costs of mood disorders are high. The cost of caring for individuals with mood disorders is about the same as caring for those with cardiovascular disease, at about $44 billion in the US during 1990. As many as 70% of psychiatric hospitalizations are for individuals with mood disorders. In addition, this subsection of the population has an increased incidence of disability and missed work. Significant morbidity and mortality are other, serious factors that raise the financial and societal costs of mood disorders. Approximately 15% of persons hospitalized with major depressive disorder eventually commit suicide, which is a significantly higher percentage than that for the general population (Depression Guideline Panel, 1993).

The percentage of the population that will require treatment for a mood disorder is high, ranging from 5 to 20%. For major depressive disorders alone the lifetime risk for women is 10 to 25% and for men is 5 to 12% (Depression Guideline Panel, 1993). Risk factors for developing these disorders include:

- Family and personal histories
- A concurrent medical disorder
- Prior suicide attempts
- Being female
- Inadequate support systems
- Life stress
- Substance abuse
- A post-partum condition.

The mood disorders are classified in the *Diagnostic and Statistical Manual of Mental Disorders, Fourth Edition,* (DSM-IV) as follows:

- Depressive Disorders (unipolar depression)
- Major Depressive Disorder
  Dysthymic Disorder
  Depressive Disorder Not Otherwise Specified
- Bipolar Disorders
  Bipolar Disorder I and II,
  Cyclothymic Disorder
  Bipolar Disorder Not Otherwise Specified

- Etiologically Based Disorders
  Mood Disorder Due to a Medical Condition
  Substance-induced Mood Disorder

This chapter focuses on the most common mood disorders: major depression, dysthymia, the bipolar disorders, and cyclothymic disorders.

■ THE CLINICAL NATURE OF BIPOLAR DISORDERS: MANIA AND DEPRESSION

MANIA VIEWED AS A MOOD STATE

In mania, the predominant mood is usually elevated and described as cheerful, euphoric, or high. The mood is judged excessive by those who know the individual well. The expansive quality of the mood disturbance is characterized by unselective enthusiasm and unceasing enthusiasm for interacting with people and for seeking involvement with the environment. If the individual is frustrated or thwarted in his attempts, the mood disturbance may change to that of irritability.

Flight of ideas is usually present. The accelerated speech may contain frequently changed topics. The individual is easily distracted and is observed through rapid changes in speech or activity in response to external stimuli, such as background noise or signs or pictures on the wall.

Characteristically, there is an inflated self-esteem, ranging from uncritical self-confidence to marked grandiosity, which may be delusional. The individual does not hesitate to start projects for which he has little aptitude, such as composing music, writing a novel, or seeking publicity for an impractical invention. Grandiose beliefs involving a special relationship to God or some well-known figure from the political, religious, or entertainment world are common.

The individual has great amounts of energy and has a decreased need for sleep. When the sleep disturbance is severe, the individual may go for days without sleep and yet not feel tired.

DEPRESSION VIEWED AS A MOOD STATE

Depression covers a broad spectrum of moods and behaviors. Depression is a common complaint, not only among psychiatric patients but also among large numbers of people who are not psychiatrically ill and may never seek psychiatric help.

The mood state of depression may occur in a normal person, in a patient with a psychiatric syndrome, or in a medical patient. Anyone can experience depression.

The mood of depression may be described as one of despair, gloom, a sense of foreboding, a feeling of emptiness, or a feeling of numbness. This mood state may be qualitatively and quantitatively different from other mood states. Whether the mood of depression in normal people differs from the mood of depression in people who have clinical depression is a matter that has not yet been decided. The same word is used, but it is not clear whether there is a clinical differentiation between the two.

When patients who have recovered from a severe depression are asked to compare the everyday kind of depression with this kind of clinical depression, they reply that the two kinds of depression are very different. Patients say that the severe depression comes over them like a very dark cloud, but the depression of everyday life is more transitory.

■ BIOLOGIC THEORIES OF DEPRESSION

Although it is believed that depression is caused by some kind of chemical imbalance in the brain, it is not known whether this imbalance is genetically triggered, what influences brain chemicals on neurotransmitters, or why antidepressant drugs work. The following sections discuss current biologic theories for depression.

GENETIC

Genetic studies and studies of the high rates of depression in first-degree biological relatives of depressed persons have led to the conclusion that most cases of recurrent depression have a biological basis. Analysis of twin studies shows a high rate of concordance for depression in dizygotic (fraternal) twins and an even higher rate in monozygotic (identical) twins. This does not mean, however, that psychological factors have no role in symptom formation or in precipitating an episode of depression (Reus, 1995); although these findings suggest a genetic link to depression, they don't explain the specific mechanism that triggers the disorder.

With regard to bipolar disorders, the rate of first-degree relatives with these disorders among patients who have such a disorder is twice as high as it is for depression. Adoption studies specifically show a greater prevalence of mood disorders among biologic than among adoptive relatives of patients with bipolar disorder (Pardes et al., 1989). There is strong support for the genetic theory but at this time there is no clearly identified gene linking to bipolar disorder. Studies comparing twins in adopted versus biological families have found that biological factors contribute significantly to the occurrence of bipolar disorder, and more so than post-natal environmental factors. Chromosome linkage studies have found pedigrees with the linkage of bipolar disorder to markers on the X chromosome, chromosome 6, and possibly chromosome 11. Yet the genetic theory cannot definitively explain the develop-

ment of bipolar illness without the identification of a consistent genetic link.

DYSREGULATION OF NEUROTRANSMISSION

The most prominent theory for the pathogenesis of mood disorders attributes them to regulatory disturbances in the neurotransmitter systems of the central nervous system, particularly those involving norepinephrine, serotonin, and dopamine (see Table 20–1). These monoamines are the principal neurotransmitters of the limbic system, which is responsible for regulating sleep, arousal, sexual function, emotional states, and appetite (see Chapter 4, Brain and Behavior). Some studies have shown that depression can arise from a functional deficit of norepinephrine at actual effector sites in the central nervous system (Schildkraut, 1978). Even more data suggest that serotonergic neurotransmission is an important factor in causing depression. Many depressed patients have decreased concentrations of serotonin in their central nervous systems. The serotonin system dysfunction is addressed by drugs that block the reuptake of serotonin thus restoring its supply. This effort at altering the serotonin system with drugs can affect other systems associated with depression such as the norepinephrine and dopamine systems. An overabundance of these transmitters can increase behavioral excitability in the patient and trigger manic behavior. This is an example of disruption of the balance between arousal and inhibition (Risby, Risch, Stoudemire, 1995).

The biogenic amine hypothesis is widely accepted as the predominant explanation for bipolar illness. Patients with such illness tend to have increased concentrations of serotonin in their brains, which could be the

TABLE 20–1. HYPOTHESES CONCERNING THE PATHOPHYSIOLOGY OF DEPRESSION

Serotonin hypothesis: Depression is associated with an absolute or functional deficiency of brain serotonin.

Catecholamine hypothesis: Depression results from an actual or functional deficiency of catecholamines.

Dopamine hypothesis: Depression is associated with changes in dopamine metabolism,

α-Adrenergic receptor theory: Depression results from an increased α-adrenergic receptor sensitivity.

Permissive hypothesis: Diminished serotonin secretion permits a mood disorder and:
    Superimposed norepinephrine deficiency results in depression
    Superimposed norepinephrine excess results in mania

Dysregulation hypothesis: Depression is caused by a failure of the inter-regulation of neurotransmitter systems.

Gamma-aminobutyric acid (GABA) hypothesis: Depression is associated with changes in GABA metabolism.

Source: Wells, B. G., (1995) Issues in the diagnosis of major depression. Formulary 30:3–9

causative factor in the manic episodes that occur in the illness. A particular paradox of this disorder is the occurrence of opposite pathological mood states within a particular individual. How one extreme of mood can give way to another can to some degree be explained by imbalances in neurotransmission. There can be rapid cycling that leads to mood instability. The cycling can occur within 12 to 24 hour periods (Risby, Risch, Stoudemire, 1995).

Another theory involving neurotransmission in bipolar disorder, and which has a connection to psychosocial theories of mood disorder, is **kindling.** According to Post (1992), kindling is a process in which neurotransmission is altered by the effects of stress. It is theorized that external stressors trigger certain internal physiologic stress responses that activate an episode of depression or mania. This then creates, within the affected parts of the brain and nervous system, an electrophysiological sensitivity to future stress. As a result, less stress is required to evoke a subsequent episode of depression or mania. The implication of this theory is that early treatment may protect the brain from serious changes in sensitivity and reduce the likelihood of future episodes of illness.

Kindling is also believed to influence other physiologic processes, such as the selective regulation of gene expression. A change in this latter process can help to activate certain genes, which may in turn initiate episodic symptoms of depression in genetically predisposed individuals.

NEUROENDOCRINE DISTURBANCES

Abnormalities in neuroendocrine regulation may show evidence of a primary disturbance in the hypothalamic-pituitary-adrenal axis (HPA) that is having an effect on physiological responses to stress. The hypothalamus controls endocrine functioning and the autonomic nervous system, which is involved in behaviors related to "fight versus flight" responses, hunger, thirst, pleasure, pain, and body temperature. These behaviors are often altered during a mood disturbance and help explain the physiological expression of vegetative symptoms of depression. Although the precise nature of the dysregulation of the HPA that causes such behavioral changes is not known, neuroendocrine dysregulation is a primary consideration in the etiology of mood disorders (Simmons-Alling, 1996).

One of the tests for neuroendocrine dysfunction is for dexamethasone suppression. Biological alterations are noted through HPA activity, which includes increased 24-hour urinary-free cortisol, dexamethasone nonsuppression (noted by increased cortisol level), a blunted adrenocorticotropic hormone (ACTH) response to corticotropin-releasing factor (CRF), and increased cerebrospinal fluid concentrations of cortisol

(Simmons-Alling, 1996). For example, the failure of the body to regulate cortisol secretion is important to the 24-hour cycle of circadian rhythms that control such physiological processes as the sleep-wake cycle and blood levels of hormones.

Chronobiological changes are another theoretical approach to mood disorders. Circadian rhythmicity allows complex physiological systems to be internally coordinated with changes in the environment. These chronobiological alterations occur over a 24-hour time period from morning when awake to night for sleep; this 24-hour rhythm is called the sleep-wake cycle. Depressive symptoms have been associated with disturbance in the sleep-wake cycle, such as early morning awakening or difficulty in falling asleep (Ryan, Montgomery, and Meyers, 1987).

Some depressed people appear to have a desynchronization in their 24-hour internal clock rhythm (Simmons-Alling, 1996). Desynchronization of the circadian rhythm is seen not only in REM sleep (see Chapter 23: Sleep Disorders) but with body temperature, melatonin and cortisol secretion cycles. Persons may start and stop releasing melatonin earlier which would lead to early morning awakening and evening sleepiness or they may start and stop releasing melatonin later than usual which would result in difficulty going to sleep and later, in awakening (Simmons-Alling, 1996).

Seasonal affective disorders (SAD) are episodes of mania or depression that recur annually at a specific season. A depressive episode may begin with the onset of winter, with persons living in climates farther away from the equator; the disorder often seems to resolve with the onset of longer days in the spring and summer. It is believed that persons with SAD are not synchronized with the day–night cycle, thereby causing a disturbance in mood.

Animal research has indicated that many typical antidepressants are effective in changing the setting of endogenous biological clocks. One hormone, for example, is melatonin, which is synthesized from serotonin and secreted by the pineal gland. Testing notes that melatonin demonstrates a circadian rhythm with highest values at night and lowest ones during the day. Because the production of melatonin is sensitive to light, it has been suggested that light modifies the melatonin circadian pattern (Simmons-Alling, 1996). Treatment has included, in some cases, the use of artificial light as a means of altering the melatonin imbalance for relieving symptoms of depression (Teicher et al., 1993).

ANATOMICAL ABNORMALITIES

Magnetic resonance imaging (MRI) has revealed lesions in the frontal or temporal lobes of the brain in some patients who were psychotically depressed (Cummings, 1993). Other methods, such as computed tomography (CT) scans, have shown evidence of enlarged ventricles, and positron emission tomography (PET) scans have shown decreased metabolic activity in the brains of patients with bipolar disorder (Simmons-Alling, 1996).

PSYCHOLOGICAL THEORIES OF DEPRESSION

COGNITIVE

One theory implicates a cognitive basis for the development of depression. The individual who has a cognitive style that focuses on what is wrong or negative in personal experience and life tends to experience depressive symptoms more often than others who focus on what is right and positive. Depressed individuals tend to attribute negative events to internal, stable, and global causes, while others attribute them to external, unstable, and specific causes (Seligman et al., 1984).

DEVELOPMENTAL

Negative resolution of a particular developmental stage in life is also hypothesized to lead to depression. If the challenges presented at the various stages of development are not successfully met, they may adversely affect identity development. Early developmental experiences within the family environment can be associated with depression. A child who experiences physical/sexual abuse, neglect, parental loss or divorce, alcoholism in the home, or other stressful life events is at a greater risk for later developing depression.

Other factors that appear to correlate with mood disorders, but which are not causative elements of them, are loneliness, low self-esteem, eating disorders (particularly among adolescents), drug abuse, and suicide.

PSYCHODYNAMIC THEORY

The psychodynamic theories for the origin and nature of depressive illness had their beginning in Freud's paper "Mourning and Melancholia," (1955), in which the gaps between grief and depression are described. Normal grief, observed Freud, shades into the abnormal, in which a complex of mechanisms such as oral dependency, identification with the lost object, inhibition, anger turned inward, and specific issues regarding loss are observed (Freud, 1955).

Extending Freud's studies, psychiatrist Edward Bibring (1953) saw depression as "a state of helplessness and powerlessness after experiences of illness, failure, and loneliness." Bibring continued his research in psychoanalytic theory and defined depression as an ego state marked by the emotional expression of helplessness and powerlessness. As an ego state, depression is characterized by a loss of self-esteem in reaction to three dynamic issues defined below. When these aspirations are threatened, they lower self-esteem and bring on depression. The psychodynamic formulation explains how a person's adherence to wishes and expectations are not tempered by reality and can play a role in depressive states.

- Wishes to be loved, to be appreciated, to be worthy versus not to be inferior or unworthy are associated with the earliest years of human social development. When these aspirations are not in an interpersonal context, the person is at risk for depression. Such persons receive their "ego supplies" for giving and care from persons who are important to them. They become depressed when someone who has cared about them leaves them or dies. In dynamic terms, this level of expectation from others and need for the self is identified as the oral stage of psychosexual development.
- Wishes to be good, to be loving, and not to be aggressive, hateful, or destructive are associated with the autonomy level of development. People with such needs struggle with issues relevant to being in control and being good versus not being in control or being bad. Depression may occur when aggressive or angry feelings within the self become too painful to acknowledge. In addition, this pattern of expectation of self is predicated on the developmental phase where nurturing and sustenance are only derived, in the individual's mind, from others. Thus, persons who cannot meet their self-expectations of perfect control are threatened with the loss of love. This core emotional state can intensify depression. For example, when someone important to the depression-prone individual dies, the individual may feel that he or she might have done something to prevent the death, or might have contributed to the death. These feelings can precipitate a depression. In dynamic terms, this level of autonomy and control is identified as the anal stage of psychosexual development.
- Wishes to be strong, superior, and secure, and not to be weak and insecure are associated with competitive issues. Some individuals, often men, become depressed when they lose in competition. They are concerned about being strong and winning rather than losing. A business failure or a poor choice in the stock market may depress this kind of person. Such persons do not talk about being not loved or about being good or bad in the moral sense, but feel defeated, and

struggle with this issue. In dynamic terms, this level of competitiveness is identified as the oedipal stage of psychosexual development.

■ SOCIOLOGICAL THEORY OF DEPRESSION

A sociological explanation for depression suggests that it is usually a response to loss. Here the problem is located at the interface of the individual and society, in contrast to psychological theory, in which the problem is viewed as being of intrapsychic origin. The sociological explanation of depression emphasizes the social system of family and peer group and its shaping and development as the primary definer of the individual. Less emphasis is placed on intrapsychic threats of loss of a nurturing other or loss of maintaining an ego-ideal as explained by Bibring (1953).

■ DEPRESSIVE DISORDERS

Depression describes a variety of conditions generally characterized by an inability to concentrate, hopelessness, sadness, dejection, disappointment, and demoralization not necessarily warranted by reality. Yet a depressive disorder encompasses more than depressive symptoms; the syndrome of depression involves a mood disturbance along with other psychological, somatic, and cognitive issues that significantly impair functioning.

MAJOR DEPRESSIVE DISORDER

A major depressive episode lasts for at least 2 weeks, is marked by a sense of sadness or a loss of interest in formerly pleasing activities, and tends to be severe and dysfunctional (Diagnostic and Statistical Manual, 4th ed.). Even though a depressed mood is the pervasive symptom of an episode of major depression, the affected individual may not actually complain of being depressed; instead, the symptoms may be of irritability, weakness, or anxiousness, or may be physical symptoms such as headaches, dizziness, or fatigue.

Diagnostic criteria for major depression (Wells, 1995) are listed below. In order to be diagnosed as having a major depression, a patient must, during one 2-week period, exhibit at least five of the following symptoms, which will represent a change from previous functioning. *At least one of the symptoms must be the first or second in the following list.*

- Depressed mood. In children and adolescents the mood can be irritable instead of depressed.
- Diminished interest or pleasure in most or all of the patient's usual activities.
- Significant weight loss or weight increase, or a decrease or increase in appetite.
- Insomnia or hypersomnia.
- Psychomotor agitation or retardation as observed by others.
- Fatigue or loss of energy.
- Feelings of worthlessness, or excessive or inappropriate guilt.
- Diminished ability to think or to concentrate; indecisiveness.
- Recurrent thoughts of death, suicidal ideation, a suicide attempt, or a specific plan for suicide.

A diagnosis of major depressive disorder is made only when symptoms are not attributable to drugs, a general medical condition, or recent bereavement.

Severely depressed individuals may also experience episodes of delusion and psychosis.

Dexamethasone Suppression Test (DST)

One of the most consistent biological findings in psychiatry is the increased concentration of cortisol found in the blood of depressed persons (hypercortisolemia). The dexamethasone suppression test (DST) is based on a theory that some depressions are associated with release of stress hormones (e.g., cortisol). Researchers have investigated the role of cortisol in depression and developed indirect tests to assess the functioning of the hypothalamic-pituitary-adrenal axis, which produces this hormone. Although the finding is not clinically reliable for the diagnosis of depression, about one-half of adults show a disruption in the system.

Epidemiology

The epidemiologic data for the mood disorders were derived from the Epidemiologic Catchment Area Study (ECA), which was initiated in 1980 by the National Institutes of Mental Health (NIMH). This study involved more than 18,000 persons living in five communities, and revealed the American community-based lifetime prevalence rates of the major psychiatric disorders. The prevalence of major depressive disorder is 5 to 9% for women and 2 to 3% for men. The risk of experiencing a major depressive disorder is low for pre-pubertal boys and girls, with an equal risk for both sexes. In nursing homes the number of persons who experience major depression is quite high, with at least 13% of residents developing new major depressive episodes. Major depressive disorder is the most common psychiatric illness experienced by the elderly (Risby, Risch and Stoudemire, 1994).

Etiological Factors and Family Patterns

Major depressive disorder has a strong familial component. First-degree biologic relatives (parents, siblings and children) of persons with depression are 1.5 to 3 times more likely to develop a major depressive disorder than relatives of unaffected individuals. Influential factors are gender and age, rather than income, ethnic background, marital status, or education. Other disorders linked to individuals who have experienced major depressive disorders are alcohol dependence in their adult first-degree biologic relatives, and attention deficit-hyperactivity disorder in their offspring.

Age of Onset and Course

The average age of onset of major depressive disorder is from the mid-20 to early 30s, although recent studies indicate that the age of onset is becoming earlier for individuals born more recently. The onset is gradual and does not necessarily follow a precipitating stressful event. If the individual is not treated for the disorder, the episode usually lasts from 6 to 24 months. The disorder is highly recurrent, with 50% of persons who experience a first episode eventually developing another major depressive episode. As the number of episodes increases, so does the likelihood that yet another episode will occur. The risk of recurrence of major depression after three episodes is as high as 90% (DSM-IV).

Impairment and Complications

The impairments seen in major depressive disorder are generally significant, including reduced social, occupational, and interpersonal functioning. Those who experience severe symptoms may not be able to maintain minimal personal hygiene or perform self-care, such as dressing and feeding themselves. Laboratory findings associated with major depression (Wells, 1995) are listed below.

- Sleep electroencephalogram (EEG) abnormalities
    - Prolonged sleep latency
    - Increased intermittent awakening
    - Early morning awakening
    - Reduced Stages 3 and 4 sleep
    - Decreased rapid-eye-movement (REM) latency
    - Increased eye movement during REM sleep
    - Increased duration of REM sleep early in evening
- Abnormal dexamethasone suppression test
- Abnormal brain imaging
- Abnormalities in evoked potential studies
- Abnormalities in the waking EEG

Complete remission of a major depressive episode can return an individual to his or her normal level of functioning. Persons who only partially recover more often experience another episode, have a poorer prognosis, need longer-term treatment, and have a greater need for both medication and psychotherapy. An individual can go for several years without an episode of depression, and some persons experience more frequent episodes as they grow older. Recovery is less likely for women, especially those who are older, have less than a high-school degree, and have an unstable marital history. Up to 43% of individuals with major depressive disorder also have one or more non-mood-related psychiatric disorders (Depression Guideline Panel, 1993).

Nursing Assessment and Diagnosis

Early diagnosis and treatment significantly improve the prognosis and quality of life of patients with major depressive disorder. Carefully interviewing the patient is important for successful diagnosis, but may not yield accurate information, since the patient may have difficulties with memory and concentration, or may deny the symptoms. The following steps are often taken to assess whether major depressive disorder exists, and to determine its cause and treatment.

- A clinical interview is performed to determine whether the nine specific symptoms of major depressive disorder are met. This interview will include a direct interview with the patient, along with self-report ratings and/or a history from the patient's spouse or a friend.
- The patient is interviewed to assess the possibility of a concurrent substance-abuse problem or the use of medications that may trigger depressive symptomatology. Substance withdrawal or intoxication can mirror depressive symptoms and require special treatment. Several medications have been implicated as causing depression, including some of the antihypertensive, steroid, and anti-inflammatory agents.
- Findings of the physical examination and medical history are reviewed to assess whether a medical disorder is causing or is associated with depressive symptoms. Several medical disorders may produce depression, including hypothyroidism, diabetes, multiple sclerosis, congestive heart failure, carcinoma, and rheumatoid arthritis.
- The patient is further evaluated to determine whether another, concurrent, non-mood-related psychiatric condition exists that could be associated with the patient's symptoms.

E CASE EXAMPLE

▶ MAJOR DEPRESSIVE DISORDER

Paula, a 25-year-old unmarried white woman, is admitted to the emergency room after taking an overdose of over-the-counter sleeping aids. She states that "life isn't worth living any more." She is accompanied by her older brother, Tom, whom she had called after taking the overdose. In the emergency room Paula is treated medically and cleared. The next day she is discharged and referred for out-patient treatment with a clinical nurse specialist.

History of Present Illness

The youngest of five children and the only daughter of a middle-class Philadelphia family, Paula asserts that she has been feeling increasingly overwhelmed and despondent since her roommate died 7 months ago. In the past 2 weeks her condition has deteriorated to the point at which she has had difficulty at work and has become uninterested in her social life and personal hygiene. Her appetite has diminished and she has lost 8 pounds. Additionally, Paula reports difficulty in falling asleep at night, and has experienced frequent awakening. Upon arising she has felt fatigued and has not gone to her job as a secretary. She was recently suspended from her job for absenteeism, and was told that she may be in danger of losing her job. As her symptoms increased in severity, says Paula, she began feeling increasingly guilty, lonely, and worthless. She asserts that she has never felt "this bad" before. She has never sought help for her problems prior to this contact. She relates that she has no medical problems, and states that she does not drink alcohol or abuse drugs.

Social History

Since her graduation from high school 7 years ago, the patient has been working as a secretary in a large law firm. She dates infrequently and prefers the companionship of her female friends. She has two close girlfriends but has not gone out socially for the past 2 months. "I really miss my roommate," says Paula, "we did everything together".

Family History

Tom, Paula's brother, was briefly interviewed and describes his sister as being "overly dependent" on the family. He says that she has always called him for advice, and that he has been controlling her finances for the past 4 years. He states that Paula has rarely argued with anyone in the family, is uncomfortable living alone since her roommate died, and is afraid of being alone. He describes Paula's mother as being overprotective of her. Her brother sees their father, a prominent businessman in the area, as very controlling.

Mental Status

Paula's appearance is disheveled. Her eye contact with the examiner is minimal and she speaks softly. She shows psychomotor retardation; her affect is blunted and her mood is depressed. However, her thoughts are clear and goal directed, and she denies suicidal ideation, saying "I guess I just didn't know how to get help." Her recent and past memory spheres are intact.

Initial Diagnosis

The initial nursing diagnosis for this patient is risk for violence to self, related to suicidal ideation and intent, as evidenced by her overdosing with over-the-counter sleeping aids. The second diagnosis is dysfunctional grieving, related to the death of her roommate, and evidenced by changes in appetite and sleep, job difficulties, and feelings of guilt, worthlessness, and loneliness.

Table 20–2 may be used to evaluate the presence of major depressive disorder as well as the other mood disorders discussed in this chapter.

TREATMENT OF MAJOR DEPRESSION

Antidepressant drugs are the primary treatment for major depression. Among the several types of antidepressants, each has different side effects and risks (Chapter 40). After careful evaluation of the patient's medical history, an antidepressant is selected that has minimal adverse side effects for the patient while addressing much of the patient's depressive symptomatology. Most often, the patient will respond positively to the drug.

Administering and monitoring antidepressant medication is a complex process. The nurse must understand the pharmokinetic and pharmodynamic actions of the different antidepressants, their beneficial and adverse effects, dosage scheduling, and drug interactions, and their contraindications and self-care implications.

Electroconvulsive therapy (ECT) is usually given to patients experiencing severe depression that has not responded to drug treatment. This therapy is much safer than it used to be, with the use of safer general anesthesia, muscle relaxants, and better machine technology. The benefit to the patient is rapid recovery, with the most common negative side effect being memory dysfunction. See p. 341–345 in this chapter for discussion of ECT.

For mild forms of depression, psychotherapy has proven to be as effective as drug therapy. Psychotherapy can be given individually or in a group setting, and is frequently used in conjunction with antidepressant drugs.

Educating patients and their families about the clinical course of major depression and its treatment enables them to overcome myths surrounding depres-

TABLE 20–2. MAJOR DEPRESSIVE DISORDER SUBGROUPS

Subgroup	Essential Features	Diagnostic Implications	Treatment Implications	Prognostic Implications
Psychotic	Hallucinations Delusions	More likely to become bipolar than nonpsychotic types. May be misdiagnosed as schizophrenia.	Antidepressant medication plus a neuroleptic is more effective than are antidepressants alone. ECT is very effective.	Usually a recurrent illness. Subsequent episodes are usually psychotic. Psychotic subtypes run in families. Mood-incongruent features have a poorer prognosis.
Melancholic	Anhedonia Unreactive mood Severe vegetative symptoms	May be misdiagnosed as dementia. More likely in older patients.	Antidepressant medication is essential. ECT is 90% effective.	If recurrent, consider maintenance medication.
Atypical	Reactive mood Overeating/ weight gain Oversleeping Rejection sensitivity Heavy limb sensation Fewer episodes	Common in younger patients. May be misdiagnosed as personality disorder.	TCAs may be less effective. MAOIs or SSRIs preferred.	Unclear.
Seasonal	Onset, fall Offset, spring Recurrent	More frequent in non-equatorial latitudes. Pattern occurs in major depressive and bipolar disorders.	Medications have ? efficacy. Psychotherapy has ? efficacy. Phototherapy is an option.	Recurs.
Postpartum psychosis/ depression	Acute onset (<30 days) in postpartum period. Severe, labile mood symptoms. 1/1,000 is psychotic form.	Often heralds a bipolar disorder.	Hospitalize. Treat medically.	50% chance of recurring in next postpartum period.

Note: ECT = electroconvulsive therapy. TCA = tricyclic antidepressant. MAOIs = monoamine oxidase inhibitors. SSRIs = selective serotonin reuptake inhibitors.
Source: Depression in Primary Care: Vol. 1. US Dept. HHS. 1993

sion, many of which claim that it is caused by a personal weakness or flaw. This education increases the patient's motivation to take a positive and active role in his or her recovery. Another benefit is being able to recognize the return of depressive symptomatology and to seek treatment for it at an early point if it does recur, possibly preventing or shortening the depressive episode.

DYSTHYMIC DISORDER

Dysthymia involves a chronically depressed mood that lasts for at least 2 years. It is often difficult to differentiate from major depressive disorder, but is less severe and of longer duration than major depression. The pervasive mood for adults is sadness, while children with dysthymia generally appear irritable. At least two of the following symptoms must be present for a diagnosis of this mood disturbance: insomnia/hypersomnia, appetite changes, low energy, low self-esteem, poor concentration/decision-making ability, and feelings of hopelessness. If a major depressive episode occurs within the 2-year period, specified as a minimum for dysthymia, the affected individual is diagnosed as having major depressive disorder.

Epidemiology

From 2.1 to 4.7% of the population of the United States has dysthymia, with the rate being twice as high among women as among men. Studies have shown that as many as 6% of women between the ages of 25 and 64 suffer from dysthymia. For boys and girls, the rates of dysthymia are the same. Fifteen percent of individuals with this disorder also experience a concurrent mood disorder.

Etiological Factors and Family Patterns

No universally accepted data exist on the etiology of dysthymia. Some clinicians believe that the disorder arises from poor self-esteem as a result of difficult early childhood experiences. Detrimental developmental experiences that might constitute risks for the disorder include neglect, sexual/physical abuse, parental death or divorce, and alcoholism in the home. Many of these factors have also been linked to major depressive disorder.

Dysthymia is more common among first degree biologic relatives of patients with major depressive disorder or bipolar disorder.

Diagnostic Category:
Major Depression.

Nursing Diagnosis: SELF-CARE DEFICIT.

Related to: (check at least one)
_____ Disabling anxiety   _____ Excessive ritualistic behaviors
_____ Withdrawal   _____ Obsessive thoughts
_____ Other

Treatment Goal: PATIENT WILL CONSISTENTLY DEMONSTRATE SUCCESS IN THE ACTIVITIES OF DAILY LIVING.

Treatment Goal Can Be Measured Using the Following Expected Outcomes:

1. Patient maintains optimal level of personal care/hygiene without assistance. (This is to include daily grooming, appropriate dressing and adequate nutrition.)

Interventions:
Date   **Date**
Initiated   **Discontinued**

_____   _____   1. Allow and encourage patient to perform normal activities of daily living (ADLs) at his/her level of ability.
_____   _____   2. Encourage independence, but intervene when patient is unable to perform.
_____   _____   3. Offer recognition and positive reinforcement independent accomplishments. (i.e., verbal praise, increased privileges.) (Identify)
_____   _____   4. Show patient how to perform activities in which he/she is having difficulty.
_____   _____   5. Keep strict records of food/fluid intake.
_____   _____   6. Offer nutritious snacks and fluids between meals.
_____   _____   7. If patient is incontinent, establish routine toileting schedule.

(Adapted from Nursing Care Plans developed by Nursing Staff at 1st Hospital Wyoming Valley, Wilkes Barre, PA under the direction of Theresa M. Croushore)

Figure 20–1. Individualized pathway nursing-care plan.

Age of Onset and Course

Dysthymia usually begins in childhood or adolescence without a clear onset, and follows a chronic course. No real history of a sustained normal mood is seen during adulthood. Many persons who suffer from this disorder go on to develop a concurrent episode of major depression, yielding what is known as "double depression." During the 2-year minimal period (1 year for children and adolescents), for dysthymia, affected individuals are not symptom-free for more than a 2-month period.

Impairment and Complications

Dysthymic individuals can often function in society, but are significantly impaired socially and occupationally. They generally experience feelings of inadequacy and insecurity, and suffer from interpersonal problems. These impairments tend to put them at increased risk for substance abuse and suicide. A dysthymic individual may suffer from an accompanying non-mood-related psychiatric disorder or a nonpsychiatric medical condition.

Treatment

Some depressive symptoms of dysthymia respond well to antidepressant medications, especially in patients with a family history of mood disorders. Generally, treatment starts with psychotherapy, which in more severe cases can be coupled with medication.

DEPRESSIVE DISORDER NOT OTHERWISE SPECIFIED (DNOS)

Depressive disorder not otherwise specified, also known as adjustment disorder with depressed mood, is a mood condition with depressive symptoms that are not as severe or long-lasting as those of the other depressive disorders. DNOS frequently occurs after some distinct stressor such as a job loss, divorce, physical illness, or natural disaster. Individuals who have poor coping skills and inadequate support systems are at a greater than average risk for this disorder.

■ BIPOLAR DISORDERS

In **bipolar disorders,** the predominant mood is usually elevated expansive or irritable, and there are associated

Diagnostic Category:
Bipolar Disorders.

Nursing Diagnosis: RISK FOR VIOLENCE, SELF DIRECTED OR DIRECTED AT OTHERS.

Related to: (check at least one)

___ Low self esteem	___ Repressed anger	___ Suicidal threats
___ Unresolved grief	___ Depressed mood	___ Hostility
___ Overt aggressive acts	___ Unmet dependency needs	

Treatment Goal: PATIENT WILL NOT HARM SELF OR OTHERS DURING HOSPITALIZATION.

Treatment Goal Can Be Measured Using The Following Expected Outcomes:
1. Patient will deny suicidal ideation.
2. Patient will deny homicidal ideation.
3. Patient will control anxiety at a level at which he/she feels no need for aggression.
4. Patient will inform staff of inability to control aggressive feelings.
5. Other _____

Interventions:

Date Initiated	Date Discontinued	
_____	_____	1. Observe patient's behavior/special treatment procedure is ordered by physician (Identify).
_____	_____	2. Assess patient for suicide potential/risk and report findings to physician. Document assessments/hospital protocol.
_____	_____	3. Obtain a verbal/written contract from patient agreeing not to harm self and to seek out staff in the event suicidal thoughts occur.
_____	_____	4. Encourage patient to recognize and accept angry or aggressive feelings.
_____	_____	5. Provide safe physical outlets for expression of anger (i.e., punching bag, play, exercise).
_____	_____	6. Remove all dangerous objects from patient's environment.
_____	_____	7. Administer prescribed medication per physician's orders. Assess for effectiveness/adverse reactions. (Identify).
_____	_____	8. Provide seclusion when necessary to decrease stimuli and agitation level.
_____	_____	9. If all other interventions fail, utilize mechanical restraints to protect patient and/or others from injury. Follow special treatment procedure/hospital policy. (Identify). (i.e., appropriate documentation and prescribed protocol for care of patient in restraints).
_____	_____	11. Other _____

(Adapted from Nursing Care Plans developed by Nursing Staff at 1st Hospital Wyoming Valley, Wilkes Barre, PA under the direction of Theresa M. Croushore)

Figure 20–2. Individualized pathways nursing-care plan.

symptoms of the manic syndrome. These symptoms include pressure of speech, hyperactivity, inflated self-esteem, flight of ideas, distractibility, a decreased need for sleep, and an excessive involvement with activities that have the potential for producing painful consequences.

The hyperactive behavior often involves excessive planning of and participation in multiple activities (e.g., occupational, political, religious, and sexual). There are efforts to renew old acquaintances, which may include telephoning friends at all hours of the night. The domineering, intrusive, and demanding nature of these interactions is not recognized by the affected individual.

Often, the expansiveness, optimism, grandiosity, and lack of judgment in the bipolar disorders lead to activities of reckless driving, buying sprees, questionable business investments, and sexual behavior unusual for the affected individual. The activities may have a bizarre quality to them, such as dressing in colorful or strange garments, wearing excessive makeup, or giving advice to passing strangers.

The speech of the affected individual is typically loud, rapid, difficult to interrupt, and filled with jokes, puns, and amusing irrelevancies. It may become theatrical, with dramatic mannerisms and singing. If the mood is irritable, there may be hostile comments, complaints, and angry tirades.

The condition is marked by great energy and a decreased need for sleep. When the sleep disturbance is severe, the affected individual may go for days without sleep and yet not feel tired.

The term "hypomania" is used to describe a clinical syndrome that is similar to bipolar disorder, but not severe enough to cause marked impairment in social or occupational functioning or to require hospitalization.

The presence of some form of mania is the key to classifying the bipolar disorders. Mania is defined as the opposite of depression, with the experience of a heightened, euphoric mood, but may also include irritability

Diagnostic Category:
Major Depression

Nursing Diagnosis: DISTURBANCE IN SELF CONCEPT (LOW SELF ESTEEM).

Related to: (check at least one) identify problem list number.
_____ Dysfunctional family system   _____ Lack of positive feedback
_____ Unmet dependency needs   _____ Repeated negative feedback
_____ Other

Treatment Goal: BY DISCHARGE, PATIENT WILL VERBALIZE POSITIVE PERCEPTION OF SELF.

Treatment Goal Can Be Measured Using the Following Expected Outcomes:

Patient will demonstrate ability to manage personal self-care, make independent decisions and use problem solving skills.

Interventions:

Date Initiated	Date Discontinued	
_____	_____	1. Convey unconditional positive regard for patient.
_____	_____	2. Spend time with patient on a one-to-one basis and in group activities.
_____	_____	3. Assist patient to establish realistic goals; plan activities in which success is likely (Identify.)
_____	_____	4. Encourage and support patient in confronting the fear of failure by attending all therapy activities. (Identify.)
_____	_____	5. Assist patient in identifying additional aspects of self and in developing plans for changing the characteristics he/she views as negative.
_____	_____	6. Do not allow patient to ruminate about past failures; withdraw attention if he/she persists.
_____	_____	7. Minimize negative feedback to patient; enforce limit setting in a matter-of-fact manner.
_____	_____	8. Encourage independence in the performance of personal responsibilities, as well as in decision-making related to own self-care.
_____	_____	9. Offer positive reinforcement for accomplishments (i.e., verbal praise, increased privileges). (Identify).
_____	_____	10. Assist patient to increase level of self awareness through examination of feelings, attitude, and behaviors.

(Adapted from Nursing Care Plans developed by Nursing Staff at 1st Hospital Wyoming Valley, Wilkes Barre, PA under the direction of Theresa M. Croushore)

Figure 20–3. Individualized nursing-care plan

and/or anger. As defined in *DSM-IV*, the three forms of bipolar disorder are bipolar I, bipolar II, and cyclothymia. Persons who have a bipolar disorder that does not fall into any of these three categories are diagnosed as having bipolar disorder not otherwise classified.

BIPOLAR I DISORDER

Bipolar I disorder is categorized by one or more manic (or mixed) episodes, usually accompanied by major depressive episodes. A true manic episode involves an abnormally and persistently euphoric or irritable mood that lasts for at least 1 week. This mood disturbance is accompanied by at least three additional symptoms, consisting of inflated self-esteem, distractibility, increased psychomotor agitation, racing thoughts, a decreased need for sleep, pressured speech, or involvement in activities that can cause harm to the affected individual or others (i.e., reckless driving or shopping sprees). Depression and hypomania (less severe manic episodes) may be regularly experienced by the individual with bipolar I disorder, but are not essential to this diagnosis. Acute mania may include hallucinations or delusions.

BIPOLAR II DISORDER

Bipolar II disorder is defined by one or more major depressive episodes accompanied by at least one hypomanic episode lasting at least 4 days. Hypomania is defined in the same way as mania, with the symptoms being less severe, and less debilitating, and not including hallucinations or delusions. If the mood is irritability instead of euphoria, four of the manic symptoms listed above must be present.

BIPOLAR DISORDERS I AND II. EPIDEMIOLOGY, ETIOLOGY, AND FAMILY PATTERNS

Males and females are equally afflicted by bipolar disorders I and II, with a prevalence of 0.4 to 1.2%. A family history of these disorders is quite common among affected individuals. First-degree biologic relatives of such individuals are 4–24 times more likely than average to develop a bipolar disorder. These same relatives

---

Diagnostic Category:
Dysthymia.

Nursing Diagnosis: IMPAIRED SOCIAL INTERACTION.

Related to: (check at least one) identify problem list number.
_____ Low self esteem   _____ Negative role modeling
_____ Unmet dependency needs   _____ Discomfort in social situations

Treatment Goal: BY DISCHARGE, PATIENT WILL BE ABLE TO INTERACT WITH STAFF AND PEERS ON THE UNIT WITH NO INDICATION OF DISCOMFORT.

Long-Term Outcome:
1. Patient will seek staff for social as well as therapeutic interaction.
2. Patient will willingly and appropriately participate in group activities.
3. Patient will verbalize reasons for inability to form close interpersonal relationships with others in the past.
4. Patient will maintain an appropriate interpersonal relationship with another patient.

Interventions:

Date Initiated	Date Discontinued	
_____	_____	1. Develop trusting relationship with patient by being honest and conveying accepting attitude.
_____	_____	2. Offer to remain with patient during initial interactions with others on unit.
_____	_____	3. Provide constructive criticism and positive reinforcement for effects (i.e., verbal praise, increased privileges). (Identify.)
_____	_____	4. Confront patient and withdraw attention when interactions with others are manipulative or exploitative.
_____	_____	5. Act as role model for patient through appropriate interactions with others.
_____	_____	6. Provide group situations for patient. (Identify.)

(Adapted from Nursing Care Plans developed by Nursing Staff at 1st Hospital Wyoming Valley, PA under the direction of Theresa M. Croushore)

Figure 20–4. Individualized nursing-care plan.

are also at greater risk for having a depressive disorder (DSM-IV).

AGE OF ONSET AND COURSE

The mean age for developing bipolar I and II disorders is the early 20s. Men with these disorders are more likely to experience a manic episode first, and women a depressive episode. One third of persons with bipolar I disorder have mixed illness, in which manic and depressive episodes occur within the same 24- to 48-hour period. Untreated manic episodes last usually 6 months, whereas untreated depressive episodes last 8 to 10 months. Full recovery usually occurs between episodes, and future episodic patterns mimic earlier such patterns. Some individuals experience rapid mood cycling, with four or more episodes of illness within a year.

IMPAIRMENT AND COMPLICATIONS

Persons with bipolar I disorder experience considerable social and occupational impairment. Morbidity and mortality from the condition are high. The unpredictability and chronicity of the bipolar disorders can lead to joblessness, divorce, legal problems, and death

by suicide. From 10 to 15% of affected individuals commit suicide if untreated, which is 10 to 20 times the suicide rate in the general population. Women are more likely to attempt suicide, with men more likely to complete the act.

Persons with bipolar II disorder do not experience the same degree of impairment, either socially or occupationally, as those with the Type I disorder. In fact, some researchers see them as having a marked increase in accomplishments, efficiency, and creativity.

NURSING ASSESSMENT AND DIAGNOSIS

Assessment of the bipolar disorders is similar to assessment of the depressive disorders, with the emphasis being to determine whether manic or hypomanic episodes exist.

In more severe stages of mania, a neuroleptic agent may be added to lithium for a brief period to help control acute psychotic symptoms. Some researchers have found that the anticonvulsant drugs are just as efficacious as the neuroleptics in rapidly controlling psychotic symptoms. The implication of this is that the psychosis can be rapidly controlled without exposing the patient to the potential side effects of neuroleptics. In the most severe stage of mania, or in mania that has not responded to medication, ECT may be necessary.

For severe cases of bipolar II disorder, lithium in combination with a tricyclic antidepressant or a monamine oxidase inhibitor (MAO) has been found efficacious. MAOs are more frequently indicated when the depression is characterized by atypical symptoms, such as increased sleep and appetite. It is imperative that the nurse carefully monitor the patient's mood cycles when tricyclic drugs are being given, in order to curtail the potential for rapid mood cycling.

Moderate bipolar II disorders have been classically treated with tricyclic antidepressant drugs alone. Because this regimen has been found to induce rapid mood cycling in some cases, lithium can be added prophylactically. Alternative medications, such as psychostimulants, bupropion (wellbutrin), anticonvulsants, and thyroid hormone, have all been used with some degree of success.

Non-pharmacologic therapy has also been used to manage bipolar depression. Sleep deprivation during the second half of the night has produced antidepressant effects, but these are generally short-lived, and the patient often relapses after a few days of normal sleep. ECT has been useful in treating acutely suicidal or delusional patients and those who have not responded to the therapies mentioned earlier.

An important nursing role in the pharmacologic management of bipolar disorder is to teach the patient the importance of maintaining his or her medication regimen, the risk of potential side effects, and how to handle such side effects if they do develop. Lithium commonly causes fine hand tremors, nausea, thirst, polyuria, fatigue, and mild muscle weakness. Psychotropic medications such as lithium can impact on major organ muscles and alter potassium levels causing muscle fatigue and cardiac arrhythmia. This toxic state can impact on the heart itself and lead to death. For this reason, patients must receive thorough instruction about all medications before being discharged from the hospital. In addition, patients who are more knowledgeable about their medications may be more compliant taking them.

Nursing care of the patient with a bipolar disorder is complex. Bipolar disorder is an illness that often challenges those who work with it as well as those who suffer from it. If not properly diagnosed and managed, bipolar disorder can be devastating to the patient and the patient's family.

CYCLOTHYMIC DISORDER

Cyclothymic disorder, the third bipolar disorder, consists of chronic and cyclical periods of hypomania and

E CASE EXAMPLE

▶ BIPOLAR DISORDER

A 28-year-old research assistant in nuclear physics is brought to the emergency room by his girlfriend, who explains that over the preceding 2 weeks he has become increasingly irritable and suspicious and has undergone a "personality change." She points out that he has not slept for the past three nights, and has become preoccupied with the belief that his research will be regarded as the "new bible of the nuclear age." His appearance is disheveled.

Because he fears that his ideas will be stolen, he has constructed an elaborate mathematical code that only he can read. He also dresses in a mismatched three-piece suit that he says is a disguise that will enable him to elude agents assigned to follow him. During the interview, he paces around the room, interrupting his responses to questions with associations to the interviewer's style of dress, a paperweight on the desk, and a book whose title he misreads.

The history obtained from his girlfriend reveals that the patient had never previously had symptoms similar to these, but that for about 3 months during the past 12 months, he had felt too tired to go to class, and spent much of the day sleeping.

A family history reveals an aunt who was hospitalized twice following the birth of her two children, and an older brother who married four times and was "quite moody."

The girlfriend is able to convince the young man to enter the hospital and begin taking neuroleptic medication, which he calls "thought pills." The medication results in a marked reduction in symptoms within 5 days. After 2 weeks of treatment with lithium, the patient's suspiciousness and grandiose beliefs diminish, but he remains excessively concerned that his research is important enough to require future protection from industrial spies (Reus, 1995).

Treatment

The nursing diagnosis in this case is a disturbance in self-concept and impaired social interaction. See Figures 20–3 and 20–4.

Lithium is the drug of choice in treating hypomanic and acute manic conditions. Hypomanias and low-grade manias usually respond to lithium alone or in combination with a sedative-hypnotic agent given at bedtime to promote restful sleep and avoid escalation of symptoms.

E CASE EXAMPLE

▶ MAJOR DEPRESSION

Although previously active in various community groups, Mrs. H., a 66-year-old attorney, stopped all her work, church, and home activities, neglected her hygiene and appearance, and stopped eating when she lost her son in an airplane crash. She would stand all day long in a corner, sobbing, wringing her hands, and praying that "God should take my life—I failed my family and caused by son's death." After 3 months of inpa-

tient psychotherapy and antidepressants, she planned to hang herself. Her husband was advised to consider legal guardianship and to investigate nursing homes for her care. As an emergency measure, ECT was initiated, and after seven treatments Mrs. H. showered, smiled, applied make-up, and requested a weekend pass to dine with her husband and conduct business. After the eighth treatment, her will to live, appetite, energy, and sense of humor returned and she began to talk sadly of her son's death (Valente, 1991).

---

mild depression that last for at least 2 years (1 year for children and adolescents). During this time there are no symptom-free periods lasting more than 2 months.

Epidemiology

The lifetime prevalence of cyclothymia is from .4% to 1%. This disorder is equally common in women and men, yet women are more likely to seek treatment.

Etiological Factors and Family Patterns

First-degree biologic relatives of individuals with cyclothymia appear to have a more frequent than average occurrence of bipolar I, bipolar II and major depressive disorders. The risk of substance abuse among the family members of someone with this disorder is also potentially greater than average.

Age of Onset and Course

Cyclothymia generally begins in adolescence or early adulthood. It has an insidious onset and a highly chronic course. From 15 to 50% of patients with cyclothymia develop a bipolar disorder.

Impairment and Complications

Like patients with bipolar II disorder, some patients with cyclothymia do function well during hypomanic episodes. Unfortunately, the chronicity and cyclical nature of the disorder can lead to unpredictable mood changes that affect functioning. Some persons may view the cyclothymic individual as unreliable, inconsistent, and temperamental. Common traits/experiences among cyclothymic individuals are marital difficulties, substance abuse problems, poor work performance, and promiscuity. See Figure 20–5.

Nursing Assessment and Diagnosis

The approach to assessing cyclothymia is similar to that for assessing the other mood disorders, with the emphasis on determining the severity of the manic/depressive episodes as well as the age of onset and duration of the disorder.

■ ELECTROCONVULSIVE THERAPY

Electroconvulsive therapy (ECT) originated in the late 19th and early 20th centuries when researchers began to study the phenomenon of mental disorders and the nature of brain dysfunction. Before the advent of electroconvulsive therapy, von Meduna induced seizures in schizophrenic patients by injecting them with oil of camphor. Later, he injected pentylenetetrazole. At about the same time, Sakel achieved a similar result by inducing insulin coma in psychotic patients as a result of the hypoglycemic state produced by insulin (Davis and Goldman, 1995).

Electroconvulsive therapy using an electrical current passed directly through the brain to produce a generalized tonic-clonic seizure was first introduced by two Italian psychiatrists, Ugo Cerletti and Lucio Bini, in 1937. The first patient to be so treated, who had been found wandering around a train station in Rome, recovered from his psychotic episode after 11 treatments and was discharged within a few months. The publicity about this treatment success spread rapidly (Davis and Goldman, 1995).

The use of ECT for psychiatric patients has had periods of both popularity and unpopularity. Initially, ECT was given with the patient in the alert and awake state. However, the procedure was often frightening to the patient and dangerous as a result of the violent

Diagnostic Category:
Bipolar Disorders.

Nursing Diagnosis: INEFFECTIVE INDIVIDUAL COPING

Related to: (check at least one)
_____ Inadequate support systems   _____ Unresolved grief
_____ Unmet Dependency   _____ Dysfunctional family systems
_____ Depressed mood needs   _____ Low self esteem depressed mood
_____ Other _____

Treatment Goal: PATIENT WILL DEVELOP AND UTILIZE EFFECTIVE AND SOCIALLY ACCEPTABLE COPING SKILLS.

Treatment Goal Can Be Measured Using The Following Expected Outcomes:
1. Patient is able to successfully resolve problems to such a degree they are able to fulfill the activities of daily living.
2. Patient is able to identify reasonable and appropriate skills or methods to be used to cope with stressors.

Interventions:
Date   **Date**
Initiated   **Discontinued**

_____   _____   1. Develop trusting relationship with patient.
_____   _____   2. Encourage patient to discuss angry feelings.
_____   _____   3. Assist patient to identify the true object of the hostility.
_____   _____   4. Provide physical outlets for healthy release of hostile feelings (i.e., punching bag, exercise, play activities, etc.).
_____   _____   5. If depressed, assess suicide potential and report findings to physician. Document assessment/hospital protocol.
_____   _____   6. Allow patient to perform as independently as possible and provide positive feedback (i.e. verbal praise, increase privileges). (Identify.).
_____   _____   7. Assist patient to identify precipitant/stressor to maladaptive coping. If a major life change has occurred, encourage expression of fears/feelings associated with the change.
_____   _____   8. Teach patient more adaptive coping skills. Document teaching/hospital protocol.
_____   _____   9. Offer positive reinforcement for use of adaptive coping skills and evidence of successful adjustment (i.e., verbal praise, increased privileges). (Identify.).

(Adapted from Nursing Care Plans developed by Nursing Staff at 1st Hospital Wyoming Valley, Wilkes Barre, PA under the direction of Theresa Croushore)

Figure 20–5. Individualized pathway nursing-care plan.

grand mal seizures it produced. Today, ECT has had a resurgence of popularity. The procedure has been greatly modified since the early days of its use: the patient is paralyzed to prevent the peripheral manifestations of seizures, and anesthesia (sleep) is induced to prevent the frightening sensations accompanying a seizure. Modern techniques have reduced morbidity and mortality from ECT allowing the procedure to gain a role as a respected and legitimate method of treatment for selected patients (Davis and Goldman, 1995).

INDICATIONS

Electroconvulsive therapy is used as a first-line treatment for patients who need rapid resolution of life-threatening symptoms or who have a poor response to other treatments. It is the recommended treatment for adults, particularly the elderly, when other treatments have not alleviated severe depression or when the risk of suicide is high (Jenike, 1985; Valente, 1991; Weiner,

1982). Although ECT is predominantly prescribed for adults with severe major depression, it also is used to treat acute mania, some compulsive disorders, catatonic conditions, and certain schizophrenic syndromes characterized by short-term illness and affective symptoms (Runck, 1985).

EFFICACY

ECT is used for inpatients and outpatients. The apparatus for ECT consists of a portable ECT instrument that requires an 110 volt power source. It can easily be carried, permits the administration of therapy in any setting.

As a rule, bilateral ECT is more effective than unilateral. In bilateral ECT electrodes are placed on both sides of the person's head, thus affecting both hemispheres of the brain. This leads to a more balanced seizure activity. The patient is usually medicated, the fear is reduced, and there is a stimulation of the various systems in the brain that re-regulate the thinking and behavior of the patient and enhances a sense of mood elevation. The point of ECT is to block out disturbing thinking patterns.

In the past, before refinement of ECT, patients had grand mal seizures often injuring an arm or a limb and causing great pain in distressed muscles. However, because there is some evidence that bilateral ECT imposes a higher risk of memory impairment, it is commonly reserved for patients in whom unilateral ECT has failed, or for whom rapid resolutions of symptoms in indicated (Davis and Goldman, 1995).

ECT is contraindicated in a variety of medical situations. Patients for whom this therapy is being considered need special evaluation if they have a history or evidence of increased intracranial pressure or a recent history of myocardial infarction, intracerebral hemorrhage, an unstable vascular aneurysm, retinal detachment, or untreated glaucoma.

Why ECT works is not clear; the underlying neurophysiological or neurochemical mechanisms by which it works are not known. It is known that ECT causes changes in the electroencephalogram (EEG), hypothalamic hormone secretion, calcium metabolism, biogenic amine levels, and neurotransmitter-receptor sensitivity. The amnesia precipitated by ECT may itself contribute to the patient's improvement (Davis and Goldman, 1995).

TECHNIQUE

Patient usually receive three ECT treatments per week. A minimum of six treatments, an average of nine treatments, and a maximum of 25 treatments are considered within a normal range for a single course of treatment.

PREPARATION

The patient is always told of the treatment. The physician generally discusses this with the patient and the patient's family. The term "electric shock" may upset some patients, and the more commonly used term is convulsive therapy, even though this is more technical. The patient is told that a transient period of memory loss will occur after the treatment, and that this memory loss may last longer for recent events. Patients who are told that they will be asleep, will receive a treatment, and will awaken before an hour has passed with no memory of the treatment are more likely to cooperate with it.

A thorough medical examination is done to determine any contraindications to ECT or whether any pretreatment or special care is needed. Informed consent is always obtained from the patient.

The steps involved in ECT are as follows:

1. Thirty minutes before treatment, the patient's temperature, pulse, respiration, and blood pressure are taken and any unusual findings are reported to the physician. At this time the patient is reminded of the treatment and should be toileted to prevent incontinence during the treatment. Dentures and eyeglasses or contact lenses should be removed and food withheld or instructions given that nothing should be taken by mouth after midnight on the night before the treatment. This will prevent any complications from aspiration during the treatment.

2. An intravenous line is inserted and 0.8 mg of atropine sulfate is administered subcutaneously 30 minutes before the treatment to decrease bronchial and tracheal secretions. This reduces the chance of respiratory embarrassment secondary to excessive secretions.

3. The electrode sites are carefully cleaned and the electrodes are placed on the patient's scalp. The patient is then oxygenated with an Ambu bag. The anesthetist next administers a quick-acting barbiturate intravenously to induce light sleep. When the patient is asleep, a bite block is inserted to protect the teeth, and an intravenous muscle relaxant such as succinylcholine chloride is given in combination with the anesthetic.

4. When paralysis is confirmed, the electrical stimulus is applied. During this process the patient is carefully monitored. The patient's pulse and blood pressure are checked before the procedure, after anesthesia, during the seizure, and periodically during and after recovery.

Since many ECT machines have a built-in EEG monitor, the seizure itself may be directly monitored. If no EEG is available, seizure duration is monitored by inflating a blood-pressure cuff on one leg after the patient is asleep and before the succinylcholine is given. The seizure can be timed by watching the tonic-clonic movements in the non-paralyzed limb. If the clinician is satisfied that an adequate seizure has been obtained, the patient is monitored carefully until alert.

The patient usually sleeps for 20 to 30 minutes after the treatment and remains confused for 30 minutes after awakening.

5. During the recovery stage the patient's respiration and blood pressure are monitored. The nurse stays with the patient until the patient is awake, able to answer simple questions, and can care for him- or herself. Since the patient will be in a confused, hazy state after the treatment, it will be necessary to have someone accompany

E CASE EXAMPLE

▶ ELECTROCONVULSIVE THERAPY

Ms. J, a 28-year-old business manager, is seriously depressed and suicidal. One year of combined medication, psychotherapy, and cognitive intervention had been ineffective. She comes to a mental health clinic and requests ECT, saying, "I can't stand this endless depression; if I can't feel like my old self, life is not worth living." Her family and

friends tell her they are appalled by her request for a treatment that passes an "electric current through the brain." The nursing staff spends time educating Mrs. J's family about ECT, and dispelling their myths.

After eight treatments, Ms. J.'s suicidal impulses decrease and she returns to work. She continues to have psychotherapy and to take antidepressants for her mild-to-moderate depression (Valente, 1991).

---

him or her back to the ward if an inpatient; or to have someone drive the patient home if an outpatient. Emotional support is needed to help the patient feel secure and relaxed as the confusion and anxiety following the treatment decrease.

Modifications of ECT produce effects other than the classic convulsions. The electrical current can be regulated so that it merely stimulates the brain (this can be useful in the treatment of severe drug intoxication). The current can also be regulated to produce a loss of consciousness and sustain muscle quivering rather than a full seizure. This kind of treatment is called electronarcosis, and usually lasts from 3 to 5 minutes.

Another type of convulsive therapy involves the use of a drug such as Hexafluorodiethyl ether (Indoklon) to induce a convulsion. In this procedure the patient is given the medication through a special vaporizer.

NURSING CARE ISSUES

Nurses are in a critical position to improve and evaluate patients' understanding of ECT, to be advocates for a patients' rights to full information and choice of treatments, and to educate patients' family members and friends about ECT.

Valente (1991) outlines the following nursing-care issues with regard to ECT.

Informed Consent

Patients are entitled to know the treatment options available to them, and the consequences of each; the risks and benefits of ECT and other available treatments; and their right to choose among these treatment options (Runck, 1985).

Patients benefit from a verbal and written explanation of treatment options and their effectiveness, side

effects, and consequences; videotapes can help to effectively inform and prepare patients and families for ECT. The nurse can explain the technical details of ECT in terms the patient understands. Because the patient's cognitive abilities and memory may be hampered by depression, family members and significant others should be enlisted to help reinforce the patient's memory. Consent obtained before ECT should be re-examined and reconsidered periodically with patients, to allow them to rescind or renew their consent. As ECT treatments progress, patients have more experience with ECT and an improved cognitive capacity, and become better able to understand and consent to this therapy (NIMH, 1985).

Educating Patients and Families

Teaching facts about ECT is important for patients and their families. Uninformed but well-meaning friends may discourage patients from consenting to ECT. Some misconceptions are that ECT can change the personality, or that it is painful. In fact, the patient is asleep during ECT, and it does not change the personality. Patients do not remember having the seizure that accompanies this treatment technique. An observer watching the treatment would notice the patient's toe twitch or eye close tightly during the few seconds of the seizure. Misperceptions of ECT may come from dramatic television portrayals or reports of those who observed it 50 years ago, before current practices made the treatment safer (Duffy and Conradt, 1989).

Teaching Points

Some of the teaching points about ECT for patients and their families are that:

- The patient should take nothing by mouth after midnight before ECT, unless medications are prescribed.

- The patient should wear loose, comfortable, nonrestrictive clothing to facilitate donning a hospital gown before the procedure.
- The patient should expect electrode paste to be placed at the temple where the electrode is positioned.
- The patient can expect confusion immediately after a seizure, since ECT produces a temporary disorientation. For instance, inpatients may be alert and awake but unable to find their way to their hospital room, cafeteria, or bathroom.
- Outpatients must be supervised after ECT.
- Outpatients should not drive, since they may be unable to find the parking lot or the way home.
- Patients generally continue to take antidepressants for 1 year after ECT, to prevent relapse. Psychotherapy is necessary to support the patient's adjustment and management of a chronic illness such as depression.

Assessing Memory and Confusion

A comprehensive assessment of the patient's mental status includes a baseline evaluation of memory and cognitive functions, and a routine evaluation of the patient's anterograde and retrograde autobiographical information and recent/current experiences. A common memory test, such as asking patients to repeat a group of digits, does not effectively assess memory loss produced by ECT. The patient's memory should be routinely monitored as ECT treatments continue.

On in-patient units, nurses monitor and evaluate a patient's memory and confusion for the first 12 hours after ECT, and observe the patient over a 48-hour period to assess the patient's supervision needs. For outpatient ECT, family members can be taught to observe the patient's activities for 24 to 48 hours after each treatment. Patients may remember that they are having ECT but forget scheduled appointments, safety precautions, and conversations with the treatment staff during treatment. In one case, a family that was aware of events only as reported by the patient during telephone conversations believed that the patient's psychotherapist had failed to monitor the patient's ECT treatment because the patient did not remember having had any therapy.

Correction of this situation required several telephone calls to the family. Help was also provided by the nurse, who before subsequent ECT sessions taught the patient to use memory aids such as notepads, lists, and telephone logs to record events. Such teaching helps to reduce the impact of any temporary memory loss from ECT.

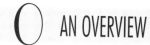

AN OVERVIEW

- Depression is believed to be caused by a chemical imbalance in the brain.
- Various theories suggest a number of reasons for the depressed mood state.
- The specific type of depression affecting a patient is diagnosed from a set of symptoms.
- Medication and psychotherapy are first-line interventions for moderate depression without suicidal thoughts.
- Electroconvulsive therapy (ECT) is recommended for patients whose severe depression is not relieved by other treatments, and for those who may be suicidal. It helps 80% of severely impaired patients.
- ECT is also used to treat some compulsive disorders, mania, and a short-term affective type of schizophrenia.
- Although refined techniques are now used to administer ECT, and extremely low morbidity and mortality levels as well as dramatic results are reported with this technique, the risks and benefits of ECT should be carefully weighed; the prevalence and duration of adverse effects are unknown.

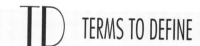

TERMS TO DEFINE

- depression
- chemical imbalance
- bipolar disorders
- bipolar I
- bipolar II
- cyclothymic disorder
- dysthymic disorder
- electroconvulsive therapy
- kindling
- major depressive disorder
- mania
- psychopharmacology
- seasonal affective disorder
- somatic treatment

Q STUDY QUESTIONS

1. According to the *DSM-IV*, in order for a diagnosis of depression to be made, a constellation of mood, cognitive, and neurodegenerative signs must be present for at least
   a. 2 weeks.
   b. 3 weeks.
   c. 4 weeks.
   d. 5 weeks or longer.

2. The mood disorder commonly characterized by the presence of manic (or hypomanic) episodes is
   a. major depressive disorder.
   b. dysthymic disorder.
   c. bipolar I.
   d. bipolar II.

3. T F Bipolar disorder is more common in first degree biologic relatives of individuals with this disorder.

4. Match the disorder with the statement that best characterizes it.

   a. major depressive disorder   1. two years of depressed mood for more days than not.

   b. bipolar I   2. one or more major depressive episodes with a hypomanic episode

   c. dysthymic disorder   3. one or more major depressive episodes

   d. bipolar II   4. one or more manic episodes, usually with a major depressive episode

   e. cyclothymic disorder   5. at least 2 years of numerous hypomanic episodes and periods of depressive symptoms

5. Which of the following symptoms is NOT included in the diagnosis of major depressive disorder?
   a. Difficulty concentrating
   b. Fatigue
   c. Sad mood
   d. Euphoric mood
   e. Sleep disturbances

6. Mood disorders pose a major health problem to society, because they
   a. lead to significant morbidity and mortality.
   b. are frequently undetected in primary health care settings.
   c. generally cause substantial social and occupational impairments.

   d. a and c
   e. all of the above.

7. T F A hypomanic episode is generally more severe and has a longer duration than a manic episode.

8. T F A hypomanic episode has symptoms that are similar to those of a manic episode, except that delusions or hallucinations cannot be present.

■ REFERENCES

Abrams R: *Electroconvulsive Therapy.* Oxford, England, Oxford University Press, 1988.

American Psychiatric Association: Diagnostic and Statistical Manual, 4th ed. Washington, DC: American Psychiatric Press, 1994.

Bibring E. The mechanism of depression. In P. Greenacre (ed.) *Affective Disorders,* New York: International Universities Press, 1953.

Cummings JL Frontal-subcortical circuits and human behavior. Proceedings of the One Hundred and Forty-sixth Meeting of the American Psychiatric Association, 1993.

Davis GC, Goldman B: Somatic therapies, in Goldman H (ed): *Review of General Psychiatry,* ed. 4. Norwalk, CT, Appleton & Lange, 1995.

Depression Guideline Panel: *Depression in Primary Care:* Vol. 1. Detection and Diagnosis. Clinical Practice Guideline, Number 5. (AHCPR Publication No. 93–0550.) Rockville, MD, U.S. Department of Health and Human Services, Public Health Service, Agency for Health Care and Policy and Research, 1993.

Duffy WJ, Conradt H: Electroconvulsive therapy: The perioperative process. *Am Oper Room Nurs J* 1989; 50(4):806–812.

Fink M: How does convulsive therapy work? *Neuropsychopharmacology* 1990; 3(2):73–82.

Frank LR: *The History of Shock Treatment.* San Francisco, CA, Leonard Roy Frank, 1978.

Freud S. Mourning and melancholia, in *Standard Edition,* London: Hogarth press, 1955 (first published in 1917).Goff DC, Jenike MA: Treatment-resistant depression in the elderly. *J Am Geriatr Soc* 1986; 34:63–70.

Goleman D: The quiet comeback of electroshock therapy. *New York Times,* August 2, 1990, p. B7.

Jenike MA: Electroconvulsive therapy. *Top Geriatr* 1983; 1(10):37.

Kramer B-A: Electroconvulsive therapy use in geriatric depression. *J Nerv Ment Dis* 1987; 175(4):233–235.

Lewy AJ Seasonal mood disorders. In DL Dunner (ed.) *Cur Psych Ther,* Philadelphia: WB Saunders, 1993.

Martin BA: Electroconvulsive therapy for depression in general psychiatric practice. *Psychiatr J Univ Ottawa,* 1989; 14(2):413–417.

National Institute of Mental Health: *Electroconvulsive Therapy.* Consensus Development Conference Statement, Vol. 5, No. 11, 1985.

Nolen WA, Haffmans J: Treatment of resistant depression. *Int Clin Psychopharmacol* 1989; 2(3):217–228.

Pardes H, Kaukmann CA, Pincus HA, and West A. Genetics and psychiatry: Past discoveries, current dilemmas, and future directions. *Am J Psychiatry* 1989; 146:435–443.

Persad E: Electroconvulsive therapy in depression. *Can J Psychiatry* 1990; 35:175–182.

Post RM: Transduction of psychosocial stress into the neurobiology of recurrent affective disorder. *Am J Psychiatry* 1992; 149:999–1010.

Reus VI: Mood Disorders, in Goldman HH (ed): *Review of General Psychiatry,* ed. 4. Norwalk, CT, Appleton & Lange, 1995, pp 246–265.

Risby ED, Risch SC, Stoudemire A: Mood disorders, in Stoudemire A (ed): *Clinical Psychiatry for Medical Students,* ed. 2. Philadelphia, JB Lippincott 1994, pp. 196–232.

Runck B: National Institute of Mental Health Report: Consensus panel backs cautious use of ECT for severe disorders. *Hosp Commun Psychiatry* 1985; 36(9):943–945.

Ryan L, Montgomery A, Meyers S: Impact of circadian rhythm research on approaches to affective illness. *Arch Psychiatr Nurs* 1987; 1:236–240.

Schildkraut JJ: Current status of the catecholamine hypothesis of affective disorders. In Lipton MA, DiMascio A, Killiam KF (eds): *Psychopharmacology: A Generation of Progress.* New York, Raven Press, 1978, pp. 1223–1234.

Seligman M, Kaslow N, Allow L, Peterson C, Tannenbaum R, Abramson L: Attributional style and depressive symptoms in children. *J Abnorm Psychol* 1984; 93:235–238.

Shuster J: The treatment of depression: A common and undertreated disorder. *Pharmacy Times,* September 1995, pp. 39–54.

Simmons-Alling S. Bipolar mood disorders, in AB McBride and JK Austin (eds) *Psychiatric-Mental Health Nursing: Integrating the Behavioral and Biological Sciences,* Philadelphia: WB Saunders, 1996.

Teicher M, Glod C, Harper D, Magnus E, Brasher C, Wren F, Pahlavan K: Locomotor activity in depressed children and adolescents: I. Circadian dysregulation. *J Am Acad Child Adolesc Psychiatry* 1993; 32:760–768.

Valente SM: Electroconvulsive therapy. *Arch Psychiatr Nurs* 1991; 5(4):223–228.

Weiner RD: The role of electroconvulsive therapy in the treatment of depression in the elderly. *J Am Geriatr Soc* 1982; 30:710–712.

Wells BG: Issues in the diagnosis of major depression, in Cohen LJ (ed): *Formulary: The Journal for Managed Care and Hospital Decision Makers* 1995; 30:3–9.

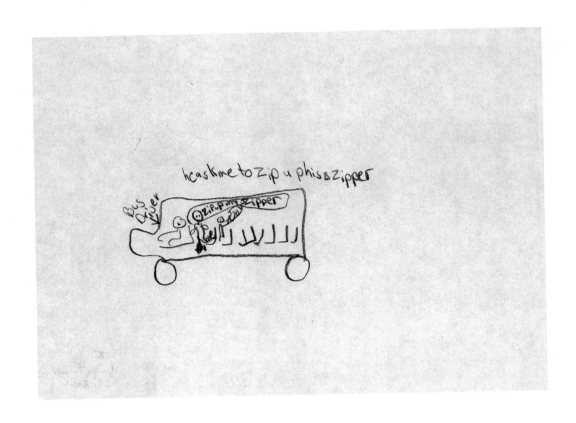

"The fact that [the interrogation of the patient rarely achieves with real consistency an aura of comfort or creates an atmosphere free of discernible prejudice toward sexual values, ideas or practices] must be acknowledged as a major factor in the clinical psychotherapy directed toward reversal of sexual dysfunction."

W. H. Masters and V. E. Johnson,
Human Sexual Inadequacy, 1970

21

Sexual Issues, Disorders, and Deviations

Ann Wolbert Burgess / June Johnson Wolf / Carol R. Hartman

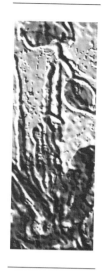

Sexuality may be a creative force or an obstacle to human development. It is a challenge to human investigation and understanding. The evolution of sexual behaviors is a critical area of study. Neuroscience provides insight into the complexity of the brain and behavior, and how that complexity connects with social systems.

The biologist views sexual behavior to be of fundamental significance because it perpetuates the species and thus the continuity of life itself. The psychologist sees in the sexual impulse of human behavior deep reservoirs of motivation that prompt people to action and provide the driving force for many day-to-day activities. Sociologists recognize the integrating, cohesive functioning of sex as contributing to the stability of the family unit and thus to the entire social structure. The ethicist finds that problems arise when people attempt to reconcile their sexual tendencies with the demands of their social group.

The expression of sexuality may be altered by personal choice, psychosocial factors, health status, or environment. Nurses encounter patients belonging to various social and cultural groups, of every age, and with various conditions that may threaten their sexual, physical, and mental well-being.

■ HUMAN SEXUAL RESPONSE AND EXPRESSION

HUMAN SEXUAL RESPONSE

The practice of diagnosing sexual disorders in order to provide interventions has a fairly recent history. With the pioneering work of Masters and Johnson in the 1960s, sexual problems became worthy of assessment and treatment.

History

There has been strong religious influence on sexual behavior dating back to biblical times. In the story of Onan in the Old Testament (Genesis 38:8–10), Onan ejaculated ("spilled his seed") on the ground rather than impregnate his deceased brother's wife. The Hebrew God disapproved of his contraceptive efforts and struck him dead for the act. Thousands of years later, boys still feel guilty for masturbating. Some modern authorities have speculated that Onan may have suffered from premature ejaculation. If so, Onan received a death sentence for having a now treatable sexual dysfunction (LaBruzza, 1994).

In the 13th century, Saint Thomas Aquinas espoused the classical theory of Natural Law. According to this theory, the goal of sexual activity in the natural order is to bear children to love and serve God. The pleasurable aspects to sex were seen as secondary.

As recently as a century ago, it was believed that frequent sexual intercourse caused infertility. Masturbation ("self-pollution") was believed to cause poor sleep, restlessness, night sweats, ringing in the ears, bad skin, headache, and poor vision. Treatment for the 19th-century self-polluter included sleeping on one's stomach on a hard bed, rising early and taking a cold sponge bath; eating light suppers; emptying the bladder before retiring; avoiding spicy foods, caffeine, and alcohol; vigorous exercise; taking iron tonic; and reading wholesome books (LaBruzza, 1994).

The next major influence on human sexuality was Sigmund Freud in the late 19th and early 20th centuries. On the basis of his clinical work, Freud wrote that sexual drives develop from infancy. He argued that sexual interest could be arrested at any stage of development as the result of psychological conflict or trauma. Freud believed that what was repressed at an early age settled into the unconscious and continued to affect adult behavior in the form of symptoms. He also believed, however, that repressed sexual desire could be sublimated into productive aspects of personality.

By 1966, Masters and Johnson made sex therapy a health care specialty, They considered sexual dysfunctions without a medical cause to be learned behaviors fostered by ignorance, performance anxiety, and poor communication. With those assumptions, they developed a system to treat sexual problems through directive psychotherapy, improved communication skills, education about sexual functioning, and desensitization through sensate focus or pleasuring activities.

Four Phases

According to William H. Masters and Virginia E. Johnson (1966), the **sexual response pattern** for males and females consists of four phases: excitement, plateau, orgasm, and resolution. (For males, immediately after orgasm and prior to resolution, there is a refractory period in which no response is possible.). Each phase brings with it a specific sex-organ response as well as a generalized body response (e.g., lubrication, erection, perspiration, tachycardia). The length of each phase varies greatly, with the longest phases being excitement and resolution.

The orgasmic response in males often differs from that in females. Generally, the male experiences one orgasm following ejaculatory demand, and requires a period of time before erection and orgasm are again possible. Three patterns of orgasmic response have, however, been reported in women. The first is similar to that in the male. The second shows a rippling effect of multiorgasms at the plateau level, and the third shows mounting excitement levels, bypassing the plateau, to orgasm and resolution.

SEXUAL EXPRESSION

Sexual expression includes both sexual arousal and behaviors deemed essential to enticing another to sexual interest. Examples are wearing a shaving lotion that is attractive to the olfactory senses, a tender gesture of presenting flowers, or a manner of dancing or dressing for the person one wishes to attract.

Sexual arousal is a term reserved for the full biological arousal for desire to express the sexual drive. Sexual arousal in humans is expressed in a variety of ways that may or may not include orgasmic discharge, and does not preclude abstinence and conscious suppression of sexually charged stimuli.

Heterosexual Modes of Sexual Expression

Petting may be defined as a continuum from simple kissing with clothes on to mutual genital stimulation and complete nudity without engaging in intercourse. Intercourse (copulation, coitus) refers to the insertion of the penis into the vagina. Oral–genital contact includes fellatio (taking the penis into the mouth), cunnilingus (mouth and tongue stimulation of the female genitalia), analingus (anal stimulation with the tongue), and mutual fellatio/cunnilingus (or "69," based on the similarity of the body configuration to this number). Anal sex usually connotes penile insertion into the anus. This is the least practiced sexual expression among heterosexuals, but is practiced by some male homosexuals.

Auto-eroticism or self-stimulation may occur by manipulating the genitals with a hand or mechanical device such as a vibrator, stream of water, or artificial phallus or vagina. Masturbation may take place in the presence of another partner, such as during intercourse to effect orgasm, or by oneself. Auto-eroticism often involves fantasy or sexually explicit materials to enhance the experience.

Abstinence may refer either to the total withdrawal of an individual from any sexual activity including masturbation, or to varying degrees of sexual activity without intercourse.

Homosexual Modes of Sexual Expression

Freedman (1971), in his study of homosexuals, describes the sexual practices of gay males and females in an attempt to clarify the "considerable confusion about what homosexually oriented men and women actually do in bed." Males engage in differentiated and preferential sexual practices as their experience increases. Among these practices are massage, mutual masturbation, fellatio, body rubbing, and anal intercourse. Body rubbing may cause painful friction if lubricant is not used. Anal intercourse may be intolerable to some males because of physical irritation or the feeling that it is depersonalizing. Multiple sex, sadomasochism (with dominance and bondage), sexual devices, and pornographic materials are also utilized. Freedman also mentions the use of "poppers" (isoamyl nitrate) or marijuana to heighten the sexual experience. Males often engage in a homosexual encounter before identifying themselves as gay; the converse is true of women. Sexual conquest in lieu of an intimate relationship is often the intent of gay males.

For the lesbian woman, emphasis is often placed on tenderness and love. The sexual practices of gay women usually involve cunnilingus and mutual masturbation. Tribadism (body-rubbing in the face-to-face position, resulting in orgasm) is less frequently practiced. A dildo or artificial penis may be used in instances in which partners wish to assume heterosexual roles. Lesbian women do not generally engage in group sex or sadomasochism, or use sexually arousing photos, but some do use stimulant drugs such as marijuana.

■ SEXUAL PREFERENCE ISSUES

Sexual preference refers to those others to whom persons are sexually attracted. Thus, a homosexual is a person whose sexual preference, or orientation, is for members of his or her own gender. The word *homosexual* is derived from the Greek root *homo*, meaning "same" (not the Latin word meaning "man"). The term *lesbian*, which is used to refer to female homosexuals, can be traced to the Greek poetess Sappho, who lived on the island of Lesbos around 600 B.C. She is famous for the love poetry she wrote to other women. Sappho was married, apparently happily, and had one daughter, but her lesbian feelings were the focus of her life (Hyde, 1990).

According to the 1948 Kinsey report entitled *Sexual Behavior in the Human Male*, 37% of American men had had at least one homosexual encounter in their lives, between 8% and 13% had been predominately homosexual for at least 3 years of their lives between the ages of 14 and 55, and 4% had been exclusively homosexual from adolescence onward. Subsequent surveys in the United States and other Western countries have confirmed these incidence figures. Studies of female sexuality indicate the incidence of exclusive lesbianism to be 2 to 3% or about one-third to one-half the rate of homosexuality in males (Kinsey, Pomeroy, and Martin, 1948).

According to physician Warren Gadpaille (1989), true incidence figures for any activity criticized by society are usually higher than reported. He states that based on the basis of various data, from 6 to 10% of adult males and 2 to 4% of adult females may be exclusively homosexual. Others dispute these figures, stating that they are influenced by the gay lobby in the United States, which has become increasingly powerful both politically and socially. These critics believe that 1 to 2% of the adult population is exclusively homosexual, and that this percentage is similar in all racial and ethnic groups at all levels of American society.

The etiology of homosexuality has long been debated and researched. Most of the research, however, has focused on males. The debate has focused on the issues of nature or nurture (i.e., physical determinism or conscious choice—or physical and psychological environment versus biology). Today much of the research on homosexuality is focused on its biology and on the part that genes may play in its development. This is in contrast to the Freudian or psychoanalytic focus on growth and development, with its particular emphasis on resolution of the Oedipal conflict.

Until 1973, homosexuality was listed in the American Psychiatric Association's *Diagnostic and Statistical Manual (DSM)* as a sexually deviant behavior. Persons diagnosed as such were described as unable to substitute normal sexual behavior for their deviant practices. Under intense pressure by gay activists and with the help of some psychiatrists, the Board of Trustees of the American Psychiatric Association removed homosexuality as a diagnosis of mental illness. Because of the discord created by this determination, it was submitted to the membership for ratification, in marked contrast to decisions made about other psychiatric illnesses. Of the 10,000 members who voted, 58% approved of the Board's decision, and when the 3rd edition of the *DSM* appeared in 1980, homosexuality had been eliminated as a mental disorder.

Today, some researchers are studying twins, both identical and fraternal, to determine the relative roles that genetics and environment may play in the development of homosexuality. Others are more focused on brain studies, some of which have shown that certain areas of the brain may exert a controlling influence on sexual orientation and behavior, which further suggests that homosexuality may be partly inherited. However, these studies are few, and other researchers have not been able to confirm these biological findings. If homosexuality is determined to have a biological basis and perhaps to be a normal variant of the human constitution, it may lose the long-standing moral stigma placed on it by many. "Gay Pride" is today a major rallying cry in many big cities in the United States and abroad. Yet despite the numbers of homosexuals in American society, their prominence in the arts, and their growing acceptance and political power, many families have difficulty accepting that a son or daughter is homosexual. Parents may blame themselves for their child's sexual orientation or believe that it is a temporary stage of their child's development. According to a 1989 study by the U.S. Department of Health and Human Services, (cited in Bass, 1994) 26% of youths who announce their homosexuality to their parents are ostracized by them. Many youths rejected in this way may end up on the streets involved with drugs or prostitution and at great risk for acquired immune deficiency syndrome (AIDS) and suicide.

NURSING INTERVENTION

What role do psychiatric nurses play in the treatment of gay people? Gay and lesbian people seek counseling for reasons as diverse as those of any other individual or group. Some prefer to see a therapist who is also homosexual and in settings that cater almost exclusively to the gay population. For others, however, the sexual orientation of the therapist does not matter. Like nonhomosexual persons, they want the best possible care in a setting in which they are accepted and treated with the dignity and respect that all human beings desire. They come for such care with the same emotional problems for which others seek help. Sexual orientation is seldom the presenting problem in such cases, since many homosexuals have already come to terms with their homosexuality and no longer view themselves primarily in that context.

Very often, gay people seek counseling for the stress involved in making a decision about their sexual preference. The stress keeps them isolated and can lead to depression. In essence, they are leading dual lives. If they are married, they have the added conflict that would result from revealing their sexual preference and possibly losing custody of their children. The stress from this is part of the necessary transition of integrating with oneself, with one's family, with a social network, and with work.

The following cases are illustrative of various stresses women have had in revealing their sexual preference to others, especially their families.

NURSING ASSESSMENT

In an out-patient mental-health setting, psychiatric nurses would conduct an initial assessment of the homosexual patient as they would with any other patient. Of first importance is a history focused on identifying information, the patient's presenting complaint and history of the complaint, past psychiatric and social history, medical history, family background, mental status, formulation of the patient's problem, and diagnosis. This process determines the nurse's interventions in diagnosis and planning of treatment.

The problems that homosexuals have in coping with the demands of life and interpersonal relationships are quite similar to those of heterosexuals (e.g., problems of self-esteem, closeness, self-assertion, impulse control, commitment, etc.). Although the presenting problem may involve a gay relationship, the issues are usually of the same nature, as in a heterosexual relationship, with the exception of the disclosure process.

Disclosure, or *coming out*, is a process that for most homosexual persons extends over many years. It commonly begins in childhood with feelings of being different from members of one's own sex. It advances through several stages, including inner acknowledgment of one's homosexuality; acceptance of a homosexual identity after disclosure to others, and ultimately the ability to develop intimate sexual relationships with members of one's own sex.

During the initial interview and in subsequent interviews, it is important to be aware of underlying feelings of social victimization, suicidal thoughts, and substance abuse in homosexual patients, particularly with those patients who appear uncomfortable with their sexual orientation. However, it is uncommon, despite such discomfort, for the patient seeking psychotherapy to want a change of sexual preference. Instead, it is essential that the patient be helped to learn and develop self-acceptance as well as helped to build self-esteem. Sustaining a sense of self-esteem is a major task for homosexuals, especially in the face of great hostility on the part of society. Positive feelings about the patient's identity must be supported and encouraged, especially during life-crisis

E CASE EXAMPLES

► MARY

Mary, a white 28-year-old teacher, seeks counseling for what she terms "feeling blah"—a lack of motivation, lack of energy, and staying up too late. Consequently, she is unable to get to work on time or does not go to work at all. She comes for treatment on the advice of friends and colleagues because she fears losing her job.

After several sessions, Mary reveals her alcoholism and the suicide of her alcoholic mother, which is a major reason for her underlying depression. She reveals her lesbianism and her inability to commit to relationships owing to her fears of physical intimacy and rejection. She uses alcohol to reduce her anxiety in both sexual and interpersonal situations. She has had many "one night stands" and only one long-term relationship, many years prior to her seeking treatment. In these situations she has to be drunk before she can become physically intimate with her partner.

Mary had her first sexual experience at the age of 17, with a 42-year-old single mother for whom she was baby-sitting. The woman had been the initiator of that encounter, but since then Mary has been the initiator even though, until she achieved sobriety, she had to be drunk to do so.

Mary knew that she was "different" from other girls by the age of 5 or 6. She prayed every night that she would awaken and find herself a boy. She stopped praying for this at menarche. She knew then that prayers were of no avail. She hated her menstrual period because it reminded her of her femaleness. Her gender identity was a source of conflict between her and her mother from the time she was a toddler. She fought with her mother about wearing a dress until she reached high school, where girls were allowed to wear slacks. The last time she wore a dress was at age 15 at her father's funeral. He had been very ill for many years and did not take any part in Mary's clothing struggle with her mother. Mary believes that this was partly due to his illness and the fact that he knew she was "different." She also believes that her father encouraged her being different, since he stressed and supported the idea that she could become anything she wanted to be with the exception of a professional athlete in such sports as baseball, hockey, and football.

Revealing her sexual orientation was not an issue. Mary was a tomboy preferring to be with boys who treated her as one of the gang; she never played with girls. In high school she gravitated toward a few females she knew to be gay. They in turn introduced her to other lesbians and most of her friends since then have been lesbians. Her few heterosexual friends accept her lesbianism. She states that her brothers knew that she was a lesbian, and that she therefore never had to tell them this directly. When her mother learned of it, she blamed herself, thinking that her forcing Mary to wear dresses might have been the cause of Mary's lesbianism. Her mother was upset that Mary would never marry nor have children. When drunk, her mother talked negatively about Mary's lesbianism.

Initially, Mary's therapy focuses on her drinking and depression. After the loss of her job, becoming homeless and sleeping in shelters, she agrees to go to an alcohol detoxification unit. She subsequently lives in a halfway home, goes to AA meetings every day, and obtains a job at which she becomes successful. After her sobriety is firmly established, issues of trust and intimacy became the treatment focus, and for the first time since age 23, she established a committed relationship with another woman.

Mary continues to struggle with what she considers society's double standards.

She is angry that heterosexuals are allowed to behave lovingly in public, and to marry, and receive health insurance and retirement benefits from their partners, while rights are granted to the gay population only in rare circumstances. However, she dislikes militant gay groups because she believes that their tactics have produced scorn and rejection in the heterosexual world, which in turn leads to further rejection and marginalization of the gay community. She also believes that there is serious drug and alcohol abuse in the gay community because of gay bars' promotion of socializing activities.

► ALLISON

Allison, a 35-year-old professional woman, is referred for treatment of anxiety and depression by the social worker at her place of employment after her supervisor complains that her work performance has deteriorated.

In early interviews, Allison focuses on her depression and its impact on her work performance. In subsequent interviews, after trust is established, she admits to being depressed about the end of a 12-year relationship with a woman. She says that she is a lesbian and has great hatred for all men, whom she characterizes as brutal, dishonest, untrustworthy, sexual predators, and abusers. She recounts a history of sexual abuse by her father and step-grandfather, beginning at the age of 4 years. Both were drug abusers as well as abusers of others in the immediate and extended family. Her sexual abuse stopped when she was 11 years old after the accidental death of her father and the departure of her step-grandfather. She thinks that her sexual orientation stemmed from these experiences, but she also wonders whether there is a genetic factor in it, since her sister told her of being bisexual. Allison says that she does not disclose her sexual orientation to others and tries to hide her aversion to men.

Allison, like Mary, complains about societal restrictions on her life as compared to that of heterosexuals. For her, the world is full of homophobic people. She is most comfortable in the lesbian world, and with a few heterosexual friends whom she believes totally accept and respect her as a lesbian woman. Respect and acceptance are what she craves and seeks in all areas of her life. As with Mary, Allison also had her first sexual experience with an older woman for whom she baby-sat. She was 13 years old and not the initiator.

In high school, Allison found a group of girls who were lesbians. They developed an informal club, and it was at that time that she disclosed her sexual orientation to other friends. She revealed it to her siblings after graduating from college, but not to her mother, who she feared would disown and ostracize her. At age 25 she finally told her mother because she knew that some members of her mother's church were making inquisitive remarks to her mother about Allison's sexual orientation. Her mother was upset by Allison's disclosure even though she herself had had suspicions of Allison's orientation for many years. Her mother's words—"I do not condone nor do I condemn; I am a Christian woman and I love you."—made an indelible and lasting impression on Allison. After her mother's unexpected and sudden death, Allison's stepfather told her never again to set foot in his home. His words also were seared into her memory, "I don't want a lesbian in my home; you are immoral and will go to hell." Allison has not seen him since that time. She never told her mother about her childhood sexual abuse for fear that it would "kill her."

Allison's sexual relationships have been long ones and monogamous. She is, however, strongly religious, and expresses her intense desire to be a respectable lesbian woman. In her past sexual activity with other women she was the initiator half of the time. She and her current partner are not sexually active.

The intervention was two-fold. The nurse-therapist focused first on symptom management of the depression and anxiety. In this situation, medication was helpful. Second, the focus of therapy was on how the loss of her mother and the condemnation by the stepfather played a role in inhibiting her natural sexual expression. Further work was aimed at dealing with past traumatic memories and their impact on her sense of self and negative thinking. This was a productive area since despite her strong positions she was open with both homosexual and heterosexual friends even though she felt alienated from others. A particular strategy of writing was used to help her express what thoughts and feelings she kept from her mother. The outcome was that she was far more self-accepting, experienced a level of comfort and peace regarding her restricted relationship with her mother, and evaluated the limits of her stepfather's response in terms of his religious affiliations and sense of entitlement to property.

▶ STEPHANIE

Stephanie, a 40-year-old professional woman, is referred by a colleague who is concerned that she might be suicidal, given her high level of anxiety, extreme irritability, fatigue, and depressive thoughts. She initially presents as a tightly controlled, wary, tense, and evasive person. After many sessions she reveals that she is a lesbian, has hidden it from her family for years, and has desperately tried to lead a "normal" heterosexual life. She had twice been engaged and broken both engagements through her fear of marriage. She felt getting married would be living a lie, and would be unfair to her spouse. Her parents' bitter disappointment on each occasion intensified her guilt and unhappiness. Her mother had died 2 years prior to her coming into therapy, and Stephanie was convinced that her mother's death had been hastened by worry and concern about her not being married and having someone to take care of her.

Shortly after her mother's death, Stephanie met and fell in love with a younger woman. This was her first lesbian relationship. After about 6 months, her partner felt they should live together and Stephanie should disclose her sexual orientation to her family, friends, and colleagues. Stephanie procrastinated for weeks about this, fearing the reaction of her father and two brothers. After her partner threatened to leave, Stephanie became increasingly depressed. Her colleague convinced her to seek help, and her partner agreed to continue the relationship, hoping therapy would have Stephanie admit her sexual orientation.

Her therapy focuses on her fears of disclosure and her ambivalence about her sexuality. After her ambivalence is resolved, she discloses her orientation to her family, which is a painful process for herself and her family. Initially her brothers are stunned and upset, but are eventually able to tell her that they still love her and want her to be part of their lives. Her father's reaction, which she had feared the most, is anger, disbelief, fury, and anguish. He wonders where he and her mother had "gone wrong"; what had they done to "deserve this"; and what friends and relatives would say. However, her father does not disown and ostracize her, as she had feared. Their relationship continues to be strained and awkward, but they strive to love and accept each other.

Stephanie understands that the disclosure has been a severe blow to her father and his hopes for her, his only daughter.

Stephanie wonders whether her mother's death was the catalyst for her first long-term lesbian relationship. At first, she feels shame and humiliation, but then exhilaration and freedom from her denial and repression of her sexuality. She is not the initiator of sexual activity between herself and her partner, "I guess I am the fem in our relationship," she says. She and her partner plan to adopt a baby through a private agency. If this occurs, Stephanie, and not her partner, will stay at home for at least a year before she resumes her career.

▶ MEGAN

Megan, referred by her partner, comes into treatment at age 39. She is depressed, not working, lacking in motivation, and seldom leaves the house. Though she does not care whether she lives or dies, she is not suicidal. She is not interested in therapy and comes only to please her lover. She is articulate but bland. She is open about her sexuality. Unlike her partner, Megan likes men and had been married and divorced twice.

Megan's first husband accused her of being a lesbian because she had a girlfriend he considered "mannish," even though the friend too was married. Knowing that Megan had enjoyed heterosexual sex bothers her lover, who fears that Megan may someday leave her for a man. Megan disputes this, claiming that she is no longer sexually interested in men.

Megan had her first lesbian relationship at age 26, with a co-worker, while married to her second husband. At that time, she and her husband were in great conflict, and their sex life was unsatisfying to her. She found herself preoccupied with her co-worker, especially when at home with her husband. Eventually her co-worker approached her and they began an affair that lasted 18 months. During that time, Megan refused sexual relations with her husband, and finally left him and moved into her lover's home.

Megan obtained a new job and promotion in another state but her girlfriend refused to move, which led to the dissolution of their relationship.

After the move, Megan disclosed her homosexuality to a close heterosexual friend, who introduced her to a lesbian with whom the friend worked. This affair lasted almost 2 years, after which Megan met Kerry, the woman with whom she has lived for the past 8 years.

Megan has not disclosed to others her orientation, but she sees no need to do so because all of her heterosexual friends know that she is gay, she says, "by the company I keep." She is an only child, and has never told her elderly widowed mother about her homosexuality, stating, "What she doesn't know won't hurt her; she avoids knowing and never asks questions." Megan's mother has visited her many times and knows Kerry, her housemate, quite well. Megan and Kerry also visit and stay overnight with Megan's mother and share a room when they do so. Even though Megan has not worked for a number of years, her mother has never asked how she supports herself.

Kerry is more militant than Megan about her homosexuality, and wanted to decorate their car and home with gay symbols. This infuriated Megan who stated, "I just want to live a normal, quiet life, and don't feel the need to advertise my homosexuality. I am a nice person. I don't need labels and just want people to accept me for

E CASE EXAMPLES   Continued

myself. I only want to be accepted as a human being. We lesbians are no different than others. We may have different likes and dislikes, different personalities, but basically we are the same. I don't hide my lesbianism. I go to gay pride marches and other gay events, but I am not a militant, angry lesbian."

This conflict and other issues between Megan and Kerry, especially Kerry's mili-

tant attitudes toward the heterosexual world, led to their seeking treatment as a couple. Ultimately, they are able to compromise on issues and to respect each other's views. Megan also realizes that she needs to work. After Megan's depression subsides, she obtains a job that reinforces her self esteem and need to be seen as no different from other persons.

---

periods, such as the loss of a relationship, family, or job. Nurses must also do a self-assessment for any homophobic feelings they may harbor and how these can affect the patient. If the feelings are more negative than can be dealt with in supervision, the obvious step is referral to another team member, as would be done with any patient to whom the nurse had an aversive response.

The nurse must be acutely aware of a common tendency to assume that patients are heterosexual. Many homosexual patients will tell of their sadness, shame, and anger in situations in which their sexual orientation was unknown and others thoughtlessly made inappropriate comments.

Psychiatric nurses can take a leadership role in advocating respect and acceptance of all people, regardless of their background, including their sexual orientation. This is a role that can make an enormous difference in the physical and mental health of patients.

■ SEXUAL DYSFUNCTION DISORDERS

Sexual dysfunction is a disruption of sexual behavior or extreme variation of sexual behavior. Sexual dysfunction as a disruption is defined by an identifiable disturbance of one or more phases of the sexual-response cycle (orgasm, excitement, or desire) by excessive pain or phobia (both simple and panic type). Avoidance of sex results. Sexual dysfunction as an extreme variation of sexual behavior is defined by the object (human or inanimate) that is required for sexual arousal and release, or by disregard for the sensitivities, rights and physical well-being of another person.

BIOPHYSIOLOGICAL ETIOLOGY

Ill health is one of the greatest detriments to sexual expression, not only because it redirects the use of energy toward recuperation, but also because it often lowers an

individual's sense of personal worth and attractiveness. Many physical conditions directly impede sexual response by interfering with endocrine levels, blood circulation, nerve transmission, and mobility, or by creating genital or generalized pain. Various surgical procedures and drugs may also affect the body. Sexual dysfunction may be a temporary concomitant of an illness or treatment, or it may be permanent. In either case, patients must be appropriately counseled so that they will know what to expect and what behavioral options they might consider.

Medical Conditions Leading to Sexual Dysfunction.

Diabetes. Millions of individuals are affected by diabetes mellitus, a condition that causes gradual impotence in almost 50% of males and orgasmic dysfunction in 35% of females. Diabetically caused sexual dysfunction is often irreversible and requires sensitive couples counseling.

Alcoholism. Alcoholism may result in impotence, decreased libido, and retarded ejaculation. Among women with alcoholism, many experience difficulties in sexual arousal, or experience loss or reduction of orgasmic frequency.

Renal Failure. Patients with chronic renal failure who receive hemodialysis have a high degree of sexual dysfunction. Among both men and women, changes in libido are reported. Hemodialysis usually does not improve sexual function, although some improvement may be seen following kidney transplantation. It is important to note that men with chronic renal failure have a very high suicide rate.

Cardiovascular Disease. When pain or weakness accompanies cardiovascular disease, sexual expression may be inhibited. Following a heart attack, however, many patients unnecessarily restrict their sexual activity because of fear or ignorance. Studies have shown that sexual activity may be resumed when the individual can tolerate climbing two flights of stairs without pain, or can walk briskly around the block. Four to 5 weeks following a heart attack are usually a sufficient period of abstinence from sexual activity.

Drugs. Numerous drugs, although effective in treating illness, have sexual side effects, such as decreased libido and erectile, ejaculatory, and orgasmic dysfunction. Antihypertensive drugs frequently affect sexual performance by interfering with nerve transmission. One such drug, guanethidine, has been shown to cause impotence in 13.6% of men, decreased libido in 59%, and retarded ejaculation in 63.6%. Of the psychotropic drugs that affect sexual capacity, monoamine oxidase inhibitors can cause impotence. Tranquilizers may create fatigue rather than decreased libido. Drug abuse with heroin and methadone decreases libido in abusers, and barbiturate abuse may result in impotence and impair sexual arousal. Thus, it is important to counsel patients about the possible effects of drug therapy on sexual functioning. Noncompliance, particularly with hypertension treatment, often occurs when patients realize that their impotence is drug-induced. Patients should be aware of the ability to reverse a sexually dysfunctional condition through stopping or changing of drug or dosage.

INTRAPSYCHIC ETIOLOGY

Sexual dysfunctions may have either immediate and specific or remote psychological causes. They reflect intrapsychic conflict, creating anxiety and blockage of erotic feelings about love-making.

Sexual dysfunction may be influenced by a fear of:

- Performance failure.
- Displeasing one's partner or being displeased.
- Abandonment or rejection.
- Loss of control.

A hurried sexual experience (e.g., an attempt at sex in the back seat of a car) may create premature ejaculation. Forced sex may be the cause of sexual aversion and vaginismus. In addition, cultural or religious taboos that consider sex to be sinful and dirty can negatively condition an individual toward nonresponsiveness.

Under conditions of severe stress or depression, sexual energy may be decreased. Low self-esteem may cause sexual dysfunction; a person with low self-esteem may be unable to accept pleasure from another, be unaware of his or her own individuality, and be unable to seek the boundaries of his or her sexual preference.

Mutilative surgery, disfigurement, or a handicap may create a poor body image. When the body is considered unattractive, anxiety and increased muscle tension are the probable responses to admiration from a sexual partner.

INTERPERSONAL ETIOLOGY

The interpersonal component of the relationship between sexual partners very often affects, to some degree, the quality of their sexual interaction. Hostility can lead to deliberately withholding pleasure through **sexual sabotage,** such as by creating tension before love-making, suggesting sex at an inopportune time, making oneself deliberately unattractive, or producing deliberate frustrations. On the other hand, lack of knowledge about sexual anatomy and poor communication about preferences may create years of sexual tension in even the most stable, loving relationships.

NURSING DIAGNOSIS AND INTERVENTION

When a behavioral matrix such as sexual functioning becomes the focus of an acute health problem, objective evidence as well as subjective data about its existence are essential. The more closely the objective evidence coincides with a definitive etiology, the more apt the intervention is to be specific. Sexual dysfunction as a diagnosis provides a broad spectrum of general data, with various possible etiologic factors. Collaboration with other professionals, as well as the specialized expertise of the nurse, are required for both the nursing diagnosis and the particular modes of intervention chosen for treating the dysfunction.

When a sexual dysfunction has a medical etiology, nursing care focuses on several areas. First is the meaning of the loss of sexual functioning; second, the concerns focusing on the type of medical intervention that is necessary; third, the ability to communicate with the partner the significance of the sexual dysfunction in the relationship; and fourth, the gradual working out of satisfying intimacy with the partner.

■ CLASSIFICATION OF SEXUAL DYSFUNCTION DISORDERS

In *DSM-IV,* disorders of sexual dysfunction are divided into four major types: those of sexual desire, sexual arousal, orgasm, and sexual pain. These divisions closely follow the description of the normal human sexual response cycle originally described by Masters and Johnson (1966). Sexual dysfunctions may be lifelong or acquired; and may be generalized or situational. Some may be due to psychological factors, others to combined psychological factors and a general medical condition.

E CASE EXAMPLE

A husband is recovering from a mild heart attack. The husband and wife are hesitant to resume their sexual relationship for fear the husband will have another heart attack. Sexual desire is present, as are prior experiences of sexual arousal and orgasmic. This couple has made a causal connection between the energy expended in the sexual act and a heart attack. Information and experience in monitoring exertion and concomitant signs such as pulse rate and any chest pain become important for the husband. Monitoring is usually done through gradual increments in physical activity. The wife's involvement is an opportunity for both partners to open communication with one another. Unrealistic expectations can be revealed and countered. In addition, the couple can become comfortable in exploring relaxing, pleasurable, and less strenuous methods for enjoying their sexual relationship.

Nursing Intervention

- Assess and establish the existence of intact sexual response patterns and rule out any extreme variation of sexual behavior.
- Establish a clear definition of the patient's primary medical problem (i.e., heart attack).
- Establish information relevant to the influence of the medical problem on the patient's sexual behavior.
- Clarify the patient's and significant other's key perceptions about the medical problem's relationship to the couple's sexual functioning.
- Provide information, counseling, and instruction about focused exercises to enhance functioning.
- Evaluate the effectiveness of the intervention.

When the etiologic factor of sexual dysfunction is psychological, education and counseling are the primary interventions. This is particularly true for minor problems. The severity of the primary psychological and relationship problems is determined in part by assessing the psychological constitution of the patient or couple, and the critical interactional components of the relationship. If the dysfunction is simple and minor, nursing care will include:

- Explaining the causal connection between an attitudinal set and behavior and its relationship to sexual concern.
- Gaining cooperation and agreement to work toward change.
- Clarifying that change is compatible, comfortable, and acceptable to the patient and his or her partner.
- Evaluating outcome. If it is unsatisfactory, reassessment is needed, and if necessary, referral for further evaluation or more specific psychiatric treatment of the psychological or relationship problem.

Resolving a sexual complaint can increase anxiety by exposing other human demands of relating, such as commitment and intimacy. Problems in these personal areas of human existence are often masked through symptoms of dysfunction. The individual may use the symptoms as defenses. In some complex relationship problems, the partner with the complaint may be a foil for the more severe psychological problems of the non-symptomatic partner. When the complaint is resolved, there is an imbalance in the relationship, and the partner's underlying psychological difficulties come to the forefront.

DISORDERS OF SEXUAL DESIRE

Disorders of sexual desire are problems in the appetitive phase described by Masters and Johnson (1966). This phase refers to sexual fantasies and the desire for sex based on inner motivation, drives, and personality factors. The sexual desire disorders described in *DSM-IV* include lack of sexual desire and aversion to sex.

Hypoactive Sexual Desire

This disorder involves a persistent and pervasive inhibition of sexual desire. Minimal sexual fantasy and desire causes distress to either the patient or the partner. Lack of sexual desire is the most common complaint of couples seeking sex counseling.

A variety of stresses have been identified as causes of lack of sexual desire. These include job conflict, religious factors, drug or alcohol use, marital disharmony, and unconscious fears about sex. Sometimes, suppressed homosexual wishes in a partner decrease heterosexual desire. The withholding of sex may be an expression of hostility between partners. Desire-phase disorders may have medical causes, for example, alteration in neural hormones that specifically mediate sexual desire.

How long sexual desire has been lacking becomes important in planning care. If the problem is chronic in a physically healthy, functioning individual without signs of severe mental illness, complex dynamic intrapsychic issues are usually considered. Psychotherapy is required, possibly combined with sex therapy. Referral is made to specialists in this area.

When the desire-phase problem is short-term and related to such factors as stress and depression, nursing intervention focuses on reducing stressors contributing to the patient's mood state, making clear their causal link with low or absent sexual desire. A pattern of avoiding sexually stimulating experiences should be explored with the patient. This is particularly true with someone who has lost a spouse and is confused about the meaning of sexual desire and anguished by the loss of a spouse.

DISORDERS OF SEXUAL AROUSAL

Disorders of sexual arousal are problems in the excitement phase described by Masters and Johnson (1966). This phase includes the physiological changes that occur with arousal and the subjective sense of sexual pleasure. Such disorders may be caused by medical or psychological problems or substance use. Many patients taking serotonin-reuptake-inhibiting antidepressants—e.g., Fluoxetine (Prozac), Sertraline (Zoloft), and Paroxetine (Paxil)—experience drug-induced problems with sexual arousal and orgasm. Some patients will not volunteer this information unless asked directly (LaBruzza, 1994).

Female Sexual Arousal Disorder

In this disorder, a woman has difficulty with the lubrication and swelling responses in sexual excitement, which leads to marked distress or problems in her sexual relationship. The patient typically reports a persistent or recurrent lack of a subjective sense of sexual excitement and pleasure during sexual activity.

Male Erectile Disorder

This disorder includes persistent or recurrent partial or complete failure by a male to attain or maintain erection until the completion of sexual activity, or persistent or recurrent lack of a subjective sense of sexual excitement and pleasure during sexual activity.

ORGASM DISORDERS

Orgasm disorders are problems in orgasm, the third phase of the sexual response cycle described by Masters and Johnson (1966). In female orgasmic disorder, or anorgasmia, orgasm is either delayed or absent following a normal excitement phase. In male orgasmic disorder, orgasm is either delayed, absent, or premature. All of these conditions cause marked problems in a relationship.

For both males and females, the orgasm phase is quite susceptible to primary organic problems. The effectiveness of nursing care for disorders of orgasm depends on proper medical intervention and an understanding of the impact of the organic problem and treatment regimen for it. Because many medical issues are irreversible or necessary for the total functioning of the individual, nursing care focuses on rehabilitative measures. If an organic problem is treatable, the nurse seeks to quell the patient's anxiety about sexual func-

tioning during the treatment period, and works with the partner as well. Education and counseling in conjunction with the patient's medical regimen constitute primary nursing intervention.

Some medical interventions greatly alter body structure and impinge on the physiology of orgasm. Special attention, therefore, is paid to the process of the patient's gaining acceptance of resulting changes in body image and regaining pleasure in sensuous, erotic, and comforting interpersonal experiences. Partners need support and counseling during this period.

When the etiology of a sexual dysfunction is immediate and psychological or an unrecognized cognitive pattern (such as visual image or internal dialogue), expectations play a large role in interfering with sexual response. In recent years, the etiology of orgasm or inhibited orgasm in a woman has been debated as has the question of whether orgasm is a necessary condition of female sexuality. In providing care, nurses should not enter such disputes, but rather present, from clinical experience, some etiologic factors that, when taken into consideration, may alter the patient's sexual-response pattern. In addition, certain dysfunctional response patterns, present or past, can contribute to a lack of perception of erotic sensation. This can result from habit and from distraction; both of which play an important role in the dysfunctions of orgasm.

SEXUAL AVERSION

Sexual aversion disorder involves an extreme, persistent or recurrent aversion to and avoidance of all or almost all genital sexual contact with a sexual partner. Avoidance of sex and sexual arousal must be evaluated carefully for underlying panic disorder. Panic disorders have been understood to be a function of intense physiological arousal that is no longer biologically inhibited. This is in contrast to interpreting panic disorder as psychologically determined through symptoms that are symbolic of some personal psychological trauma. It is thought that such behavior has a genetic precursor. At any rate, experiments with drug treatment have demonstrated a reduced panic response. When the response is reduced and psychotherapy and sex therapy are combined, there have been favorable results.

Simple phobic responses are usually amenable to psychotherapy or to behavior therapy combined with instruction. When panic or phobic avoidance of sex is evident, referral is the appropriate nursing intervention.

SEXUAL PAIN DISORDERS

Sexual pain disorders involve genital pain associated with sexual activity. Two types of pain are described: dyspareunia and pain caused by a traumatic event.

Dyspareunia

Dyspareunia, distressing genital pain and vaginismus, refers to painful involuntary spasms of the muscles of the outer third of the vagina that interfere with sexual intercourse.

More often than not, pain associated with sex has an organic cause. Nursing intervention is primarily directed toward making sure the patient is thoroughly evaluated for such a source of pain.

Nursing interventions for sexual disorders often involve the cognitive technique of thought-stopping and re-education, best accomplished with the patient and the patient's partner. Special knowledge, techniques, and counseling skills are necessary to identify and change sexually dysfunctional thought patterns. Some clinical specialists in psychiatric nursing provide this type of sex therapy, as do nurse clinical specialists in the areas of dysfunctional or neurological diseases. Sex therapy provokes anxiety and its success requires motivation on the part of the patient. People with problematic psychological functioning and precarious relationships may not withstand the therapy and can decompensate under its stress. On the other hand, a patient with a known psychiatric problem who has had periods of undisputed sexual functioning can be assisted with an approach that focuses directly on sexual functioning. In these situations, the dysfunction is not a defense against the underlying psychological problem.

Traumatic Events

Traumatic events may precipitate a psychologically based sexual dysfunction. Particularly important is to identify whether the patient has been the object of rape, incest, or a brutalizing abusive situation.

In cases of unresolved sexual trauma, counseling would be the primary intervention. Focused sex therapy may be required when the traumatic event is resolved.

In counseling for underlying psychological or relational problems, it must be remembered that pain can be a defense against pleasure, and that efforts to eliminate pain may provoke intense anxiety and cause withdrawal from counseling until an acceptance of pleasure is established.

In general, the first step in nursing intervention for disorders involving sexual pain is to determine whether the disorder has a medical or psychogenic cause. If there is doubt, the patient is referred for more specialized evaluation. If a medical or psychogenic cause of pain is established, the most appropriate of the following nursing interventions is undertaken, depending on the cause and level of the patient's sexual dysfunction: education; general counseling about personal and relationship issues; or focused exercises to alter cognitive sets or physical behavior that impedes sexual and erotic behavior. The patient's sexual partner is included in these interventions.

Nursing diagnoses in cases of trauma may be sexual dysfunction or altered sexuality patterns. In the case of forced, non-consenting sex, a diagnosis of rape trauma syndrome is made. There are two additional diagnoses of rape trauma: compound reaction. That includes additional psychosocial problems and silent reaction where the rape has not been disclosed (Burgess and Holmstrom, (1974).

■ SEXUAL DEVIATIONS

Sexual deviation is an extreme variation in sexual behavior in which there is little or no regard for the welfare of another person. The behavior is highly compulsive and repetitive, and intervention in such cases requires a specialist.

Nurses are in contact with sexually deviant individuals in many settings, including prisons, the home, and the health-care system. Nurses often provide services to the victims of sexually deviant individuals or refer them for services. In some cases the victim may be hospitalized.

Sexually deviant individuals need access to victims, especially persons they can control. In seeking victims, they may target the workplace or even a health-care setting. In a 1994 San Antonio, TX, case, a 32 year-old nursing home patient who had been in a coma for more than 14 years was found to be 6 months pregnant. In a similar 1996 case, a 29 year-old nursing home patient, comatose for 10 years, became pregnant.

PARAPHILIAS

The **paraphilias** are characterized by arousal in response to sexual objects or in situations that are not part of normative arousal activity patterns, and which may interfere in varying degrees with the capacity for reciprocal, affectionate sexual activity.

The essential features of disorders of this subclass are recurrent, intense sexual urges and sexually arousing fantasies that generally involve nonhuman objects; the suffering or humiliation of oneself or one's partner (not merely simulated); or children or other nonconsenting persons. The diagnosis is made only if the individual has acted on these urges or is markedly distressed by them. In other classifications, the paraphilias are referred to as sexual deviations. The term *paraphilia* is, however, preferred, because it correctly emphasizes that the deviation (para) lies in the object to which the individual is attracted (philia).

E CASE EXAMPLE

The following case involves patients as victims of sexual deviance and a nurse as the perpetrator. The daughter of a 57-year-old woman hospitalized in a coronary intensive care unit for a myocardial infarction, reports to the nursing supervisor that her mother had called her nurse a "pervert" and said that he had sexually assaulted her three times. A hospital investigation reviews the matter and notes that co-workers of this 32-year-old nurse support him and emphasize the impossibility of such an incident since the unit was extremely busy on the day of the report; many of the staff were in contact with the patient, and the patient's room was directly across from the nursing station. The nurse is characterized as competent and professional and is well-liked by peers and patients. Moreover, the report notes that a time study had been conducted on the day of the alleged violation. As a result, a surveyor was documenting the activities of every staff member at 5 to 10-minute intervals, and noted no unusual occurrences. The nurse on the subsequent shift did not notice anything out of the ordinary, nor did the patient express any concern or exhibit any behavior suggesting a problem with her care. It is also noted that the nurse accused of the violation handles the matter very well and receives tremendous support from the Risk Management and Administration Staff. No further action is taken.

Five months later, the husband of a 66-year-old woman hospitalized at the same coronary intensive care unit reports that the same nurse had attempted to sexually assault his wife. This time the nurse is immediately placed on investigative suspension. The results of the investigation note that the nurse had lied several times. The nurse had, for example, told the husband that a female nurse had been present during the time he was providing care to the patient, and documented this in his nursing notes. He had also claimed to have administered procedures and medications that were not recorded in the nursing record, and had given medication when the patient had not complained of pain. The nurse's written statements contradicted his charting entries in the medical record.

Within a week of the second complaint, a 52-year-old mentally retarded woman reports to her case manager that the male nurse, making a home visit, had asked her to engage in sexually explicit acts (similar to those he forced on the critically ill patients in the coronary care unit.)

CASE ANALYSIS

We learn from this case that the nurse is sophisticated about medications. He exercises control over his work environment; his peers like him and see him as bright and competent. They do not believe the allegations against him. He selects victims in a critical life situation, whose credibility can be challenged in terms of memory. He gives them mind-altering medications that will further interfere with their ability to remember and identify him. These patients are considered low-risk victims because they can not identify him. In contrast though, he abuses these people in the context of a work setting where the potential for discovery by others is relatively high. Thus, he commits a high-risk offense in terms of being caught. This paradox is tied in to the arousal pay-off for the offender. He requires a certain level of environmental threat to achieve arousal, and over time this organization of criminal activity needs to increase the danger to induce and sustain his emotional arousal. This belies his ability to have a normal sexual response. What is replacing the response is this complex activity and the accompanying fantasies of power, control, and even discovery. Over time, his behavior escalates because it is much harder to achieve arousal. At this point, the danger increases to the victims as well as his potential for discovery. The court outcome for this nurse defendant was a hung jury who later commented that they could not understand why there was no evidence of the sexual assault; no semen had been detected on the women. However, the State Board of Nursing revoked his license and he currently is not practicing as a registered nurse.

The specific paraphilias include: (1) exhibitionism; (2) fetishism; (3) frotteurism; (4) pedophilia; (5) sexual masochism; (6) sexual sadism; (7) transvestic fetishism; and (8) voyeurism.

Persons with paraphilia commonly suffer from several varieties of this disorder and may have additional mental disorders. The criteria for severity follow:

- Mild. The person is markedly distressed by the recurrent paraphilic urges but has never acted on them.
- Moderate. The person has occasionally acted on the paraphilic urge.
- Severe. The person has repeatedly acted on the paraphilic urge.

Definition

Paraphilia is predominantly a male psychiatric disorder. The term paraphilia literally means "beside-love," which suggests a critical pathognomonic feature comprising a multiplicity of cognitive, affective, and behavioral patterns. In cases of paraphilia, the establishment and maintenance of intimacy between two adults has been interfered with or displaced. Common features among the paraphilias are an inability to cope with

---

This section on paraphilias (through page 364) is written by Mark F. Schwartz and William H. Masters from the Masters & Johnson Institute, St. Louis, Mo.

closeness and attachment to other adults and the inevitable loneliness that is an integral part of social separation. Persons with paraphilias usually cope with their social pathology by withdrawing into the secretly comfortable world of fantasy.

Paraphilia involves obsessive-compulsive behavioral patterns and appears to have a number of clinical similarities to addiction. The paraphiliac engages in obsessional sexual thinking and compulsively "acts out" his fantasies. The illicit compulsion may involve cross-dressing; fetishes for leather, undergarments, inanimate objects, or pornography; exposing the genitals; making obscene telephone calls; peeping into windows; or fondling children. Generally the paraphiliac is unresponsive to nondeviant, affectional sexual stimuli and becomes dependent on highly specific imagery or socially inappropriate external stimulation to achieve sexual arousal.

Addictive Components

Like other addicts, the paraphiliac experiences almost a "trance-like" sense of relaxation, relief, and homeostasis when involved in the illicit sexual activity, and conversely, exhibits social distress when not sexually "acting out." "Acting out" becomes an escape from distasteful aspects of life. The paraphiliac usually evidences adolescent-like narcissism, which results in his frequently attempting to extract unrealistic demands from his environment. Because he usually fails in this effort, he is continually frustrated and frequently angry. Other errors in cognition and thinking add to his continuing frustration. Beyond this, chronically low self-esteem, a preoccupation with self-deprecation, and poor assertiveness skills cause the paraphiliac to repeatedly feel victimized, as in the case of a male pedophile who became enraged that the parking lot near a clinic was closed, preventing him from participating in a therapy session. These individuals feel an overwhelming sense of inadequacy and lack of control. When frustrated, paraphiliac's "acting out" behavior becomes an expression of rage or an attempt at control, giving him a temporary sense that "he is calling the shots."

Paradoxically, this illusion of control is rapidly abated, leaving an overwhelming feeling of inadequacy. Pushed by their problem, persons with paraphilia spend hours each day seeking the right situation in which to "act out." They become unable to make decisions based on personal morality, and rarely recognize the potential harm of their acts to themselves or others. Their continued internalization of feelings of a lack of mastery and self-responsibility eventually generalize and result in other manifestations of self-sabotage, such as alcohol abuse.

PEDOPHILIA

For the paraphiliac who is uncomfortable in sociosexual interaction with adult males or females, eroticism may emerge either in response to an object (fetishism), through sexual interaction at a distance from another adult (voyeurism, exhibitionism, obscene telephone calling), or in the form of a sexual act with a nonthreatening child (pedophilia). Because the pedophile's social development has been impeded, he typically verbalizes a sense of uneasiness with other adults. The only time at which the pedophile can feel comfortable and "be himself" is with a child. In pedophilia, psychosocial trauma has caused a fixation of or an impediment to cognitive maturation, causing the pedophile to often think, feel, and act like a child.

INCEST OFFENDERS

Incest offenders may or may not have paraphilia; however, because many are pedophiles, and those who are not are clinically similar, to the latter, the incest family is included in this discussion. Many incest offenders are pedophiles who have married and continued their pedophilia with greater safety by sexually approaching their own child or a stepchild. Although most male incest offenders deny being sexually aroused by children, plethysmographic studies suggest that many experience greater arousal by children than they are willing to admit even to themselves. A plethysmograph measures penile erection to visual observation of slides of adult and child figures.

Another reason for the inclusion of incest in this discussion is that incest offenders require treatment similar to that for the patient with paraphilia, with the major difference being that intervention for the incest offender also includes a family-therapy component. In the incestuous family, the husband-and-wife relationship evolves into an immature, undifferentiated couple, creating confusion, conflict habituation, and other types of destructive dependent relationships. The homes of these men and women reflect any combination of chaos (few rules are consistently followed), enmeshment (all family members are involved in one another's business), disengagement (no one cares what the others say or do), and rigidity (extreme authoritarianism). In about 40% of reported cases, the incest offender or wife suffers from alcoholism. According to recent data and clinical experience, the nonalcoholic offender may actually display more psychopathology than the alcoholic.

Some incest offenders are extremely rigid and authoritarian, and sometimes even physically abusive to other family members. The rigidity protects the of-

E CASE EXAMPLE

▶ VOYEURISM

Mr. L., a 32-year-old carpenter, reports a 15-year history of voyeurism. He goes to public parks looking for young women not wearing brassieres and follows them for as long as he can. On other occasions he goes to a public beach and video tapes the chests of women. At work he climbs into the ceiling and peers through ventilation ducts into the women's bathroom. He begins to worry that he will lose his job if discovered, and tries to stop his behavior. He is unsuccessful and seeks psychiatric intervention. Because of the obsessive-compulsive features of his deviation, he is successfully treated with fluoxetine. His intrusive urges and compulsive voyeurism are reduced within 3 months.

---

fender from overwhelming feelings of inadequacy in dealing with daily transactions. The male incest perpetrator is often intimidated by other men, and uneasy in his work and social interactions. One perpetrator who had dropped out of school at age 16 and recently been promoted to an administrative position said that he felt he had "to fake it every day," and felt "uneasy, inadequate, and incompetent" with his wife yet was unbearably lonely without her. At times, he was overtly acquiescent with her, and other times, particularly when drinking, his rage manifested itself with physical violence.

VOYEURISM

The voyeur becomes sexually aroused through observing unsuspecting persons, usually strangers, who are either naked, in the process of disrobing, or engaging in sexual activity. The act of looking (peeping) is done for the purpose of achieving sexual excitement; no sexual activity is sought with the person who is being watched. Orgasm, usually produced by masturbation, may occur during this voyeuristic activity, or later, in response to the memory of what was witnessed. Voyeurs often enjoy the fantasy of having had a sexual experience with the observed person when in reality this has not occurred.

TRANSVESTIC FETISHISM

Transvestic fetishism includes recurrent, intense, sexual urges and sexually arousing fantasies of at least 6 months duration, involving cross-dressing. The affected individual usually keeps a collection of women's or men's clothes that he or she intermittently uses to cross-dress when alone. While cross-dressed, the individual usually masturbates and imagines other members of the

E CASE EXAMPLE

▶ TRANSVESTIC FETISHISM

Syd was 12 years old when he first ran away from home because he had difficulty in concentrating at school and because his mother and stepfather were unable to accept his fetishism and cross-dressing. Syd says that he had wanted to dress like and be a girl from the age of 5. He thought about being a girl, preferred playing with dolls, and would often use his mother's makeup. This latter behavior upset his father to the point at which the father would tear the boy's mattress apart looking for cosmetics. Until age 5, Syd had been raised by his mother, an aunt, and his grandmother. His aunt encouraged his feminine interests and often put makeup on him. Syd has strong positive memories of his female caretakers. His mother's remarriage when he was 5 was very upsetting to Syd.

Syd's first sexual experience was at age 11, when he was approached by an adult male for oral sex while in a public bathroom. When he ran away, he was given refuge by the manager of a men's clothing department. This man talked openly of gay clubs and "queens" who cross-dressed, and in exchange for sex, the man bought Syd his first woman's wardrobe and makeup. After the man tired of him, Syd earned money hustling at gay bars and on the street. At age 14, he had tried all of the available street drugs and had been treated for sexually transmitted diseases. His hope is to be able to afford a sex-change operation.

same sex being attracted to him or her in the attire of the opposite sex.

EXHIBITIONISM

The individual with exhibitionism, typically a heterosexual male, becomes sexually aroused by exposing his genitals to an unsuspecting stranger, usually a woman or girl. About a third of sexual offenders referred for treatment are exhibitionists. The more timid individual with exhibitionism will expose a flaccid penis. The more aggressive exhibitionist may masturbate to erection and delight in shocking an unwary female.

FROTTEURISM

A frotteur is an individual who derives sexual stimulation by rubbing against a nonconsenting person. The touching and rubbing, rather than any coercion, is the sexually arousing aspect of the act. Both rubbing and fondling are included within this category. The frotteur usually rubs in crowded places, such as on public transportation or a busy sidewalk, from which he can easily move to escape arrest. The act usually involves rubbing the genitals against the victim's thighs and buttocks, or fondling her genitalia or breasts with the hands. While doing this the frotteur usually fantasizes an exclusive, caring relationship with his victim. The victim may not initially protest the frottage because she cannot imagine that such a provocative sexual act would be committed in such a public place.

FETISHISM

The person with fetishism becomes sexually aroused by inanimate objects such as shoes or women's clothing. Among the common fetish items are brassieres and women's underpants, stockings, shoes, boots, or other wearing apparel. The fetishist may masturbate while holding, rubbing, or smelling the fetish object, or may ask his sexual partner to wear the object during their sexual encounters. Usually the fetish is required or strongly preferred for sexual excitement, and in its absence there may be erectile failure.

SEXUAL MASOCHISM

Sexual masochism involves the derivation of sexual pleasure from being humiliated, beaten, bound, or otherwise made to suffer. Masochistic acts may be fantasized, such as being raped while being held or bound by others so that there is no possibility of escape. Other individuals act on their masochistic sexual urges through binding themselves, sticking themselves with pins, shocking themselves electrically, or seeking self-

mutilative or masochistic acts with a partner. Such acts include restraint (physical bondage), blindfolding (sensory bondage), paddling, spanking, whipping (flagellation), pinning and piercing (infibulation), and humiliation (such as being urinated or defecated on, being forced to crawl and bark like a dog, or being subjected to verbal abuse). Forced cross-dressing may be sought for its humiliating associations. The term *infantilism* is sometimes used to describe the desire to be treated as a helpless infant and clothed in diapers.

One particularly dangerous form of sexual masochism is hypoxyphilia, which involves sexual arousal by oxygen deprivation. The individual with this disorder produces oxygen deprivation by means of a noose, ligature, plastic bag, mask, chemical (often a volatile nitrate that produces a temporary decrease in brain oxygenation by peripheral vasodilation), or chest compression, but allows the person the opportunity to escape asphyxiation before consciousness is lost. People engaging in such behavior report that the activity is accompanied by sexual fantasies in which they asphyxiate or harm others, others asphyxiate or harm them, or they escape near brushes with death. Oxygen-depriving activities may be used when the individual is alone or with a partner.

When cases of hypoxyphilia are correctly identified, conservative estimates suggest that the condition causes from 500 to 1,000 deaths annually, with the majority among adolescents and young adults. In a Federal Bureau of Investigation study of 132 cases of autoerotic asphyxial death, 127 involved males and 5 females, with the mean age being 26.5 years. Four victims were preadolescent, 37 were teenagers, 46 were in their twenties, 28 in their thirties, 8 in their forties, 6 in their fifties, 2 in their sixties, and 1 in his seventies. There were 124 white victims, 5 black victims; 2 victims were Native American and 1 was Hispanic. Most of the victims were not married at the time of death (Hazelwood, Dietz, and Burgess, 1983).

In the majority of cases in this study, the victim was found dead by a family member or friend. Persons learning of such a death are typically stunned and shocked. The victim is usually described as having been in good spirits, good physical health, active, and having a future orientation. There is rarely any suspicion of suicidal ideation. The sensation of shock is often due to a short time interval between having last seen the victim and the victim's death.

Death resulting from the use of an injurious agent during a masturbatory ritual is considered unusual because many persons—including professionals—have never previously heard of it. Although many people are familiar with autoeroticism involving manual stimulation, a significantly smaller number seem to be aware of techniques for reducing oxygen delivery to the brain as the source of an altered state of consciousness and for the enhancement of erotic sensation and fantasy.

Forensic Nursing Implications

The clinical relevance for nursing is that autoerotic deaths are accidents; they are not suicides. Therefore, psychiatric nurses provide education about this fact and counsel families in their grief.

The nurse may be consulted by the police investigating a case of hypoxyphilic death for any observations suggesting that the death was autoerotic. For example, if the victim is brought into the emergency room of a hospital, the nurse may observe the body; and if pertinent information is heard regarding the life-style of the victim, the nurse can bring it to the attention of police officials. The nurse may also be part of a crisis-intervention team that provides care to the families of suicide or accidental death victims.

The emotional response to the death of a family member is particularly traumatic when the body is discovered by a family member or associate, when the death is sudden and untimely, when the decedent is young, and especially when the death is sexually related. These factors are generally present in autoerotic fatalities. The families of victims of autoerotic death have many feelings about the nature of the death. The nurse should encourage the family members to talk about and share their feelings, and should provide referrals for counseling, since the family members of such victims are considered to be at high risk for unresolved grief.

SEXUAL SADISM

Sexual sadism refers to sexual arousal by the suffering of another. This disorder may be associated with antisocial personality disorder. When the sadistic urges are strong, there is danger of serious harm or death to the victim. Sadistic fantasies or acts may involve activities that indicate the dominance of the sadist over the victim (e.g., forcing the victim to crawl, or keeping the victim in a cage), or restraining, blindfolding, spanking, whipping, pinching, burning, electrically shocking, raping, cutting, strangling, or killing the victim. The sadistic fantasies are likely to have been present since childhood.

■ GENDER AND SEXUALITY

To illustrate how complicated gender is, Money (1987, cited in Hyde, 1990) distinguishes among eight variables of gender, as follows:

- *Chromosomal gender.* XX in the female; XY in the male.

- *Gonadal gender.* Ovaries in the female; testes in the male.
- *Prenatal hormonal gender.* Estrogen and progesterone in the female; testosterone in the male before birth.
- *Internal accessory organs.* Uterus and vagina in the female; prostate and seminal vesicles in the male.
- *External genital appearance.* Clitoris and vaginal opening in the female; penis and scrotum in the male.
- *Pubertal hormonal gender.* At puberty, estrogen and progesterone in the female; testosterone in the male.
- *Assigned gender.* The announcement at birth, "It's a girl" or "It's a boy," based on the appearance of the external genitals; the gender that the parents and society believe the child to be; the gender in which the child is reared.
- *Gender identity.* The individual's private, internal sense of maleness or femaleness, expressed in personality and behavior, and the integration of this sense with the rest of the personality and with the gender roles prescribed by society.

The variables listed above can be subdivided into biological variables (the first six) and psychological variables (the last two). In most cases, all of the variables are in consonance in any individual, and the individual is a "consistent" female or male. If the individual is female, she has XX chromosomes, ovaries, a uterus and vagina, and a clitoris; she is reared as a female; and she thinks of herself as a female. If the individual is male, he has the parallel set of appropriate characteristics.

Although there is clear differentiation between the sexes, and adult men and women have very different reproductive anatomies, their reproductive organs have similar origins. When a male sexual organ and a female sexual organ develop from the same embryonic tissue, they are said to be *homologous*. The following discussion reviews prenatal biologic influences in the sexes and identifies two genetic deficiencies that illustrate biological problems of gender identity.

BIOLOGICAL INFLUENCE

Certain hormones bring about the differentiation of the embryonic sex-cell mass into female or male genitalia. Hormonal signals initiated by the specific chromosomal pattern established in the embryo at conception determine the sex of the resulting fetus. Each ovum produced by the female carries an X chromosome, whereas each sperm produced in the male carries either a single X (female) or a single Y (male) chromosome. Only one of the

200-million sperm cells contained in a single ejaculate will penetrate and fertilize the female ovum. An X-bearing sperm fertilizing the ovum will produce an XX, or female, child. A sperm bearing a Y chromosome will produce an XY, or male, child.

The complex human sexual system, under the control of hormones, begins with the differentiation of the gonads into male testes or female ovaries. The reproductive system of the embryo is simply an undifferentiated genital thickening on the posterior outer layer of the embryonic cavity. This internal sexual transformation is visible at about 6 weeks' gestation.

During this embryonic phase of sexual development, the gonads emerge as ridges of tissue. They are not differentiated sexually, and can become either testes or ovaries. At this same point in development, two duct systems develop. These wolffian and mullerian duct systems are primitive precursors of specific genital structures. The primitive gonads transform into testes when the chemical substance known as H-Y antigen initiates this process. This antigen, controlled by the Y chromosome, must be present for the male to develop; otherwise the primitive gonads will always develop into ovaries.

Once the sex of the embryo has been established by gonadal development, the ducts of the opposite sex remain undeveloped or degenerate. In the male, a chemical called mullerian duct-inhibiting substance causes the mullerian ducts to shrink and virtually disappear. Testosterone, an androgen, is produced, and the wolffian ducts develop into the epididymis, vas deferens, seminal vesicles, and ejaculatory ducts. Testosterone is converted to dihydrotestosterone, another androgen, which in turn is responsible for the development of the penis, scrotum, and prostate gland. The female organs are not dependent on hormones for their development. Ovaries develop around the 12th week after gestation, and the mullerian duct system evolves into the uterus, fallopian tubes, and inner third of the vagina. The wolffian duct system shrinks because of the absence of androgens. By the 14th week the fetus is clearly differentiated into either a male or female, with visible internal sex structures.

The external genitalia of males and females are identical until the 7th week of development. Initially the ovaries and the testes are formed in the abdomen, with the testes moving into the scrotum under the influence of androgen. The lack of androgen stimulation results in clitoral, vulvar, and vaginal development, with the ovaries eventually settling into the pelvis. The external genitalia are initially located between the umbilical cord and the tail of the embryo. The area called the genital tubercle eventually becomes the clitoris in the female and the glands of the penis in the male. A groove that forms in front of the genital tubercle around the 4th week of life produces a separation known as the perineum.

Although genetic sex is fixed at the time of fertilization, it is not until the 5th or 6th week of development that the genes actually influence the embryo. Normal development depends on the presence of androgen, and if the male is deprived of androgen the mullerian system regresses, the wolffian system does not develop, and hermaphroditism results. The hermaphrodite is born with both testicular and ovarian tissue. Pseudohermaphrodites have gonads that match their sex chromosomes, but genitals that represent the opposite sex.

Other genetic defects may occur during gestation. Klinefelter's syndrome, a common chromosomal abnormality, occurs when an extra X chromosome is present in the male. This condition occurs about once in every 500 live male births but is often not discovered until the male reaches maturity. Testosterone production is reduced, the testes are abnormal, and sperm production does not occur. A reduced sexual drive and impotence have been noted, although the condition may improve with regular testosterone injections.

Turner's syndrome is the absence of an X chromosome. It results in nonfunctioning ovaries and the subsequent absence of menstruation. The syndrome is accompanied by infertility, shortness of stature, and a variety of abnormalities that may involve facial appearance and internal organs. Turner's syndrome occurs in about one of every 2,500 live female births. Besides sex-chromosome disorders and genetic conditions, exposure of the fetus to drugs taken by the mother can also influence its sexual development.

Both biology and learning influence sexuality. Their interaction throughout life affects sexual behavior and emotions. The separation of these two influences is impossible, as noted in the following two case examples.

THEORIES ABOUT GENDER AND SEXUALITY

The biologic influences of one's sexuality interact with the psychological and social factors that operate from birth forward. Psychosocial development in human sexuality is concerned with sex identity (a biologically assigned classification), gender identity (the personal perception of being male or female), and gender role (the outward expression of socially accepted masculine or feminine traits).

The sexual classification assigned at birth generally guides the roles, relationships, and behaviors that an individual will assume throughout life. Gender-identity formation occurs during early childhood, beginning between 18 months and 3 years of age. The development of gender identity and gender role is shrouded with controversy, and several theories have been advanced to explain their sequence and interrelationships.

E CASE EXAMPLES

▶ GENDER IDENTITY AND ROLE

When identical twin brothers underwent circumcision at 7 months of age, surgical error led to loss of the penis of one twin. After considerable anguish and consultation with various medical experts, the parents were finally referred to Johns Hopkins University, and a decision was made that the twin missing a penis would be raised as a girl. At 17 months, the child's name, clothing, and hair-style were changed, and four months later the first of a series of surgical procedures designed to reconstruct the child's genitals as female was begun. Family members were provided with the best available advice on how to cope with gender re-assignment.

The parents took great care to treat their twins as a son and daughter, even while knowing that both were biologically male. As a result, the daughter quickly began to prefer dresses to slacks, and showed other "typical" signs of femininity. The twins were encouraged to develop play patterns and interests in toys along traditional lines, with dolls for the girl and cars and tools for the boy. The mother also reported that her son and daughter imitated their parents' behavior differentially, with the son following his father's example and the daughter imitating what the mother did. According to sex researchers reporting the case (Money and Ehrhardt, 1972), these two children achieved normal (and different) gender identities and gender roles, although both were of the same chromosomal, anatomical, and hormonal sex during prenatal development and for the first 7 months of life.

The adjustment of the girl, however, was not sustained. According to interviews with her psychiatrist (Diamond, 1982), she developed problems as a teenager and became un-feminine in appearance and behavior, resulting in classmates calling her "cavewoman." While this problem may have reflected a need to adjust the child's estrogen dose during adolescence, this case does not lend support to the position that gender development depends primarily on learning.

▶ SEXUAL IDENTITY

A research study by Imperato-McGinley and associates (1979) supports an opposite conclusion to that in the case study described above. In 1974, 38 male pseudohermaphrodites were discovered in four rural villages of the Dominican Republic. Although they had normal sex chromosomes, an inherited enzyme defect had caused improper formation of their external genitals, even though their prenatal testosterone production had been normal. At birth, the babies had an incompletely formed scrotum that looked like labia, a very small penis that looked like a clitoris, and a partially formed vagina. As a result, many were raised as females. Then, during puberty, normal male testosterone production began and definite masculine changes occurred. The children's voices deepened, male-pattern muscles developed, the "clitoris" grew into a penis, and the testes descended into the scrotum. Normal erections occurred and intercourse was possible.

Of the 18 genetically male children with this condition who were raised as girls, 17 changed to a male gender-identity and 16 of 18 shifted to a male gender-role during or after puberty. Imperato-McGinley and associates (1979) interpreted these findings as showing that when the sex of rearing is contrary to the biological sex, the biological sex will prevail if normal hormone production occurs during puberty.

The social-learning model suggests that gender development is learned from the personal role models and cultural influences that the child experiences during growth. The child imitates and models the parents' behavior and is rewarded for this imitation. A child learns sex-typed behavior as he or she learns any other type of behavior, through a combination of reward, punishment, and observation of what other people are doing. Role conditioning is reinforced by praise or criticism: "He's built just like his father," or, "little girls don't climb trees and get dirty," or, "that's women's work." The child thus learns which behaviors will be sanctioned through specific direction and imitation of the same-sex parent or a surrogate role model.

The cognitive-development theory posits that children form a firm gender identity around the ages of five or six, when they understand that gender is constant (e.g., that dressing up in Mommy's shoes does not change a boy into a girl). This theory suggests that children learn by observation and imitation, not for parental reward as the learning theory suggests, but rather simply to obtain self-identity.

The biosocial interaction theory stresses critical periods in sexual development that influence gender development. This comprehensive concept of sexual development includes prenatal programming, psychology, and social norms and their interactions with biologic factors.

GENDER-IDENTITY DISORDER

Gender-identity disorder refers to a persistent and powerful identification with the opposite sex, accompanied by a discomfort with one's gender role or identity. Individuals with gender-identity disorder are uncomfortable with their true sex and its gender roles, and have a fervent desire to be a member of the other sex. For the diagnosis to be given to a child, the following five criteria must be met:

- A wish to be of the opposite sex.
- A preference for clothing of the opposite sex.

- Fantasies of being of the opposite sex, or a preference for roles of the opposite sex.
- Wishes to engage in opposite sex play.
- A preference for playmates of the opposite sex.

Adults with this disorder state that they feel they were born as members of the wrong sex. They wish to be and to be treated as members of the opposite sex. They may request surgery to become more like the opposite sex. They may have symptoms of self-loathing or disgust at their genitals.

Gender-identity disorder in adults is recognized by a strong and consistent cross-gender identification. It is not a simple desire to be a member of the other sex because of the latter's perceived social advantages, nor is it a matter of sex-role identification, in which an individual identifies with dressing patterns and activities usually associated with the other sex (e.g., a tomboy), nor cross dressing for the arousal of sexual desire. Rather, it is a marked preoccupation of being: (1) of the wrong sex; (2) in the wrong body; and (3) belonging to the other sex.

In childhood, the manifestations of gender-identity disorder may consist of a real reluctance to adhere to the dress and behavior patterns of the existing gender. Small children are often not articulate, and therefore often do not express the deep sense they have of being forced to be who they do not desire or think they are.

E CASE EXAMPLE

▶ GENDER-IDENTITY DISORDER

Bob Maines, a 20-year-old man in counseling with a clinical specialist in psychiatric nursing, says at his next-to-last session, "I know it is close to our last session, but what I have to tell you is nothing I have ever told anyone else. I want to be a woman. I have been aware of this since I was 5 years old."

How did this young man keep this feeling to himself for 15 years?

Bob came to therapy at the request of his mother. She was concerned by his isolation, his passivity in pursuing college, and his quiet behavior at home.

Bob is a dark haired, brown eyed, handsome young man. He is 5-feet, 1 inch in height, and a bit overweight. He arrived for his first session wearing a black tee shirt with a purple, outlined figure of a young man looking out of a window into a dark and infinite night.

The marked impression of loneliness and emptiness that this created was overwhelming to the nurse. Bob did not agree to be in therapy, but he acquiesced to his mother's request. Once in treatment he did admit to being rather sad, having a lot of anger, and above all feeling very protective of his parents and sad that he was not pleasing them.

Bob comes from a warm and academically achieving family. He shares a passion for cars with his father, but his deepest passion is with ancient history and arms used in both ancient and current warfare. He is most guarded in telling of these passions for fear that they will cause disapproval.

Acceptance of his position and a comment about his tee shirt set the stage for a warm and trusting relationship. Bob agreed that he needed to clarify what made him angry, and needed help to overcome his isolation and move on to college.

For a year and a half Bob worked on these issues, and was accepted at a prestigious college. His social life increased through his joining several groups that dealt with the customs and warring behaviors of the ancients. His social network included some peers, but many of the people whose company he enjoyed most were older than he. His parents were pleased with his progress but were still distressed that he did not par-

ticipate as did his younger, athletic brother, with groups of friends closer to his age and more identified with conventional activities.

Bob did not want to terminate his therapy during the first year he went to college. He kept in touch by telephone and letter. Despite some academic shakiness, he finished his first year and entered his second year of college. While on summer break he resumed his regular counseling sessions. It was in the context of discussing dating that Bob came to a session near the end of the summer and told the nurse that there was something he was keeping from therapy: a strong preoccupation and desire to be a woman. In part, he kept this to himself because he knew that to act on it would be devastating to his parents. He loved his parents and was pained by their worry for him and his need to keep his secret. Through his remaining sessions, Bob expressed sadness but was resolute in his decision not to address this issue in therapy. The nurse respected this decision and discussed with him options he might consider in the future. He also knew it would be important to do more focused work on the formative development of his sense of identity in order to better understand the basis of his wish. He relaxed more as he had a place to talk about how he felt. He explained how he wanted long hair to brush and run his fingers through, and how he felt free when imagining himself in women's attire. More importantly, he talked about how, from the age of 4 or 5, he had felt he was in the wrong body.

Bob recognized the paradox of his interests in warrior activity. He was strongly identified with masculine might and roles, yet confused by his strong sense of being the wrong sex.

Bob knows he can continue in therapy if he chooses. He decides that he would rather not. Relieved of the anger and anxiety that plagued him when he began counseling, he has gained confidence and socialized with peers. He finished college; got a job as a librarian; and began graduate work in history.

The clinical import of this case is that when it comes to issues of transsexuality therapists must be cautious in not pushing their own agenda. Patients can choose what and when to discuss their issues in treatment.

O AN OVERVIEW

- Sexual behavior is viewed from a different perspective by the biologist, psychologist, sociologist, and ethicist.

- Gay persons who seek counseling have the same emotional problems for which heterosexual persons seek help. Sexual orientation is seldom the presenting problem, since many gay persons have come to terms with their homosexuality.

- Sexual dysfunction as a disruption of sexual behavior is defined by an identified disturbance in one or more phases of the sexual response cycle (orgasm, excitement, or desire phase disorders), by excessive pain, or by phobic (simple or panic-related) avoidance of sex.

- Sexual dysfunction as an extreme variation of sexual behavior is defined by the object (human or inanimate) that is required for sexual arousal and release or by disregard for the rights and sensitivities of another person.

- Lack of sexual desire is the most common complaint of couples seeking sex counseling. How long the problem has persisted is important in planning care.

- Sexual deviation is an extreme variation in sexual behavior in which there is little or no regard for the welfare of another person.

- Paraphilias are characterized by arousal in response to sexual objects or situations that are not part of normal arousal-activity patterns and that in varying degrees may interfere with the capacity for reciprocal, affectionate sexual activity. The disorders include exhibitionism, fetishism, frotteurism, pedophilia, sexual masochism, sexual sadism, transvestic fetishism, and voyeurism.

- Gender-identity disorder refers to a persistent and powerful identification with the opposite sex, accompanied by a discomfort with one's gender role or identity.

TD TERMS TO DEFINE

- dyspareunia
- gender identity disorder
- orgasm disorders
- paraphilias
- sexual arousal disorders
- sexual aversion disorder
- sexual desire disorders
- sexual deviation
- sexual expression

- sexual pain disorders
- sexual response pattern (Masters and Johnson)
- sexual sabotage

Q STUDY QUESTIONS

1. Masters and Johnson considered the etiology of sexual dysfunction without a medical cause to be
   a. psychological.
   b. learned behavior.
   c. sociological.

2. One of the greatest detriments to sexual expression is
   a. sexual dysfunction
   b. illness
   c. attitude

3. A critical part of nursing assessment for sexual dysfunction is to
   a. interview the patient and partner together.
   b. establish information relevant to any health cause.
   c. establish information relevant to sexual knowledge.

4. DSM-IV classification of sexual dysfunction disorders includes
   a. desire, arousal, orgasm, and pain.
   b. expression, arousal, orgasm, and pain.
   c. orientation, arousal, orgasm, and pain.

5. Evaluation of a sexual aversion should reveal
   a. an underlying panic disorder.
   b. an underlying sexual deviation.
   c. an underlying sexual perversion.

6. Dyspareunia is a
   a. sexual aversion disorder involving avoidance of genital contact with a sexual partner.
   b. sexual pain disorder involving genital pain associated with sexual activity.
   c. sexual arousal disorder encountered during the excitement phase.
   d. sexual desire disorder involving the appetitive phase of sexual relations.

7. Match vocabulary in Column A with its definition in Column B:

COLUMN A	COLUMN B
1. exhibitionism	a. rubbing a nonconsenting person
2. frotteurism	b. sexual preference is a child
3. pedophilia	c. observing unsuspecting persons
4. voyerism	d. exposing one's genitals
5. fetishism	e. arousal by suffering
6. masochism	f. aroused by clothing or objects
7. sadism	g. aroused by being beaten/humiliated
8. autoerotic asphyxia	h. accidental death

8. The paraphilias are characterized by arousal in response to objects or situations that are not normal arousal activity patterns. How are paraphilias like obsessive compulsive disorder?

9. List Money's eight variables of gender.

10. T   F   Hermaphrodites are born with both testicular and ovarian tissue.

11. T   F   Patients choose the topics to be discussed in counseling.

■ REFERENCES

Bailey JM, Pillard R., Neale M, Agyei Y: Factors influencing sexual orientation in women, *Arch Gen Psychiatry* 1993; 50 (3):217–223.

Bass A: Moment of truth: When a child says I'm gay. *Boston Globe,* 1994; July 11, 1994, 20.

Bell AP, Weinberg MS, Hammersmith SK: *Sexual Preference.* Bloomington, Indiana University Press, 1981.

Burgess AW and Holmstrom LL. Rape trauma syndrome, Am J Psychiatry, 131, 1974, 981–986.

Dew RF: *The Family Heart: A Memoir of When Our Son Came Out.* Boston, Addison-Wesley, 1994.

Diamond M. Sexual identity, monozygotic twins reared in discordant sex roles, and a BBC followup, Archives of Sexual Behavior, 11, 181–186.

Freedman M: *Homosexuality: A Changing Picture.* Belmont, CA, Brooks/Cole, 1971.

Gadpaille W: Homosexuality. In Kaplan & Sadock (eds) Textbook of Psychiatry, 1989, Baltimore: Williams and Wilkens.

Hyde JS: *Understanding Human Sexuality.* New York, McGraw Hill, 1990.

Hazelwood RR, Dietz PE, Burgess AW. Autoerotic Fatalities. Lexington, MA: Lexington Books, 1983.

Imperato-McGinley J, Peterson R: Androgens and the evolution of male-gender identity among male pseudohermaphrodites with reductase deficiency. *N Engl J Med* 1979; 300 (22):1233–1237.

Kinsey AC, Pomeroy WB, Martin CE, Gebhard P: *Sexual Behavior in the Human Female,* Philadelphia; WB Saunders, 1953, pp. 468–474.

Kinsey AC, Pomeroy WB, Martin CE: *Sexual Behavior in the Human Male.* Philadelphia; WB Saunders, 1948.

LaBruzza AL: *Using DSM-IV.* Northvale, NJ, Jason Aronson, 1994.

Martin HP: The coming out process for homosexuals. *Hosp Commun Psychiatry* 1991; 42(2):158–162.

Masters WH, Johnson VE: Human Sexuality. Boston, Little Brown, 1966.

Masters WH, Johnson VE, Kolodny RC: Human Sexuality, ed. 2. Boston, Little Brown, 1985.

Money J, Ehrhardt AE: *Man and Woman, Boy and Girl.* Baltimore, Johns Hopkins University Press, 1972.

Money J. Sin, sickness, or status? Homosexual gender identity and psychoneuroendocrinology, Am Psychologist, 42, 384–399.

Small M: The gay debate: Is homosexuality a matter of choice or chance? *American Health,* March, 1993, pp. 70–77.

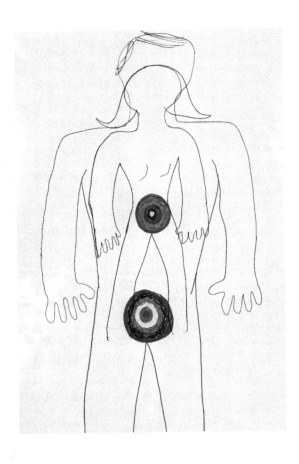

"My anorexia is a form of self-knowledge. People think that anorexics imagine ourselves fat and diet away invisible flab. But people are afraid of the truth: we prefer ourselves this way, boiled down bone, essence . . . I know exactly what I look like, without hyperbole. Every inch of skin, each muscle, each bone. I see where and how they connect. I can name the tendons and the joints. I finger the cartilage. When I eat, I follow the food as it digests, watching the lump of carrot or rice cake diminish, until, finally, elimination."

Stephanie Grant, *The Passion of Alice.*

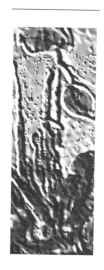

22
Eating Disorders

Ann Wolbert Burgess / Laureen M. Burgess

Eating disorders were first described in the 1870s but were not commonly diagnosed until the 1970s. Since then, between 4 to 8% of the population of the United States, predominately women, has experienced an eating disorder (Kendler et al, 1991). An important factor in the high rate of eating disorders is believed to be our emphasis on beauty and fashion. Women often feel pressured to mirror today's image of the ideal woman, who is thin. This stereotype creates stressors that can lead to guilt and shame and, for some, a pattern of self-harmful dieting behavior. Given these and many other stressors women experience as they strive to be successful in marriage, the workplace, motherhood, and homemaking, some women develop eating disorders in an effort to gain control of their lives.

The primary symptoms of eating disorders are a preoccupation with weight and a strong desire to be thinner, which generally involve a psychological struggle to maintain a sense of personal autonomy and self-control. Although the disorders are classified as psychiatric conditions, considerable morbidity and mortality can arise from the consequent physical problems, many of which are difficult to diagnose in isolation. This is why assessment of the individual patient's psychological condition is important to the development of a successful treatment program for an eating disorder.

The two eating disorders classified in DSM-IV are anorexia nervosa and bulimia nervosa. Binge eating disorder and obesity are not included in the Manual, but are discussed in this chapter along with anorexia nervosa and bulimia nervosa.

■ EPIDEMIOLOGY

Eating disorders are more common in women than men; 90 to 95% of those who have an eating disorder are female. From 1 to 5% of the United States population suffers from anorexia nervosa, and 6 to 18% from bulimia nervosa (Yager 1994). A broader range is estimated for bulimia because this disorder is much easier to hide and may often go undiagnosed. Athletic women are more likely to suffer from one of these disorders, especially those who participate in activities that require "leanness," such as ballet, gymnastics, and long-distance running.

■ ETIOLOGICAL FACTORS AND FAMILY PATTERNS

The multidimensional nature of the eating disorders has made it difficult to determine their precise etiology Since no single cause has been identified, one must understand the interrelationship between biological, psychological, and sociological factors in assessing and treating the patient with an eating disorder.

BIOLOGICAL THEORIES

For many of the biological theories for eating disorders, it is difficult to prove whether physiological responses are triggered by the starvation process or whether they precede, and cause, the disorder.

Hypothalamic Abnormality

A popular theory for eating disorders in women is that a hypothalamic or suprahypothamic abnormality produces: low serum estrogen levels; disturbances in the secretion of follicle-stimulating hormone (FSH), luteinizing hormone (LH), and cortisol; and deviations in opioid and catecholamine metabolism. The problem with this theory is that it is based on data obtained from patients who are already or have nutritional im-

balances. It is a question whether these abnormalities precede the onset of the disorder or result from starvation.

Genetic Basis

There is a division over the theory that the eating disorders have a genetic basis. One position is that a much higher concordance exists between monozygotic twins (50%) than among dizygotic twins (14%) in the incidence of these disorders. Although a familial pattern is seen, studies have not shown to what extent it is influenced by genetic or environmental factors (Yager, 1994).

Relationship to Mood Disorders

The neurobiological origin of mood disorders seems to be strikingly similar to that of eating disorders, especially the bulimic syndromes. Resemblances in neuroendocrine dysfunction, neurotransmitter dysregulation, and patient response to antidepressant medication have shown researchers that a link exists between mood and eating disorders (Laessle, et al., 1988). Moreover, major depression frequently occurs prior to the onset of an eating disorder or after a long remission, suggesting that the two have some psychobiological connection (Pope and Hudson, 1989). Additional supporting factors are a recurrent co-morbidity of affective disturbance withf eating disorders and a greater prevalence of mood disorders in the biological first-degree relatives of patients with bulimia nervosa.

Autointoxication

Exercising and dieting may cause auto-intoxication by endogenous opioids. This produces an altered state of consciousness, which leads to an auto-addiction to internally generated opioids. These opioids can initially produce pleasurable feelings, prompting the individual to try to reproduce this response by repeating the antecedent behaviors.

■ PSYCHOLOGICAL THEORIES

COGNITIVE DISTORTIONS

Socially awkward adolescents may misperceive what others think of their physical appearance. The adolescent at risk for an eating disorder sees their own self-worth on the basis of how they look. Cognitively, they tends to overgeneralize, take things too personally, overmagnify events, and view the world in absolutes.

PERCEPTIVE DISTORTIONS

A greater than normal perceptive distortion about body width may create a sense that the individual is fat, even when she or he is below normal weight. Other perceptual problems have to do with difficulty in identifying various emotional states and hunger/satiety.

MALADAPTIVE STRESS RESPONSES

The individual may react to anxiety by means of an inappropriate "learned" response. In the case of the anorexic individual, the response is a food or weight phobia. For the bulimic individual tension is relieved through excessive eating, which produces a feeling of guilt or shame. As a result, this individual purges herself.

DEVELOPMENTAL CONFLICT

Adolescent discord over "growing up" can lead to regression to a pre-pubertal state. The adolescent is unable to deal with issues such as identity formation, separation from the family, sexual urges, and peer pressures. This manifests itself through difficulty in making decisions and accepting responsibility for actions taken. Often, but not always, this response is preceded by some crisis or significant loss, such as entering high school or college, the onset of puberty, the break-up of a relationship, or the death of a friend or relative.

LOW SELF-ESTEEM

A child may have a weak sense of self for her particular developmental level, such that the only characteristic she likes about herself is her ability to lose weight. This individual may also be taken for granted by parents and attempt to meet their needs at the expense of her own. This weakness may be masked by achievement in such areas as sports or academics.

FAMILIAL FACTORS

In the past, it was believed that family dynamics could cause an eating disorder in an individual. This has not proven to be true. Yet certain parental characteristics, such as over-involvement with the child's life/activities, overprotectiveness, rigid communication patterns, and an avoidance of conflict have tended to be present in some cases. It is hypothesized that parents with these characteristics are seeking fulfillment of their own unresolved dependency issues. In addition, a family history of depression, alcoholism, or chronic dieting may predispose some individuals to an eating disorder.

■ SOCIOLOGICAL THEORIES

Maturational differences between the sexes may be a factor in the development of eating disorders. Girls tend to reach their psychosexual maturation approximately 2 years earlier than boys. Consequently, they must deal with this issue at a young age, with a greater vulnerability to conflict with boys.

Societal ideals are another factor in eating disorders. As noted previously, our society is obsessed with beauty and fashion, resulting in a shift in the cultural standard to steadily decreasing weights for individuals' respective heights.

■ AGE OF ONSET AND COURSE

Eating disorders generally start in adolescence or young adulthood. Patients range in age from 13 to 69 years, although onset is rare after the age of 40. As noted previously, the onset of an eating disorder is generally triggered by a stressful life event.

Approximately 30 to 50% of anorexic patients recover fully within a few years. The prognosis is better if the onset of the condition occurs at a younger age and the anorexia is of the restricting subtype (see the section on anorexia nervosa). The course is variable, comprising a single episode or multiple episodes that end spontaneously or through treatment. For patients with bulimia, the disorder is usually chronic and, if untreated, can last from years to decades. Brief periods of remission can occur, and approximately 40% of patients recover fully.

■ NURSING ASSESSMENT AND DIAGNOSIS

The key to diagnosis and treatment of the eating disorders is recognizing the psychophysiological impact of associated medical and psychological conditions. Assessment of these disorders comprises a thorough history, physical examination, and laboratory studies. The history involves asking the patient questions about her pattern of daily living. Common inquiries concern sleep patterns, weight changes, exercise levels, elimination patterns, meal times and meal frequency, and menstruation history. The tests performed can include physical observations and physiological analyses such as electrolyte levels, endocrine studies, urinalysis, electrocardiograms, evaluations for blood-pressure changes (provided a baseline measurement is available), examination for dental disease, and measurement of the percentage of body fat and of weight changes.

Obesity and **binge-eating,** not classified in DSM-IV as eating disorders, are not consistently associated with behavioral or psychological syndromes. Binge eating has recently been recognized as similar to bulimia nervosa without the purging.

■ ANOREXIA NERVOSA

Anorexia nervosa is a complex disorder involving behavioral, physiological, and psychological changes related to an obsession with thinness. It is characterized by a refusal to maintain the body weight at a minimum normal level for one's age and height, or by maintaining a body weight that is 15% below normal. For children and young adolescents, anorexia is defined as an inability to gain sufficient weight during growth, with a body weight 15% below that expected. This weight loss results in significant physical problems that, left untreated, can lead to death.

In persons with anorexia, eating behaviors such as the following become bizarre in the effort to lose weight:

- A tendency to eat alone.
- The use of unusual spices and food flavorings.
- A low caloric intake (300 to 600 calories per day).
- Excessive, compulsive exercise.
- Avoidance of certain groups of foods.

Anorexic individuals often see themselves as fat even when they are thin, and have an intense fear of weight gain; this fear worsens as they continue to lose weight. Ironically, their obsession with food involves enormous amounts of time spent thinking about and preparing it, without much eating.

Low self-esteem is a common issue for anorexics and is highly dependent on their body shape and weight. Other psychological problems, frequently compounded by drug and alcohol abuse, include depression, emotional lability, erratic behavior and an irritable mood.

Anorexia nervosa can be broken down into two different subtypes: restricting and bulimic. The individual with **restricting anorexia** dramatically limits food intake, is socially withdrawn, and exhibits obsessive and ritualistic behaviors in areas not related to food. The person with **bulimic anorexia** experiences food binges and/or purges by self-induced vomiting or by misusing laxatives, enemas or diuretics. The bulimic anorexic has a higher incidence of comorbid psychiatric conditions and a greater risk of medical problems.

IMPAIRMENTS AND COMPLICATIONS

The physical consequences of anorexia nervosa can include significant morbidity and mortality, with studies reporting 5 to 10% of patients dying within 10 years from starvation, suicide, and electrolyte imbalances (Norman, 1995). The harmful physical effects of the disorder include muscle wasting, bradycardia and other arrhthymias, fat depletion, abdominal pain, constipation, lethargy, leukopenia, osteoporosis, and in severe cases, cachexia and lanugo. All females with prolonged anorexia nervosa stop menstruating and experience alterations in thyroid and reproductive functioning.

Anorexic individuals have a higher incidence (60%) of major depressive disorder, and 20% have diagnoses of anxiety disorder (Normal, 1995). Other psychological impairments are depressed mood, social withdrawal, irritability, insomnia, and a decreased interest in sex. It is unclear whether these symptoms are secondary to the effects of starvation or are attributable to the disorder itself.

TREATMENT

A multidisciplinary approach must be taken to effectively treat anorexia nervosa. The dysfunctional and life-threatening physical problems and psychological disturbances affecting the patient must be addressed along with the behavioral issues surrounding food and exercise. Focusing on one area alone dramatically increases the likelihood of recidivism. (See Table 22–1).

Initially, the patient's physiological needs are met through planning an adequate diet and establishing an eating program. In doing so, the physical problems can begin to be resolved as the negative impact of starvation on cognitive functioning is reduced. However, psychological intervention is also necessary to help the patient consistently meet the basic requirements of nutrition, normal elimination, and safety. Psychodynamically oriented psychotherapy is effective, since it supports the patient and focuses on the attainment of autonomy and self-control. Psychoeducation is also important. It enables patients to understand why an adequate nutritional state helps them to feel better and to have enough energy to deal with the deeper psychological issues associated with overcoming their anorexia disorder.

TABLE 22–1. TREATMENT APPROACH TO ANOREXIA NERVOSA

1. Assess and treat the medical complications of starvation. Determine whether purging is present, and treat for dehydration and electrolyte imbalance as necessary.

2. Decide whether hospitalization is necessary. If dizziness, light-headedness, or fainting from bradycardia or hypotension is reported, if any sign of congestive heart failure is present (including reports of dyspnea on exertion), fluid and electrolyte balance cannot be maintained, excessive exercise presents a risk of congestive heart failure and cannot be monitored safely on an outpatient basis, cognitive impairment from starvation precludes the utility of outpatient psychotherapy, or the patient reports mental exhaustion from battling food and eating issues, hospitalization is essential. Hospitalization is also indicated when reasonable outpatient efforts have failed.

3. Complete laboratory investigation. This includes a full electrolyte profile including potassium, magnesium, calcium and phosphates, glucose, complete blood count (CBC), erythrocyte sedimentation rate (ESR), total protein, albumin, liver function tests, renal function tests, thyroid function tests, iron, folate, B$_{12}$, electrocardiogram (ECG), chest X-ray, and bone-density studies.

4. Restore nutritional balance through normal eating, and encourage weight gain. This often involves setting up a behavior-modification protocol. Low-dose neuroleptics or benzodiazepine-class anxiolytics may be used if fear of weight gain is excessive. Cyproheptadine may be useful to encourage weight gain in cases where weight loss is extreme.

5. Diagnose and treat psychiatric co-morbidity. The presence of affective disorder may warrant the use of antidepressant medications. These medications may not be especially effective when patients are significantly underweight, but may be very effective when weight gain has occurred. Issues stemming from personality disorders should be addressed in psychotherapy.

6. Identify and treat underlying ideas, attitudes, and psychological conflicts. Treat with cognitive and/or psychodynamically based psychotherapy.

7. Assess the family. Utilize family therapy to facilitate support for the patient and to address family dynamics that may be contributing to the patient's development of illness.

8. Provide ongoing support. Support healthy diet and exercise habits, constructive approaches to self, family, and interpersonal problems, enhanced self-esteem, and a sense of autonomy with ongoing psychotherapy.

From: Norman, K: Eating disorders, in Goldman HH (ed): *Review of General Psychiatry*, ed. 4. Stamford, CT; Appleton & Lange, 1995.

Antidepressants can be used for patients with co-morbid psychiatric conditions, but are generally not effective until the individual gains weight. It should be noted that some of these medications do cause weight gain and therefore engender a lower level of compliance in patients to whom they are administered. Certain medications have adverse effects; one is fluoxetine, which tends to cause appetite suppression early in treatment. Bupropin, which can increase seizure susceptibility, should not be given.

For patients who exercise, guidelines must be established. The type, frequency and site of exercise are controlled to prevent physical activity from exceeding the caloric value of the food being consumed. When setting this plan, the psychiatric nurse should also factor in the role of exercise in reducing anxiety and increasing the sense of wellness.

How well a patient complies with the treatment plan for anorexia nervosa is closely connected to the trust relationship developed between the psychiatric nurse and the patient. Because of the nature of the illness, this early relationship will involve some secretive behavior on the patient's part. The following measures help create a safe environment that discourages such behavior:

- Have the patient eat meals in the presence of others.
- Carefully check the eating tray and record what is eaten.

- Have the patient remain in a public area for at least one hour after eating.
- Conduct regular room checks.

This type of environment fosters trust by helping the patient to comply with treatment and enabling the nurse to avoid "spying" on the patient. Nevertheless, some patients view the nurse as a jailer who makes them eat, administers punishment for not eating, and in other ways disrupts their sense of control.

Family therapy may also be needed to help family members better understand and support the patient with anorexia nervosa through recovery. It may also address the family dynamics that have led to the development of this disorder. Ongoing psychotherapy should focus on developing and maintaining healthy eating and exercise habits, positive approaches to the self and to interpersonal problems, and self-esteem and a sense of autonomy.

■ BULIMIA NERVOSA

Patients with bulimia nervosa are predominately weight-preoccupied females who have had major eating binges and purging episodes at least twice a week for 3 consecutive months. The binges involve an uncontrollable consumption of 5,000 to 10,000 calories per episode. These episodes last up to 2 hours and often oc-

E CASE EXAMPLE

▶ ANOREXIA NERVOSA

An 18-year-old high school senior begins dieting to improve her appearance. Her family becomes concerned when she continues to lose weight, her exercising increases, she becomes obsessed with food, ignores her friends, and has her grades plummet from As to Cs and Ds. She begins to have mood swings, and although everyone tells her that she is too thin, she sees herself as severely obese. She resents her family's pressure for her to gain weight and perceives them as controlling and manipulative. Although she tries to continue dieting, she begins to complain that she always feels cold, has trouble sleeping, cannot concentrate, and cannot keep still. When persistent bradycardia develops, with hypotension and episodes of fainting, the patient is hospitalized in a psychiatric unit.

A diagnosis of anorexia nervosa is made. The initial goal of treatment is to counteract the effects of starvation by promoting weight gain and restoring a normal nutritional balance. Two nursing diagnoses are made: a disturbance in self-concept and a fluid-volume deficit (see Figures 22–1 and 22–2). A behavior-modification protocol is implemented and family therapy initiated. In individual therapy the patient reveals that she is frightened about graduating from high school and leaving home to attend college. She has no confidence that she can manage by herself. She worries that her parents, who quarrel constantly, might separate. Her life feels out of control.

She gains weight in the hospital and after discharge continues with individual and family therapy. She goes to a college within 100 miles of home and adjusts quite well.

DSM-IV Diagnosis: Anorexia Nervosa

Nursing Diagnosis: Disturbance in self-concept (low self-esteem).

Related to: (check at least one):
  ___ Lack of positive feedback.
  ___ Preoccupation with appearance and how others perceive them.
  ___ Unmet dependency needs.
  ___ Perceived failures.
  ___ Threat to security secondary to dysfunctional family dynamics.

Short-Term Outcome: Patient will verbalize three positive aspects of self and exhibiting decreased preoccupation with own appearance.

Long-Term Outcomes: 1. Patient will verbalize five positive aspects of self.
              2. Patient will express interest in welfare of others and decreased preoccupation with own appearance.

Interventions:

Date   Date
Planned   Discontinued
_____   _____   1. Assist patient to recognize positive attributes.
_____   _____   2. Offer positive reinforcement for independent decision making (i.e., verbal praise, encouragement, increased privileges).
_____   _____   3. Offer positive reinforcement when honest feelings related to autonomy/dependency issues remain separated from maladaptive eating behaviors (i.e., increased privileges, verbal praise and encouragement).
_____   _____   4. Assist patient to develop a realistic perception of body image and relationship with food.
_____   _____   5. Promote feelings of control within the environment through participation, independent decision making, and offering reasonable choices whenever possible.
_____   _____   6. Help patient realize that perfection is unrealistic, and explore this need.
_____   _____   7. Teach patient to claim angry feelings and to recognize that expressing them is acceptable if done so in an appropriate manner.

(Adapted from Nursing Care Plans developed by Nursing Staff at 1st Hospital Wyoming Valley, Wilkes Barre, PA under the direction of Theresa M. Croushore.)

Figure 22–1. Nursing pathway plan of care.

DSM-IV Diagnosis: Anorexia Nervosa.

Nursing Diagnosis: Fluid volume deficit (actual or potential).

Related to (check at least one):
_____ Decreased fluid intake.
_____ Excessive use of diuretics.
_____ Self-induced vomiting.
_____ Electrolyte and/or acid/base imbalance.
_____ Excessive use of laxatives or enemas.

Short-Term Outcome: Patient will exhibit no signs and symptoms of dehydration by discharge.

Long-Term Outcomes: 1. Vital signs, blood pressure, laboratory serum studies are within normal limits.
2. Patient verbalizes knowledge about consequences of fluid loss due to self-induced vomiting.

Interventions:

Date   Date
Planned   Discontinued
_____   _____   1. Input and output.
_____   _____   2. Teach patient importance of daily fluid intake of 2000 to 3000 ml.
_____   _____   3. Daily weights immediately upon arising and following first voiding.
_____   _____   4. Assess and document condition of skin turgor and any changes in skin integrity.
_____   _____   5. Teach patient to avoid using hot water and soap when bathing if skin is very dry.
_____   _____   6. Monitor laboratory serum values and notify physician of significant changes.
_____   _____   7. Observe patient 1 hour after eating.
_____   _____   8. Assess and document moistness and color of oral mucous membranes.
_____   _____   9. Encourage frequent oral care.
_____   _____   10. Assist patient in identifying true feelings and fears that contribute to maladaptive eating behaviors.
_____   _____   11. Other _____

(Adapted from Nursing Care Plans developed by Nursing Staff at 1st Hospital Wyoming Valley, Wilkes Barre, PA under the direction of Theresa M. Croushore.)

Figure 22–2. Nursing Pathway Plan of Care

cur one or more times a day. Immediately prior to a binge, the individual has dysphoric mood, interpersonal stress, or intense hunger that is temporarily relieved during the binge. Yet shortly after the binge ends, the depressed mood returns, along with feelings of guilt and shame.

The two subtypes of bulimia are **purging** and **non-purging.** Individuals with purging bulimia use self-induced vomiting or laxatives or diuretics to rid themselves of what they eat. Vomiting is the most common method selected for purging, and usually occurs at least once a day. Eventually, the individual becomes skilled enough to vomit at will. Laxatives are taken to reduce or maintain weight, and the majority of individuals who use them take about 18 pills a day. The most widely used laxatives are Senokot, Correctol, and Ex-Lax, because they act rapidly and are easy to purchase. Diuretics are taken by up to one-third of individuals with purging bulimias; diuretics are also easy to buy. Individuals with non-purging bulimia exercise excessively or fast instead of purging.

Typical behavior involves avoiding social eating situations, secretive eating, compulsive exercise, disap-

pearance after meals, and unrelenting over-concern about weight and body shape.

IMPAIRMENTS AND COMPLICATIONS

Seventy-five percent of persons with bulimia have a concurrent major depressive or anxiety disorder (Yager, 1994). They also experience high rates of chemical dependency and personality disorders. The situation for a bulimic individual can often be dire, as significant morbidity and mortality exist and the disorder is not easily detected. The resultant physical problems are difficult to diagnose, because they are generally nonspecific and sometimes linked to psychogenic problems. Yet knowledge of the multitude of physical symptoms can aid the practitioner in the diagnosis and treatment of bulimia.

The physical problems of bulimia include:

- **Fluid and electrolyte abnormalities.** Fluid abnormalities stem from the volume depletion that occurs with the frequent diarrhea, diuresis, and vomiting in purging bulimia. As a result, arterial and venous blood pressure can be lowered. Metabolic acidosis from diuretic and laxative abuse, or alkalosis from excessive vomiting, can also occur. The most common electrolyte imbalance involves bicarbonate ($HCO3^-$). Such an imbalance can reduce the seizure threshold, causing more frequent seizures in those already prone to such attacks.

- **Gastrointestinal tract problems.** Repeated laxative abuse can lead to cathartic colitis, which is manifested in constipation, bloating, and lower abdominal pain. Stimulant-type laxatives can trigger bleeding, which, if chronic, can lead to anemia.
- **Dental enamel erosion and decay.** Those persons with bulimia who induce vomiting may develop dental disease (Clark, 1985). Highly acidic vomitus erodes the teeth, resulting in lost enamel and diminished dentine sensitivity to temperature and foods. This symptom can often be an early indicator of bulimic behavior. In addition, a patient who has halitosis with a stomach-acid odor may be bulimic instead of neglectful of hygiene.
- **Parotid and salivary gland hypertrophy.** Painless swelling of the cheeks, along with painless parotid and salivary gland enlargement, may be seen in patients with bulimia.

Many bulimic patients deny their physical problems to avoid detection, and the outward signs of this disorder are much less obvious than those of anorexia nervosa. Bulimia is an insidious disorder, and can often go undetected for long periods. The health-care professional must be knowledgeable about the nature of this disorder and how it manifests itself physically so that the appropriate diagnostic tests can be ordered, and the disorder can be effectively diagnosed.

TREATMENT

The treatment program for bulimia nervosa is similar to that for anorexia nervosa, with medical complications being treated first, followed by psychoeducation about the detrimental effects of purging, diagnosis and treatment of co-morbid conditions, and utilization of psychotherapy to help change attitudes and behavior (see Table 22–1 and 22–2). The most encouraging reports of treatment success in bulimia nervosa come from studies using pharmacological therapies. Antidepressant therapy has shown dramatic efficacy, with a patient response ranging from decreased binging and purging to complete remission. The psychotherapeutic approach with a strong success rate is cognitive behavioral therapy. The patient focuses on the thoughts and feelings that precede binge/purging behavior and on a change in attitude with respect to body shape and weight. A useful tool in treatment is a food diary, which is used to track what has been eaten and what feelings were present prior to, during, and after eating. By keeping a diary, the patient learns to identify what triggers bulimic behavior and eventually learns how to cope with it.

■ OBESITY

A person weighing at least 20% above ideal weight, as listed in standard height and weight tables, is defined as obese. One subgroup of obesity is defined by emotionally based patterns of overeating. For these individuals, dieting creates substantial biological and psychosocial stress, which can cause agitation, irritability, and emotional reactivity.

TABLE 22–2. TREATMENT APPROACHES TO BULIMIA NERVOSA

1. Evaluate and treat the medical complications associated with bulimia nervosa. Replace fluid and electrolytes as necessary. Monitor electrolytes on a regular basis. Refer for dental evaluation.

2. Ascertain the mechanism of purging. Educate patients about the medical dangers of chemical purgatives such as ipecac and baking soda, as well as of diuretic and laxative abuse.

3. Hospitalize when necessary. If fluid and electrolyte balance cannot be maintained, episodes of fainting occur, concentration impairment makes employment or schoolwork impossible to perform, or binge eating and purging behavior are the dominant activities in the patient's life, a brief hospitalization is necessary to break the cycle and initiate treatment.

4. Diagnose and treat co-morbidity. The presence of an affective disorder is an indication for treatment with an antidepressant medication if such treatment has not already been initiated on the basis of bulimic symptoms alone. Indeed, a trial of antidepressant medication is generally indicated for bulimia nervosa and is often effective even in the absence of concurrent affective disorder. Issues pertaining to personality disorders, when present, should be addressed in psychotherapy.

5. Identify and address psychological and cognitive underpinnings of bulimic behavior. Psychodynamically oriented and cognitive behavior therapy that addresses attitudes and feelings related to self and body images are effective treatment modalities. Such treatments may be especially effective for many patients when combined with antidepressant medications. Support groups are also often helpful in the treatment of bulimia nervosa.

From: Norman, K: Eating disorders, In Goldman HH (ed): *Review of General Psychiatry*, ed. 4. Stamford, CT; Appleton & Lange, 1995.

E CASE EXAMPLE

► BULIMIA NERVOSA

A 22-year-old woman is admitted to the emergency department following 3 days of binge eating and vomiting. Her symptoms began when she was a college freshman and she was worried that she was too heavy. She went on a diet with her roommate, who suggested vomiting after meals.

The patient reports bingeing three or four times a week, usually in the evening and always when alone. She usually feels depressed and anxious when the urge to binge overcomes her. She typically binges on sweets and breads. It is not unusual for her to eat half a gallon of ice cream, a box of cookies, and a loaf of bread during a binge, which typically lasts 30 to 45 minutes. Eating gives her relief from her depression, and she reports sensations of warmth, safety, security, and unconditional acceptance when eating. She ends her binges with her stomach aching, and feels guilty after vomiting. She takes large doses of laxatives daily and occasionally uses diuretics. She

spends up to $60 on a single binge and reports stealing food from grocery stores. She tells of having superficially cut her wrists on two occasions. She was brought to the emergency department by her concerned roommate.

Two nursing diagnoses are provided for this patient (see Figures 21–3 and 21–4), and include alterations in nutrition and ineffective individual coping. The patient is admitted to an inpatient unit, where her weight and eating are stabilized. On an outpatient basis she begins individual psychotherapy and attends a support group for women with bulimia. Her symptoms improve in the first 6 months of treatment, with the frequency of binges dropping to once a week. A trial dose of fluoxetine is begun which results in complete remission of the patient's binge eating and purging behavior. She continues in therapy to better understand her eating disorder and to work on some long-standing problems related to low self-esteem and difficulty in social relationships (Norman, 1995).

DSM-IV Diagnosis: Bulimia Nervosa.

Nursing Diagnosis: Ineffective individual coping.

Related to (check at least one): identify problem list number.
_____ Unfulfilled tasks of trust
_____ Excessive overeating, followed by vomiting.
_____ Self induced vomiting and/or abuse of laxatives.
_____ Dysfunctional family system.
_____ Laxatives and diuretics.
_____ Refusal to eat.
_____ Obsession with food.
_____ Feelings of helplessness and lack of control.
_____ Low self esteem.
_____ Chronic depression.

Short Term Outcome: Patient will verbalize three adaptive coping mechanisms that can be realistically used in his/her life by discharge.
Long Term Outcomes: 1.   Patient will accurately assess three maladaptive coping behaviors.
                      2.   Patient will be able to utilize five adaptive coping strategies that can be utilized in the home environment.

Intervention:

Date Planned	Date Discontinued	
_____	_____	1. Establish a trusting relationship with patient by being honest and accepting.
_____	_____	2. Acknowledge patient's anger and feelings of loss of control.
_____	_____	3. When nutritional status has improved, explore feelings associated with fears of gaining weight.
_____	_____	4. Explore family dynamics (i.e., assist patient to identify specific concerns within family structure and ways to relieve those concerns).
_____	_____	5. Discuss with patient the importance of patient's separation of self as an individual within the family system.
_____	_____	6. Initially, allow patient to maintain dependent role.
_____	_____	7. Encourage independence in self-care activities as trust is developed and physical condition improves.
_____	_____	8. Offer positive reinforcement for independent behavior and problem solving/decision making. (i.e., increased privileges, verbal praise, encouragement.)
_____	_____	9. Explore with patient ways in which she/he may feel control within the environment without resorting to maladaptive eating behaviors.
_____	_____	10. Other: _____

(Adapted from Nursing Care Plans developed by Nursing Staff at 1st Hospital Wyoming Valley, Wilkes Barre, PA under the direction of Theresa M. Croushore.)

Figure 22–3. Nursing Pathway Plan of Care

DSM-IV Diagnosis: Bulimia

Nursing Diagnosis: Alteration in nutrition: less than body requirements.

Related to: (check at least one):
_____ Refusal to eat.
_____ Ingestion of large amounts of food, followed by self-induced vomiting.
_____ Abuse of laxatives, diuretics, diet pills.
_____ Physical exertion in excess of energy produced through caloric intake.
_____ Loss of 15% expected body weight.

Short Term Outcome: Patient will exhibit no signs or symptoms of malnutrition by discharge.

Long Term Outcome: 1. Patient verbalizes importance of adequate nutrition.
                      2. Blood pressure, vital signs, laboratory serum studies are within normal limits.
                      3. Patient has achieved and maintained at least 90% of expected body weight.

Interventions:

Date Planned	Date Discontinued	
_____	_____	1. In collaboration with dietician, determine number of calories required to provide adequate nutrition and realistic weight gain.
_____	_____	2. Prescribed behavior-modification program as outlined by treatment team; explain details of program to patient (i.e., contingencies, rewards, consequences. (Identify)
_____	_____	3. Sit with patient during mealtime for support and to observe amount ingested.
_____	_____	4. Reasonable limit time allotted for meals (i.e., 30 minutes).
_____	_____	5. Observe patient for at least 1 hour after meals.
_____	_____	6. Input and output.
_____	_____	7. Daily weights immediately upon arising and following first voiding.
_____	_____	8. Once protocol has been established, do not discuss food/eating with patient.
_____	_____	9. Offer support and additional reinforcement for improvements in eating behaviors. (i.e., verbal praise, encouragement, increased privileges.)
_____	_____	10. Explore the feelings of fear associated with gaining weight, until nutritional status improves and eating habits are established.
_____	_____	11. If patient is unable or unwilling to maintain adequate intake, notify physician of patient's status and carry out physician's orders. (i.e., transfer to medical facility).

(Adapted from Nursing Care Plans developed by Nursing Staff at 1st Hospital Wyoming Valley, Wilkes Barre, PA under the direction of Theresa M. Croushore.)

Figure 22–4. Nursing Pathway Plan of Care

EPIDEMIOLOGY

Estimates are that 15 to 50% of the population of the United States is obese. The prevalence of obesity increases with age up to age 50, when the rate drops off sharply because of an increased mortality rate. More women are obese than men, and 25% of children are significantly overweight. Socio-economic, ethnic, and religious backgrounds can be related to the development of obesity. Persons in lower socioeconomic classes tend to have a greater likelihood of being obese. Certain ethnic groups and religious groups, have a higher prevalence of obesity, and research is needed to further clarify this observation (Norman, 1995).

ETIOLOGICAL FACTORS AND FAMILY PATTERNS

High rates of obesity occur in adolescents with obese parents; as many as 80% of obese adolescents have two obese parents. Twin studies suggest a genetic influence in such obesity, but environmental factors are present as well.

Weight studies indicate that there is a biological "set point" for body weight. For obese individuals who are dieting, their weight-loss efforts work against the natural biological processes that maintain their bodies at a certain weight. Weight gain is seen through an increase in the numbers of fat cells or in the size of these cells. The number of fat cells in the body cannot be reduced; only the size of the fat cell can decrease. It is believed that even fat cells have a set point that determines their "natural" size. Because of this, weight gain tends to stop once an individual's fat cells have reached the normal size.

Persons who experience juvenile-onset obesity have a greater-than-normal number of fat cells. Adult-onset obesity is usually connected with a normal number of larger-sized fat cells. Children experience two periods of cellular proliferation: from birth to 2 years of age and from 10 to 14 years of age. Many obese children have a longer initial period of cell growth.

Other possible etiological factors in obesity include anomalies in triglyceride metabolism; disturbances within the central and peripheral nervous systems; disturbances in chemical regulators of appetite; and unresolved dependency needs that are fixated at the oral level of psychosexual development.

AGE OF ONSET AND COURSE

Obesity can develop at any time from childhood to adulthood. The amount of body fat increases with age, even when an individual's weight is kept constant. The course of obesity is usually chronic and progressive.

The odds of a person's losing excess weight and keeping it off are not good. If obese children do not reach a normal weight by the end of adolescence, the chances are poor that they'll ever reach such a weight.

Mortality increased by about 90% occurs for severely obese individuals (50% greater weight than the ideal weight for height). This is not true for persons who are moderately obese, weighing up to only 30% over their ideal weight.

IMPAIRMENTS AND COMPLICATIONS

Complications of obesity are numerous, and range from psychological disturbances to physical impairments. Some of the psychological problems experienced are major depression, anxiety disorders, social phobias, and drug/alcohol abuse problems. These problems sometimes result from the conditions that precede its onset.

Generally, the physical impairments that result from obesity are low back pain, huge calluses on the feet, aggravated osteoarthritis, amenorrhea, increased sweating, impaired heat loss, edema in the hands and feet, intertrigo in tissue folds, a reduced respiratory capacity, and dyspnea upon exertion. Other associated medical conditions include diabetes mellitus, hypertension, renal dysfunction, pulmonary disorders, and cardiovascular disease. Surgery, anesthesia, and pregnancy pose additional risks for obese persons.

NURSING ASSESSMENT AND DIAGNOSIS

Assessment of the obese patient involves measurement of the patient's weight along with measures of body fat. Other medical conditions that cause this condition, such as hypothyroidism, need to be ruled out.

TREATMENT

Obesity is treated similarly to the eating disorders. The medical conditions accompanying the condition need to be assessed and treated. A diet and exercise program is established. Any co-morbid psychiatric conditions, such as binge eating and anxiety disorders, should be treated with antidepressants and cognitive behavioral therapy. Appetite suppressants may be given and, as a last resort, surgery involving intestinal bypass and gastric stapling may have to be performed.

■ BINGE EATING

Binge eating is a newly recognized medical condition that involves recurrent episodes of uncontrollable eating in which the inappropriate compensatory behaviors characteristic of bulimia are usually absent. This behavior typically involves the binge consumption of about 20,000 calories in less than 2 hours. It must occur at least twice a week for a 6 month period to be classified as binge eating.

The binge-eating process entails eating rapidly, even when not hungry, until uncomfortably full, and then experiencing shame and guilt after the binge. Binge eaters often eat alone to prevent embarrassment over the quantity of food they consume.

EPIDEMIOLOGY

From 23 to 46% of persons in weight-control programs have binge-eating problems. Women are one-and-one-half times more likely to suffer from this condition than men. Estimates of the United States population that eats in binges vary from 0.7 to 4%. Approximately 36% of young adults engage in some sort of binge eating (Norman 1995).

ETIOLOGICAL FACTORS AND FAMILY PATTERNS

The etiologic factors related to binge eating have not yet been determined. What is known is that the binge is often triggered by a dysphoric mood, depression, or anxiety. Some binge eaters do not have any precipitant feelings, but find some relief of tension from a binge-eating episode.

IMPAIRMENTS AND COMPLICATIONS

Persons who have the pattern of binge eating reach varying degrees of obesity. They often have a long history of dieting with minimal success. Their eating problems tend to interfere with relationships, work, and the ability to feel good about themselves. Other impairments include weight gain and an increased risk of high blood pressure, heart attack, stroke, diabetes; bone and joint problems; and some cancers.

NURSING ASSESSMENT AND DIAGNOSIS

Like bulimia nervosa, binge eating is difficult to assess. The binge eater can easily hide the problem from others, and may not have any serious complications that warrant immediate medical attention. A thorough interview of the patient's daily patterns, along with an examination to identify resultant medical conditions, will aid in uncovering the problem.

TREATMENT

The best approach to treating binge eating involves cognitive behavioral therapy, and for some patients, antidepressants. The nurse must work with the patient to re-establish regular eating habits and promote the keeping of an eating journal like those used in treating bulimia nervosa. As with the other eating disorders, the medical conditions and co-morbid psychiatric conditions accompanying obesity need to be treated as well as the primary disorder.

O AN OVERVIEW

- The psychiatric eating disorders, anorexia nervosa and bulimia nervosa, have been seen in 4-8% of the United States population since they began to be commonly diagnosed in the 1970s. That eating disorders occur predominantly in women is not a surprising finding, given modern western society's emphasis on thinness as the ideal female body image.

- The primary symptoms of eating disorders are a preoccupation with weight and a strong desire to be thin, which generally involve a psychological struggle to maintain a sense of personal autonomy and self-control.

- Because no single cause of the eating disorders has been identified, it is important to understand the relationship between biological, psychological, and sociological factors when assessing and treating patients with these disorders.

- Nursing assessment and diagnosis of the eating disorders centers on recognition of the psychophysiological impact of related medical and psychological conditions.

- In treatment, the patient's physiological needs are met first. Once the negative effects of starvation on cognitive functioning have been reduced, early psychological interventions, such as psychoeducation and psychotherapy, can begin.

- Anorexia nervosa is characterized by refusal to maintain body weight at a minimum normal level for one's age and height (i.e., body weight 15% below normal), and has two subtypes: restricting and bulimic.

- Bulimia nervosa involves episodes of binge eating in which 5,000 to 10,000 calories may be consumed; the aftermath of these episodes differs by bulimic subtype. In purging bulimia, self-induced vomiting, laxatives, or diuretics are used to purge the food from the body. Excessive exercise and fasting characterize non-purging bulimia.

- Obesity and binge eating are medically recognized eating conditions; however, the *DSM IV* does not classify them as eating disorders because they are not consistently associated with behavioral or psychological syndromes.

TD TERMS TO DEFINE

- anorexia nervosa
- binge eating
- bulimia nervosa
- bulimic anorexia
- non-purging bulimia
- obesity
- purging
- purging bulimia
- restricting anorexia

Q STUDY QUESTIONS

1. The rate of recovery from eating disorders is generally
   a. 80 to 100%.
   b. 50 to 80%.
   c. 30 to 50%.
   d. less than 30%.

2. Which family characteristic increases the risk of an individual developing an eating disorder?
   a. History of depression
   b. Chronic dieting patterns
   c. History of alcoholism
   d. All of the above
   e. None of the above.

3. Describe the signs and symptoms of bulimia nervosa and explain why it is referred to as the "most insidious" of eating disorders.

4. T F   The restricting anorexic experiences food binges and/or purges by self-induced vomiting or with the misuse of laxatives and diuretics.

5. T F   Anorexic individuals have a better prognosis for recovery if they are of the restricting subtype and develop it at a young age.

6. Which of the following statements about obesity is considered true?
   a. Men suffer from obesity more than women.
   b. Approximately 50% of children are classified as obese.
   c. Certain ethnic groups exhibit a higher prevalence of obesity.
   d. The prognosis of someone losing excess weight and keeping it off is good.

7. How is binge eating different from bulimia?

8. T F People who are binge eaters often reach varying degrees of obesity.

9. Discuss the benefits of keeping an eating journal for patients with eating disorders, especially bulimics and binge eaters.

■ REFERENCES

American Psychiatric Association: Diagnostic and Statistical Manual, 4th ed. Washington, DC: American Psychiatric Press, 1994.

Beumong PJV: A comprehensive, multidisciplinary approach for the management of patients with anorexia nervosa, in Touya SW, Beumont PJV (eds): *Eating Disorders: Prevalence and Treatment.* Sydney, Williams & Wilkins, 1985, pp. 11-22.

Clark DC: Oral complications of anorexia nervosa and/or bulimia with a review of the literature. *J Oral Med* 1985; 40:134-138.

Hofland SL, Dardis PO: Bulimia Nervosa—Associated Physical Problems. *J Psychosoc Nurs,* 1992; 30(2):23–27.

Irwin EG: A focused overview of anorexia nervosa and bulimia. I: Etiological issues. *Arch Psychiatr Nurs* 1993; 7(6):342–346.

Irwin EG: A Focused Overview of Anorexia Nervosa and Bulimia: Part II—Challlenges to the Practice of Psychiatric Nursing. *Arch Psychiatr Nurs* 1993; 7(6):347–352.

Kendler KS, MacLean C, Neale M, Kessler R, Heath A, Eaves L: The genetic epidemiology of bulimia nervosa. *Am J Psychiatry* 1991; 52:464–471.

Laessle RG, Schweiger U, Fichter MM, Pirke KM: Eating disorders and depression: Psychobiological findings in bulimia and anorexia nervosa, in Prike KM, Vandereycken W, Ploog D (eds): *The Psychobiology of Bulimia Nervosa.* Berlin, Springer-Verlag, 1988, pp. 90–100.

Michielli DW, Dunbar CC, Kalinski MI: Is Exercise Indicated for the Patient Diagnosed as Anorectic? *J Psychosoc Nurs* 1994; 32(8):33-35.

Norman K: Eating Disorders, in Goldman HH (ed): *Review of General Psychiatry,* ed. 4. Stamford, CT: Appleton & Lange, 1995, pp. 355–367.

Pope HG, Hudson JI: Eating disorders, in Kaplan H, Sadock BJ (eds): Comprehensive textbook of psychiatry/V. Baltimore, Williams & Wilkins, 1989; pp. 1854–1864.

Tunick B. When food is the enemy. *First for Women,* 1996; 8(5):106–111.

Yager J: Eating Disorders. In Stoudemire A (ed): *Clinical Psychiatry for Medical Students,* ed. 2. Philadelphia, JB Lippincott, 1994, pp. 355–371.

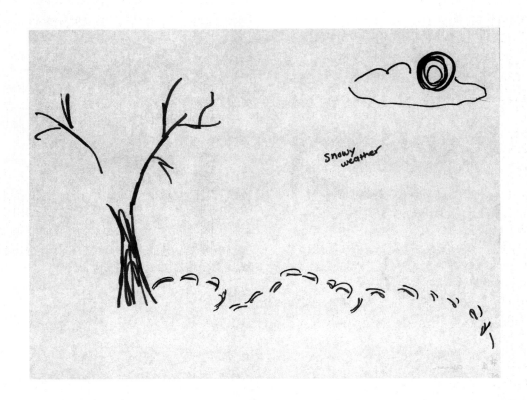

snowy weather

Huge and mighty forms that do not live
Like living men, moved slowly through the mind
By day, and were a trouble to my dreams.

William Wordsworth (1770–1850)

The Tables Turned

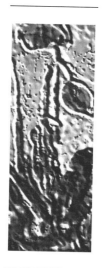

23
Sleep Disorders
Carole-Rae Reed

People spend nearly one third of their lives sleeping. A human behavior that is under both conscious and autonomic control, sleep is sensitive to physiological, pathological, behavioral, and environmental changes. It is well established in the research literature that sleep is affected in most psychiatric disorders, as well as in numerous medical conditions. Sleep may be further compromised by the effects of medications and environmental conditions.

Sleep disturbances are associated with numerous mental disorders. The psychiatric nurse must have an understanding of sleep, sleep-related phenomena, sleep hygiene, sleep disorders, and the relationship between disturbed sleep and psychiatric illness in order to provide optimum care and patient education in inpatient and outpatient settings.

This chapter includes a tool that nurses may use to perform an in-depth assessment of sleep history. In addition, sleep-related symptoms and phenomena are defined, and nursing diagnoses and interventions related to sleep are discussed. The chapter concludes with a summary of sleep disorders described in the (DSM-IV) along with specific sleep alterations associated with selected mental disorders.

■ OVERVIEW OF NORMAL SLEEP

Behaviorally, sleep is defined as "a reversible behavioral state of perceptual disengagement from and unresponsiveness to the environment" (Carskadon and Dement, 1994, p. 16). Physiologically, sleep is "a state of active, heterogeneous, neurophysiological functioning, synchronized with the light-dark cycle of the environment and characterized by the cycling of the stages of sleep throughout the sleep period" (Shaver and Giblin, 1989, p. 73).

STAGES

Sleep is a human behavior that is currently measurable by direct means (polysomnography). Sleep can be divided into separate and distinct stages and sub-stages based on physiological parameters.

Non-Rapid Eye Movement Sleep

Non-rapid eye movement (NREM) sleep is conceptualized as involving a "relatively inactive yet actively regulating brain in a moveable body" (Carskadon and Dement, 1994, p. 16). NREM sleep may be divided into four sub-stages representing a continuum of depths of sleep: Stage 1 represents the lowest arousal threshold (or lightest sleep) and Stage 4 represents the highest arousal threshold (or deepest sleep). NREM stages 3 and 4 are often referred to as slow-wave sleep, or delta sleep, due to the characteristic delta waves seen on electroencephalograms (EEGs) during these stages.

Rapid Eye Movement Sleep

Rapid eye movement sleep (REM) is conceptualized in terms of a "highly activated brain in a paralyzed body" (Carskadon and Dement, 1994, p. 17). The mental activity of REM sleep is associated with dreaming. REM sleep is characterized by EEG activation, muscle atonia, and episodic bursts of rapid eye movements.

SLEEP CYCLE

Onset of human sleep normally occurs with the NREM stage. Sleep usually proceeds through NREM stages 1 through 4 and then progresses to REM sleep. NREM and REM sleep alternate throughout the sleep period in a cyclic fashion, with episodes of REM increasing in duration as sleep progresses. NREM stages 3 and 4 usually become shorter in the second cycle of sleep and may be absent from later cycles (Carskadon and Dement, 1994).

Carskadon and Dement (1994) provided the following general description of the normal young-adult sleep cycle:

- Sleep is entered through NREM sleep.
- NREM sleep and REM sleep alternate within a period near 90 minutes.
- Slow-wave sleep predominates in the first third of the night and is linked to the initiation of sleep.
- REM sleep predominates in the last third of the night and is linked to the circadian rhythm of body temperature.
- Wakefulness within sleep usually accounts for less than 5% sleep time.
- NREM Stage 1 sleep generally comprises about 2 to 5% of sleep.
- Stage 2 sleep generally comprises about 45 to 55% of sleep.
- Stage 3 sleep generally comprises about 3 to 8% of sleep.
- Stage 4 sleep generally comprises about 10 to 15% of sleep.
- NREM sleep, therefore, is usually 75 to 85% of sleep.
- REM sleep usually comprises 15 to 25% of sleep, occurring in four to six discrete episodes.

SLEEP AND AGING

According to Carskadon and Dement (1994, p. 21) "The strongest and most consistent factor affecting the pattern of sleep stages across the night is age." The following generalizations can be made about sleep and aging; however, numerous factors can affect a person's sleep. Individuals, therefore, may vary greatly in their sleep patterns and still be normal. The sleep of children, depending on their age, is very different from that of adults, and is not addressed in this chapter.

- The capacity to initiate sleep at any time of the day is greatly diminished after the age of 25 years (Zarcone, 1994).
- The number and length of awakenings during the night increases with age, dramatically so after age 45 years (Zarcone, 1994). This is true of both conscious and transient (those of which the individual is unaware) arousals (Carskadon, Brown, and Dement, 1982).
- It is a myth that older people need less sleep, but with age there may be changes in the sleep-wake pattern or sleep architecture. Some of these changes may reflect an age-related change in circadian rhythm.
- The incidence of sleep apnea increases with middle age in men, and after menopause in women.

- A progressive reduction and sometimes disappearance of Stages 3 and 4 sleep (deepest NREM levels) occurs during old age, especially in men (Carskadon and Dement, 1994; Bliwise, 1994).
- The percentage of Stage 1 sleep increases greatly during old age (Bliwise, 1994).
- Periodic leg movements (PLMs) during sleep may be more frequent in the elderly.
- Napping is common in the elderly, and may be beneficial (Evans and Rogers, 1994). (Hauri and Linde, 1990; Zarcone, 1994).

MEASURING SLEEP

The Polysomnogram

Polysomnographic recordings are used to objectively measure human sleep in sleep-disorder centers and laboratories. Polysomnographs monitor and record brain-wave activity during sleep, as well as eye movements, chin movements, leg movements, breathing, and heart rate. Oxygenation is usually measured simultaneously through a pulse oximeter placed on one finger. A small video camera allows the technician to watch the patient sleep; this may be recorded on videotape. As with any procedure, patients must be thoroughly informed about what will be done during polysomnography and must give their consent to it.

Conductive paste and small electrodes (about a quarter-inch in diameter) are placed on the patient's head; with two being placed under the chin, one beside each eye, one above the nose, one behind each ear, and two on the top of the head. These scalp electrodes are attached with collodion-soaked gauze and dried with compressed air. Other electrodes, similar to those used for electrocardiograms, are attached to both legs to record leg movements and to the chest to record heart rate. Thermistors may be placed near the mouth or bands may be placed around the chest to record breathing. The wires from the various electrodes are gathered into a bundle to prevent tangling, and lead to a single plug that may easily be unplugged when the patient wants to get up and go to the bathroom. Most patients do not find the equipment for polysomnography uncomfortable or disruptive to sleep. The patient is usually asked to arrive at the sleep laboratory at least an hour prior to his or her normal bedtime, and is usually allowed to go to bed at his or her normal time and to awaken spontaneously. If the sleep study is being recorded as part of a research project, it is customary to set aside at least one adaptation night to allow the patient to adjust to the laboratory setting. Only data collected on subsequent nights are used in the research. For a clinical sleep study, one night may be sufficient.

After the **polysomnogram** is recorded it must be scored, or staged. Computerized scoring systems are available, or the polysomnogram may be hand-scored. Rechtschaffen and Kales' (1968) criteria are the accepted standard method for staging sleep, that is, determining when a particular stage of sleep begins and the length of time spent in each stage. It is important to stage sleep, regardless of the reason for a sleep study, because physiological regulatory systems are state-dependent (Carskadon and Rechtschaffen, 1994). For example, body-temperature-regulating responses are barely altered during NREM sleep, but are almost totally lacking during REM sleep (Carskadon and Rechtschaffen, 1994).

Standard polysomnographic calculations include sleep continuity, sleep architecture, and REM measures. The following list of measurements is based on Rechtschaffen and Kales' (1968) scoring method. Although some controversy surrounds how best to calculate certain measures, this list is useful in understanding terminology. It may also help nurses better interpret published sleep research (Different researchers or sleep laboratories may use slightly different calculations or criteria.)

- Sleep Continuity Measures
  1. Total Period Recorded: the total time from the start to the end of polysomnographic recording.
  2. Sleep Latency: the time period from lights out to onset of the first cycle of Stage II sleep.
  3. Sleep Period Time: the length of time between sleep latency and wake-up at the end of the total recording period.
  4. Time Spent Asleep: the difference between sleep period time and time awake; also referred to as total sleep time.
  5. Sleep Efficiency: the time spent asleep divided by the total recording period.
  6. Awake Percentage: the waking time divided by the sleep period time.
- Sleep Architecture. There are five measures of sleep architecture, each of which is expressed as the percentage of sleep time spent in that stage (number of minutes in the stage divided by time spent asleep). The stages are NREM 1,2,3,4, and REM.
- REM Measures.
  1. REM Latency. This is the period of time from sleep onset to the start of the first REM period.
  2. Number of REM Periods. This is the number of REM periods noted throughout the total recording period. There are usually three to five REM periods in a normal recording.

3. REM Percentage. This is also a measure of sleep architecture, and consists of the total percent of time spent in REM sleep throughout the time spent asleep.
4. REM Activity. This is the total number of rapid eye movements during sleep.
5. REM Density. This measures the total eye movements during sleep, and is calculated by dividing REM activity by the total REM time in minutes.
6. Average REM Period Duration. This is calculated by dividing the total minutes spent in REM sleep by the number of REM periods. It measures the average duration of REM periods.
7. Average REM Cycle Length. This is calculated by dividing the time separating REM onsets by the total number of REM periods.

Sleep Histograms

The sleep histogram is a visual summary of polysomnographic data. The data are collapsed into the his-togram, which provides a graphic display of sleep stages and transitions throughout the sleep-recording period. Sleep stages are labeled on a left-hand vertical axis and time elapsed in hours is labeled along the bottom horizontal axis. Other data may be displayed as well.

Figure 23–1 is the sleep histogram of a 35-year-old female with initial insomnia. The histogram displays the characteristic "stair-step" pattern of entry into sleep, from wakefulness, to stage 1, then stage 2, and then stages 3 and 4. After this, however, the patient departs from normal in that she has several awakenings during the first third of sleep, and does not enter REM sleep until nearly 4 hours after falling asleep.

Note the additional data displays. This subject consistently had an oxygen saturation (SO_2) level in the upper nineties throughout the night. Continuous positive airway pressure (CPAP) and carbon dioxide (CO_2) levels were not recorded. She remained positioned on her right side throughout the night.

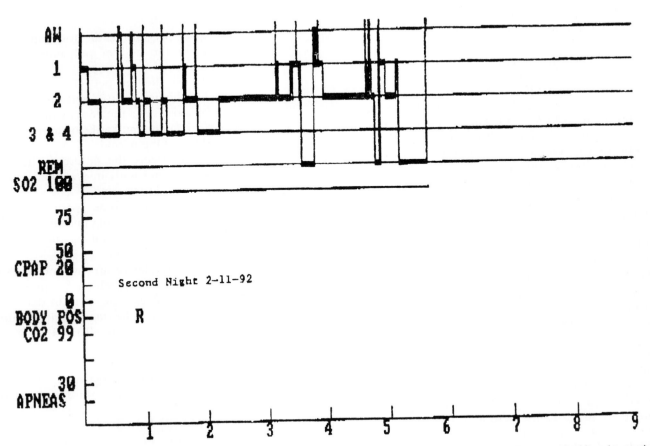

Figure 23–1. Sleep Histogram: 36 year old Female with Initial Insomnia. On the left axis AW = awake; 1 = NREM stage 1; 2 = NREM stage 2; 3 & 4 = NREM stages 3 and 4 (delta or slow wave sleep); REM = REM sleep. The patient is lying on her right side. The stars indicate awakenings during the first 2 hours of sleep. Note the inability to sustain stage 3 & 4 sleep in the beginning of the night and the absence of REM sleep until after hour 3.

Multiple Sleep Latency Test

The Multiple Sleep Latency Test (MSLT) is the most commonly used polysomnographic test for daytime sleepiness. After electrodes are attached, the patient is placed in a quiet, darkened room and asked to lie down and not resist falling asleep. This procedure is repeated at five separate times during the day. The sleep latencies, or amount of time it takes to fall asleep, are calculated, as is an average of the five latencies. The MSLT is considered a measure of physiological sleepiness (*DSM-IV*, 1994).

■ SLEEP HISTORY ASSESSMENT

A sleep history assessment designed to gather comprehensive patient information about sleep, sleep hygiene, sleep habits, and the presence of sleep-related symptoms or phenomena is shown in Fig. 23-2. As with any patient interview, open-ended questions and a nonjudgmental approach will yield the best information. Do not appear rushed, and allow the patient to talk and explain. Some of the information needed for the assessment may be contained in the patient's record or in

---

PATIENT NAME:
DATE:
TIME:
INTERVIEWED BY:

1. ENVIRONMENT: Usual sleeping arrangements, setting, bed, pillow(s), room temperature, noise level, pets.

2. USUAL BEDTIME:

3. PRE-SLEEP RITUALS/HABITS:

4. SLEEP AIDS: Medication, alcoholic beverage, how successful, how often needed.

5. LENGTH OF TIME NEED TO FALL ASLEEP:

6. UNUSUAL SLEEP ONSET EXPERIENCES: Sleep paralysis, hypnic jerks, hypnogogic hallucinations, how frequent.

7. NOCTURNAL AWAKENINGS: Frequency, duration, precipitants, ease of falling back asleep.

8. USUAL WAKING TIME: With/without alarm clock.

9. WAKING EXPERIENCES: Condition of bed, rested/refreshed, tired, dry mouth, sleep drunkenness, hypnopompic hallucinations.

10. HISTORY/FAMILY HISTORY OF SLEEP SYMPTOMS OR PHENOMENA:

    SNORING
    BRUXISM
    SLEEP APNEA SYNDROME
    NARCOLEPSY
    CATAPLEXY
    EXCESSIVE DAYTIME SLEEPINESS/FATIGUE SLEEP ATTACKS RESTLESS LEGS/KICKING
    REM BEHAVIOR SYNDROME
    SLEEP-WALKING
    SLEEP-TALKING
    SLEEP TERRORS
    AUTOMATIC BEHAVIOR
    HEADBANGING (JACTATIO CAPITUS NOCTURNA)

11. DREAMS: Recall, recurrent, nightmares, vividness, traumatic

12. NAPS: Frequency, environment, duration, effect on nocturnal sleep

13. PAIN, DISCOMFORT, STIFFNESS, HEADACHE, TMJ DISEASE

14. CAFFEINE/NICOTINE INTAKE

15. ALCOHOL INTAKE: How much, how often, what type, time of last drink, how long

16. MEDICATIONS, OVER THE COUNTER DRUGS: dosage, timing, when last taken, how long taking, for what condition, history of side effects, allergies

17. PSYCHIATRIC HISTORY

18. MEDICAL HISTORY

19. PSYCHOSOCIAL AND LIFESTYLE HISTORY: Resources/supports—how reliable, stress reduction and coping strategies—how successful, current sources of stress

20. IS THERE ANYTHING ELSE THE PATIENT (OR FAMILY) THINKS IS IMPORTANT TO MENTION OR WOULD LIKE TO DISCUSS?

Fig. 23–2. SLEEP HISTORY ASSESSMENT

other patient assessments. If the patient agrees, it may help to have the patient's bed-partner, a close family member, or a house-mate be present to clarify or add to the information. Most of the items in a sleep-history assessment are self-explanatory. Explanations and definitions of sleep-related symptoms and phenomena are provided at the end of this section.

The sleep history assessment can also uncover important information not necessarily related to sleep. For example, a patient who describes drinking a pint of whiskey nearly every night in an attempt to get to sleep most likely has a substance-related problem. Knowledge of pre-sleep rituals can be useful in pediatric settings, and following them as closely as possible can add to the pediatric patient's sense of comfort and security, thereby promoting rest.

■ SLEEP-RELATED SYMPTOMS AND PHENOMENA

BRUXISM

Bruxism is "the forcible grinding or gnashing of the teeth, produced by rhythmic contraction of the masseter and other muscles, that occurs without the patient's awareness during sleep" (Hartmann, 1994a, p. 598). About 20% of the population grind their teeth at night. Bed-partners of those with bruxism are often awakened by the sound. Most persons with bruxism are told about it by bed-partners or as a result of dental examination. Soreness of the jaw is often present upon awakening. Bruxism usually begins in late childhood or adolescence, and is less common after the age of 40. Its etiology is unknown, but the fact that bruxism runs in families suggests that it has a genetic component. Local anatomic factors, such as jaw malformation or malocclusion, may be implicated in some cases of bruxism. Nervous system and psychological factors are also thought to play a role. A thorough dental examination is recommended to determine whether there are correctable or anatomic factors involved. In rare cases, central nervous system lesions are responsible for bruxism. In most cases, however, neither anatomical nor neurological factors are found. Psychotherapy may be helpful in some cases in which suppressed anger and conflict are present. The most common treatment for bruxism is the use of mouthguards, worn during sleep, which do not prevent bruxism but do prevent damage to the teeth (Hartmann, 1994a)

HEADACHES

Morning headaches are associated with several sleep disorders as well as with many medical disorders. About 20% of people with obstructive sleep apnea complain of a dull headache upon awakening (Aldrich and Chauncey, 1990). According to Wooten (1994), the following three types of headaches may be triggered by sleep:

- Migraine headache—"an episodic and initially hemicranial headache that may be accompanied by nausea, vomiting, and in some cases, special sensory disturbances, hemianesthesia, and hemiparesis" (Wooten, 1994, p. 510).
- Cluster headache—characterized by "constant, severe pain in and around one eye and involving the malar area and temporal area" (Wooten, 1994, p. 51), with long periods of remission.
- Chronic paroxysmal hemicrania—a one-sided headache that occurs more often than cluster headaches and is without periods of remission.

If a patient complains of morning headaches, it is important for the nurse to gather further information about the nature of the headache, its onset and duration, and other possible associated symptoms, such as excessive daytime sleepiness. Monitoring or observing for sleep apnea may be indicated, along with appropriate medical consultations or referrals. The symptom of headache should not merely be medicated and ignored. Repeated headaches require full evaluation.

HYPNIC MYOCLONIA (HYPNIC JERKS)

Hypnic myoclonia occurs at the onset of sleep. People may report a sensation of falling and then suddenly being jerked or startled into full wakefulness. According to Carskadon and Dement (1994, p. 19) hypnic myoclonia is "experienced as a general or localized muscle contraction, very often associated with rather vivid imagery." Most people have experienced this symptom at one time or another, and it is not considered pathological. However, it may be associated with stress or irregular sleep schedules (Carskadon and Dement, 1994).

INSOMNIA AS A SYMPTOM

Insomnia is defined as "a perception by patients that their sleep is inadequate or abnormal" (Zorick, 1989, p. 431). It is a common subjective complaint and is associated with a variety of medical disorders, psychiatric disorders, and specific sleep disorders. As a group, patients complaining of insomnia show longer sleep latencies and less total sleep time than asymptomatic controls. In normal sleepers, there is a good correlation between self-estimates of sleep and polysomnograms. Patients with insomnia show wide variation in their own estimates of sleep onset and duration and a poor correlation of these with polysomnogram data (Zorick, 1989).

According to Aldrich (1994, p. 419), "timing determines the three main types into which insomnia is classified: delayed sleep onset, impaired sleep continuity, and early morning awakening." Others include non-restorative sleep in this category (Zorick, 1989).

It is important to ask patients whether they have difficulty falling asleep (initial insomnia); staying asleep, as evidenced by several awakenings with difficulty resuming sleep (middle insomnia); or awaken earlier than they want to, with an inability to go back to sleep (early morning awakening). Each of these symptoms should be reported and documented in the patient record.

JACTATIO CAPITUS NOCTURNA (HEAD-BANGING)

Jactatio capitus nocturna, or head-banging during sleep, is more common in infants and children than in adults. It consists of "rhythmic forward-and-back head movements, sometimes accompanied by rocking body movements, occurring just before sleep and during stages 1 and 2" (Aldrich, 1994, p. 424). The occurrence of head-banging at sleep onset, and its long duration (up to 1 hour or more), help to differentiate this condition from seizure activity (Aldrich, 1994). The nursing concern with this symptom is to prevent injury.

NARCOLEPSY

Narcolepsy is a sleep disorder that tends to run in families. Its cardinal symptoms are excessive daytime sleepiness, with sleep attacks and either cataplexy or recurrent intrusions of REM sleep into the waking state. Associated symptoms are excessive sleepiness, hypnogogic or hypnopompic hallucinations, and sleep paralysis. Narcolepsy is usually treated with central nervous system stimulants (for excessive daytime sleepiness) and tricyclic antidepressants (for cataplexy, sleep paralysis, and hypnogogic and hypnopompic phenomena).

A great deal of patient and family education is needed to assist with adjustment to narcolepsy. Community education is also necessary. If the patient is a child, education of school personnel may be indicated.

NIGHTMARES

A **nightmare** is a "long frightening dream that awakens the sleeper from REM sleep" (Hartmann, 1994b, p. 407). Most people easily recall nightmares upon awakening. Nightmares are common in children. Hartmann (1994b), a leading researcher of nightmares, estimated that over 50% of children, and nearly all children aged 3, 4, and 5 years, experience nightmares. Women report more frequent nightmares than men (Hartmann, 1984). It is important to determine the onset, frequency, and content of nightmares, and to differentiate nightmares from night terrors (which will be discussed subsequently). Did the onset of nightmares follow a stressful or traumatic event? Nightmares that replay a traumatic event are called traumatic dreams (Hartmann, 1994b), and may be indicative of traumatic stress disorder. A sudden increase in frequency of nightmares along with insomnia over a period of a few weeks may be a precursor to a psychotic episode (Hartmann, 1994b). Some people report a life-long history of frequent nightmares. In one study, over half of life-long nightmare sufferers expressed no desire to get rid of the nightmares; some even used them creatively in their artistic endeavors (Hartmann, 1984). Hartmann (1984) theorized persons who experience that life-long nightmares have thin or permeable boundaries that may leave them vulnerable to mental illness or letting others take advantage of them. Nightmares do not always require treatment (Hartmann, 1994b), especially if they are not distressful to the individual and do not impair sleep. Psychotherapy and behavioral interventions can be useful in treating nightmares. Moreover, discussion of nightmare content and meaning can be useful in the psychotherapeutic process.

Nursing care for the patient who awakens from a nightmare includes gentle reassurance and a willingness to listen and assist the patient to process and integrate the nightmare experience. Repeated or recurrent severely distressing nightmares may warrant further evaluation.

SLEEP TERRORS AND CONFUSIONAL AROUSALS

Sleep terrors are also referred to as *pavor nocturnus,* or night terrors. They typically occur during stages 3 and 4 of NREM sleep and are characterized by signs of increased sympathetic activity, such as dilated pupils, sweating, increased heart and respiratory rates, and increased blood pressure. The patient typically screams, appears terrified, is inconsolable for several minutes following the episode, and then relaxes and returns to sleep. The following morning there is little to no recall of the event. Sleep-walking may occur simultaneously with a sleep terror. Milder episodes, called confusional arousals, may involve only moaning, thrashing movements, or muttered vocalizations (Aldrich, 1994). Sleep terrors are different from nightmares and traumatic dreams.

SLEEP-TALKING

Sleep talking is common at all ages, and occurs during NREM stages I, 2, and REM. More females than males talk in their sleep. Sleep-talking in itself is not abnormal, and is of no particular concern (Aldrich, 1994).

However, if it occurs in conjunction with other parasomnias (abnormal behaviors during sleep), such as sleep-walking, or if there is also excessive daytime sleepiness, sleep-talking may indicate a more serious problem and should be evaluated.

SLEEP-WALKING (SOMNAMBULISM)

Sleep-walking, or **somnambulism,** is more common in children, but does happen in adulthood. It usually occurs during the first third of the night. The affected individual does not respond to verbal commands, but usually can be easily led back to bed without waking, and does not remember the episode. Sleep-walking can cause injury. Nurses should make sure that windows are closed, doors are locked, and stairways are blocked. Sleep-walking has been associated with nocturnal complex partial seizures, but this is rare. In elderly persons, what appears to be sleep-walking may be disorientation rather than true somnambulism (Aldrich, 1994).

SLEEP APNEA

Apneic episodes are intervals during which breathing ceases for at least 10 seconds. There are three types of sleep apnea syndromes: obstructive sleep apnea, caused by upper airway obstruction; central sleep apnea, associated with cardiac or neurological problems affecting ventilation; and mixed sleep apnea, which is a combination of obstructive and central sleep apnea. Obstructive sleep apnea is by far the most common form of the condition, and is often treated with a device worn during sleep that promotes continuous positive airway pressure (CPAP), thereby preventing upper airway obstruction. Other oral devices used to treat obstructive sleep apnea include those that thrust the lower jaw forward, thereby opening the airway.

Apneas noted in sleep (or at any other time) should be reported to the physician. Patients with apneas should be closely observed, and any such episode documented in the patient record.

SNORING

Snoring is a relatively common symptom, but should not be ignored. A recent epidemiological study indicated that about 19% of the population comprising more men than women, snore every or almost every night (Lugaresi et al., 1990). Snoring progressively increases in both men and women after age 35, but gradually decreases in men after age 65 (Lugaresi et al., 1990). Although quiet snoring is not of concern, loud snoring may be the first apparent symptom of obstructive sleep apnea, occurring in about 80% of apneic individuals. Snoring is caused by the vibration of soft tissues in the upper airway. Loud snoring is not a benign symptom; an increase in the volume or character of snoring strongly suggests sleep apnea (Aldrich, 1994).

Nurses should carefully observe loudly snoring patients for possible apneas. Suspected apnea is reported to the physician. A sleep history assessment may be done by the nurse. Patient education describes sleep hygiene and obstructive sleep apnea syndrome. Appropriate referrals are made.

HYPNOGOGIC AND HYPNOPOMPIC HALLUCINATIONS

Hypnogogic hallucinations are visual, auditory, or tactile hallucinations appearing at the onset of sleep, at the transition from wakefulness to sleep. They may be pleasant or frightening, and last for seconds to minutes, often ending with a hypnic jerk. Coupled with a complaint of excessive daytime sleepiness, they may suggest narcolepsy. Otherwise, they are not diagnostic and may occur in anyone with a disrupted sleep schedule. Unlike the hallucinations associated with psychosis, people experiencing hypnogogic hallucinations do not confuse them with reality, and are aware that they are hallucinating (Aldrich, 1994).

Hypnopompic hallucinations are essentially the same as hypnogogic hallucinations, but occur at the termination of sleep, at the transition from sleep to wakefulness.

SLEEP PARALYSIS

During an episode of sleep paralysis, the individual feels partially or fully awake but unable to move, and may describe struggling to move or wake up. Sleep paralysis starts suddenly and lasts for a few minutes at the onset or end of sleep. It can end gradually or abruptly, and may be terminated by a sound or a touch. It consists of complete or total flaccid paralysis of skeletal muscles, with the absence of reflexes, and can be differentiated from seizure activity, syncopal episodes, or periodic paralysis by its onset at the beginning or end of sleep, termination by noise or touch, and the patient's immediate return to full consciousness at the end of an episode. It is common in narcolepsy, but may occur in anyone, especially at times when sleep and circadian rhythms are disrupted. However, sleep paralysis at sleep onset may indicate narcolepsy or familial sleep paralysis (Aldrich, 1994).

AUTOMATIC BEHAVIOR

Automatic behavior consists of episodes of seemingly purposeful, repetitive activity performed by sleepy persons. The affected individual usually has no memory of the episode. Automatic behavior is associated with impaired vigilance and attention. Repeated "microsleeps" have been noted in tests of people involved in boring tasks, and may be partly responsible for automatic behavior. Soldiers who fall asleep while marching provide an example of automatic behavior (Aldrich, 1994). A night-shift nurse reported observing a co-worker writing in a patient chart, but the writing consisted of unintelligible scribbles. When alerted, the co-worker had no recollection of the event, and was surprised to see the writing. Automatic behavior is also common in narcolepsy, in which it is often accompanied by hallucinations.

SLEEP DRUNKENNESS

Sleep drunkenness, usually occurs in the morning and is marked by an inability to attain full alertness for some time after awakening. There may be feelings of grogginess, disorientation, incoordination, and automatic behavior, such as repeatedly turning off the alarm clock. The affected individual may report very deep sleep with difficulty in awakening. Sleep drunkenness is often associated with sleep apnea or central nervous system disorders, but can occur in anyone after severe sleep deprivation (Aldrich, 1994).

CATAPLEXY

Cataplexy is a cardinal symptom of narcolepsy. It consists of the sudden loss of muscle tone triggered by intense emotional stimuli, such as laughter, anger, surprise, fright, joy, or intense concentration. It may range from transient muscle weakness, noticed only by the patient, to weakness in the knees or sagging of the jaw or eyelids, to complete collapse in which the patient falls to the ground. The patient remains fully conscious during the attack, although if the episode lasts longer than a minute, REM sleep may occur (Aldrich, 1994).

RESTLESS LEGS SYNDROME

This consists of unpleasant crawling, pulling, or painful sensations in the legs, especially the calf areas, while sitting or lying down. There is an almost irresistible urge to move the legs. Symptoms commonly appear at bedtime while the patient attempts to lie still, but may occur during daytime periods of inactivity. Relief is associated with movement, especially walking. Insomnia is associated with restless legs syndrome. However the syndrome is considered medically benign, except for the disruption of sleep and daytime function (Fredrickson and Kreuger, 1994).

REM BEHAVIOR SYNDROME OR REM WITHOUT ATONIA

In normal REM sleep, muscle atonia limits movement to minor twitches. In REM behavior syndrome, muscle tone, and therefore movement, is preserved during REM sleep. This allows patients to literally act out their dreams. The behaviors associated with this syndrome are complex, vigorous, and sometimes violent. They can cause injury to the sleeper and sometimes to bedpartners. Vivid imagery often accompanies episodes of REM without atonia. Persons with REM behavior syndrome are usually middle-aged or elderly. About one-third have a neurological disorder of some sort.

Nursing responsibilities for patients with REM behavior syndrome include documentation of the actual behaviors observed and of the patient's account of the event; notification of the physician; facilitation of appropriate referral for evaluation; and patient and family education.

EXCESSIVE DAYTIME SLEEPINESS

The symptom of excessive daytime sleepiness (EDS) is almost ubiquitous in sleep disorders and disturbances. Patients may complain of decreased concentration and a proclivity to fall asleep during the day, often at inconvenient times or during boring activities. EDS reflects nocturnal sleep of poor quality and/or a disrupted sleep-wake cycle. If EDS is a persistent symptom, the patient should be fully evaluated for a medical, psychiatric, or sleep disorder. A sleep history assessment is useful in identifying associated symptoms that may aid in the eventual diagnosis of such disorders. EDS can severely impair social and occupational functioning and functioning in other important areas of life. Persistent EDS should not be ignored. The physician should be notified and the nurse should facilitate appropriate referrals for further evaluation. Patient and family education about principles of sleep hygiene is indicated.

■ PRINCIPLES OF SLEEP HYGIENE

Principles of sleep hygiene are essentially simple behavioral interventions that promote sleep and decrease awakenings. A full sleep and life-style assessment can indicate additional behavioral interventions that may improve sleep. If an individual's sleep problems are severe enough to affect functioning or persist for several months, a complete medical and psychiatric work-up and referral to a sleep disorders center are advised.

The principles of sleep hygiene are as follows:

- Establish and maintain a regular bedtime and awakening time. Try to awaken at the same time each day, even if sleep is poor the night before. This strengthens the individual circadian rhythm and leads to regular times of sleep onset.
- Sleep only as much as needed in order to feel refreshed the next day. The amount of sleep re-

quired varies among individuals, and may have a genetic component. Some people need more than 9 hours of sleep to feel rested, others do well with 6 hours. The idea that everyone requires a minimum of 8 hours of sleep is not supported by research.

- Reserve the bedroom for sleep. Avoid bill-paying, studying, exercise, and important discussions in the bedroom. In this way the bedroom becomes associated with calm, relaxing, pleasant activities rather than stressful ones thus promoting sleep.
- Don't go to bed hungry, but don't eat a large meal before bedtime. A light snack, such as warm milk and crackers, is best. Hunger can disturb sleep.
- Avoid caffeine-containing foods or beverages in the evening. Caffeine can cause more frequent awakenings and decreased total sleep time, even in people who feel that caffeine does not affect them. Sensitivity to the effects of caffeine can last from 8 to 14 hours.
- Avoid alcohol intake prior to sleep. Alcohol may help induce sleep, but the resulting sleep is usually disturbed. Alcohol can further decrease ventilation in people at risk for sleep apnea, including post-menopausal women, middle-aged men, the obese, and heavy snorers. Alcohol is metabolized at the rate of approximately 1 drink per hour. Wait until the alcohol has been metabolized before attempting sleep.
- Regular moderate exercise is healthy and may deepen sleep over time, but occasional, "one shot" exercise will not have an effect. Strenuous exercise late in the evening can stimulate the body and make it difficult to get to sleep.
- Naps can disrupt night-time sleep if taken at the wrong time. The natural tendency to sleep is biphasic, with the second peak coming approximately 8 hours after morning awakening. Napping at any time other than during this peak, especially 10 to 12 hours after morning awakening can disrupt nocturnal sleep. Discourage napping except in the elderly, who may benefit from periodic naps.
- Clear the mind prior to sleep. Relax with a book or soft music, or do relaxation exercises. Thinking about what happened during the day, what has to be done tomorrow, or worrying about problems will make it more difficult to fall asleep.
- Don't struggle to fall asleep. If unable to sleep after 15 or more minutes, turn on the light, get up, and do something relaxing. Reading, listening to music, having a light snack, or doing relaxation exercises may help. Covering the bedroom clock may be beneficial in reducing the stressful "hurry up and sleep" syndrome, in which one calculates, "If I go to sleep right now I'll only get 4 hours and 17 minutes of sleep."
- The bedroom environment should be kept dark, quiet, and at a moderate temperature to promote sleep and decrease awakenings. Occasional loud noises can disturb sleep, even in those who do not wake up. Keep the bedroom as quiet as possible. Consider using sound attenuation techniques such as insulation, heavy drapes, carpeting, or using a fan, air conditioner, or other source of "white noise" if sleeping close to excessive noise. An excessively warm or cool room temperature can disturb sleep.
- Allowing pets to sleep in the bedroom or on the bed can disrupt sleep, even in persons who are unaware of the disruption. Try sleeping without pets in the room if suffering from disturbed sleep.

(Hauri and Linde, 1990: Zarcone, 1994).

■ NURSING DIAGNOSIS

The recommended nursing diagnosis for sleep disturbances is "sleep pattern disturbance related to" a specific cause or associated factors (Carpenito, 1995). This diagnosis denotes the state in which the individual experiences or is at risk of experiencing a change in the quantity or quality of his rest pattern that causes discomfort or interferes with desired lifestyle (Carpenito, 1995, p. 865).

According to Carpenito (1995, p. 866), "The nursing diagnosis *Sleep Pattern Disturbance* must be differentiated from sleep disorders, chronic conditions (e.g., sleep apnea, narcolepsy) usually not treatable by a nurse generalist. *Sleep Pattern Disturbance* should be used to describe temporary changes in usual sleep patterns and/or those which a nurse can prevent or reduce, e.g., disruptions for treatments, anxiety response" To make this diagnosis, the nurse must gather information about the patient's lifestyle, environment, fears, and circadian rhythms (Carpenito, 1966).

Conditions that require monitoring and co-management by nurses and physicians should be considered as collaborative problems. An example is: Potential Complication: Obstructive Sleep Apnea (Carpenito, 1995).

When giving the reason for a sleep-pattern disturbance, it is important to be specific. The diagnosis should indicate the treatment needed, as in the following example: "Sleep Pattern Disturbance related to changes in usual sleep environment, unfamiliar noises, and interruptions for assessments" (Carpenito, 1995, p. 866).

■ NURSING INTERVENTIONS

Nursing interventions should be based on the principles of good sleep hygiene, and these should be incorporated into the plan of care. Each patient's care plan should be individualized and take into account the patient's specific needs and condition.

In the inpatient setting, the environment should be kept as quiet as possible at night in order to minimize disruption and promote sleep. Turning down the volume level of paging systems and patient call boards, for example, reduces noise. Putting padding on equipment, such as intravenous poles, that is moved during the night reduces the noise produced by equipment hitting the patient's bed or chair. Rubber bumpers are available for this purpose, or padding can be improvised from towels, foam, or other such material. One of the most frequently heard inpatient complaints is an inability to sleep because of noise made by the care staff. One patient stated, "It sounded as if they were having a party out there all night, laughing and shouting. I couldn't sleep a wink." There is no excuse for this type of staff behavior. Keep conversations low, and save jokes and loud talking for breaks. Set limits for patients who may be awake and making noise. Take patients or staff into a room other than the nurses' station to talk during night hours.

Pain is a major cause of disturbed sleep. Evaluate the effectiveness of the pain-control regimen of patients who awaken frequently during the night. Collaborate with the physician in developing a plan for effective pain control. Longer-acting analgesics may be indicated for use during the night.

Patients who awaken at frequent intervals to go to the bathroom should be evaluated for urinary retention. Placing a commode near the bed for elderly or unsteady patients may decrease the possibility of falls during a longer walk to the bathroom. A regular toileting schedule can minimize night-time bathroom trips.

Keep the patient's environment as safe as possible in order to minimize the possibility of injury when the patient gets up at night. Keep a night light turned on, and make sure there is no equipment or furniture blocking the patient's path to the bathroom or door. Keep the lower side rails down at night to minimize injury caused by patients' attempts to climb over them.

Learn the patient's pre-sleep habits and rituals, and allow the patient to follow them as much as possible. This is especially useful with pediatric patients. The nurse may need to allow a longer time for pediatric patients to get ready for bed. Do not rush such patients through their bedtime rituals, and encourage them to bring comforting objects from home, such as a stuffed animals or favorite pillows.

Extremes of temperature can disrupt sleep. Keep the patient's room at a moderate temperature. Lower the room temperature if the patient complains it is too hot, or provide extra blankets if the patient is cold.

Provide extra pillows if requested. If no extra pillows are available, improvise a pillow by placing a bath blanket in a pillowcase.

Try to plan nursing assessments, routine treatments, and medication administration so that the patient gets a minimum of 4 hours of uninterrupted sleep at night ("anchor sleep"). Coordinate nursing activities with those of other departments such as the laboratory and the respiratory therapy unit so that the number of sleep interruptions is kept to an absolute minimum. For patients who require frequent vital-sign measurements during the night, consider the use of automatic blood pressure cuffs or monitors to decrease disruptions. Consider moving patients who require frequent observation or treatment closer to the nurses' station.

When frequent checks are required during the night in psychiatric settings, enter the patient's room as quietly as possible. Avoid bumping into furniture or equipment, use a flashlight rather than turning on the room light, and avoid shining the flashlight directly on the patient's eyes.

Make sure the call bell is within the patient's reach. Reassure patients that you will be checking on them during the night and that you will be available. Answer call bells promptly and in person whenever possible, and avoid using the intercom, which may disturb other patients. If there is a commotion on the unit during the night, such as a code call or a disruptive patient, close the doors to other patient's rooms and assign staff members to reassure and check on them.

Spend some time with patients who awaken during the night. Try progressive relaxation techniques or tapes, guided imagery, warm milk (it works!), or other calming approaches before resorting to hypnotic medications for patients. Some nurses have found it helpful to read to the patient for a short while, and they keep children's books available (even in adult units) for this purpose.

Evaluate the need for and effectiveness of hypnotic and other medications. Observe the patient for side effects of medications, such as increased confusion or morning "hangover." Timing of medications can be as important as their dosage. Many medications can affect sleep. Collaborate with physicians about the patient's medication regimen. Plan patient and family education sessions about sleep hygiene, identified sleep disturbances, successful interventions, and medications.

Communicate with other care-givers and members of the health-care team about patients' sleep-related symptoms, interventions, and care plans. If disturbed sleep is expected because of surgery, medical procedures or treatments, or the nature of the patient's illness, include interventions and goals for the patient's return to a normal sleep pattern or discontinuation of hypnotic medications in critical-path documents or care maps. Document sleep-related observations and sleep interventions in the patient record. Be specific about the behavior observed. "Slept well" is an inappropriate statement.

Finally, nurses themselves should practice good sleep hygiene. Adequate rest and a healthy life-style on the part of the nurse contribute to the ability to provide high-quality patient care.

■ PRIMARY SLEEP DISORDERS

The *The Diagnostic and Statistical Manual of Mental Disorders,* Fourth Edition (DSM-IV), published by the American Psychiatric Association (1994), defines primary sleep disorders as those in which the etiology cannot be attributed to a mental disorder, medical disorder, or chemical substance. Primary sleep disorders are divided into the **dyssomnias** and **parasomnias.** Almost all sleep disorders described in *DSM-IV* include the following diagnostic criteria:

- The sleep disturbance must cause clinically significant distress or impairment in social, occupational, or other important areas of functioning
- The disorder is not better explained by mental disorder
- The sleep disorder is not due to the physiological effects of a general medical condition
- The sleep disorder is not due to the effects of a substance

DYSSOMNIAS

Dyssomnias are "characterized by abnormalities in the amount, quality, or timing of sleep" (*DSM-IV,* 1994, p. 551).

Primary Insomnia

The essential feature of this primary insomnia is a complaint of "difficulty initiating or maintaining sleep or non-restorative sleep that lasts for at least one month . . . and causes clinically significant distress or impairment in social, occupational, or other important areas of functioning. . . ." (*DSM-IV,* 1994, p. 553).

The true prevalence of primary insomnia is unknown. Its onset is usually sudden and associated with psychological, social, or medical stress. The disorder typically begins in young adulthood or middle age, and

rarely begins in childhood. There is often a combination of difficulty in falling asleep and intermittent wakefulness during sleep. Primary insomnia is associated with negative conditioning or negative associations related to sleep. The patient gradually often develops these negative associations in relation to the unsuccessful attempt to sleep and becomes negatively conditioned. Preoccupation and distress may lead to the "development of a vicious cycle: the more the individual strives to sleep, the more frustrated and distressed the individual becomes and the less he or she is able to sleep" (*DSM-IV,* 1994, p. 553).

Polysomnography may show poor sleep continuity, increased muscle tension, or increased alpha-wave activity in sleep electroencephalograms. Some patients report sleeping better at the sleep laboratory than at home.

Primary Hypersomnia

The essential feature of primary hypersomnia is excessive sleepiness for at least 1 month, as evidenced by prolonged sleep or daytime sleep episodes that occur almost every day. Persons with primary hypersomnia usually sleep 8 to 12 hours per night and have difficulty awakening in the morning, although the quality of their sleep is good. However, prolonged sleep is not necessarily restorative. Excessive daytime sleepiness is marked by intentional or inadvertent naps. Unintentional sleeping typically occurs during times of low stimulation or low activity, such as while attending a lecture. Sleep drunkenness may be present during the transition from sleep to wakefulness. The persistent daytime sleepiness may lead to automatic behavior.

Polysomnography usually shows normal to prolonged sleep duration, shortened sleep latency, and normal to increased sleep continuity. The MSLT provides physiological evidence of excessive daytime sleepiness with shortened latencies.

The true prevalence of primary hypersomnia is unknown. The onset of the condition normally occurs between the ages of 15 and 30. The disorder gradually progresses over weeks to months, and becomes chronic and stable if left untreated.

If primary hypersomnia is recurrent, it should be specified as such. Hypersomnia is considered recurrent if "there are periods of excessive sleepiness that last at least three days occurring several times a year for at least 2 years" (*DSM-IV,* 1994, p. 558). In recurrent hypersomnia, daytime alertness and nighttime sleep are normal between the periods of excessive sleepiness.

Narcolepsy

Narcolepsy is characterized by repeated, irresistible attacks of refreshing sleep occurring daily for at least 3 months. In addition, the patient experiences either cataplexy, with episodes of sudden loss of muscle tone usually precipitated by intense emotional stimuli, or recurrent intrusions of elements of REM sleep into the transition between sleep and wakefulness (such as paralysis of voluntary muscles or dreamlike hallucinations).

Sleep episodes or attacks of narcolepsy typically last 10 to 20 minutes, but can last for as long as an hour. They can occur at any time, and can therefore be dangerous if the individual is driving, for example. If the condition is untreated, there may be from two to six episodes per day of intentional or unintentional sleep. Cataplexy may be manifested subtly, by a sagging jaw or drooping eyelids, or more severely, by falling to the ground. The affected individual is fully alert and conscious during the cataplectic episode, and full muscle strength returns afterwards. Approximately 70% of patients with narcolepsy have cataplexy. About 20 to 40% of persons with narcolepsy report hallucinations occurring during sleep onset (hypnogogic hallucinations) or just after awakening (hypnopompic hallucinations). The hallucinations are usually visual, but may be auditory or tactile. From one-third to one-half of patients with narcolepsy experience sleep paralysis when falling asleep or just after awakening. Sleep-related hallucinations and sleep paralysis may occur simultaneously and can be frightening. Both are thought to be intrusions of elements of REM sleep into the waking state. Polysomnograms may show sleep latencies of less than 10 minutes and sleep-onset REM periods (SOREMPs). MSLT results include latencies of 5 minutes or less, and REM sleep during two in every five naps.

Narcolepsy has been associated with mood disorders, substance-related disorders, and generalized anxiety disorder. A history of parasomnias, such as sleepwalking, bruxism, and enuresis, may also be associated with this condition. Narcolepsy occurs with equal frequency in males and females. The adult prevalence rate ranges from 0.027% to 0.16%. Daytime sleepiness is the first symptom, and is usually noted in adolescence, but may be traced to early childhood. Onset of narcolepsy after the age of 40 is rare. There may be a genetic component to narcolepsy, with up to 35% of first degree relatives also having the disorder. From 30 to 50% of first-degree relatives of individuals with narcolepsy have disorders characterized by excessive sleepiness.

Breathing-Related Sleep Disorder

The essential feature of breathing-related sleep disorder is sleep disruption caused by abnormalities of ventilation. Excessive daytime sleepiness, due to frequent awakenings associated with attempts to breathe normally may precipitate episodes of sleep during relaxing or boring situations. Naps are not experienced as refreshing, and a dull headache may be present on waking. Some affected individuals may complain of difficulty in breathing while supine or sleeping. According to the *DSM-IV* (1994, p. 568), "abnormal respiratory events during sleep in Breathing-Related Sleep Disorder include apneas (episodes of breathing cessation), hypopneas (abnormally slow or shallow respiration), and hypoventilation (abnormal blood oxygen and carbon dioxide levels)." Three forms of breathing-related sleep disorder have been identified: obstructive sleep apnea syndrome, central sleep apnea syndrome, and central alveolar hypoventilation syndrome. All are medical diagnoses, which is why breathing-related sleep disorder is also coded on Axis II in *DSM-IV*.

Obstructive sleep apnea syndrome, the most common form of breathing-related sleep disorder, consists of repeated episodes of upper-airway obstruction during sleep. It is associated with above-normal weight and loud snoring, or "brief gasps that alternate with episodes of silence that last 20-30 seconds" (*DSM-IV*, p. 568). Breathing sometimes stops for a minute to a minute and a half, and the patient becomes cyanotic, although respiratory movements continue. The condition usually has a gradual onset, gradual progression, and chronic course.

In children, obstructive sleep apnea is the most common breathing-related sleep disorder; however, its symptoms may be subtle. Agitated arousals, unusual sleeping positions, and bed-wetting are common. Polysomnography is recommended for definitive diagnosis of the condition in children. Obstructive sleep apnea is also common in overweight, middle-aged males (*DSM-IV*, p. 571.) The prevalence of obstructive sleep apnea syndrome ranges from 1 to 10% in adults and may be even higher in the elderly. Among adults, it is eight times more frequent in men than women.

In central sleep apnea syndrome, the patient stops breathing episodically, but does not have airway obstruction. This syndrome is more common in the elderly as a result of cardiac and neurological conditions that affect respiratory regulation. Mild snoring may be present but is not a major complaint.

Central alveolar hypoventilation syndrome is characterized by "an impairment in ventilatory control that results in abnormally low oxygen levels further worsened by sleep (*DSM-IV*, p. 568). There is hypoventilation without apneas, hypopneas, or mechanical abnormalities of the lung. Central alveolar hypoventilation syndrome occurs mainly in very overweight persons. Affected individuals complain either of excessive sleepiness or insomnia.

Individuals with breathing-related sleep disorder often awaken feeling more tired than they did before going to sleep. They are often described as restless sleepers. Dryness of the mouth is common, as is nocturia. The condition may be accompanied by sleep drunkenness or headaches lasting for up to 2 hours after awakening. Memory disturbance, poor concentration, irritability, and personality changes may result from the excessive sleepiness. Mood disorders, anxiety disorders, and dementia are also associated with sleep-related breathing disorder. Erectile dysfunction and decreased libido may occur. Children may exhibit developmental delay or learning problems.

Each breathing-related sleep disorder is associated with specific polysomnographic and physiological findings related to the specific ventilatory problem involved. There may also be a shortened sleep latency, frequent arousals, short duration of sleep, increased stage 1 sleep, and decreased slow-wave and REM sleep. Evidence of excessive daytime sleepiness is found with the MSLT, which typically shows latencies of less than 5 or 10 minutes. Mild hypertension and reduced oxygen saturation are common.

Obstructive sleep apnea can cause death. Obstructive sleep apnea syndrome may show a familial tendency.

Circadian Rhythm Sleep Disorder

The essential feature of circadian rhythm sleep disorder is "a persistent or recurrent pattern of sleep disruption that results from a mismatch between the individual's circadian sleep-wake system . . . and exogenous demands on the timing and duration of sleep . . ." (*DSM-IV*, 1994, p. 573. Many people with circadian rhythm related disturbance do not seek treatment or have sub-clinical symptoms. Diagnosis is primarily based on the clinical history. The pattern of naps, work, sleep, free time, and attempts to cope with symptoms are important to assess. The following subtypes of circadian rhythm disorder are listed in DSM-IV and must be specified in the diagnosis.

Delayed-Sleep-Phase Disorder. In this disorder, the internal sleep-wake cycle is delayed relative to social norms. The affected individuals are sometimes called "night owls." They keep late hours and are unable to move their bedtime forward (phase advance). However, their sleep cycle is stable, and if left to their own schedule, they will keep regular hours of sleep, although they are later than those considered socially acceptable. There is consequent difficulty in arising at a socially acceptable time. Persons with this disorder may be sleep-deprived by attempting to adhere to a schedule dictated by societal custom, and may therefore complain of excessive sleepiness.

In delayed sleep-phase disorder, people go to bed and wake up later on their days off and during vacations, and they experience a reduction in symptoms on those days. Sleep drunkenness may be observed if awakening occurs earlier than the internal schedule dictates. Performance is also phase delayed and usually peaks in the late evening.

Jet-Lag-Type Sleep Disorder. In this disorder, the internal body clock is normal, but conflict occurs between the individual's sleep-wake cycle and the pattern demanded by a different time zone. The greater the number of time zones crossed, the more severe are the symptoms, with the most severe symptoms occurring when eight or more time zones have been crossed within 24 hours. Adjustment is more difficult when traveling from east to west (advancing sleep-wake hours) than when traveling from west to east (delaying sleep-wake hours).

Shift-Work-Type Circadian Rhythm Sleep Disorder. In this condition the internal sleep-wake cycle is normal but there is conflict between the internal cycle and the pattern of sleep and wakefulness required by shift work. Rotating sleep schedules are the most disruptive because they preclude adjustment to a consistent sleep-wake schedule. Night and rotating-shift workers have shortened sleep and frequent disturbances in sleep continuity. They may experience sleepiness during work hours.

Unspecified-Type Circadian Rhythm Sleep Disorder. This category encompasses sleep-wake patterns, other than those previously described, that vary from normal. Examples include an advanced sleep-phase pattern (the opposite of a delayed sleep phase), a non-24-hour sleep pattern (based on a 24- to 25-hour day, despite an environment with 24-hour time cues), and an irregular sleep-wake pattern (absence of an identifiable pattern).

Subtype Features and Test Findings. The jet lag and shift work subtypes of circadian rhythm sleep disorder may be more common in so-called "morning people." Jet lag is associated with headache, fatigue, and gastrointestinal symptoms that may be related to travel conditions. Occupational, social, and family dysfunction may occur with the shift work syndrome. Individuals with any Circadian Rhythm Sleep Disorder are at risk for substance-related disorders, since they may use alcohol, sedatives, hypnotics, or stimulants to control symptoms. The delayed phase type and certain unspecified types of sleep disorder (non-24-hour and irregular pattern) have been associated with schizoid, schizotypical, and avoidant personality features. The jet lag and shift work types of sleep disorder may bring on or worsen a manic or major depressive episode.

Polysomnograms in the various types of sleep disorder vary, depending on when they are recorded.

When individuals with the delayed phase type disorder are studied during their preferred hours of sleep and waking, findings are normal; when they are studied on a socially normal sleep-wake schedule, there is usually prolonged latency, late spontaneous awakening, shortened REM latency, and normal sleep continuity. Core body temperature measurements verify the phase delay.

When studied during a conventional sleep–wake schedule, polysomnograms of persons with shift work type sleep disorder are normal. When studied during work hours, however, these individuals show a normal or shortened sleep latency, shortened duration of sleep, and disturbances in sleep continuity. There is often a reduction in stage 2 and REM sleep. The MSLT reveals sleepiness during desired times of wakefulness.

Middle-aged and elderly persons are more vulnerable to the shift work and jet lag types of sleep disorder, and their symptoms may be more severe than those of young adults. The prevalence of these disorders is not well-established, but "surveys suggest a prevalence of up to 7% for Delayed Sleep Phase Type in adolescents and of up to 60% for shift work type in night-shift workers" (*DSM IV*, 1994, p. 576). The delayed sleep phase type circadian rhythm disorder lasts for years or decades, but may correct itself with age. The shift work type disorder typically lasts as long as the individual does shift work, but symptoms disappear within 2 weeks after resuming a normal sleep-wake schedule. In jet-lag-type sleep disorder, 1 day per time zone traveled is generally needed for the circadian system to become synchronized to local time.

Dyssomnia Not Otherwise Specified

This category of sleep disorder is reserved for "insomnias, hypersomnias, and circadian rhythm disturbances that do not meet criteria for any specific dyssomnia" (*DSM-IV*, 1994, p. 579).

PARASOMNIAS

Parasomnias are "characterized by abnormal behavioral or physiological events occurring in association with sleep, specific sleep stages or sleep-wake transitions" (*DSM-IV*, 1994, p. 551).

Nightmare Disorder

Essential to nightmare disorder are repeated, frightening dreams that lead to awakening with full alertness. The nightmare content typically involves perceived physical danger or, less commonly, personal failure or embarrassment. Nightmares following traumatic events tend to replay the actual event, but most nightmares do not involve actual experiences. Nightmares occur during the REM stage of sleep, and can therefore occur periodically during sleep. Since REM sleep periods generally become longer during the last half of the night, nightmares are more likely to occur at that time. A sense of fear or anxiety following a nightmare often causes difficulty in returning to sleep. If there are frequent awakenings or if sleeping is avoided through fear of nightmares, excessive daytime sleepiness, decreased concentration, irritability, or symptoms of depression or anxiety sufficient to impair daytime functioning may occur. On awakening from a nightmare, sweating and increased heart and respiratory rates may be noted.

Polysomnograms show abrupt awakenings from REM sleep that correlate with patients' self-reports of nightmares. The REM period in which the nightmare occurs typically lasts for more than 10 minutes and may show an increased number of eye movements. The heart rate and respiratory rate may increase or become more variable before the awakening. Persons with Posttraumatic Stress Disorder (PTSD) usually have a normal sleep continuity and sleep architecture. Traumatic nightmares may occur during NREM sleep (especially stage 2) as well as during REM sleep.

Nightmares are frequent in childhood, and often begin in childhood between the ages of 3 and 6, but most children subsequently outgrow nightmare problems. Women report nightmares more often than men, but this may reflect a reporting bias rather than a true gender difference. The true prevalence of nightmare disorder is unknown. Some persons report life-long nightmare disturbances, but there may be a tendency for nightmares to decrease with old age. Diagnostically, it is important to differentiate nightmare disorder from sleep terror disorder.

Sleep-Terror Disorder

The essential features of sleep-terror disorder are recurrent abrupt awakenings that typically occur during the first third of the night, begin with a panicky scream, and are accompanied by intense fear and autonomic arousal, tachycardia, tachypnea, and sweating. The affected individual is "difficult to awaken or comfort" (*DSM-IV*, 1994, p. 583), "no detailed dream is recalled and there is amnesia for the episode" (*DSM-IV*, 1994, p. 587). The patient may suddenly sit up in bed, crying or screaming, but usually does not fully awaken.

In children, sleep terror disorder is not associated with other mental disorders; however, the opposite is true of adults. In adults, the disorder occurs more frequently in persons with PTSD and generalized anxiety disorder (GAD). Dependent, schizoid, and borderline personality disorders have also been associated with sleep-terror disorder. Sleepwalking can occur simultaneously with sleep-terror disorder.

Polysomnograms reveal that sleep terrors begin in NREM sleep associated with delta wave activity, especially in stages 3 and 4 sleep, and therefore occur more often in the first third of sleep. The onset of a sleep terror episode is marked by very high voltage delta wave activity on the electroencephalogram, and by increases in muscle tone and heart rate. Partial arousals may be noted, as may sudden arousals from NREM sleep with an increased heart rate that do not progress to a sleep terror episode. Sleep terror can occur during daytime naps.

In children, the disorder is more common among boys than girls, but in adults it occurs equally in males and females. Sleep-terror disorder in children usually begins between the ages of 4 and 12 years and resolves during adolescence. In adults, its onset is between the ages of 20 and 30. The disorder has a chronic course, with a waxing and waning severity and frequency of sleep terrors. There is a familial tendency toward the disorder, and often a history of sleepwalking in the families of affected individuals.

Sleepwalking Disorder

The essential feature of sleepwalking disorder is "repeated episodes of complex motor behavior initiated during sleep, including rising from bed and walking about" (*DSM-IV*, 1994, p. 587). During sleepwalking, affected individuals typically have a blank stare and are relatively unresponsive to the attempts of others to communicate with or awaken them. On awakening from the episode or on the following morning, the sleep-walker has little or no recall of the episode. Although there may be a brief period of confusion if the person awakens directly after the episode, there is no impairment of cognition or behavior.

Sleepwalking disorder is equally frequent in males and females. The true prevalence of the disorder is unknown, but up to 30% of children have had at least one episode of sleep walking. Episodes commonly begin between ages 4 and 8, with a peak prevalence at about 12 years. Sleepwalking usually resolves spontaneously by about age 15. Less commonly, sleepwalking episodes may recur in adulthood. Sleepwalking rarely begins in adulthood without prior childhood episodes, and in adults, the disorder usually has a chronic waxing and waning course. Up to 80% of sleepwalkers report a family history of sleepwalking or sleep terrors. The risk for sleepwalking increases when both parents have a positive history of the disorder, suggesting a genetic component.

Many types of behavior have been observed during sleepwalking episodes, including talking, urinating, running, going up and down stairs, eating, and even operating machinery. Sleepwalkers may injure themselves during episodes and inappropriate behavior, especially children. Affected individuals may awaken spontaneously during the episode, or return to bed and continue sleeping.

Internal or external stimuli can trigger sleepwalking episodes. Psychosocial stressors and alcohol or sedative use can increase the likelihood of sleepwalking. The frequency of sleepwalking episodes can increase with sleep deprivation or fever. Migraine headaches are associated with sleepwalking disorder, as are obstructive sleep apnea and disorders that disrupt stages 3 and 4 sleep. Adults are more likely to exhibit violent behavior during sleep walking episodes. In children, sleepwalking disorder is not associated with other mental disorders, but in adults the disorder may be associated with personality disorders, mood disorders or anxiety disorders. Sleep-terror disorder can accompany sleepwalking disorder.

Polysomnograms and audiovisual monitoring show that sleepwalking episodes usually begin during stages 3 and 4 sleep in the first part of the night. Just prior to the episode there is rhythmic, high voltage delta wave activity that continues during the episode. Alpha waves may also be seen. Heart and respiratory rates may increase at the onset of the arousal. An increased number of transitions from stages 3 and 4 sleep and decreased sleep efficiency may also be found.

Parasomnia Not Otherwise Specified

This category of sleep disorders comprises "disturbances that are characterized by abnormal behavioral or physiological events during sleep or sleep-wake transitions, but do not meet criteria for a more specific Parasomnia" (*DSM-IV*, 1994, p. 592). Examples include REM sleep behavior disorder and sleep paralysis.

SUMMARY

The preceding discussion provides an overview of the primary sleep disorders. The nurse should refer to *DSM-IV* for full diagnostic criteria and more detailed information. The remaining sleep disorders are secondary to other mental or medical conditions or are substance induced. The following section provides an overview of sleep disturbances associated with selected mental disorders.

◼ SLEEP AND SELECTED MENTAL DISORDERS

Disturbed sleep is a symptom of virtually all psychiatric disorders. A major nursing concern in the care and treatment of psychiatric patients is the promotion of adequate rest, and medical treatment of mental disorders addresses sleep-related symptoms such as insomnia. Understanding the sleep disturbances related to psychiatric illness enhances the nurse's ability to observe, assess, plan, and evaluate effective nursing care and to collaborate with others in the overall treatment of mentally ill patients.

In 1992, Benca et al. performed a meta-analysis of 177 studies of sleep and psychiatric disorders. They found that "Overall, the results did not suggest that any individual sleep variable was either sensitive or specific enough for the diagnosis of a particular mental disorder, although some variables appeared to be helpful for distinguishing certain patient groups from controls" (Benca et al., 1992, p. 661). Thus, mental disorders cannot be diagnosed from sleep findings; however, such findings do provide a better understanding of these illnesses.

MOOD DISORDERS

Disturbed sleep (either insomnia or hypersomnia) is part of the diagnostic criteria for all mood disorders (formerly known as affective disorders). It is extremely rare to find a patient with a mood disorder who does not have difficulty initiating or maintaining sleep. Most patients with mood disorders report insomnia. Among the mental disorders, mood disorders have been the best researched with regard to sleep.

Major Depressive Disorder

In a comprehensive review of research on electroencephalographic sleep and depression, Reynolds and Kupfer (1987), two leading researchers of sleep and depression, reported:

> Approximately 90% of depressed patients show some form of EEG verified sleep disturbance. The most predictable abnormalities of endogenous depression include (a) sleep continuity disturbances (i.e.) prolonged sleep latency, multiple nocturnal awakenings, and early morning awakening); (b) diminished slow wave sleep (Stages 3 and 4), with a shift of slow wave activity from the first to the second NREM period; (c) an abbreviated first NREM sleep period leading to earlier appearance of the first REM sleep period (earlier, that is, with respect to sleep onset but not with respect to clock time itself . . .): and (d) altered intranight temporal distribution of REM sleep, with increased REM sleep time and REMs earlier in the first half of the night. All of these features tend to become more marked with advancing age (p. 203).

The foregoing changes are stable over time and are seen even when the depressive illness is in remission. Although there are several conflicting reports in the literature on sleep and depression, most consistently support the above findings. Age is an important variable with regard to sleep disturbance in depression.

In one study, about 10 to 15% of patients with depressive disorders showed high sleep efficiencies and reported spending more time in bed. This finding was associated with complaints of anergia and psychomotor retardation (Reynolds & Kupfer, 1987). Additionally, there is considerable night-to-night variability in REM latency associated with depression. Sleep onset REM periods (SOREMPS) have been seen in some patients with depression (Coble, Kupfer, and Shaw, 1981; Annseau et al., 1984).

Initial work by Vogel and associates (1975, 1977) demonstrated that sleep deprivation had an antidepressive effect in depressed individuals, but subsequent studies indicated that the effect was transient and affected by even short naps (Knowles, et al., 1987). Although the use of total sleep deprivation, partial sleep deprivation, and REM sleep deprivation initially showed promise as clinical modalities in the treatment of depression, the difficulty of administering these treatments, their short-lasting effects, and their poor tolerance by patients made them generally impractical (Fleming, 1989).

Currently, polysomnograms are used primarily in research on depression, in attempts to better understand the biophysiological basis of this disorder. However, the sleep changes described are not unique to depression, and therefore do not provide specific diagnostic information. For example, shortened REM latencies not significantly different from those seen in mood disorders have also been seen in schizophrenia and narcolepsy (Benca et al., 1992). Sleep latency has been found to be prolonged in alcoholism, anxiety disorders, borderline personality disorder, eating disorders, dementia, and insomnia (Benca et al., 1992). However, EEG sleep studies confirm depressed patients' reports of difficulty with going to sleep, frequent awakenings, early morning awakening, and a reduction of total sleep time. These are the symptoms that should be of concern to the nurse.

Bipolar Disorder

Most patients with bipolar disorder report insomnia while in the depressive cycle of the illness, but some report symptoms of hypersomnia. During manic phases, patients with bipolar disorder report reduced amounts of sleep coupled with a subjective sense of needing less sleep. In many cases, entry into a manic phase of the illness is preceded by periods of sleeplessness (Benca, 1994).

Few polysomnographic studies have been done on patients with bipolar disorder. One study compared the sleep of patients with unipolar depression or bipolar depression with the sleep of normal controls (Duncan, Pettigrew, and Gillin, 1979). The bipolar group had lower REM efficiency than the unipolar group, with more fragmented REM periods. Otherwise, the sleep of patients with bipolar disorder did not differ significantly from that of those with unipolar depression. However, patients with unipolar or bipolar depression differed significantly from normal controls on several measures, with the sleep of those with unipolar disorder differing more from normal than the sleep of bipolar-disorder patients. Sleep deprivation can induce mania in patients with bipolar disorder. (Wehr, 1992; 1989).

Although research is sparse, it appears that the sleep of patients with bipolar disorder depends on whether they are in the depressive or manic phase of the illness. When depressed, their sleep is similar to that of patients with major depression.

ANXIETY DISORDERS

Anxiety is a symptom associated with almost all psychiatric disorders, but it is the predominant symptom in the anxiety disorders. Sleep disturbance is a diagnostic criterion for GAD, PTSD, and acute stress disorder. However, very little research has been done on the relation between sleep and the anxiety disorders.

Posttraumatic Stress Disorder

That sleep disturbances, nightmares, and/or repetitive dreams are common symptoms reported by victims of psychic trauma is well established. These disturbances have been reported by rape victims (Larsen and Pagaduan-Lopez, 1987; Mezey and Taylor, 1986), concentration camp survivors (Krystal and Niederland, 1968; Niederland, 1968), and combat veterans (Ross et al., 1989). Among combat veterans, sleep disturbance has been considered by some a hallmark of PTSD (Ross et al., 1989; Brett and Ostroff, 1985).

Although many studies report sleep disturbances or nightmares following psychological trauma, few describe these phenomena further. Most rely on self-reports by subjects. Because of methodological problems, it is difficult to determine which, if any, sleep disturbances are related specifically to trauma response or PTSD. In fewer than a dozen studies polysomnograms used to measure sleep in people diagnosed as having PTSD; all were limited to male subjects, with the exception of two studies that did not report the subjects' gender. Research that compared polysomnograms of people with and people without PTSD found that those with PTSD had more insomnia, a poorer sleep efficiency, and fewer REM periods (Astrom, et al., 1989;

Greenberg, Pearlman, and Gampel, 1972; Kramer and Kinney, 1985; Lavie, et al., 1979; Schlosberg and Benjamin, 1978; Mikulincer, et al., 1989). One study reported the absence of stage 4 sleep in PTSD (Astrom et al., 1989). The work of Ross and associates suggests that PTSD may involve a dysregulation of REM sleep as well as some general motor dyscontrol during sleep. Interestingly, one combat veteran who reported an anxiety dream after awakening from REM sleep in the laboratory (Ross et al., 1990a) also reported having anxiety dreams approximately 3 times a week.

Although polysomnographic research in patients with PTSD is a relatively recent area of inquiry, and many of the results are conflicting, it appears that REM sleep parameters are most often affected in PTSD (Ross et al., 1989; 1990b). PTSD (at least in males) is associated with more insomnia, less efficient sleep, and a shorter total sleep time than normal.

Panic Disorder

Sheehan reported that 77% of patients with panic disorder described having restless and disturbed sleep, and that 68% described difficulty in falling asleep. Recent research has verified the existence of so-called sleep panic attacks that are quite similar to daytime panic attacks (Mellman and Uhde, 1990). Uhde (1994) theorizes that patients with sleep panic attacks develop secondary anxiety and avoidance behavior regarding sleep that is similar to the development of agoraphobia in patients with daytime panic attacks. He suggests that the following profile develops chronologically: (1) sleep panic attacks; (2) conditioned fear of sleep; (3) delayed sleep and chronic-intermittent sleep deprivation; (4) sleep deprivation-induced and/or relaxation-induced precipitation or exacerbation of waking and sleep panic attacks; and (5) worsening of fears and avoidance behaviors (Uhde, 1994, p. 873). After a comprehensive review of research related to sleep and panic disorder, Uhde (1994) concluded the following:

> Taken together, the observations of several research teams indicate that the complaints of insomnia and sleep panic attacks are reported by a majority of patients with panic disorder. The sleep EEG generally corroborates complaints of restless or broken sleep, although, as a group, the sleep architecture of patients with panic disorder is surprisingly "normal." Sleep panic attacks (when evaluated in patients with pure panic disorder under controlled conditions) appear to be linked in most cases to late stage 2 or early stage 3 sleep (p. 880).

Uhde's review indicates that sleep panic attacks may be a type of parasomnia that differs from sleep terrors.

Patients with sleep panic attacks may develop bizarre sleep habits and try to hide their illness (Uhde, 1994). Careful nursing observations in the inpatient setting, and gentle, non-judgmental questioning of outpatients with panic disorder may help to uncover the presence of sleep panic attacks. An understanding of the dynamics of panic disorder and of the nature and development of sleep (as well as daytime) panic attacks is essential in the treatment of patients with panic disorder.

Generalized Anxiety Disorder

Little research has been done on sleep and GAD, and what has been done has typically included patients with other anxiety disorders in a mixed group (Akiskal et al., 1984; Sitaram et al., 1984, cited in Uhde, 1994). However, the findings of such studies were similar to those of Reynolds, and colleagues (1983), whose polysomnographic research showed increased sleep latencies, increased time awake, and decreased delta sleep in GAD out-patients as compared with depressed outpatients. Therefore, the major sleep problems associated with GAD appear to be difficulty initiating or maintaining sleep (initial or middle insomnia), and restless, fragmented sleep (Uhde, 1994).

SCHIZOPHRENIA

In a review of polysomnographic research with schizophrenic patients, Benson and Zarcone (1989, p. 915) noted that "the most consistently reported sleep abnormality in empirical studies of sleep patterns in schizophrenia is a marked increase in sleep onset latency." In other words, patients with schizophrenia take longer to get to sleep after going to bed. The amount of stage 4 sleep is reduced (Benson and Zarcone, 1989). REM sleep is reduced early in the course of an acute exacerbation of schizophrenia with a return to normal as the illness improves (*DSM IV*, 1994). Slow wave sleep is also reduced in exacerbations of the disease (*DSM IV*, 1994). A meta-analysis indicated a reduced REM latency, decreased total sleep time, reduced sleep efficiency, and prolonged sleep latency in schizophrenia, but these effects were also seen in affective disorders, anxiety disorders, dementia, and insomnia. (Benca, et al., 1992)

DEMENTIA

Moderate to severe sleep disturbances are associated with dementia. It has been theorized that these sleep disturbances are an exaggeration of the deterioration of sleep seen with normal aging. There is a flattening of the sleep–wake cycle with episodes of wakefulness during nocturnal sleep and decreased alertness as well as sleep during the day. Wandering at night is common and may lead to institutionalization (Walsh, Moss, and Sugarman, 1994).

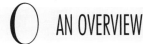

AN OVERVIEW

- Sleep is affected in most psychiatric disorders and many medical conditions; it may be further compromised by the effects of medication and the environment.

- On the basis of physiological parameters that can be directly measured by polysomnography, sleep is divisible into non-rapid eye movement (NREM) sleep, which has four stages, and rapid eye movement (REM) sleep.

- A sleep history assessment gathers comprehensive patient information about sleep patterns, sleep hygiene, sleep habits, and the presence of sleep-related symptoms or phenomena such as bruxism, headaches, insomnia, or nightmares.

- The principles of sleep hygiene are behavioral interventions that promote sleep and decrease awakenings. Maintaining a sleep schedule, avoiding alcohol and caffeine prior to sleep, and relaxing immediately before bedtime are examples of sleep-hygienic practices.

- The nursing diagnosis of sleep-pattern disturbance should be specific with regard to the cause or factors associated with the disturbance. Nursing interventions should be based on the principles of sleep hygiene as well as the patient's specific needs and condition.

- Primary sleep disorders are those in which the etiology cannot be attributed to a mental disorder, medical disorder, or substance. They are divided into dyssomnias, which are characterized by abnormalities in the amount, quality, or timing of sleep, and parasomnias, in which abnormal behavioral or physiological events occur in association with sleep, specific sleep stages, or sleep–wake transitions.

- Disturbed sleep is a symptom of virtually all psychiatric disorders, and is one of the diagnostic criteria for all mood disorders.

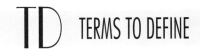

TERMS TO DEFINE

- bruxism
- cataplexy
- dyssomnias
- hypnic myoclonia

- hypnogogic hallucinations
- hypnopompic hallucinations
- insomnia
- narcolepsy
- nightmare
- parasomnias
- polysomnogram
- somnambulism

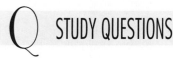

STUDY QUESTIONS

Multiple Choice

1. Rapid eye movement (REM) sleep is best conceptualized as
   a. a highly activated brain in a moveable body.
   b. a relatively inactive brain in a moveable body.
   c. a highly activated brain in a paralyzed body.
   d. a relatively inactive brain in a paralyzed body.

2. In adults, sleep is normally entered through which of the following?
   a. NREM stage 2.
   b. Slow-wave sleep.
   c. REM period 1.
   d. Sleep onset REM periods (SOREMPS).

3. Which of the following statements is true about the effect of NREM sleep?
   a. Strenuous exercise late in the evening will promote sleep.
   b. Regular moderate exercise will deepen sleep over time.
   c. Occasional, "one shot" exercise during the day will lead to deeper sleep during the night.
   d. For people over the age of 60, exercise has no effect on nocturnal sleep.

4. During a Monday morning group meeting on the inpatient unit, P.B., a 36-year-old patient with borderline personality disorder, complains that she could not sleep during the past weekend because the night staff was laughing and talking loudly. Several of the more vocal patients agree. The nurse would be justified to recognize that

   a. this is a clear attempt at splitting the staff.
   b. the patient has abandonment issues that intensify at night and stem from early childhood experiences.
   c. the patient probably did not receive her PRN sleep medication over the weekend.
   d. this is a potentially valid complaint that requires further investigation.

5. M.K., a 32-year-old patient with major depressive disorder, was admitted to the inpatient medical-psychiatric unit 3 weeks ago. He has AIDS, peripheral neuropathy, and a history of substance abuse. He states he has been drug-free for about a year. During the past 3 nights he has awakened frequently, complaining of pain. The nurse recognizes that this indicates
   a. drug-seeking behavior.
   b. the treatment team must be notified to evaluate the patient's pain, behavior, and the need for analgesia.
   c. the patient does not yet have a therapeutic blood level of antidepressants.
   d. the patient is using attention-getting behavior to manipulate the night nurse to spend more time with him.

6. P.J., a 50-year-old man in the partial hospitalization program, has been complaining of morning headaches several times a week for the past few weeks. He has a headache again this morning. The best nursing interventions would be to
   a. institute seizure precautions, hold all psychotropic medications, and call the psychiatrist.
   b. give the patient his PRN headache medication, document its effectiveness, and educate him about principles of sleep hygiene.
   c. give the patient his PRN headache medication, assess his sleep history, and notify the psychiatrist that he has been having recurrent morning headaches.
   d. give the patient his PRN headache medication and enter into a therapeutic discussion to help him see how his behavior the night before relates to his present symptoms.

7. Following a class about the principles of sleep hygiene that you teach at a community senior center, a 90-year-old woman mentions that for as long as she can remember she has seen strange things right before going to sleep. She denies other sleep-related problems, except that she wakes up more often at night than she used to. She says she knows that these visions aren't real, and because they only come right before sleep they don't bother her. In

later discussing this with your colleagues, you explain that

   a. the visions are a classic example of mild schizophrenia that has probably gone undiagnosed because the woman is highly functional.

   b. such hallucinations are a cardinal symptom of dementia, and because of the effects of age on long-term memory, the patient probably cannot accurately recall her age at the onset of symptoms.

   c. the woman probably has a long history of alcohol or substance abuse.

   d. the patient has given a classic description of hypnogogic hallucinations, which are benign in the absence of other symptoms. There may be a family history of narcolepsy.

Essay Questions

1. L.G., a 70-year-old man who attends the bereaved-spouse-support group you facilitate, complains to you that he has not slept well lately. He has a doctor's appointment next week but wants you to suggest something to help him sleep. He also asks you why you think he is having this problem.

   • What further information would you want to gather?

   • What are some possible causes of his problem?

   • What would you suggest to help him sleep?

2. You have been asked by the nurse manager to conduct a class on sleep-related issues for staff being oriented to the night shift. They have already had a class on normal sleep and principles of sleep hygiene. What specific major points would you want to include in your class from a nursing perspective? Explain your rationale for including each point.

■ REFERENCES

Akiskal H, Lemmi H, Dickson H, King D, Yerevanian B, Van Valkenberg C: Sleep EEG differentiation of primary dysthymic disorders from anxious depressions. *J Affect Disord* 6:287–295.

Aldrich MS: in Kryger M, Roth T, Dement W (eds): Cardinal manifestations of sleep disorders. *Principles and Practice of Sleep Medicine, 2nd ed.*, Philadelphia, WB Saunders, 1994, pp. 413–425.

Aldrich MS, Chauncey JB: Are morning headaches part of obstructive sleep apnea syndrome? *Arch Intern Med* 1990; 150:1265-1267.

Diagnostic and Statistical Manual of Mental Disorders, 4th ed. Washington, DC, American Psychiatric Association, 1994.

Annseau M, Kupfer DJ, Reynolds CF, McEachran AB: REM latency distribution in major depression: Clinical characteristics associated with sleep onset REM periods (SOREMP's). *Biol Psychiatry* 1984; 19:1651–1666.

Astrom C, Lunde I, Ortmann Boyce G, Trojaborg W: Sleep disturbances in torture survivors. *Acta Neurol Scand* 1989; 79:150–154.

Becker J, Skinner L, Abel G, Tracey E: Depressive symptoms associated with sexual assault. *Arch Sex Behav* 1984; 10(3):185–192.

Benca RM: Mood Disorders, in Kryger M, Roth T, Dement W (eds): *Principles and Practice of Sleep Medicine, 2nd ed.*, Philadelphia, WB Saunders, 1994, pp. 899–913.

Benca RM, Obermeyer WH, Thisted RA, Gillin JC: Sleep and psychiatric disorders: A meta-analysis. *Am J Psychiatry* 1992; 49:651–668.

Benson K, Zarcone V: Slow wave sleep deficits: Their magnitude, distribution and reliability. *Sleep Res* 1989; 18:165.

Bliwise DL: Normal aging, in Kryger M, Roth T, Dement W (eds): *Principles and Practice of Sleep Medicine, 2nd ed.*, Philadelphia, WB Saunders, 1994, pp. 26–39.

Borbely AA: The S-deficiency hypothesis and the Two-process model of sleep regulation. *Pharmacopsychiatry* 1987; 20:23–29.

Brett E, Ostroff R: Imagery and posttraumatic stress disorder: An overview. *Am J Psychiatry* 1985; 142(4):417–425.

Borbely AA, Wirz-Justice A: Sleep, sleep deprivation and depression: A hypothesis derived from a model of sleep regulation. *Hum Neurobiol* 1982; 1:205–210.Carskadon M, Brown ED, Dement WC: Sleep fragmentation in the elderly: Relationship to daytime sleep tendency. *Neurobiol Aging* 1982; 3:321–327.

Carskadon M, Dement W: Normal human sleep: An overview, in Kryger M, Roth T, Dement W (eds): *Principles and Practice of Sleep Medicine, 2nd ed.*, Philadelphia, WB Saunders, 1994, pp. 16–25.

Carskadon M, Rechtschaffen A: Monitoring and staging human sleep. in Kryger M, Roth T, Dement W (eds): *Principles and Practice of Sleep Medicine, 2nd ed.*, Philadelphia, WB Saunders, 1994, pp. 943–960.

Carpenito LJ: *Nursing Diagnosis: Application to Clinical Practice,* (6th ed.), Philadelphia, JB Lippincott, 1995.

Coble PA, Kupfer DJ, Shaw DH: Distribution of REM latency in depression. *Biol Psychiatry* 1981; 16:453–466.

Duncan WC, Pettigrew KD, Gillin JC: REM architecture changes in bipolar and unipolar depression. *Am J Psychiatry* 1979; 136(11):1424–1427.Evans D, Rogers A: 24-hour sleep/wake patterns in healthy elderly persons. *Appl Nurs Res* 1994; 7(2):75–83.

Fleming J: Sleep architecture in depression: Interesting finding or clinically useful? *Neuropsychopharmacol Biol Psychiatry* 1989; 13:419–429.

Forman B: Cognitive modification of obsessive thinking in a rape victim: A preliminary study. *Psychol Rep* 1980; 47(3 pt. 1):819–822.

Frank E, Stewart B: Depressive symptoms in rape victims: A revisit. *J Affect Disord* 1984; 7(1):877–895.

Frank E, Turner S, Duffy B: Depressive symptoms in rape victims. *J Affect Disord* 1979; 1(4):269–277.

Frederickson PA, Krueger BR: Insomnia associated with specific polysomnographic findings, in Kryger M, Roth T, Dement W (eds): *Principles and Practice of Sleep Medicine, 2nd ed.*, Philadelphia, WB Saunders, 1994, pp. 523–533.

Gillin J, Sitaram N, Duncan W: Muscarinic supersensitivity: A possible model for sleep disturbances of primary depression? *Psychiatr Res* 1979; 1:17–22.

Greenberg R, Pearlman C, Gampel D: War neuroses and the adaptive function of REM sleep. *Br J Med Psychol* 1972; 45:27–33.

Hartmann E: Bruxism, in Kryger M, Roth T, Dement W (eds): *Principles and Practice of Sleep Medicine, 2nd ed.*, Philadelphia, WB Saunders, 1994a, pp. 598–601.

Hartmann E: Nightmares and other dreams, in Kryger M, Roth T, Dement W (eds): *Principles and Practice of Sleep Medicine, 2nd ed.*, Philadelphia, WB Saunders, 1994b, pp. 407–410.

Hartmann E: *The Psychology and Biology of Terrifying Dreams.* New York, Basic Books, 1984.

Hauri P, Linde S: *No More Sleepless Nights.* New York, John Wiley & Sons, 1990.

Knowles JB, Southmayd SE, Delva N, MacLean AW, Cairns J, Letemendia FJ: Five variations of sleep deprivation in a depressed woman. *Br J Psychiatry* 1979; 135:403–410.

Kramer M, Kinney L: Is sleep a marker of vulnerability to delayed posttraumatic stress disorder? *Sleep Res* 1985; 14:181.

Krystal H, Niederland W: Clinical observations on the survivor syndrome, in Krystal H, (ed): *Massive Psychic Trauma.* New York, International Universities Press, 1968, pp. 327–348.

Larson H, Pagaduan-Lopez J: Stress-tension reduction in the treatment of sexually tortured women—an exploratory study. *J Sex Marit Ther* 1987; 13(3):210–218.

Lavie P, Hefez A, Halperin G, Enoch D: Long-term effects of war-related events on sleep. *Am J Psychiatry* 1979; 136(2):175–178.

Libow J, Doty D: An exploratory approach to self-blame and self-derogation by rape victims. *Am J Orthopsychiatry* 1979; 49(4):670–679.

Lugaresi E, Cirignotta F, Coccagna G, Piana C: Some epidemiological data on snoring and cardio circulatory disturbances. *Sleep* 1980; 3:221–224.

McCarley RW: REM sleep and depression: Common control mechanisms. *Am J Psychiatry* 1982; 139:565–570.

Melman TA, Uhde TW: Sleep in panic and generalized anxiety disorders, in Ballenger JC (ed): *Neurobiology of Panic Disorders (Frontiers in Clinical Neuroscience, vol. 8,* New York, Alan R. Liss, 1990, pp. 365–376.)

Mezey G, Taylor P: Psychological reactions of women who have been raped. *Br J Psychiatry* 1988; 152:330–339.

Mikulincer M, Glaubman H, Wasserman O, Porat A: Control-related beliefs and sleep characteristics of posttraumatic stress disorder patients. *Psychol Rep* 1989; 65:567–576.

Miles LE, Dement WC: Sleep and aging. *Sleep* 1980; 3:1–220.

Nadelson C, Notman M, Zackson H, Gornick J: A follow-up study of rape victims. *Am J Psychiatry* 1982; 139(10):1266–1270.

Niederland W: An interpretation of the psychological stresses and defenses in concentration camp survivors and the late aftereffects, in Krystal H, (ed): *Massive Psychic Trauma.* New York, International Universities Press, 1968, pp. 60–70.

Norris J, Feldman-Summers S: Factors related to the psychological impacts of rape on the victim. *J Abnorm Psychol* 1981; 90(6):562–567.

Rechtschaffen A, Kales A (eds): *A Manual of Standardized Terminology: Techniques and Scoring System for Sleep Stages of Human Subjects.* Los Angeles, UCLA Brain Information Service/Brain Research Institute, 1968.

Reynolds CF, Kupfer DJ: Sleep research: State of the art circa 1987. *Sleep* 1987; 10(3):199–215.

Reynolds CF, Shaw DH, Newton TF, Coble PA, Kupfer DJ: EEG sleep in outpatients with generalized anxiety—A preliminary comparison with depressed outpatients. *Psychiatr Res* 1983; 9:81–89.

Ross R, Ball W, Dinges D, Kribbs N, Morrison A, Silver S: REM sleep disturbance as the hallmark of PTSD. *American Psychiatric Association New Research.* American Psychiatric Association 143rd Annual Meeting, New York, 1990a.

Ross R, Ball W, Dinges D, Mulvaney F, Kribbs N, Morrison A, Silver S: Motor activation during REM sleep in posttraumatic stress disorder. *Sleep Res* 1990b; 19:175.

Ross R, Ball W, Sullivan K, Carroff S: Sleep disturbance as the hallmark of PTSD. *Am J Psychiatry* 1989; 146(6):697–707.

Shaver JL, Giblin EC: Sleep. *Annu Rev Nurs Res* 1989; 7:71–93.

Schlosberg A, Benjamin M: Sleep patterns in three acute combat fatigue cases. *J Clin Psychiatry* 1978; 39:546–549.

Uhde TW: The anxiety disorders, in Kryger M, Roth T, Dement W (eds): *Principles and Practice of Sleep Medicine, 2nd ed.*, Philadelphia, WB Saunders, 1994, pp. 871–898.

Vogel GW, McAbee R, Barker K, Thurmaond A: Endogenous depression improvement and REM pressure. *Arch Gen Psychiatry* 1977; 34:96–97.

Vogel GW, Thurmond A, Gibbons P, Sloan K, Boyd M, Walker M: REM sleep reduction effects on depression syndromes. *Arch Gen Psychiatry* 1975; 37:247–253.

Vogel GW, Vogel F, McAbee RS, Thurmond AJ: Improvement of depression by REM sleep deprivation. *Arch Gen Psychiatry* 1980; 32:765–777.

Walsh JK, Moss KL, Sugarman J: Insomnia in adult psychiatric disorders, in Kryger M, Roth T, Dement W (eds): *Principles and Practice of Sleep Medicine, 2nd ed.*, Philadelphia, WB Saunders, 1994, pp. 500–508.

Wehr TA: Improvement of depression and triggering of mania by sleep deprivation. *JAMA* 1992; 267(4):548–551).

Wehr TA: Sleep loss: A preventable cause of mania and other excited states. *J Clin Psychiatry* 1989; 50(suppl 12):8–16.

Wehr T, Wirz-Justice A, Goodwin F: Phase advance of the circadian sleep-wake cycle as an antidepressant. *Science* 1979; 206:210–213.

Wiegand M, Berger M, Zulley J, Lauer C, von Zerssen D: The influence of daytime naps on the therapeutic effect of sleep deprivation. *Biol Psychiatry* 1987; 22:389–392.

Wooten V: Medical causes of insomnia, in Kryger M, Roth T, Dement W, (eds): *Principles and Practice of Sleep Medicine, 2nd ed.*, Philadelphia, WB Saunders, 1994, pp. 509–522.

Zarcone VP: Sleep hygiene, in Kryger M, Roth T, Dement W (eds): *Principles and Practice of Sleep Medicine, 2nd ed.*, Philadelphia, WB Saunders, 1994, pp. 542–546.

Zorick F: Overview of insomnia, in Kryger M, Roth T, Dement W (eds): *Principles and Practice of Sleep Medicine*, Philadelphia, WB Saunders, 1989, pp. 431–432.

3

Level 3

Traumatic Stress Crises

Crises precipitated by strong, externally imposed stresses compose Level 3 of the stress–crisis continuum. These crises may involve experiencing, witnessing, or learning about a sudden, unexpected, and uncontrolled life-threatening event that overwhelms the coping capacity of the individual. Examples of traumatic crises are crime-related victimization by assault, rape and sexual assault, arson, and hostage taking. Level-3 crises are also experienced by victims of serious vehicular accidents or airplane crashes; they are caused by the sudden death of a partner or family member; accidents resulting in physical dismemberment; and diagnoses of serious medical illness.

The individual's response is intense fear, helplessness, and behavioral disorganization. Usual coping behaviors are rendered ineffective by the sudden, unanticipated nature of the stress. This may be followed by a refractory period in which the individual experiences emotional paralysis, and cannot mobilize coping behaviors.

The etiology of traumatic stress involves activation of the limbic system, which is the part of the autonomic nervous system responsible for the "fight-or-flight" response. Cognitive processing of traumatic information is interrupted.

Cognitive behavioral therapy (cognitive processing therapy) is recommended to help patients process trauma-related information. Pharmacotherapy is used to treat traumatic stress. Anti-anxiety medication is given for the long-term physiological symptoms of PTSD. Following individual trauma therapy, patients may be referred for stress reduction/relaxation treatment, to crisis or self-help groups, and to psychoeducation groups.

Traumatic stress crises are discussed in the following two chapters:

- *Treating Child Sexual Trauma*
- *Victims of Sexual Assault*

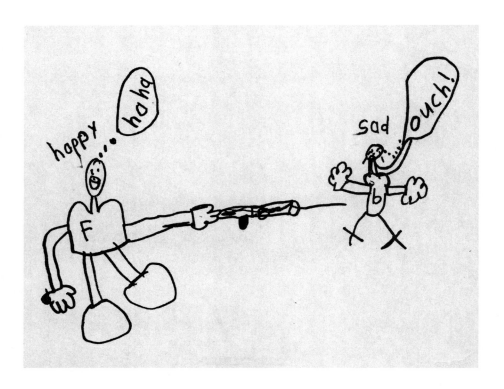

Canst thou not minister to a mind diseas'd,
Pluck from the memory a rooted sorrow,
Raze out the written troubles of the brain,
And with some sweet oblivious antidote
Cleanse the stuff'd bosom of that perilous stuff
Which weighs upon the heart?

William Shakespeare, *Macbeth*

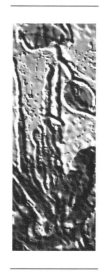

24

Treating Child Sexual Trauma

Ann Wolbert Burgess / Carol R. Hartman / Paul T. Clements, Jr.

The question "Where do childhood memories go?" has been debated in terms of infantile amnesia for decades. Do failures to recollect early events in life come from problems of memory retrieval, problems of memory storage, or some combination of the two? The fate of childhood memories launched Freud's psychoanalytic career. Although Freud (1953, 1963) argued passionately that early autobiographical memories persist, albeit repressed in the unconscious, and influence daily behavior in a disguised manner, he and others (Anthony, 1961; Isakower, 1938) questioned the recoverability of early memory. Even so, psychoanalysts believed that a favorable therapeutic outcome for psychological disorders hinged on the successful retrieval and analysis of early childhood events.

The importance of childhood traumatic memories stemming from rape and molestation and their relationship to acting-out behavior is for the early identification of hypersexual or aggressive sexual perpetrating behavior among teenagers. This chapter presents a theoretical framework for the information processing of trauma model, the outcome patterns of sexual trauma, their effects on the processing of memories, and the sequelae of these memories on psychological function.

■ INFORMATION PROCESSING OF TRAUMA (IPT)

The conceptual framework of traumatic event processing was developed for a research project (Burgess, Hartman and McCormack, 1987) because of the lack of explicit, tested frameworks for understanding the link between child sexual victimization and level of adjustment. During the research design phase, we were not aware of any related models and our confidence in this model came from clinical and interview experiences with victims and victimizers (Burgess, et al., 1984; Burgess, et al., 1986). Further work on the model included posttrauma outcomes in DSM-IV terminology (Burgess, Hartman, and Clements, 1995).

CONCEPTUAL FRAMEWORK

The Information Processing of Trauma Model assumes the basic constructs of information processing in a living system: experiences are processed on a sensory, perceptual, and cognitive level (see Chapter 5). The sensory level is the basic registrant of experience in the individual. The perceptual level is the beginning classification of sensory processing. The cognitive phase represents the larger organization of experience into meaning systems. The construct of memory is applicable to each level of information processing.

Horowitz (1976) began to research the impact of trauma and the response to stressful stimuli. A general stress response syndrome was identified by a clustering of disturbing psychological phenomena of intrusive imagery (e. g., flashbacks to sights, thoughts, sounds, feelings, and odors) associated with the memories of the traumatic event. Avoidant strategies were employed to keep the memories and associations to the trauma out of awareness with the presumption that traumatic information is kept in active awareness until it can be placed in distant memory. Trauma resolution occurs when there is sufficient processing for the information to be stored. The event is remembered, attendant feelings are neutralized, and the anxiety generated by the event is controlled. When a traumatic event is not resolved and either remains in active memory or becomes defended by a cognitive mechanism—such as denial, dissociation, or splitting—the diagnosis is generally posttraumatic stress disorder (PTSD). The central feature of PSTD, which is the stress pattern resulting from traumatization, is that the individual reexperiences the original trauma both unconsciously and consciously.

The four major phases of the Information Processing of Trauma Model (see Figure 24–1) gives a rationale to the various response patterns identified in child victims (Burgess, et al, 1984; Hartman and Burgess 1988). Intervention is an optional phase.

1. The **Pretrauma Phase** identifies parameters of the child's make up and social context that might affect the child's management and resolution of sexual abuse (e.g., development in terms of age, personality, sociocultural factors, family structure and interaction with child, and history of prior trauma).

Research on the influence of the parameters is not definitive in predicting outcome. Rather, these parameters serve to mediate that which is particular to the general stress response syndrome.

2. The **Trauma Encapsulation Phase** focuses on the mechanisms used by the child to regulate ongoing sexual activities and responses. The INPUT is derived from the offender's behavior (e.g., victim relationship to offender, entrapment and access to child, use of force, control used, occurances and sexual activities, and method of insuring secrecy). Offender behaviors are received, transmitted, and processed by the sensory, perceptual, and cognitive domains of the child. THRUPUT includes the coping and defensive mechanisms employed by the child to deal with the anxiety, fear, and danger invoked by the abuse. During the encapsulation phase, various defenses are put into play. They are dissociation, denial, fragmentation of self, arousal disharmony, repression, and splitting. These defenses with their particular behavioral and experimental dimensions are noted by clinicians.

Dissociation is a general process in which the mind fragments psychic integrity in the service of survival by disengaging from an ongoing trauma. Sensory dissociation is marked by a total numbing of a body part; perceptual dissociation is noted in dimming of sensory cues such as a muffling of sound, a narrowing and distancing of the perceptual field; cognitive dissociation is noted in the experience of being somewhere else, floating above the trauma scene.

Denial is the total discounting that something has happened, that one has a negative emotional reaction to an event. In children, there is this denial of abuse, the event itself, or denial that it was upsetting in any way.

Repression is keeping from conscious awareness all aspects of a traumatic event. It is more comprehensive and basic than denial. Most dramatic is the lifting of repression, with the child having full recollection of the abuse.

Fragmentation of a sense of self implies disruption of integrative personality functions that result in knowledge of self. For example, an awareness of one's capacity to aggress is blocked; consequently the child is unaware of assaulting another child. A sense of competency is compromised, the child identifies with his inability to master a particular situation but does not recognize the ability to handle other situations. Self-appraisal is distorted. The ability to move from experience in a flexible manner, using memory, making con-

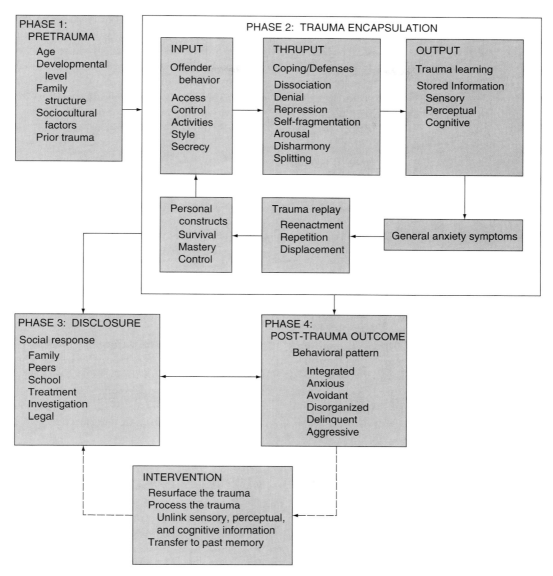

Figure 24–1. Information Processing of Trauma Model

nections between different levels of experience and evolving an integrated sense of self are compromised.

Arousal disharmony is the disruption of the capacity to regulate states of excitement and calmness. This phenomena is noted in the numbness state that ensues to block sensory overload during the traumatic event. This leaves the individual blocking a massive state of anxiety generated by the trauma, and at the same time the person is cut off from regulated ranges of arousal generated in nontraumatizing situations. In sexual abuse of children a premature excitation of sexual sensations is compounded by fear and confusion. Incongruent commands from the offender disrupt the child's naturally unfolding, sensory regulating capacities. One

consequence of this is excessive masterbation without awareness.

Splitting is the polarization of complex units of behavior, perceptions, and cognitions manifested in responses to self and other. In psychoanalytic terms, it is a conflict between the demand of the instinct and command of reality. The rift never heals, but instead increases with time. In the sexually abused child splits are noted in the good vs bad parent, the good child, the loved vs hated child, the trusted other the betraying other.

During the THRUPUT component of the Encapsulation Phase, these defensive operations shape the primary meaning of the abuse as well as shape the structure of how the abuse information is processed, stored, and represented through affect and nonverbal behavior.

The third component of the trauma encapsulation phase, OUTPUT, is the primary trauma learning which is the charged sensory, perceptual, and cognitive memory base of the event. Trauma learning is an important anxiety-management mechanism. Of the three domains the sensory and perceptual often override the cognitive in registering the abuse. All of the information associated with the trauma learning results in an important feedback loop of intermediate outputs. These looping outputs have a reinforcing quality because of short-term anxiety reactions—they do not neutralize the anxiety; they are general anxiety symptoms. For example, the child develops new fears, and there is an onset of bedwetting and soiling, irritability, regressive behavior, tics, startle response, and physical complaints. *Trauma replay* is the manifestation of specific actions, reactions, and activities that directly represent the trauma learning linked to the behaviors developed during the trauma itself. A series of fixed behaviors emerge and the three manifestations of trauma replay presented in the model are descriptions to sensitize an observer to this phenomena. *Reenactment* is reliving the event. *Repetition* is a repeating of acts onto another person, usually a child, that resembles the abusive event. *Displacement* is the symbolic representation of the abusive act as in doll play, drawings, dreams, or fantasy construction.

The feedback loop also contains *the dynamic individual meaning* that the trauma holds for the child. Dynamic underscores the shifting meanings which arise from the victim as well as the victimizer's behaviors. The interplay of cognitive mediation efforts of the trauma are grounded in person constructs. First are constructs dealing with the recognition of danger and survival strategies associated with the reenactment of the trauma. The second level of construct and meaning formation deals with preliminary mastery over actions, reactions, and transactions that occur during the trauma and is represented in the various replay patterns. The third level of construct formation centers around control over anxiety induced by specific memories of the trauma and is more often manifested in displacement replay of the trauma. This third level construct contains the conscious recollection of the event. This is the conscious reconstruction memory of what happened.

Nondisclosure presumes encapsulation of the primary trauma learning. Over time, the child left to his own devices, reformulates the trauma through the defensive operations used to survive, the general anxiety symptoms, and the emerging meaning structures the child attaches to the trauma. Behavior and learning problems are not associated by others with the sexual abuse and often compromise the child's development. The event is sealed from ongoing daily life. However,

to the degree that the anxiety remains charged (non-neutralized), relationships, social and academic achievements, and a sense of right and wrong and of self can be distorted. There is disturbance in the self-comforting, caring, and protective functions of the child's self-system. Attachment to others and social values is distorted and/or weakened. There is distortion in a personal sense of pleasure.

Phase Two (Trauma Encapsulation) emphasizes the looping back principle in an active system. Continued abuse is registered and modified in this process. We theorize that the powerful aspects of this primary trauma learning are linked to dominance of the sensory and perceptual domains over the cognitive domain.

3. The **Disclosure Phase** of the model contains the social, or secondary, meaning. What happens if the child tells someone of the abuse or if the abuse is kept secret? This phase heralds the child fielding the reactions of his social network by revealing the sexual abuse. This learning can result in a reformulation of the trauma.

4. During the **post-trauma outcome phase** the victim of a traumatic experience exhibits a progression of symptoms and behaviors. Six behavioral patterns are noted: integrated, anxious, avoidant, disorganized, delinquent, and aggressive. These patterns have been refined to the diagnostic language of the DSM-IV (see Figure 24–2).

■ OUTCOMES PATTERNS OF TRAUMA LEARNING

The victim of a traumatic experience exhibits a progression of symptoms and behaviors. A traumatic event is defined as a stressor that overwhelms biological systems for managing stimuli. After the traumatic event is encountered, various memory and learning patterns may occur, including integration of trauma, post-traumatic stress disorder (PTSD), or delayed PTSD.

INTEGRATION OF TRAUMA

The optimal response to a traumatic event results in its integration into the victim's life experience; post-traumatic stress disorder (PTSD) does not occur. In the integrated pattern of response to sexual trauma, the patient can relate to the traumatic experience but is not compelled to dwell on it or avoid it through psychological defenses.

POST-TRAUMATIC STRESS DISORDER

In a classic PTSD, a bi-phasic response is noted: the victim may exhibit intrusive thoughts and/or avoidant behaviors. Exposure to stimuli can induce a state of hy-

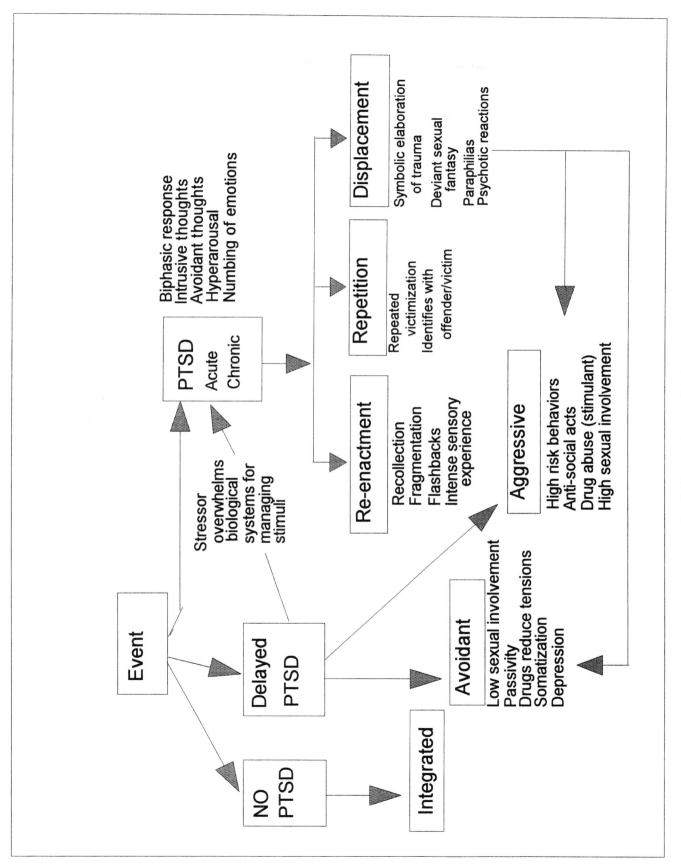

Figure 24.2: Post-trauma: Outcomes and PTSD Outcomes

perarousal and numbing, which may cause the victim to experience highly emotional states with lower levels of thinking. Rainey et al. (1987) describe visual and motoric reliving of the traumatic event, with nightmares and flashbacks that are generally preceded by physiological arousal. These disruptions may also affect sensory, perceptual/cognitive and interpersonal performance. Symptoms of sensory disruption, for example, may include hyperactivity, headaches, stomachaches, back pain, genitourinary distress, and nightmares; perceptual and cognitive disruptions may include intrusive images and auditory and kinesthetic information associated with the traumatic experience, set off by internal and external cues. These may be related to future concerns about repeated danger. Symptoms of disruption in interpersonal performance include avoidant behaviors, such as excessive fear of others, and an inability to assert and/or protect oneself. Other disruptions may be manifested as aggressive behaviors, including agitation, aggression toward peers/family/pets, and potentially sexualized behavior toward others.

Several patterns of symptoms are noted in PTSD, as follows:

- The **anxious pattern** is characterized by generalized fears that have to do with developmental tasks as well as with the abuse experience. There is anxious recollection of the abuse experience if the patient is probed or asked. Anxiety disorder, eating disorder, phobic disorder, and obsessive–compulsive disorder have been associated with unresolved trauma.
- The **avoidant pattern** is characterized by denial or recanting of the abusive event. The patient appears distant and alienated. There is a lack of energy for living and learning. Often the patient has a preoccupied, "day-dreamy" quality. Adolescents with a history of sexual trauma may have a substance-abuse history, depression, suicidal thoughts, phobic behavior, an adjustment problem, or conduct disorder.
- The **aggressive pattern** of symptoms is characterized by excessive sexual and/or aggressive behavior. This acting out may be bold or secret. Minimal acknowledgment or frank denial of prior abuse is typical. Rules are tested and broken. The patient is impulsive and fights with peers. Anxiety is also evident in fears and somatic concerns. Diagnostic labels of "hyperactive," "learning disabled," "conduct disorder," or "impulse disorder" are sometimes used. The disorganized pattern of reaction is characterized by fragmented and sometimes bizarre behavior. Dissociative states need to be ruled out. There may be denial or frank amnesia for prior sexual abuse.

DELAYED POST-TRAUMATIC STRESS DISORDER

Because of the neurobiology of trauma, the victim's typical response pattern is not manifested. Van der Kolk (1989) warns that the victim who does not integrate the trauma is doomed to repeat the repressed material as a contemporary experience, rather than remembering it as something that belongs to the past.

Some victims of trauma may not initially develop PTSD, but may rather progress to delayed PTSD, displaying no visible sequelae of the traumatic event. Van der Kolk (1988) notes that persons with this type of PTSD continue to live in the emotional atmosphere of the traumatic event, with an enduring vigilance for and sensitivity to environmental threats.

Avoidant behaviors include infrequent sexual involvement, passivity, the use of substances to reduce tension, somatic complaints, and depression. Aggressive patterns include participating in high-risk behaviors and anti-social acts, use of stimulant substances, and excessive sexual involvement.

Delayed PTSD is activated either through another trauma or some symbolic event such as the anniversary of the original trauma. Van der Kolk (1988) points out an intertwining of psychological and biological reactions to trauma.

■ TYPES OF TRAUMA LEARNING

Trauma learning emphasizes the repetition of a pattern of behavior a notion Freud (1939) discussed in his book *Moses and Monotheism*. This repetition can be observed in traumatized children as a reenactment of the traumatic event, reflecting positive and negative effects of a traumatic experience—repetition of the trauma as its victim or perpetrator, or displacement of the aggression (Hartman and Burgess, 1988).

RE-ENACTMENT

In **re-enactment,** the patient first recollects a traumatic event. This may be indicated by flashbacks, which may contain fragmented detail, and intense sensory experiences. Young children may engage in repetitive play in which themes or aspects of the trauma are expressed. The verbal or play behaviors reveal the child is re-experiencing the trauma. During this stage, identification with the role of the victim continues.

REPETITION

During the **repetition** stage of the trauma learning process, behavior patterns are generally noted in the victim's play with others. These patterns involve mimicking the abusive act with another person, who is usually

E CASE EXAMPLE

▶ REENACTMENT

Diana, a 7-year-old child of mixed African–American and Caucasian racial background, is the only child of her biological parents. She was removed from her home after the parents were unable to maintain a safe living environment. Because Diana's father was reportedly abusive to both Diana and her mother, foster-home placement of the child was effected. While in the foster home, Diana began to report that she was engaging in sexual activity with her foster mother and other children (both male and female) at the home.

Diana was returned to her mother, who began to observe her exhibiting aggressive and uncontrolled behaviors. She kicked, scratched and banged her head, and ran away from school. These behaviors escalated to the point at which hospitalization was required to maintain Diana's safety.

During her inpatient stay, Diana was evaluated by both her school psychologist and the hospital psychiatrist. She told the psychologist she had not wanted to shut the bathroom door, stating: "I was scared to be in there alone, it's where Tim [one of the children in her foster home] humped me."

Diana was observed to be excessively fearful both during the day and night, needing a light on at all times and the bedroom and bathroom doors kept open while she was at home. She reported nightmares in which she was being killed, but was then saved by the Teen-age Mutant Ninja Turtles. Nightmares without the recall of relevant material are usually viewed as a re-enactment of trauma.

During a videotaped interview, Diana was seen to express re-enactment in clinging behavior with the interviewer, interspersed with episodes of agitation and incoherence. In therapy, Diana had many episodes of acting-out, with themes of danger, violation, and assault noted in her play.

Diana, once out of the abusive home, demonstrated an almost continuous state of fear and re-enactment. Her aggressive outbursts appeared to be more focused on escape and protection than on the perpetrative behavior she had previously reported to her mother.

The instability of Diana's behavior required her hospitalization. It was feared that she was self-destructive. The constant intrusion of thoughts related to terrorizing abuse, coupled with the early demand to participate in the abusive act or be gravely harmed has split her sense of her emerging self. This split represents a disruption of the basic functions of explicit memory and learning; Diana views others as potential aggressors or turns the aggression on herself.

Nursing Intervention

Diana's treatment begins with teaching her to self-soothe and calm herself. Her environment must be safe from abuse. Her intrusive memories and their distorted presentations in her daily life can then be linked to the trauma and fear that disrupts her integrative capacities. Learning to identify disruptions as related to traumatic memories rather than to the present, and the development of strategies to modulate the fear response, become the first steps in dealing with traumatic information. The focus of treatment is on altering the patient's response patterns to the recollection of initially overwhelming, fearful experiences.

---

also a child if the victim is a child (Hartman and Burgess, 1988). The behavioral repetition of the trauma may be played out in the role of either the victim or the victimizer. Repetition of the victimization with the victim in the role of the aggressor is a major cause of violence. It is suggested that replay of the trauma through the repetition of sexual act with younger and weaker children gives the child victim a sense of mastery and superiority without concern for the fear, pain, shame, or degradation of another (Burgess, Hartman, and McCormack, 1987). This may in turn create a high risk for prostitution, drug abuse, and suicide attempts in the children who are the objects of the re-enactment (van der Kolk, 1989, p. 391).

DISPLACEMENT

During the **displacement** stage of the trauma learning process, behaviors related to the trauma and thoughts about it are symbolically elaborated. This elaboration may manifest itself as a restorative dream or fantasy, and may include symbolic representation of the abusive act, as in doll play, drawings, dreams, or fantasy construction. Other patterns of elaboration may be deviant sexual fantasies, paraphilias, and ultimately psychotic reactions in cases in which patterns of the original trauma have become embedded in the patient's mental processes.

During the trauma encapsulation (which means before disclosure) several levels of defense begin with dissociation. Dissociation is a biologically adaptive process arising from physiological changes associated with the response to a trauma. Clinically, this response may range from numbness to hyperarousal. A further level of cognitive and behavioral organization occurs out of the disruption in the internal organization of psychic structures in existence prior to the traumatic event. The patient develops schemas that either avoid internal tension or attempt to contain higher levels of internal tension.

Externalizing of these schemas is seen in patterns of aggressive behavior, and internalizing of the schemas is seen in patterns of avoidance and withdrawal (Achen-

E CASE EXAMPLE

▶ REPETITION

Kevin, almost 4 years old, lived with his mother in a rented room at a private residence. Kevin was placed temporarily in the same bedroom with a boy named Tony, the 12-year-old son of the proprietor of the rental property. Over a period of several weeks, Kevin began to display an increasing frequency of masturbation, constant erections, and trying to have "sex" with his teddy bear.

One day, Kevin's mother found that he had emptied all of the toys from his toy box, had removed all of his clothing, and had climbed into the toy box and closed the lid. His distraught mother removed him from the toy box, re-dressed him, and asked him about his actions. Kevin reported that "Tony" had taught him to do that. He also indicated that Tony had touched both his genital and anal regions.

Kevin shows a propensity to identify both with role of the victim and that of the victimizer. In this specific scenario, Kevin has returned to the probable scene of his molestation, has removed all of his clothing, and is recreating his role in the sexual acts of which he was the victim. He has recreated his precarious position by returning to the confines of the toy box, and supports this concept by reporting that this is something that Tony, his victimizer, has "taught" him to do. In his role identification with the vic-

timizer, Kevin has re-created the details of his victimization scenario as he remembers them. The newest factor in his repetition of his traumatization is the addition of his teddy bear, which he is now using in his attempts to act out the role of the perpetrator.

Nursing Intervention

Kevin, with the cooperation of his mother and nurse, can be helped through play to link his aggressive, acting-out behavior to his abuse at the hands of Tony. This is not an easy process because the identification with Tony protects Kevin against the fear he experienced during his victimization and his diminished sense of self as he was overpowered. Instruction about how to survive without becoming a perpetrator will be a key aspect of his therapy.

When a child is forced into actual perpetration, the task is for the child to acknowledge that its behavior was wrong and hurtful. This is a highly difficult process and requires repeated re-working. The therapist attempts to reverse the identities that the victim attributes to him- or herself (e.g., good self, bad self) and to acknowledge that in order to survive, he or she made decisions that do not match the desired, idealized self (Burgess, Hartman, Clements, 1995).

---

bach and Edelbrock, 1978). The complex of trauma learning during the encapsulation phase, in a social context that either encourages or does not deal positively with the externalizing of schema patterns, increases the likelihood that the victim will adapt to the role of aggressive perpetrator. A child's denial of vulnerability and helplessness as a victim, or a child's dissociation from the terror of vulnerability, enhances identification with the aggressor. This reformulation of the original traumatic experience creates the link between being abused and becoming the abuser (Burgess, Hartman, and McCormack, 1987).

■ PRINCIPLES OF EVALUATION AND INTERVENTION

Several evaluation and intervention principles are used in play therapy to help elicit the structure of the trauma learning.

ANCHORING FOR SAFETY

Safety must be established when working with traumatized children. In introducing the child to the interview, clinicians use the skills that are necessary for the child to view the therapist as warm, safe, trusting, and sincere. The context of safety has to be reinforced by

those caring for the child. Parents need to be advised about how to begin to establish safety with their child when it has been eroded by the abuse experience.

This principle has its roots in the encapsulation phase of the IPT model. Associations that the child might have to a safe, caring protective world are loosened. The energy that has been used in attachment to others and to the world of people and values is ruptured. The description in the model alerts the therapist to the difficult task of reestablishing a connection between caring adults and the child. The protest behaviors noted in the child guide the therapist in recognizing the power of what has been learned during the trauma and its primacy over ongoing environmental efforts to reduce the anxiety and terror. Children often sense the efforts of caring adults and will attempt to reduce tension by adopting a quasi-positive state. When this occurs, the dissociation of the trauma is noted in the child's almost automatic fear reactions to stimuli associated with the trauma event.

ESTABLISHING STRESS-REDUCING RESOURCES

The personal inner resources of the child need to be established, recovered, and strengthened. These resources address the sensory, perceptual, and cognitive domains and include relaxation, humor, separating

E CASE EXAMPLE

▶ DISPLACEMENT

Michael was a 10-year-old white child who had witnessed a neighborhood fire that caused the death of a friend. Michael's behavior decompensated during the following year, including agitated depression and hyperactivity resulting in admission to an inpatient child psychiatric facility. During his hospitalization, Michael reported to his mother that an adolescent boy, hospitalized on his unit, had exposed his genitals to him and told him to pull his pants down. On interview, Michael indicated that he was not a willing participant, and had been forced to do what the older boy wanted him to do.

Michael required numerous subsequent hospitalizations. His mother reported that he had stabbed her with a fork and had threatened to kill his siblings. He also displayed violent outbursts at bedtime and refused to sleep in his own bedroom. He showed significant sleep-pattern disturbances, with reports of frequent nightmares. He also developed incontinence of the bladder and then of the bowel, particularly at bedtime. Michael also showed aggression toward his peers and siblings both at home and while hospitalized; his boundary control was poor; he was observed to have minimal concern for others' feelings. The hospital documentation noted that he engaged in frequent episodes of lying, with periods of inability to acknowledge the truth. He shifted blame to others, refusing to take responsibility for his own actions.

Michael began to create tales of fantasy, which frequently included encounters with the police, or the injury or murder of some unknowing victim. He would brag about how he had stabbed his mother in the hand. His gender identity began to blur and he expressed confusion about the roles of boys and girls.

Michael continued to decompensate, with progressive episodes of aggression and behaviors increasingly predicated on fantasy. Ultimately, long-term hospitalization was required to maintain him at an optimal level of safety.

Michael demonstrated displacement in the extreme of acting out behavior. He verbalized homicidal impulses to his mother and siblings. He took the position that no one could control him, but that instead he could control others. The compounded trauma of the fire, his hospitalizations, and the dominance of the older boy in his encounter while at the hospital totally disrupted his sense of attachment to others and that part of himself that was vulnerable.

Nursing Intervention

Taking control of Michael is the initial therapeutic task until, through negotiation and self control, he learns that the primary caretakers in his external world are consistent, safe, and not intent on harming him. Work can then be done on his destructive behavior, and on his defensiveness caused by the overwhelming anxiety he experienced from his trauma.

Michael's acting-out behavior and pattern that "nobody can control me" suggest missing pieces of information about an adult abuser. His background history did not reveal abuse suggestive of his level of aggression. However, further investigation revealed a pattern of family violence, including pathological lying. Medications for Michael may include serotonin-reuptake inhibitors, which enhance serotonin, re-establish the behavioral inhibitory system, and help modulate the catecholamines released during states of potential threat. With this, he will be capable of a more accurate appraisal of his situation, and his aggressively assaultive behavior can be reduced. (Burgess, Hartman, Clements, 1995).

---

past from present, positive imagery, and developing mastery, control, and self-confidence.

This principle acknowledges the arousal and disharmony in the encapsulation phase. It requires that the therapist attend to the pattern of disruptive behavior manifested by the child. For example, in dealing with hyperactive or acting-out behavior, the child is helped to learn that activity can be increased and then relaxed. This skill will help the child manage the tension associated with more direct recall and recounting of the trauma itself. For the child who is avoidant and anxious, quiet music and relaxation help the child deal with anxiety.

SURFACING THE TRAUMA

The principle of surfacing the trauma is applied within the ability of the child to control the degree of detail. Safety parameters and personal resources are used to comfort and reduce anxiety.

Various defenses have been employed by the child to survive the abuse; the child made decisions to inhibit certain behaviors and to produce others. Surfacing the trauma is done to resurrect those behaviors inhibited by the child. The inability to neutralize the trauma rests in part on the child's lack of recognition that what he or she did was important, rather than a reconstructed assumption that he did nothing or was responsible for what happened. The non-neutralized aspects of memory constructs are "fixed" because the cognitive appraisal is limited by the age of the child or the distortion perpetrated by the offender. Consequently, the sensory and perceptual domains dominate the learning, and the child is unable to move from a highly noxious affective state induced by any cue associated with the event. The child and the therapist need to institute any stress-reducing resources that have been developed.

PROCESSING THE TRAUMA

In trauma processing, what happened during the abuse is to be recalled, as well as what did not happen but went on in the mind of the child: what the child did and what he did not do but wanted to do and why he was unable. This processing helps to integrate the fragmented experiences of the trauma and underscores the resourcefulness of the child to survive. Part of the processing is to assist the child in recognizing that the behaviors used to protect are no longer necessary because the child is now safe. This unlinking is done at the sensory, perceptual, and cognitive levels. The trauma experience is neutralized in regard to its fear-induced symptoms and later in the aggressive behaviors manifested in repetition and displacement.

TRANSFERRING THE PROCESSED, OR INTEGRATED, TRAUMA TO PAST MEMORY

The child is introduced to strategies to reduce and categorize what is necessary to remember, what to forget, and how to remember and recall from memory, controlling the associated anxiety.

TERMINATIONS

Finally, the child's verbal reformulation of the trauma is reviewed. This includes terminating the therapeutic relationship and planning telephone follow-up to monitor the child's progress.

O AN OVERVIEW

- Trauma learning patterns of behavior include re-enactment, repetition, or displacement—the symptom complex of post-traumatic stress disorder.

- Although dissociation has been considered a psychological defense, it may better be understood as a first-line biological adaptation to trauma.

- In the encapsulation phase following a traumatic event, symptoms present themselves, but the event itself remains undisclosed.

- Trauma-specific behavior patterns, general hyperarousal symptoms, and avoidant, numbing symptoms persist; however, the emerging disruptive behaviors are not linked to the traumatic event.

- When a child cannot link ongoing, self-defeating, disruptive behavior to a traumatic experience, the underlying fear created by the experience persists; fear interferes with the child's ability to modulate emotions.

- The ability of a traumatized child to discriminate new from old information may be lost; the child is either numb to new information or hyperalert and perceives danger.

- In treatment, consideration is given to children's distress about memories of a traumatic experience and to their incapacity to learn and develop from new interpersonal experiences.

- Nurses must first help the traumatized child to re-learn flexibility through self-observation, pursuing self-soothing and calming behaviors, processing new information, and strengthening social relationships. With new, strengthened personal resources, the child becomes able to begin processing its memories of the trauma.

TD TERMS TO DEFINE

- integration of trauma
- limbic system
- post-traumatic stress disorder
- aggressive pattern
- anxious pattern
- avoidant pattern
- trauma learning
- re-enactment
- repetition
- displacement
- traumatic event

Q STUDY QUESTIONS

Multiple Choice Questions

1. During which of the following phases does a traumatized child display behaviors that reflect identification with both the roles of the victim and the victimizer?
   a. Re-enactment
   b. Repetition
   c. Displacement
   d. Post-traumatic stress disorder

2. In which region of the brain is a person's "alarm system" located?
   a. Cerebellum
   b. Hypothalamus
   c. Frontal lobe
   d. Limbic system

3. Traumatic memories are encoded
   a. bioelectrically.
   b. psychosomatically.
   c. neurohormonally.
   d. naturally.

4. The optimal response pattern following a traumatic event is
   a. no memory of the event.
   b. frequent flashbacks of the event.
   c. delayed post-traumatic stress disorder.
   d. integration of the trauma.

5. All of the following sequelae are associated with post-traumatic stress disorder EXCEPT
   a. intrusive behaviors.
   b. avoidant behaviors.
   c. seizures.
   d. numbing.

6. Denying the occurrence of a traumatic event is typically associated with what dynamic of trauma learning?
   a. Aggressive pattern of behavior
   b. Avoidant pattern of behavior
   c. Integrated pattern of behavior
   d. Delayed post-traumatic stress disorder

7. During which stage of trauma learning would the child's behavior patterns mimic the traumatic event?
   a. Re-enactment
   b. Repetition
   c. Displacement
   d. Aggression

8. During which stage of trauma learning is there a symbolic elaboration of the thought of the trauma?
   a. Re-enactment
   b. Repetition
   c. Displacement
   d. Post-traumatic stress disorder

Essay Questions

1. Briefly describe the concepts of implicit memory and explicit memory, listing the common characteristics of each.

2. Briefly describe the role of the limbic system in human functioning.

3. Briefly describe the function of the fight/flight response pattern to trauma.

4. Briefly describe how nurses can help children through teaching self-soothing and calming behaviors. List 2 realistic interventions for nurses to pursue.

■ REFERENCES

Achenbach T, Edelbrock C: The classification of child psychopathology: A review and analysis of empirical effects. *Psychol Bull* 1978; 85:1275–7307.

Anthony EJ: A study of screen memories, in Eissler RS et al (eds): *The Psychoanalytic Study of the Child,* Vol 16. New York, International Universities Press, 1961; pp. 211–245.

Burgess AW, Hartman CR, Clements PT: Biology of memory and childhood trauma. *J Psychosoc Nsg* 1995; 33:16–26.

Burgess A, Hartman C, McCormack A: Abused to abuser: Antecedents of socially deviant behaviors. *Am J Psychiatry* 1987; 144(11)

Burgess A, Hartman C, Kelly S: Assessing child abuse: The TRIADS checklist. *J Psychosoc Nurs* 1990; 28(4):13.

Chi MTH, Koeske RD: Network representation of a child's dinosauer's knowledge, *Dev Psychol* 1983; 19:29–39.

Flapen D: *Children's Understanding of Social Interaction.* New York, Teachers College Press, 1968.

Freud S: *Moses and Monotheism.* In Strachey J (ed): *The Standard Edition of the Complete Psychological Works of Sigmund Freud.* London, Hogarth Press (original work published in 1905), 1939.

Freud S: Three essays on the theory of sexuality, in Strachey J. (ed): *The Standard Edition of the Complete Psychological Works of Sigmund Freud,* (Vol. 7, pp. 135–243) London: Hogarth Press (original work published in 1905).

Freud S: Introductory lectures on psychoanalysis, in Strachey J (ed): *The Standard Edition of the Complete Psychological Works of Sigmund Freud* (Vol. 15–16, 243–496) London: Hogarth Press. (Original work published in 1916–1917)

Goelet P, Kandel E: Taking the flow of learned information from membrane receptors to genome, *Trends Neurosci* 1986; 9:492–499.

Harlow HF: The development of affectional patterns in infant monkeys, in Foss B (ed): *Determinants of Infant Behavior.* London, Tavistock Institute of Human Relationship, 1961, pp. 75–100.

Harris J, Liebert R: *The Child.* Englewood Cliffs, NJ, Prentice Hall, 1991.

Hartman C, Burgess A: Information processing of trauma. *J Interpers Violence* 1988; 3(4):443.

Hess EH: Imprinting. *Science,* 1959, 130, pp. 133–141.

Horowitz MJ: *Stress Response Syndromes.* New York: Jason Aronson, 1976.

Howe ML, Courage ML: On resolving the enigma of infantile amnesia, *Psychol Bull* 1993; 113(2):305–326.

Isakower O: A contribution to the patho-psychology of phenomena associated with falling asleep, *Int J Psa* 1938; 19:331–345.

Lorenz K: *On Aggression.* New York: Harcourt, Brace and World, 1966. Maser JD, Seligman MEP (eds): *Psychopathology: Experimental Models.* San Francisco, WH Freeman, 1977.

McEwen BS, Mendelson S: Effects of stress on the neurochemistry and morphology of the brain: counter regulation versus damage., In L. Goldberger and S Breznetz, *Handbook of Stress: Theoretical and Clinical Aspects,* 2nd ed., 1993; 101–126.

Pynoos RS, Nader K: Children's memory and proximity to violence. *J Am Acad Child Adolesc Psychiatry* 1989; 28:236–241.

Rainey J, Aleem A, Ortiz A, Yaragani V, Pohl R, Berchow R: Laboratory procedure for inducement of flashbacks. *Am J Psychiatry* 1987; 144:1317–1319.

Squire LR: *Memory and Brain.* New York: Oxford University Press, 1987.

Teicher MH, Glod CA, Surrey J, Swett C Jr: Early childhood abuse and limbic system ratings in adult psychiatric outpatients, *J Neuropsychiatr Clin Neurosci* 1993; 5:301–306.

van der Kolk B: The trauma spectrum: The interaction of biological and social events in the genesis of trauma response. *J Traumatic Stress* 1988; 1(3):274.

van der Kolk B: The compulsion to repeat the trauma: Re-enactment, revictimization, and masochism. *Psychiatr Clin North Am* 1989; 12(2):389.

van der Kolk B, Saporta J: Biological response to psychic trauma. In JP Wilson, B Raphel (eds): *International Handbook of Traumatic Stress Syndromes.* New York: Plenum Press, 1993; pp. 25–33.

Yehuda R, Resnick H, Kahana B, Giller EL: Long-lasting hormonal alterations to extreme stress in humans: Normative or maladaptive? *Psychosom Med* 1993; 55:287–297.

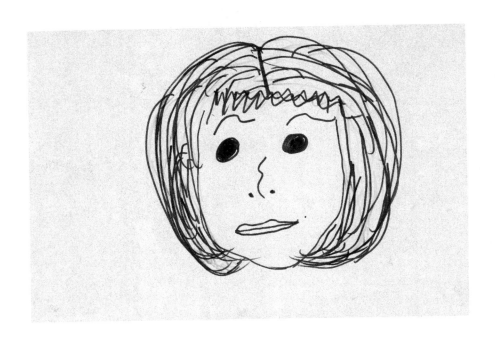

She drew back; he was calm:
 "It is this that had the power."
And he lashed his open palm
With the tender-headed flower.
He smiled for her to smile,
But she was either blind
Or willfully unkind.

He eyed her for a while
For a woman and a puzzle.
He flicked and flung the flower,
And another sort of smile
Caught up like fingertips
The corners of his lips
And cracked his ragged muzzle.

The Subverted Flower, Robert Frost

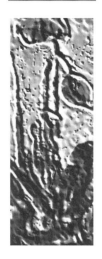

25

Victims of Sexual Assault

Ann Wolbert Burgess / Carol R. Hartman

Rape and incest disrupt the lives of thousands of people every year. In the United States, more than 100,000 cases of forcible rape are reported to the Federal Bureau of Investigation annually. In about half of these cases an assailant is identified and a criminal legal suit follows. Many more cases of incest are known to exist than are reported, owing to pressure applied to an abused child by a family member to keep the abuse secret.

Sexual victimization includes direct and indirect physical and sexual contact. Psychological trauma (an indirect act) is a major component of the psychological aftermath of sexual victimization. The terms describing sexual victimization—rape, incest, and harassment—denote the relationship of the offender to the victim and the location of the assault. Thus, incest implies that the offender is a family member; rape implies that the offender is a stranger or acquaintance; and harassment implies sexual victimization in the workplace. All victimizations, however, are traumatic life events, and all have the capacity to disrupt the normal life patterns of the victim.

The symptoms of stress response to victimization vary. Nurses are key health professionals in providing early intervention and care for victims of sexual assault.

■ RAPE

Rape is forced, violent sexual penetration of a body orifice without the victim's consent. Rape trauma—a clinical nursing term—describes a clustering of bio-psycho-social and cognitive symptoms exhibited by the victim following a rape. Most victims of forcible rape develop a pattern of symptoms described as **rape trauma syndrome** (Burgess and Holmstrom, 1974). This syndrome is an acute reaction to an externally imposed situational crisis. The initial crisis phase of the syndrome, lasting from a few days to several weeks, is followed by a longer phase during which the victim attempts to reorganize her or his disrupted life-style and return it to its precrisis status.

The acute phase of rape trauma syndrome includes many physical symptoms, especially skeletal muscle tension, gastrointestinal irritability, and genitourinary disturbance. Marked disruption may be noted in eating and sleeping patterns ("I have no appetite . . . tried sleeping with the lights on and can't.") as well as a wide range of emotional reactions are reported. ("I'm so jumpy and nervous . . . . cry a lot."). The reorganization phase includes increased motor activity ("Took a trip . . . . just had to get away.") and is characterized in many cases by changes of telephone number and place of residence. There may be an increased need and request for family and social network support ("Visited my family . . . didn't tell them about the rape . . . just wanted to see them.") The development of fears and phobic reactions to the circumstances of the assault is common, as are repeated frightening and disturbing episodes of daytime anxiety and nightmares ("I keep jumping when I walk anywhere . . . so many things scare me . . . never used to be like this."). One victim said, "I lived in a shell for 6 months after the rape. I didn't go anywhere or see anyone. I finally forced myself to find another job, and now two years later I have applied to school."

■ INCEST

Incest has been a social issue and problem throughout the history of civilization, and in the United States has been a growing problem with every successive generation. Like rape, incest is a legal term. It usually refers to sexual intimacies between two persons so closely related that they are forbidden by law to marry. The early feminist literature cites two major dilemmas that confront the incest victim: role/identity confusion and divided loyalty. In terms of role/identity confusion, Herman and Hirschman (1977) describe the situation as follows: A woman who has been raped by someone who is not a

family member can cope with the experience by reacting to it as an intentionally cruel and harmful attack. She is free to hate the rapist because she is not socially or psychologically dependent upon him. In a case of father–daughter incest, however, the daughter is dependent on her perpetrator-father for such parental functions as protection and care. Her mother frequently is not an ally, and the daughter therefore has no recourse to her for protection. Herman and Hirschman point out that the daughter in such a case often does not dare express, or even feel, the depths of her anger at being used. She must comply with her father's demands or risk losing the parental love that she needs. She is not an adult. She cannot walk out of the situation (though she may try to run away). She must endure it, and find in it what compensation she can.

The issue of family loyalty is very important in sexual assault cases in which the assailant is a family member. The question that the family must face is: Should we be loyal to our child and react to the offender as we would react to any perpetrator, basing this decision on our duty as community members to bring such a person to the attention of the law? The alternative to this choice is to make an exception for the family member perpetrator and be loyal to family ties, rather than bring him to an outside group's attention. The family must choose one of the two courses of action.

Decision making involves a cognitive thought process. It may also involve an emotional reaction to completing the process. When a person must decide whether to side with one or two family members over an issue, the psychological reaction may be experienced as a sense of divided loyalty.

■ SEXUAL HARASSMENT

Sexual harassment is a serious offense that generally occurs in the workplace. It may involve sexual language, job discrimination, and physical contact. Whether or not it entails physical contact, the sexual attention is unwanted and forced on the victim.

■ NURSING RESEARCH AND A TYPOLOGY OF SEXUAL TRAUMA

In the early 1970s little was known about sexual trauma or a victim's response to such injury. Feminist groups had just begun to raise the issue of rape, and the 1971 New York Speak-Out on Rape had been held. Only a few academic publications and special services relevant to the subject existed. The research was designed by Ann Wolbert Burgess and Lynda Holmstrom in an attempt to correct this oversight. Burgess and Holmstrom were called by the nurses at the Boston City Hospital Emergency Room every time a rape victim was admitted. The sample included 146 individuals admitted with a complaint of rape during a one-year period. In addition to 25 articles and chapters, the study yielded a book on the clinical assessment, diagnosis, and treatment of rape victims (Burgess & Holmstrom, 1986) and a book on the institutional treatment of victims (Holmstrom & Burgess, 1983).

One of the major clinical findings was a typology of sexual trauma. The analysis of both clinical and follow-up interviews of the victims yielded three types of sexual trauma based on the issue of consent: rape trauma or no consent; pressured sex or the inability to deny consent; and sex-stress or consent followed by significant distress (Burgess and Holmstrom, 1986). The first two categories are described below.

RAPE TRAUMA

Rape trauma involves a sexual assault that is clearly against the victim's will and generates a potentially life-threatening situation. The following case example illustrates the victim's fear for her life and the control exerted by the assailant.

In this type of rape, known as a power rape, the offender achieves control over his victim by intimidation with a weapon or by physical force, with the threat of bodily harm. The aim of the assault is to gain power by effecting sexual intercourse; to accomplish this, the assailant renders the victim helpless.

PRESSURED SEX: INABILITY TO DENY CONSENT

In pressured sex, the victim—most often a child or young adolescent is pressured into sexual activity by a person who holds a position of power over them through age, authority, or in some other way. Because of her or his age and stage of personality or cognitive development, the victim is unable to make a responsi-

ble decision of consent. Incest victims fall into this group.

The victim's emotional reaction to this situation results from violation of the self and pressure to keep the act secret. In incest, this chiefly involves the betrayal of a parent, accompanied by the underlying failure of the parent to psychologically recognize the victim's needs. In essence, the parent discounts the victim's needs, emotional and otherwise. In effect, the child victim is viewed as a sex object by the incestuous parent.

The offender gains access to the victim in one of three ways: by offering material rewards (e.g., candy, money); by offering the psychological rewards of attention, affection, and interest; or by misrepresenting moral standards ("It's OK to do this—your mother and I do it.")

This trauma syndrome that develops in the victim often manifests itself through a gradual social and psychological withdrawal from the latter's usual activities, especially when the sexual offense is repeated over an extended period. Such withdrawal is especially prominent when the victim has been pressured into secrecy by the offender. The burden of carrying the secret creates considerable tension in putting the victim constantly on guard to maintain her or his secret. How and when the secret is revealed becomes a key diagnostic factor. The following example is from a 23-year-old therapy patient and illustrates her confrontation with her mother at age 10, whereby the mother ignores the grandfather's incest.

> One time when I came back from a weekend with my grandparents, my mother wouldn't talk with me . . . she finally said she was disgusted with me and that she knew what my grandfather and I were doing and that I would have to tell a priest in confession. She wouldn't talk to me for days and I was upset and mad at her. It was her father and he told me to and I was supposed to obey elders. . . . So why was she mad at me? Why wasn't she mad at him?

E CASE EXAMPLE

▶ RAPE TRAUMA

A 19-year-old woman was leaving a restaurant at 6 P.M. to go to her car. On the stairway to the parking garage, two young men, one of them holding a knife to her throat, pushed her against the wall and asked for her money. She was then forced to leave the

parking lot in their car. Over the next 2 hours, the woman was raped by both men. They threatened to kill her if she reported them to the police. She was pushed out of the car near a shopping mall. She flagged down a police car and was taken to a local hospital.

■ TYPES OF OFFENDERS

Four types of offenders—compensatory, exploitative, angry, and sadistic—were empirically derived from a large sample of convicted male rapists examined at the Bridgewater, Massachusetts Treatment Center (Knight & Prentky, 1990).

In the case of the *compensatory offender* the assault is primarily an expression of rape fantasies, the core of which is that the victim will enjoy the experience and perhaps even "fall in love" with the offender. The rapist's motivation derives from the belief that he is so inadequate that no woman would voluntarily have sex with him. The offender usually has a history of sexual preoccupation typified by the living out or fantasizing of a variety of perversions, including bizarre masturbatory practices, voyeurism, exhibitionism, obscene telephone calls, cross-dressing, and fetishism.

In the case of the *exploitative offender* sexual behavior is expressed as an impulsive, predatory act. The sexual component is less integrated into the assailant's fantasy life than in the case of the compensatory offender, and has far less psychologic meaning to the assailant. The rape is determined more by situation and context than by conscious fantasy. The offender is "on the prowl" for a victim. Offenders of this type tend to have a distinctive "macho" style and cannot believe that a woman can or should say "no" to their sexual advances.

In the case of the *displaced anger offender,* sexual behavior is an expression of anger and rage, with the victim representing, in a displaced fashion, a hated individual. The assailant has a persistent, angry, negative attitude toward women. The aggression may take a wide range of forms, from verbal abuse to brutal murder.

The sexual behavior of the *sadistic offender* is an expression of sadistic fantasies. As sexual arousal increases, so do aggressive feelings. The sadistic offender's violence is usually directed at parts of the body having sexual significance, and may kill the victim.

■ INITIAL INTERVIEW OF VICTIMS

The initial interview of a victim of sexual assault is considered a primary therapeutic tool. It provides the nurse with an opportunity to assess the extent of the victim's psychological distress, and to identify those people in the social network who may be of greatest support to the victim in the days and weeks that follow the assault. In conducting the interview, it is important to remember that the victim has already experienced two stressful events: coping with the traumatic event itself and disclosing the event.

COPING BEHAVIOR OF THE VICTIM

The experience of sexual assault varies with the modus operandi of the rapist and the reactions of the victim. The mode of attack has important implications for how the victim copes in the attack situation. Burgess and Holmstrom (1976) studied the victim's **coping behavior** at three points relative to the attack: during the early awareness of danger, during the attack itself, and after the attack.

Appraisal of danger, threat, or harm is a psychological process that intervenes between a stressful event and coping behavior. This early awareness may be cognitive, perceptual, or affective. The coping task during this phase is to react quickly to this warning.

The threat of attack is the point when the person realizes that there is definite danger to his or her life. The coping task at this stage is to attempt to avoid or escape the danger. Coping behavior depends on the amount of time between the threat of attack and the attack, on the type of attack, and on the type of force or violence used. Victims cope by cognitive assessment ("I thought about ways to escape."), verbal tactics ("I tried to engage him in conversation."), and physical action ("I hit him.").

The third coping phase is escaping from the assailant. Victims have to secure help by notifying others such as police, family, and/or friends. The victim may have to negotiate with the assailant for her release or cope with physically freeing herself ("I lay still for a while and then realized that the faster I got myself untied, the faster I could get to the police and my friends.").

It is important for the nurse to understand that the psychological processes used to cope with the trauma play a dominant role in the victim's subsequent adjustment, whether the trauma is rape or incest. Assessment of the coping behaviors at the three points of the attack can be used in the therapeutic recovery of the victim to know he or she did take action.

DISCLOSURE

Superimposed on a traumatic sexual event is the stress of disclosure—the act of telling someone else what has happened to oneself. This process has its own dimensions of anxiety. The anxiety may come simply from anticipating the response of others; (e.g., fear of a judgmental, non-accepting response). The response of the victim's immediate family is of paramount importance in the victim's subsequent adjustment. The nurse must remember that the victim's family members as well as the victim will be traumatized by the assault. In the case of incest, the non-involved parent is likely to be thrown into confusion, often being challenged to choose between the veracity of the involved parent and the child. The disclosure of incest must always be accompanied by the provision of safety for the child, and in many situations for the non-involved parent as well. Most often the father is accused of incest. He may respond with denial and rage directed at either the child, the mother, or both.

In the case of rape, family members are initially faced with considering the role of the victim. As the dynamics of rape have become more widely known, there is less inclination to blame the victim, but this is a possible response, with deleterious effects. Husbands and boyfriends have a particularly difficult time with their range of reactions, to the victim, as well as with the ways in which they believe themselves capable of helping the victim over time. Of equal importance to the family is the response of the nurse and others who have contact with the victim. Even though the victim is a stranger, to the health worker, the emotional impact of rape and incest breaks through professionalism and evokes different levels of social and moral judgment. The nurse must take account of these personal biases in reflecting on the questions asked by victims of sexual trauma, how they can affect the thoroughness of the examination, and how they may influence the manner in which the nurse conveys information to others.

Given these points about the issues that must be dealt with by the victim and others, the assessment of sexually traumatized individuals follows several accepted general principles.

Establish Rapport

It is essential for the nurse to establish rapport with the victim. The formalities of introduction are important. The victim has the right to be told the purpose of the interview, the identity of the nurse, and the procedure of the clinic in treating victims of sexual trauma. Providing safety, comfort, and step-by-step guidance about what will be done for the victim assists in establishing rapport. The victim also needs to be treated with respect and honesty in order to feel and believe that her treatment will be helpful and meaningful for her recovery. Additionally, the victim needs to be made to feel as relaxed and comfortable as possible.

Evaluate the Victim's Sense of Self

Following the establishment of rapport, the next step is to tell the victim that it is important for her treatment that she reveal in detail what happened to her. In the case of children, the nurse can use anatomical dolls, puppets, games, and drawings to gain this information. In this phase of the evaluation, the nurse can assess the victim's emotional demeanor in terms of whether it is expressed (e.g., by crying, anger, extreme agitation) or controlled (the victim appears emotionless, calm, and quiet).

It is not unusual for victims of sexual trauma to resist telling what has happened to them. More often, the desire to forget about what happened, is overtly expressed as the reason for not talking. At a deeper level, the victim will complain that talking about what happened is uncomfortable. Sleeplessness, weight loss, stomachaches, and other somatic complaints reveal the stress of the event. Sometimes a victim will disclose the immediate surface memories of what happened, and will have considerably greater recall of the event after the passage of days or weeks. What the nurse is assessing in this recall is the meaning the victim attributes to the traumatic experience and her or his beliefs about it. These verbalizations provide some clues about how the victim coped with the assault. Does the victim recall feeling confused or helpless; or express fear of dying? These statements reflect the loss of sense of self. Does the victim attribute the event to bad luck, chance, or not know why it happened?

Does the victim blame herself for what happened? Does she express self-blame for her feelings? Although self blame has a dimension of distress, it does acknowledge a sense of self. Here the nurse is assessing whether the victim is developing a sense of total helplessness or complete self-blame, either of which will curtail effective recovery. A sense of helplessness divorces the victim from her ability to be self-assertive and in charge of her life. Self-blame leads to fragmentation of the sense of self, divorcing the victim from sexual and aggressive capacities essential for living and relating to others.

The following sections address several important details that the nurse should gather and confirm in evaluating a victim of sexual trauma.

Medical Issues

What are the victim's physical signs and symptoms of trauma? Did the hospital emergency record (or private physical record) note bruises, lacerations, and laboratory tests for evidence of sexual intercourse? What other general statements did the victim make about personal health? For children and adolescents or adults who have not had previous pelvic examinations, special preparation must to be made to ease the normal anxiety associated with such intrusive procedures.

Circumstances of the Assault

When and where was the victim approached? Why was the victim there, and where did the assault occur? Who was the assailant(s); was he of the same race as the victim? Was he a stranger, acquaintance or relative of the victim? What conversation did the assailant make before, during, and after the assault? What humiliating remarks were made? What methods of control did the assailant use in the assault? Were there threats, weapons, physical force?

Behavioral Issues

What types of sex were demanded and obtained? What other degrading acts were demanded?

Psychological Issues

What coping strategies did the victim use before, during, and after the assault in terms of cognitive, verbal, and physical behavior? What signs and symptoms suggest emotional trauma?

CLOSURE TO THE INITIAL INTERVIEW

In completing an initial interview with a victim of sexual trauma, the nurse should keep a constant focus on how the victim felt and what she or he thought about every detail of the assault. The nurse should then explore in detail the victim's expectations of and encounters with her or his family with regard to the assault, and the family's responses to the victim. In addition to the assessment of the event itself, the nurse should evaluate the victim for potential self-harm. Care must be exercised in conferring any type of psychiatric diagnosis at this time. The trauma of rape and incest, and the stress of disclosure, have such powerful disorganizing effects that they pre-empt psychiatric classification.

In completing the assessment, it is imperative that the nurse determine from the victim and important others the identities of those persons immediately available to assist the victim when she or he leaves the hospital or clinic. Networking is also important for establishing the victim's safety. In the case of rape, the assailant may have threatened the victim about returning and attacking once again. If the assault took place in the victim's home, it is important to ensure that the victim returns to a safe environment, either a family member's or friend's home. In addition to these precautions, it is useful for the nurse to review with the victim how she felt about the interview itself and any other hospital or clinic procedures. Referrals, telephone follow-up arrangements, and crisis-center services are all important in closing the interview and assessment process.

■ TREATMENT AND FOLLOW-UP

The nursing care of victims of sexual trauma in the follow-up phase includes integrating treatment that focuses on their physical health, social needs, and behavior, and on psychological issues.

PHYSICAL HEALTH

The nurse should carefully review any physical symptoms or alterations in the victim's body systems. For example, the status of the circulatory system can be assessed for the presence of headache, flushing, perspiration, and sensations of coldness or heat; the respiratory system for breathing pattern, sighing, respirations, and dizziness; the gastrointestinal system for abdominal pain, nausea, lack of appetite, diarrhea, and constipation; and the genitourinary system for urinary frequency and interference with sexual functioning. The nurse needs to carefully document the victim's symptom picture over time in terms of the nature and intensity of the symptoms occurring within a 24-hour period. The victim should have a gynecological and medical follow-up examination after she completes her first menstrual period after the assault. All victims—male and female—should have blood studies done for sexually transmitted diseases (STDs), including microbiological cultures that are repeated every 4 to 6 weeks following the assault, or as advised by the clinician and by laboratory guidelines.

SOCIAL NETWORK

Treatment that makes use of the victim's social network calls upon family and friends of the victim to assist in strengthening the victim's self-confidence, which, in turn, will help her resume her normal style of living. Whether the victim chooses to tell family or friends about the rape is not the point, but rather that she seeks support from her network.

The victim is encouraged to resume normal activity according to her ability to pace herself. The longer a victim avoids a normal activity such as school or work, the greater the difficulty she will later encounter in trying to return to it. The victim usually has specific decisions to make, and seeks advice about such issues as whether to press charges against the assailant, whether to quit work or school, or how to tell people about the incident.

BEHAVIORAL THERAPY

Therapeutic intervention into the behavior of a victim of sexual trauma is aimed at desensitizing the victim to the painful aspects of the assault. One method for accomplishing this is to encourage the victim to talk about the assault as a means of providing psychological control over the memory of it, and stripping it of its power to distress the victim. During this treatment, the victim is encouraged to master her fears by thinking back through the traumatic experience with support from the nurse and/or friends. Gradually, this method desensitizes the victim and allows thoughts of the assault to enter the victim's mind without the accompanying emotional reactions.

PSYCHOLOGICAL ISSUES

In managing the psychological issues involved in sexual trauma, the nurse attends to the emotional response of the victim and assesses the negative effects of the assault. It is essential that the nurse make the victim aware of the need to describe her symptoms in working through the trauma. Any other technique encourages isolation of the symptoms and increases the possibility of the rape remaining an unsettled issue. Although repression may be a protective process, it absorbs valuable psychic energy that the victim needs to resolve her crisis. The nurse should also carefully review the victim's mental functioning in terms of impaired attention, poor concentration, poor memory, changes in outlook, and future planning. The victim's emotional reactions should also be reviewed in terms of irritability, mood changes, disturbances in dreaming, and changes in relationships with family and friends.

Talking with a victim as soon as possible after the assault is essential to repairing the emotional damage it inflicts. This is also important for minimizing the psychological after-effects of the trauma by providing emotional support of a non-judgmental nature. Talking with the victim works toward establishing an alliance and provides an opportunity for maximum assessment of the impact of the assault and the victim's reactions.

The overwhelming impulse of victims of sexual trauma is to avoid dealing with the experience. In such situations, the nurse encourages the victim to talk about the incident and supports the expression of fear by pointing out that it is a natural reaction to danger and violation of the self.

Talking about the assault and bearing the distressing feelings that accompany it are essential steps in the process of resolving the victim's crisis and regaining confidence. The goal of treatment is to help the victim re-establish her style of living and restore her equilibrium. A supportive person, such as the nurse, can help to validate the victim's feelings. Working with family and social networks is encouraged to provide the victim with added emotional support during her recovery.

E CASE EXAMPLES

▶ SEXUAL HARASSMENT

Elaine F. is 28 years old. She was born in the Middle East and moved to the United States in 1982, where she lived with 4 brothers and attended a local high school. She has a strong employment history, having worked part-time as a clerk in various food markets while attending high school. Before her current employment, she describes herself as having been happy, energetic, and healthy. She slept well at night and maintained a desirable weight. In 1989 she returned to the Middle East, and became engaged in 1994, before returning to the United States. She witnessed bombing in her home country and saw dead bodies. She describes feeling sad about what she saw, but was not preoccupied or otherwise upset.

When she returned to the United States she was in good health. She underwent a physical examination before taking a job at a convenience store. She saw the new job as a way to earn money for her wedding, and to continue her schooling. She was not afraid of people, and would walk home alone at night from work.

The Event: Sexual Harassment, Sexual Discrimination and Employment Termination

About a week after Elaine had been hired, the supervisor who had hired her, a man in his 60s, began to call her at work, telling her that he loved her and wanted to go out with her. He then talked about sexual acts. He would call at least 10 to 15 times a day.

Her manager became angry with the repeated telephone calls. Elaine was afraid to say anything for fear of losing her job, and the supervisor continued his telephone calls, phoning her at home as well as at work.

During this time, Elaine became nervous, had stomach pains, was unable to sleep at night, and became fearful of being alone and of walking alone. The supervisor occasionally came to the store, called her into his office, and attempted to expose himself at which point she would run out of the office. He persisted with lewd language and vivid descriptions of sexual acts despite her protests. He claimed that he liked her, wanted to date her, and wanted to take her to a hotel where he could have sex with her. He also said that he wanted to watch her have sex with a woman. Her pleas were met with threats of losing her job. Her responses were to work harder, to be polite to him, to say he was like a father to her, and to question why he was harassing her. These responses did not stop his actions.

In the fall, Elaine returned to the Middle East because her father was hospitalized. In asking another manager for permission to leave, she told him about the sexual harassment, but he said that he did not believe her, and told her to be back at work within a month. When she did return, she learned that she had been dismissed. She was first told that she had been terminated because of a "bad cashier performance record." When she inquired further about this, she was told by the company's regional

E CASE EXAMPLES—Continued

supervisor that she had been terminated because her visit to her native country had not been authorized.

Even after her termination, the supervisor continued to call her at home. He claimed that she could again have her job, at another location, if she would do with him what he wanted. She refused, and reported that she had been both fearful of the supervisor and of the new work location.

In detailing the supervisor's sexual expressions and behavior, which included his wish to participate in and observe oral sex, masturbatory acts, lesbian acts, and sex acts with vegetables; attempts to open Elaine's blouse and to fondle her genitals, and rub against her; and exposure of his genitals, Elaine chokes back tears and appears extremely depressed. She was confused about why her descriptions of the supervisor's behavior had not been believed. She is despondent; and believes that her experience has cost her her future. When her fiancee had approached her or tried to hold her hand, she had been flooded with the sound of the supervisor's voice repeating his lewd and sexually threatening acts and language. Her fiancee then broke their engagement when Elaine decided to return to the United States. Elaine believes that the strain of her experience led to the end of her engagement, and since returning to the United States has been to several hospital emergency rooms with nervousness, stomach upset, vomiting of blood, and an irregular menstrual cycle. She was treated with medication for anxiety. She is in need of dental and health care as well as finances for daily living.

Diagnosis
DSM-IV: Post-Traumatic Stress Disorder, DSM IV 309.81

Nursing diagnosis: Rape trauma syndrome

Elaine has intrusive recollections of her supervisor's behavior, ("I can't get it out of my mind"), recurrent dreams in which men come after her, threatening to commit sexual acts; and feelings that traumatic events were recurring even when she was with her fiance. She also has physical symptoms of anxiety and depression, and a foreshortened future ("I lost my future").

Elaine is suffering from the trauma of extended psychological abuse and sexual threat. In addition her livelihood has been threatened and she has lost a fiancee and is threatened with the loss of her father through illness. Her offender would be classified as a compensatory offender.

His abuse is compounded by Elaine's cultural background. In her native country, a woman defiled in any way is socially outcast. Moreover, as a matter of family honor and her religion, families handle such interpersonal transgressions through retaliation and punishment of the offender. This cannot be done in the United States, which isolates Elaine from a natural social-support system. Her family does not know of her sexual harassment, and she fears that if her brothers did learn of it, they would punish the offender severely. She is protective of her family, fearing that it would get into trouble for such aggressive behavior in the United States.

In this case the patient needs a supportive and trauma-counseling program, with therapeutic efforts made in two major directions:

- To maintain the patient's physical health.
- To strengthen her self-esteem and sense of self-worth.

The counseling program should have two goals: (1) to deal actively with the current trauma of the harassment, with the specific purpose of reducing the patient's intrusive symptoms, numbing phenomena, and disharmony surrounding sexual arousal; and (2) to deal with the patient's hopelessness about the future. This second area would also involve educational efforts and the identification of other skills and abilities.

▶ ABDUCTION AND RAPE AT A MALL

In January 1992, two high-school juniors and best friends, Rachel and Joan, went to a mall to shop after having dinner. Neither girl wore any heavy outdoor clothing. They bought several items, talked briefly with several friends at the mall, and walked to the mall parking lot at about 8 P.M. Joan's father's van was in front of a store entrance. As Joan unlocked the driver's door and entered the car, Rachel heard someone coming. He looked as if he were passing the car when he turned toward her, holding a gun in his left hand. He grabbed Rachel around the waist. Joan saw the man and pressed on the horn; and both girls screamed. The man told them to shut up or he would kill them. He pushed Joan into the front seat of her car and got into the rear seat, telling Joan to drive. When they passed a security car in driving out of the parking lot, the abductor advised them not to do anything "stupid." He then gave directions to Joan and they proceeded onto an interstate highway. Rachel could feel the gun being pushed into her back. She heard the man moving around in the middle seat; he had a large bag with him and metal objects could be heard clinking.

The abductor was white, with shoulder length dark curly hair parted in the middle, no accent, about 5'8", wore dark sweat pants, looked dirty, and his fingers smelled of cigarette smoke. He told the girls that he would hold them for a couple of days and then return them to the mall. He also said that he would take their car and blow it up. He asked many questions about who owned the car, what time the girls were due home, and whether the car had fire and theft insurance. When Rachel asked the man why he was doing this, he said that he wanted the car and would not harm them.

Rachel, sitting next to Joan, suggested getting into an accident. Joan was not wearing a seat belt and indicated she was too scared to try. The man felt Rachel's face and then wrapped an ace bandage around her face and eyes. After passing a toll booth, the man made Rachel get into the back seat of the car. He pushed her down and fondled her breasts, and then put a bag over her. He then made Joan stop the car at the side of the road, made her get into the back seat, and put her under the bag with Rachel. The man then drove the car, stopping for gas at one point. He pulled onto a dirt road and both Joan and Rachel thought they were going to die. They prayed and said they loved each other; Rachel told Joan she was her best friend.

The abductor pulled the two girls out of the back seat, taped Rachel's mouth shut and her wrists behind her back, and again put her in the hatchback of the van, pushing Joan into the middle seat. Rachel could hear the assailant raping Joan. She tried to tell herself it wasn't happening. Then Rachel heard the man walk Joan out into the snow. She could hear the sound of tape. The man then came back to the van. When he tried to push Rachel down she fought with him and he said that he was not going to rape her. He then pulled her into the snow and faced her to Joan. He asked Rachel if she

E CASE EXAMPLES—Continued

wanted a drink, which she refused. She heard him go back to the car and a rustling sound. The girls thought they were going to be shot, but the abductor then drove off in the car. They feared he was still present. The girls then freed themselves of their wrist bindings and mouth gags, and began running through the woods. Joan told Rachel that she had been raped. Finding a house, they were afraid to knock on the door, fearing that it might be the abductor's house. When they nevertheless knocked on the door, a man opened it and called the police. After a police interview and hospital examination, the girls' parents came to take them home.

Crisis Response of the Victims

Following an abduction and rape, the two major time phases that can be noted in the victim's response are (1) the disruptive phase and (2) the reorganization phase. Generally victims travel through these two phases and, in various degrees, display characteristic symptoms directly related to the assault. In this case, the trauma represents the abduction, physical and sexual assault molestation and the auditory witnessing of the rape.

In the disruptive phase, which can last as little as a few days to several weeks or months, in which the victim needs time to recover to the degree necessary to resume daily activities, the two victims in this case experienced many symptoms, including fear of being alone, constant intrusive thoughts of their traumatic experience, and nightmares related to it.

Both girls then continued to have symptoms that persisted in the reorganization phase and were pronounced for more than 4 years. Many of the symptoms displayed during the disruptive phase were present.

A year after the abduction, Rachel developed an eating disorder in which she lost more than twenty pounds.

She had difficulty concentrating in school, and her grades dropped. She had to take time off from her work as a sales clerk, since she became nervous when she perceived people who seemed suspicious. Although she had planned to go to the college, she was unable to leave home. She took courses part time at a local school and only passed one course.

When the police found the girls' car, which had been abandoned and burned, but did not find the abductor, Rachel became very frightened, worrying that the abductor knew their names and addresses. When she is in public she sometimes thinks she sees him. Last year she was at a restaurant with her mother and she thought she saw him; had her mother call the police who came and determined he was not the assailant. Rachel's parents divorced when she was very young and she and her 21 year old brother have been raised by the mother. She earned average grades, liked sports and played varsity sports. She was active in school committees and was a class officer prior to the crime.

Joan, the only daughter and middle child of five children, came from an intact family. Her parents were both professionals in the educational field. Joan was an honor roll student and in varsity sports, active in school clubs and on the Yearbook staff prior to the crime.

Joan found it difficult to continue her schooling because of the extensive media coverage and classmates quickly learned that Joan and Rachel were the victims of this crime. Her school provided her with a pass to use if she felt upset and wanted to leave class. She had trouble concentrating but was able to pass her courses due to her previously high academic standing. She did not work that summer, deciding to stay home; she does not remember what she did that summer. She believes she passed her senior year because many of her science courses required lab partners and joint papers were written and teachers were understanding of her situation. The summer before college she worked one week as a substitute at a Day Care. She did not work the rest of the summer because she did not feel well.

Her first year of college was dismal. She had wanted to go to the college to which many of her high-school classmates were going, but decided to go to a local college where she could live at home. She failed several courses and has not done well in others.

Her mother describes her current behavior as resembling that of her pre-adolescence. She does not like to go out alone, calls home frequently when out, and is unable to leave home for college. Her critical development in terms of self-differentiation, separation from her nuclear family, and mastery of independence has been seriously curtailed. Because she was blindfolded during her abduction and rape, and could not see, her imagination of events that might occur often becomes the focus of her attention, and she shows the fear response of persons blindfolded during an experience of trauma. She isolates herself in her house because she does not know how to manage outside. Blindfolding the victim keeps an assailant from being identified, reducing the probability that he will kill the victim.

Impact on Victim

The evaluation of the impact of an abduction and rape may be conducted in three ways:

- Reviewing the details and circumstances of the assault and noting any unusual or extraordinary features. In this approach there are many details and circumstances that contribute to evaluating the impact of the assault on the victim's life. In this case they include: (1) The abrupt nature of the crime. There was no warning. The girls were getting into a car when an assailant, brandishing a gun, surprised them (2) The terrorizing and life-threatening aspect of the assault. The girls' lives were threatened verbally as well as physically. A gun was used to control and terrorize them, and to create fear that the assailant would kill them. (3) The assailant's sexual and aggressive demands. The assailant forced Rachel into the back seat of the car, where she was molested. She was abducted, verbally abused, and physically restrained. Joan was raped.
- Listing the symptoms that reflect the post-traumatic state. This approach to evaluating the after-effects of sexual trauma involves documenting the symptoms that the victim develops as a result of the attack. In this case both victims had many symptoms.
- Classifying the crime and citing the assailant's behavioral dynamics and motives. This third approach to evaluating the impact of an attack is directed at understanding the specific aspects of the assault that victimized the patient. The crime is classified as a primary felony rape; abduction rape; and exploitative rape.

E CASE EXAMPLES—Continued

In a primary felony rape, the major offense is a non-sexual felony, such as car theft. The victims are at the scene and are sexually assaulted as a second offense. Abduction rape involves forcibly moving the victim from one location to another, at which the sexual assault occurs. In exploitative rape, sometimes called opportunistic rape, the assailant's expressed aggression generally does not exceed what is necessary to force the victim's compliance. Callous indifference to the victim is evident. Investigative research indicates the offender usually has limited formal schooling; poor job record; short-term, unstable relationships. He is usually very impulsive; has a long record of serious behavioral problems; may have been arrested several times for criminal offenses starting in adolescence and through most of adult life. Offenses are highly impulsive with minimal planning, e.g., opportunistic in vulnerable environments; and alcohol/drug use is common (Douglas, Burgess, Burgess & Ressler, 1992).

In the case of Rachel and Joan, the primary felony was car theft, followed by sexual assault. The assailant exerted his need for domination and control by use of a weapon and abduction. The subsequent car arson and assailant's conversation about burning and blowing up the car indicates a high level of dangerousness.

The crime occurred in a vulnerable environment; it was a bold act by the assailant and led to the commission of the crime. He abandoned the girls in a isolated location, tied them, and left them blindfolded, without adequate clothing, terrorized and exhausted.

Diagnosis: Chronic Post-Traumatic Stress Disorder
The abduction and molestation of Rachel and Joan occurred at a critical developmental period in both girls' lives. They were beginning the process of separation, differentiation, and mastery of independence from their families. This normal process has in their case been seriously curtailed, and the process and dynamics of their assault will have to be dealt with in therapy. Rachel was terrified that she and her friend would be killed. The assailant said he would keep them for days. She had a clear image of him. While blindfolded she heard the rape and she dissociated and feared this would happen to her. She was helpless to assist her friend.

Rachel uses obsessive-compulsive defenses to manage underlying, traumatic anxiety and depression. Her memory of a gun being held to her stomach needs to be explored for its connection to her anorexia, as it is potentially life threatening. The symptoms Rachel describes are consistent with a severe post-traumatic response. Currently, she is depressed and paranoid, has the numbing response of dissociation and uses avoidant defenses. Her treatment will have to be conducted slowly and cautiously because her defenses are very weak (see the later discussion of testing). The anxiety of her trauma is locked within her body. The trauma is still unresolved psychologically. Her coping style of avoidance makes it difficult for her to express her feelings. She continues to have to deal with extraordinary stress in order to maintain her equilibrium.

The prognosis for Joan is guarded. The structure of her trauma is a result of the terror and anxiety associated with an abduction and rape at gun point. Her continued apprehensions and flashbacks to her abduction and rape, set off by environmental cues, represent the neurobiology of trauma and the persisting nature of chronic post-traumatic stress disorder.

Both Rachel and Joan have been significantly altered by their abduction, and Joan by her rape. They are now both essentially "different" persons psychologically than they were before their trauma. Treatment for both victims must consist of a multimodal approach and be implemented according to their ability to tolerate the stress and anxiety of dealing with their traumatic experience. Educational material about psychological trauma will be necessary for both victims to understand the reasons for their symptoms. Their distress is so severe that medication will probably be needed in the early phases of their treatment. They will also have to be monitored for any prescribed medication. When they are ready, a program of supportive therapy should be begun and should alternate with sessions of trauma therapy to re-build their ego defenses and control their anxiety. Stress management and relaxation techniques will have to be taught and mastered. Cognitive re-framing will be essential for reversing the pre-suppositions that both girls have developed as a result of their abduction and rape (e.g., blame, guilt, and thoughts about the post-traumatic self). This approach will begin to reduce the girls' avoidant responses and allow the self-confidence necessary for their continued development.

▶ INCEST OF 10-YEARS' DURATION

Abby is a 32-year-old divorced mother of two. Because of her father's military career, her family moved several times during her childhood, and she remembers her parents having frequent arguments. When her parents divorced, Abby and her brother, four years younger, were boarded while their mother worked. The family was reunited when a boyfriend began living with the mother. The two subsequently married.

After graduating from high school in 1978, Abby enlisted in the military. She was married in 1981, and has two sons. In 1990 she began experiencing severe fatigue and bowel irritability, and sought medical help. The doctor asked if she were depressed. While she thought about this, her husband made an appointment for her to see a psychotherapist. She began therapy and was given an antidepressant drug. It was during therapy that her incest trauma was revealed.

Description of Incest
Abby's 10 year period of incest began in 1967, when her stepfather told her to watch him and her mother having intercourse so that she would know how it was done. While having sex, he would look at her, grin, and wink. When her mother made noises, Abby became frightened and ran to her bedroom shaking, got into bed, and pulled the covers over her head. Later, the stepfather would go into the bathroom, look at Abby, laugh and make humping motions. Abby would close her eyes, trying to make him disappear.

Nude photographs were taken of Abby at age 12 in the basement. The stepfather once told her that her mother had found the photographs and that Abby should say that a friend had taken them. Her mother, however, never mentioned the photographs.

Her stepfather's sexual activity with Abby began initially in her mother's bedroom, while the mother was working. The stepfather would fondle Abby through her underpants, advancing to digital penetration. The molestation eventually advanced to full intercourse. The stepfather also showed Abby pornographic books. The sexual abuse

E CASE EXAMPLES—Continued

began when the stepfather joined the family as mother's boyfriend. Abby tried to stop the incest verbally, but her stepfather continued it. While in high school, she told two close friends about it.

In 1981, while preparing for her wedding, Abby consulted a military associate, who had a social-work background, about her history of incest. The associate advised Abby to tell her mother about her experiences. Abby, after refusing to invite her stepfather to her wedding, disclosed the abuse to her mother, who came to see her. When hospitalized in 1992, Abby sent a confrontation letter to her stepfather, who denied his sexual abuse of her.

Dynamics of Childhood Sexual Abuse

Several questions need to be answered: Why did Abby not report the childhood and adolescent sexual assaults at the time of occurrence; Why was she unable to recognize her injuries; What is the causation of her injuries; and What prevented her from understanding or acting on her legal rights? Abby did not report her incest when it occurred because of: (1) having been told not to tell about it; (2) her fear of her stepfather; (3) her fear of the consequences if she did reveal it; and (4) her fear of damaging her new family. Her stepfather used strategies that confused her and inhibited her from telling about her abuse.

Adults usually pressure children into sexual activity through various lures and manipulations; they then intimidate the children so that the abuse will remain a secret, with the implication that in some way the abuse has been the child's fault. These are among the offender's dynamics for controlling a child victim in the case of incest. Thus, immediate disclosure following abuse by a family member is not the norm. The Abby's disclosure of her abuse to her mother, years after leaving her home and in the context of a major life event such as marriage, is not unusual. Abby was threatened and intimidated by the stepfather to ensure secrecy. Abby's reports of her forced sexual activity with her stepfather are consistent with reports noted in many cases of incest. The additional supporting evidence is the history of her telling peers and her mother. Only with the encouragement of professionals, e.g., the staff at the hospital, is she able to confront the stepfather.

Abby was led into sexual activity with her stepfather by the latter's compelling her to watch parental intercourse and showing her pornographic books, implying that this was expected behavior. In high school, Abby had to give sex in order to get anything. The stepfather stalked her at school. She joined clubs in school in order to avoid him.

Injuries of Incest

Abby was unable to recognize the injuries from her forced incest because she was dissociated from her feelings. She did not understand the effect of the incest on her, and her experience was not cognitively integrated. She blocked her emotions and repressed the effect associated with the incest. She can report the incest, but is numb to its emotional aspect. Her distress is expressed in physical symptoms. When in therapy, she becomes highly symptomatic as she begins to understand and experience her feelings.

Abby's symptoms of the incest experienced during her childhood and adolescence include sexual fantasies of her 4th grade male teacher (e.g., wondering about his penis and comparing it with her stepfather's). She is sexually precocious, and does not understand her preoccupation as being connected to her incestuous experience. Her hypersexuality begins to be manifested as sexual fantasy. She remembers numerous vaginal infections and trauma to her genitals.

Victim Response to Incest

Abby has significant trauma as a result of her forced incest. Her persisting symptoms include depression, mood swings, irritable bowel syndrome, and sexual dysfunction.

Testing revealed a symptom profile of high level of somatization evidence of self-depreciation, feelings of inferiority, and a sense of inadequacy and self doubt. Depression is evident, as is mild social alienation.

Impact of Incest

Abby's description of her incestuous experience reveals feelings of betrayal as well as helplessness and humiliation. She is isolated; finds work stressful and intimacy impossible, and feels chronically tired and irritable. She trusts few people, her marriage has failed, and she finds parenting stressful.

Only recently has the widespread nature of incest been realized, along with the parental and familial dynamics that keep its victims from talking about it. Abby, like many other incest victims, was conditioned not to talk about her abuse. This programming prevented her from recognizing any link between her psychological symptoms and her abuse, and also helps to explain why she did not previously see her abuse as a cause of her problems.

The recent study of incest has provided better understanding of how its prolonged effects can resurface throughout the victim's life span. Briere (1992) has written about its numbing effect on its victims, and Finkelhor (1995) has described the symptoms of depression, anxiety, substance abuse, and self-destructive behavior (including suicide attempts and sexual maladjustment) that can come from incest. Gelinas (1983) has written about chronic traumatic neurosis and continuing relational imbalances as the result of incest, and the increased intergenerational risk of incest. Herman (1992) emphasizes the many symptoms to be addressed in the treatment of incest victims, and Russell's (1986) work demonstrates that more severe forms of sexual abuse produce higher levels of trauma than fondling and molesting. Current research on the neurobiology of trauma, including Putnam & Trickett (1993) observation of increased levels of cortisol in sexually abused children, may explain the increased incidence of attention deficit—hyperactivity disorder (ADHD) in children.

Abby did not act on her legal rights at the time of her forced incest because she had no conscious awareness of its link to her psychological and physical distress. Once in therapy, she was able to assert her legal rights. She filed a civil suit, the stepfather admitted the incest, and she received a financial settlement.

O AN OVERVIEW

- The psychological processes that a victim of sexual trauma invokes to handle the trauma of victimization will play a dominant role in the victim's subsequent adjustment.

- In telling another person about the traumatic event, the victim is engaged in an activity that has its own dimensions of anxiety.

- The impact of the trauma on the victim's immediate family is paramount in the adjustment of the victim.

- For the nurse to establish rapport during an interview, the victim must feel safe and comfortable, and be given step-by-step guidance about what is going to happen.

- The victim often resists recounting the details of the traumatic event; surface memories may be related first, and after days or weeks the victim will have considerably more recall.

- During the interview, important details for the nurse to question include what physical signs and symptoms of trauma are medical issues; when and where the victim was approached, what conversation occurred and other circumstances of the assault; the types of sex and other acts were demanded (behavioral issues); and what coping strategies the victim used before, during, and after the assault.

TD TERMS TO DEFINE

- compensatory offender
- coping behavior
- displaced-anger offender
- exploitative offender
- incest
- rape
- rape trauma syndrome
- sadistic offender
- sexual harassment

Q STUDY QUESTIONS

1. The legal definition of rape does NOT include:
   a. forced sexual penetration.
   b. oral, anal, or vaginal penetration.
   c. lack of consent.
   d. psychological trauma.

2. Rape trauma syndrome is a:
   a. nursing diagnosis.
   b. psychiatric diagnosis.
   c. medical diagnosis.
   d. legal term.

3. In disclosing incest, a dilemma faced by the victim is:
   a. telling the family.
   b. divided family loyalty.
   c. keeping the secret.
   d. making a legal report.

4. Categorizing sexual trauma focuses on:
   a. consent.
   b. victim-offender relationship.
   c. extent of injury.
   d. psychological trauma.

5. During the assault, the compensatory rapist:
   a. is expressing anger.
   b. is expressing rape fantasies.
   c. is pressuring the person for sex.
   d. is expressing his macho image.

6. Emotional demeanor may be classified as
   a. happy or sad
   b. expressive or controlled
   c. open or closed
   d. present or absent

7. Initially it would be helpful to say to a victim:
   a. "I'm here to help."
   b. "I'm sorry this happened to you."
   c. "You must be very upset."
   d. "I will call your family."

8. Counseling helps the victim to
   a. report the rape
   b. talk about the victimization
   c. reunite the family
   d. get medical attention

9. A *DSM-IV* psychiatric diagnosis to consider with rape trauma is:
   a. depression
   b. rape trauma syndrome
   c. post-traumatic stress disorder
   d. adjustment reaction

10. Identify and describe the level of stress-crisis for rape trauma.

11. Describe the psychological issues often faced by an incest victim that are not faced by someone who has been raped by a stranger.

12. Which rape offender(s) would be most likely to kill the victim?
    a. Displaced anger offender
    b. Compensatory offender
    c. Sadistic offender
    d. Exploitative offender

13. Why is disclosing the rape to others so difficult for rape victims?

14. All of the following are true about sexual harrassment EXCEPT it:
    a. may involve job discrimination.
    b. generally occurs at the workplace.
    c. does not involve physical contact.
    d. is unwanted and forced on the victim.

15. T F Rape trauma syndrome has two phases: acute disorganization and reorganization.

16. Which of the following is NOT true about the initial phase of rape trauma syndrome?
    a. lasts a few days to several weeks
    b. is usually of delayed onset
    c. involves physical symptoms like gastrointestinal irritability
    d. may involve dramatic changes in eating and sleeping patterns

17. All of the following statements is NOT true about incest?
    a. It usually refers to sexual relations between 2 persons so closely related that they cannot legally marry.
    b. Victims frequently don't report the crime to authorities.
    c. Incest is forbidden in every state.
    d. Incest is often considered consental on the part of the victim.

18. T F The perceived power that the victimizer has over the victim and how the victimizer uses it greatly impacts how the victim copes with the event, before and after.

19. Which of the following statements is NOT true about treating a victim of rape trauma?
    a. The victim is encouraged to take time off from usual activities, like work, to aid in the healing process.
    b. Support from the victim's network is important for strengthening self-confidence.
    c. The victim is encouraged to "mentally review" the assault with support from the nurse and/or friends.
    d. The victim must be made aware of the link from the physical symptoms to the rape trauma.

■ REFERENCES

Briere J: *Child Abuse Trauma: Theory and Treatment of the Lasting Effects.* Newbury Park, CA, Sage, 1992.

Burgess, AW and Holmstrom LL: Rape trauma syndrome, *Am J Psychiatry* 131, 1974, 981–986.

Burgess, AW and Holmstrom, L.L. Coping behavior of the rape victim, *Am J Psychiatry* 133 (4), 1976: 413-417.

Burgess AW, Holmstrom LL: *Rape: Crisis and Recovery,* West Newton, MA: Awab, Inc., 1986.

Burgess AW, Hartman CR, Clements PT Jr.: Biology of memory and childhood trauma, *J Psychosoc Nurs* 1995; 33(3):16–26.

Douglas JE, Burgess AW, Burgess AG, and Ressler RK: *The Crime Classification Manual,* San Francisco, CA: Jossey-Bass, 1992.

Finkelhor D: The victimization of children: A developmental perspective. *Am J Orthopsychiatry,* 1995; 65, 177–193.

Gelinas D: The persisting negative effects of incest. *Psychiatry* 1983, 43:312–332.

Herman JL: *Trauma and Recovery,* New York: Basic Books, 1992.

Herman JL, Hirschman L: Father-daughter incest, signs: *J Women Culture and Soc,* 2 (4), 1977:745–746.Holmstrom, LL, Burgess AW: *The Victim of Rape,* New Brunswick, N.J.: Transaction Books, 1983.

Knight, RA, Prentky RA: Classifying sexual offenders: The development and corroboration of taxonomic models. In Marshall WL, Laws DR, Barbaree HE: (eds.) *The Handbook of Sexual Assault: Issues, Theories and Treatment of Offenders,* New York: Plenum, 1990, pp. 23–52.

Putnam FW, Trickett PK: Child sexual abuse: A model of chronic trauma, *Psychiatry: Interpersonal and Biological Processes,* 1993, 56:82–95.

Russell DEH: *The Secret Trauma,* New York: Basic Books, 1986.

Herman JL: *Trauma and Recovery.* New York, Basic Books, 1992.

Putnam FW, Trickett PK: Child sexual abuse: A model of chronic trauma. *Psychiatry: Interpers Biol Proc* 1993; 56:82–95.

Russell DEH: *The Secret Trauma.* New York, Basic Books, 1986.

4

Level 4

Relational and Family Crises

Emotional crises that result from attempts to deal with interpersonal situations are the types of crises included in Level 4. The situations may be relational, such as between associates or friends, or familial involving family members.

The etiology of such crises relates to the neurobiology of chronic trauma, and generally reflects a struggle with a deeper, but usually circumscribed, developmental issue that was not resolved adaptively at an earlier time.

The developmental issues that lead to relational crises include dependency, value conflicts, sexual identity, emotional intimacy, issues of power, or the attainment of self-discipline. Those who present with this type of crisis have often repeated a pattern of specific relationship difficulties over the course of time. The crisis may be internally or externally directed, with chronic abuse an example of the latter. In the context of the family, such abuse includes child abuse, the use of children in pornography, parental abduction of children, adolescent runaways, and domestic battering and rape. Child abuse and domestic battering are interpersonal crises occurring in long-term relationships. The psychological response to such abuse is chronic fear, an inability to protect self and others, and learned helplessness.

Interpersonal problems are the defining characteristics of personality disorders.

Every type of emotional crisis involves an interaction between an external stressor and a personal vulnerability of an individual. In an interpersonal crisis, the locus of the resulting stress is primarily internal, and determined by the unique psychodynamics of the individual and/or a pre-existing mental illness, which becomes manifest in particular problematic situations.

The goals of intervention in interpersonal crises are to help the involved individuals to restabilize their lives, strengthen their interpersonal relationships, and avoid psychiatric symptom illness. This first involves resolving the crisis state, such as by stopping abuse, and promoting adaptation to changes in life-style. Dysfunctioning within the family system must be addressed.

Interventions in interpersonal crises are designed to prevent or manage stress and eliminate or reduce the potency of the causative stressors. Techniques might include physical activity to discharge repressed energy; nutrition to enhance physiological recovery; spiritual support for persons who value religious beliefs to promote a sense of integrity with the natural world; relaxation to counter hypervigilance; pleasure activities to promote a sense of fun and humor; and expressive activities such as reading, art, and music.

Both therapeutic and psychoeducational interventions have been developed to change dysfunctional behavior; many have decreased violent or exploitative behavior. Such interventions generally include elements designed to increase communication and knowledge with regard to family roles.

Conditions representative of relational and family crises are discussed in the following three chapters:

- Personality Disorders
- Child Abuse and Neglect
- Violence in Families

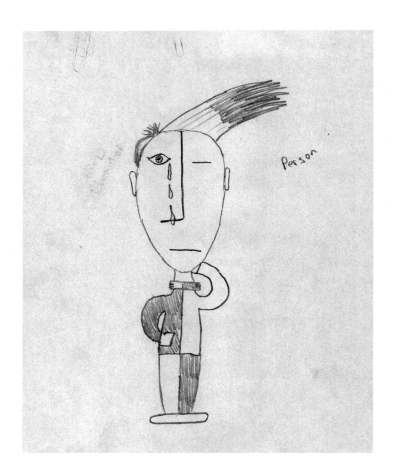

*One might compare the relation of the ego to the id with that
between a rider and his horse. The horse provides the locomotor
energy, and the rider has the prerogative of determining the goal
and of guiding the movements of his powerful mount towards it. But
all too often in the relations between the ego and the id we find a
picture of the less ideal situation in which the rider is obliged to
guide his horse in the direction in which it itself wants to go.*

Sigmund Freud (1856–1939)

"The Anatomy of the Mental Personality"

in *New Introductory Lectures on Psychoanalysis*

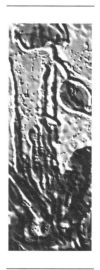

26

Personality Disorders

Pamela E. Marcus

Personality structure determines how a person thinks and feels about him- or herself, evaluates his or her environment, and interacts with family members and others in the community. Personality structure also determines how much information an individual will disclose to a nurse providing care, how an individual interprets personal problems, and what information an individual can learn during professional intervention. It is important to assess all patients for personality disorder, since the nursing-care plan and outcome statements in cases of such disorder must be tailored to each type of disorder.

The Diagnostic and Statistical Manual of Mental Disorders, Fourth Edition (DSM-IV) outlines a number of features that indicate a personality disorder. Among these are the personality traits of inflexibility and maladaptiveness, which cause significant difficulty in functioning and create subjective distress. Moreover, the thoughts, feelings, and behavior of individuals with a personality disorder differ markedly from those of others in the same culture.

■ *DSM-IV* DESCRIPTION OF PERSONALITY DISORDERS

The criteria given for personality disorder in DSM-IV are as follows:

- Marked differences in thought processes, emotional reactivity, interpersonal relationships, and impulse control from those of others in the individual's culture and peer group.
- The different patterns of thought, emotionality, and behavior are enduring and inflexible, and are demonstrated consistently in most personal and social situations.
- Significant personal distress and/or impairment is evident during interactions within the family and with others in a social or occupational setting.
- The patterns of enduring thoughts, emotions, and behavior become evident during adolescence and early adulthood.
- The cognitive, emotional, and behavioral patterns are not due to any other psychiatric disorder, the physiological effects of a substance such as alcohol, the side effects of medications, or exposure to toxic chemicals.

Three clusters, or groups of related personality disorders, known as Clusters A, B, and C, have been classified in *DSM-IV* (1994) as follows:

CLUSTER A comprises personality disorders in which the behavior of the individual appears odd or eccentric. These disorders are **paranoid personality disorder**—a pattern of distrust and suspiciousness such that others' motives are interpreted as malevolent; **schizoid personality disorder**—a pattern of detachment from social relationships and a restricted range of emotional expression; and **schizotypal personality disorder**—a pattern of acute discomfort in close relationships, cognitive or perceptual distortions, and eccentricities of behavior.

CLUSTER B comprises personality disorders in which the behavior of the individual appears dramatic, emotional, or erratic. These disorders are **antisocial personality disorder**—a pattern of disregard for, and violation of, the rights of others; **borderline personality disorder**—a pattern of instability in interpersonal relationships, self-image, and affects, and marked impulsivity; **histrionic personality disorder**—a pattern of excessive emotionality and attention seeking; and **narcissistic personality disorder**—a pattern of grandiosity, need for admiration, and lack of empathy.

CLUSTER C consists of personality disorders in which the behavior of the individual appears anxious or fearful. These include **avoidant personality disorder**—a pattern of social inhibition, feelings of inadequacy, and hypersensitivity to negative evaluation; **dependent personality disorder**—a pattern of submissive and clinging behavior related to excessive need to be taken care of; and **obsessive-compulsive personality**—a pattern of preoccupation with orderliness, perfectionism, and control.

■ THEORETICAL PERSPECTIVES

Theorists such as Freud, Erickson, Kernberg, and Mahler have thought about why individuals with personality disorders have cognitive, emotional, and behavioral reactions that vary from those of other individuals in the same population. Freud began to postulate about how the personality develops and what causes problems by conceptualizing developmental stages and the internal psychic structures known as the id, ego, and superego. Erickson studied Freud and expanded his theory by labeling stages marked by explicit conflicts that must be resolved if an individual is to relate to others in a healthful manner. Erickson's personality development theory includes stages of adult development. Recently, several theorists have studied object relations, or the issue of how the individual views him- or herself in relation to significant others.

Freud's Tripartite Model hypothesizes that a person's internal psychic structures consist of the id, ego, and superego. These three structures provide a stable psychic organization with which to experience the world, and provide information to an individual about his or her emotional milieu. The id is an unconscious structure that houses primitive thoughts, feelings, and impulses in the adult. The Id operates and stores repressed material. The ego, part of which exists in the conscious realm and part in the unconscious, is the observant component of the psyche that watches reality and attempts to understand its observations within the context of earlier experiences. The ego mediates the primitive demands of the id and the restraints imposed by the superego. The ego keeps primitive impulses, such as sexual desires, aggressive fantasies, and/or unconscious conflicts from entering into conscious awareness. The superego is the guilt center, which develops during the phallic stage of psychosexual evolution, is based on culturally acquired mores, values, and restrictions. Like the ego and the id, it has both conscious and unconscious elements. (Freud, 1923a; Tyson and Tyson, 1990)

■ DEVELOPMENTAL STAGE THEORIES OF FREUD AND ERICKSON

This section examines the work of two major theorists, Sigmund Freud and Eric Erickson, and their theories about the developmental stages of the psyche. The stages of psychosexual development were described by

Freud in his "Three Essays on the Theory of Sexuality." (Freud 1905b). Erickson viewed development as a life-long process and elaborated Freud's theory by including three additional adult stages of psychic development (Erickson, 1950; Tyson and Tyson, 1990). These consecutive stages do not follow a strict chronological timetable. Erickson thought that each child has an individual timetable of development. He theorized that the specific stages in this timetable are not passed through and then left behind, but rather that each stage contributes to the total personality.

ORAL STAGE: TRUST VERSUS MISTRUST

Freud's oral stage, which he considered the earliest stage of psychosexual development, occurs from birth to 18 months of age. During this stage the infant's needs, perceptions, and modes of expression are primarily centered around the mouth, lips, tongue, and other organs related to the oral zone. The child who successfully works through this stage learns to give, receive from others, and trust without excessive dependence or envy. Conflicts during this stage result in dependency, envy, and jealousy of others. Narcissism develops and the individual is self-absorbed and unable to empathize with others. These traits are often seen in patients with Cluster A and Cluster B personality disorders.

Erickson called this oral-sensory stage the period of basic trust versus basic mistrust. In it, the infant learns trust and hope by receiving the consistent care of parents who provide such satisfying experiences as tranquillity, nourishment, and warmth. Its lack can cause the infant a sense of separation and abandonment. In its positive aspect, it is characterized it by the infant's capacity to sleep peacefully, to take nourishment comfortably, and to excrete without negative feedback.

ANAL STAGE: AUTONOMY VERSUS SHAME AND DOUBT

The anal stage, between ages 1 and 3, occurs when neuromuscular control over the anal sphincter matures and control over the bowels becomes voluntary. During this stage, toilet training takes place. The child begins to strive for independence and separation from dependence on the parent and the parent's control. There is some degree of ambivalence in that struggle to accomplish this separation. The child tries to achieve some degree of autonomy and independence without excessive shame and doubt about the loss of control. Conflicts during the anal stage result in the character traits of ambivalence, messiness, defiance, rage, frugality, and orderliness. These traits are often seen in the patients in Cluster C.

Erickson called this stage the period of autonomy versus shame and doubt, and characterized it as the period during which the child learns parental expectations, obligations, privileges, and limitations on behavior. Adults help the child to understand these limitations by exercising control over the child in a firmly reassuring manner, thereby preventing secretive, sneaky, and sly behaviors. Failure of self-control can cause feelings of shame and doubt.

During this stage, the child's gradual acceptance of adult limit-setting shapes the child's later understanding of societal rules. Judgment begins the differentiation between right and wrong.

PHALLIC STAGE: INITIATIVE VERSUS GUILT

Freud's phallic stage occurs between the ages of 3 and 5 years, when the child begins to express genital interest. There is curiosity, exploration, stimulation, and excitement in the genitals. Freud described "penis envy," or the female infant's perception of the lack of a penis as evidence of castration, as developing during this stage. Tyson and Tyson (1990) have described the phallic stage in a more modern approach as the "infantile genital stage" in which both boys and girls discover their genitals. During this stage, there is an increase in genital masturbation, with unconscious fantasies of sexual involvement with the parent of the opposite sex. Part of the development of the individual's perception of castration, called *castration anxiety,* was theorized as comprising feelings of guilt about masturbating and having fantasies of involvement with the parent of the opposite sex. By working through these conflicts the child develops the superego, or guilt center, while also beginning to lay the foundation for its gender identity. Formation of the superego is postulated as being based on identification with the parent figures; the child's emerging gender identity begins to give it a sense of mastery over persons and objects in its environment, as well as over its own internal processes and impulses, ultimately leading to impulse control. Disturbances often seen in patients who did not successfully master the phallic stage or infantile genital stage include extreme guilt for events and circumstances that were not under the patient's direct control. Patients with conflicts in gender identity have had difficulty in working through this stage of development. Freud and his followers theorize that conflict in this stage can be responsible for nearly all aspects of neurotic development. Patients with antisocial personality disorder, for example, exhibit no remorse for behavior that would normally cause feelings of guilt.

LATENCY STAGE: INDUSTRY VERSUS INFERIORITY

Freud's latency stage takes place from ages 6 or 7 through puberty (the first menses in girls, the first seminal emission in boys). It is a period of quieting of the sexual focus and sublimation of the libidinal and aggressive drives into learning and play activities. Children learn how to control their instinctual impulses while dealing with their environment. As it begins to be able to function in a more autonomous fashion, the child develops a sense of mastery. Persons who have difficulty completing the tasks of this stage have difficulty with impulse control, exhibiting a diminished capacity to sublimate their energies into task completion. Some individuals become too adept at controlling their impulses, and develop obsessive character traits.

Erickson called the task to be mastered during this stage industry versus inferiority. Formal education leads to control of the imagination and produces a sense of industry. Competence, perseverance, and diligence emerge. Failure in this stage may lead to a sense of inferiority.

GENITAL PHASE: IDENTITY VERSUS IDENTITY CONFUSION

During Freud's genital stage, there is an intensification of the sexual drives as the hormone systems develop and adult genital functioning occurs. This is accomplished by a regression in personality organization that reopens conflicts that were unresolved in its environment. Disturbances often seen in patients who did not successfully master the phallic stage or infantile genital stage include extreme guilt for events and circumstances that were not under the patient's direct control. Patients with conflicts in gender identity have had difficulty in working through this stage of development. Freud and his followers theorized that conflict in this stage can be responsible for nearly all aspects of neurotic development.

Erickson called the task to be mastered during this stage industry versus inferiority. Formal education, leads to control of the imagination, and produces a sense of industry. Competence, perseverance, and diligence emerge. Failure in this stage may lead to a sense of inferiority.

The primary tasks in this stage of development are separation from the parents and the establishment of lasting relationships, that satisfy the need for affection and dependency with other individuals. A mature sense of the self (personal identity) develops during this stage, as the individual struggles to accept and integrate adult roles and functions that are consistent with social and cultural expectations. This involves the ability to enjoy meaningful participation in work, love, and the ability to solve problems, in a creative manner. Individuals who cannot resolve the conflicts of this stage develop multiple psychological and personality deficits (Freud 1905b, Freud, 1923a; Tyson and Tyson, 1990)

Erickson called this stage identity versus identity confusion. During this stage, when adolescents become aware of their individual characteristics, such as their likes and dislikes, anticipated goals for the future, and

their control over their own destiny. The activating agent in the formation of identity is the ego, in both its conscious and unconscious aspects. The adolescent's behavior during this chaotic period is inconsistent and unpredictable. Adolescents who experience confusion of roles, or identity confusion, can feel isolated, empty, anxious, and indecisive. They may feel that society is pushing them to make decisions, to which they respond with resistant behavior.

The task during this stage of development is to resolve an identity crisis, in the form of the transitory failure to form a stable identity or a confusion of roles. The most common defense used by children and adolescents who are developing a negative identity is projection (e.g., "They are bad, not me").

The virtue of this stage of development is fidelity. The individual's behavior shuttles from impulsive, thoughtlessness, sporadic actions, to compulsive restraint. During this difficult time, the adolescent seeks an inner knowledge and understanding of him- or herself, and attempts to formulate a set of values.

INTIMACY VERSUS ISOLATION

Erickson called the sixth stage intimacy versus isolation. In it, the young adult prepares to unite his or her identity with that of another person, seeking relationships of intimacy, partnerships, and affiliations. There is a commitment to developing the strengths needed to fulfill these relationships despite the sacrifices they may involve. The individual develops sexual intimacy with a loved partner. Persons who experience difficulty in developing intimacy may isolate themselves, avoiding relationships because they are unwilling or unable to commit themselves to intimacy.

GENERATIVITY VERSUS STAGNATION

Erickson called the seventh stage of development generativity versus stagnation. This stage is characterized by the concern for ensuring that the next generation has access to information, products, and ideas. Erickson believed that if generativity is weak or not given expression during this stage, the personality regresses and takes on a sense of impoverishment and stagnation (Erickson, 1950) One means of expressing generativity is through caring. This is expressed by showing concern, by wanting care for those who need it, and sharing one's knowledge and experience with others. Caring and teaching are responsible for the survival of cultures.

INTEGRITY VERSUS DESPAIR

The final stage in Erickson's theory of development is integrity versus despair. Integrity is achieved after one has taken care of people and managed events and has adapted to the successes and failures of life. The essential counterpart of integrity is despair over the ups and downs of the individual's life cycle. This can aggravate a feeling that life is meaningless and that death is near, with a fear of and wish for death. Time is perceived as being too short to turn back and attempt alternative styles of life.

The virtue of this stage is wisdom. Wisdom maintains and conveys the integrity of accumulated experience from the individual's previous years. A feeling of wholeness can counteract the feeling of despair, alleviating the feeling of helplessness and dependence that can mark the very end of life.

■ OBJECT RELATIONS

Object relations, another theoretical framework, explores how an individual views him- or herself and his or her relationships with others. This framework is particularly useful when working with patients who have a severe personality disorder. These individuals have grave disturbances in their self-concepts and problems in relating to others. These relational problems are evident in the therapeutic relationship, and sometimes can block the patient's progress in problem solving. Using the theory of object relations helps the therapist to understand the patient's self-concept and interaction with others, thereby facilitating interventions that will be useful and understandable to the patient.

Psychiatrist Otto Kernberg defines object relations as the "stability and depth of the patient's relations with significant others as manifested by warmth, dedication, concern, and tactfulness. Other qualitative aspects of this concept are empathy, understanding, and the ability to maintain a relationship when it is invaded by conflict or frustration" (Kernberg, 1984). Kernberg used his study of object relations to develop an understanding of borderline personality disorder and to define this disorder in depth. He also used this theory to understand narcissistic personality disorder. Kernberg developed a list of symptoms and behaviors that underlie the interactive and inner thought and feeling processes of individuals with both these diagnoses. Splitting is one symptom that is particularly useful to understand when providing care to such individuals. Splitting occurs when the individual cannot integrate "good" and "bad" images of him- or herself and others. An individual with borderline personality disorder may, for example, view the self and others as either all good or all bad. Such an individual may describe his mother as the most positive influence in his life, but when discussing his wife be unable to discuss any of her positive characteristics.

Another symptom that is important to understand when caring for individuals with severe personality disorders is their inability to achieve object constancy,—the ability to maintain a relationship, even during times of frustration and changes in the relationship. Margaret Mahler (1963) observed mothers and their infants in a laboratory setting and began to identify patterns of interaction between the two. Mahler developed a theory of separation and individuation that helps to define the child's intrapsychic self-representation and the separate representation of the mother. The child's task during the first 3 years of life is to develop a unique identity. Inherent in this process is the development of object constancy, which occurs around 25 months of age. The child learns that when the mother does not directly meet its needs, it can achieve comfort by soothing itself with something that represents the mother, such as a stuffed animal. Individuals with a severe borderline personality disorder have not fully developed object constancy. When someone significant to them leaves for work, for example, they cannot picture that person's return at the end of the work day. The individual with a severe borderline personality disorder may call the significant other multiple times during the day, become very emotional, and think that the other person will never return. They cannot use any self-soothing mechanism to calm their fears. Emotions take over their behavior.

■ STUDIES IN THE DEVELOPMENT OF PERSONALITY DISORDER

As studies continue to investigate the roles of the brain and genetics in psychiatric disorders, one finding in the area of family studies is that of a strong genetic influence in several personality disorders, suggesting ties between biological factors and personality organization (Siever and Davis, 1991; Kavoussi and Siever, 1991; Siever, 1992). Biological tests used to study individuals with schizotypal personality disorder have demonstrated the role of the brain in abnormal interpersonal relations. One of these tests, known as smooth-pursuit eye tracking, examines the ability of the eyes to track a smoothly moving target (Siever, 1992). Smooth-pursuit eye tracking is important for the cognitive interpretation of information in the environment. Individuals with schizophrenia demonstrate difficulty with smooth-pursuit eye movements, which is thought to reflect disrupted neurointegrative functioning of the frontal lobes. (Siever, 1992). The studies indicating impaired eye tracking are associated with the "deficit" traits of schizophrenia: social isolation, detachment, and inability to relate to others. Lencz et al. (1993) studied eye tracking in undergraduate students with schizotypal personality disorder, and found that they demonstrated an impairment in eye-tracking movements.

Backward masking, another biological test, is indicative of cognitive-perceptual difficulties often seen in patients with schizotypal personality disorder. In this test of neurointegrative functioning, the individual is shown a visual stimulus, which is immediately followed by different visual stimulus. The individual is then asked to identify the object that served as the first visual stimulus (Kavoussi, Siever, 1991). Siever (1985) noted that individuals with schizotypical personality disorder have test results similar to those noted in individuals with schizophrenia, but not as severe.

Measurement of the concentration of homovanillic acid in the cerebrospinal fluid was used in two studies, one by Siever (1992) and the other by Kavoussi and Siever, (1991). Both studies reported an increase in homovanillic acid in the cerebrospinal fluid among patients with schizotypal personality disorder that correlate with positive psychotic-like criteria for this disorder. Schultz et al. (1988) reported that patients with borderline personality disorder and those with schizotypal personality disorder both showed evidence of an exacerbation of psychotic-like symptoms in response to an infusion of amphetamines.

The role in personality disorders of neurotransmitters, and especially serotonin, has also been studied. Several studies in this area have demonstrated disturbances in central serotonergic neurotransmission. Brown et al. (1982) found that aggressive and suicidal behaviors in individuals with a personality disorder correlated with reduced levels of 5-hydroxyindoleacetic acid, a major metabolite of serotonin, in the cerebrospinal fluid. This reduction indicates decreased serotonergic neural activity in these individuals. Mann (1986) found increased numbers of post-synaptic serotonergic receptors in suicide victims, and Stanley and Stanley (1990) found a reduction in serotonin neurotransmission, which is interpreted as biochemical risk factor for suicide. Marin et al. (1989) and Kavoussi and Siever (1991) hypothesize that there seems to be a reduction in serotonergic neural activity in such behaviors as impulsiveness, motor aggression, and suicidal tendencies. Brown and Linnoila (1990) demonstrated a relationship between reduced serotonergic activity and aggressive, impulsive behavior.

Siever and Davis (1991) suggest that individuals with antisocial personality disorder may have dysfunction in the brain system's ability to modulate and inhibit aggressive responses to environmental stimuli. They found EEG slow-wave activity and reduced thresholds of sedation among such individuals, but not among those with long-term depression (Siever, Davis 1991).

■ LEVELS OF STRESS-CRISIS

People with personality disorders, particularly those in Cluster A, (paranoid, schizoid, and schizotypal disorders) and Cluster B (antisocial, borderline, histrionic, and narcissistic disorders) have a variety of crises in their lives. Those with Cluster C-type disorders (avoidant, dependent, and obsessive compulsive) tend to not seek help from mental health providers to the same extent as individuals with other personality disorders. In addition to utilizing critical pathways for planning nursing care, it is helpful to consider the levels of stress and crisis precipitants (Burgess and Roberts, 1995) in planning appropriate interventions. Many individuals with personality disorders caused by incomplete mastery of a developmental task or stage can be classified under Level 2: transition stress. Because partial mastery results in a wide range of personality problems and disturbed functioning, such individuals may be classified as falling within any of the stress-crises levels. Some individuals with long-standing difficulty in identifying the self and maladaptive relationships with others may be classified as falling within Level 4 if there is family dysfunction, or Level 5 if there is an ongoing psychotic process. Often, the individual with a Cluster B-type personality disorder may become suicidal and/or homicidal, exhibit stalking behavior, or commit rape. These behaviors would be classified as falling within Level 6, or psychiatric emergencies. Occasionally, individuals with Cluster B-type disorders have a Level 7 or catastrophic crisis when they have many unresolved psychiatric problems and exhibit life-endangering behavior, such as planning to kill a business partner or themselves as revenge for a poor business decision, and taking physical steps to accomplish this. Case examples of individuals with personality disorder illustrate the types of stress-crises.

■ AN INTERDISCIPLINARY APPROACH TO PLANNING CARE FOR PATIENTS WITH PERSONALITY DISORDERS

Assessment is an essential part of an interdisciplinary approach to the planning of care for patients with personality disorders. A thorough assessment lays the foundation for the *DSM-IV* and nursing diagnoses of these disorders, expected patient outcomes, interventions, and evaluation of the care provided for the patient. Multiple interviews and input from the treatment team, including nurses, psychiatrists, psychologists, social workers, and activities therapists, are necessary to provide a complete picture of the patient. All of these members of the team bring observations and insights critical to making medical and nursing diagnoses and effective planning of care.

ASSESSMENT

Patients with personality disorders, particularly those falling within Cluster B, are often seen several times over the course of their lives in a mental-health setting. Comprehensive assessments may reveal their most significant symptoms, which will establish the foundation for a plan of their care.

To identify those questions that will yield significant data during an assessment of such patients, it is important to review the characteristics that mark a personality disorder. These include difficulty in identifying the self; interpersonal relationships that are often affected by the disorder; and behavioral patterns, views, and expressions of emotions that differ from those of the patient's cultural milieu. The *DSM-IV* (1994) definition of a personality disorder as "an enduring pattern of inner experience and behavior that deviates markedly from the expectations of the individual's culture, is pervasive and inflexible, has an onset in adolescence or early adulthood, is stable over time, and leads to distress or impairment" serves as a guideline for the assessment questions.

The following questions assess the areas of disturbance in an individual with a personality disorder. These questions framed after the individual has identified the problems that prompted his or her visit to the treatment setting. The individual's past experiences and history can provide further information.

- Assessment of the identification of self
  1. How does the individual take care of his or her physical needs? Does the individual appear clean and appropriately dressed? Is the individual getting sufficient sleep, nourishment, exercise?
  2. Does the individual exhibit an inappropriate facial expression or have flat, constricted affect?
  3. Ask the individual to describe him- or herself, elaborating on strengths and weaknesses. Does the individual often focus on weakness in a critical manner without acknowledging strengths? Does the individual inflate his or her importance? What are the individual's likes and dislikes? (This question indirectly assesses self-esteem and view of self.)
  4. How anxious is the individual? Are vital signs elevated? Is the individual pacing, glancing about, or fidgeting? What is the individual worrying about, how often do they think about these worries?

5. Ask the individual to describe what calming measures are used when he or she is feeling anxious, upset, or sad. Does the individual ever use alcohol or other drugs, engage in sex with multiple partners, eat excessively, or harm him- or herself in anyway?
6. Ask the individual if he/she has ever felt like committing suicide or killing anyone else. Does the individual feel that way now? Do they have a plan for accomplishing it? How often does the individual think about this plan? Is a weapon available? How does the individual prevent him- or herself from acting on these thoughts?
7. Ask the individual if there has ever been a time when they have mutilated themselves, such as cutting the skin until it bled, burning the skin with cigarettes, or pulling out significant amounts of hair. When did these incidents occur? Are the behaviors ongoing?
8. Does the individual deny strong emotions, such as anger and joy?
- Assessment of interpersonal relationships
  1. How does the individual interact with family members? Does he or she have friends? How does the individual interact with friends? Can he or she tolerate frustrations and disappointments in a relationship without resorting to vindictive behavior, or hurting others either verbally or by exhibiting aggressive behavior?
  2. How does the individual function in the work place? Does he or she need constant supervision to complete a task? Does the individual complain about his or her boss or supervisor? Are the complaints centered around resenting assignments and having to provide accountability for work performance? (These questions can help in understanding the individual's view of authority figures)
  3. Can the individual identify with other people? Does he or she lack empathy? Does the individual constantly behave in a manner that places him or her in the center of attention? Does the individual demonstrate critical behavior toward others? Is he or she concerned about how others will evaluate him/her?
  4. Does the individual demonstrate a low tolerance for frustration? What does the individual do when frustrated with others? (Ask how he or she reacts when driving and is suddenly stuck in a traffic jam as an example of a commonly experienced frustration.)
  5. Does the individual identify him- or herself in the context of a relationship? (A woman may identify herself as Mrs. John Jones, and dis-

cuss most issues in the manner of how she and her husband would respond to them). Does the individual indicate a dependence on family members or a significant other to meet most of his or her needs? (A 40-year-old unmarried man may live alone but have most of his meals at his parents' home.)

6. Does the individual have any friends? What is the nature of the friendship? Does the individual have an intimate relationship? Ask him or her to describe that relationship. Does the individual have multiple sexual relationships? (This question will help the nurse to assess the individual's ability to form intimate relationships, and whether these relationships are intense, stormy, or supportive and reciprocal).

- Assesment of Behavioral Patterns

1. How does the individual describe the problem areas that caused him or her to seek help? Does the individual demonstrate the ability to identify these problems and discuss some possible options to solving them? Does he or she blame others and/or indicate a plan of retaliation? Does the individual indicate a sense of entitlement when discussing the problem areas?

2. Does the individual engage in illegal activities? How does he or she view these activities? Has he or she ever been arrested? If so, have they ever been convicted? What did the individual do as punishment? How did they handle the sentence emotionally?

3. Has the individual experienced a lack of consensual validation? Has the individual ever experienced any ideas of reference? During the assessment interview, does the individual discuss any odd beliefs or magical thinking that influences his or her behavior?

4. Does the individual read hidden meanings into benign remarks by others? Is he or she suspicious of others? Does he or she question the fidelity of his or her significant other?

5. Is the individual impulsive? Does he or she have difficulty in learning from mistakes? (This would be reflected by repeated experience of the same problem without further understanding of the problem or how the individual reacted to the issues.)

6. Does the individual have a history of failing to honor financial obligations? Does he or she plan ahead, such as securing a new job prior to quitting a current position?

7. How does the individual view parenting responsibilities? Is there a history of child neglect, abuse (physical, verbal, sexual)? Does the individual (parent) provide adequate care for his or her children?

8. Does the individual use drugs or alcohol? Has he or she ever been in trouble with the law because of drug or alcohol use (including driving when intoxicated)?

NURSING DIAGNOSIS

The nursing diagnosis depends on the patient's presenting clinical state, evolving from the in-depth nursing assessment. It is formulated on the basis of the clinical examples illustrating the various *DSM-IV* diagnoses. Determining the nursing diagnosis in cases of personality disorder serves several functions. It defines the patient's problem from a behavioral perspective; identifies problems to be examined with the patient; and therefore becomes a guidepost for the outcomes of care.

PLANNING CARE

In planning strategies for the care of a patient with a personality disorder, the nurse determines the expected outcome criteria for the patient based on the diagnosis. The nurse and other members of the care team then select the most appropriate interventions for helping the patient to achieve the outcome expectations of the care plan (Fortinash and Holoday-Worret, 1991). The plan is integrated with critical pathways, and identifies the expected length of treatment. The patient is consulted and given a review of his or her identified problem areas, the desired outcomes, and the interventions that will be used to achieve them. The patient's feedback about the plan of care is carefully evaluated to determine his or her ability to collaborate in the plan, and the assistance patient needs in order to further understand his or her problem areas. Goals set for patients with personality disorders must be within the patient's ability to successfully achieve. Because these patients' symptoms have become chronic, interventions focus on highlighting their repeated problem areas, and offer new options for problem solving that are easy to implement and can yield rapid success.

EXPECTED OUTCOME CRITERIA

The expected outcome criteria for the plan of care in cases of personality disorder are included in a statement that is used to determine the success or failure of the evaluation portion of the nursing diagnosis. These outcome criteria are measurable, and based on the symptoms described in the nursing diagnosis.

Statements of outcome criteria are provided below for the nursing diagnosis specific to the personality disorders.

INTERVENTIONS AND RATIONALE

Interventions help the patient to meet the planned outcomes of nursing care. Each intervention is followed by an explanation of its rationale.

The components of care planning—assessment, *DSM-IV* and nursing diagnoses, critical pathways, expected outcome, intervention, and rationale—are illustrated in the following section with a case example for each of the personality disorders.

■ THE NURSE'S ROLE IN IMPLEMENTING CARE

The primary context for implementing a care plan in psychiatric nursing is the therapeutic relationship. In this relationship, it is important that the psychiatric nurse maintain a non-judgmental posture and promote the patient's problem-solving capacity. This can be done by asking strategic questions of patients so that they can arrive at the best options for problem solving within their belief system. If the nurse lectures the patient rather than asking well-thought-out questions, the onus of responsibility for the patient's outcome may shift from the patient to the nurse. Individuals with personality disorders have difficulty in relating to others, and often distort information. If patients discover their own patterns of thought and behavior through therapeutic interventions, their therapeutically developed coping skills will remain with them longer.

Another aspect of implementing care is patient teaching. Books, movies, television, and news broadcasts may be used for this. Such teaching broadens the patient's experience to include new coping skills by examining a main character in a movie and suggesting behavioral changes that might be helpful to that character. The nurse can then ask the patient to identify a similar problem in his or her life and discuss whether these suggestions would be helpful in resolving it.

An important aspect of psychoeducation is to teach patients about psychotropic medications they may be taking. Davis, Janicak, and Ayd (1995) surveyed the literature to determine the best psychopharmacotherapy for the population of patients with personality disorders. They suggested that small doses of antipsychotic drugs are helpful for patients who have transient psychosis or paranoia; that antidepressants, such as the selective serotonin response inhibitors are useful for treating concurrent panic attacks, phobias, and compulsive symptoms with depressive syndromes; and that mood stabilizing drugs (carbamazepine, tegretol) are useful for treating cyclothymic disorders.

Nurses play an important role in case management (Chapter 44). In this context, the nurse coordinates services that are available to the patient. These services help the patient to learn the coping skills necessary to solve an identified problem. Case management may entail coordination with the primary psychotherapist, social worker, family members and others who provide the patient's support system.

Cluster A: Behaviors Appearing Odd or Eccentric

E CASE EXAMPLES

▶ PARANOID PERSONALITY DISORDER

Aaron, age 36, has always been suspicious. He does not trust anyone, even his family members. All who knew him were surprised when Aaron married; he decided to marry Delores so that she would not date anyone else. Within a month after their marriage, he began to suspect that she was being unfaithful. He began going through her mail, checking the telephone numbers she called with the "caller identification" system, and to look through her purse for clues pointing to an affair. He became angry and vindictive when interacting with Delores. The more she tried to prove her innocence, the more suspicious and angry he became. Delores begged him to come with her to a couples-therapy session to save their marriage.

Critical Pathway for Level 4 Stress-Crisis

Nursing diagnosis: Altered thought processes

Related to: Inability to trust,

As Evidenced by: Aaron's inaccurate interpretation of his wife's behavior, suspiciousness, and hypervigilance.

Outcome: Aaron will attend couples-therapy sessions with Delores.

Interventions:

The nurse suggests that Aaron keep a journal of his suspicious thoughts, including the circumstances under which these thoughts occur, and their frequency. When they are repeated, does Aaron find that he is more watchful? What behavior does he exhibit when he has these suspicious thoughts?

continued

E CASE EXAMPLES   Continued

The nurse and Aaron will discuss his journal, identifying the patterns of his thoughts and behavior, as well as the pattern of the content of his repeated ideas.

Rationale

When Aaron identifies a thought and/or behavioral pattern, he can determine how useful the pattern is to solving his recognized problems, and can further determine the changes in his thinking that may be more helpful to solving these problems.

Intervention

A discussion between the nurse and Aaron can help him to highlight other actions he can take to decrease his anxiety and suspicious, hypervigilant behavior toward his wife.

Rationale

Often, individuals become repetitive in their pattern of thought and behavior, and do not discuss other means of problem solving. A discussion often assists the patient to think through new ways of tackling an issue.

Intervention

Using a character in a movie or a television program who is suspicious of his wife, ask Aaron how he would have reacted if he were the husband character.

Rationale

When people view movies or television dramas, they often identify with one or several characters in the plot. Selecting this media for therapeutic purposes utilizes this process in a constructive manner.

Pathway

Date Planned	Date Completed	
____	____	1. Aaron will be able to recognize thoughts that increase his internal anxiety, to which he reacts with suspiciousness and hypervigilance, within 2 weeks.
____	____	2. Aaron will be able to identify two actions he can take to decrease his anxiety and suspicious, hypervigilant behavior toward his wife within 2 weeks.

▶ SCHIZOID PERSONALITY DISORDER

Steve is 40 years old, unmarried, lives alone, and has no friends. He is quiet and rarely speaks to his co-workers or neighbors. He visits his parents' home when his mother invites him, but he rarely participates in the family's conversations. He looks down at the ground when other people are present. His face shows no emotion. Steve works hard as a maintenance engineer, but rarely responds to complements. His hobbies are solitary. After work, he goes home and watches television or plays computer games. He has never dated. If you ask Steve about how he views his life, he describes, in as few words as possible, that he is satisfied with it.

Critical Pathway for Level 2 Stress-Crisis

Nursing Diagnosis:

Impaired Social Interactions

Related to: Inability to establish a relationship with others due to a disruption in development of interpersonal skills.

As evidenced by: Rarely interacting with others, including family members and co-workers, rarely looking at others when they are present, and solitary interests.

Outcome

Steve will be able to select one item of information to discuss briefly with an individual of his choice. He will also join one community social activity group.

Interventions

Discuss with Steve several activities that he enjoys.

Ask him to select one in which to engage with a person who is least threatening.

Rationale

To assist Steve to experience a pleasant experience in the presence of another person.

Intervention

Steve agrees to discuss, for five minutes, the activity in which he chooses to engage with another person, with that individual and with the nurse.

Rationale

To assist Steve to socialize in a limited manner.

Pathway

Date Planned	Date Completed	
____	____	1. Steve will be able to identify one activity in which he can engage in the presence of others within 2 weeks.
____	____	2. Steve will be able to select one item of information to discuss briefly with an individual of his choice within 2 weeks.

▶ SCHIZOTYPAL PERSONALITY DISORDER

Alice is a 27-year-old, unmarried woman who works as a computer information analyst. She has a reputation of being hard to approach because many of those who know her describe her as "weird." She has a different interpretation than others of events that occur in her environment. She often states that she has a sixth sense and can tell what is going to happen before it does. She is hesitant in her speech and thinks that when people near her are talking, they are discussing her. Her face is usually devoid of emotion. When Alice meets with her fellow workers, in a social milieu, such as at a luncheon, or meets with fellow workers to "brainstorm," she becomes very anxious. Her anxiety builds as the meeting continues, and she feels overwhelmed by it. Her verbal responses become disjointed and her thought process deteriorates. She recently experienced a major depression after her cat died. She interpreted the cat's death as a warning from the spirit world.

Critical Pathway for Level 5 Stress-Crisis

Nursing Diagnosis:

Altered Thought Processes

Related to: Panic level of anxiety and stress sufficiently severe to threaten Alice's work performance, as evidenced by inability to think in a clear manner and inflexible social behavior that reflects inaccurate thinking.

Disturbance in self-esteem.

Related to: a perceived threat to the patient's self-concept, as evidenced by suspiciousness of others and distortion of events, such as believing that others are talking about

CASE EXAMPLES   Continued

Outcome:

Alice will be able to identify two situations that increase her anxiety sufficiently to make her unable to think in a clear manner.

Intervention:

The nurse suggests to Alice that she keep a journal outlining her anxious thoughts, including when these thoughts occur, their frequency, and when she finds it difficult to think clearly. The nurse and Alice will discuss the journal in order to identify her patterns of thought and behavior, as well as the pattern of content of her repeated ideas.

Rationale:

To help the patient to determine when a thought and/or behavioral pattern increases her anxiety to such a high level that abstract thinking becomes impossible.

Outcome:

Alice will be able to identify one action that she can take to reduce her anxiety adequately to enable her to think clearly.

Intervention:

During a discussion with the nurse, Alice and the nurse will outline actions that she can take to decrease her anxiety, such as taking a deep breath and/or using a positive affirmation instead of attending to repetitive anxious thoughts.

Rationale:

This intervention will provide Alice with concrete behaviors and thoughts that she can utilize to reduce her anxiety.

Pathway:

Date Planned	Date Completed	
_____	_____	1. Alice will identify two situations that increase her anxiety sufficiently to make her unable to think in a clear manner within 2 weeks.
_____	_____	2. Alice will be able to identify one action that she can take to reduce her anxiety adequately to enable her think in a clear manner within 2 weeks.

Cluster B: Behaviors Appearing Dramatic, Emotional, or Erratic

CASE EXAMPLES

▶ ANTISOCIAL PERSONALITY DISORDER

Larry, age 34, is a patient in a forensic psychiatric unit. He was committed to this unit after beating two men and resisting arrest. Larry has a record of breaking and entering dating to when he was 14 years old. At the time of his first arrest he was living in a foster home, since his mother felt that she could not control his truancy from school or his propensity to start small fires. Larry is angry, threatening, and intimidating to the care staff and patients, and believes that he was unjustly arrested. "Those men approached me first," he says when asked. "They started the fight. The cop wouldn't listen, so I thought I'd teach him a lesson, but he arrested me and made me come here. I don't think you can help. You don't know anything about me, and you don't care. I'm just a prisoner to you."

Critical Pathway for Level 6 Stress-Crisis

Nursing Diagnosis:

Risk for Violence directed at others.

Related to: Overt and aggressive acts as evidenced by beating two men and resisting arrest, provocative behavior (angry, threatening, intimidating to staff and patients), and a history of violent behavior (truancy from school, a prior record of breaking and entering, and a history of arson when younger).

Outcome:

Larry will identify two thoughts or events that cause his angry reactions.

Intervention:

The nurse will encourage him to discuss the beating incident that caused his confinement to the hospital unit, and will highlight his thoughts prior to his actions that led to the fight.

Rationale:

To assist Larry to connect his thoughts and behaviors with anger-producing stimuli in order to prevent future aggressive behavior.

Outcome:

Larry will demonstrate control of his aggressive impulses during his hospitalization.

Intervention:

Discuss with the patient a contract for safety that specifies the patient's responsibility for preventing any aggressive or violent outbursts.

Intervention:

Discuss techniques that the patient can utilize to maintain control over his aggressive impulses, such as walking away from situations that cause him to feel angry, taking a 10-minute period in a quiet area as a "time out," asking for a medication that may assist him with impulse control, taking slow deep breaths, coupled with thoughts such as "I can maintain control over my anger; the staff will hear my complaint without my yelling."

Rationale:

The patient can learn new ways in which to deal with the overwhelming feeling of anger, which are not aggressive and/or violent.

Pathways:

Date Planned	Date Completed	
____	____	1. Larry will identify two thoughts or events that cause him to have angry reactions within 1 week.
____	____	2. Larry will demonstrate control of his aggressive impulses during his hospitalization within 2 weeks.
____	____	3. Larry will be able to discuss two methods to assist him to control his aggressive impulses when feeling anger and/or frustration within 1 week.

▶ BORDERLINE PERSONALITY DISORDER

Cheryl, age 28, was admitted to a psychiatric unit after taking an overdose of Valium (diazepam) when her husband left her after an intense verbal and physical fight. Cheryl said that her husband had refused to listen to her, that she had then grabbed his collar, and that he then threw her against the wall. Her marriage has a history of verbal and physical fights since she became married. She interpreted her husband's leaving as the end of their relationship and took the overdose of Valium on the belief that she could not live without him. Cheryl has a history of problems in her relationships. In the nursing exploration of whether she had any family or friends who would help her during her marital crisis, she told of relationships that had ended because the significant other had not satisfied her needs. Her mother has a history of suicidal ideation and depression; her father has alcoholism and was abusive when Cheryl was a child.

Critical Pathway for Level 6 Stress-Crisis

Nursing Diagnosis:

a. Risk for Violence: Self-Directed

Related to: marital conflict, as evidenced by a threat of abandonment by her husband, a family history of suicide attempts, abuse during childhood, and depression and inadequate coping skills.

Nursing Diagnosis:

Ineffective Individual Coping

Related to: to ongoing marital conflict and a perceived threat of abandonment by her husband, as evidenced by a suicidal gesture in response to her husband's leaving her after a fight, inability to differentiate her own sense of self from that of her husband, and inability to identify any individuals who could assist during her marital crisis, as the result of difficulty in relating to others.

Outcome:

Cheryl will be able to identify the factor that precipitated her suicidal gesture.

Intervention:

Discuss the suicidal gesture with Cheryl and help her to identify what caused this action. Encourage her to discuss her marital crisis, including her feelings when her husband walked out the door, what she wanted to tell him, and how she could communicate this verbally rather than with suicidal behavior.

Rationale:

This intervention will help the patient to recognize the link between her feelings of anger and abandonment and her suicidal gesture.

Intervention:

Ask Cheryl to contract to ensure her safety in a written statement that includes information about any increase in suicidal thoughts, and an agreement to discuss these with a member of the nursing staff and her psychotherapist.

Rationale:

To assist the patient to maintain impulse control and safety, as well as encouraging her to take responsibility for preventing future suicidal gestures.

Outcome:

Cheryl will be able to list one purpose in life that is not related to her role as a wife.

Intervention:

Ask Cheryl to describe the activities that constitute her usual day.

Help her to recognize the purposes of these activities and how they contribute to her life.

Rationale:

To help the patient to identify a purpose in her life that enhances her self-esteem.

Outcome:

Cheryl will be able to identify two methods of decreasing her anxiety about abandonment, which could be utilized to stop her from any further suicidal gestures.

Intervention:

Help Cheryl to determine the pattern in her marital relationship that results in arguments followed by her husband's leaving her for short periods; discuss communication methods she can use instead of arguing with her husband; teach her several different ways of self soothing herself when she is feeling alone, such as listening to music, reading a comforting short story or book (including the Bible), watching a television program or movie that is soothing to her, and exercising.

Rationale:

If the patient begins to master some of her abandonment anxieties, her behavior will be less impulsive and self destructive.

Outcome:

Cheryl will be able to identify the causal factor that precipitated the argument with her husband.

Interventions:

Encourage Cheryl to discuss the argument between her and her husband. What was she angry or upset about? How did she communicate this feeling? Why did the argument escalate to her aggressive act of grabbing his collar? How did she feel when he walked out the door? How could she communicate this in a verbal way rather than by a suicide attempt?

E CASE EXAMPLES Continued

Outcome:

Cheryl will be able to recognize two problem-solving options rather than a suicidal gesture when faced with her husband's leaving her after an argument.

Interventions:

Discuss ways in which Cheryl can release her emotional tension after a serious argument rather than making a suicidal gesture, such as writing a letter to her husband telling him her thoughts and feelings about the argument (not a letter to send, but one to ventilate and clarify her feelings).

Rationale:

This intervention affords Cheryl an alternative means of discussing her feelings without harming herself or others.

Intervention:

Have Cheryl employ the self-soothing techniques described above.

Rationale:

By learning self-soothing techniques to use when feeling abandoned, Cheryl may decrease some of her impulsive behavior.

Outcome:

Cheryl will be able to list individuals she can contact if she becomes suicidal.

Intervention:

Assist Cheryl to list people she can contact if she feels suicidal. The list can be modeled after the contract for safety described above, and can be generated by asking Cheryl about who she talks to and spends time with in activities.

Give Cheryl the telephone number of the suicide "hot line" as well as the telephone number of the clinic's primary psychotherapist.

Rationale:

Cheryl is less likely to make a suicidal gesture if she is able to identify people she can contact for help.

Pathways:

Date Planned	Date Completed	
＿＿	＿＿	1. Cheryl will be able to identify the causal factor that precipitated her suicidal intent within 2 weeks.
＿＿	＿＿	2. Cheryl will be able to discuss her suicidal intent, the argument between her husband and herself, and how she felt when he walked out the door within 2 weeks.
＿＿	＿＿	3. Cheryl will be able to list one purpose in life that is not related to her role as a wife within 2 weeks.
＿＿	＿＿	4. Cheryl will be able to identify two methods of decreasing her abandonment anxiety, which could be utilized to stop her from any further suicidal gestures.
＿＿	＿＿	5. Cheryl will be able to recognize within 2 weeks two problem-solving options rather than a suicidal gesture when faced with her husband's leaving her.
＿＿	＿＿	6. Within 2 weeks, Cheryl will be able to list individuals she can contact if she becomes suicidal.

▶ HISTRIONIC PERSONALITY DISORDER

Robert is a actor with a local Shakespeare company. He is 27 years old and was reviewed as an excellent Hamlet, his current role. He has recently had difficulty in his relationship with his girlfriend, Karen. He craves being the center of attention both on and off stage. He tells Karen that he is an "entertainer" and will always want attention. He recently had an intense argument with her when he criticized another actor's work while they were attending a play. During the play, Karen told Robert that she would never again accompany him to a live entertainment event. Robert became enraged with Karen and yelled so that the whole theater knew he was an actor and that he and his girlfriend were having an argument. Robert turned to the people in the foyer of the theater as though they were an audience, and told them the story of his relationship problems with Karen.

Critical Pathways for Level 2 Stress-Crisis

Nursing Diagnosis:

Disturbance in self-esteem

Related to: Perceived occupational and relationship problems, as evidenced by approval-seeking behavior (Robert's view of himself as an "entertainer" always wanting attention), emphasizing other's deficits (involving the audience in Robert's personal argument with Karen), and difficulty in forming close relationships.

Outcome:

Robert will be able to identify three positive aspects of himself without seeking affirmation from others.

Intervention:

Encourage Robert to list three strengths of his personality; determine how often he acknowledges his character strengths to himself; encourage him to regularly use affirmations in his thought processes as a healthy way to build self-esteem.

Rationale:

These interventions will help Robert to enhance his self-esteem and decrease his need for affirmation from others.

Outcome:

Robert will recognize when his behavior is aimed at seeking attention from others.

Intervention:

Ask Robert to discuss two of Karen's typical responses when he is behaving in an attention-seeking manner. Ask Robert to determine the frequency and intensity of the behavior he utilizes to gain attention from others.

Rationale:

If Robert can identify the pattern of behavior that indicates a need for attention from others, he may be able to plan healthier methods of meeting this demand.

Pathways:

Date Planned	Date Completed	
＿＿	＿＿	1. Robert will be able to identify three positive aspects of himself without seeking affirmation from others within 1 week.
＿＿	＿＿	2. Robert will recognize when his behavior is aimed at seeking attention from others within 2 weeks.

E CASE EXAMPLES   Continued

▶ NARCISSISTIC PERSONALITY DISORDER

Martha, age 43, is an accountant in a large firm. She is known for asking people to help her and having them end by completing the project for her, while she gets the credit for it, and sometimes a pay raise. Martha is highly verbal at most office staff meetings, usually bragging about what she has accomplished. She never acknowledges the persons who have assisted her. She views herself as one of the top accountants in the region, and expects to be treated as such. When other staff members assist her by completing a project, Martha sees this as though they were interning under her supervision. She sees herself as entitled to an expensive automobile, large house, jewelry, a housekeeper, and gardener. Martha is married, but seems to have lost the spark in her marital relationship. When she mentions her husband, it usually is followed by a criticism and an explanation of how she could do better.

Critical Pathways for Level 2 Stress-Crisis

Nursing Diagnosis:
Defensive Coping
Related to: Unrealistic expectations of self and others, as evidenced by denial of obvious problems, projection of blame and responsibility, rationalization of failures, and a superior attitude toward others.
Outcome:
Martha will be able to list two strengths and two weaknesses of her behavior.
Intervention:
Through discussion and a journal, help Martha to list and describe two strengths and two weaknesses of her behavior.

Rationale:
This will help Martha to view both the positive and negative aspects of her behavior.
Outcome:
Martha will be able to identify the times at which she is blaming another person for her behavior by recognizing two key words that she uses when relinquishing responsibility for her actions.
Intervention:
Encourage Martha to keep a journal of her daily activities, including her thoughts and feelings about the day's events. Utilize the journal to help Martha to identify redundant, blaming thoughts. Point out the key words Martha uses when conversing with her.
Rationale:
This may help Martha to determine the pattern of her behavior and its negative impact on others.
Pathways:

Date Planned	Date Completed	
____	____	1. Martha will be able to list two strengths and two weakness of her behavior within 2 weeks.
____	____	2. Martha will be able to identify when she is blaming another person for her behavior by recognizing two key words she uses when relinquishing responsibility for her actions within 2 weeks.

Cluster C: Behaviors Appearing Anxious or Fearful

E CASE EXAMPLES

▶ AVOIDANT PERSONALITY DISORDER

Beth is a 39-year-old woman who works as a bookkeeper in a small printing company. She has worked in this same company since she graduated from high school. Prior to this year, all of her company's financial records were kept by hand, using a calculator. Because of the advantages of computer programs, Beth's boss bought a computer and a software package to keep track of the company's expenditures and profits. Beth views the computer as the end of her job. Even though her boss has assured her that he is not planning to terminate her job, Beth remains emotionally paralyzed by fear and unable to learn how to use the new computer system. Beth is certain that she will make mistakes that will make her "look dumb," and she is certain that she will then be fired. She also worries that if she is fired, she will lose her condominium, since she lives alone. She sees herself as worthless and unable to try anything new. She is often anxious, particularly around people. Beth has only two friends to whom she speaks, and she has not shared her problem with them for fear that they will label her as stupid.

Critical Pathways for Level 2 Stress-Crisis

Nursing Diagnosis:
Disturbance in self-esteem

E CASE EXAMPLES   Continued

Related to: Repeatedly negative feedback, resulting in diminished self-worth, as evidenced by self-negating verbalization, evaluation of the self as unable to deal with a new computer system, rejection of positive feedback (Beth's boss's support for learning the new skill), and exaggeration of negative thoughts about the self (will never learn to use the computer system, sees self as stupid).

Outcome:
Beth will list two tasks that she does well in the office.

Intervention:
During discussion, question Beth about her job and the types of tasks she does that contribute to the accomplishment of her work. Suggest that she keep a list of her accomplishments at work.

Rationale:
The acknowledgment of what Beth has accomplished will enhance her self-esteem.

Outcome:
Beth will discuss one recent project in which she learned something new. She will then outline how the learning took place.

Intervention:
Discuss with Beth something that she learned by reading and following directions, such as following a cooking recipe.

Rationale:
Beth will be able to transfer something she has accomplished into the new learning situation.

Outcome:
Beth will transfer a learning skill (such as reading) into learning how to use the new computer system (reading how to turn on the machine and enter her identification number).

Intervention:
Through discussion, the nurse will demonstrate to Beth how she can transfer a learning skill she has mastered (cooking a new recipe) to turning on the computer and entering her password.

Rationale:
Beth may feel more secure in a new learning situation if she employs some of the techniques she has used in other areas of her life.

Pathways:

Date Planned	Date Completed	
_____	_____	1. Beth will list two tasks that she does well in the office within 1 week.
_____	_____	2. Beth will discuss one recent project in which she had learned something new within 1 week.
_____	_____	3. Beth will outline how this learning took place within 2 weeks.
_____	_____	4. Beth will transfer a learning skill (such as reading) into learning the computer system (reading how to turn on the machine and enter her identification number) within 2 weeks.

▶ DEPENDENT PERSONALITY DISORDER

Jake is 47 years old, unmarried, and living with his parents. He is unable to sustain a relationship with a woman for more than a couple of months. He expects a woman to make most of the couple's decisions, do all the driving when they go somewhere, make all arrangements for entertainment, and pay half the fee for the entertainment. He tends to compare the woman he is dating with his mother, with whom he has a very close relationship. His mother prepares the family meals, washes all of Jake's laundry, and cleans up Jake's room and the family common areas. Jake works in a corporate mail room and prepares copies of reports for corporate meetings. He occasionally contributes money to his family with which to buy groceries. Jake moved out of the family house once, 10 years ago, when he was offered a job in another state. He felt so alone and upset at the new job that he left the job and moved back to his parents' home. He often worries about what will happen when his parents, particularly his mother, die.

Critical Pathways for Level 4 Stress-Crisis

Nursing Diagnosis:
Ineffective individual coping

Related to: inadequate psychological resources due to an immature developmental level, as evidenced by failure to maintain a close, intimate relationship because of excessive dependency on his partner, inability to move out of the parental home due to inability to recognize and meet adult role expectations, and inappropriate use of defense mechanisms to maintain this level of dependency.

Outcome:
Jake will begin to list the types of tasks he does to contribute to his family's household.

Intervention:
Through discussion and use of a paper and pencil, encourage Jake to list tasks he can do to contribute to his family's household.

Rationale:
Jake will be more likely to complete these tasks if he identifies their importance.

Outcome:
Jake will plan to take on one new task of self care, such as washing his own clothing. His mother will support this by not laundering his clothing.

Intervention:
Once Jake has identified the task he is willing to do, ask him to contract with the nurse and his mother for a date by which the task will be completed. Involve his mother in this intervention so that she agrees to change her pattern of doing the task for him.

Rationale:
Jake will be more likely to attempt the task if he agrees to a date for its completion and how he will do it. It is important to involve his mother, since this supports his performing this assignment.

Outcome:
Jake will describe his feelings of apprehension when faced with the problem described above, and will describe how he will accomplish the task.

Intervention:
Encourage Jake to describe his feelings when he is attempting to identify a task that he

E CASE EXAMPLES   Continued

will do, how he will do it, when he will do it, when contracting with the nurse and his mother to perform the task, and when completing it.

Rationale:

By having Jake understand the feelings generated by his trying something new, he can later utilize this accomplishment to solve another problem.

Pathways:

Date Planned	Date Completed	
_____	_____	1. Jake will begin to list what types of tasks he does to contribute to his household within 1 week.
_____	_____	2. Jake will plan to take on one new task of self care, such as washing his own dirty clothing. His mother will support this by not laundering his clothing. Both will be done within 2 weeks.
_____	_____	3. Jake will describe his feelings of apprehension when faced with the problem described above, and will describe his next action, within 2 weeks.

▶ OBSESSIVE-COMPULSIVE PERSONALITY DISORDER

Vince, age 53, is a dentist who has a large private practice. He is known as a good, careful dentist. His personal life, however, presents some degree of conflict. Vince is married and has three children. He and his wife decided early in their marriage that she would stay home after the children were born, and take care of the child rearing. Vince is frustrated and angry with his wife, feeling that she is not setting a good example for their children. He thinks that they spend too much time playing when they should be studying or practicing the piano or ballet. He thinks their world should be more disciplined and structured. Vince is particularly upset with how his wife spends money. He gives her a $20 allowance weekly and expects her not to ask for more money. She has been using her bank card in an automatic teller machine (ATM) to obtain money to purchase gasoline for the car and groceries, and occasionally to pay for an activity with the children. Vince handles his anger with his wife by refusing to speak to her, and she becomes upset and tearful about this. He then tells her to control her emotions, "particularly in front of the children."

Critical Pathways for Level 2 Stress-Crisis

Nursing Diagnosis:

Impaired Social Interactions

Related to: Unmet dependency needs, and a knowledge deficit about ways in which to enhance mutuality in the marriage, as evidenced by an inability to establish and/or maintain a stable, supportive marital relationship, rigid expectations of others, and unsuccessful social-interaction behaviors (refusing to speak to his wife when angry with her).

Outcome:

Vince will recognize three unrealistic expectations that he has for his wife.

Intervention:

Discuss how Vince describes his marriage. How does he view his role? How does he regard his wife's role? How do his expectations compare to the current behavior of both spouses? How does he cope with the differences between his expectations and his family's actual behavior?

Rationale:

Helping Vince to identify his beliefs and expectations of his marriage versus its true interactive status may help him to understand the dynamics of his familial relationship.

Outcome:

Vince will acknowledge two instances of anger in which he became silent and withdrew, refusing to discuss the source of his anger.

Intervention:

Help Vince to identify when he is feeling angry; question him about the behavior he exhibits when he is feeling angry; and encourage him to understand that his silence and withdrawal increases the probability of his dysfunctional marital dynamic repeating itself.

Rationale:

Recognizing his typical pattern of behavior and emotion may help Vince to plan a healthier way of expressing his feelings.

Outcome:

Vince will plan one scenario of a subject that has concerned him, but which he has not addressed in a verbal, thoughtful manner with his wife.

Intervention:

Encourage Vince to discuss a scenario of a subject that has upset him but which he has not discussed with his wife. This scenario can be "acted out" by asking Vince to approach the nurse as if she were his wife and having the nurse respond in kind. Discuss what Vince expects his wife to say in order to anticipate her reaction, and how he can reply with a constructive comment to keep the discussion on course.

Rationale:

If a problematic subject is discussed in a "rehearsed" manner, Vince may be able to utilize the resulting information to promote a constructive conversation with his wife.

Pathways:

Date Planned	Date Completed	
_____	_____	1. Vince will recognize three expectations that he has for his wife that are not realistic within 1 week.
_____	_____	2. Vince will acknowledge two instances of anger in which he became silent and withdrew, refusing to discuss the source of his anger and will do this within 2 weeks.
_____	_____	3. Vince will plan one scenario of a subject that has concerned him but which he has not addressed in a verbal, thoughtful manner with his wife, and will do this within 2 weeks.

Inpatient psychiatric nurses utilize the therapeutic ward milieu to assist the patient in effecting the changes necessary to facilitate discharge. The inpatient milieu consists of patient groups that explore universal issues, such as socialization, intense feelings such as anger, (Anderson-Malico, 1994), and psychoeducation about psychiatric illness and medications.

■ EVALUATION

Evaluation is an important part of the treatment process, as it asks the clinician to compare the patient's current symptoms with what was described in the outcome statements. If the outcome statements reflect the patient's current status, the plan of care was successful. If that is not the case, however, further exploration is necessary. Often, nurses set outcome goals at a level that patients cannot achieve. Patients with personality disorders have enduring patterns of maladaptive behavior. This is an important consideration when setting outcome criteria as well as during the evaluation of the patient's clinical course. An important consideration is whether the patient felt that he or she was consulted and involved in the plan of care. A care plan often fails when the patient views the care as having been imposed rather than incorporating the patient as an active participant. If the patient's behavior continues to demonstrate target symptoms, each step of the nursing process should be reassessed in conjunction with the patient.

■ NURSING CARE CONSIDERATIONS

Patients with personality disorders have difficulties in identifying themselves as well as in understanding the concept of personal boundaries. In working with this population, it is particularly important that the nurse understand the concept of professional boundaries and use them therapeutically. These boundaries blur when the nurse helps patients beyond their needs and desires, controls patients by asserting authoritarian rules and structures that are not part of the therapeutic milieu, or focuses on the patients' negative symptoms to the exclusion of their strengths. (Pilette, Berck, and Achber, 1995)

When working with patients who have problems with impulsivity, it is important to think about limit setting. This concept is often taken to mean the strict communication of a set of rules with which the patient must comply in order to remain in the treatment milieu. Morrison (1994, 1995) suggests that nurses begin to explore when they are communicating in a coercive inter-actional manner. This type of interaction increases patients' impulsive and possibly aggressive behavior. Limit setting can be accomplished by discussing behavior that is inappropriate for the milieu and contracting with the patient to prevent this conduct. An example of this intervention was presented earlier in the chapter in the case example of Larry, the patient with an antisocial personality disorder, where it was used to assist him in controlling his aggressive impulses.

Patients with borderline personality disorder are a very challenging group. This diagnostic category is extensively covered in the literature, owing to the complexity of the symptoms manifested by individual patients and the reactions of the professionals who provide their care. It is the personal responsibility of nurses to know when they are becoming overly emotionally invested in a patient. This can take the form of anger, withdrawal from interaction with the patient, or protecting or defending the patient within the care setting and in contacts between care providers. Clinical supervision is helpful when the patient is complex and generates strong internal feelings in the nurse. Such supervision involves a structured meeting with either an expert practitioner or a peer group to discuss the patient's presentation and care plan, as well as to utilize theoretical information in order to formulate a new treatment approach. In this setting, nurses benefit from the opportunity to openly and honestly discuss their feelings about patients, and the patient profits from the new treatment approach.

O AN OVERVIEW

- Patients with personality disorders have inflexible, maladaptive personality traits.

- These patients have difficulty in establishing relationships that incorporate trust and problem-solving efforts.

- The symptoms of patients with personality disorders involve patterns of thoughts, emotionality, and behavior that differ from the norm, and that are demonstrated consistently in most of these persons' personal and social situations.

- In planning outcome statements and interventions, expectations of the patient must be realistic.

- Patients with personality disorders must take an active part in their own treatment if it is to be successful.

- Nurses must monitor their reactions to patients with personality disorders, and seek clinical supervision if they begin to see a patient in a negative or excessively positive light.

TD TERMS TO DEFINE

CLUSTER A

- paranoid personality disorder
- schizoid personality disorder
- schizotypal personality disorder

CLUSTER B

- antisocial personality disorder
- borderline personality disorder
- histrionic personality disorder
- narcissistic personality disorder

CLUSTER C

- avoidant personality disorder
- dependent personality disorder
- obsessive-compulsive personality

Q STUDY QUESTIONS

1. Amy is a psychiatric patient who has been admitted to a medical unit with pneumonia. She is screaming, swearing, and refusing to allow the nursing staff to start an intravenous unless her boyfriend is consulted. Her mother has accompanied Amy to the hospital and tells the nurse that Amy is "lost" without her boyfriend and often becomes upset to the point of suicidal ideation if they are apart for even a short period. A psychiatric liaison nurse informs the nurse on the medical unit that Amy has a borderline personality disorder. When considering care for Amy's pneumonia, what principles of psychiatric nursing must be considered?

    a. Amy is on a medical unit for pneumonia, and her psychiatric disorder has no relevance for the unit's nurse or other care team members.

    b. The psychiatric liaison nurse can attend to Amy's emotional needs while the medical nurse treats her physical needs.

    c. Understanding Amy's emotional needs, resulting from her personality disorder, helps the nurse to attend to her physical needs.

    d. Amy should be transferred to a psychiatric unit to prevent a suicidal gesture because of her inability to cope without her boyfriend.

2. Malher and associates observed infants and their mothers in order to determine how emotional attachments between the infant and the parent assist personality development. Which of the following best describes their findings?

    a. The infant and mother have a symbiotic relationship until age 5, when the child begins formal education.

    b. The infant and mother have a tension between giving and withholding during the anal phase of development.

    c. The infant develops a separate identity that is unique to him or her during the first 3 years of life.

    d. The infant learns to deal with his or her sexual identity on the basis of the mother's sense of self.

3. Which individual described below has a personality disorder?

    a. Dana is often described as a loner, rarely shows emotion, has ideas that are different from those of others, and has no relationship with his family of origin.

    b. Jamie is consistent, dependable, loyal, but is easily upset and emotionally sensitive, often expressing this in art, poetry, and music.

    c. Diane describes her marriage as one that is based on trust and understanding; however, she is concerned that her husband will grow tired of her as she becomes older and less attractive.

    d. Edward is often thoughtful and easily engages in conversation, but describes himself as shy and retiring although he has several friends and interests.

4. An individual with a borderline personality disorder has which of the following characteristics?

    a. Ability to have relationships with others, including a close family system; is able to identify problem areas but often has a fear of abandonment and failure.

    b. Has relationships with others that are stormy, with frequent arguments and concerns of abandonment; problems are avoided, denied, or reacted to with impulsive behavior.

    c. Avoids relationships and prefers to be alone and involved in solitary activities; problems are either denied or are approached with a sense of failure.

    d. Has exploitative relationships with others; often has a criminal record; problems are avoided or blamed on others.

5. It is important to include questions in the initial patient assessment that may help the nurse to determine whether a patient has a personality disorder. Which kinds of questions should be included?

   a. Those that identify the patient's perception of self; the quality of the patient's interpersonal relationships; and the patient's behavioral patterns, views, and expressions of emotions.

   b. Those that identify the patient's view of the world around him or her, the patient's reaction to these outside stimulations, and the patient's relationship with his or her family system.

   c. Those that identify the patient's ability to solve problems, his or her use of alcohol and/or drugs, and any suicidal ideation or impulsive behavior directed toward others.

   d. Those that identify the patient's role in his or her family system and in other personal interactions, whether the patient participates in family events, and whether the patient is close to either parent.

6. Rita has been a neighbor of one of the nurses on the inpatient unit for 7 years. Last night Rita slashed her wrists in a suicide attempt and was admitted to the in-patient unit for stabilization. When the charge nurse made the assignments for the shift, she assigned the care of Rita to her neighbor. What steps should the nurse take?

   a. Accept the assignment and provide care for Rita that is directed toward reducing her suicidal ideation.

   b. Accept the assignment and delegate Rita's care to the psychiatric techician.

   c. Renegotiate the assignment by disclosing to the charge nurse that Rita is a neighbor.

   d. Renegotiate the assignment by making a point in rounds that assignments never are fair.

7. Sally is a 29-year-old patient who has been admitted to the psychiatric unit for a drug overdose after her boyfriend told her he no longer wanted to continue their relationship. This suicidal gesture was due to which theoretical construct?

   a. Projection
   b. Failure in achieving object constancy
   c. Emptiness
   d. Problems with identification of self

8. Often, patients do not meet the outcome criteria that were formulated while writing a nursing-care plan. Describe two reasons why this may occur and what action the nurse would take to assist the patient.

9. Under what circumstances is limit setting appropriate? What is the best way to convey the limit-setting statement?

10. Describe the role clinical supervision has in the treatment of individuals with personality disorders.

■ REFERENCES

Akhtar S: *Broken Structures: Severe Personality Disorders and Their Treatments*, Northvale, NJ, Jason Aronson, 1992.

Akhtar S: *Quest for Answers: A Primer of Understanding and Treating Severe Personality Disorders*, Northvale, NJ, Jason Aronson, 1995.

Anderson-Malico R: Anger management using cognitive group therapy. *Perspect Psychiatr Care* 1994; 30:17–20.

Diagnostic and Statistical Manual of Mental Disorders, Fourth Edition, Washington, DC, American Psychiatric Association, 1994.

Brown GL, Ebert MHM, Goyer PF, et al.: Aggression, suicide and serotonin relationships to CSF amine metabolites, *Am J Psychiatry* 1982; 139:741–745.

Brown GL, Linnoila MI: CSF serotonin metabolite (5-HIAA) studies in depression, impulsivity, and violence, *J Clin Psychiatry* 51 1990; (Suppl.):31–43.

Burgess AW, Roberts AR: Levels of stress and crisis precipitants: The stress-crisis continuum, *Crisis Intervention*, 1995; 2:31–47.

Carpenito LJ: *Nursing Diagnosis: Application to Clinical Practice*. Philadelphia, JB Lippincott, 1992.

Cauwels, JM: *Imbroglio: Rising to the Challenges of Borderline Personality Disorder*, New York, WW Norton, 1992.

Davis J, Janicak PG, Ayd, FJ: Psychopharmacotherapy of the personality-disordered patient. *Psychiatr Ann* 1995; 25:614–619.

Erikson EH: *Childhood and Society*, New York, WW Norton, 1950.

Fortinash KM, Holoday-Worret PA: *Psychiatric Nursing Care Plans*. St. Louis, MO, Mosby-Year Book, 1991.

Freud S: Three essays on the Theory of Sexuality. *Standard Edition*. 7:125–243, London, Hogarth Press, (1905b).

Freud S: The Development of the Libido and the Sexual Organizations. *Standard Edition* 16:320–338, London, Hogarth Press, (1917a).

Freud S: The Ego and the Id. *Standard Edition*. 19:3–66, London, Hogarth Press, (1923).

Freud S: The Dissolution of the Oedipus Complex. *Standard Edition* 19:72–79 London, Hogarth Press, (1924).

Harris D, Morrison EF: Managing violence without coercion. *Arch Psychiatr Nurs* 1995; 9:203–210.

Kavoussi RJ, Siever LJ: Biologic validators of personality disorders, in Oldham JM (ed): *Personality Disorders: New Perspectives on Diagnostic Validity*. Washington, DC, American Psychiatric Press, 1991.

Kernberg OB: *Severe Personality Disorders: Psychotherapeutic Strategies.* New Haven, CT, Yale University Press, 1984.

Kreisman, JJ, Straus H: *I Hate You—Don't Leave Me: Understanding the Borderline Personality.* Los Angeles, The Body Press, 1989.

Mahler MS: Thoughts about development and individuation. *Psychoanal Study Child* 1963; 18:307–324.

Mahler MS: A study of the separation-individuation process and its possible application to borderline phenomena in the psychoanalytic situation. *Psychoanal Study Child* 1971; 26:403–424.

Mahler MS: On the first three subphases of the separation-individuation process. *Int J Psychoanal* 1972a; 53:333–338.

Mahler MS: Rapprochement subphase of the separation-individuation process. *Psychoanal Q* 1972b; 41:487–506.

Manfield P: *Split Self Split Object: Understanding and Treating Borderline, Narcissistic, and Schizoid Disorders.* Northvale, NJ, Jason Aronson, 1992.

Mann JJ, Stanley M, McBride, PA, et al. Increased serotonin-2 and beta-adrenergic receptor binding in the frontal cortices of suicide victims. *Arch Gen Psychiatry* 1986; 43:954–959.

Morrison EF: The evolution of a concept: Aggression and violence in psychiatric settings. *Arch Psychiatr Nurs* 1994; 8:245–253.

Lencz, Raine, and Scerbo, et al. Impaired eye tracking in undergraduate students with schizotypal personality disorder. *Am J Psychiatry* 1993; 150:152–153.

Marin D, De Meo M, Frances A, Kocsis J, Mann J: Biological models and treatments for personality disorders. *Psychiatr Ann* 1989; 19:143–146.

Masterson JF: *Psychotherapy of the Borderline Adult: A Developmental Approach.* New York, Brunner/Mazel, 1976.

Pilette PC, Berck CB, Achber LC: Boundary management. *J Psychosoc Nurs Mental Health Serv* 1995; 33:40–47.

Siever LJ: Biologic markers in schizotypal personality disorder. *Schizophr Bull* 1985; 11:564–575.

Siever LJ: Schizophrenia spectrum personality disorders, in Tasman A, Riba MB (eds): *American Psychiatric Press Review of Psychiatry,* vol 11, Washington, DC, American Psychiatric Press, 1992.

Siever LJ, Davis KL: A psychobiological perspective on the personality disorders. *Am J Psychiatry* 1991; 148:1647–1658.

Stanley M, Stanley B: Postmortem evidence for serotonin's role in suicide. *J Clin Psychiatry* 1990; 51 (Suppl.):22–27.

Townsend MC: *Nursing Diagnoses in Psychiatric Nursing: A Pocket Guide for Care Plan Construction,* ed. 3. Philadelphia, FA Davis, 1994.

Tyson P, Tyson R: *Psychoanalytic Theories of Development and Integration.* New Haven, CT, Yale University Press, 1990.

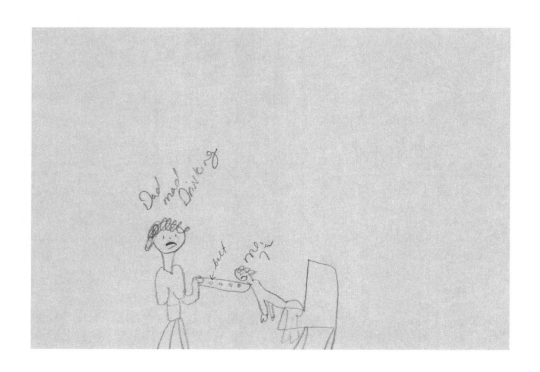

Tap. Tap. Smash. The pain. I'm not here. I'll go away. Can't leave. The pain. My teeth. My teeth. Choking. Can't breathe. Gurgle. Can't scream. My teeth—stuck in my throat. I'll die. Good! I'll die. Far away. I'll go far away. Tape is ripping. My head—rip! Choke! Gag! Spit the blood and teeth out. My teeth are gone! Oh! My teeth! Tongue feels cut, sharp edges. Electric pain. Is my face gone? Is my whole face smashed in? I can't feel my face. Maybe no face. I can see. Do I have a nose? Emily come back. Take this face and run away. We'll hide in our room forever. Too ugly to be seen. Maybe we can die now. The pain. Oh! It hurts!

Marcia Cameron, *Broken Child*, 1995

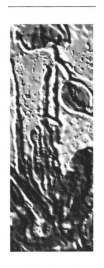

27

Child Maltreatment

Susan J. Kelley / Elizabeth B. Dowdell

Child maltreatment is one of the most serious mental-health problems in the United States, yet its comprehensive identification and treatment are relatively recent developments. In 1962 Dr. C. Henry Kempe and colleagues (Kempe et al., 1962) introduced the concept of the battered child syndrome. It was not until 1967, however, that all states had passed child-abuse reporting laws.

The true scope of child maltreatment is difficult to ascertain, since definitions of child maltreatment and investigative procedures for revealing it vary among states. In addition, reported cases of child maltreatment represent only the tip of the iceberg, because many maltreated children remain unidentified.

Nurses need to be aware that child abuse occurs on a frequent basis. In 1994, an estimated 3,140,000 children were reported to child-protective services (CPS) in the United States as alleged victims of maltreatment (Wiese and Daro, 1995). This reflects a 63% increase in reports from 1985, the first year in which the National Committee for the Prevention of Child Abuse (NCPCA) began its annual, 50-state survey. Factors to which this dramatic increase are attributed include increased reporting due to public awareness of the problem, *and an actual increase in maltreatment as a result of poor economic conditions and fewer resources for parents (Wiese and Daro, 1995).*

In 1994, the following prevalences of maltreatment were reported by type: neglect, 45%; physical abuse, 26%; sexual abuse, 11%; emotional abuse, 3%; and other, 16% (Wiese and Daro, 1995). While fathers and mothers' partners are frequently the perpetrators, the majority of child maltreatment is committed by mothers. The most likely explanation for this is that mothers spend more time with children than any other care-givers; in addition, many children are raised by single mothers. Abuse involving day-care centers and foster homes accounts for only 1% of all cases of child maltreatment (Wiese and Daro, 1995).

Following an overview of the definition, etiology, and impact of child maltreatment, the chapter treats this subject in two main sections. The first considers physical abuse, psychological abuse, and neglect, together with approaches to nursing assessment of the abused child. The second section discusses child sexual abuse and its assessment. The chapter concludes with an examination of the nursing interventions appropriate to these different types of child maltreatment.

■ DEFINITIONS OF CHILD MALTREATMENT

Child maltreatment is generally divided into four major categories: (1) **physical abuse;** (2) **sexual abuse;** (3) **psychological abuse;** and (4) **neglect.** Each state's reporting law provides definitions of physical abuse, sexual abuse, and neglect, with these definitions varying slightly from one state to another (Myers, 1992). The following are generally accepted definitions:

- Physical abuse—physical injury intentionally inflicted on a child by a parent or caretaker through the use of excessive and inappropriate physical force.
- Sexual abuse—any sexual contact between a child and an adult (or considerably older child),

whether by physical force, persuasion, or coercion. Sexual abuse can also include acts such as exhibitionism, sexually explicit language, showing children sexually explicit materials, and voyeurism, which do not involve physical contact.
- Psychological abuse—parental behaviors that are degrading, terrorizing, isolating, or rejecting.
- Neglect—failure to meet a child's basic needs, including its needs for food, shelter, clothing, health care, education, and safety. Unlike physical abuse, neglect typically involves acts of omission rather than commission.

Although the behaviors that characterize these forms of maltreatment are distinct from each other, it is important to note that the types of abuse often occur together. Thus, a child may experience several types of maltreatment simultaneously.

ETIOLOGY OF CHILD ABUSE AND NEGLECT

A number of theoretical frameworks have been used to explain the complex phenomenon of child maltreatment. Psychological or psychopathologic conceptualizations focus on care-giver characteristics, while sociological perspectives are based on factors such as poverty and low educational attainment. More recent theoretical models of child maltreatment are multi-factorial and take into account parental, child, and ecological variables. An example of a complex multi-factorial model of child maltreatment is the developmental-ecological perspective (Belsky, 1993). It conceptualizes child maltreatment as a social and psychological phenomenon determined by multiple forces acting within the individual, family, community, and culture. According to Belsky (1993), the balance of stressors and supports—that is, the balance of potentiating (risk) and compensatory (protective) factors, determines whether maltreatment takes place. When stressors outweigh supports, or when potentiating factors are not balanced by compensatory ones, the probability of child maltreatment increases. Thus, there is no single cause of child abuse and no single solution to the problem.

Another example of a comprehensive approach to child maltreatment is the stress-and-coping model (Figure 27–1) proposed by Hillson and Kuiper (1994). This model documents the various ways in which stress levels may become increased in care-givers and thus contribute to child maltreatment. In this model, the care-giver's cognitive appraisals and coping strategies are believed to play an important role in the occurrence of child maltreatment.

The four major components of the stress-and-coping model are:

- Potential stressors (parental, child, and ecological)
- Cognitive appraisals (primary and secondary)
- Coping resources
- Care-giver behaviors (facilitative behavior, neglect, and abuse)

These components are linked by multiple pathways, reflecting the interactive and dynamic nature of the various elements of the stress-and-coping process (Hillson and Kuiper, 1994). The model acknowledges the multi-determinate nature of maltreatment, beginning with the need for continuous monitoring of parental, child, and ecological factors as potential stressors. Whether these factors are stressful is determined by primary cog-nitive appraisals. If these primary appraisals indicate the presence of a stressor, secondary appraisals are used to determine what internal and external resources are available to the care-giver to cope with it.

The type of coping behavior that is sought from the care-giver depends on the outcome of the primary and secondary appraisals, with the coping response determined in part by the care-giver's coping dispositions or tendencies. Care-givers' coping strategies may be facilitative and not result in maltreatment, or may be less facilitative and result in child neglect. Coping responses such as focusing on and venting emotions may be quite maladaptive and result in child abuse (Hillson and Kuiper, 1994).

CHARACTERISTICS OF MALTREATING PARENTS

A combination of individual, familial, and societal factors contributes to the likelihood that a care-giver will abuse a child. Stress factors such as economic difficulty, crowded or inadequate housing, and unemployment can enhance a parent's potential for abuse. Parental factors that contribute to the potential for abuse include unrealistic expectations of children, lack of preparation for the parenting role, lack of empathy, and poor parental role models. Psychological factors may include poor impulse control, substance abuse, and depression. Neglectful parents are often socially isolated, lack adequate social support, and experience loneliness and low self-esteem. Children whose mothers are physically abused by their husbands or live-in partners are themselves at increased risk of physical abuse (O'Keefe, 1995).

Physical abuse may consist of excessive corporal punishment. Parents who over-discipline their children cross the fine line between what some would consider acceptable forms of physical discipline and what the law would consider a reportable case of abuse. The abuse may take place while parents are attempting to "teach the child a lesson" in order to change what they perceive as unacceptable or bad behavior. Unrealistic and distorted expectations of children can lead to abuse through a care-giver's lack of knowledge of normal, age-appropriate child behaviors. For example, some abusive parents believe that young infants cry for attention because they are "spoiled."

Another major factor that contributes to the potential for abuse is the type of parenting that a care-giver received as a child, since most people internalize this experience to some degree. Many abusive parents were themselves physically abused as children and relate to their children as their parents related to them, with rejecting and mistreating behaviors. However, it is important to note that a history of mistreatment in childhood does not necessarily lead to parents who are

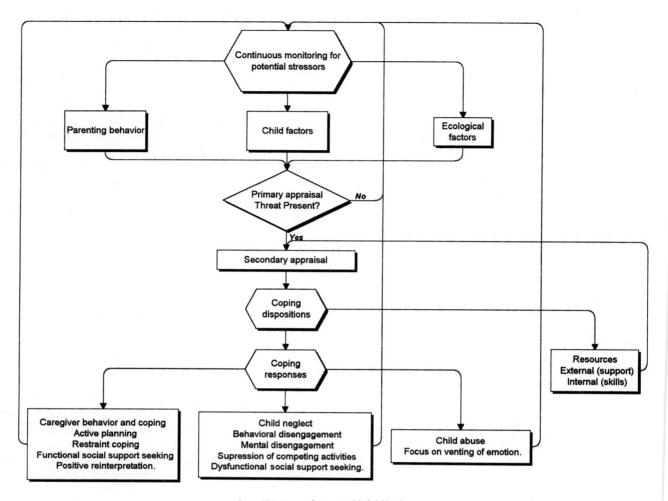

Figure 27-1: Stress-and-Coping Model of Child Maltreatment

abusive or neglectful of their own children. It is estimated that only 30% of abused children become abusive parents (Kaufman and Zigler, 1989). Subsequent involvement in emotionally supportive relationships decreases the likelihood that a maltreated child will become a maltreating parent.

Parental risk factors for physical abuse as identified by Milner (1995) are:

- Non-biological parent present in home
- Single parent
- Lower level of parental education
- Social isolation
- Negative social support
- Child-health problems
- Parent-health problems
- Parental anxiety, depression, anger, or distress
- Substance abuse
- Reliance on corporal punishment for discipline

- Negative parent–child interactions
- Parental childhood history of abuse
- Lack of economic resources
- Inadequate living conditions
- Spousal/partner abuse

Clearly, each abusive parent does not have all of these characteristics, nor is it necessary to possess any of these characteristics to physically abuse a child. Which combination of characteristics puts parents at greatest risk for mistreating children remains unknown.

Substance-Abusing Families

Research findings indicate that substance-abusing caregivers are clearly at increased risk for maltreating their children (Chaffin, Kelleher, and Hollenberg, 1996; Jaudes, Ekwo, and Voorhis, 1995; Kelley et al., 1991; Kelley, 1992). Characteristics of substance-abusing women that interfere with their parenting abilities include depression (Boyd, 1993; Coles and Platzman, 1993), increased parenting stress (Kelley, 1992), inadequate social support (Coles and Platzman, 1993), and low educational attainment (Kelley, 1992). A national survey indicated that substance abuse is a factor in approximately 35% of all cases of substantiated reports of child maltreatment (Wiese and Daro, 1995). Substance-abusing families are less likely than non-substance-abusing families to comply with interventions aimed at protecting their children. Because substance abuse, including alcohol abuse, is a common problem in our society, all parents should be screened for a history of substance abuse.

CHILD RISK FACTORS

Several factors that are believed to put children at increased risk for maltreatment are:

- Premature birth
- Congenital defect
- Product of a multiple birth
- Developmental disability
- Physical disability
- Chronic illness

It is important to note that many children who are maltreated who do not have any of these characteristics, and that many children who have one or more of these characteristics are not maltreated. Moreover, although these factors may put a child at increased risk for abuse, they do not cause a parent be abusive. Rather, the factors listed above may cause increased stress in the family system.

■ IMPACT OF CHILD MALTREATMENT

Research has clearly established that child maltreatment has serious immediate and long-term consequences. Maltreatment negatively affects the cognitive, emotional, social, and in some instances physical development of children, and often has long-term implications.

Numerous studies have documented the relationship between various types of child maltreatment and psychological harm in childhood (Claussen and Crittenden, 1991; Famularo et al, 1990; Kelley, 1992). Child maltreatment is also associated with lower intelligence, developmental delays, and poor academic performance (Allisandir, 1991; Eckenrode, Laird, and Doris, 1993; Kendall-Tackett and Eckenrode, 1996; Sawyer and Dubowitz, 1994). Cognitive and language deficits

are also noted. Childhood physical abuse has consistently been linked to aggressive and antisocial behaviors in the victim (Prino and Peyrot, 1994; Kelley, 1992; Kolko, 1996). Physically abused children also tend to have poorer self-esteem, which could be the result of the abuse *per se* or of broad aspects of personal and family dysfunction (Kolko, 1996). Neglect in childhood is associated with withdrawn and submissive behaviors (Prino and Peyrot, 1994). Children seek increased attachment to a care-giver when they perceive external danger, such as occurs during child maltreatment. This is true even when the threat emanates from the attachment object (e.g., the care-giver). Van der Kolk (1994) describes the behavioral problems of children at risk for and vulnerable to child maltreatment as:

- Temperamental abnormalities (e.g., fearfulness, shyness, and clingingness)
- Fear of new situations, vacillation between anxious and socially withdrawn behavior and hyper-aggressiveness and insensitivity to other children's needs
- Chronic anger and anxiety (e.g., in children exposed to excessive threats of separation and abandonment by their parents)

Long-term effects of child maltreatment abuse include depression (Carlin et al., 1994); reduced intelligence and reading performance (Perez and Widom, 1994); and psychopathology, sexual difficulties, decreased self-esteem, and interpersonal problems (Mullen et al., 1996). In cases of severe abuse, the sequelae often include symptoms of post-traumatic stress disorder (PTSD) and dissociation (Briere, 1996). Problematic school performance (e.g., low grades, poor standardized test scores, and frequent retention in school) is a fairly consistent finding in studies of physically abused and neglected children. Physically harmed children may also be less attentive to social cues, more inclined to attribute hostile intent to others, and less able to manage personal problems.

■ NEGLECT, PSYCHOLOGICAL ABUSE, AND PHYSICAL ABUSE

NEGLECT

Although it receives considerably less attention than other forms of maltreatment in both the professional literature and public media, neglect is the most prevalent form of child maltreatment. Child neglect involves acts of omission, or failure to meet the basic needs of a child for nutrition, health and safety. Neglect often involves inadequate financial resources, lower parental educational attainment, lack of parenting skills, and poor parental problem-solving skills. Physical neglect tends to be chronic, whereas physical abuse is typically episodic. In addition to physical neglect, a child may be subjected to emotional or educational neglect.

Neglect is often not obvious, and many cases go undetected for long periods. Because neglect is sometimes difficult to distinguish from poverty, its recognition often involves skilled clinical judgment. Therefore, when neglect is suspected, it is important to consider what the family should be doing, as opposed to what it is economically capable of doing.

Physical indicators of neglect in children include malnourishment, poor hygiene, and inappropriate dress, such as light clothing in the winter, or very soiled clothing. Bald patches on the scalp of an infant may be the result of its lying in a crib in one position for extended periods. The child may have evidence of inadequate medical care, including unattended medical and dental problems, and lack immunizations. Neglected children may have a history of numerous accidental injuries due to inadequate supervision. With educational neglect there may be a history of truancy and school avoidance, which may lead to an adolescent's failing to complete high school. Because failure to complete high school is practically a guarantee of life-long poverty, educational neglect must be addressed aggressively.

Behavioral indicators of neglect include developmental delays, particularly in the area of language development. Malnourished children generally do poorly in school because they have a low energy level and an inability to concentrate. Neglected children also often fall asleep during class because they have inadequate sleep at night. Neglected infants and toddlers may appear dull, inactive, and excessively passive.

Failure-to-Thrive Syndrome

Failure to thrive (FTT) **syndrome** is a clinical diagnostic term used to describe a lack of growth according to expected norms for age and sex (Frank and Drotar, 1994). The term non-organic failure to thrive was formerly used to describe poor weight gain without apparent physical cause, and was therefore believed to be related to environmental or psychosocial factors. The concept of organic failure to thrive was used to refer to a failure to grow adequately as the result of an identified medical condition. According to Frank and Drotar, however, this distinction is overly simplistic and obsolete, since the proximate cause of growth failure is malnutrition.

Failure to thrive typically occurs in the first 2 years of life. The criteria for the diagnosis of failure to thrive are usually based on an infant's or child's weight being below the fifth percentile for its age on an anthropometric chart.

Infants and young children who show failure to thrive and who are below the fifth percentile for weight and height should be referred to their primary-care providers or to a specialist for evaluation. Some infants who show failure to thrive are admitted to the hospital for a comprehensive evaluation, especially if they are younger than 6 months of age. Infants who have received an inadequate caloric intake at home often gain weight while hospitalized.

Frank and Drotar (1994) note several parental and child characteristics that are risk factors for failure to thrive. Parental characteristics associated with this condition include a history of a difficult childhood, including abuse, emotional rejection, and a significant loss. Child risk factors include problems of physical health that increase parental stress, and lack of a good response to the parents. Poverty is considered the greatest single risk factor for failure to thrive.

PSYCHOLOGICAL ABUSE

Psychological abuse of children involves behaviors that are emotionally harmful to them. Although physical abuse, neglect, and sexual abuse are inherently accompanied by psychological harm, psychological maltreatment can occur independently of these other forms of abuse. Psychological maltreatment can be just as damaging, and in some instances more so, than other forms of maltreatment. Like neglect, psychological maltreatment is often a chronic impediment to normal development. Of all the forms of child maltreatment, psychological abuse has received the least attention in research and clinical practice, possibly because it is difficult to define and is not as readily observable as other kinds of maltreatment.

Many studies have documented that maltreated children have negative thoughts. Chronic perceptions of helplessness and danger are believed to come from maltreatment occurring when children are unable to resist or defend themselves from the abuser. A child's assumption that there is no recourse from such treatment leads to hopelessness about the future. The expectation of such injurious treatment may also lead to hyperactivity or overreaction to real threats.

Other effects of psychological maltreatment may include:

- Failure to thrive syndrome
- Developmental delays
- Speech disorders
- Poor appetite
- Enuresis
- Encopresis
- Sleep disorders
- Low self-esteem

E CASE EXAMPLE

▶ CHILD NEGLECT

Robbie is an 8-year-old boy who arrives at the emergency room of a community hospital in the company of a social service worker for a complaint of abdominal pain. Upon examination, Robbie is found to be in the 10th percentile for weight and 50th percentile for height on a pediatric growth chart. He has gum disease with dental caries, poor finger- and toenail growth, pale skin, poor skin turgor, and an overall gaunt appearance. Additionally, the nursing staff observes that he has social-interactional and developmental delays. Robbie is admitted for 3 days to a general medical floor for re-hydration and a nutritional consultation.

A social history reveals that Robbie is the oldest of three children, all of whom lived with both of their parents until the latter's divorce, which occurred when Robbie was 4 years old. At that time Robbie remained with his mother, while his father gained custody of the younger two siblings. When the divorce became final, the mother became very reclusive. She withdrew Robbie from pre-school and kept him at home. When the mother would go to her part-time job, the store, or an appointment, she would lock Robbie in the walk-in closet of the main bedroom with toys and books. He was often in the closet for hours; an old coffee can was left as his toilet. During the 4 years that Robbie lived with his mother, he received no medical or dental care and no education (other than what the mother taught him), and had no contact with his father or younger siblings. He was allowed contact with no one except his mother. If someone came to the door, Robbie was placed into the bedroom closet. His mother was never physically or sexually abusive toward Robbie; her greatest fear was that if she let the "outside" world see him, then he too would be taken away from her. She wanted Robbie to be 100% dependent upon her. As he grew older and bigger, one way in which she would control him was with food. Because of his lack of medical care (no immunizations, etc.), his mother felt that Robbie needed to be on a strict health diet, which

included no meat; limited fluids (one glass of milk a day and no fruit juices); rationed fruits, breads, and carbohydrates; and no sweets.

In the emergency room, Robbie is quiet. He often appears anxious when new people enter the room. He speaks in simple sentences with a pronounced stutter; he knows his ABC's but is unable to read or count past 20. However, he can dress himself without assistance and has appropriate hygiene habits for an 8-year-old child. He is fearful of questions involving his mother and his removal from her home. He is suspicious of social workers, law enforcement officials, and physicians.

On the basis of all these observations, the following nursing diagnosis is made:

- Altered growth and development of child as evidenced by regressed physical and emotional growth.
- Altered parenting as evidenced by the mother's reclusive behavior and social isolation of her child.
- Fluid-volume deficit as evidenced by poor skin turgor.
- Anxiety (child).

After his hospital stay, Robbie is placed in foster care until a custody hearing can take place. During this time he is evaluated to determine the type and extent of the services he will need to treat his delays. The court rules in favor of the father, and Robbie is then moved out of state to his father's home.

The primary concern with regard to nursing intervention is Robbie's fluid/dehydration status. Fluids are encouraged immediately, and teaching is initiated about how many glasses of water, milk, and other liquids Robbie should have per day. A primary nurse is assigned to care for Robbie so as to establish a therapeutic alliance with him and decrease the number of strangers with whom he will have to interact. A calm, gentle approach is used to begin to decrease his anxiety. Multidisciplinary communication is initiated through team meetings with the social service department as plans are made for Robbie's foster care placement.

- Developmental delays
- Speech disorders
- Aggressive behavior
- Depression
- Suicidal behavior

Psychological abuse may be classified into five types (Hart and Brassard, 1993).

Spurning is a type of maltreatment, primarily verbal, that combines rejection and hostile degradation. The parent or caretaker may refuse to help the child or even to acknowledge the child's request for help. Spurning includes: (1) belittling, denigrating, or other non-physical forms of overtly hostile or rejecting treatment; (2) shaming and/or ridiculing a child for showing normal emotion, such as affection, grief, or sorrow;

(3) consistently singling out a particular child to criticize and punish, perform most of the household chores, or receive fewer rewards from among several siblings; and (4) public humiliation of a child.

Terrorizing involves threatening to physically hurt, kill, or abandon a child for misbehavior. It also means exposing a child to violence or threats directed toward a child's loved ones, and leaving a young child alone. Terrorizing includes: (1) placing a child in unpredictable, chaotic circumstances; (2) placing a child in recognizably dangerous situations; (3) setting rigid or unrealistic expectations with the threat of loss, harm, or danger if they are not met; (4) exploiting a child's fears and vulnerabilities by threatening to isolate or spurn the child, become emotionally unavailable to it, or exploit and corrupt it; (5) threatening or perpetrating violence against the child; or (6) threatening or perpetrating violence against a child's loved one or personal objects.

Isolating includes confining a child or setting unreasonable limits on the child's freedom or movement within his or her environment, the child's social interactions within the home, and social interactions with peers or adults in the community. It also includes isolating a child from nondangerous sources of information or ideas.

Exploiting and corrupting involve modeling antisocial acts and unrealistic roles for a child, or encouraging and condoning deviant standards or beliefs. Exploiting and corrupting include permitting or encouraging antisocial behavior (such as prostitution, pornographic media performances, or substance abuse) or inappropriate behavior (such as parentification, or infantalization of the child or having it live the parent's unfulfilled dreams).

Denying emotional responsiveness is to ignore a child's attempts to interact with a care-giver, or to interact with a child in a mechanical manner devoid of affectionate touch or conversation. Through acts of omission, parents or caretakers who deny emotional unresponsiveness communicate that they are not interested in the child and are emotionally unavailable. This form of maltreatment includes: (1) failing to be sensitive to the child's health and social-emotional development; (2) being detached from and uninvolved with the child, either through incapacity or a lack of motivation; (3) interacting only when absolutely necessary; and (4) failing to express affection, caring, and love for the child.

PHYSICAL ABUSE

Factitious Disorder by Proxy

Factitious disorder by proxy (FDBP), also known as Munchausen syndrome by proxy (MSBP), is a rather rare form of child abuse in which a parent falsifies an illness in a child by fabricating or creating symptoms and then seeks medical care for the child. Named after Baron Von Munchausen, an 18th-century story teller, the term Munchausen syndrome was first applied to adults who fabricated illnesses with false medical histories and altered laboratory and physical findings. Only later was the term Munchausen syndrome by proxy applied to children with a fabricated medical problem. The factitious disorder by proxy is now used to describe this phenomenon.

Victims of FDBP usually range in age from infancy to six years, although school-aged children may be abused in this manner. Older children may aid in the parents' deceptions in order to protect themselves or to avoid retribution. False histories given by parents in cases of FDBP often include seizures, apnea, cardiopulmonary arrest, hematuria, and hematemesis. Parents may induce physical findings in their children by suffocation, administration of drugs or toxic substances, or placing their own blood in the child's urine, vomitus, or stool specimens. Drugs often used in cases of FDBP include laxatives, to induce severe diarrhea; insulin, to induce hypoglycemia and seizures; ipecac, to induce vomiting; and drugs or alcohol, to alter a child's level of consciousness. Salt may be added to an infant's formula to induce hypernatremia. Clinical indicators of factitious disorder by proxy include:

- Recurrent illnesses for which no cause is identified.
- Unusual symptoms that do not make clinical sense.
- Symptoms that are observed only by the parent.
- Frequent visits to various hospitals, resulting in normal findings.
- The finding of drugs that induce specific symptoms in a toxic screen.
- Discrepancies between the child's history and physical findings.
- Numerous hospitalizations at many different hospitals.

In the vast majority of identified cases of FDBP, mothers are the perpetrators. Frequently, the mother herself is found to have Munchausen syndrome, with physical complaints similar to those she fabricates for her child. In some instances the mother has had training in one of the health-care professions, and is therefore adept at making falsified information appear credible. The mother often appears genuinely concerned about her child's illness, and when the child is hospitalized, rarely leaves the child's bedside.

Rosenberg (1987) reviewed 117 cases of factitious disorder by proxy and found that the most common presentations were bleeding, seizures, central nervous system depression, apnea, diarrhea, vomiting, fever, and a rash. In these cases the mortality was 9%, the long-term morbidity rate was 8%, and the short-term morbidity rate was 100%. Failure to thrive was associated with FDBP in 14% of the children. In all cases the perpetrators were the victims' mothers.

Alexander et al. (1990) have reported cases in which multiple children in a family have been victimized by induced or false illness, a condition referred to as serial Munchausen syndrome by proxy. These cases were found to be associated with a high mortality (31%) and a high incidence of maternal psychiatric illness.

Child Maltreatment Fatalities

One of the most tragic clinical situations encountered by nurses is the death of a child from abuse or neglect. The true number of fatalities from child abuse is difficult to determine with certainty. According to the National Committee on the Prevention of Child Abuse, an estimated 1,271 children died of abuse or neglect in 1994 (Wiese and Daro, 1995). This represents a 48% increase from 1985 to 1994. The 1994 figures indicate that more than three children died each day from abuse or neglect.

Homicide is the second leading cause of death among children. While almost two-thirds of deaths due to injury occur among 15 to 19 year olds, 23% occur among children younger than five years of age (Centers for Disease Control, 1990). The high rate of homicide among children under five years of age is primarily due to caretaker abuse and neglect (Christoffel, 1990). About half of all maltreatment fatalities among children from birth to four years of age result from inflicted blows, and approximately 10% of children in this age group are killed by firearms (Centers for Disease Control, 1990).

Children are at greatest risk of being killed during the first month of life; the rate of child homicide decreases as the child's age increases (Crittenden and Craig, 1990). The most likely explanations for the inverse relationship between age and the risk of fatal child abuse are the greater biologic vulnerability of infants to assault because of immaturity of their brains and other organs, the limited mobility of younger children, and the annoying nature of some child behaviors (Christoffel, 1992). Victims of child homicide from abuse are generally the youngest or next to youngest children in a family (Christoffel, 1992). After the first year of life, boys are at greater risk than girls for fatal child maltreatment; among children younger than one year, the incidences of fatal maltreatment may be similar for the two sexes (Christoffel, 1992). Most fatal child abuse among infants is committed by mothers (Crittenden and Craig, 1990), and mothers who begin child-bearing at an early age are considered to be at increased risk for fatally maltreating their children.

Most children who die as a result of abuse or neglect have experienced maltreatment before the fatal incident; in the vast majority of cases the fatal incident is not the first occurrence of abuse, but is rather the culmination of a series of abusive incidents. Between 1992 and 1994, 45% of the children who died of maltreatment had current or prior contact with child protective service agencies (Wiese and Dara, 1995). These findings highlight the importance of detecting maltreatment at an early point and reporting maltreating families to the proper authorities before fatal incidents of maltreatment occur.

Most states have interagency, multidisciplinary review teams at the local or state level for systematically evaluating and managing cases of suspicious child fatalities. These child death review teams typically comprise representatives of the medical examiner's office, law enforcement agencies, and child protective service agencies, as well as prosecutors, pediatricians, and nurses with child-abuse expertise. Among the advantages of such review teams are improved communication and cooperation among agencies, increased knowledge of risk factors for child homicide, systematic evaluation of agency actions and inactions, and the identification of surviving siblings at risk for maltreatment.

Assessment of Physical Abuse

Nurses need to be knowledgeable about possible indicators of child abuse and neglect, especially those that are manifested before a child suffers serious injury, emotional impairment, or developmental delay. Early recognition and intervention are the keys to preventing subsequent abuse and negative sequelae.

History It is essential to elicit a careful, detailed history of all injuries from both an injured child and its caregivers and to compare the given explanation with the observed injury. Abusive parents may give an implausible explanation for an injury, or a vague account of the events surrounding it, or they may deny any knowledge of how the injury occurred. If a discrepancy exists between the reason given for an injury and the physical findings, abuse should be suspected. Whenever possible, the child and each caretaker who is present should be interviewed separately, since discrepancies may exist between the caretakers' and the child's accounts. Also, when interviewed alone, the child is more likely to accurately report the cause of an abusive injury and the identity of the abuser. Evoking as many details as possible helps to reveal any inconsistencies between the child's and the caretakers' accounts. The child's past medical history, including any previous injuries, should be carefully elicited. When available, the child's medical record should be reviewed for previous suspicious injuries. Information indicated in histories that should alert nurses to the possibility of child abuse (Kelley 1994) is summarized below.

- A history inconsistent with an existing injury.
- Denial of any knowledge of the cause or mechanism of an injury.
- Reluctance of the caretaker to give information about an injury.

- A caretaker who blames a child for its own injury.
- A child who is developmentally incapable of having incurred a specified self injury.
- Delay in seeking medical attention for a child injury.
- Inconsistencies in the history of an injury.
- A history of repeated child injuries or hospitalizations.
- A response inappropriate for the severity of an injury.
- Previous placement of a child in foster care.
- Previous involvement with a child protective services agency.

A delay in seeking medical attention for an injury to a child should raise the suspicion of abuse; some abusive parents and other caretakers ignore the seriousness of an injury in the hope that it will heal without medical attention, thereby avoiding detection and legal action. Another important factor to consider is the distance over which the caretaker has traveled to seek care for an injured child. If the caretaker has traveled an unusual distance for medical attention, bypassing care facilities closer to home, the caretaker may be trying to avoid detection by staff members who have suspected him or her of abuse on previous occasions. Abusive parents often seek medical care at many different treatment facilities in order to avoid being identified.

Knowledge of normal child growth and development is essential when assessing for possible abuse. One must consider whether it is developmentally possible for a child to have injured him- or herself in a particular manner. For example, if the mother of a 1-month-old infant with a skull fracture states that the baby rolled over in its crib and fell out and onto the floor, abuse should be suspected, because infants are not capable of rolling over until 3 to 5 months of age. Likewise, fractures of the limbs are unusual in infants who have not yet learned to walk.

Physical Examination A complete physical assessment should be done on all children for whom abuse or neglect is suspected. It is important to be aware that many cases of abusive injury in children are identified while a child is being treated for a condition other than the injury. Thus, for example, inflicted rib fractures may be found during a chest X-ray done to rule out pneumonia in an infant who presents with an upper respiratory infection. Similarly, previously undiagnosed fractures of an extremity may be detected on X-rays made to assess a recent, unintentional injury. Table 27-1 summarizes indicators of physical abuse in children.

Cutaneous Lesions. Cutaneous lesions are the most common manifestations of physical abuse in children, and the most easily recognized signs of abuse. Cutaneous lesions caused by maltreatment include contusions, abrasions, lacerations, burns, bite marks, and hair loss. The most important aspects of such lesions are their location, configuration, and age. The size, shape, location, distribution, and color of all injuries should be carefully documented.

Bruises change color with time as blood is reabsorbed from the skin. It is therefore important to compare the reported date of an injury with the color or age of the reportedly associated bruises in order to detect any discrepancies. Table 27-2 provides a guide for estimating the age of bruises. Multiple bruises in various stages of healing should raise concern.

The pattern of an abusive bruise typically reflects the method or instrument used to inflict the abuse. Bruises consisting of straight lines are uncommon in uninflicted injuries, and injury from a man-made object should therefore be considered when linear contusions or contusions of unusual configuration, such as those having sharp angles, are noted. Evidence of the objects frequently used to strike children include the characteristic loop-shaped mark made by an extension cord; linear marks from a belt, strap, or stick; and imprints from a spoon, buckle, paddle, spatula, hair brush, or hand.

Linear marks, often found over curved body surfaces, generally indicate injury with a belt. In some cases, an imprint of the belt buckle is noted. If a hand is used to strike a child, characteristic parallel linear marks may be noted, representing the fingers and the spaces between them. The characteristic loop-shaped marks made by a doubled electrical extension cord or lamp cord are typically found on the back, buttocks, upper arms, and thighs. In contrast, marks from a coat hanger leave a wider loop mark, caused by the flat base of the hanger. Circular or oval marks on the upper arm may be the result of forcible grasping of a child and the application of pressure to the site. Cords or rope used to bind ankles and wrists leave thin, circumferential bruises; thicker marks may indicate tying of the child with sheets.

Infants and young children may be gagged or have clothes or objects stuffed in their mouths to stop them from crying. Gag marks leave down-turned lesions at the corners of the mouth. Other types of oral trauma include burns caused by excessively hot food or fluids placed in the child's mouth, and injuries to the labial frenulum and lingual frenulum caused by forcing a bottle or spoon into the mouth. Missing or loosened teeth and oral lacerations may be signs of direct blunt trauma to the face.

TABLE 27–1. INDICATORS OF PHYSICAL ABUSE

Cutaneous injuries
 Bruises
  In various states of healing
  Bilateral, linear, or geometric injuries
  In configuration of object
  Pinch marks, pair of crescent bruises
  Located on face, neck, thighs, genitals, back, inner upper arms, thorax
  Grip marks on upper arms
 Human bite marks
  Oval shape pattern of teeth marks
 Traction alopecia
  Irregular areas of hair loss
  Broken hair
  Subgaleal hematoma
 Abrasions, lacerations
  Circumferential abrasions or friction burns from ropes at neck, wrist, ankles, torso
  Chain imprints
  Linear puncture marks from fork
Burns
 Immersion burns
  Uniform in depth, sharp lines of demarcation
  Bilateral burns of feet, hands, and buttocks
  Flexion creases spared because child flexes extremities
 Contact burns
  Resemble configuration of object In various stages of healing
  Circular crater the diameter of a cigarette
  Commonly located on face and dorsum of hands and feet
Head trauma and central nervous system injuries
 Bilateral skull fractures
 Multiple skull fractures
 Skull fractures with widths greater than 5 mm
 Subdural hematomas

Separation of sutures due to chronic subdural hematoma
Subgaleal hematoma
Decreased level of consciousness
Grip marks on upper arms
Spinal cord injury
Ophthalmic injuries
 Hyphema
 Retinal detachment
 Dislocated lens
 Retinal hemorrhage
 Subconjunctival bleeding
 Periorbital ecchymosis
Neck trauma
 Subluxation or dislocation
Skeletal injuries
 Multiple fractures, especially bilateral
 Fractures of various ages
 Spiral fractures of humerus (forcible twisting)
 Transverse fractures (blunt trauma)
 Rib fractures, especially if multiple, bilateral, or posterior
 Fractures of the sternum, spinous processes, scapula
 Fractures of femur in children younger than 3 years
 Fractures of the epiphyseal–metaphyseal junction
 Digital fractures
Blunt abdominal trauma
 Abdominal distention, tenderness, bruising
 Absent bowel sounds
 Peritoneal or mesenteric bleeding
 Persistent vomiting or abdominal pain
 Bilious vomiting
 Hypovolemic shock
 Injury to liver, spleen, pancreas, duodenum, jejunum, kidneys
 Signs of peritonitis

Adapted from Kelley SJ (ed): *Pediatric Emergency Nursing*, ed. 2. Norwalk, CT, Appleton & Lange, 1994.

TABLE 27–2. GENERAL GUIDE TO ESTIMATION OF AGE OF BRUISES

Color	Age of Bruise
Red-blue	1–2 days
Blue-purple	2–4 days
Greenish yellow	5–7 days
Yellow-brown	7–14 days
Normal skin color	14–21 days

Reproduced with permission from Kelley SJ (ed): *Pediatric Emergency Nursing*, ed. 2. Norwalk, CT, Appleton & Lange, 1994.

Examination for cutaneous lesions may reveal bite marks or evidence of hair pulling. Human bite marks may resemble a double horseshoe or have an irregular doughnut shape, and can be measured in order to determine whether they were inflicted by an adult or a child. Adult bite marks have a 3-cm or greater distance between the canine teeth. Unlike dog bites, human bites typically do not leave puncture marks.

Areas of baldness on the scalp may result from a child's being pulled by the hair, a condition referred to as traction or traumatic alopecia. Such cases are marked by irregular areas of hair loss. Hair pulling may also cause bleeding under the scalp.

Burns. Inflicted burns are seen in approximately 10% of substantiated cases of child abuse, and are the third leading cause of death from child abuse. From 10% to 25% of burns of children are deliberately inflicted by adults. Two-thirds of these cases involve children under 3 years of age.

Children who repeatedly suffer burns should be carefully evaluated for abuse. Suspicion should be raised when treatment of a child's burns is delayed for more than 24 hours. Intentionally inflicted burns may involve hot liquids or objects, and often leave identifiable patterns on the skin. Although burn injuries result from a wide variety of causes, most inflicted burns are caused by hot water.

Intentional scalding is often the result of a child's being immersed in hot water. The resulting injury is typically uniform, and has sharp lines of demarcation. Inflicted immersion burns are typically symmetric, whereas accidental burns are usually asymmetric. These burns are often bilateral, involving both feet, hands, and buttocks, and often appear sock-like on the feet, glove-like on the hands, and doughnut-like on the buttocks or genitalia. Flexion creases are usually spared because the child flexes his or her extremities in the hot water. Immersion burns of the hands can be caused by the exploratory behavior of a child, though tap-water scald burns are often inflicted; an immersion burn of the buttocks and lower extremities of an infant is more likely to have been deliberately caused by the caretaker. Accidental hot water burns are usually not as clearly demarcated on their edges as inflicted immersion burns. Moreover, inflicted burns tend to be full thickness burns, whereas unintentional burns are often of partial thickness.

Patterned burns result from contact with cigarettes and other hot objects. Accidental cigarette burns typically occur on or around the face of a child who walks into a lighted cigarette being held by an adult at waist height. Cigarette burns found on the soles of the feet, palms of the hands, buttocks, or back are often inflicted. Inflicted cigarette burns are typically 8 to 10 mm in diameter and are indurated at their margins. Accidental cigarette burns are usually shallower, more irregular, and less circumscribed than deliberately inflicted burns.

Contact burns in the configuration of a heated object are often inflicted on children. Objects often involved in intentional contact burns include steam irons, electric stove burners, hot plates, forks, knives, curling irons, automobile cigarette lighters, conventional cigarette lighters, radiators, hair dryers, and candles. Caretakers have been known to place toddlers in the process of being toilet trained on radiators to dry their wet diapers, resulting in burns to the buttocks.

Fractures. Abuse-related bone injuries are more common in children younger than 4 years of age than among older children, whereas accidental fractures occur more commonly among school-age children. Fractures and dislocations that are inconsistent with the mechanism of injury are highly suspect as indicators of abuse. Because caretakers often delay in seeking medical treatment in cases of inflicted injury, manifestations typically seen in the acute phase of skeletal injury, such as swelling and tenderness, may not be present in children with abuse-related bone injuries.

Transverse fractures of bones may result from inflicted, blunt trauma, whereas spiral fractures of long bones may result from the intentional twisting of an extremity. Spiral fractures of the humerus are particularly suspicious for such abuse. Fractures of the femur in infants and toddlers, and fractures of the skull, nose, or facial structures, are often also the result of abuse. Rib fractures, common in abused children, are frequently multiple and bilateral, often reflecting a squeezing of the chest. Multiple fractures in various stages of healing may indicate repeated abuse.

On the other hand, the possibility that multiple fractures in a child are related to an underlying disease, such as osteogenesis imperfecta, scurvy, syphilis, rickets, neoplasia, or osteomyelitis, should be considered. These rare disorders can be ruled out by appropriate diagnostic procedures.

Head Injuries. Inflicted head injuries are the leading cause of death from child abuse. Such injuries may result from direct trauma, vigorous shaking, or a combination of the two. Most deaths from head trauma among children younger than two years are the result of maltreatment.

Subdural hematomas in children also often come from abuse, such as direct trauma to the head from a blow or being thrown, dropped, or severely shaken. Accidental falls usually result in single linear fractures of the skull, whereas non-accidental trauma is more likely to cause multiple or complex fractures and depressed fractures.

The term **shaken baby syndrome** is used to describe an intracranial injury in an infant who may have no external evidence of head trauma. These injuries are the result of rapid acceleration and deceleration from vigorous shaking, which may or may not include blunt trauma to the head. The findings may include retinal hemorrhages, subdural or subarachnoid hemorrhages, cerebral edema, grip marks on the chest and upper arms, and rib fractures. The major precursor to the occurrence of shaken baby syndrome is persistent infant crying, which triggers abusive behavior in a care-

E CASE EXAMPLE

▶ PHYSICAL ABUSE/SHAKEN BABY SYNDROME

Shanna, a 6-month-old baby girl, arrives at the Emergency Department of an urban Children's Hospital via paramedic helicopter in respiratory distress. Her father states that the morning began in its usual way and that he dressed Shanna, and gave her a bottle in her car seat while he got ready for work. He says that when he finished doing this, he found Shanna asleep, removed the bottle, and dressed her 3-year-old sister. The father reports that he then checked Shanna at 10:15 A.M. and found that she was not breathing, at which point he called the police at 911. When paramedics arrived, says the father, Shanna was totally unresponsive and needed assistance in breathing with an ambu bag and oxygen; peripheral intravenous infusions were started. Shanna was then transported to an emergency room. While in the emergency room, she went into full respiratory arrest requiring intubation and mechanical ventilation. Neurological signs indicate that she responds only to deep pain stimuli; her pupils deviate to the left, and are dilated and unreactive. Additionally, retinal hemorrhages are seen in an eye examination. A computed tomographic scan indicates a subdural hemorrhage. Shanna is then transported to a children's hospital, where she is admitted directly to the intensive care unit. Further X-rays and a physical examination indicate severe neurological damage. A central line is started for access and blood drawing, and Shanna is connected to a ventilator. A cerebral blood flow test, performed 5 days later, indicates that she had only brain stem function. She is weaned from the ventilator on day 7 of her hospital stay, and is breathing completely on her own by day 10, without respiratory complications. However, Shanna cannot swallow or suck, and a feeding tube is therefore inserted into her stomach. Subsequent investigation leads the police to arrest the father for shaken baby syndrome.

The nursing diagnosis includes an alteration in neurological status, potential for an alteration in respiratory status, potential for a nutritional deficit, and parental anxiety related to Shanna's status. The nursing interventions in Shanna's case are to maintain an open and clear airway, provide pulmonary care every 4 hours, maintain appropriate nutritional balance via feeding tube, remain alert to possible aspiration risks. Interaction with Shanna's mother involved helping her with psychosocial issues related to Shanna's compromised neurological status. She was offered support and encouraged to be an active participant in her daughter's care. Convenient referrals were set up to facilitate the mother's participation in care-giving.

Shanna's father received a suspended 11-month sentence with community time to be served after he plead guilty to having shaken the baby. He confessed that he had lied. He said she had been crying during the night before her injury and that he had picked her up in an effort to stop the crying. He had then shaken her and she stopped crying, after which he put her to bed until the morning, when he could not arouse her. By the time the father called 911, Shanna had been bleeding intracranially for a minimum of 16 hours.

---

giver who has lost control of his or her emotions and behaviors.

Ocular Injuries.
Inflicted eye injuries may leave no external evidence of trauma. A funduscopic examination is therefore essential in suspected cases of such Eye injuries that can result from physical abuse include periorbital hematomas, fractures of the orbital or facial bones, subconjunctival hemorrhage, dislocation of the lens, retinal detachment, retinal hemorrhage, hyphema, corneal abrasion, and optic atrophy.

Ear Injuries.
The external ear may show evidence of contusions. Ecchymoses on the internal surface of the pinna may be the result of boxing the ear and crushing it against the skull. A direct blow to the ear may also cause hemotympanum and perforation of the tympanic membrane. Discoloration behind the ear (Battle sign) may indicate a basilar skull fracture.

Abdominal Trauma.
Abdominal injuries, although infrequent, rank second to head trauma as the leading cause of death from child abuse. Blunt abdominal trauma, the most common type of inflicted abdominal trauma in abused children, usually results from their having been punched or kicked in the abdomen. It may produce intraabdominal hemorrhage with few external signs of trauma. The blow is usually to the midabdomen.

The child may present for treatment with persistent bilious vomiting, abdominal pain, or hypovolemic shock. Internal organs that may be injured by blunt trauma include the pancreas, duodenum, jejunum, mesentery, liver, spleen, and kidneys. The high mortality resulting from these injuries may be due to exsanguinating intra-abdominal hemorrhage, delay in seeking medical attention, or failure of emergency personnel to make the correct diagnosis when lifesaving surgery is still possible. Severe internal injuries may not be immediately detected because of the parent's or other caretaker's failure to give an accurate history of the trauma, and because there may be little or no external evidence of abdominal trauma at the time of examination.

■ SEXUAL ABUSE

Sexual abuse of children encompasses a wide range of actions, including exhibitionism; fondling or manipulation of the genitals; digital penetration, orogenital contact; vaginal or rectal penile penetration; insertion of foreign objects in the genitals, penis, or rectum; and the use of children in pornography or prostitution (Kelley, 1994). Sexual abuse also includes non-contact sexual activity, such as sexually explicit language directed toward a child; obscene telephone calls; the showing of pornographic materials to a child; and voyeurism. Most sexually abused children experience multiple types of sexually abusive acts. The legal definition of sexual abuse varies by state jurisdiction. Most states define sexual abuse as any sexual contact or sexual activity between a child and an adult, whether by force or coercion.

The nature of the sexual victimization of a child is important to understand. Typically, sexual activity between an adult and a child involves a steady progression or escalation in the severity of the sexual activity. Often, the activity is initially presented to the child as a "game," "secret," or "something special." The sexual abuse may begin with the offender exposing him- or herself to the child or viewing the child naked. The activity may then involve masturbation by the offender in front of the child, followed by encouragement of the child to imitate this behavior. Very often the activity progresses to fondling, digital penetration of the vagina or rectum, and orogenital contact. The activity may also involve vaginal or rectal intercourse. In some cases the offender does not attempt vaginal intercourse but instead simulates intercourse by rubbing his penis against the genitorectal region of the child.

PERPETRATORS

Most adults who sexually abuse children are relatives, friends of the family, or other trusted adults who are well known to the child victims. According to Faller (1990), the sexual abuse of children has two prerequisites: sexual arousal of the adult in the presence of children, and the willingness to act on this arousal. Although most reported cases of child sexual abuse involve male offenders, women are perpetrators in approximately 10% of cases. Many offenders commit their first offenses during adolescence.

PREVALENCE AND RISK FACTORS

Research has indicated that sexual abuse of children occurs quite commonly in American society. In a large, nationally representative survey of 2,626 American adults, a childhood history of sexual abuse was disclosed by 27% of women and 16% of men (Finkelhor et al., 1990).

The following are considered risk factors for sexual abuse: presence of a stepfather, children who are living without one or both of their biological parents; a mother who is disabled, ill, or extensively out of the home; poor parenting; and paternal violence (Finkelhor, 1993). It is important to note that race, social class, and ethnicity have not been found to be risk factors for child sexual abuse (Finkelhor, 1993).

IMPACT OF SEXUAL ABUSE

Immediate

The immediate, or short-term, sequelae of child sexual abuse include behavioral problems (Burgess et al., 1996; Kelley, 1989; Kelley, 1992; Waterman et al., 1993); low self-esteem (Waterman et al., 1993), anxiety and depression (Kelley, 1989; Kelley, 1992; Waterman et al., 1993), fears (Kelley, 1989; Waterman et al., 1993), increased sexualized behavior (Friedrich, 1993; Friedrich et al., 1992; Kelley, 1989) and post-traumatic stress disorder (Waterman et al., 1993).

Factors associated with the impact of sexual abuse during childhood include the frequency and duration of the abuse; the use of physical force; sexual acts involving penetration; and abuse by a biological father or a stepfather (Kelley, 1995). Lack of maternal support, family conflict, and self-blaming by the child following sexual abuse exacerbate the negative sequelae of such abuse (Kelley, 1995).

Long-Term Impact

Besides having short-term effects, sexual abuse is also associated with long-term sequelae. A meta-analysis of 38 studies examining the relationship between childhood sexual abuse and psychological problems in adult women revealed a significant association between child sexual abuse and symptomatology (Neumann et al., 1996). A history of childhood sexual abuse was strongly associated with the following problems in adulthood: anxiety, anger, depression, re-victimization, self-mutilation, sexual problems, substance abuse, suicidality, impairment of self-concept, interpersonal problems, obsession and compulsion, dissociation, post-traumatic stress disorder, and somatatization (Neuman et al., 1996).

Traumagenic Dynamics Model

A comprehensive conceptual model to explain the multi-faceted effects of child sexual abuse is the Traumagenic Dynamics Model formulated by Finkelhor and Brown (1986). According to this model, child sexual abuse has a variety of effects. These depend on the characteristics of the abuse and on four major areas of children's development: sexuality, ability to trust, self-esteem, and sense of an ability to affect the world. Four distinct mechanisms account for differences in the effects of sexual abuse in childhood: **traumatic sexualization,** betrayal, stigmatization, and powerlessness.

Traumatic sexualization refers to the aspects of sexual abuse that affect a child's sexuality in inappropriate ways. Examples include fondling; oral, anal and vaginal penetration; and the insertion of objects into the child. Betrayal refers to a child's discovery that someone in whom it trusts has caused it harm. Betrayal also refers to a child's perception that one or more non-offending relatives have failed to protect it from abuse. Stigmatization refers to the negative messages about the self, such as guilt and shamefulness, that are communicated to a child by a sexually abusive experience. Repeated violations of the child's sense of control and efficacy, as well as intrusion upon its body space and coercion and threats, lead to a feeling of powerlessness.

ASSESSMENT OF CHILD SEXUAL ABUSE

History

A sexually abused child may be referred for evaluation and therapy because of a known history of sexual abuse, behavioral problems or disturbances, depression, or medical indicators of sexual abuse in the absence of its disclosure. Referrals may come from primary-care providers, law-enforcement agencies, or child protective workers, or may be initiated by a parent.

A careful, detailed history is important in cases of suspected sexual abuse. Obtaining separate histories from the child and parents is preferable to obtaining a history in the presence of all three for several reasons. First, many children are hesitant to disclose abuse in the presence of a parent or other care-giver, especially if the offender is a family member or friend of the family. Some children are threatened by a parent or caretaker to not disclose sexual abuse or identify the abuser. It is common for the responsible parties to attempt to protect the identity of the offender. Embarrassment may prevent some children from disclosing abuse in the presence of a parent. Another reason for interviewing children and parents separately is that parents need a private opportunity to express their feelings in relation to a suspected abuse, which may include

shock, disbelief, and anger, as well as any other concerns they may have.

Interviewing Parents. The information needed from parents or other caregivers in a case of suspected sexual abuse of a child includes, when appropriate, their reasons for believing that their child has been abused and who they suspect as the abuser. If the parent does not know who the abuser may be, he or she should be asked who has access to the child, such as a baby-sitter, day-care worker, teacher, relatives, or family friends. Parents may be hesitant to reveal their suspicions or to identify the offender, especially if the offender is a family member or friend. Parents should be carefully questioned about any family history of sexual victimization. It is usual for more than one child in a nuclear or extended family to be victimized by the same offender, or for a child to be abused by more than one relative. The possibility of multi-generational sexual abuse should be explored, especially if the offender is a grandparent.

Physical and behavioral indicators of child sexual abuse should be elicited in the history obtained from the parent or caretaker. Physical indicators (Kelley 1994) of child sexual abuse include:

- Trauma to the genitals or rectum.
- Chafing, abrasions, or bruising of the inner thighs.
- Scarring or tears of the hymen.
- A decreased amount of hymenal tissue.
- Vaginal or rectal bleeding.
- Vaginal, penile, or rectal lacerations.
- A vaginal or penile discharge.
- Foreign bodies in the urethra, vagina, or rectum.
- Pregnancy, especially in young adolescents.
- Complaints of vaginal or rectal pain.
- The presence of a sexually transmitted disease, including chlamydial infection, gonorrhea, syphilis, herpes genitalia, condyloma acuminata (anogenital warts), and *Trichomonas vaginalis* infection.

Pregnancy in a young adolescent (10 to 14 years of age) should raise concern, especially if the adolescent attempts to conceal the pregnancy for an extended period. The issue of paternity should be pursued in such cases to determine whether an adult or older adolescent forced or coerced the adolescent into the sexual activity that resulted in the pregnancy.

Behavioral changes are more common than physical complaints in a child subjected to sexual abuse. Therefore, a careful history should be elicited for behaviors that could be associated with sexual abuse. Sexually abused children often exhibit sexual behavior with peers, siblings, and adults. Sexual behaviors seen

E CASE EXAMPLE

A mother returns home unexpectedly to hear her 6-month old daughter screaming. She runs up the stairs and catches the 17-year-old son of her baby-sitter tucking his shirt into his pants. The infant is lying naked on the changing table, crying uncontrollably. The mother and her son provide baby-sitting services to a church nursery, and an investigation into the situation elicits a confession from the youth that he has molested all of the children in his mother's care. The number of child victims grows as the investigation continues, with the son admitting to physically pinching the children, inserting his fingers or a thermometer into the children's anus or vagina, exposing himself, and anally penetrating the children. A search of the family home reveals Vaseline, thermometers, baby aspirin, a wide range of magazines including family-oriented ones, soft- and hard-core pornographic magazines, and children's videos. Pornographic pictures are found hung on the son's bedroom wall.

Interview and examination of 11 children in this case one year later reveals symptoms of rape trauma. Interviews with the parents reveal symptoms of ineffective and compromised family coping. An outline of the nursing diagnosis and intervention in such cases follows.

Nursing Diagnosis
- Ineffective family coping: compromised.

Defining Characteristics
- The parents are unable or unwilling to provide emotional support to the child victim.
- Some parents are in denial of their child's abuse.

Nursing Interventions
- Ensure that the child is protected from subsequent sexual abuse.
- Provide support to the parents.
- Assist the parents in referring their child for play therapy.

Expected Outcomes
- The parents demonstrate supportive actions toward their child.
- The parents verbalize distress over betrayal by the babysitter.

---

more often in sexually abused children than in those not subjected to sexual abuse include placing the mouth on another child's genitals; asking others to engage in sexual acts; masturbating with objects; inserting foreign objects into the vagina or rectum; imitating intercourse; and making sexual sounds (Friedrich et al., 1992). Sexually abused children often make precocious remarks or ask questions that indicate their increased awareness of adult sexual behavior. There also may be a history of frequent and compulsive masturbation.

■ INTERVENTION

THERAPY

Although research has documented that children suffer short- and long-term consequences of maltreatment, most abused children do not receive therapy. Children who have experienced any form of maltreatment should be referred for a psychological evaluation to determine whether there is a need for therapy; those who have been severely abused may need in-patient treatment. Because child maltreatment most often occurs in the family setting, therapy for it must address not only the child's individual needs, but family dysfunction as well.

Treatment modalities frequently used with abused children include individual therapy, group therapy, family therapy, play therapy, and art therapy. A core tenet of modern approaches to therapy for abused children, adolescents, and adults is that it should be abuse-focused (Chaffin et al., 1996). **Abuse-focused therapy (AFT)** borrows from a wide variety of behavioral, cognitive, systemic, and dynamic therapeutic techniques. It is based on the concept that abuse is a form of victimization by the powerful of the relatively powerless and that the sequelae of abuse are readily understandable if not expected "normal" adaptations to abnormal experiences. Abuse-focused therapy emphasizes describing, exploring, and comprehending the individual's experience of the abuse (Chaffin et al., 1996).

LEGAL ISSUES

Careful documentation in all cases of suspected child abuse and neglect is of the utmost importance. It is not enough to write "multiple bruises in various stages of healing noted." Rather, each bruise, lesion, or burn needs to be described in detail according to its size, location, color, and shape. Color photographs of all injuries should be taken with a 35-mm camera and an instant camera whenever possible. In some jurisdictions parental permission to take a child's photograph is needed, whereas in others photographs can be taken without parental consent.

Even the most severely abused children are often physically healed by the time of a court hearing. The photographs help the judge or jury to understand the extent of the child's injuries. All significant statements made by parents and children during a nursing interview should be carefully recorded, with as many direct quotations as possible. The behavior of the child and parents should be described carefully. Medical records, including the nurse's notes, are often subpoenaed and introduced as evidence in cases of child abuse. Consequently, the nurse has an important responsibility to carefully report all facts, omitting subjective opinions.

The disposition in cases of child abuse depends on many variables, such as the severity of the presenting injury and the circumstances under which it occurred. The most important single factor to assess is whether the child is at immediate risk of further abuse if returned home. If such a risk exists, the child may be temporarily removed from the home through admission to the hospital, placement in the home of a relative, such as a grandparent or aunt, or placement in an emergency foster home. Often, temporary removal from the home allows time for the parent to receive necessary support services.

All states provide a mechanism for protecting children in emergencies (Myers, 1992). If a parent refuses to allow a child to be admitted to the hospital or placed with a relative or in foster care, an emergency care and protection order can be obtained by telephone from a judge in most jurisdictions. This gives the hospital authority to temporarily remove the child from the home, pending further investigation into the child's safety; it also allows time for arrangement of support services for the family.

REPORTING SUSPECTED CHILD ABUSE AND NEGLECT

Legislation in each of the 50 states mandates the reporting of suspected child abuse and neglect by professionals who work with children. The list of mandated reporters includes educators, physicians, nurses, mental-health professionals, social workers, and day-care providers. In most states, mandated reporters have no discretion about whether to report cases of suspected abuse or neglect (Myers, 1992).

The conditions for reporting child abuse are defined by individual state statutes: the identity of the mandated reporters, the agency to which one reports, and protection for those who report such abuse in good faith. In most states, nurses are identified as mandated reporters. It is important to be knowledgeable about child-abuse laws in the jurisdiction where one practices. The statutes of many states include penalties for those who fail to report suspected abuse and neglect. Those who report abuse or neglect in good faith are usually immune from criminal and civil liability.

It is important to understand that only a suspicion of abuse or neglect is necessary for reporting a case; actual proof or evidence is not required by law. According to Myers (1992), reporting is mandatory when a professional has evidence that would lead a competent professional to believe that abuse or neglect is reasonably likely. A professional who postpones reporting until all doubt has been eliminated probably violates the reporting law (Myers, 1992). The ultimate decision about whether abuse or neglect has occurred is the responsibility of investigating officials, not mandated reporters (Myers, 1992).

Reporting of suspected abuse should never be viewed as an accusation or punitive action, but rather as a referral for further investigation into a child's environment and well-being, as well as for the provision of social services for the child's family or other caretakers. Reporting should never be used as a threat to force parental or care-giver's cooperation, nor should parents or other caretakers ever be told that they will be given a second chance and that no report will be filed. If a report is not made immediately after suspicion of child abuse has been raised, there may be subsequent injury to the child and a delay in services for the family. Also, if a professional had reason to suspect child abuse and fails to report it, and the child is re-injured, the professional can be held liable for those injuries.

Parents and other caretakers should always be informed that a report of child abuse is being made, and should be told the purpose of the report. Parents need to know that the report is not a criminal complaint but rather a referral for services. They should also be told to expect a telephone call or home visit from a caseworker from the reference agency as a follow-up to the report. Nurses' responsibilities in cases of child abuse are listed below.

- Having knowledge of indicators of child abuse and neglect.
- Case identification.
- Obtaining a careful history and comparing it with a child's existing injury.
- Observing of interactions between the parent(s) and child.
- Collaborating with other members of the health-care team.
- Carefully documenting of all objective data.
- Reporting all suspected cases of abuse and neglect to child-protective services.
- Assessing of the immediate risk to a child if child is returned home.
- Protecting child from subsequent abuse through hospitalization or foster placement of the child.

- Referring 479the family for support services.
- Giving emotional support to the child and parents.
- Preventing of child maltreatment.

MULTIDISCIPLINARY APPROACH

A multidisciplinary approach to child maltreatment involving nurses, physicians, therapists, attorneys, and social workers is imperative. The problem of child maltreatment is complex, and thus cannot be addressed by any single discipline. Nurses concerned with the problem of child abuse should become involved in the American Professional Society on the Abuse of Children (312-554-0166). This interdisciplinary society for professionals supports research, education, and advocacy that enhance efforts to respond to abused children, those who abuse them, and the conditions associated with child abuse.

O AN OVERVIEW

- Child maltreatment is generally divided into four categories: physical abuse, sexual abuse, emotional abuse, and neglect. It is not unusual for more than one of these types of abuse to be present in a given case.

- Understanding the complex causes of child maltreatment requires a multi-factorial approach that takes individual, familial, socio-economic, and cultural variables into account. Stress and coping behavior are also thought to be important in the etiology of child maltreatment.

- Parents who maltreat their children may do so because of stress (e.g., economic difficulties, inadequate housing, unemployment), lack of parenting skills and role models, inappropriate expectations for their children, or psychological conditions such as depression, poor impulse control, low self-esteem, or substance abuse.

- Maltreatment negatively affects the cognitive, emotional, social, and in some instances physical development of children, and often has long-term implications. Lower intelligence, developmental delays, poor academic performance, aggressive and antisocial behavior, low self-esteem, depression, and in severe cases symptoms of post-traumatic stress disorder are among the sequelae of abuse.

- Child neglect, or failure to meet basic needs for food, shelter, clothing, medical care, and a safe environment, is the most prevalent form of child maltreatment, and if severe may lead to the syndrome of failure to thrive.

- The syndrome of failure to thrive may also result from psychological maltreatment, or behaviors directed toward a child that are psychologically harmful. Sleep and speech disorders, low self-esteem, aggressive behavior, depression, and even suicide are among the effects of psychological maltreatment.

- Factitious disorder by proxy, also known as Munchausen syndrome by proxy, is a rare form of child abuse in which a parent creates the appearance of an illness in a child and then seeks medical attention for it. This disorder is associated with a high rate of child mortality and a high incidence of maternal psychiatric illness.

- Assessment of physical maltreatment of a child requires a detailed history, preferably taken in separate interviews with the child and each parent or caretaker, as well as a carefully documented examination for cutaneous lesions, burns, fractures, and injuries of the head, eyes, ears, mouth, and abdomen.

- Although assessment for child sexual abuse is similar to that for physical maltreatment, it is important to note that behavioral changes are more common than physical complaints in cases of sexual abuse.

TD TERMS TO DEFINE

- abuse-focused therapy
- denying emotional responsiveness
- emotional abuse
- exploiting and corrupting
- factitious disorder by proxy
- failure to thrive syndrome
- isolating
- neglect
- physical abuse
- sexual abuse
- shaken baby syndrome
- spurning
- terrorizing
- traumatic sexualization

Q STUDY QUESTIONS

1. The hallmark clinical indicators of shaken baby syndrome are
   a. retinal hemorrhage and intracranial injury.
   b. raccoon eyes and skull fractures.
   c. nasal fractures.
   d. intracranial injury and low self-esteem.

2. Munchausen syndrome by proxy is
   a. a genetic disorder characterized by psychological impulses.
   b. a violent act against a child by a father.
   c. when a parent falsifies illness in a child.
   d. when a parent produces psychological trauma in a child.

3. The four major types of child neglect are
   a. physical, emotional, medical, and educational.
   b. physical, emotional, nutritional, and educational.
   c. physical, emotional, nutritional, and medical.
   d. physical, medical, psychosocial, and educational.

4. T F Crisis theory examines the internal and external stressors that may precipitate child abuse and neglect in a family.

5. T F No legal protections are included in the mandating report system for professionals who report child maltreatment.

6. T F A systematic approach to identifying indicators of child abuse is crucial.

7. T F The majority of sexual abuse occurs outside the child's family unit or by someone unknown to the child.

8. Two basic ways in which an offender gains sexual access to a child are
   a. pressure and sadistic situations.
   b. power and control situations.
   c. pressure and forced situations.
   d. anger and sadistic situations.

9. Child sexual abuse can be described as consisting of
   a. repeated assaults on the same child, growing more severe the longer the abuse continues.
   b. a one time assault upon the child.
   c. physical assault and damage to the child in each instance.
   d. all of the above.

10. Grounds for a nurse reporting suspected child maltreatment or neglect does not include
    a. direct evidence and/or personal feelings.
    b. parental confession and/or knowledge base.
    c. direct and/or circumstantial evidence.
    d. instincts and/or intuition.

Questions 11 thru 13 Refer to the Following Case Study:

Jamie is a 6-month-old girl brought to the hospital by her mother. In your assessment of Jamie you find multiple bruises in different stages of healing and a decreased range of motion of the left leg.

11. Following the nursing assessment of Jamie, the nurse would
    a. call the hospital's department of human services.
    b. maintain confidentiality of the physical data until all of the paper work in the case is completed by the mother.
    c. obtain a thorough patient and family history.
    d. have the mother leave the room so that Jamie may be interviewed alone.

12. Jamie has been diagnosed as having a fractured femur. During your interview with Jamie's mother about the fracture, which of the following statements by the mother would cause you to suspect abuse?
    a. "Jamie got her leg caught in the crib and twisted it."
    b. "Jamie hurt herself while crawling."
    c. "I can't remember Jamie falling or hurting herself."
    d. "Jamie fell out of her car seat because I didn't have it secured properly."

13. The most important criterion by which the nurse may suspect child abuse is
    a. appropriate parental concern for the degree of injury.
    b. absence of the parents for questioning about the child's injury.
    c. parental concern about other health problems than those associated with the possible abuse.
    d. incompatibility between the history given and the observed injury.

14. Child abuse can be defined as
    a. something that happens occasionally to a child.
    b. a willful injury of a child.
    c. a one-time intentional injury to a child.
    d. a premeditated and planned event.
    e. all of the above.

15. T   F   When the evidence strongly suggests child abuse, it is the role of the nurse to report the evidence.

16. T   F   A report to the proper authorities includes both verbal and written explanations.

17. T   F   A nurse's report of child abuse should include feelings and thoughts about the abuse.

18. T   F   All 50 states (and the District of Columbia) provide immunity to professionals who report child abuse in honesty and good faith.

■ REFERENCES

Alexander R, Smith W, Stevenson R: Serial Munchausen syndrome by proxy. *Pediatrics* 1990; 86:581–585.

Beitchman J., Zucker KJ, Hood JE, DaCosta CA, Arkman D, Cassavia E: A review of the long-term effects of child sexual abuse. *Child Abuse Neglect* 1992; 16:101–118.

Belsky J: Etiology of child maltreatment: A developmental-ecological analysis. *Psychol Bull* 1993; 114:413-434.

Briere J: A self-trauma model for treating adult survivors of severe child abuse, in Briere J, Berliner L, Bulkley JA, Jenny C, Reid T (eds): *The APSAC Handbook on Child-Maltreatment,* Newbury Park, CA, Sage, 1996; pp. 140–157.

Burgess AW, Baker T, Hartman C: Parents' perceptions of their children's recovery 5 to 10 years following day-care abuse. *Schol Inq Nurs Pract: Int J* 1996; 10

Burgess AW, Hartman CR: Children's drawings. *Child Abuse Neglect* 1993; 17:161–168.

Carlin AS, Kemper K, Ward NG, Sowell H, Gustafson B, Stevens N: The effect of differences in objective and subjective definitions of childhood physical abuse on estimates of its incidence and relationship to psychopathology. *Child Abuse Neglect* 1994; 18:393–399.

Centers for Disease Control Childhood injuries in the United States. *Am J Dis Child* 1990; 144:627–646.

Centers for Disease Control and Prevention: Sexually transmitted diseases treatment guidelines. G25 MMWR; 1993; 42 (No. RR-14):1–102.

Chaffin M, Kelleher Kelly, Hollenberg J: Onset of physical abuse and neglect: Psychiatric, substance abuse, and social risk factors from prospective community data. *Child Abuse Neglect* 1996; 20.

Christoffel KK: Violent death and injury in U.S. children and adolescents. *Am J Dis Child* 1990; 144:697–706.

Christoffel KK: Child abuse fatalities, in Ludwig S, Kornberg AE (eds): *Child Abuse: A Medical Reference.* New York: Churchill Livingstone, 1992; pp. 49–59.

Claussen AH, Crittenden PM: Physical and psychological maltreatment; Relations among types of maltreatment. *Child Abuse Neglect* 1991; 15:5–18.

Crittenden PM, Craig SE: Developmental trends in the nature of child homicide. *J Interpers Violence* 1990; 5:202–216.

Eckenrode J, Laird M, Doris J: School performance and disciplinary problems among abused and neglected children. *Dev Psychol* 1993; 29:53–63.

Faller KC: *Understanding Child Sexual Maltreatment.* Newbury Park, CA 1990; Sage, pp. 38–67.

Finkelhor D: Epidemiological factors in the clinical identification of child sexual abuse. *Child Abuse Neglect* 1993; 17:67–70.

Finkelhor D, Hotaling G, Lewis IA, Smith S: Sexual abuse in a national survey of adult men and women: Prevalence, characteristics, and risk factors. *Child Abuse Neglect* 1990; 14:19–28.

Frank DA, Drotar D: Failure to thrive, *Child Abuse: Medical Diagnosis and Management.* Malvern, PA, Lea and Febiger, 1994, pp. 298–324.

Friedrich WN: Sexual victimization and sexual behavior in children: A review of recent literature. *Child Abuse Neglect* 1993; 17:59–66.

Friedrich WN, Grambsch P, Damon L, et al: The sexual behavior inventory: Normative and clinical findings. *Psychol Assess* 1992; 4:303–311.

Hart SN, Brassard MR: *Psychological Maltreatment. Violence Update,* Newbury Park, CA, Sage, 1993.

Hillson JMC, Kuiper NA: A stress and coping model of child maltreatment. *Clin Psychol Rev* 1994; 14:261–285.

Jaudes PK, Ekwo E, Voorhis JV: Association of drug abuse and child abuse. *Child Abuse Neglect* 1995; 19:1065–1075.

Kaufman J, Ziegler E: Do abusive children become abusive parents? *Am J Orthopsychiatry* 1987; 57:186–192.

Kelley SJ: Parental stress responses to sexual and ritualistic abuse of children in day care centers. *Nurs Res* 1990; 39:25–29.

Kelley SJ: Child maltreatment, stressful life events, and behavior problems in school-aged children in residential treatment. *J Child Adolesc Psychiatr Mental Health Nurs* 1992; 5:5–13.

Kelley SJ: Child sexual abuse: Initial effects. *Ann Rev Nurs Res* 1995; 14:63–85.

Pediatric Emergency Nursing, ed 2. Norwalk, CT, Appleton and Lange, 1994.

Kelley SJ, Walsh JH, Thompson K: Prenatal exposure to cocaine: Birth outcomes, health problems, and child neglect. Pediatr Nurs 1991; 17:130–135.

Kendall-Tackett K, Eckenrode J: The effects of neglect on academic achievement and disciplinary problems: A developmental perspective. *Child Abuse Neglect* 1996; 20:

Kempe CH, Silverman FN, Steel BF et al: The battered child syndrome. *JAMA* 1962; 181:17–24.

Kolko DJ: Child physical abuse in Briere J, Berliner L, Bulkley JA, Jenny C, Reid T. (eds): The APSAC Handbook on Child Maltreatment, Newbury Park, CA, Sage, 1996, pp. 21–50.

Milner JS: Physical child abuse assessment: Perpetrator evaluation. In Campbell JC (ed): *Assessing Dangerousness: Violence by Sexual Offenders, Batterers, and Child Abusers,* Newbury Park, CA, Sage, 1995, pp. 41–67.

Mullen PE, Martin JL, Anderson JC, Momans, SE, Herbison GP: The long-term impact of the physical, emotional, and sexual abuse of children: A community study. *Child Abuse Neglect* 1996; 20:7–21.

Myers JEB: Legal issues in child abuse and neglect practice. Newbury Park, CA, Sage, 1992.

Neumann DA, Houskamp BM, Pollock VE, Briere J: The long-term sequelae of childhood sexual abuse in women: A meta-analytic review. *Child Maltreat* 1996; 1:6–16.

O'Keefe M: Predictors of child abuse in maritally violent families. *J Interpers Violence* 1995; 10:3–25.

Perez CM, Widom CS: Childhood victimization and long-term intellectual and academic outcomes. *Child Abuse Neglect* 1994; 18:617–633.

Prino CT, Peyrot M: The effect of child physical abuse and neglect on aggressive, withdrawn, and prosocial behavior. *Child Abuse Neglect* 1994; 18:871–884.

Rosenberg DA: Web of deceit: A literature review of Munchausen syndrome by proxy. *Child Abuse Neglect* 1987; 11:547–563.

Sawyer RJ, Dubowitz H: School performance of children in kinship care. *Child Abuse Neglect* 1994; 18:587–597.

Sperber ND: Bite marks, oral and facial injuries: Harbingers of severe child abuse? Pediatrician 1989; 16:207–211.

Waterman J, Kelly RJ, Oliveri MK, McCord J: *Beyond the Playground Walls: Sexual Abuse in Preschools*. New York, Guilford, 1993; pp. 79–165.

Wiese D, Daro D: Current trends in child abuse reporting and fatalities: Results of the 1994 annual fifty state survey. Chicago, National Committee to Prevent Child Abuse, 1995.

Wilkinson WS, Han DP, Rappley MD, Owings CL: Retinal hemorrhage predicts neurologic injury in the shaken baby syndrome. *Arch Ophthalmol* 1989; 107:1472–1474.

Van der Kolk BA: The behavioral and psychobiological effects of developmental trauma, in Stoudemire A (ed): *Human Behavior*. Philadelphia, JB Lippincott, 1994.

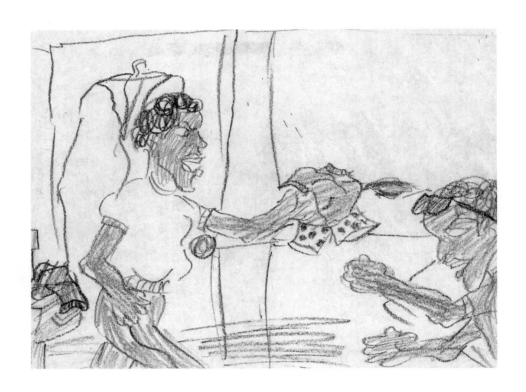

What happens to a dream
deferred?
Does it dry up
like a raisin in the sun?
Or fester like a sore—
And then run?
Does it stink like rotten meat?
Or crust and sugar over—
like a syrupy sweet?
Maybe it just sags
like a heavy load
Or does it explode?

Langston Hughes (1902–1967)

Harlem, 1951

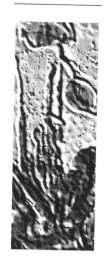

28

Violence in Families

Ann Wolbert Burgess / Albert R. Roberts

The possibility of injury or having one's home invaded by strangers is a frightening one. Yet hundreds of thousands of Americans face an even more devastating reality: they are harmed not by strangers, but by someone they have trusted. Vicious crimes of violence are committed by family members against children, parents or grandparents, spouses, and other close relatives.

The family is still viewed as the center of society. To be abused by a spouse, parent, trusted adult, or one's own child, or to witness such abuse, leaves deeply ingrained memories and has other serious consequences, such as substance abuse. Victims of domestic violence must wrestle with myriad emotions not experienced by persons victimized by strangers, including simultaneous feelings of fear, loyalty, love, self-blame, guilt and shame. They become torn between the desire to shield and help a loved one and their fear for their own safety and the stability of their household. Children are harmed by those who should protect them. For most people, home represents security; to victims of domestic violence, it is a place of danger.

This chapter presents definitions of and current statistical trends in family violence from a developmental perspective. It covers courtship abuse, threats and violence by spouses and partners, domestic homicide, child abuse, neglect, and sexual assault, and elder abuse. It also discusses key concepts of family violence, such as socialization into violence and learned socialized violence; the psychodynamics of violent behavior including altered attachment, jealousy, guilt, and revenge; and the biology of trauma.

The problem of family violence is as old as humankind itself. Women have been battered by their male partners in almost every society in history. In some countries, killing one's wife is not even a crime. In 1885, the Chicago Protective Agency for Women, established to help women who were victims of physical abuse, provided legal aid, court advocacy, and personal assistance to such women. The agency could provide an abused woman with up to four weeks of shelter at a refuge operated by the Women's Club of Chicago. It also helped women to secure legal separations, divorces, and equitable property distributions. Over five years, 25 cities followed Chicago's lead in developing protective agencies for women. By the 1940s few shelters remained, partly because of marital separations caused by World War II.

Similarly, the history of childhood, from biblical times to the present, is replete with suffering. In 1874, the Wilson case opened America's eyes to the plight of many children: Eight-year-old Mary Ellen Wilson lived with her adoptive parents in New York City. They held her in their home in chains, starving and beating her. The police responded but could do nothing because it was a "family matter," and parents held the "rights" (Zigler and Hall, 1989). A man named Henry Berg was contacted. He was able to extricate Mary Ellen from her family torture chamber. Who was Henry Berg, and why was he called? Henry Berg had founded a protective group the preceding year: The Society for the Protection of Cruelty to Animals.

■ EPIDEMIOLOGY OF FAMILY VIOLENCE

Just as the term *family* has no universal definition, neither does violence. The definition of violence published in the report entitled Understanding and Preventing Violence (Reiss and Roth, 1993) may be useful, however. It states that interpersonal violence is "behavior by persons against persons that intentionally threatens, attempts, or actually inflicts physical harm."

Nowhere in the criminal law and its administration is the social construction of violent crime changing more rapidly than in what constitutes family violence and society's response to it (Reiss and Roth, 1993). Because of the myriad state and local laws and regulations, there is no national legal definition of a family in the United States. Data on family violence are therefore classified by current marital status (married, separated, divorced, or single), spousal status (spouse/ex-spouse), or by relationships among members of a household (co-habitants, child/parent, sibling, parent). On the basis of these categories, statistics can be generated on changes in family structure over time. For example, the Bureau of Census (1990, 1991) has reported that the proportion of all households consisting of two-parent families declined from 40% in 1970 to 26% in 1990. The number of unmarried-couple households almost tripled between 1970 and 1980, and grew by 80% between 1980 and 1990, from 1.6 to 2.9 million. The proportion of children under 18 years of age living with two parents declined from 85% in 1970 to 73% in 1990, with an estimated 15 percent of these children being stepchildren. And in 1990, 19% of white, 62% of black, and 30% of Hispanic children under age 18 lived with only one parent.

Trends in family violence, according to Reiss and Roth (1993), must be interpreted against a decline in the percentage of households consisting only of married couples and their biologic children. Violence between growing numbers of same-sex and opposite-sex cohabiting partners is increasingly being regarded as family violence regardless of the partners' legal marital status. Violence between divorced or separated ex-couples is also listed as family violence.

The National Research Council's Panel on Understanding and Preventing Violence (Reiss and Roth, 1993) considered all violent behavior within a household as family violence; this behavior consisted specifically of spouse assault, physical and sexual assault of children, sibling assaults, and physical and sexual assaults of other relatives who resided in the household. Psychological trauma, or indirect harm, includes such events as verbal abuse and threats, harassment or humiliation, and stalking.

DYNAMIC NATURE OF FAMILY VIOLENCE

Several characteristics distinguish family violence from violence by strangers (Reiss and Roth, 1993 pp. 222–223). Although there is a continuing relationship among the members of a family, just as in many other relationships (e.g., teacher-student; employer-employee; child-caretaker, etc.), daily interaction and a shared domicile increase the opportunities for violent encounters within families. Because the members of a family are bound together in a continuing relationship, it is quite likely the offender will repeat violations. An unequal power relationship between partners or parents and children makes one more vulnerable to aggression and violence by the offender. Moreover, the offender often threatens further violence if the incidents of violence are disclosed. The victim may refrain from disclosure through fear of stigmatization and denigration. Finally, episodes of family violence often occur in private places, are invisible to others, and are less likely to be detected or reported to police than are episodes of violence by strangers.

■ DEVELOPMENTAL ASPECTS OF FAMILY AND ITS STRUCTURE

The family may be viewed as progressing through three developmental phases, just as a child matures through developmental stages to adulthood. The first phase begins with dating, courtship, and marriage; the middle phase includes partnership and work, with childbearing and parenting being an option; the third phase continues a work focus, optional grandparenting, and retirement. Types of family violence are discussed within these three developmental phases.

PHASE I: ASSAULTS ON PARTNER

The first phase of family life includes dating, courtship and marriage. Although dating does not necessarily lead to courtship or marriage, it is instructive to review data on early problems in relationships and aggression during dating (Riggs, 1993). Theories of both marital aggression (Gelles and Straus, 1979) and aggression during dating (Riggs and O'Leary, 1989) identify conflict as an important factor in such aggression. Violence during dating appears to begin as early as age 15 or 16 (Durst, 1987); Henton et al., 1983). This typically includes slapping and pushing, beating, and threatening with or using weapons. Recurring and escalating episodes of violence in a relationship are quite common if the relationship is not terminated. About 50% of the victims do terminate the relationship (Cate et al., 1982; Henton et al., 1983; Laner, 1983; Roscoe and Benaske, 1985).

Research indicates that a large number of college students experience physical aggression in dating relationships. Estimates of the prevalence of dating aggression among college students range from 20% (Cate *et al.,* 1982; Makepeace, 1981) to as high as 50% (Sigelman, Berry, and Wiles, 1984).

Research also provides a better understanding of relationship problems that lead to violence during dating. In Riggs' study (1993), although aggressors reported more problems in general than did non-aggressive individuals, the difference appeared to result from specific problem areas including jealousy; interference by persons outside the relationship, such as friends and parents; and more fighting and conflict within the couple. Riggs (1993) states that if one conceptualizes jealousy as a reaction to the threat of loss, such a threat may also result in anger that could lead to aggression. Other issues often related to jealousy, such as possessiveness and control, may also lead to aggression.

Violence can continue within marriage. According to Stark and Flintcraft (1991:139), spousal assault is the single most common cause of injury for which women seek emergency medical attention. In a study of emergency treatment of women in a metropolitan hospital, Stark and Flintcraft report that battered women were 13 times more likely than other women receiving emergency care to be injured in the breast, chest, and/or abdomen, and three times as likely to be injured while pregnant (Stark and Flintcraft, 1991:140 and 1982).

In 1988, the National Crime Survey (NCS) (Bureau of Justice Statistics, 1990) began to report annual estimates of the extent of family violence for persons age 12 and older. The NCS, however, lacks the information necessary to determine the full extent of family violence. For example, the 1990 survey's data-collection process excludes violence among co-inhabitants and information about violence against children under age 12. Despite these limitations, the survey's victimization statistics are still useful. These show, for example, that 59% of assaults within families were by a spouse (41%) or ex-spouse (18%), while 29% were by other relatives. Seven percent were by parents and 5% by children (Bureau of Justice Statistics, 1990). The Conflict Tactics Scale developed by Straus (1979) is the measure of domestic violence used most often in surveys. This scale includes verbal and aggressive acts, among which are violent acts ranging in severity from hurling objects to the use of a deadly weapon such as a gun or knife. Using the Conflict Tactics Scale in an initial national telephone survey of couples in 1975, Straus, Gelles, and Steinmetz *(1980)* found that 16 of every 100 couples reported at least one incident of physical aggression during the year before the survey, and the prevalence of severe violence to a victim in both surveys was 4 per 100 among females and 5 per 100 among males. These statistics are believed to be low because the sample excludes unmarried couples and misses segments of the population that do not have telephones (Reiss and Roth, 1993).

What factors place a woman at risk for being physically abused? Asking why a particular woman is targeted by violence is the wrong question according to the National Research Council Panel on Research on Violence Against Women (Crowell and Burgess, 1996). They suggest asking why men use violence and what conditions support and maintain current levels of victimization of women. This conclusion is in response to the dismal record of success in identifying women's risk factors for violence. One interpretation is that of the confounding that occurs when traits and behaviors are assessed at some point post-victimization and assumed to represent the previctimization state. For example, factors that have been at one time or another linked to women's likelihood of being raped or battered are passivity, hostility, low self-esteem, alcohol and drug use, violence in the family of origin, having more education or a greater income than one's partner, and violence toward children. On the other hand, Hotaling and Sugarman (1986), in a review of 52 studies that included comparison groups, found that the only risk marker consistently associated with victimization by physical abuse was having witnessed parental violence as a child. This marker characterized both victimized women and their male assailants.

PHASE II: ASSAULTS ON CHILDREN

Within the phase of partnerships and work, family members can assault children. Various commissioned government studies have investigated assaults on children. The U.S. Advisory Board on Child Abuse and Neglect, a government advisory board created by the 1988 amendments to the Child Abuse and Prevention and Treatment Act, estimated that in 1989 at least 1,200 and perhaps as many as 5,000 children died from maltreatment, and that more than 160,000 children were seriously harmed (U.S. Department of Health and Human Services, 1990, p. 15). The advisory board noted that in 1974 there were about 60,000 cases of reported child maltreatment. This figure rose to 1.1 million in 1980, and more than doubled to 2.4 million in 1988 (U.S. Department of Health and Human Services, 1988:X). These increases may, however, be partly due to the use of more inclusive definitions of abuse and neglect, and to an increase in the professional recognition of maltreatment, rather than to an increase in its incidence *per se* (U.S. Department of Health and Human Services, 1988:xxv). It is also likely that cases of child maltreatment are reported to public health or educational agencies that do not in turn report to the social services agencies that provide case figures. Moreover, many cases of intrafamilial or third-party assaults on children are never reported to any professionals involved in the health or welfare of children (Reiss and Roth, 1993, p. 228).

Family violence can escalate to homicide. Assessments of the risks of intrafamilial homicide are considered more accurate than of those for other forms of assault (Reiss and Roth, 1993, p. 234). Several patterns are noteworthy: newborns, infants, and children aged 1 to 4 years are more likely to be victims of familial homicide than are children aged 5 to 9 years (Federal Bureau of Investigation, 1990, p. 11); infants and small children are more likely to be killed by their mothers than by their fathers, perhaps partly as a result of differential risk exposure. Also, according to a case control study, the risk of homicide for children under age 5 is greater for male than for female children, (Winpisinger *et al.,* 1991, pp. 1053–1054). Although the overall risk of homicide for men is three times that for women, women face a greater risk of homicide by their spouses than do men (Federal Bureau of Investigation, 1990, p. 8); intrafamilial violence was responsible for 15% of all family homicides in 1989; 44% involved husbands and wives.

PHASE 3: ASSAULTS AGAINST THE ELDERLY

Within the phase of grandparenting and retirement, family members can assault the elderly.

The National Research Council (1993) recommends that priority be given to the collection of more precise information about the prevalence and incidence of violence toward the elderly, and its consequences. Surprisingly little is known about the occurrence of violence toward the elderly in families, for several reasons. First, most studies do not distinguish between elder abuse and elder neglect. Second, families are unlikely to report such abuse, since the perpetrator may be a son or daughter. Moreover, many elderly people are homebound, with no one to see what is happening to them.

In a stratified random-sample study of all persons 65 years of age and older in the Boston metropolitan area, Pillemer and Finklehor (1988) estimated that from 2.5 to 3.9 persons within this age group had experienced physical violence, verbal aggression, or neglect. A national survey of elder abuse in Canada found similar results (Podnieks and Pillemer, 1989).

■ EXPLANATIONS OF FAMILY VIOLENCE

Most theories about the causes of family violence are only partial explanations. They either attempt to explain a single type of family violence, or a few types, such as partner assault, or seek to identify a particular factor or set of factors that account for some of the observed differences in behavior leading to violent as opposed to nonviolent acts (NRC, 1993). The leading explanations for family violence are derived from social, cultural, and biopsychosocial analyses.

THE SOCIAL AND CULTURAL PERSPECTIVE

Gelles (1983) developed an integrated theory of cultural and structural determinants and social learning factors to explain family violence. He points out, for example, that feminist theory asserts that the unequal distribution of power between men and women subjects women to male dominance in all spheres of life (work, family, and community life). This inequality of power extends to the sexual relationship, as well as to work and social relationships (Russell, 1982). The various ways in which men use coercion in families depends on their pattern of use of physical and social power to maintain a dominant family position (Finklehor, 1983).

The unequal distribution of power is also the basis for parental physical and sexual abuse of children. Parental power renders the child helpless in the face of demands by the parent (Finklehor and Browne, 1986:183).

Within this framework of a patriarchal society that emphasizes male dominance and aggression and female victimization, children are socialized into their respective sex roles (Dobash and Dobash, 1979). They also learn these roles through family experience or through the media. This learning becomes reinforced in the larger community, where male and female roles similarly rest on elements of male cultural domination.

Recent changes in family organization and structure may explain some intrafamilial aggression. Changes that affect social and moral bonding among family members are probably most significant in this respect. One such change, evolving since the 1970s, is the deinstitutionalization of children without families, the mentally ill, the homeless, and the disabled. Adoption, the temporary placement of children in foster homes, or the informal placement of children with relatives exposes them to risks of violence from caretakers for whom the minimal moral constraints of a biological parent are less salient (Reiss and Roth, 1993, p. 241).

A second major change in family organization is the increased number of children who are not living with their natural parents. This number is substantial, owing to serial cohabitation, divorce, and desertion (Reiss and Roth, 1993), as well as to caretakers' incarceration, substance abuse, or death.

SOCIAL ISOLATION

Social isolation has been identified as a characteristic of some families in which there is a high risk for physical and sexual abuse of a spouse or children (Garbarino and Crouter, 1978; Pike, 1990). The isolation may be forced on the partner by the abuser by screening telephone calls and restricting visitors. On the other hand, shame may prompt the visibly battered spouse to even further withdrawal. Victims often become isolated from friends, their families of origin, neighbors, or anyone who could become acquainted with their abuse. Some families isolate themselves in subtle ways, using unlisted telephone numbers or having no telephone. Some lack a means of transportation, so that they cannot visit others, and the homes of some families in which abuse occurs may be physically shuttered from the gaze of outsiders. Many such families lack community ties of any kind (Garbarino and Sherman, 1980). Risick and Reese (1986) suggest that violent families rarely invite others to their homes, avoiding engagement in social and recreational activities. They put little emphasis on personal growth and development.

GENERATIONAL TRANSMISSION OF VIOLENCE

The transmission of the behavioral basis for violence from one generation to the next is as much a component of subculturation as any other learned behavior. Straus and colleagues (1980) reported that of adults who were abused as children, more than one-fifth later abuse their own children. Although Widom (1989, p. 161) cautions that the methodologic limitations in studies of the intergenerational transmission of abusive behavior, especially in terms of their retrospective design, restrict the validity of conclusions about the long-term consequences of abuse in childhood, most professionals are concerned about the generational transmission factor in family violence.

BIOPSYCHOSOCIAL PERSPECTIVE

Children's perceptions of and interactions with family members are important factors in their development. Essentially, attachments early in life (sometimes called bonding) translate into a blueprint of how a child will perceive situations outside the family. Positive attachment, based on warmth, affection, caring, protective behaviors, and accountability, leads to basic trust (Erickson, 1950). It is the basis for human socialization. Through attachment, an individual gets feedback for the emergence of the self. At about 18 months of age, there is consolidation of a sense of self. Early development of the ability to soothe oneself provides an inner core of calmness and to avoid being overwhelmed by stimuli.

Social bonding can fail or become narrow and selective. Caretakers can ignore, rationalize, or normalize various behaviors in the developing child, or through

their own problems (such as violent behavior), can support the child's developing distortions and projections.

The child who lacks protection by a caretaker experiences strong interpersonal anxiety and may survive by dissociating him- or herself from the trauma of witnessing or experiencing abuse. This dissociation produces a feeling of numbness and inhibits a sense of connectness to other persons and the outside world. In the earliest manifestations of this numbing, children may be observed to be cruel to animals, siblings, and friends, and even to parents or grandparents. There is a lack of sensitivity to the pain of others, and there can be a distorted association of pain with various events. In a Massachusetts case, a 14-year-old youth took a 7-year-old retarded boy into the woods and beat him to death. He had told people that he was going to do this, but no one intervened.

Cruel and detached behavior can also be seen in date abuse occurring in junior and senior high schools. Gang rape may occur, as happened in a New Jersey case, in which several male high school students inserted objects into the vagina of a developmentally retarded girl while other male students watched (State v. Archer et al., 1993). The youths had no sense of the impact of their actions on the victim, or of social responsibility.

Although **attachment theory** was intended as a revision of psychoanalytic theory, it has been infused by biological principles, control-systems theory, and cognitive psychology (Crittenden and Ainsworth, 1989). Although attachment theory began with an attempt to understand the disturbed functioning of individuals who had suffered early separations or traumatic losses, it is a theory of normal development that suggests explanations for some types of atypical development (Bowlby, 1969, 1973, 1980). Since Bowlby's preliminary formulations (1958), attachment theory has stimulated research into socio-emotional development and the growth of interpersonal relationships. For example, the theory suggests a causal relationship between the lack of attachment in the parent and abuse of the child (Ainsworth, 1980).

Family violence has been linked to mental illness and personality disorders, although the links have been established for clinical populations rather than by using case-control methods or general population surveys.

Persons prone to depression may be more prone to violence. A number of studies report that abusive mothers as well as men who physically abuse their partners show signs of depression (Zuravin, 1989). While some sources of depression (e.g., repressed anger toward others) may cause such abuse, the depression may result from being labeled abusive, or other consequences of the violent act (Reiss & Roth, 1993:238). Studies of populations in women's shelters (Frieze and Browne, 1989, p. 197) have found that depression is common among women who are repeat victims of domestic violence.

ASSAULTIVE AND HOMICIDAL BEHAVIOR

It is difficult to explain **interpersonal violence,** especially violence and homicide between partners, because it involves the transgression of a seemingly fundamental connectedness.

In courtship violence, the perpetrator cannot tolerate separation and often does not want the relationship to end. He or she feels abandoned, angry, and depressed. Often, rage is behind the depression. Rejection is an attack on the ego. Such persons often feel that they cannot manage on their own. The limbic system is affected by the activation of stress hormones on the brain structure and neurotransmitters.

In a study of murderers, Ressler, Burgess and Douglas (1988) identified three formative events that contributed to the development of hostility: early childhood trauma, developmental behavior, and interpersonal failure. Early childhood trauma occurs as psychological, physical, and/or sexual abuse. The developing child encounters a variety of life events, some normative and others unusual and extraordinarily negative. Disturbances in early attachment and the impairment of self-regulation are a major problems with traumatized children (van der Kolk and Fisler, 1994). Within the context of the child's dysfunctional social environment, the distress caused by the trauma is probably neglected or mishandled. The child is neither protected nor assisted in recovery from the trauma; his or her external environment does not address the negative consequences of the traumatic events. A second important factor in the formative background of murderers is developmental failure. For some reason, there is failure to positively attach to the primary adult caretaker during childhood. As a result of this negative social attachment, the caretaker has no influence over the child, or later over the adolescent.

Interpersonal failure, the third formative event in the development of a murderer, is the inability of the child's primary caretaking adult to serve as a role model for the child. There are various reasons for this failure, including the caretaker's absence or inadequacy as a role model, (e.g., an abusive parent). The child may witness a violent home environment in which he or she sees aggression in the form of fights and aggressive sexual behavior.

In domestic murders, the killing may be **spontaneous,** occurring without planning. For example, in June 1995, two young boys died of hyperthermia after being buckled in car seat belts for 8 or 10 hours while their 20-year-old mother partied and fell asleep at a Tennessee motel (Boston Globe, June 20, 1995). This case does not involve intentional killing. Some domestic murders, however, are staged and involve careful planning, as in the case example.

ELDER ABUSE

Aggression toward the elderly is multifaceted. Grown children may abuse parents who were themselves abusive and exploitative. There is also elder spousal abuse. Although child and spousal abuse have received growing attention in research into family violence, little is known about the nature of elder abuse. The characteristics of individuals and families who are associated with abuse of the elderly require study as do other forms of

E CASE EXAMPLE

In a 1983 case in Oregon, Diane drove into the emergency department of a local hospital with a gunshot wound in her arm, screaming for help for her three children, who had also been shot. Her 7-year-old daughter was dead on arrival; her 8-year-old daughter had two bullet wounds in her left chest and a third bullet wound through the base of her left thumb, and her 3 year-old son had a bullet wound to his spinal column. Diane said that she had been driving in her car when she noticed a man standing in the middle of the road. She said that she had stopped and gotten out, at which point the man had pulled out a gun and shot the children and herself. She said that she had then pushed and kicked him in the leg, jumped into her car, and sped to the hospital. The story fell apart when Diane's wounded daughter said that she had seen her mother go to the trunk of the car, retrieve a gun from it, come back around the car, and shoot her sister,

her brother, and herself. Another witness testified to seeing Diane's car moving slowly rather than speeding along the road just after the shooting, apparently as Diane waited for her children to die before going to the hospital. Diaries and unmailed letters to a married letter carrier with whom she was having an affair contained such incriminating statements as, "You know I don't want a daddy for my kids . . . you would never be left alone with them." The motive was to eliminate her children for the sake of a fantasized relationship with her lover.

A history of Diane's background revealed child abuse, neglect, and incest. She developed little, if any, attachment to her caretakers. The result was clearly a flaw in human development and attachment. She was sentenced to prison for killing her child.

family violence and the features of interventions that might be adapted to this problem.

■ INTERVENTIONS

The problems of family violence have no easy answers. A comprehensive set of family-support programs or a continuum of services for families at each of the developmental phases of family life does not exist. Although services are needed for ongoing cases of abuse, it is first critical to identify families at risk for violence. Rather than waiting for incidents of violence, counseling and education need to build on an integration of existing interventions and design initiatives that are responsive to community needs and feasible with community resources. Issues within this area include police responses to family violence, shelters, **primary prevention programs,** medication, foster care, and home nursing visits.

POLICE RESPONSES

Police arrest of persons responsible for domestic abuse has the immediate goal of stopping the abuse. Research findings, however, are mixed with regard to whether this prevents the recurrence of domestic violence. Arrest, in replication studies, has not proven to be an effective deterrent in all cases. Some partners may increase their violent behavior (Sherman, 1992).

SHELTERS AND OTHER SERVICES

The last few decades have seen programmatic efforts toward providing shelters for battered women where they and their children can reside safely and receive emotional support. Approximately 1,200 shelters now offer temporary emergency housing to more than 300,000 women and children each year. Typically families stay from 2 days to 3 months. (Reiss and Roth, 1993).

The primary goal of such shelters is to provide safety. Other services are designed to help the women housed in such shelters to become self-sufficient. These include relocation assistance, day care for children, and welfare advocacy. Services directed at increasing self-esteem include support groups and courses on parenting, job readiness, and budgeting. Services for children who have witnessed family violence are often also incorporated into shelter programs.

The **Duluth, Minnesota, Domestic Abuse Intervention Project (DMIP)** conducted a 12-month follow-up study in which battered women were asked their opinion of the interventions the Project had used in an effort to have their abusive partners abandon violent habits. When surveyed as to "what helped"; women said they sensed improvement when the abusive partner took part in education and group counseling. Women

also stated that the improvement had resulted from a combination of involvement by the police, courts, group counseling, and the shelter (Pence and Paymer, 1993).

PRIMARY PREVENTION PROGRAMS

Primary programs for reducing partner assault include public education and awareness programs for the assailants. Such programs emphasize that family violence is a crime and that help is available. Courts also mandate that batterers attend programs that teach them alternative ways of behaving. Alcohol and drug abuse programs are required for batterers whose substance abuse is an issue. Educational programs help children as well as parents develop nonviolent ways of coping with anger and frustration.

MEDICATION

Pharmacological interventions may be useful in reducing family violence. If a significant subgroup of abusive parents or caretakers have major depression and other affective disorders, chemical and other forms of treating these disorders may be a means of controlling family violence. This approach assumes that reasonably effective means are available for controlling affective disorders, and particularly volatile mood swings associated with them (Reiss and Roth, 1993:239).

FOSTER CARE

Placement into **foster care** is a major intervention in cases of child abuse. As in the case of shelters for battered women, this intervention has the immediate goal of stopping abuse. An estimated 15% of victims of child maltreatment are put into foster homes outside their families (American Humane Association, 1979; Runyan et al., 1981). However, research into the negative long-term effects of this on such children has had mixed findings. Several studies have found that the more changes in residence a child experiences, the greater the likelihood of adult criminality and violent criminal behavior (Hensey et al., 1983; Lynch and Roberts, 1982; Widom, 1990).

HOME NURSE VISITATION

Home nurse visiting is a primary means of detecting maltreatment of infants and pre-school children. Olds and Henderson (1988, 1989) have studied this intervention in high-risk groups consisting of economically deprived, unmarried, teen-age mothers having a first child, and have found that home nursing visits decrease but do not totally eliminate the incidence of child abuse in comparison with groups not receiving this intervention. In this study, there was a 5% rate of child abuse or neglect in the high-risk group despite home nursing visits, suggesting the need for additional pre-

E CASE EXAMPLE

▶ SOMATIC DISTRESS

Doris is a 23-year-old divorced mother of two children, aged 2 and 4 years. Her husband's abusive behavior has caused her to make multiple visits to an emergency room. While Doris was pregnant, her husband would repeatedly punch her in the stomach, throw her to the ground, and tell her how she repulsed him. Her terror of him grew when he began to periodically attempt to strangle her and she noted "his eyes were popping out." After a divorce and during visits to his former home, his abuse occurred in the presence of the children. Although Doris sought medical assistance, she had previously never reported that she was being abused, but instead provided a reason for each of her injuries. At her most recent emergency room visit, she reports, "He knocked the front teeth out of my mouth. I was in a bar and I never went to a bar while we were married. But, he started rejecting me and telling me I was ugly and stuff. He found me there and said, "What are you doing here with all these guys looking at you?" I wasn't even looking at them. He called me a slut and punched me in the mouth with a glass

and broke my teeth and bashed my head in front of everyone in the bar. I went to the emergency room but they really couldn't do anything for me but stop the bleeding. They told me to go to a dentist. I had to get two false teeth. The doctors' were helpful but I lied to them because he was standing over me. I told them I fell and did it to myself."

Nursing intervention:

- Treat injuries, identifying and confirming her abuse.
- Assess safety; refer victim to a shelter and to law enforcement for protection orders.
- Monitor by telephone the implementation of legal intervention.
- Ensure home nursing visits to assess both the patient and children, teaching basic content about domestic violence.
- Refer the patient to a stress-reduction group.
- Refer the children to a play group for children who have witnessed family violence.

---

ventive or ameliorative interventions. However, home nursing intervention had additional positive effects beyond reducing the incidence of maltreatment. At 12 and 24 months, infants of mothers in the high-risk group showed improved intellectual functioning on development tests, and there was some evidence of improved family functioning, with less evidence of conflict and scolding and less punishment of infants. Olds and Henderson (1989) also concluded that although the visiting nurse can link families to community and social services, in order to ameliorate the effects of poverty, vi-

olence, and drug use, the lack of employment opportunities in the neighborhoods in which these families live imposes severe constraints on their continued improvement, especially when the intervention stops.

■ LEVELS OF SEVERITY OF FAMILY VIOLENCE

This section provides case examples of family violence according to the seven levels of the stress-crisis continuum (Burgess and Roberts, 1995).

E CASE EXAMPLE

▶ TRANSITIONAL STRESS

A 2-day-old infant was abducted from his hospital bassinet while his mother was in the shower. The hospital security staff was notified immediately and a search for the infant was initiated. Local police were called into the investigation within an hour of the abduction. A search of the apartment of the mother's former boyfriend revealed the infant. He was returned unharmed after being kept for 14 hours. The abductor told the police that his girlfriend—the infant's mother—had acknowledged that he was the baby's father, but said that she had refused him visiting rights.

Intervention

- Refer case to a family court for legal resolution.
- Train staff in planning for critical incidents, in order to provide guidance and define staff roles and instant means of communication (portable radio, dedicated telephone line, and closed-circuit television with taping and monitoring).
- Debrief staff members after the crisis.
- Refer mother and infant for follow-up in order to ensure their continued safety.

E CASE EXAMPLE

▶ TRAUMATIC STRESS

A college sophomore and her roommate take the campus bus to the school library to study. After the young women have been studying for 3 hours, two male students invite them to the dormitory to play cards. The game requires the loser to drink a glass of beer. Over the new few hours, the four become intoxicated and the women miss the bus back to their dormitory. The young men say that they will sleep on the couch, and offer their beds to the women. One young woman falls asleep immediately but is awakened by the presence of one of the young men, who removes her clothing and proceeds to force sex on her despite her protests. The next morning the women return to their own dormitory. The one who was assaulted becomes increasingly anxious and distressed. She cannot forget the rape. She is unable to concentrate in class, do homework assignments, continue her part-time job, or attend social functions. By the end of the semester she has failed two courses and is on academic probation. Her roommate encourages her to report the rape to the college's Women's Health Center, where she is interviewed by a nurse.

Intervention
- Assess physical and emotional health.
- Report the rape to law enforcement (e.g., college police and local police).
- Refer the victim for short-term counseling for rape trauma syndrome.
- Refer the victim for group sessions at the local rape crisis center.

SOMATIC DISTRESS

Patients with somatic distress of Level 1 are generally seen in primary-care facilities for medical presentations of symptoms. Examples of this type of symptoms in cases of domestic violence include bruises, fractures, and bleeding. The patient's response to this level of stress is generally fear, anxiety, or masked depression. Emergency staff personnel generally diagnose and treat this level of stress.

TRANSITIONAL OR ALTERED SELF-REGULATORY PATTERNS

Level 2 abuse within families may occur during pregnancy or after the birth of the infant. Such abuse may occur when family members visit a maternity, pediatric,

E CASE EXAMPLE

▶ FAMILY CRISES

Emily died at the age of 9 months. She had been the youngest member of a family known to her city's department of children and families for more than 3 years. Three weeks before the injuries that led to her death, Emily had suffered a broken leg without a reasonable explanation for this.

Intervention
- Review case for failures in the systems designed to assist abusive families.

A review of Emily's case revealed several points at which the extreme danger to children in her family might have been recognized. First, the multiple injuries to a sibling during the sibling's first year of life were never recognized as suggestive of abuse by the medical staff at a local hospital during sporadic clinic appointments. When severe medical neglect of another child in Emily's family had been reported to the city department of children's services, its serious consequences had not been sufficiently understood, and medical information about the other siblings in the family was not sought (which would have revealed a pattern of possible abuse). Instead, the case was closed. Four years before Emily's death, the police arrested her mother for risk of injury. The arrest record states that the investigating police officers had found two children hanging out of an open, third-story window. There were no adults in the unheated apartment, there was animal excrement on the beds, and no food was available. The police officers had taken the children to a relative after arresting the mother, and had not called the department of children's services until the next day. A final opportunity to avert tragedy occurred just weeks before Emily's death when she presented at a local hospital emergency room with a spiral fracture of her leg. The hospital reported this injury to the department of children's services 6 days after the injury was treated by an emergency care physician and orthopedist. This referral was handled by a social worker who believed the inconsistent explanation of an "accidental injury" given by the mother. Emily remained in her home until her fatal injury.

E CASE EXAMPLE

▶ SERIOUS MENTAL ILLNESS

The editor of a federal government magazine was shot and killed at his home in Virginia because he happened to arrive home at the wrong time, according to police. The 34-year-old editor and two of his roommates were killed by an emotionally disturbed man who was a cousin of one of his roommates. According to reports, the man arrested in the triple slaying went to the house intending to kill two of the victims, his cousin and her boyfriend. The killer was believed to have had ongoing problems with the two. The killings were triggered by an argument over a bicycle, living arrangements, and other problems.

Intervention

- The prevention of murder in this case would have required case monitoring and management for homicidal thoughts in this man and an assessment for his hospitalization or sheltered care before his symptoms became manifest. Monitoring medication is critical for psychotic thinking. Continuity of care is accomplished through the case manager. Other services should include referral for vocational training and group work.

---

or nursery unit and an argument ensues about paternity, infidelity, or custody.

TRAUMATIC CRISES

Level 3 or traumatic crises are precipitated by externally imposed stress that overwhelms the individual. Examples of this in cases of domestic violence include physical assault, rape, and sexual assault. The response is intense fear, helplessness, and behavioral disorganization.

In the case described, criminal charges were not filed by the local authorities, but a civil suit was filed against the university and later settled out of court.

FAMILY (RELATIONAL) CRISES

Family crises of Level 4 reflect serious disruption in partner or care-giver relationships. These crises involve failure to master such developmental issues such as dependency, value conflicts, emotional intimacy, power and control, and self-discipline. Examples of family crises at this level include child abuse, the use of children in pornography, parental abduction, adolescent running away from home, battering and rape, homelessness, and domestic homicide.

E CASE EXAMPLE

▶ PSYCHIATRIC EMERGENCIES

Mindy, age 22, a visiting nurse with a five-year-old son, described vivid scenes of battering wherein her boyfriend would hit her with a lead pipe and empty beer bottles. In an attempt to cope with the abuse, she took drugs and attempted suicide. In the words of Mindy, "I O-D'ed on cocaine intravenously. Purposely. I couldn't take it anymore. I was real depressed and upset and afraid that he was going to beat our son. I went to the hospital. They pumped my stomach and then told me I was a drug addict."

Intervention

- Rapidly assess the patient's psychological and medical condition.
- Clarify the situation that produced or led to the patient's condition.
- Mobilize all mental health and/or medical resources necessary to effectively treat the patient.
- Arrange for follow-up or coordination of services to ensure continuity of treatment as appropriate.

Follow-up indicated that Mindy had been entered into a 90-day inpatient drug program that she hadn't completed. She had been started on antidepressant drug therapy and had completed a course of short-term counseling. Her son was enrolled in play therapy and his behavior is improving.

E CASE EXAMPLE

► CATACLYSMIC CRISES

The police received an emergency call that a pregnant woman and her husband had been shot by an unknown assailant while driving home from a childbirth class. Police located the couple and rushed them to a local hospital. Surgeons were unable to save the young woman. Her baby was born by cesarean section but died 10 days later. Following a lengthy investigation, the police identified the prime suspect as the husband. Prior to his arrest, however, the husband jumped off a bridge and drowned. The husband's brother was arrested and charged with aiding in a felony; he had disposed of two bags containing jewelry and the murder weapon. Police divers located the evidence. This case qualifies as a cataclysmic crisis because of the deaths of the mother and her infant, the disclosure of the wife as a silent battered woman during the marriage and pregnancy, and the suicide of the abuser.

SERIOUS MENTAL ILLNESS

Crises of Level 5, involving serious mental illness, reflect pre-existing psychiatric problems causing disorganized thinking and behavior.

PSYCHIATRIC EMERGENCIES

Crises of Level 6, involving psychiatric emergencies, are situations in which an individual's general functioning has been severely impaired. There is a threat of harm or actual harm to the self and/or others. Such emergencies often result from drug overdosing or entail suicide attempts, stalking, personal assault, rape, and homicide. The psychiatric nurse needs to be confident of her or his skills in order to manage the patient's uncontrolled behavior or have adequate assistance available for this.

Dangerous and volatile situations should be handled by police and local rescue squads, who can provide rapid transportation of the potential or real assailant to a hospital emergency room.

CATACLYSMIC CRISES

Crises of Level 7, or interpersonal cataclysmic crises, as contrasted with mass disasters, consist of a Level 3 traumatic crisis in combination with Level 4, 5, or 6 stressors. In cases of domestic violence, the victim is often a battered wife and there is real or threatened escalation that includes the partner as well as the children.

An example is Lila, the second oldest child in a family of 10. Her father had been stabbed to death when she was 13. She had moved out of her home at age 16, pregnant with her first child. She did not complete high school or engage in social activities because she had to work to support her child. She married at age 20 and had four more children. Her husband was physically abusive, punching, kicking, and burning her with a lit cigarette. He threatened during the year they were separated that he would burn the house down with her and the children in it.

In a second example, an estranged husband lured his wife and three children into his car under the pretense of driving them to a local mall to buy school clothes and supplies. He detonated a car bomb while parked at the mall, killing himself and his family and injuring a number of other persons.

O AN OVERVIEW

- Most theories about the causes of family violence offer only partial explanations; valid explanations can be derived only from social, cultural, and biopsychosocial perspectives.

- Positive early-life attachments lead to basic trust, the core of human socialization.

- Counseling and education services for victims and perpetrators of family violence must build on existing programs and new approaches that are responsive to community needs, such as police responses, shelters, primary prevention programs, medication, foster care, and home nursing visits.

- Early intervention is the management technique of choice for family violence.

- Public education encourages people to come forward to report abuse.

TD TERMS TO DEFINE

- attachment theory
- Duluth, Minnesota Domestic Abuse Intervention Project (DMIP)
- foster care
- interpersonal violence
- primary prevention programs

Q STUDY QUESTIONS

1. Which of the following statements does not characterize family violence?
   a. It is more likely to be repeated than violence committed by a stranger.
   b. It has greater stigmatization if the acts are disclosed.
   c. It often occurs in public places.
   d. When family members live in the same home, violent interaction can increase.

2. T   F   Aggressors in dating violence situations generally do not report more relationship problems than nonaggressive individuals, only different types of problems in the relationship.

3. Battered women are more likely to seek emergency medical attention and are more often injured on the
   a. face or head region
   b. breast or chest region
   c. abdomen
   d. all of the above
   e. b and c

4. What age groups are more vulnerable to child homicide?
   a. Newborns and infants
   b. Ages 1 to 4 years
   c. ages 5 to 9 years
   d. a only
   e. a and b

5. Who is most likely to kill children in the vulnerable group(s)?
   a. A stranger
   b. The mother
   c. The father
   d. b and c are equally likely

6. Why is attachment (bonding) to a caretaker so important to human development?

7. Describe how social isolation can put a person at a high risk for physical and sexual abuse.

8. T   F   Violent behavior is commonly transmitted from one generation to the next.

9. Which psychological disorder is most common in those prone to violence?
   a. Schizophrenia
   b. Depression
   c. Mental retardation
   d. Panic disorder

10. T   F   Arresting a domestic abuser may serve as a deterrent to further violence.

11. Match each level of stress crisis in family violence with its description.

    A. Somatic distress

    B. Transitional self-regulatory patterns

    C. Traumatic stress crisis

    D. Family crisis

    E. Serious mental illness

    F. Psychiatric emergencies

    G. Cataclysmic crisis

    1. General functioning is severely impaired and there is actual threat or harm to self and/or others.
    2. Abuse that usually occurs during pregnancy
    3. Is a traumatic stress crisis with the additional stressors of a family crisis, serious mental illness, and psychiatric emergency.
    4. Generally seen in medical primary-care facilities.
    5. Precipitated by externally imposed stress that overwhelms individual.
    6. Serious disruption in partner relationships.
    7. Pre-existing psychiatric problems interact with patient's disorganized thinking and behavior.

■ REFERENCES

Ainsworth, M.D.S. attachment and child abuse, *in* Gerber G, Ross CJ, and Zigler E (eds): *Child Abuse Reconsidered: An Agenda for Action.* New York, Oxford University Press, 1980.

National Center for Child Neglect and Abuse Reporting. Denver, American Humane Association, 1979.

Baldwin BA: A paradigm for the classification of emotional crises: Implications for crisis intervention. *Am J Orthopsychiatry* 1978; 48:538–551.

Burgess AW, Hartman MP, McCausland MP, Powers P: Response patterns in children and adolescents exploited through sex rings and pornography, *Am J. Psychiatry,* 1984; 141(5):656–662.

Burgess AW, Roberts AL: A stress-crisis continuum: A crisis typology. *Crisis Intervent Time-Limited Treatment,* 1995; 2:31–47.

Bowlby J: The nature of the child's tie to his mother. *Int J Psychoanal* 1958; 39:359–373.

Bowlby J: *Attachment and Loss,* Vol. I: *Attachment.* New York, Basic Books, 1969.

Bowlby J: *Attachment and Loss,* Vol. II: *Separation.* New York, Basic Books, 1973.

Bowlby J: *Attachment and Loss,* Vol. III: *Loss.* New York, Basic Books, 1980.

Bureau of Justice Statistics, U.S. Department of Justice: Criminal Victimization in the United States, 1988. A national crime survey report, December, NCJ-122024. Washington, DC, U.S. Government Printing Office, 1990.

Catalano R: Violence in the workplace, *Psychiatr Serv* 1995; 46(1):85–86.

Catalano R, Dooley D, Novaco R, et al.: Using ECA survey data to examine the effect of job layoffs on violent behavior. *Hosp Commun Psychiatry* 1993; 44:874–879.

Catalano R, Dooley D, Wilson G, et al.: Job loss and alcohol abuse: a test using data from the Epidemiologic Catchment Area project. *J Health Soc Behav* 1993; 34:215–225.

Cate CA, Henton JM, Koval J, Christopher FS, Lloyd S: Premarital abuse: A social psychological perspective. *J. Fam Iss* 1982; 3:79–90.

Conte JR: Progress in treating the sexual abuse in children, *Social Work* 1984; 3:258–263.

Crittenden PM, Ainsworth MDS: Child maltreatment and attachment theory, in Cicchetti D, Carlson V (eds): *Child Maltreatment.* Cambridge, MA: Cambridge University Press, 1989, pp. 432–463.

Crowell N, Burgess AW: *Understanding Violence Against Women.* Washington, DC: National Research Council.

Durst M: Perceived peer abuse among college students: A research note. *Nat Assoc Stud Pers Adm J* 1987; 24:42–47.

Federal Bureau of Investigation: Uniform Crime Reports for the United States: 1990. Washington, DC, U.S. Government Printing Office, 1991.

Finklehor D: Common features of family abuse, in Finklehor D, Gelles RJ, Hotaling GT, Straus MA (eds): *The Dark Side of Families.* Newbury Park CA, Sage, 1983.

Finklehor D, Williams LM, Burns N: *Nursery Crimes: Sexual Abuse in Day Care/* Newbury Park, CA, Sage, 1988.

Frieze IH, Browne A: Violence in marriage. *in* Ohlin L, Tonry M (eds): *Family Violence.* Chicago, University of Chicago Press, 1989, pp. 163–218.

Garbarino J, Crouter K: Defining the community context of parent-child relations: the correlates of child maltreatment. *Child Dev* 1978; 43:604–616.

Garbarino J, Sherman D: High-risk families and high-risk neighborhoods. *Child Dev* 1980; 51:188–198.

Gelles RJ: An exchange social control theory, *in* Finklehor D, Gelles RJ, Hotaling, GT, Straus MA (eds): *The Dark Side of Families.* Newbury Park CA, Sage, 1983.

Gelles RJ, Straus MA: Determinant of violence in the family: Toward a theoretical integration. In Hill RB, Nye FI, Reiss IL (eds): *Contemporary Theories About the Family,* New York, Free Press, 1979, pp. 549–581.

Hensey OJ, Williams JK, Rosenbloom L: Experiences in Liverpool. *Dev Med Child Neurol* 1983; 25:606–611.

Henton J, Cate R, Koval J, Lloyd D, Christopher D: Romance and violence in dating relationships, *J Fam Iss* 1983; 4:467–482.

Karr A: Labor letter. *Wall Street Journal,* Apr. 14, 1992, p. 1.

Laner MR: Courtship abuse and aggression: Contextual aspects. *Sociol Spectr* 1983; 3:69–83.

Lynch MA, Roberts J: *Consequences of Child Abuse.* London, Academic Press, 1982.

Makepeace, JM: Courtship violence among college students. *Fam Relat* 1981; 30:97–102.

Olds DL: The prenatal/early infancy project, *in* Price RH, Cowen EE, Lorion RP, Ramos-McKay, R (eds): *Fourteen Ounces of Prevention: A Casebook for Practitioners.* Washington, DC, American Psychological Association, 1988, pp. 9–32.

Olds DL, Henderson CR: The prevention of maltreatment, *in* Cicchetti D, Carlson V (eds): *Child Maltreatment: Theory and Research on the Causes and Consequences of Child Abuse and Neglect.* Cambridge, England: Cambridge University Press, 1989, pp. 772–763.

Pillemer K, Finklehor D: Prevalence of elder abuse: A random sample survey. *Gerontologist* 1988; 28:51–57.

Pike KM: Intrafamilial sexual abuse of children. Paper prepared for the National Research Council Panel on the Understanding and Control of Violent Behavior, Washington, D.C.

Podnicks E, Pillemer K: *Final Report on Survey of Elder Abuse in Canada.* Ottawa, Canadian Department of Health and Welfare, 1989.

Pynoos RY, Eth S: Developmental perspective on psychic trauma in childhood. In Figley CR (ed): *Trauma and its Wake,* New York: Brunner/Mazel Psychological Stress Series, 1985.

Reiss AJ Jr, Roth JA (eds): *Understanding and Preventing Violence,* Vol. 1. Washington, DC, National Academy Press, 1993.

Reiss AJ Jr, Roth JA (eds): *Understanding and Preventing Violence,* Vol. 3, *Social Influences.* Washington, DC, National Academy Press, 1993.

Resick PA, Reese D: Perception of family social climate and physical aggression in the home. *J Fam Violence* 1986; 1:71–83.

Ressler RK, Burgess AW, Douglas JE: *Sexual Homicide.* New York, Free Press, 1988.

Riggs DS: Relationship problems and dating aggression, *J Interpers Violence* 1993; 8(1):18–35.

Riggs DS, O'Leary KD: A theoretical model of courtship aggression, *in* Pirog-Good MA, Stets JE (eds): *Violence in Dating Relationships: Emerging Social Issues.* New York, Praeger, 1989, pp. 53–71.

Roscoe B, Benaske N: Courtship violence experienced by abused wives: Similarities in patterns of abuse, *Fam Relat* 1985; 34:419–424.

Runyan DK, Gould CL, Trost DC, Loda FA: Determinants of foster care placement for the maltreated child. *Child Abuse Neglect* 1981; 6:343–350.

Russell D: *Rape in Marriage.* London and New York, MacMillan, 1982.

Sedlak AJ: *National Incidence and Prevalence of Child Abuse and Neglect: 1988.* Washington, DC, Westat, Inc. (Revised September 5, 1991), 1991a.

Sedlak AJ: *Supplementary Analysis of Data on the National Incidence of Child Abuse and Neglect.* Washington, DC, Westat, Inc. (Revised August 30), 1991b.

Sherman LW: *Policing Domestic Violence: Experiments and Dilemmas.* New York, Free Press, 1992.

Sigelman CK, Berry CJ, Wiles KA: Violence in college students' dating relationships. *J Appl Soc Psychol* 1984; 5:530–548.

Stark E, Flintcraft A: Medical therapy as repression: The case of the battered woman. *Health Med* 1982; 1:29–32.

Stark E, Flintcraft A: Spouse abuse, *in* Rosenberg M, Fenley MA (eds): *Violence in America: A Public Health Approach.* New York, Oxford University Press, 1991.

Straus MA: Measuring family conflict and violence: The conflict tactics scale, *J Marriage Fam Living* 1979; 36:13–19.

Straus MA, Gelles RJ: Societal change in family violence from 1975 to 1985 as revealed in two national surveys. *J Marriage Fam* 1986; 48:465–479.

Straus MA, Gelles RJ, Steinmetz SK: *Behind Closed Doors: Violence in the American Family.* Carden City, NY, Doubleday, 1980.

U.S. Bureau of the Census: Household and family characteristics: March 1990 and 1989. Current Population Reports, Population Characteristics. Series P-20, No. 447. Washington, DC, U.S. Government Printing Office, 1990.

U.S. Bureau of the Census: Marital status and living arrangements: March 1990. Current Population Reports. Series P-20, No. 450. Washington, DC, U.S. Government Printing Office, 1991.

U.S. Department of Health and Human Services: Study Findings: Study of National Incidence and Prevalence of Child Abuse and Neglect. National Center on Child Abuse and Neglect, Washington, DC, U.S. Government Printing Office, 1988.

U.S. Department of Health and Human Services: Child Abuse and Neglect: Critical First Steps in Response to a National Emergency. Washington, DC, U.S. Government Printing Office, 1990.

Whiteside N: Unemployment and health: an historical perspective. *J Soc Policy* 1988; 17:177–179.

Widom CS: The cycle of violence. *Science* 1989; 244:160–166.

Widom CS: Research, clinical and policy issues: Childhood victimization, parent alcohol problems and long-term consequences. National Forum on the Future of Children, Workshop on Children and Parental Illegal Drug Abuse, National Research Council: Institute of Medicine, March 8, 1990.

Winpisinger KA, Hopkins RS, Indian RW, Hosteler JR: Risk factors for childhood homicides in Ohio: A birth certificate-based case-control study. *Am J Public Health* 1991; 81:1052–1054.

Zigler, E, Hall N: Physical child abuse in America: Past, present and future. In D. Cicchetti and V. Carlson, (eds) *Child Maltreatment* Cambridge, Eng.: Cambridge University Press, 1989, pp. 38–75.

Zuravin SJ: The ecology of child abuse and neglect: Review of the literature and presentation of data. *Violence Victims* 1989; 4(2):101–120.

5

Level 5

Serious Mental Illness

Crises at this level reflect serious mental illness in which pre-existing problems have been instrumental crisis precipitants. Alternatively, the severity of the illness may significantly impair or complicate adaptive resolution of the situation and precipitate a crisis. Examples of serious mental illness include continued schizophrenia or other psychoses.

The patient response is disorganized thinking and behavior. The etiology is neurobiological.

In intervening, psychiatric nurses respond primarily to the patient's immediate problem, emphasizing problem-solving skills and environmental manipulation. The nurse is supportive, but careful not to produce or reinforce dependency or regression by allowing the therapeutic process to become diffuse. The nurse acknowledges the deeper problems of the patient, and assesses them to the degree possible within the crisis therapy context. No attempt, however, is made to resolve problems representing deep emotional conflict. Crisis intervention helps the patient stabilize his or her functioning to the fullest possible extent. The process of intervention also prepares the patient for referral to other services.

Case monitoring and management are indicated, as is assessment of the need for hospitalization or sheltered care. Medication will be needed for psychotic thinking. Continuity of care is critical for this level of crisis, and is generally accomplished through the case manager. Other services should include referral for vocational training and group work.

Conditions representative of Serious Mental Illness are discussed in the following two chapters:

- *Schizophrenia*
- *The Seriously Mentally Ill, Homeless Population*

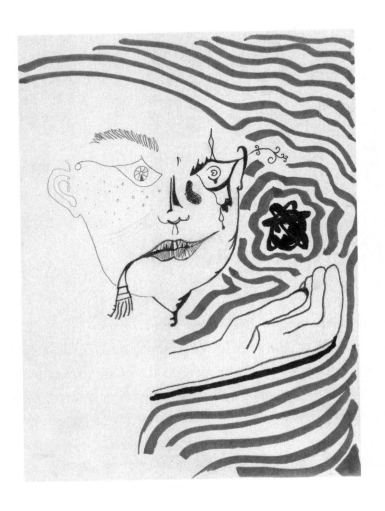

The mind is its own place, and in itself
Can make a heaven of Hell, or a hell of Heaven.

John Milton (1608–1674)

Paradise Lost

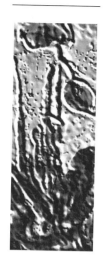

29

Schizophrenia

Doris Vallone

Schizophrenia, an illness often synonymous with madness, connotes both mystery and fear. Prior to the advances in technology that enabled researchers to assess the functioning brain, the odd behavioral manifestations of schizophrenia were attributed to various spiritual, psychological, and social causes (Kales, Kales, and Vela-Bueno, 1991). The distorted reality perception of the person with schizophrenia was misunderstood, feared, and regarded as evil or a punishment for some wrong-doing (See Table 29-1). Removal of these individuals from society and alienation of their families resulted in a profound social isolation of persons whose only crime was the misfortune of having developed a chronic brain disease.

Currently, the political consequences of decreased social functioning and participation by individuals with schizophrenia have resulted in low levels of interest in the disease and its low priority for allocation of resources. Advocates for individuals with schizophrenia include associations for the mentally ill, the families of these individuals, and committed health professionals. Nurses have a dual role in caring for these individuals. First, because persons with schizophrenia will continue to make extensive use of mental-health services, nurses can provide compassionate and supportive care and education to these patients and their families. Second, nurses are in a position to be advocates for research funding and expanded nursing roles in the care of patients with schizophrenia and in dispelling the prevailing myths about the illness itself. Following are some of the common myths—and realities—of schizophrenia:

- Schizophrenia means split personality. Reality: The term schizophrenia derives from the Greek schizein, to cut or cleave, and phren, meaning mind. The schizophrenic individual suffers from a shattered or fragmented mind. The schizophrenic process causes a fragmentation of many facets of the personality, according to psychiatrist Anthony LaBruzza (1994), and affects most aspects of human functioning.

- Schizophrenia is caused by "inadequate mothering." Reality: Psychoanalysts hypothesized that early separation from the mother or overdependence on the mother resulted in both inadequate ego development and a consequent failure of reality testing.

- Schizophrenia is caused by lysergic acid diethylamide (LSD) and street drugs. Reality: Hallucinogenic and stimulant drugs such as LSD, phencyclidine (PCP), and cocaine are associated with psychotic symptoms that can mimic schizophrenic symptoms, but do not cause the disease.

- Persons with schizophrenia are mentally retarded. Reality: Persons with schizophrenia are not mentally retarded, but experience difficulties in mental and social functioning.

- Schizophrenia is uncontrollable and disabling. Reality: Symptoms of the disease can be controlled, and many persons with schizophrenia lead productive lives (Muesser and Gingerich, 1994).

■ EPIDEMIOLOGY

Schizophrenia has an incidence of 1 in 100,000 persons, but because of the chronic nature of the illness it affects from 0.5 to 1% of the population in the United States and worldwide. At present, between 2 million and 3 million individuals in the United States have schizophrenia. The median age of onset is the early to late twenties in males and the late twenties in females. The disease appears with equal frequency in males and females, but its earlier onset and increased severity in males result in higher hospitalization rates for males with schizophrenia (Group for the Advancement of Psychiatry, 1992). Persons with schizophrenia currently occupy 268,000 beds in psychiatric hospitals, a reduction from over 500,000 beds prior to the de-institutionalization movement of recent years. Because many persons who are no longer in hospitals have lost their social-support systems, from 33 to 50% of homeless Americans have a diagnosis of schizophrenia (Carpenter and Buchanan, 1995).

■ DIAGNOSTIC CRITERIA

The importance of nurses' awareness of diagnostic criteria for schizophrenia cannot be overstated. There is no known biological marker or laboratory test for the disease, and many of its manifestations also appear in other mental illnesses, medical illnesses, and toxic syndromes. An accurate report of a patient's behavioral manifestations, history, social functioning, and cognitive status is critical to the differentiation of schizophrenia from these other entities.

Throughout history there are descriptions of seriously deranged or psychotic individuals who would be today diagnosed as suffering from schizophrenia. Efforts toward the diagnosis and classification of schizophrenia have evolved for over a century and a half. Benedict Morel, Emil Kraeplin, Eugen Bleuler, and Kurt Schneider were the first scientists to identify symptoms associated with what has come to be called schizophrenia (Igbal, et al., 1993).

In 1852 Benedict Morel reported cases of *demence precoce*—that is, progressive intellectual deterioration beginning in adolescence. In 1896 Emil Kraepelin used a similar term, *dementia praecox,* to designate individuals who developed chronic progressive functional impairment in early adulthood, often accompanied by intellectual deterioration, hallucinations, and delusions. Kraepelin distinguished dementia praecox from manic-depressive psychosis and from paranoia or delusional disorder. In Kraepelin's view, dementia praecox had an early onset and chronic deteriorating course (LaBruzza, 1994).

In 1911 Eugen Bleuler coined the term schizophrenia to emphasize the splitting of psychic processes that he believed to be at the core of the group of disorders. Bleuler emphasized four primary features: ambivalence, affect (flat), associations (loose), and autism. Bleuler's definition broadened the concept of schizophrenia and allowed persons who did not follow the chronic deteriorating course to be diagnosed with schizophrenia (LaBruzza, 1994).

In 1959 Kurt Schneider, reacting to the overly broad Bleulerian concept of schizophrenia, suggested a narrower definition based on a set of specific hallucinations and delusions, called Schneiderian "first-rank" symptoms. He sought to define a set of symptoms that reflected the core schizophrenic experience of a loss of sense of autonomy over the self and a blurring of the boundaries between the self and reality. According to Schneider's conception, schizophrenic individuals suffer a fundamental loss of a sense of who and what they are and of where they end and outside reality begins (LaBruzza, 1994).The contributions of Kraeplin, Bleuler, and Schneider are summarized in Table 29–2. Current diagnostic criteria continue to incorporate some of these concepts.

The *Diagnostic and Statistical Manual of Mental Disorders, Fourth Edition* (DSM-IV, 1994) contains the current diagnostic criteria for schizophrenia. These criteria must be met for the diagnosis of schizophrenia or one of its many subtypes (See Table 29–3). Schizophrenia must also be differentiated from other psychiatric illnesses, drug reactions, and medical syndromes that can present with symptoms similar to those of schizophrenia (Table 29–4).

TABLE 29–1 HISTORICAL CONCEPTS OF SCHIZOPHRENIA

Period		Concept
Prehistoric		Malignant, supernatural force creates symptoms
Classical		
Hippocrates		Madness is excess of bodily humors
Aristotle		Described emotions
Galen		Identified four humors
Medieval	10–15th Century	Religious and superstitious beliefs leading to persecution of mentally ill. Demonology and witch-hunting
Renaissance	16th Century	Mental illness due to natural rather than supernatural causes
Enlightenment	18th Century	Mental disorders are a focus of medicine
Pinel		Introduced moral treatment
Esquirol		Classified mental illness
Modern	20th Century	Schizophrenia is a distinct entity called "dementia praecox"
Kraepelin		
Bleuler		Introduced the term "schizophrenia"

TABLE 29–2 HISTORICAL CLASSIFICATION OF MANIFESTATIONS OF SCHIZOPHRENIA

Kraeplin (1896)

"Dementia Praecox"
Early onset of mental deterioration. Kraeplin made the distinction from the dementia of the elderly and those with brain damage

Bleuler (4 A's) (1911)

Ambivalence:
Simultaneous experience of conflicting feelings.

Affect (flat):
Minimal change in emotional expression

Associations (loose):
Disconnection between thoughts and ideas

Autism:
Preoccupation with inner experiences

Schneider (First Rank)* (1959)

Delusions:
False belief that is maintained in spite of evidence to the contrary

Hallucinations:
A false perception not accounted for by any external stimuli

Thought insertion and thought withdrawal:
The experience of having someone else control the thoughts by putting them into the mind or removing them from the mind

Thought broadcasting:
The belief that one's thoughts are spread to others

*Pathonomonic for schizophrenia

Another useful classification scheme is Andreasen's positive and negative dimensions of schizophrenia (Andreasen et al., 1994). These are outlined in Table 29–5. In this model, **positive symptoms** of schizophrenia are manifestations considered to be psychotic, such as hallucinations, delusions, and dissociative thought, as well as disorganized and bizarre behavior. They are labeled "positive" because of their unique presence in schizophrenia. **Negative symptoms** are con-

TABLE 29–3 DSM-IV KEY FEATURES OF SCHIZOPHRENIA

- Psychotic symptoms, at least two, present for at least a month:
    Hallucinations
    Delusions
    Disorganized speech
    Disorganized or catatonic behavior
    Negative symptoms (flat affect, lack of motivation)
- Impairment in social or occupational functioning
- Duration of the illness for at least 6 months
- Symptoms are not primarily due to a Mood Disorder;
    Schizoaffective Disorder; Medical, Neurologic or Substance-Induced Disorder.

TABLE 29–4 IMITATORS OF SCHIZOPHRENIA-LIKE PSYCHOSES

Brain disorders	*Drug reactions*
Embolism	Alcohol withdrawal
Ischemia	Amantadine
Trauma	Amphetamines
Tumor	Atropine
Epilepsy	Bromide
Encephalitis	Bromocriptine
Narcolepsy	Carbon Monoxide
Systemic disorders	Cocaine
Vitamin B-12 deficiency	Corticosteroids
Acquired immune deficiency	Dexatrim
syndrome (AIDS)	Ephedrine
Syphilis	Levodopa
Tuberculous meningitis	Levodopa
Pellagra	Lidocaine
Hypoglycemia	LSD
Hepatic encephalopathy	MAO inhibitors
Hyperthyroidism	Phencyclidine
Lead poisoning	Propranolol
Lupus	Tricyclic antidepressants
Multiple sclerosis	

---

sidered deficit symptoms and include poverty of speech, blunted affect, anhedonia, and avolition.

Crow (1980) suggested a two-disease classification scheme, with Type I schizophrenia characterized by eccentric behavior and Type II by withdrawal behavior and apathy. Crow also correlated the two subtypes with neurological changes. This classification has been abandoned, since many patients with schizophrenia exhibit both negative and positive symptoms.

■ ETIOLOGY

Schizophrenia is a brain disease of unknown etiology. It is heterogeneous: it manifests with a variety of symptoms and has a variable course. Andreasen and Carpenter (1993) suggest that most explanatory models fall into one of three categories that define schizophrenia as:

1. A single process leading to diverse manifestations. A medical illness that exemplifies such a process is multiple sclerosis.
2. Multiple disease entities leading to the illness. An example of such a process is mental retardation.
3. Specific symptom clusters reflecting different disease processes that combine in different ways in different patients.

TABLE 29–5 POSITIVE AND NEGATIVE SYMPTOMS OF SCHIZOPHRENIA

Positive Symptoms

Hallucinations
A false perception not accounted for by any verifiable stimuli. May be visual (seeing images), auditory (hearing voices or sounds), tactile (feeling sensations on the skin), olfactory (smelling odors), gustatory (experiencing tastes), or somatic (believing that organs are missing).

Delusions
A belief that is maintained in spite of evidence to the contrary. May be persecutatory (beliefs that one is in danger or being pursued) or grandiose (beliefs that one is an important or historical person)

Formal thought disorder
The presence of looseness of associations or concreteness

Bizarre behavior
Odd or eccentric mannerisms

Disorganization
Difficulty structuring activities

Negative Symptoms

Alogia
Inability to express oneself through speech

Affective blunting
Minimal change in emotional expression

Anhedonia
Inability to experience pleasure

Attention impairment
Inability to focus the attention; distractibility

Avolition
Difficulty making choices

These assumptions have guided much of the research into the cause of schizophrenia. While there is greater understanding of the disease process and the pathophysiological changes in schizophrenia, the definitive cause has not been determined. However, several theories have been proposed.

■ THEORIES

The theories of schizophrenia have reflected the nature-versus-nurture or biological-versus-psychological dichotomies for the origin of the illness. More recently, integrative models have been proposed.

PSYCHOANALYTIC AND FAMILY-INTERACTION THEORIES

Psychoanalytic theories explain schizophrenia as being caused or precipitated by dysfunctional family interactions and deficient parenting. Care-givers who continue to subscribe to these theories seek the origins of the illness in the history of family communication patterns; as a result, families may feel blamed and alienated from the health-care community. Since the biological breakthroughs in understanding schizophrenia, however, most such theories have been discarded. They are mentioned only for historical interest.

BIOLOGICAL THEORIES

Genetic

The search for specific genetic transmission factors in schizophrenia has intensified over the past 20 years. These studies have involved blood relatives of persons with schizophrenia, twins, and adopted children whose biological mothers had schizophrenia. The studies have verified that schizophrenia runs in families. First-degree relatives of individuals with schizophrenia have a tenfold greater risk of developing the disease than the general population. This rate increases to 15% in dizygotic twins and nearly 50% in monozygotic twins. Children born to women with schizophrenia but reared by others were found to develop schizophrenia at the same rate as children born to and reared by mothers with schizophrenia. Adoption studies are most frequently cited as evidence of the role of genes in the transmission of some predisposition to the disorder.

Prenatal and Environmental

Children born during the winter months are at greater risk for schizophrenia than those born at other times of the year, possibly because of a viral infection that increases genetic vulnerability to the disease. Prenatal factors in schizophrenia may include the mother's nutritional state at delivery, complications during delivery, and post-natal apnea and hypoxia (Lehmann, 1983).

Neurophysiological

The development of brain-imaging techniques has advanced the understanding of schizophrenia by enabling researchers to make functional as well as structural assessments of the living brain. Consistent structural findings in schizophrenia have included ventricular enlargement, cerebral asymmetry, and decreased cell density.

Biochemical

A relative excess of dopamine in the limbic system has been hypothesized to account for the psychotic symptoms of schizophrenia, and evidence that neuroleptic medications alleviate symptoms by blocking dopamine receptors lends support to this view. Additionally, drugs such as amphetamines, which increase dopamine activity, induce psychotic symptoms. An excess of dopamine can produce an increased number of dopamine receptors, increased receptor sensitivity, or an increased rate of neurotransmission, perhaps mediated by another neurotransmitter. The excess of dopamine is believed to be responsible for many of the cognitive dysfunctions observed in schizophrenia.

INTEGRATIVE: STRESS VULNERABILITY

The **stress-vulnerability model** has evolved over the past 20 years as a framework for understanding the factors that determine the severity of the symptoms of schizophrenia. No single scientist is credited with developing the model, since many have contributed to it (Muesser and Gingerich, 1994). The dopamine dysfunction previously described as being thought to exist in schizophrenia can be the beginning point for discussion of the stress-vulnerability model, which has utility for nursing practice and research (O'Connor, 1994). As can be seen in Figure 29–1, the stress-vulnerability process is clearly circular, with multiple feedback loops and interactions with the environment (Neuchterlein, Dawson, Ventura et al., 1994).

Vulnerability

Dopamine Dysfunction. The individual with schizophrenia has an inherent vulnerability to **dopamine** dysfunction. Where and how this dysfunction arises are the questions researchers are striving to answer. There is some defect in the neurotransmission of dopamine to the prefrontal or learning areas of the brain. This defect is accompanied by decreased blood flow during challenging cognitive tasks. Reduced cognitive performance is suggested as a possible result of decreased

processing capacity in the prefrontal areas (O'Connor, 1994). The prefrontal dopamine system also plays a regulatory role in the inhibition of dopamine in the mesolimbic system. Increased secretion of dopamine in the mesolimbic system is responsible for the psychotic symptoms of schizophrenia. Stress increases dopamine release in the mesolimbic system, and when the excess dopamine is unmodulated by properly functioning inhibitors, symptoms of the illness increase during stress. Stress also reduces the ability to process cognitive information, which makes the management of stress more difficult.

Cognitive Processing Deficits. Deficits in cognitive processing are important in understanding some of the thinking difficulties exhibited by persons with schizophrenia. Cleghorn and Albert (1990) summarized some of these deficits as seen in experimental settings. The deficits occur in selective attention, active and long-term memory, and a central executive function responsible for the "switching" that occurs in processing information from one perceptual mode to another. Persons with schizophrenia experience delays in switching modes or "channels" of perception, such as from sight to hearing. They demonstrate lapses of attention when performing complex tasks, and they have difficulty in selectively focusing their attention on stimuli, a tendency also found in families of persons with schizophrenia. The cognitive deficits in schizophrenia are also demonstrated in problems with motor responses. For example, in response to a new request, persons with schizophrenia will repeat an action prompted by a previous request. New theories of "cognitive modules" of brain function, borrowed from computer terminology, are being applied to explain how such symptoms of schizophrenia as delusions and hallucinations may be formed.

Stress

Three classes of potentiators or stressors have been implicated in the stress-vulnerability model of schizophrenia: stressful life events and daily annoyances, environmental stimulation, and critical family or residential-staff attitudes.

Life Events. For persons with schizophrenia, the stresses of daily life often correlate with exacerbation or onset of the illness. There is little control over life events such as losses, financial problems, deaths, disasters, and forced relocation.

Environment. Environmental stimulation, such as noise, crowds, and moving objects, is a part of daily existence. This stimulation demands adequate cognitive processing ability and selective attention or focus in order

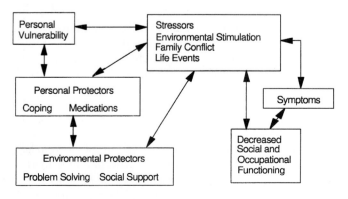

Figure 29-1: Stress-vulnerability Interaction

for one to perform daily activities. These abilities are decreased or lacking in persons with schizophrenia. One might imagine being in a classroom where every small environmental noise occurs at the same volume as the instructor's voice. It would be difficult to concentrate.

Family Conflict.
A critical or emotionally overinvolved family climate is the third category of stress in the stress-vulnerability model of schizophrenia. There has been much discussion of the role of a **high level of expressed emotion** in exacerbating schizophrenic symptoms (Stirling, 1994). A high level of expressed emotion is the tendency to respond in a critical, unsympathetic, and overinvolved manner in times of trouble. In families with a member who has schizophrenia, these responses may be reactions to the problematic behavior exhibited by that family member, resulting in negative and stressful interactions that further exacerbate symptoms (Bellak and Mueser, 1993). Family members who are not educated about schizophrenia may respond to the behaviors of a relative with the illness as though they were deliberate or under that individual's control.

Protectors

Antipsychotic Medication.
Antipsychotic medication is thought to raise the threshold for psychotic symptoms, reducing their frequency and severity. Compliance with antipsychotic medication regimens is a factor in preventing relapse, of the illness, and so must become part of the affected individual's life.

Coping Skills.
Coping skills are a second personal protector. Symptom monitoring is particular useful. This technique enables the patient to identify early symptoms of relapse and to seek adjustments in medication and intensive treatment to prevent hospitalization.

Family Education, Problem-Solving, and Social Support.
There is considerable evidence that family education about schizophrenia and the way emotional reactivity contributes to it can assist in the prevention of highly charged interactions that can exacerbate the illness (Muesser, Gingerich, and Rosenthal, 1993). Family education programs have been designed to provide basic information about the pathology of and medication for schizophrenia, relapse prevention, and resource utilization. These programs include stress and crisis management techniques for family members. Increased social support, such as intensive case management and drop-in centers, give the individual with schizophrenia a network and a place to which to turn for help.

■ TREATMENTS

PSYCHOPHARMACOLOGICAL

Before the discovery in 1956 of the neuroleptic medication chlorpromazine, the characteristic agitation of schizophrenia was managed with sedatives. The neuroleptic drugs showed great promise in alleviating the psychotic symptoms of schizophrenia and decreasing the agitation that characterizes the illness. Since the discovery of chlorpromazine, several other neuroleptic agents have been introduced. The most common include thioridazine (Mellaril), fluphenazine (Prolixin), perphenazine (Trilafon), thiothixene (Navane), and haloperidol (Haldol). Chlorpromazine and thioridazine are considered low potency agents and fluphenazine, perphenazine, thiothixine and haloperidol are considered high potency agents as lower dosage achieves the desired effect on psychotic symptoms. There is agreement (Breslin, 1992) that these medications have similar effects on psychotic symptoms and differ only in their potency and side-effect profile. Generally, the high-potency agents have a greater likelihood of producing extrapyramidal symptoms, while the lower potency agents have greater sedative and anticholinergic effects. Side effects are considered when a specific drug is selected.

Newer trends in psychopharmacological treatment include use of the minimum drug dosage necessary to produce an effect and, in selected patients, intermittent targeted treatment. This typed targeted treatment is medication begun when patients become symptomatic alternating with drug free periods during remission (Breslin, 1992).

A relatively new agent, clozapine, is classified as an antipsychotic rather than a neuroleptic drug because it more specifically targets the positive and negative symptoms and does not cause movement disorders. The drug is reserved for treatment resistant to other drugs or treatments, because of its potential for causing life-threatening blood dyscrasias. Evidence suggests that environmental adjustment and coping skills are crucial in maintaining symptom control in schizophrenic patients with minimal-medication regimens.

ENVIRONMENTAL

Crisis Intervention

Short-term hospitalization is an intense form of both environmental manipulation and social support often necessary for acutely disturbed psychiatric patients. Recent health-care trends have shown a decrease in the number of days of in-patient hospitalization across all groups of in-patients, with no exception for the mentally ill. Patients may have to be hospitalized involuntarily if they are a danger to themselves or others, or exhibit an inability to maintain their basic needs. In addition to maintenance of safety, the goals of hospitalization include diagnostic assessment and evaluation. The patient is also assessed for non–schizophrenia-related causes of symptoms and started on medication and psychosocial programming. Ideally, the patient is rapidly moved to a less intensive treatment environment, such as a partial hospitalization or assisted-living program, outpatient treatment, or home care. However, schizophrenia is a chronic illness, and various factors may lead to further hospitalizations for acute exacerbations of its symptoms. These occasions should not be viewed as treatment failures, but as acute crises that require brief, intensive treatment.

Social-Skills Training

Social-skills training (SST) is effective in countering the deficits that result from the social isolation and alienation brought on by schizophrenic symptoms. Social-skills training is initiated when acute symptoms of the illness have been controlled with medication. In a highly structured format, patients engage in basic conversational, assertiveness, heterosocial, and medication-management skills. Training groups are often formed within a structured treatment setting, such as a partial hospital.

■ NURSING ASSESSMENT

For nurses, learning the diagnostic criteria for schizophrenia is important so that patient behavior consistent with these criteria can carefully documented. Nursing care of the patient with schizophrenia is directed toward the patient's responses to an illness that drastically alters one's experience of the environment and of other persons. Nurses understand the individual manifestations of schizophrenia from the patient's point of view, and recognize that the patient's responses are quite consistent with the world as he or she perceives it. A patient's particularly puzzling behavior or verbalization reflects an altered perception of reality and a decreased ability to coordinate and sort information. An individual with schizophrenia is compromised in the way he or she can function both mentally and socially. Environments and persons intolerant of individuals with the processing difficulties characteristic of schizophrenia create further emotional distress, compound the painful experience of the illness, and add to the patient's dysfunction.

The nurse's task is to recognize responses that are consistent with impaired mental processing and to initiate both verbal and environmental interventions that

decrease the need for patients to function in ways beyond their capabilities. No one would think of asking a patient with a congenital limb weakness to sprint or run, yet sometimes patients with impaired mental processing are expected to perform complex tasks of organization. Much of the emotional distress created by the schizophrenic patient's inability to perform what others consider a simple task can be alleviated by providing support during the acute phase of the illness and education following the cessation of symptoms.

From a nursing perspective, the phenomenology of schizophrenia manifests itself in the form of alterations in thinking, alterations in feelings, and alterations in movement and behavior. Nurses consider the experience of the patient as well as the objective signs of the illness. Torrey (1988), a champion of persons with schizophrenia, developed a manual for these persons' families and classified the symptoms of the disease from the patient's point of view. These patient experiences of schizophrenia fit the model of altered thoughts, feelings, and behaviors. Considering patients' experiences instills compassion and empathy, and serves as a guide for developing patient-centered nursing interventions.

All of the manifestations discussed here do not appear in every patient with schizophrenia. The intensity of each symptom increases with continued stress or decreases with successful treatment.

ALTERATIONS IN THINKING

Alteration of the Senses

The patient with schizophrenia feels a sensory overload, may feel flooded with perceptions of light and color, and may be overwhelmed and awed. There may be an acuity of smells, sounds, and colors. Background sounds come forward and are indistinguishable from a focus of attention. Later in the illness, senses are dulled and the world seems flat. The following passage is an example of the subjective experience of sensory alteration:

> My focus was a bit bizarre. I could do portraits of people who were walking down the street. I remembered license numbers of cars we were following coming into Vancouver. We paid $3.57 for gas. The air machine made eighteen dings while we were there (Vonnegut, 1975, p. 107).

Patients' observed behavior may include pacing and moving about. There may be an inability to concentrate or remain in an area, particularly a noisy one. Patients may state that they are having a mystical experience or express the belief that they possess god-like powers.

Inability to Interpret Incoming Sensations

Patients with schizophrenia describe difficulty in understanding the meaning of sentences. Instead, they hear individual words and attempt to derive meaning from them. They may have difficulty connecting visual and auditory perceptions, such as in television viewing. They cannot hold strings of sequences together. Patients with the illness state that they must keep specific steps of a process in their head in order not to forget them, or that they feel stupid because they cannot perform simple tasks such as making a bed, playing cards, or assembling a puzzle. This same difficulty is what results in the loss of ability to perform activities of daily living and to function even in simple jobs. Patients' subjective experiences may resemble the following example:

> If I do something like going for a drink of water, I've got to go over every detail—find cup, walk over, turn tap, fill cup, turn tap off, drink it. I keep building up a picture. I have to change the picture each time. I got to make the old picture move. I can't concentrate. I can't hold things. Something else comes in, various things. It's easier if I stay still.
> (Torrey, 1988, p. 32)

In their observed behavior, patients with schizophrenia may appear to be unable to make a decision and seem apt to freeze when called upon to do so. This behavior might have been labeled "ambivalence" in the past. Patients may respond to fragments of sentences, refuse participation, and withdraw from others. Linen may remain in a pile on the bed, clothing go unwashed, and self-care deteriorate.

Loose Associations

The inability to distinguish concepts by meaning produces **loose associations** in the mind of the patient with schizophrenia. Words become associated through some common characteristic, often known only to the patient. In the following example, the patient was asked to define contentment.

> Contentment? Well uh, contentment, well the word contentment, having a book perhaps, perhaps your having a subject, perhaps you have a chapter of a reading, but when you come to the word "men" you wonder if you should be content with men in your life and then you get to the letter "T" and you wonder if you should be content having tea by yourself or be content with having it in a group or so forth
> (Sass, 1992, p. 179).

Concreteness

Often seen in responses to simple proverbs, **concreteness** is the ability to abstract meaning from a situation. The following example reflecting concreteness of thinking in schizophrenia is a patient's response to the proverb "people who live in glass houses shouldn't throw stones":

> Because they might be put out for the winter.
> Because it might bust the wall and people would see you
> People who live in glass houses shouldn't forget people who live in stone houses and shouldn't throw glass.
> (Torrey, 1988, p. 34).

Hallucinations

Hallucinations are defined as sensory perceptions (sight, sound, smell, taste or touch) that occur in the absence of an external stimulus to the corresponding sensory organ. Hallucinations in schizophrenia are most often auditory (hearing voices or sounds), but may also be visual (seeing objects or persons), gustatory (tasting foods or chemicals), olfactory (sensing smells), or tactile (feeling skin sensations). An example of hallucination in schizophrenia is provided by the following statement:

> "Sometimes more and more Voices [sic] chimed in, until all the Voices joined into a horrendous crowd, an appalling cheering section that had suddenly turned into a riot. These crowds of voices were loud, painfully loud. When I heard them coming, I would run for my Walkman. But often it was no use. They would scream and shout over even a rock tape turned up to 10.
> (Schiller, 1994, p. 150).

In their observed behavior, patients with schizophrenia may be seen mouthing words when no one else is immediately present. They may have animated conversations, react in fear and anger to some internal stimulus, take actions in response to internal vocal commands, or glance around suspiciously.

Delusions

A **delusion** is "a fixed false belief maintained despite experience and evidence to the contrary" (Rosenthal and McGuiness, 1986). Individuals with persecutory delusions feel that they are being victimized. Beliefs that one is evil or worthless are called negative delusions, and beliefs that one is special, important, or has special powers are called grandiose delusions. The beliefs that outside forces are manipulating the mind or body are called delusions of control. Beliefs involving manipulation of body parts or organs are called somatic delusions. The following example is of early delusion formation in schizophrenia:

> A patient noticed the waiter in the coffee-house; he skipped past him so quickly and uncannily. He noticed odd behaviour in an acquaintance which made him feel strange; everything in the street was so different, something was bound to be happening. A passer-by gave such a penetrating glance, he could be a detective. then there was a dog who seemed hypnotised, a kind of mechanical dog made of rubber . . . (Sass, 1992, p. 53)

Compare this to an advanced delusion:

> We were never born. My sister and I were made by a machine. She is not my sister, but she is nearer than a sister and we belong together by machine rules. . . . The machine is called the "invisible." We do not know how it works. . . . We do not see the machine. Sometimes it changes to a person and back again. (Sass, 1992, p. 309)

The observed behaviors of patients who have delusions are guided by false beliefs. For example, a patient who thinks he is being poisoned will not eat. Persons with schizophrenic delusions may perform strange rituals with food, objects, or clothing. A belief that others are trying to hurt the patient may result in defensive aggression.

ALTERATIONS IN FEELINGS

Altered Sense of Self

The sense of body boundaries and personal space is disrupted in schizophrenia. People with the illness frequently need increased personal space, and sometimes need hardly any at all. Most nurses have known patients who move very close to them when making a request or, conversely, demand that staff members keep their distance. Additionally, patients with schizophrenia sometimes experience alienation of body parts. The following example illustrates the altered sense of self that is often seen in the illness:

> That's the rain. I could be the rain. That chair . . . that wall. It's a terrible thing for a girl to be a wall (Sass, 1992, p. 311).

Changes in Emotions

Inappropriate, flat, or exaggerated affect is commonly seen in persons with schizophrenia. They also report fear and excessive guilt. In late stages of the illness, however, there is no observable affect. Following are two examples of affect in schizophrenia:

> I had to die to keep from dying: I know that sounds crazy but one time a boy hurt my feelings very much and I wanted to jump in front of a subway. Instead I went a little catatonic so I wouldn't feel anything (Sass, 1992, p. 310).

> I used to feel emotions like physical pain and I couldn't stand it. So I blocked off. I can't empathize with people. I can't work because there is nothing in me. Perhaps my nervous tissue has been destroyed . . . I used to think everyone else was an automaton. Then I saw them relating to one another and I realized I was the automaton (Sass, 1992, p. 310)

ALTERATIONS IN MOVEMENT AND BEHAVIOR

In schizophrenia, **catatonia** is the most dramatic change in movement. The patient remains motionless and demonstrates a phenomenon called "waxy flexibility": for example, if one moves the arm of a catatonic patient, it remains in the new position. Neuroleptic medications may be responsible for many of the movement alterations seen in schizophrenia; these alterations must be differentiated from movements caused by the illness itself. Brain involvement can also result in repetitive ritualistic movements, tics, and general awkwardness or clumsiness.

■ NURSING INTERVENTIONS

GENERAL PRINCIPLES

- Maintain a non-judgmental attitude. Be aware of your own fears, biases, and prior beliefs about individuals with odd or eccentric speech. Identify patient strengths and successes as soon as possible.
- Maintain a curious attitude. Attempt to understand the speech and behavior of patients from the perspective of their world. Recognize that these responses make sense to patients with schizophrenia, given the distortion of their perceptions.
- Develop trust by being honest and keeping agreements with the patient. Recognize that the patient's heightened perceptions and inability to filter out stimuli may make the patient aware of staff members' subtle facial and body movements.
- Present your reality without challenging the patient's reality. Once trust is established, patients are more willing to accept a reality they can't experience. Acknowledge their experience and ask them to consider the possibility of distortion caused by their illness.

- Promote and create structure. Avoid making demands for the performance of complex tasks or problem solving. Use written and verbal cues to help patients organize time and space. Provide assistance with self-care.
- Carefully assess patients for side-effects of neuroleptic medications and distinguish bizarre behavior, mannerisms, flatness, and catatonia from dystonic or slowed movements and muscular rigidity caused by medications.
- Maintain awareness of personal space and body boundaries. Set limits on intrusive behavior. Monitor the environment.
- Advocate increased or reduced medication doses, as appropriate, and treatment of medication side-effects.

Alterations of the Senses

Environmental Interventions. Environmental interventions for patients with schizophrenia include decreasing stimuli, monitoring the noise level in the room (e.g., television, stereo systems, loudspeakers), and reducing unnecessary noises. Remove the patient from a noisy, busy area, and reintroduce the patient to the area when activity in the area decreases.

Verbal Interventions. Speak directly and softly to patients, and assess whether they can focus on the sound of your voice. Use therapeutic listening. Express one thought or request at a time.

Inability to Synthesize and Respond

Environmental Interventions. The first step for patients whose thinking is slowed or confused is to simplify the environment. Perform tasks with the patient and assess his or her level of functioning. Allow the patient to remain on the periphery of groups, be sure that schedules are posted and followed, and provide the patient with a personal schedule that allows for quiet time. Assign a team member to help the patient follow the schedule.

Verbal Interventions. Simplify sentences to one complete thought, and allow the patient time to respond. Interact in quiet areas that are free from distractions. Use restatement and reflection to emphasize and clarify your thoughts.

Loose Associations

Attempt to clarify what you hear. Emphasize the most relevant theme and direct the patient back to it. Let patients know you do not always see the connection between their expressions, and let them know what you do understand that they are trying to express something.

Delusions

Environmental Interventions. Assess the patient's responses to environmental stimuli. Be alert for suspiciousness. If the patient is paranoid, be aware of spatial distances in groups and activities. Allow the patient to sit on the periphery and leave an activity if necessary. Be aware of potentially dangerous objects that might be used as weapons by a patient who feels highly threatened. Observe and treat increased levels of anxiety with PRN medication. Allow the patient an appropriate degree of choice (e.g., opening medication packets in the patient's presence; giving unopened food packets).

Verbal Interventions. Do not challenge patients' delusions. Rather, respond to their expressed feelings. Acknowledge that their beliefs may be very frightening to them.

Altered Sense of Self

Assess the patient's use of personal space: set limits if the patient is intrusive, and maintain distance if the patient is fearful. Be very judicious with the use of touch; it can be misinterpreted and create fear and anxiety. Always ask permission to touch patients. When used appropriately, touch can be highly therapeutic, since patients with schizophrenia are often socially isolated.

Changes in Emotions

Recognize that patients with schizophrenia may not be able to express emotions appropriately; assess their feelings and respond to the expressed content. Assess the environment for emotional stimulation, and monitor and manage others' inappropriate responses to the patient. For example, set limits on negative comments and ridicule.

Changes in Movement and Behavior

Provide opportunities for the patient to have movement and exercise. Assess rituals performed at specific times (e.g., meals, medication times, bedtime). Promote privacy and set limits if the patient displays inappropriate sexual behavior (e.g., public masturbation, inappropriate touching). Explore the meaning of the patient's behavior to the patient, and assess the patient for medication side-effects.

■ NOTES FROM A STUDENT'S JOURNAL*

DAY 1

I arrive on the fourth floor of the psychiatric unit and am told to report to the east wing, which is the locked ward. My assigned patient is Pam, a 20-year-old college student for whom everybody on the staff has expressed fondness. I look through her chart first. It shows a record of an acute psychotic episode and an evaluation to rule out paranoid schizophrenia. We haven't covered that yet; what if I say the wrong thing and make her worse? I can't stay here in the nurses' station any longer. I must go find Pam.

I introduce myself to Pam. Is this the patient of whom everyone is so fond? I see a young, disheveled woman. Her face is a mask and her eyes are penetrating. She paces the hall as if she must get somewhere.

E CASE EXAMPLE

Ron is a 21-year-old pre-medical student who was brought to the emergency center 3 days ago for bizarre behavior and property destruction. He smashed all of the electronic equipment in his dormitory room, screaming that the "viruses must be destroyed." He is currently taking only one college course, because during the previous semester his grades dropped significantly. He stated that he had trouble concentrating. He visited the campus counselor briefly and refused to continue, stating that his problems had been caused by stress and that a decreased course load was the answer. During that time, his girlfriend of 6 months transferred to another college and expressed a desire to discontinue their relationship. This semester, Ron isolated himself and spent many hours reading books about surveillance and viral warfare.

Ron's personal care deteriorated about three months ago, and he sometimes wore the same clothes for 3 days at a time. He stopped making his bed and his side of his dormitory room became littered with trash and uneaten food. His roommate would clean the room, but became disgusted and moved to an off-campus apartment with a group of friends.

About a week ago, Ron began warning other students that enemies had planted deadly viruses in electronic equipment and that the viruses would be activated when music with certain notes would be played. He had elaborate explanations for this and stated that the voice of Lister had told him that he was "chosen" to save the world. Prior to his admission he began smashing radios and stereo equipment and was restrained by fellow students when he attempted to smash a portable stereo that was playing at a party. He was brought to the emergency room in leather restraints and involuntarily committed to the psychiatric unit. Following the admission interview, he was sedated and placed in restraints in a quiet room. Based on his history and presenting behavior Ron was diagnosed with a psychosis. All screens for drug reactions were negative. He was assessed by the internist and cleared for treatment with medication. He was begun on sedatives and neuroleptic medications and was in physical control of himself by the second hospital day. He was still fearful and suspicious of electronic equipment, but did not display any destructiveness.

DSM-IV Diagnosis: Schizophrenia

Nursing Diagnosis: Potential for harm to self or others

Goal: Ron will not hurt self, others or property, while hospitalized.

Interventions:
- Assess the patient's level of agitation.
- Attempt to determine the source and meaning of the patient's fears.
- Maintain an environment free of harmful objects.
- Model appropriate problem-solving behavior.
- Model appropriate tone of voice, maintain personal distance.
- Set limits on aggressive behavior: use verbal interventions and time-outs as appropriate. Use seclusion or restraints if milder measures fail or if danger is imminent.
- Evaluate the patient's anxiety level and administer a sedative PRN if one has been ordered.
- Encourage appropriate physical activity

Outcomes:
- The patient will demonstrate relaxed body posture
- The patient will verbalize alternatives to aggression
- The patient will cooperate with limit-setting even if he doesn't agree.
- The patient will verbalize feelings, rather than act out
- The patient will remain safe

Nursing diagnosis: Altered sensory perception: auditory hallucinations.

Goal: Patient will question validity of hallucinatory voices and report to nurse.

Interventions:
- Observe for listening behavior and ask patient if he is hearing voices.
- Assess for effect of external stimuli.
- Decrease stimuli: provide quiet space; or increase stimuli: engage patient in alternative activities, particularly those that require talking.
- Verbalize your understanding that the patient hears voices, but that you do not share them with him.
- Assist patient to identify situations that provoke hallucinations.

Outcomes:
- The patient will question validity of voices.
- The patient will verbalize precipitating stressors.
- The patient will engage in alternative activities when hearing voices.
- The patient will report hallucinatory voices to nurse.

But there is nowhere to go. The doors at both ends of the long hallway are locked. Pam is stuck here, whether she wants to be or not.

We talk, but we don't have a conversation. I ask questions. Sometimes she answers; sometimes she doesn't. I want to get to know the real Pam, the college student who majored in dance. But she's answering questions that I'm not asking. "How are you feeling now?" I ask. "I was dead and they brought me back to life," she answers. "How long did you study ballet?" "I'm a vampire and I'm ready to fly," she replies. We pace down the hallway and I try repeatedly to reach her. But we are in two different worlds. Suddenly, for a moment, Pam the college student emerges. She holds on to the hall railing and shows me ballet steps: first position, second position. But the young student is soon gone. Pam the patient returns.

I leave the locked doors and attend an activity. I am discouraged. I return to Pam to say goodbye for the day, and I am amazed: She holds out her hand to shake mine. She says "Thank you" and almost smiles. This, then, is the person of whom everybody is fond: the young girl who they want to heal. We finally have a connection!

DAY 2

I am anxious to see Pam. I'm sure she'll be better today. Didn't she shake my hand and say thank you? I check the chart; nothing new. I find Pam. She is agitated. "They" are out to get her. Video cameras are following her. "Someone" tried to kill her yesterday. Oh Pam, where are you today? Yesterday you looked me in the eyes and saw me. Come back to my world. But no, there is nothing today but lying down, smoking, and intense agitation.

Today, I am present but not in the same reality as Pam. I am tolerated because I am not a threat, but I am useless. I cannot help her out of her world, wherever that is. She is agitated about making a choice, but doesn't know what the choices are. As I leave for the day, I realize that I have not even seen a glimpse of the Pam who smiled and shook my hand yesterday.

DAY 3 (1 WEEK LATER)

I am again assigned to Pam. I noticed from her chart that she has been started on a new medication. But I remember my last visit and expect nothing. I am greeted by a stranger. Pam is actually looking at me. She asks about my college. Perhaps she will transfer to it, she says. She has friends there. She knows that she was having delusions; she knows that she has to find a way to cope with stress and that she has to forget about her former boyfriend. She wants to go home. Pam, welcome back! You are emerging from a depth from which I thought it was impossible to climb out. Come back just

a little bit more. Goodbye, Pam, for today. I am so happy for you.

---

*From: JoAnne Dow, Allentown College of St. Francis de Sales, BSN, 1996.

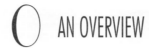 AN OVERVIEW

- Schizophrenia is a complex and often misunderstood illness that manifests in disturbances of cognitive and social functioning. Its cause is unknown, but it is believed to result from a combination of genetic and environmental factors.

- Symptoms of schizophrenia result from biochemical alterations in the limbic system of the brain. An excess of dopamine results in problems in cognitive processing, perception, and mood.

- Stressors contributing to the development of symptoms of schizophrenia include major life events, family conflict, and environmental noise.

- Personal and environmental protectors can reduce some of the disturbing manifestations of schizophrenia. These protectors include coping mechanisms, compliance with medication, family regimens, education, problem solving, and social support.

- Schizophrenia has no cure. Psychopharmacological medications alleviate many of the symptoms and enable the patient to live a productive life. These medications have many undesirable side effects. Environmental adjustment and coping skills contribute to adjustment.

- Hospitalization may be periodically necessary for crisis intervention. Treatment is provided in partial hospital, residential, and outpatient settings.

- Nursing assessment considers the patient's experience. Interventions are directed toward decreasing the stress resulting from attempting to adapt to the world while experiencing disturbances in thoughts and feelings.

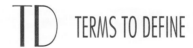 TERMS TO DEFINE

- catatonia
- concreteness
- delusions
- dopamine
- hallucinations

- high level of expressed emotion
- loose associations
- negative symptoms
- positive symptoms
- schizophrenia
- social skills training
- stress-vulnerability model

Q STUDY QUESTIONS

1. Which of the following is NOT one of Bleuler's "4As"?
   a. Association
   b. Autism
   c. Attitude
   d. Affect

2. Which of the following is a negative symptom of schizophrenia?
   a. Loose association
   b. Anhedonia
   c. Delusion
   d. Hallucination

3. Biologic theories state that the symptoms of schizophrenia are in part caused by dysfunction of which of the following neurotransmitters?
   a. Dopamine
   b. Norepinephrine
   c. Epinephrine
   d. GABA

4. In the stress-vulnerability theory, which of the following is considered an environmental protector?
   a. Coping skills
   b. Family education
   c. Antipsychotic medication
   d. Symptom monitoring

5. Which of the following outcome statements would be appropriate for a patient who is hearing voices?
   a. Client will be totally free of voices.
   b. Client will question the reality of voices.
   c. Client will identify the source of the voices.
   d. Client will learn to enjoy the voices.

6. In caring for a patient who has a disturbance of body boundaries, it is important to
   a. speak clearly.
   b. monitor personal distance.
   c. repeat to the client what you have heard.
   d. close the door when entering a room.

7. Match each phrase in the first column with an illustrative statement in the second column.

   a. loose association
   b. delusion
   c. hallucination
   d. concrete thinking

   1. People who live in glass houses should not forget people who live in stone houses and shouldn't throw glass.
   2. I am a prince from another country; I was kidnapped.
   3. The voice of Buddy Holly is calling me.
   4. The theater is not life. I know the customs of the theater. The theater becomes a habit. Life does not. I do not like the theater with a square stage, I like a round stage . . . like an eye.

■ REFERENCES

Andreasen NC, Carpenter WT: Diagnosis and classification of schizophrenia. *Schizophr Bull* 1993; 19(2):199–214.

Andreasen NC, Nopolos P, Schultz S, Miller D, Gupta S, Swayze V, and Flwum M: Positive and negative symptoms of schizophrenia: Past, present and future. *Acta Psychiatr Scand,* 90 (Suppl 384) 1994; 384):51–59.

Bellack AS, Mueser KT: Psychosocial treatment for schizophrenia. *Schizophr Bull* 1993; 19(2):317–336.

Bowden WD: First person account: The onset of paranoia. *Schizophr Bull* 1993; 19(1):165–167.

Breslin NA: Treatment of schizophrenia: Current practice and future promise. *Hosp Commun Psychiatry* 1992; 43:877–885.

Cleghorn JH, Albert ML: Modular disjunction in schizophrenia: A framework ofr a pathological psychophysiology, *in* Kales A, Stefanis CN, Talbott JA (eds): *Recent Advances in Schizophrenia.* New York, Springer-Verlag, 1990.

Clements K, Turpin G: Vulnerability models and schizophrenia: The assessment and prediction of relapse, *in* Birchwood M, & Tarrier N, (eds): *Innovations in the Psychological Management of Schizophrenia.* New York, John Wiley & Sons, 1993.

Group for the Advancement of Psychiatry: *Beyond Symptom Suppression: Improving Long-term Outcomes of Schizophrenia.* Washington, DC, American Psychiatric Press, 1992.

Hoffman RE, McGlashan TH: Parallel distributed processing and the emergence of schizophrenic symptoms. *Schizophr Bull* 1993; 19(1):119–140.

Iqbal N, Schwartz BJ, Cecil A, Zahid I, Canal C: Schizophrenia diagnosis. *Psychiatr Ann* 1993; 23:105–110.

Kales A, Stefanis, CN, Talbott JA (eds): *Recent Advances in Schizophrenia.* New York, Springer-Verlag, 1990.

LaBruzza A.L. *Using DSM-IV: A Clinician's Guide to Psychiatric Diagnosis,* Northvale, N.J., Jason Aronson Inc, 1994, pp. 259–260.

Lehman HE: Current perspectives on the biology of schizophrenia. In Menuck MN, Seeman MV (eds): *New Perspectives in Schizophrenia.* New York, Macmillan, 1985.

Malone, JA: Schizophrenia research update: Implications for nurses. *J Psychosoc Nurs Mental Health Serv* 1990; 28(8):4–6, 8–9.

Muesser KT, Gingerich S: *Coping with Schizophrenia: A Guide for Families.* Oakland, CA, New Harbinger Publications, 1994.

Muesser KT, Gingerich S, Rosenthal CK: Educational family therapy for schizophrenia: A new treatment model for clinical service and research. *Schizophr Res* 1994; 13:99–108.

Neuchterlein, K.H., Dawson, M.E., Ventura, J., Gitlin, M., Subotnik, K.L., Snyder, K.S., Mitz, K., and Bartzokis, G. (1994). The vulnerability/stress model of schizophrenic relapse: A longitudinal study. *Acta Psychiatrica Scandinavica,* 89(Supp. 382), 58–64.

O'Connor FW: A vulnerability-stress framework for evaluating clinical interventions in schizophrenia. *Image* 1994; 26:231–237.

Sass LA: *Madness and Modernism.* New York, Basic Books, 1992.

Shapiro RM: Regional neuropathology in schizophrenia: Where are we? Where are we going? *Schizophr Res* 1993; 10:187–239.

Schiller L, Bennett A: *The Quiet Room.* New York, Warner Books, 1994.

Stirling J: Schizophrenia and expressed emotion. *Perspect Psychiatr Care* 1994; 26(3):18–23.

Torrey EF: *Surviving Schizophrenia: A Family Manual* (Revised edition). New York, Harper & Row, 1988.

Vonnegut M: *The Eden Express.* New York, Praeger Publishers, 1975.

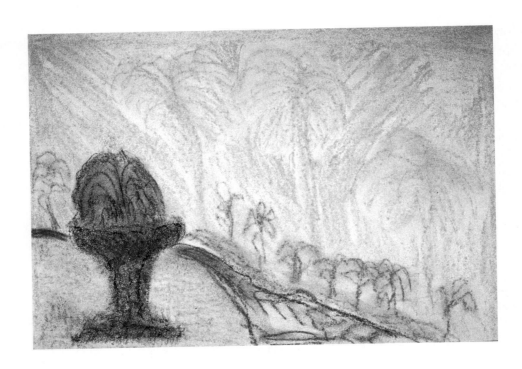

She belonged to no club and was a member of nothing in the world. Frankie had become an unjoined person who hung around in the doorways, and she was afraid.

Carson Smith McCullers (1917–1967)

The Member of the Wedding, 1946

30

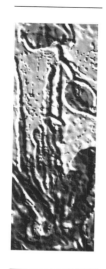

The Seriously Mentally Ill, Homeless Population

Victor A. McGregor

Seriously mentally ill, a term used by the National Center for Mental Health Services, is synonymous with the term severely and persistently mentally ill (SPMI) and the older term chronically mentally disabled. This nomenclature groups together patients with significant functional impairment both socially and occupationally. Many persons in this group suffer from co-morbid disorders of psychotic disorders and substance abuse.

Seriously mentally ill patients—some 500,000 in the United States—were discharged from state hospitals providing long-term care over a period of 20 years as a result of the Community Mental Health Centers Act of 1963. The Act promoted mental-health care in the least restrictive environment, emphasizing comprehensive services and local service delivery. Early intervention and comprehensive services were intended to reduce psychiatric hospitalization and thus reduce its attendant costs.

The mental-health-care delivery system was not prepared for the needs that the Community Mental Health Centers Act imposed on care providers. A structure did not exist to implement the Act, and monies were insufficient to cope with the substantial reorganization of mental-health care that the Act created. Rather than early treatment and services, the shift resulted in a loss of focus on services for seriously mentally ill persons. Thousands of persons were prematurely discharged into communities unprepared to house and manage individuals with serious mental illness (VanderStaay, 1992).

The community mental health movement fostered expansion of the role of the nurse to include individual and group psychotherapy, primary prevention of mental illness, consultation with other nurses in non-psychiatric settings, and helping the families of patients released from psychiatric institutions to understand the nature of serious mental illness. Linda Aiken (1987) emphasized that psychiatric nurses working in a primary-care setting and knowledgeable about anti-psychotic drug management would be the ideal professional for the seriously mentally ill. Nurses could maximize individual psychiatric patients' capacity to function, which is an essential component in caring for patients with incurable illnesses.

The Community Mental Health Centers Act (CMHC) overestimated the seriously mentally ill patient's ability to function in the community, such as keeping psychiatric appointments, taking medicine, calling crisis lines in times of need, applying for services and funds, and engaging in other activities of daily living and self-care. The predictable outcome for these difficult-to-treat clients was often homelessness.

Persons with severe, persistent mental illness are often described in terms similar to those used for homeless persons, as having high rates of unemployment, physical disability, victimization, substance abuse, severe social disaffiliation, frequent contact with the criminal justice system, and subsistence level incomes. Because the numbers in both groups continue to increase, homelessness imposes a considerable additional burden on the lives of severely mentally ill individuals (Amussen, 1994; Cohen and Thompson, 1992).

■ THE SERIOUSLY MENTALLY ILL

Many seriously mentally ill individuals suffer from continuous schizophrenia, which means there has been no remission of symptoms during the recorded period of their illness. Schizophrenia is a seriously disabling psychiatric disorder. Kay (1991) suggested that schizophrenia be viewed along four dimensions: a positive syndrome, a negative syndrome, a depressive syndrome (feelings of guilt and depression), and an excitement/impulsivity syndrome (excitement, tension, and poor impulse control). The positive symptoms are identified as persecutory delusions, delusions of reference, delusions of being controlled, delusions of mind reading, tangential thinking, loose associations, hearing voices commenting or conversing, and visual hallucinations. The negative symptoms include an unchanging facial expression, a paucity of peer relationships, few recreational interests or activities, lack of persistence at school or a job, poor grooming and hygiene, lack of expressiveness, low energy, and difficulty in forming close personal relationships.

Seriously mentally ill persons refer to enduring (usually lasting more than a year) self-care deficits in all of the biopsychosocial spheres. These deficits fluctuate according to the effect of treatment. However, although the causes are probably multifactoral, neurobiological changes in the brains of persons with schizophrenia and other serious psychiatric illnesses have been confirmed through the following advanced technologies:

- Computed tomography (CT scan). A sophisticated x-ray of brain structures, which has revealed larger ventricles in schizophrenia.
- Nuclear magnetic resonance imaging (MRI). A three dimensional image without exposure to radiation; and which is expensive, but is replacing CT scans.
- Positron emission tomography (PET scan). A technique in which radioactive atoms are introduced into the brain and produce images reflecting metabolic activity in specific areas of the brain. In schizophrenia there is low activity in the prefrontal lobes, which govern planning, abstract thinking, and expression of feeling. The PET scan is highly flexible and sensitive, but very expensive. One observation based on PET scans is that schizophrenic patients who are right handed have greater cerebral blood flow to the left hemisphere of the brain when they perform tasks that ordinarily produce greater flow in the right hemisphere. This suggests more rationality, but may be less related to the disease itself.

■ MANAGED CARE

The concept of managed care has developed from models of health maintenance organizations (HMOs), which aim to provide comprehensive health care services at reduced cost. The principles of managed care are based on prevention services, early intervention, and continuity of care. These concepts are very similar to those promoted in the 1960s as outcomes of Community Mental Health Centers and the deinstitutionalization of psychiatric patients (Kane, 1995). To avoid the pitfalls of deinstitutionalization, Kane (1995) recommends that programs be developed to educate health-care teams in interdisciplinary collaboration; that safeguards be placed in the system to prevent the usurpation of mental-health-care money in favor of other health-care services; and that strategies be developed for supporting and maintaining psychiatric patients in the community (Kane, 1995).

CASE MANAGEMENT AS INTERVENTION

Case management is a multidisciplinary strategy that the National Institute of Mental Health (NIMH) identified in the mid-1970s for ensuring the continuous availability of appropriate forms of assistance through the Community Support System (CSS).

Case managers are public-health advocates and agents through whom the seriously mentally ill can find and obtain appropriate resources in the community. As community mental health workers, case managers make assessments, home visits, and referrals. They coordinate resources, provide crisis intervention, and provide specific psychoeducation such as social-skills training and family support. In 1980 Lamb recommended that the case manager also be the primary psychiatric therapist for homeless mentally ill patients in the community in order to obtain in-depth knowledge of these persons' needs and strengths. This recommendation was a result of the finding that homeless mentally ill men had fewer long-term therapists than their domiciled counterparts (Lamb, Bachrach and Kass, 1992).

The case load for case managers varies according to intensity of need and program resources. Case managers have to be well informed about the procedures needed to procure entitlements and other disability benefits for which their patients may be eligible. (See Chapter 44, Case Management.)

NURSE CASE MANAGERS

Nurse case managers represent about 10% of all case managers, and are trained in psychiatric and community mental-health nursing. They perform all of the therapeutic activities described above as well as providing health and mental-health education and health teaching, and leading educational groups on topics such as substance abuse and medication. The medication-related activities of nurse case managers include being responsible for ordering stock supplies of medication; administration of medication, particularly long-acting depot injections of antipsychotic drugs; record keeping; and monitoring for drug side-effects and adverse reactions. Because of the high cost of the newer antipsychotic medications, the nurse case manager assists in the application process for Medicaid so that patients can have their prescriptions filled at a community pharmacy.

Case managers, nurses, and community mental-health workers including physicians have often had to deal with the expected feelings of frustration and even powerlessness in working with a system that has serious flaws in terms of the needs of patients with serious mental-health problems. Nurse case managers are new to this field, and their salaries will need to be addressed in settings in which city and state employees are not paid on a salary scale competitive with that of in-patient nursing. In 1988 the American Nurses Association (ANA) recommended the merging of case management with nursing as an effective tertiary preventive service for the homeless mentally ill population. Nurses are well prepared in the collaborative practice model for case management (Bower, 1992). They bring to their practice a theoretical background in the biological and social sciences and humanities, as well as in health maintenance, disease processes, and medication administration.

ASSERTIVE COMMUNITY TREATMENT (ACT)

A treatment model that emphasizes strong collaboration between service providers is the program of **assertive community treatment** (PACT). It was developed by Stein and collegues, in 1993, and has been shown to be effective for the seriously mentally ill. It is becoming a "gold standard" for out-patient services for this population; however, when the burden of homelessness is added to serious mental illness, the odds of achieving the same success as with inpatients decrease. Little outcome research has been applied to its use of the Program of Assertive Community Treatment with the homeless seriously mentally ill population.

Complicating the problem of homelessness is distrust of authority among this population, and disenchantment with mental-health service providers. Dato and Rafferty (1985) argues that a model for care of the ill is insufficient if the staff are not empathically attuned to the patients. Program effectiveness depends on the quality of both the staff and patient relationships that develop over time. Collaboration is therefore not only a vital ingredient of the nurse–patient relationship, but

also an essential characteristic of the nurse's interaction with the care team and the team's interaction with the numerous organizations in the community. The Assertive Community Treatment team interfaces with organizations such as universities, governmental health agencies, medical clinics, state and community hospitals, community support programs, and the local Alliance for the Mentally Ill.

The Baltimore PACT project underscores the importance of a joint effort in community mental-health care. Using a multi-disciplinary team of physicians, nurses, social workers, family outreach workers, and people familiar with the experience of the seriously mentally ill, the project's staff-to-client ratio is 1:10. The project offers continuous availability, no limitation on treatment duration, strong linkages to housing, medical care, and continuity of care even when the patient is admitted to the hospital. Its philosophy is to be flexible and its primary goal is to engage this patient.

The PACT model does not replace the case-management model. Rather, it is adapted to complement and enhance the case-management model. Its effectiveness can be measured in the reduced rate of hospital recidivism, psychiatric emergency room visits, substance abuse relapses, increased medication compliance, and socialization among the patients it treats.

RECIDIVISM AND THE SERIOUSLY MENTALLY ILL

The mental-health system is haunted by what is known as the "revolving door syndrome." This phenomenon is a pattern of repeated hospitalizations with short discharges into the community. **Recidivism,** or relapse, happens for a variety of reasons.

The first reason is the patients' non-compliance with medication regimens and lack of insight into their mental illness. The second reason is a lack of careful discharge planning, follow-up calls, and linkages between institutions and community placement agencies. Many in-patient staff members (and probably many policy makers as well) are unfamiliar with the resources in their community and such problems as easy access to street drugs. Shortages of affordable supervised housing and reductions in single-room occupancy housing (80% in New York City between 1970 and 1990) are additional reasons for relapse of the seriously mentally ill.

MEDICATION ISSUES

Patients' attitudes about medication are a critical issue with the seriously mentally ill. Because patient attitudes vary, it is beneficial in medication groups to let those patients with positive attitudes toward pharmacotherapy explain how it has helped them. The seriously mentally ill appreciate personal disclosure as a method of teaching. They are more influenced to continue taking their medications if a peer with whom they can identify talks during group sessions. They often feel that experts lack credibility in terms of life experience with serious psychiatric illness. For this reason, peer counselors are highly valued in teaching and group work with the seriously mentally ill.

Many psychiatric patients associate medications with attempts to control them. They have seen peers with the side-effect called the "thorazine shuffle," uncontrollable mouth writhing, or the over-sedated look of a "zombie." The distorted movement of the hands or feet known as tardive dyskinesia is iatrogenic and a major side-effect of thorazine and similar drugs. Patients may therefore feel some ambivalence about neuroleptic medications. Fortunately, newer antipsychotic medications such as clozaril (Clozapine) and risperidone do not have as many extrapyramidal side effects.

Psychiatric nurses must be sensitive to the feelings of the seriously mentally ill about having to take medications for long periods. Open communication with the prescriber must be encouraged, whether the latter is a nurse practitioner or a psychiatrist. The seriously mentally ill often need an intermediary person to help them understand the purpose of the medication prescribed for them. If possible, switching roles with the prescriber in medication groups is a recommended technique for fostering such understanding.

Titration of medication dosages is ideally done by mutual agreement, although the nurse often has more success in weighing the risk-benefit ratio of various dosages and explaining this to the patient. This is best done on an individual teaching basis, so that personal connection with the patient supports the content of the nurse's message. The timing of the teaching can make a difference in patients' comprehension and retention of knowledge, and such teaching is therefore done when the patient is most receptive.

Nurses' interdisciplinary training in the bio-psycho-social aspects of health care equips them to provide this teaching, which is vital in reducing recidivism (Connolly, 1991).

The methods and patterns of communication of the seriously mentally ill make it extremely difficult for anyone to understand their subjective experiences (Watzlawich, 1967). Schizophrenia, for example, can affect such individuals' communication with health-care personnel to the extent that both parties are convinced that the other is in another realm. When this happens, power struggles emerge over the opposing positions, crisis ensues, and the patient usually has to move out or is moved out for the protection of the others. It is at this point that patients often slide into the downward spiral that leads to homelessness. Families in these situations must weigh the benefits of petitioning for an involuntary admission if the patient is a danger to him- or herself or to others.

Psychiatric emergency services, homeless outreach programs, and mobile crisis teams evaluate the homeless mentally ill for evidence of homicidal or suicidal ideation; a history of physical violence to the self, others, or property; and other key factors revealing their mental status. Questions to be answered are whether the affected individual has understandable speech, is responding to internal stimuli, or is paranoid or hypervigilant. Persons who clearly cannot take care of themselves can be involuntarily committed to a hospital for evaluation. Sometimes a case can be made on the grounds that they such a person is a danger to him- or herself by reason of extreme neglect. Most patients recognize their own irrational behavior after being medicated, and do not hold a grudge. Law enforcement and security officials need to be educated in dealing with the human side of the patient whose thinking and emotions are disorganized. Such education assists in avoiding degrading involuntary commitment, which can result in a strong distrust of the mental-health-care system.

■ CRISIS INTERVENTION

Seriously mentally ill patients may not have the communication skills necessary to ask for the help they need. Moreover, their self-esteem is often too low for them to admit to inner weakness. Yet such patients have high levels of unspoken fear. In order to be a source of emotional security to the seriously mentally ill nurses need to assess their own feelings about working with this population. Although this is easier said than done, it is important for the nurse to be genuine and warm in calming the patient. Because the nature of schizophrenia interferes with patients' ability to block out stress, they may internalize any emotional disturbance in their environment. Their stress can then build unless some lines of communication are kept open. Approaching the patient in a sensitive manner in the early stages of a perceived problem usually helps reduce the intensity of their emotions.

If a gentle human approach fails in a crisis situation, and the patient feels isolated and threatened, a "show of force" (as in numbers of uniformed officers) alone is sometimes enough to enlist cooperation. The nurse must make a decision in conjunction with other available staff members, including the patient's primary therapist and the supervisor. The supervisory nurse makes the final judgment about the course of action to be taken. Crisis management of the seriously mentally ill patient will often demand further steps toward control and safety, according to institutional or organizational procedures. The principle of least restrictive measures is the basis for this. Usually, the seriously mentally ill are not as dangerous as the uninformed public believes, and a trigger to their emotions can often be identified and avoided before their emotions escalate to rage. It is important to watch for the early, non-verbal signs of agitation (e.g., rapid respiration, avoidance of eye contact, or an intense tone of voice).

■ SUBSTANCE ABUSE

The seriously mentally ill have a high incidence of substance abuse. In major metropolitan shelters, this is probably higher than currently estimated, and suggests the need for expertise and programs to address this issue. Nurses must try to understand the motivating factors behind these individuals' use of alcohol or drugs.

If the purpose of the abuse can be identified (e.g., to relieve depression), alternative options can be identified for satisfying that need. The counterproductive effects of the individual's negative behavior can be explained to him or her in a way that communicates care and support. Given the state of mind of a person taking illicit drugs or abusing alcohol, it is understandable that he or she is highly vulnerable to risk-taking behaviors. Substance abuse can lead to loss of control and the risk of violence.

With nowhere to go, and profound feelings of loneliness and sorrow, many homeless persons find substance abuse a temptation hard to resist. When such an individual is engaged in a health-service program, the nurse can set limits to such behavior. The collaborative team approach is critical for fair, firm, caring and consistent treatment of the substance-abusing individual. The team can provide mutual peer review and supervision that is essential when working with the seriously mentally ill. The purpose of such supervision is to help with countertransference feelings when a patient ignores or refuses treatment or relapses.

Working with the seriously mentally ill population will test the nurse's assumptions about her or his ability to effectively help those most in need. High expectations are not to be imposed on the treatment; however, an attitude of confidence in the patient's ability to eventually help him- or herself is necessary. Taking urine specimens for drug screening may be helpful in day-care programs, but the psychiatric nurse's role may be better served by focusing on building positive therapeutic alliances. Continuing education and a good mentor can be an invaluable support for the nurse in coping with the challenges posed by the homeless, seriously mentally ill population.

Statistically, the Twelve Step Program Alcohol Anonymous or Narcotic Anonymous has achieved the best outcomes for those seriously mentally ill individuals who have a substance-abuse problem and are willing and able to try this program (Chapter 31). Unfortunately, many of the mentally ill homeless do not have adequate communication skills for this. In New York State, however, detoxification programs are not allowed to turn a patient away. Specialized longer-term rehabilitation programs are harder to find and usually have a waiting list. If the client is willing and able to get to and participate in an AA Clubhouse, such referrals are recommended. The Clubhouse Program provides a structured opportunity for learning new skills in socializing, and for possible vocational training. Skills such as cooking, typing, computer literacy, and semi-sheltered employment are sometimes available. No state has yet provided adequate community services for the long-term treatment of chronic substance abusers in the seriously mentally ill population.

■ FAMILIES OF THE SERIOUSLY MENTALLY ILL

Families of the seriously mentally ill suffer enormously in trying to cope with such severe illness. Even a high familial tolerance for frustration is often exceeded by the persistent nature of the illness, which not only thwarts progress but may even include relapse when the patient is fully complying with treatment. Support for family members of these patients is available from a patient advocacy organization called the **National Alliance for the Mentally Ill** (NAMI). Founded in 1984, it has more than 140,000 members across the United States. NAMI members lobby to prevent budget cuts for mental health services and to actively promote biological research in mental illness.

NAMI members are committed to decreasing the stigma of serious mental illness because of their own mental anguish in caring for family members with such illness. Their group meetings help families to understand the biological basis of serious mental illness. This prevents parents from self-blame for poor parenting in early childhood. The labeling of parents as "schizophrenogenic," with a high level of expressed emotion, has caused untold harm to parents and families.

Because the emotional cost of having a family member with schizophrenia is incalculable in any event, support groups and psychoeducational groups for these individuals' families are recommended. Family therapy is recommended for understanding the role of the patient in maintaining the family system. The focus on the entire family system prevents blaming any individual member. Unfortunately, not many families of patients in the shelter system have so far been available for family therapy.

The cost of treatment for mental disorders is a focus of great concern for the health-care system, but the economic challenges that families face in caring for a relative with severe mental illness are often overlooked. When someone with a mental illness also has a problem with alcohol or other drugs—as do more than half of all people with schizophrenia at some point in their lives—the economic burden may be even greater (Clark, 1994a,b).

■ HOMELESSNESS

Homelessness, like other issues in mental health, requires definition, and has a theoretical and clinical history. For epidemiological purposes, researchers have defined homelessness as sleeping in public places, bus or train stations, streets, abandoned buildings, parks, beaches, or shelters for any number of nights.

Homelessness may also be viewed in a broader, more abstract perspective as disaffiliation. Disaffiliation refers to a lack of social support structures or friends to whom one can turn in time of need (Breakey, 1992). This definition does not assume that the homeless do not have emotional attachments; most such individuals do not choose to be homeless.

Cohen and Thompson (1992) argue that there is a false dichotomy between the mentally ill homeless and other homeless persons. Recent socio-economic data and political shifts have raised concern for homelessness regardless of whether the affected individual also has a mental illness or not. Advocates for the homeless have recommended focusing on community-level interventions, consumerism, entitlements, and empowerment to combat the problem.

Without minimizing the affected individual's or society's responsibility for homeless, its nature can be viewed at an abstract, meta-psychological level. Postmodern theorists (Foucault 1973; Deleuze and Guattari, 1986) maintain that a transient state of being is an authentic representation of the self. According to this concept, homelessness carries a spiritual meaning that is absent in mainstream, materialistic society. This perspective highlights the extent of spiritual illness in the structure of society that perpetuates the suffering of the poor.

The similarities between modernism and madness are well articulated by Sass (1992). He compares the art of seriously mentally ill individuals (from museums and his own professional practice) with famous art to help the reader develop insight into the ways in which the destiny of "the self" and "the world" are intertwined with homelessness and serious mental illness. In refusing to romanticize schizophrenia, Sass rigorously argues that it echoes the most alienating aspects of modern life.

DEMOGRAPHICS AND STATISTICS ON HOMELESSNESS

It is generally agreed that the number of homeless persons grew dramatically during the 1980s (Link, Phelan, Bresnahan et al., 1995). Hombs and Snyder (1982) claim that the number of homeless in the United States could be as high as 3 million. This is a staggering figure, especially when one knows that the numbers keep increasing. Recent findings on the prevalence of homelessness suggest that the numbers of homeless persons have been seriously undercounted because earlier studies of homeless people did not include persons with a history of homelessness (Link, Susser, Stueve et al., 1994). On any given night there are 24,000 people in New York City's Shelters. In 1992 alone 86,000 different individuals were sheltered within the city's shelter system (CMHS, 1995). Another study found that 239,425 people, or 3.3% of the residents of New York City and 3% of those in Philadelphia had spent some time in a shelter between 1988 and 1991 (Culhane, 1991).

From 1988 to 1992 in New York City, the number of homeless families rose by 32%. The rental subsidy to families on welfare fell by 42% from 1972, while the real cost of housing rose. This alone forced many persons to leave their homes. The epidemiology of homelessness has also being changing in recent years, from the stereotypical "skid row" single or divorced middle-aged male to younger persons of both sexes; 23% were homeless before the age of 18. At least 41% reported physical assault in the home before the age of 18 (not all the projects asked this). Nearly 30% had had an out-of-home placement before the age of 18 and 63% reported they been incarcerated at least once. The cities in which these data were compiled were Baltimore, Boston, New York, and San Diego.

In 1995, the McKinney Demonstration Project found that of homeless persons, 72% were black, 22% Hispanic, 2% white, and 3% other; 60% had not completed high school; 73% had never married; and 21% were veterans, but only 3.9% were receiving Veterans Administration benefits.

The McKinney Demonstration Program Interim Report (CMHS, 1995) on Homeless Adults with Serious Mental Illness described 78% as having had a psychotic disorder and 20% had an affective disorder, 80% reported depressive symptoms in the past 30 days; 55% were on Medicaid, and the usual monthly income was $343.

This population is not homogenous and it is expected that the demographics and personal strengths of this population will vary even more greatly in the future.

It has been estimated that about 30% of the homeless have mental illness (Tessler and Dennis, 1989), although experts in epidemiology report that it has been almost impossible to obtain accurate numbers for this. Many homeless individuals are simply "invisible" to researchers (Dear and Wolch, 1987; Rossi, 1989), either because they cannot be found or are unwilling or unable to cooperate with research studies. Nevertheless, it would seem reasonable to assume that the prevalence of mental illness among the homeless will continue to increase at unprecedented rates, especially if recent reductions in social benefits continue, rents continue to rise, and Medicare is threatened with bankruptcy by the beginning of the 21st century.

Moreover, an increased frequency of physical health problems is being seen in homeless shelters, such as tuberculosis. From 1990 to 1993, about 40% of men in the Columbia Presbyterian Psychiatric Shelter Program tested positive for tuberculosis and about 20% tested positive for human immunodeficiency virus (HIV).

■ SHELTERS AND PRINCIPLES FOR NURSING PRACTICE

Homelessness, housing instability, and inadequate housing are common problems for the seriously mentally ill, especially those with a substance-abuse problem. Many factors contribute to homelessness among the seriously mentally ill. A federal task force studying the problem of homelessness among the seriously mentally ill identified deinstitutionalization, the loss of low-income housing units, fragmentation of responsibility among health-care providers, and limited resources as major contributors to this problem (Outcasts on Main Street, 1992).

Providing housing to the homeless, seriously mentally ill is fraught with problems. They suffer from tremendous stress, social isolation, poverty, frequent contact with the law, and generally poor health (Gounis and Susser, 1990; Isaac and Armet, 1990).

Two conceptual frameworks have been described for organizing housing for persons with persistent and severe mental illness. One such framework is the residential or "level of care" model, which calls for assignment to residences for mentally ill persons. These facilities are linked to treatment centers providing different levels of care and with varying degrees of professional supervision. The assumption is that patients progress through different levels of care until they acquire the skills necessary for independent living (Dixon et al., 1994).

The second framework is that of "supported housing," which is generally independent and not linked to services or treatment. Patient choice and housing availability dictate where patients live, and support services are provided as needed to help patients maintain the housing they choose (Kane, 1995; Torrey, 1988).

CRITICAL TIME INTERVENTION MODEL

The **Critical Time Intervention** (CTI) project in New York was one of five that received funds from the McKinney Research Demonstration Program pool of more than $26.8 million between 1990 and 1994. CTI found that intensive time-limited services during the period of transition from the shelter to permanent housing, and community-based mental health services, produced significantly fewer homeless nights than were found for a control group that received regular treatment (i.e., no special follow-up in the 9-month period after housing placement).

The critical period of adjustment for the homeless and mentally ill is the first several months in community housing, when new relationships have to be forged. Because this is an obviously stressful time for such individuals, extra services are provided to help "bridge" the transition period. Specialists in Critical Time Intervention are case managers who know the patient and the community's resources, which enables them to provide a stable linkage between the shelter and small community care agencies. The case manager follows a client for 9 months after the latter leaves the shelter, calling weekly and checking with the contact personnel at the care agency until the client is stable. The case manager helps not only the client but also the client's new caregivers to understand what the client has learned while in the shelter program. The case manager is then available for any crisis that may arise. He or she may be called by the client or the new staff for assistance.

THE FORT WASHINGTON MEN'S SHELTER

The Fort Washington Men's Shelter in New York City is based on a Critical Time Intervention model. Referrals for community mental-health support services are made from the intake interview. The shelter program provides a day program with case management and follow-up during the critical period. It has a census of about 200 men with serious mental illness, who attend the day program on a voluntary basis.

Any shelter resident who has a history of mental illness or otherwise seems disturbed is referred to the program for screening. The resident attends for one week while being informally observed; during this time, the program team decides whether to enroll the resident. The resident is accepted if it is felt that he can benefit from the program. Once accepted, he is assigned a case manager. The psychiatric nurse then sets up an appointment for a physical examination and ensures that follow-up appointments are kept. Sometimes this is not as easy as might be expected, since psychotic clients may insist that they are in good health, and therefore see no need for an examination. City policy, however, requires that all clients be tested for tuberculosis. Documentation of test results and those of the physical examination in the client's chart is the responsibility of the nurse. If a client refuses any injections, including the purified protein derivative (PPD) test for tuberculosis, an effort is made to obtain a chest X-ray.

The psychiatric nurse, with the psychiatrist or prescribing nurse practitioner, must first determine which residents of the shelter have the greatest need for immediate care and medication. During the assessment, the nurse inquires whether the client has been taking any medication or recalls where and when he last received medication. Nurses verify the medication name, dose, and frequency of dosing. They also inquire about the client's insurance coverage, and specifically about Medicaid. Those who have coverage that pays for medication from a local pharmacy have the opportunity to receive the newer anti-psychotic agents. Many mental-health programs cannot afford to pay for risperidone (Risperdal) for many psychotic clients, and a less costly medication may therefore be ordered until entitlements are procured. Homeless seriously mentally ill clients are usually not prescribed clozapine (Clozaril) until a more stable housing placement is arranged for them so that their weekly white blood cell counts can be monitored to prevent dyscrasia. Two percent develop agranulocytosis.

Initially, clients are more willing to take oral than injectable medication, but as the therapeutic alliance develops, they became more willing to try injections of long-acting antipsychotic medications. The independence that these afford by obviating daily dosing usually elicits a favorable response from the client. The nurse case manager writes up short treatment goals and documents medication compliance and any side effect. That will foster the client's full engagement in the program. The program has four weekly groups covering medication, money management, housing, and substance abuse.

A psychosocial summary of the client's history is completed and an assessment of the client's living skills is made in order to suggest the appropriate level of supervision needed in housing placement. A New York City Housing application form is completed, since the city must approve this before the client can be considered ready for housing placement. The placement locations range from apartments for more highly functional

clients through single room occupancies (SRO) quarters, structured community residences, and transitional living communities. The latter, although only temporary residences, are considerably better than a shelter. They provide substance-abuse counseling and a variety of community services in preparation for permanent placement.

Most often, housing begins with a well-structured community residence that will ensure that the client's basic needs are being met. The residence supervises the client's cleaning duties, laundering, meal preparation, and other essential activities, common social activities such as sharing telephones and television watching. Most community residences of this kind will automatically deduct a third to a half of the client's income for rent and services. Clients are told that they will have an opportunity to work their way up to more independent housing placements as their functioning improves.

Nurse case-management services are necessary for planning and structuring clients' activities while they are still in the shelter. The nurse case manager completes application forms for entitlements such as Social Security, Supplemental Security Income, Social Security Disability Benefits, food stamps, and Medicaid, all of which help the client after placement in the community.

Supplemental Security Income is paid to persons who are both poor and disabled (or elderly or blind). Social Security Disability Benefits are in some cases applicable to dependents too, for persons who have worked for usually 10 years or 40 quarters. In New York, if clients receive over $550 they are not eligible for Medicaid and will need to pay for their own medication or presumably buy into a private insurance. Medicare is deducted from anything over $550 but it only covers inpatient hospitalization (some cases cover up to $48 of a private psychiatrist's fee, which is usually around at least $150) so domiciled clients are expected to be serviced in their catchment area clinic. Some clients from the shelter who do not have any public assistance are given tokens to go to the nearest public hospital outpatient clinic and pharmacy.

Some clients are eligible for Medicare coverage after 2 years of persistent serious mental illness. While the client is in the shelter, the nurse makes referrals to outpatient clinics for follow up of infectious diseases such as human immunodeficiency virus infection. The care team relies on the nurse for this, since most case managers do not have any medical training. Client education is conducted throughout the placement process and even afterward. The nurse responsible for critical time intervention may provide simple reminders to the client about "paying the rent as soon as he get receives his support check."

ENTRY PROCEDURE

Link, Susser, Steuve and colleagues (1994) have written about winning the confidence of the homeless seriously mentally ill. Identifying a positive attribute in the client facilitates this process. The timing of efforts to gain the client's attention can also facilitate the process. The most vulnerable point for a homeless, mentally ill individual is at the time of entry into a shelter, when he or she often feels demoralized and may be most receptive to outreach (Susser, 1990).

The second step needed to engage the seriously mentally ill requires warmth and the creation of a positive impression. Such individuals are often timid and introverted. The nurse must initially compensate for this by initiating contact and establishing communication. The content is not as important as the emotional exchange. A respectful nodding of the head may be more effective than a superficial cliché about the weather. Because the homeless and seriously mentally are typically not used to verbal praise, positive reinforcement is effective in strengthening their self-esteem. Residents of the Fort Washington men's shelter, for example, value being treated with respect, as do all people. More likely than not, they have had little experience with being respected, since many are not only homeless and seriously mentally ill, but also have a substance abuse problem and perhaps a criminal record. This is where an understanding nurse can make a vital difference in helping a highly introverted client to risk opening up and re-experiencing human feeling. Susser and colleagues (1990) underscore that working with this population requires a significant modification of traditional interactive techniques and clinical strategies. The nurse's role is to facilitate an emotional connection with the client without violating professional boundaries or the institution's policies.

E CASE EXAMPLE

Alex is a 26-year-old single, homeless black male who was referred to the Fort Washington men's shelter after stays at other shelters over the previous year. He received psychiatric services at one of these shelters and reports being given a prescription for Thorazine. However, he never had this prescription filled. He states that he was transferred to the second shelter after an argument with staff at the first shelter, but cannot supply details about this. Prior to entering the shelter system, Alex lived in the street for one year, sleeping in subways and tunnels. He denies any current substance abuse. Following his admission, he was begun on oral haloperidol (Haldol) four times daily, followed by a dose increase.

Past History

Alex has no history of psychiatric hospitalizations. His only prior contact with a psychiatrist was in the evaluation done of him at his first shelter.

He denies any history of substance abuse and denies having any medical problems. His family has no known history of mental illness. He reports that both of his parents were multiple-substance abusers.

Psychosocial History

Alex was born and raised in New York City. He reports that his father managed a liquor store and sold drugs, and that his mother worked as a baby nurse. He has no siblings, but does have three step-siblings. He has no contact with any of his family members. His parents worked long days and were unavailable to him.

Alex attended special education classes until the 10th grade. After dropping out of school he worked for a stapler-manufacturing company and then went to trade school in Boston, where he studied electronics repair for a year. He then returned to his parents' home in New York. After an argument with his father "because he was selling and using dope," Alex went into the streets for about a year before entering the shelter system.

Alex has never married. He claims to have a couple of friends but has lost contact with them. He has no military or criminal history. However, he does have a history of fighting and being argumentative in numerous previous shelters. In many of these cases Alex had a legitimate complaint (e.g., he objected to other men smoking in the dormitory). Unfortunately, he did not have interpersonal skills needed to report this in a manner that would not jeopardize his welfare. He also had feelings about male sexuality that prevented him from having a man stand closer than two arms lengths behind him. This occasionally led him to overcompensate by challenging others to a fight, in a manner more typical of adolescent boys. Alex has a physically solid build that enables him to hold his own, but this was becoming increasingly risky in his previous environment.

Assessment

The client, a homeless, 26-year-old black male with an undiagnosed psychotic disorder, was referred for evaluation by the community service office of the Fort Washington men's shelter after causing disturbances in the dormitory at night. He is stocky, neatly dressed and groomed, and is alert, attentive, and cooperative during his interview, but tends to be isolative and guarded with other shelter residents. His motor activity is normal. He speaks softly, stutters, and has difficulty expressing himself. His mood is euthymic and his affect is guarded. There are some loose associations. He is quite paranoid, often believing that people standing directly behind him with the intent of harming him. He refuses a physical examination and any injections because of his paranoia. He denies having hallucinations.

The client is in the low-average or borderline range of intelligence. He is oriented to time, person, and place. His memory is intact. There is some impairment of his judgment. His insight is limited, but he is willing to accept treatment. He has no suicidal ideation, but does make threats against others when angry. He is easily provoked to fighting, but rapidly calms down when reassured, and can be contained.

Alex came from an economically poor background and a broken home, with a long history of intense conflict between his parents. His father had a drinking problem and his mother, who lived with her sister, was dependent on this sister. Alex was raised by an extended family without any male role models. He had a learning disability and completed school through the 9th grade, in a special class. He has no significant work history and a brief history of using crack cocaine.

Alex's personality is basically reserved, his eye contact poor, and he has a stutter that can test the listener's patience. His speech is of low volume, underproductive, and very slow. He seems to have a communication problem, with difficulty in expressing himself. On closer examination, however, he appears to be more intelligent than initially suspected. He can do simple mathematics and can spell, read, and write. He has some knowledge of current events. However, in addition to his language problems, he suffers from paranoia and poor impulse control, perhaps suggesting some underlying, probably non-focal organic deficit. This may come from maternal substance abuse during his pre-natal period.

Initially, his affect was predictably depressed and somewhat hostile. It is understandable that having to rely on a program for homeless men with severe and persistent mental illness might compromise his self esteem. His referral must therefore have induced some initial defensiveness that may nevertheless be viewed as a strength.

DSM-IV Diagnosis

Axis I: Psychotic Disorder, NOS
Expressive Language Disorder
Learning Disability

Nursing Diagnoses

Ineffective coping
Altered thought process

Progress in Shelter

Since entering the program, Alex has had three arguments or fist fights with other clients, but all have been contained before anyone was hurt.

Although Alex refused to talk in the first week of his being at the Fort Washington shelter, the nurse was sensitive to his distress, did not feel rejected, and maintained an interested and genuine approach to him. As Alex began to realize that the nurse did not personalize the negative feelings that he was projecting, he began asking what the nurse could do for him. Initially, Alex behaved somewhat like a young child, expecting his "parent"—the shelter—to feed, clothe, and house him without his having to work for this. However, one of his requests was noteworthy: While completing his application for housing and entitlements, Alex boldly said that he wanted a car. The nurse sensed his sincerity and thought that his request for a car was symbolic of his wish for an acceptable male identity. Keeping this perception in mind, while continuing to express respect for Alex as worthy of making such a request, the nurse told him that he needed to take one small step at a time. The task at hand was to complete his lengthy housing application and the medical follow up tests for his positive tuberculin skin test. The nurse said that there was a good chance that he could eventually have what he wanted, feeling it important to allow some hope for the realization of Alex's wish. In this way rapport was maintained.

Case Evaluation

The case manager must inevitably confront issue of transference. Clients try to make the provider meet their wishes for childhood as well as current needs. The nurse in Alex's case faced the challenge of dealing with his most important need and convincing him of

its priority, since he would have to accomplish it. This meant taking medications to improve his logical thinking and reduce his paranoia and excessive defensiveness. The medication slowed Alex's movements significantly, but he was receptive to the nurse's reasoning. He began to see that the benefits of his medication would outweigh its uncomfortable side effects until he was accepted for community placement. He had no fights in the shelter after complying with his medication regimen. He was able to complete several interviews for housing placement and social security benefits. He valued talking and sharing stories with the nurse.

Alex was able to identify the nurse as someone who cared and whose recommendations he trusted. His affect brightened when he spoke of his aspiration to obtain a driver's license. As he became more self-confident he made contact with his mother, and her ongoing collaboration assisted his treatment plan. Because the Fort Washington Men's shelter program is the founding model for critical time intervention, Alex was assured that the nurse would provide him with 6 to 9 months of follow-up after his placement in the community. This support provided the confidence he needed to bridge the gap between the shelter and the community, and to replicate the working alliance he had developed with the nurse.

Plan of Care

1. Continue on Haldol. Add valproic acid to help control the client's aggressive behavior. Increase the dosage as tolerated, while checking blood levels of the drug.
2. Set limits on the client's behavior.
3. Order a physical examination, including a neurological and neuropsychological work-up if possible.
4. Manage the client's case with regard to housing and benefit applications.

Updated Psychiatric Assessment

Alex now regularly attends the shelter's community support system. He generally complies with his medication regimen, and takes his injected medications. He has refrained from substance abuse.

Since beginning his medication, Alex is notably calmer, with better impulse control. The addition of valproic acid seems to have helped him to control his aggression. He has slightly more spontaneous speech and expressive affect, but continues to demonstrate prominent negative symptoms. He also has parkinsonian side effects from his Haldol, and an apparent learning disability that compounds his drug-related psychomotor retardation.

Outcome

Alex has a complicated presentation of psychotic symptoms and cognitive deficits. He has clearly improved with his current medication regimen, but suffers from residual negative and extrapyramidal symptoms. He seems to have a learning disability, but is probably in the low-normal or borderline range of intelligence. He has done surprisingly well in the shelter's community support program, attending regularly and becoming much more in control of his behavior. He appears ready to move into supervised housing.

For information on:
The National Alliance for the Mentally Ill (NAMI): call (800)950-NAMI.
Clozapine: call (800)950-FACT
Friends and Advocates of the Mentally Ill, monthly report: write to 432 Park Ave. South, NY, NY 10016.
National Resource Center on Homelessness and Mental Illness: call (800)444-7415 or write to 262 Delaware Ave., Delmar, NY 12054.

O AN OVERVIEW

- Under the managed health-care system, job opportunities will increase for psychiatric nurses, especially those certified in addiction counseling. Opportunities will be in homeless outreach programs, mobile crisis centers, shelter-associated day programs, transitional living communities (TLC), and community residences for the dually diagnosed.

- Working with seriously mentally ill individuals requires nursing committment and good psychiatric skills. It is expected that the nurse will recognize help-rejecting behavior as an individual strength, rather than a poor prognostic factor.

- The great challenge of working with seriously mentally ill individuals reflects its rewards.

TD TERMS TO DEFINE

- assertive community treatment (ACT)
- Critical Time Intervention Model (CTI)
- homelessness
- National Alliance for the Mentally Ill (NAMI)
- nurse case manager
- recidivism
- seriously mentally ill (SMI)

Q STUDY QUESTIONS

1. In assessing an individual with a chronic mental illness, such as schizophrenia, which of the following data is probably most important from a holistic nursing perspective to determine the individual's readiness for community living?
   a. Patient has a history of being drug free for at least six weeks
   b. Patient has growing rapport with staff and peers
   c. Patient is compliant with medication regimen
   d. Patient manages money entitlements well

2. The writings of Talbott, Lamb, Bachrach, Drake, and Gudeman about the homeless population provide authoritative citations supporting which of the following statements?
   a. Eighty percent of homeless people use illicit drugs
   b. Deinstitutionalization caused increased homelessness among the mentally ill
   c. Poverty is the chief cause of increased homelessness among the mentally ill
   d. Homelessness can be a voluntary unconventional living arrangement

3. The most likely reason homeless people lose their entitlements is
   a. their illness makes them too paranoid to go for an interview.
   b. usually they have no means of transportation to the social security office.
   c. the letter requesting a recertification interview does not reach them.
   d. their attention span and memory are too short to remember the date and time of the appointment.

4. A homeless individual may experience an overwhelming hopelessness that can spiral into even greater passivity. Which of the following responses to the individual's situation by the nurse would be best initially?
   a. Offer the individual vocational counseling
   b. Identify the syndrome and be empathetic
   c. Refer the individual for antidepressant medication
   d. Give the individual the Hot Line telephone number to inquire about assistance

5. Mobile outreach teams often find that the most effective initial engagement with a resistant homeless individual involves
   a. using the harm reduction model.
   b. using milieu therapy.
   c. offering cigarettes or some other concrete service.
   d. arranging involuntary hospitalization certified by two physicians.

6. In 1996, the most common diagnoses among mentally ill homeless individuals was
   a. head injury and organic disorders.
   b. major depression with melancholia.
   c. psychotic disorders.
   d. posttraumatic stress disorder and dissociative disorders.

7. According to the outreach psychologist Dr. Thomas L. Kuhlman, clinicians working with the homeless population can be most effective if
   a. strict limit setting contracts are enforced.
   b. "resistance and rejecting" behaviors are viewed as adaptive, not untreatable.
   c. a policy of random drug testing is implemented.
   d. a 12-step program philosophy is used.

8. Assertive community treatment (ACT) teams are currently a state of the art method for community mental health. Which of the following statements about ACT is NOT true?
   a. It is a 24-hour unlimited service.
   b. It has been tested for at least 10 years and shows positive outcomes.
   c. It is flexible and its services coordinated.
   d. It provides individuals with the same primary care provider.

9. Demographic and prevalence rates for homelessness and mental illness are difficult to obtain. Which of the following statements does NOT explain why that situation is true?
   a. The homeless have poor visibility.
   b. A hidden political hostility is directed toward the homeless population.
   c. Mental disorganization among the homeless is incompatible with answering survey questions.
   d. Political motivation works to maintain status quo.

10. Because the homeless population is increasing and because more women and children are among the homeless, it is suggested that during the next millennium homelessness will be a social problem second only to
   a. AIDS.
   b. heart disease.
   c. cancer.
   d. smoking.

11. Which of the following statements is least helpful for clinicians trying to understand the homeless individual's distrust of authority figures?
   a. Previous negative experiences with medical personnel are not uncommon among the homeless population.
   b. Homeless individuals have experienced involuntary hospitalizations and restraint application.
   c. Stories circulate among the population about tardive dyskinesia and other iatrogenic conditions.
   d. Homeless individuals often have experienced abuse in their family of origin.

12. Which of the following would NOT be information that a nurse case manager would need in working with homeless people?
   a. Public health and community mental health policy
   b. Entitlement descriptions and the procedures required for eligibility and follow-up
   c. Cultural needs and differences of marginalized and oppressed population groups
   d. Interdisciplinary team members working in substance abuse, infectious disease, and psychopharmacotherapy
   e. Early signs of organic dementia and head injuries

13. Which of the following does NOT explain the high incidence of substance abuse among the homeless population?
   a. Members of the population tend to have highly addictive personality styles.
   b. Drugs are accessible within the shelter system.
   c. Stressful life circumstances predispose the homeless population to trying substances that might lift their spirits.
   d. The drug subculture provides the population, particularly males, with an experience similar to that of earlier ceremonial initiation rites; e.g., a sense of bravado.

14. Which of the following is the most likely cause of burnout among staff persons working with the homeless population?
   a. A fatalistic attitude toward substance abuse
   b. An inadequate education and awareness of cultural issues
   c. Demoralization due to the societal stigma of working with mentally ill, homeless persons
   d. A resignation to the idea that the population will remain mentally ill and homeless

15. The most effective way to prevent burn out is to
   a. commit to building team spirit among team members.
   b. pursue professional advancement in clinical skills to qualify as an advanced practice nurse.
   c. write case studies, present them in small groups, and get supervision.
   d. participate in interdisciplinary discussions about the best clinical approaches and legislated public health policies.

■ REFERENCES

Aiken LH: Unmet needs of the chronically mentally ill: Will nursing respond? *Nursing* 1987; 19:121–125.

Amussen SM: Old answers for today's problems: integrating individuals who are homeless with mental illness into existing community based programs. A case study of Fountain House. *Psychosoc Rehab J* 1994; 18(1):75–93.Bower KA: Case management by nurses. Washington, DC: American Nurses Publishing, 1992.

Baier, M: Case management of the chronically mentally ill. In Judith T. Maurin (ed.) *Chronic Mental Illness: Coping Strategies*. Thorofare, NJ: Slack, Inc; 1989.

Breakey WR: Health and mental health problems of homeless men and women in Baltimore. *JAMA 262*(10), 1352–1357.

Clark RE: Family costs associated with severe mental illness and substance use, *Hosp Commun Psychiatry* 1994a; 45(8):808–813.

Clark RE, Drake RE: Expenditures of time and money by families of people with severe mental illness and substance use disorders, *Commun Mental Health J* 1994b; 30:145–163.

CMHS, Center for Mental Health Services *Making a Difference. Interim Status Report of the McKinney Demonstration Program for Homeless Adults with Serious Mental Illness*. Rockland, MD: U.S. Department of Health and Human Services, 1995.

Cohen CI, Thompson KS: Homeless mentally ill or mentally ill homeless. *Am J Psychiatry* 1992; 149(6):861–822.

Culhane DP: Images of the homeless. [letter] *Hospital and Community Psychiatry* 1991; 92(2):200–1.

Connolly PM: Services for the underserved: A nurse-managed center for the chronically mentally ill. *J Psychosoc Nurs* 1991; 29(1):15–20.

Dato C, Rafferty M: The Homeless mentally ill. *Int Nurs Rev* 1985; 32(6):170–173.

Dear MJ, Wolch JR: *Landscapes of despair: From deinstitutionalization to homelessness*. Princeton, NJ: Princeton Press, 1987.

Deleuze G, Guattari F: *Nomadology and the War Machine*. (Massumi B, Trans.). New York, Columbia University Press, 1986.

Dixon L, Kernan E, Krauss, N. *Assertive Community Treatment for Homeless Adults with Severe Mental Illness in Baltimore*. Baltimore University School of Medicine, Dept. of Psychiatry, Baltimore, 1994.

Drake RE, Osher FC, Wallach MA: Homelessness and dual diagnosis. *American Psychologist*. 1991; 46(11),1149–1158.

Federal Task Force on Homelessness and Severe Mental Illness: *Outcasts on Main Street*. Washington, DC, Interagency Council on the Homeless; 1992, p. 18.

Foucault M: *The birth of the clinic*. (A.M.S. Smith, Trans.) London: Tavistock, 1993.

Gounis K, Susser E: Shelterization and its implications for mental health services. In: N. Cohen (ed), *Psychiatry takes to the streets*. Guilford Press, 1990.

Hombs, ME, Snyder M: *Homeless in America: A forced march to nowhere*. Washington, DC: Community for Creative Nonviolence, 1982.

Isaac RJ, and Armat VC: *Madness in the streets: How psychiatry and the law abandoned the mentally ill*. New York: Free Press, 1990.

Kane CF: Nursing update: Deinstitutionalization and managed care: Deja vu?, *Psychiatr Serv* 1995; 46(9):883–884.

Kay SR: Positive and Negative Symptoms in Schizophrenia. New York, Brunner/Maazel, 1991.

Lamb HR, Bachrach L, and F Kass (eds.) *Treating the Homeless Mentally Ill*. Washington, DC: American Psychiatric Association, 1992.

Link BG, Susser E, Stueve A, Phelan J, Moore RE, and Streuning E: Lifetime and five year-year prevalence of homelessness in the United States. *American Journal of Public Health*. 1994; Dec;84(12):1907–12.

Link BG, Phelan J, Bresnahan M, Stueve A, Moore R and Susser E: Lifetime and five-year prevalence of homelessness in the United States: New evidence on an old debate. *American Journal of Orthopsychiatry*. 1995; 65(3):347–54.

Kuhlman T: *Psychology of the Streets*. NY: John Wiley & Sons, 1994.

Rossi PH: *Down and out in America: The origins of homelessness*. Chicago: University of Chicago Press, 1989.

Stein, L. et al. A Systems approach to reducing relapse in schizophrenia. *J Clin Psychiatry* 1993; 54(Suppl.):7–12.

Susser E, Goldfinger SM, White A: Some clinical approaches to the homeless mentally ill. *Commun Mental Health J* 1990; 26(5):463–479.

Sass LA: *Madness and Modernism. Insanity in the Light of Modern Art, Literature, and Thought*. New York, Basic Books, 1992.

Tessler RC, and Dennis DL: *A synthesis of NIMH-funded research concerning persons who are homeless and mentally ill*. Rockville, MD: National Institute of Mental Health, 1989.

Torrey E. Fuller: *Nowhere to go: The tragic odyssey of the homeless mentally ill*. New York: Harper & Row, 1988.

Valencia E, Susser E, Caton C, and Felix A: *Critical time Intervention Manual*. NY, NY: Columbia University, 1994.

VanderStaay S: *Street Lives, an oral history of homeless Americans*. Philadelphia, PA: New Society Publishers, 1992.

Warren CAB: New forms of social control: the myth of deinstitutionalization. *American Behavioral Scientist*, 1981; 24, 727

Watson J: Postmodernism and knowledge development in nursing. *Nursing Science Quarterly*, 1995; 8(2):60–64.

Watzlawich, P. *Pragmatics of Human Communication*. New York, WW Norton, 1967.

Wilkinson L: A collaborative model: Ambulatory pharmacology for chronic psychiatric patients. *J Psychosoc Nurs* 1991; 29(12):26–29.

6

Level 6

Psychiatric Emergencies

Psychiatric emergencies involve crisis situations in which general individual functioning has rapidly deteriorated, such as through drug overdosing. The individual is rendered incompetent, unable to assume personal responsibility, and unable to exert control over his or her feelings and actions. There is threat or actual harm to the self and/or others.

The individual presents with a loss of personal control. An assessment is made immediately. The level of cooperation of the patient with emergency intervention is affected by the patient's level of consciousness and orientation, rationality, rage, and anxiety.

The etiology of these crises involves the self-abusive component of suicide attempts and drug overdoses. Aggression toward others suggests the need for dominance, control, and sexualized violence.

In intervening, psychiatric nurses must be confident in their skills for managing patient behavior that is out of control, or adequate assistance should be available. When an emergency occurs, cooperative efforts are made to locate the patient, determine what the patient has done, and identify the availability of significant others. If serious physical danger exists or if data are insufficient to determine the danger, emergency medical attention is required. Police and rescue squads should handle situations in which there is immediate danger, and should ensure rapid transportation to a hospital emergency room.

Psychiatric emergencies are the most difficult type of crises to manage. Information about these situations may be incomplete; the patient may be disruptive or minimally helpful; and there is an immediacy to understand the situation in depth in order to initiate effective treatment. Patient assessment is facilitated if the patient is accompanied by informants who have knowledge of the precipitating events. In addition, informants are often helpful in planning appropriate psychological and medical interventions.

The basic intervention strategy for Level 6 psychiatric crises involves:

- Rapidly assessing the patient's psychological and medical condition.
- Clarifying the situation that produced or led to the patient's condition.
- Mobilizing the mental-health and/or medical resources necessary to treat the patient effectively.
- Arranging follow-up or coordination of services to ensure continuity of treatment.

The psychiatric nurse must work effectively and quickly in highly charged situations, and perhaps intervene when there are life-threatening implications for the patient.

Conditions representative of Psychiatric Emergencies are discussed in the following three chapters:

- Substance Abuse
- Managing Suicidal Patients
- Managing Assaultive Patients

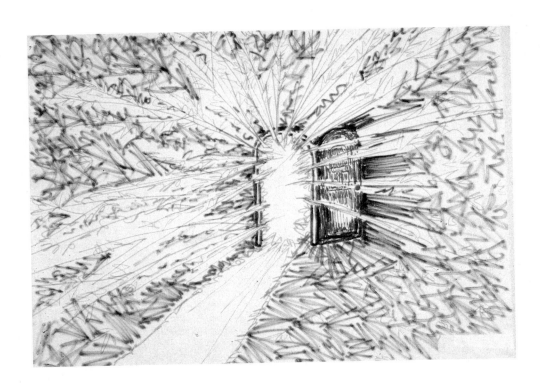

"One night, returning home much intoxicated, from one of my haunts about town, I fancied the cat avoided my presence. I seized him; when, in his fright at my violence, he inflicted a slight wound upon my hand with his teeth. The fury of a demon instantly possessed me. I knew myself no longer. My original soul seemed, at once, to take its flight from my body; and a more than fiendish malevolence, gin-nutured, thrilled every fiber of my frame. I took from my waistcoat-pocket a pen knife, opened it, grasped the poor beast by the throat, and deliberately cut one of its eyes from the socket! . . . I again plunged into excess, and soon drowned in wine all memory of the deed."

Edgar Allan Poe (1809–1849)

The Black Cat

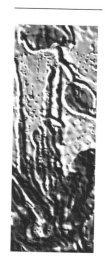

31
Substance Abuse

Linda S. Cook

Humans seem to have a need to periodically alter their states of consciousness. This alteration in consciousness has been produced by music, fasting, meditation, dancing, sex, religious experience, and other activities that alter an individual's perception of reality. This behavior is not limited to adults; Weil and Rosen (1993) describe the blissful state that rocking produces in infants and the way in which small children spin in circles until they collapse with dizziness. Weil and Rosen conclude that altering one's level of consciousness is a societally accepted and desirable behavior.

With regard to drug use related to religious observance, marijuana was used in ancient India, peyote by some Native American tribes, and alcohol in Christian, Judaic, and Greek Dionysian cultures as part of religious rites and ceremonies. Most of the time, society accepts (if not approves) such drug use. This acceptance becomes disapproval when drugs are used for recreational purposes.

Substance abuse and dependence tend to provoke strong emotional reactions from health-care providers as well as the general public. Very few persons' lives have not been touched by at least one of the consequences or correlates of substance abuse, such as accident and trauma, crime, low birth rates, birth *defects, and infections. This emotional reaction is influenced by whether one understands addiction as originating from physical illness, learned behavior, genetics, or moral failing.*

This chapter will discuss addiction as a complex problem that cannot be understood through a single explanatory theory. Effective treatment of addiction requires a holistic approach that incorporates medical, psychosocial, and family theories.

■ THE PROCESS OF ADDICTION

Addiction is a process of psychoactive substance use ending in the user's physical and/or emotional dependence on the substance being used. This process usually has five phases: experimentation, recreation, habituation, abuse, and dependence. Experimentation involves a personal trial of a drug to assess its effects. The typical introduction to drugs and alcohol occurs in the presence of peers or significant others. The recreational phase of addiction is marked by use of a drug expressly for entertainment and/or relaxation. Habituation involves the use of a drug on a routine basis and apart from diversional or recreational activities. At this point in the addiction process, the drug of choice begins to assume an increased importance to the individual. As he or she moves into drug abuse and dependence (defined below), increasing time and energy are invested in seeking and using the drug of choice. The time required to progress from experimentation to dependence varies greatly and is influenced by the drug and the individual using it. (See Table 31–1).

The *Diagnostic and Statistical Manual of the American Psychiatric Association,* Fourth Edition *(DSM-IV)* lists specific criteria for the diagnosis of both abuse and dependence.

Substance abuse is the use of a psychoactive chemical despite the significant physical, psychological, and social problems that result from its use. **Substance or chemical dependence** is the use of a psychoactive chemical that produces the following effects:

1. Tolerance of the substance.
2. Continued use of the substance in spite of its producing problems with employment, the law, or relationships.
3. The occurrence of withdrawal symptoms when the substance or chemical is discontinued.

Depressant drugs activate and/or exaggerate the effects of the parasympathetic nervous system, or repress the sympathetic nervous system to produce physical, emotional, or cognitive feelings of calm and euphoria. **Stimulant drugs** activate and/or exaggerate the effects of the sympathetic nervous system or repress the effects of the parasympathetic nervous system to produce a sense of excitement and euphoria. **Hallucinogenic drugs** are chemicals that interfere with the sensation and perception of reality by producing visual, tactile, olfactory, or aural hallucinations. These drugs may also alter the user's ability to distinguish reality from delusional thinking.

Impairment refers to the alteration of judgment and/or physical responses by a psychoactive substance. **Intoxication** is the elated, excited, or exhilarated physical and emotional state produced by the ingestion of chemicals. **Tolerance** is the need for increasing amounts of a chemical to maintain its effects. **Withdrawal** refers to a cluster of signs and symptoms experienced when a chemical upon which one is dependent is removed. The cluster reflects hyperactivity of the opposite system affected by the chemical of dependence; i.e., when heroin (a parasympathetic stimulator) is stopped, the individual experiences symptoms of sympathetic stimulation.

■ EPIDEMIOLOGY

Substance abuse is at epidemic levels in the United States, and has been termed the country's leading health problem (Volpiecelli, 1995). There is a 13% prevalence of alcohol dependence (Volpicelli, 1995) in

TABLE 31–1: SUBSTANCE ABUSE AND DEPENDENCE

DSM-IV Criteria: Substance Abuse
The person must have experienced one or more of these in the past 12 months:
- failure to fulfill role obligations at home, school, or work
- recurrent drug or alcohol use in physically dangerous settings
- recurring drug-related legal problems
- continued use despite recurring interpersonal problems

DSM-IV Criteria: Substance Dependence
The person must have experienced three or more of these in the past 12 months:
- drug tolerance
- drug withdrawal
- drug use is greater in amount and frequency of use than intended (i.e., loss of control)
- persistent desire and unsuccessful attempts to stop or control drug use
- increasing time and energy spent in obtaining the drug
- lifestyle changes (social, recreational, or occupational) due to drug use
- drug use is continued despite knowledge of life problems

American Psychiatric Association (1994) Diagnostic and Statistical Manual of Mental Disorders, 4th Edition: Washington, D.C.: American Psychiatric Association

the United States, and more than half of the American population uses alcohol, with 15% using a disproportionately large amount (Ray and Ksir, 1993). A national survey published in 1993 demonstrated that 10.3% of men and 4.1% of women in the United States were alcohol dependent, and that another 3.9% of men and 1.0% of women were severely dependent (Rice, 1993). Another survey found that approximately 18-million Americans have significant alcohol-related problems (U.S. Department of Health and Human Services, 1992).

After reaching a high point in the mid-1980s with 30-million users (Gawin and Ellinwood, 1988), the use of cocaine has since been steadily dropping. The National Institute on Drug Abuse reports a decline of cocaine use by young adults from 9% in 1980 to 2% in 1991 (Childress, Ehrman, Robbins, Kung, & O'Brien,

1992). Despite the overall decrease in the numbers of persons using cocaine, the number of regular users of cocaine increased from 600,000 in 1980 to 800,000 in 1990 (Weinreib and O'Brien, 1993). This smaller but potentially more dependent group may help to explain a mortality rate related to cocaine use that remained stable over the same time frame (National Institute on Drug Abuse, 1991).

Opiate addiction includes the use of heroin and morphine, as well as synthetic derivatives of these drugs. The use of heroin seems overshadowed by the attention given to cocaine in terms of both research and media exposure during the past two decades. However, the actual numbers of persons who were and are heroin-dependent may not have been reflected by the data. Significant numbers of persons addicted to opiates returned to the United States at the end of the Viet Nam conflict. Popular wisdom held that heroin users were primarily from this group and from poor urban populations. Both groups became heavy users of opiates in environments in which opiates were cheap and easily available. Another population of opiate-dependent persons are those who become dependent upon narcotics inappropriately prescribed for medical problems (O'Brien, 1994).

Because of the focus on cocaine and the relative dearth of research on opiate addiction in the past two decades, reliable figures for the prevalence of heroin addiction are not available. Surveys of high-school students reveal that only 5% of high-school seniors have experimented with nonprescription narcotics, as compared with the 86% who have experimented with alcohol (Volpicelli, 1995). New populations of users, however, have in the past decade developed "black tar," a very pure form of heroin, and "China White," a synthetic narcotic (Ray and Ksir, 1993).

Hallucinogens have remained fairly constant in their appeal and popularity, although the substance of choice has varied. Lysergic acid diethylamide (LSD)

E CASE EXAMPLE

Melissa is a 21-year-old college junior. She had her first drink of alcohol as a high-school senior at a graduation party, when all of her friends had a drink. As a college freshman, she began drinking on weekends with her friends. In her sophomore year, she began drinking every evening after studying. Over the summer, she received two citations for driving while intoxicated, and has repeatedly been late for classes. She and her

boyfriend have been drinking together and then fighting on a regular basis. Her parents want Melissa to get help, but she tells them she is all right and "just doing what the rest of the kids do." When she stopped drinking to prove to them that she could do it, she experienced a grand mal seizure.

was extraordinarily popular through the 1960s and early 1970s. Much of the popular drug subculture was focused on the use of LSD to "tune in, turn on, and drop out." The past two decades have seen an increase in the popularity of phencyclidine (PCP) as the hallucinogenic drug of choice.

DIVERSITY AND SOCIOCULTURAL ISSUES

The use of psychoactive agents is common to all cultures and ethnic groups, and attitudes toward their use vary within cultures and ethnic groups. This variance makes it difficult, if not impossible, to generalize specific drug use to specific groups of people.

Use of specific drugs may be geographically defined apart from the factors of culture and ethnicity. For example, use of inhalants such as toluene may be extremely popular in a neighborhood composed of a cultural group (Caucasians from low socio-economic background) that, in terms of nationwide averages, usually uses alcohol as its drug of choice.

Research has shown significant differences in the way specific drugs are metabolized by genetically similar groups. This implies that some genetically similar groups will tend to be more or less susceptible to specific drugs.

SPECIAL POPULATIONS

Women

Women constitute from 25 to 30% of the addicted population. During much of the period of early research on alcoholism, women were excluded from the research sample because the variance created by differences in physiology and socialization made data difficult to interpret. Thus, much of what we "know" about addiction applies to men, without necessarily applying to women.

Based on the research done thus far, the following are some facts about women addicts:

- Women tend to begin using drugs and alcohol when with partners or mates, while men tend to start using them when with other men.
- Fewer women than men enter into treatment for substance abuse.
- Women tend to have more problems in physical health as a result of using drugs and alcohol than do men.
- Women tend to have stronger cravings for drugs and to relapse in the week before menstruation.
- Up to 70% of women addicts were sexually abused as children.
- Pregnant addicts do not seek drug treatment during their pregnancies because they fear being

jailed and having their children removed by Child Protective Services.
- Women become drunk more rapidly than do men because they have proportionately less body water.

More research must be done to evaluate the specific needs of addicted women and women in recovery. In the meantime, it is important to realize that recommendations routinely made to men to aid in their recovery may not be appropriate for women.

Children and Adolescents

Alcohol use has always been common among adolescents as they begin to experiment with adult behaviors. In the past decade, statistics have reported declining drug use by adolescents. It is important to remember that these figures are based on surveys done with high-school seniors. The United States has an overall high-school drop-out rate of 29.6%; Black and Latino urban youth have a drop-out rate of 50%. It is highly unlikely that these young people were included in the survey figures. Rather, it is more likely that we do not know how many children and adolescents are using drugs and alcohol.

The Impaired Professional

The health-care professional is in no way immune to the problems of substance abuse and dependence. The impaired professional is described as typically working during the night or evening shifts when there are fewer people present. Such individuals show unexplained and sudden mood swings and an overall decline in job performance. Finally, there are either discrepancies in the narcotics count at the site of employment or patients who continue to complain of unchanging pain after receiving supposed analgesics.

The highly punitive attitude toward addicts that used to be prevalent remains in many settings with regard to addicted health-care professionals. It is somehow assumed that these people should know better or should have more sense about drugs. Until recently, state boards of nursing routinely withdrew licensure from nurses with addiction problems.

Most state boards of nursing now move toward rehabilitation rather than punishment. Working with the employing agency, these state boards now instead mandate treatment and have the nurse return to work in areas that do not involve handling narcotic drugs. Ongoing treatment is demanded in the form of support groups; most urban areas have 12 Step programs specifically for impaired professionals, which address the concerns of that population. It is important that nurses working with an addicted professional population be aware of these resources for referral.

The Dually Diagnosed

Dual diagnosis is the term used for patients who have both a psychiatric and a substance-abuse disorder. Providing care to these patients is very complex, since most of them have a cluster of problems produced by the interaction of a severe mental illness with substances of abuse. The employment, financial, legal, and relationship problems found with substance abuse are compounded by the coping difficulties and disorganized behavior found with mental illness. In addition, drug use can exacerbate some symptoms of mental illness. For example, cocaine used by persons with schizophrenia can produce psychotic symptoms, assaultiveness, and disorganized thinking.

Dual diagnosis is thought by some to be self-medication on the part of mentally ill persons; that hallucinations may lose some of their intensity when dulled by chemicals, or that severely depressed persons may feel somewhat better during the euphoric phase of intoxication. Others propose that certain factors may produce both substance abuse and mental illness. Some of these proposed factors include trauma and genetic predisposition. A third explanation posits that substance abuse may produce mental illness. This is exemplified by the person who becomes psychotic after using hallucinogens.

The dually diagnosed face exceptional difficulty in finding treatment. The physiological needs of those in withdrawal are beyond the means of many psychiatric facilities. Similarly, the bizarre behaviors of many psychiatric patients are not conducive to the therapeutic process in drug-treatment centers. Also, the advice given to the dually diagnosed in one setting may be contraindicated in the other—many Twelve-Step programs advocate avoiding any psychoactive medication.

The nurse caring for the dually diagnosed must avoid rescue fantasies with this patient population. As one becomes aware of the many stressors facing the patient, one can become overwhelmed by his or her needs. It is critical to have access to referral agencies in the community in order to assist in meeting such patients' many needs.

■ THEORETICAL FRAMEWORKS

MEDICAL MODEL

Much research has been directed at establishing physical correlates of chemical dependence. Neurophysiology has provided a greater understanding of drug dependence with the discovery of specific neurotransmitters that are affected by drugs of abuse. To produce dependence, a drug must inhibit or stimulate cerebral neurotransmitters. Alterations in specific neurotransmitters have been identified as underlying the effects of most of the common drugs of abuse.

A second medical framework holds that all addicting drugs activate the pleasure or reward center in the limbic region of the brain. The dopamine pathway is the common pathway stimulated by food, sex, and addicting drugs. Some researchers think that all addicting drugs eventually act to stimulate the release of or inhibit the reabsorption of dopamine in this pathway.

Another area of research is the identification of specific genes carrying a trait for chemical dependence. No evidence has been found thus far of a specific genetic dysfunction common to all chemically dependent persons.

Research into the metabolism of drugs has produced interesting findings. Four variants of the enzyme aldehyde dehydrogenase have been found. The most common variant is that shared by most of the population. The metabolism of alcohol begins in the stomach, through the action of alcohol dehydrogenase. This

E CASE EXAMPLE

Larry is a 26-year-old white male who lives with his parents. He was unable finish high school because of increasingly bizarre behavior that culminated with his screaming and jumping out of a second-story classroom at the age of 16, convinced that demons were pursuing him. Larry had begun drinking at the age of 15, when he was encouraged to do so by classmates with whom he had cut class. His alcohol intake gradually increased when he realized that alcohol intoxication dulled the voices in his head. He refuses to take chlorpromazine (Thorazine) because it makes him "feel dead," and drinks whenever he can get enough money to buy beer. He steals money from his parents, sneaks out of the house, and disappears for days at a time. His parents are too frail to restrain him, and he is not overtly dangerous to himself or others; therefore, he can't be committed. Larry is unable to work and uninterested in therapy. As his case worker, what would you recommend to him and his parents?

converts some of the alcohol to acetaldehyde. The alcohol and the acetaldehyde are then both dumped into the circulation. The remaining metabolism of the alcohol occurs in the liver. Here the acetaldehyde entering in the blood is further metabolized by aldehyde dehydrogenase to produce acetic acid, which is then excreted. About 2% of the alcohol is excreted unchanged through respiration and perspiration. In most people, this process leads to the excretion of acetaldehyde over the 24-hour period following alcohol intake. A second variant of alcohol dehydrogenase appears to differ chemically, from the first and most common variant, but behaves functionally in the same way.

A third variant of aldehyde dehydrogenase is found primarily in some Asian subgroups. This variant is much less efficient than the first, and allows an accumulation of acetaldehyde. An individual with this variant of the enzyme becomes ill with palpitations, facial flushing, diaphoresis, and nausea following the intake of alcohol. Drinking for such persons is a less pleasurable experience.

A fourth variant of aldehyde dehydrogenase is found primarily in some Native American populations. This variant is extraordinarily efficient and permits copious alcohol metabolism and, thereby, potentially greater alcohol intake. This variant is, not surprisingly, found in persons with more severe addiction to alcohol and concomitant physical illness.

PSYCHOSOCIAL MODEL

Social learning theory holds that people learn to use specific drugs in specific settings. The "teachers" may be peers or family members. The common ground for such learning is an environment that either supports or at least allows drug use. This learning of addiction as coping is reinforced if feelings of low self-esteem and/or the effects of poverty and hopelessness are blunted by the effects of the drug.

A second psychological theory states that people use drugs to relieve anxiety. Several facts support this theory. Anxiety has a tendency to pre-date drug use. Stimulation of the pleasure center, such as by certain drugs, has a dampening effect on sympathetic arousal and therefore on anxiety. Finally, persons who have stopped drinking tend to relapse after experiencing trauma or crisis. In this theory, the use of drugs or alcohol becomes a maladaptive means of coping.

A formerly popular theory held that there was an "addictive personality." Although a great many addicts will indeed test positively for antisocial personality disorder while still addicted, these traits tend to disappear after sobriety has been achieved and maintained. No specific personality disorder can be ascribed to addicted persons.

FAMILY-SYSTEMS THEORY

Family-systems theory views the use of drugs and alcohol as a response to increased anxiety within the family. In the family system, the person(s) with the least power display(s) symptoms (e.g., using drugs or alcohol) when anxiety within the family increases. As a consequence of abusing drugs or alcohol, the addict underfunctions emotionally; more powerful persons in the family overfunction, and act to protect the weak member and preserve the family structure.

This pattern is most readily exemplified when the addicted family member is an adolescent. Consider the following example:

In a now classic study, Stanton and Todd (1982) reported that substance abuse within the family was a function of the loss of family members, either through death or immigration. With the loss of a family member, the family "script" is disrupted. This disruption increases family anxiety, which in turn has the effect of increasing substance abuse.

Approximately 54% of the families interviewed in Stanton and Todd's study named newborns after family members who died or immigrated. When the deceased or absent family member had an alcohol or addiction problem, the newborn was three times as likely to also be addicted. In this way, the family script of chemical dependence as a response to anxiety was maintained. See Chapter 8 for a more detailed discussion of systems theory and family systems theory.

■ SUBSTANCES OF ABUSE

ALCOHOL

History

Alcohol appears to be universal in its appeal—all cultures have used alcohol in some form. Evidence of alcohol use appears in archeological findings worldwide. Fruit wines and beer date to approximately 6400 B.C. The oldest brewery found thus far was in Egypt and was built in 3700 B.C. Mead, made of fermented honey, is probably the oldest alcoholic beverage; historians place its origins in the Paleolithic Era at about 8000 B.C.

Alcohol has an ambivalent history in America. When they arrived, the Pilgrims found the Native American tribes using beer. The Pilgrims, while veering away from the gin epidemic in England, themselves made and consumed hard cider. They perceived alcohol as one of God's blessings; it was immoderation and inebriate behavior that was perceived as sinful. This acceptance of alcohol while condemning its effects has remained as a prevailing attitude toward alcohol in America.

E CASE EXAMPLE

A married couple have been thinking about getting divorced. Each time the couple fights, their teen-aged son comes home drunk. After the couple visits a divorce attorney, their son causes a serious accident in which he is injured, and is charged with driving un-

der the influence of alcohol. The couple postpones their divorce plans in order to take care of their sick child.

Pharmacokinetics

As described earlier, the metabolism of alcohol begins in the stomach with the enzyme alcohol dehydrogenase. A small amount of the alcohol is then converted to acetaldehyde and the remainder transported unchanged into the small intestine. From the small intestine, the alcohol is absorbed into the circulatory system and is disseminated to all body tissues, including cerebral tissues. About 10% is excreted unchanged via perspiration and respiration, and the remainder is converted in the liver by aldehyde dehydrogenase into acetic acid and water.

The alcohol that is disseminated to cerebral tissue acts similarly to narcotics and endorphins, in that it stimulates the dopamine pathway. The dopamine pathway is the same pleasure center in the brain that is stimulated by food and sex. With the research available at this time, it is still unclear whether individual mechanisms of alcohol metabolism are inheritable or even primarily responsible for alcoholism.

One drink—12 ounces of beer, 4 ounces of wine, or one shot of whiskey—contains approximately one-half ounce of ethyl alcohol, or ethanol. An average-size

adult male is able to metabolize approximately one-half ounce of alcohol per hour; women have proportionately less body fluid than men and have greater blood alcohol levels after consuming less alcohol.

The blood alcohol level represents the concentration of alcohol in the blood. Blood alcohol levels are measurable approximately 20 minutes after alcohol ingestion, and reach a peak in one and a half hours. If an individual drinks faster than the alcohol can be metabolized, the concentration of blood alcohol rises. Table 31–2 demonstrates the correlation between blood alcohol levels and the resulting physiological/behavioral effects.

As a drug that produces dependence, alcohol leads to the development of tolerance. As the individual progresses in the process of addiction, greater amounts of alcohol are needed to achieve the desired effects. Tolerance also develops behaviorally. The individual is able to walk, talk, and function with higher blood alcohol concentrations.

As the liver becomes less functional, however, this tolerance reverses, so that less alcohol is needed for intoxication. With less alcohol being metabolized and excreted, the individual has higher blood alcohol levels, which also last for longer periods.

A sudden decrease in blood alcohol level can result in withdrawal symptoms. For most persons with alcoholism, withdrawal symptoms begin from 6 to 8 hours after the last drink. For the individual who maintains a chronically increased blood alcohol level, however, a sudden 25% decrease in that level (such as following rapid intravenous fluid infusion in an emergency setting) will produce withdrawal symptoms.

Assessment of the Alcoholic Patient

Psychiatric/Psychological Factors. It is critical for the nurse to assess his or her own underlying beliefs, values, and attitudes about alcohol before attempting to care for the patient with an alcohol problem. Because the alcoholic individual experiences difficulty in maintaining

TABLE 31–2 BLOOD ALCOHOL CONCENTRATIONS (BAC) AND BEHAVIORS

BAC (ounces)	Behaviors
0.05	Impaired judgment, reduced alertness, loss of inhibitions, euphoria
0.10	Slower reaction times, decreased caution in risk-taking behavior, impaired fine-motor control
0.15	Significant and consistent losses in reaction time
0.20	Gross impairment in sensory and motor function
0.25	Severe sensory and motor impairment
0.30	Stuporous
0.35	Surgical anesthesia
0.40	Respiratory depression, lethal in approximately half of population

sobriety, some health-care providers maintain an attitude that they perceive to be "realistic" but which is in reality punitive.

This punitive attitude is easy to understand when one considers that persons with addictions use two defense mechanisms to excess: **denial** and **rationalization.** In the early development of the addiction, it is very threatening to the ego to allow the possibility of addiction into one's awareness. Thus, the affected individual tends to deny the existence of the problem. Denial becomes ego-preserving in that the individual is spared conscious knowledge of the extent to which alcohol has control over his or her life.

Health-care providers tend to become impatient with denial, and even perceive it to be lying on the patient's part. Patients whose denial is challenged with the truth become more anxious and defended. This defensiveness is frequently hostile, thereby blocking the possibility of a therapeutic relationship.

The patient using rationalization as a defense mechanism is aware of his or her drinking behavior but either minimizes the extent and effects of the behavior or offers logical reasons for it. The alcoholic businessman may tell the nurse that he drinks at lunches with other businesspeople while working; the college student may say that she drinks only to fit in with the group with which she socializes. The reasons given for drinking to excess may sound plausible until one examines the patient's behavior in the context of an addiction model and discovers that the patient is continuing to drink despite problems caused by the drinking.

In addition to their use of defense mechanisms, alcoholic patients engage in manipulative behaviors as a part of their addictive illness. It is often necessary for the alcoholic individual to manipulate his or her environment in order to keep functioning and prevent withdrawal. Most people dislike being manipulated and come to resent the persons who behave in a manipulative manner. This is no less true for health-care providers than for the general public. It is necessary to evaluate one's feelings about being manipulated in order not to act them out when dealing with the addicted or alcoholic individual.

Once the nurse understands his or her reactions to alcoholism, it is possible to be a source of acceptance, concern, and strength to patients with this problem. These patients may be frightened, fearful of rejection, and desperate.

The nurse should pay close attention to the patient's presenting problems. As one seeks more information about the circumstances leading to the patient's current problem, questions about alcohol intake should be included with questions about dietary intake, smoking, and the use of both prescription and nonprescription medications. It is important to be aware that the patient who admits to a pattern of drinking may minimize the amounts of alcohol used. Asking questions about the frequency of drinking, the amounts of alcohol consumed in each episode, and the length of time since the last episode of drinking allows the patient to begin to look objectively at his or her behavior.

If the questioning reveals a problematic pattern of alcohol use, it is appropriate to ask further questions drawn from the criteria set forth in *DSM IV.* Have problems with work or school increased (i.e., has work or school performance declined or has there been an increase in tardiness or absenteeism)? Have family members or significant others begun to approach the patient with their concerns about his or her drinking? Has the patient begun to use alcohol at obviously inappropriate times, such as early in the morning or during school or work? Has the patient tried to cut down the amount consumed? Positive responses to these questions may lead both the patient and the nurse to greater concerns about the possibility of alcoholism.

Physical Factors. During the initial assessment, the nurse should observe the patient for physical signs of alcohol use, abuse, and dependence. These may include an odor of alcohol on the patient's breath, skin, or clothing; an unsteady gait; slurring of speech; and the presence of ecchymotic areas on the arms and legs. These signs would alert the nurse to recent alcohol ingestion. Tremors of the hands; generalized irritability; and increased blood pressure, pulse, and temperature could signal a lack of alcohol in an alcohol-dependent client. The withdrawal syndrome is discussed in more depth in a later section of this chapter.

The nutritional status of the alcoholic patient should always be assessed. Although alcohol does contain calories and can be classified as a food, its calories are "empty" or devoid of any nutrient value. In addition, heavy alcohol intake acts as an anorectic stimulus by increasing the release of cholecystokinin from the intestinal mucosa, which results in ketosis, diminishing the ability to taste one's food, and in high rates of gastritis and pancreatitis. The alcoholic individual thus has fewer protein and glycogen stores to use for times of healing and/or increased stress.

Metabolism of alcohol occurs in the liver. The liver produces alcohol dehydrogenase, which combines with ethyl alcohol to begin the process of converting it to acetaldehyde, water, and carbon dioxide. This process has as a side effect the increased production of and decreased oxidation of lipids. These excess lipids are stored in the liver and inhibit liver function. In some alcoholic individuals, the liver tissue becomes inflamed, resulting in **alcoholic hepatitis.** This hepatitis differs from viral hepatitis in that it is not contagious, but produces the same type of long-term liver damage. The chronic inflammation produces scarring and loss of functional liver tissue—the defining characteristics of cirrhosis. Alcoholic liver disease is characterized by pain in the right upper quadrant, anorexia, jaundice, elevation of temperature, leukocytosis, and an enlarged liver mass.

As the liver becomes increasingly sclerotic, blood pressures in the hepatic portal circulation become very high. These high pressures produce backflow into the venous circulation, resulting in enlarged veins. The veins most often affected are those of the esophagus. The affected veins become varicose and bleed easily.

Chronic high levels of alcohol intake affect other organ systems than the gastrointestinal system. The two organ systems typically affected are the cardiovascular and neurological systems. Alcohol affects cardiac tissue in such a way that its contractile force is decreased. The heart thus functions as a less efficient pump. With time, the heart enlarges as its muscle tissue is forced to work ever harder to maintain cardiac output. Cardiomyopathy and heart failure are the eventual results.

The most glaring physical effect of alcoholism on the neurological system is cerebral atrophy. Chronic alcohol use produces tissue destruction visible as a loss of cerebral mass on a computed tomographic (CT) scan. The concomitant cognitive losses do not return with abstinence from alcohol.

Withdrawal from alcohol is a potentially lethal phenomenon. Approximately 8 hours after the last drink, the alcoholic individual begins to experience initial symptoms of central nervous system irritability. These symptoms include restlessness, anxiety, nausea, and tachycardia; they are common on awakening in the morning, and are relieved by an "eye-opener"—or a drink early in the morning. The affected individual may complain of feeling "shaky" inside.

If these symptoms are not treated by alcohol ingestion or a sedative, the restlessness progresses to visible tremors, increased anxiety, tachycardia, mild systolic hypertension, diaphoresis, insomnia, anorexia, nausea and vomiting, confusion, and transient hallucinations. Convulsions may begin at this stage of withdrawal. The alcoholic individual is obviously ill; treatment with sedatives to reduce autonomic reactivity must be started emergently in order to prevent severe symptoms.

Without treatment, severe withdrawal symptoms— also known as delirium tremens—occur within 72 hours. These symptoms include severe, uncontrollable shaking, restlessness, and agitation. The affected individual is intensely fearful. Food and fluids are refused because of marked nausea and vomiting; even with no food or fluid intake the individual experiences dry heaves. Other symptoms are disorientation, confusion, and terrifying hallucinations. All vital signs are markedly elevated, as is the metabolic rate. Grand mal seizures are common.

Medical and nursing care of the patient in withdrawal from alcohol focuses on rehydration and decreasing autonomic reactivity. These goals are met by encouraging oral fluid intake when possible, and providing fluids intravenously when necessary. Autonomic reactivity is decreased chemically, usually with benzodiazepenes. The drug most commonly used for outpatient detoxification in alcoholism is oxazepam (Serax), owing to its relatively short half-life of 5 to 15 hours. Should the alcoholic individual begin to drink alcohol after taking a benzodiazepene such as oxazepam, the combined effects of the two substances may be lethal. Patients treated for alcoholism on an in-patient basis may be appropriately given one of the longer-lasting benzodiazepenes.

Alcohol withdrawal has a mortality rate of 10 to 15%. Death is caused by the drastic reduction in glucose available to cerebral tissue following or during grand mal seizures, as well as by electrolyte imbalances from dehydration and prolonged vomiting. Delirium tremens is treated with sedation (or alcohol ingestion), intravenous fluids, and reduction of stimulation. Successful recovery from alcohol withdrawal depends on the early recognition of the symptoms of withdrawal and appropriate treatment.

DEPRESSANTS

History

Depressant drugs are those that depress the sympathetic nervous system or that stimulate the parasympathetic nervous system. Categories of drugs includZed in the depressant class are sedatives, hypnotics, and narcotic-analgesics. **Sedatives** are drugs used for calming or relaxation, **hypnotics** are used to promote sleep, and **narcotic-analgesics** are used to relieve pain.

Sedative and hypnotic drugs have been used since the early 19th century. The classic "Mickey Finn" used to shanghai sailors consisted of chloral hydrate mixed with alcohol. Chloral hydrate was developed in 1832, and its therapeutic use as a sleep-inducing agent began in 1870. Paraldehyde was developed in 1829 and was the first sedating agent used in mental hospitals.

Narcotic-analgesics have been used for centuries in the form of opium. Early Greek, Roman, and Egyptian cultures used opium for recreation as well as pain relief. The use of opium diminished during the Middle Ages. Arabic and Asian cultures, however, refined and promoted the use of opium. By the 19th century, opium was used in American and European cultures as it had been used in Arab and Asian cultures for centuries, in the form of laudanum solution.

The use of opium in the form of laudanum was both legal and widespread. All that was necessary to obtain a bottle of laudanum was to visit a pharmacy and request it. No social stigma was attached to its use. The demographic study of opium addiction during this period, in the late 18th and 19th century, revealed the average opium addict of the time to be white, middle or upper class, and female.

The primary active ingredient in opium, morphine, was isolated in 1831; this was followed in 1832 by the identification of codeine. The invention of the hypodermic syringe in 1853 in conjunction with three major wars stimulated the worldwide use of opiates as analgesics. Addiction to the opiates was commonplace, and was called the "army disease."

The end of the 19th century saw the development by the Bayer company in 1896 of heroin as a nonaddicting substitute for codeine. Heroin is approximately three times more powerful than morphine. Because it was administered orally, however, several years passed before its addictive potential was realized.

A groundswell of feeling against the recreational use of drugs and alcohol began with the Temperance Movement in the mid-19th century in America. This culminated in the passage of the Harrison Act in 1914 and the Volstead Act in 1920. The Harrison Act made it possible to secure narcotics only from a physician. The Volstead Act made the manufacture, distribution, and consumption of alcohol illegal.

With physicians generally unwilling to prescribe narcotics in order to maintain addiction, and prevent withdrawal from these drugs, the demographics of addiction changed quickly. As opiates became illegal, their use shifted from the mainstream population to "people in the life—show people, entertainers, and musicians; racketeers and gangsters; prostitutes and pimps" (Preble and Casey, 1969).

Current attitudes and beliefs about narcotics and the people who use them remain relatively unchanged in the United States. Narcotics are considered appropriate only for medicinal purposes, and recreational or abusive narcotics users are individuals distinctly outside the law.

Pharmacokinetics

Depressant drugs suppress the sympathetic nervous system by altering neurotransmitter levels. Opiate drugs (morphine, codeine, heroin, and the synthetic opiates such as meperidine, hydromorphone, and fentanyl) occupy endorphin receptors, producing euphoria and analgesia. This effect is particularly marked in the medulla, and is the cause for respiratory depression and the cessation of breathing in cases of opiate overdose.

In addition, chronic users of narcotic drugs deplete serotonin at a more rapid rate than do non-users. Serotonin is an inhibitory neurotransmitter regulating pain perception and anxiety. Without a narcotic drug occupying endorphin receptors at the synapse, the addicted individual perceives greater pain and anxiety in response to less stimulation than does the non-addicted person.

As addicting drugs, narcotic analgesics produce tolerance. Progressively greater amounts are needed to produce the desired effects. Logically, the addicted individual who is ill or injured and in need of analgesia will require far greater doses of medication before experiencing relief of pain. This tolerance to drugs, with loss of the normal effect of serotonin and ongoing complaints of pain (sometimes for relatively minor medical problems) leads health-care providers to ascribe the addicted person's request for analgesia to drug-seeking behavior.

Withdrawal from opiates produces very uncomfortable symptoms in the addict. Approximately 6 to 8 hours after the last use of an opiate, the addict begins to feel nervous and edgy. This is followed within a short time by a runny nose, tearing, and piloerection. Muscles, joints, and bones begin to ache. Nausea, vomiting, and diarrhea begin. These symptoms last from 4 to 7 days. These symptoms are extremely unpleasant (keep in mind the increased pain and anxiety that result from low serotonin levels), but have never been documented as lethal. The symptoms are relieved with the ingestion of opiates or other central nervous system depressants.

Sedative-hypnotic drugs enhance the effects of gamma-aminobutyric acid (GABA) at the synapses. GABA has an inhibitory effect on synaptic activity in the central nervous system, producing a sense of calm and relaxation. Sedative-hypnotic drugs also produce tolerance in the individual, who requires ever-increasing doses to achieve a sense of calm.

The broad category of sedative-hypnotic agents includes several different types of drugs. The most commonly abused are the benzodiazepenes, a family of drugs that includes diazepam (Valium), lorazepam (Ativan), alprazolam (Xanax), chlordiazepoxide (Librium), oxazepam (Serax), and triazolam (Halcion). Historically abused sedatives include the barbiturates, meprobamate, and methaqualone. Although there are still individuals who use and abuse these latter drugs, excessive use of the benzodiazepines constitutes by far the most prevalent problem.

The benzodiazepenes are relatively safe when compared with the opiates. However, they still carry some very real dangers.

It is almost impossible to orally ingest a lethal dose of benzodiazepenes. One falls asleep before a lethal oral dose can be consumed. This changes dramatically when benzodiazepenes are combined with alcohol. In this case the respiratory center of the brain can become depressed and breathing can stop. The affected individual can die from a lethal overdose of benzodiazepenes, sometimes unintentionally.

Another danger associated with the benzodiazepenes is withdrawal. As the individual who misuses these drugs becomes tolerant of them and increases their dose, the seizure threshold of the brain is raised. Raising the seizure threshold means that greater stimulation is required to cause a seizure. Abrupt cessation of benzodiazepenes lowers this threshold in a sudden manner and causes seizures, frequently in the form of status epilepticus. Benzodiazepene withdrawal must be gradual, and is best done with the dependent individual hospitalized for careful monitoring.

Nursing Assessment

Persons addicted to depressant drugs may or may not fit the common stereotype of an addict. Those who are users of intravenous heroin may indeed be emaciated and have large inflamed areas of the body surface from recurrent cellulitis. In a person who uses heroin intranasally, however, there may be few obvious signs of addiction.

In taking a history, all medication use should be considered. The nurse should inquire about current prescriptions, over-the-counter (OTC) medications, and recreational drug use. Past illnesses and traumatic injuries should be listed, since there are correlations between some illnesses and addiction (Table 31–3), as well as between trauma and addiction.

Nutritional status should also be assessed, since drug dependence and nutritional deficits are strongly correlated. This is due not only to the direct effects of some addictive drugs, but also to economics. A person attempting to avoid withdrawal tends to spend whatever money is available on drugs rather than on food. Further, the food that is consumed tends to be inexpensive and low in nutrient value.

The infection status of the addict should also be assessed. Intravenous drug users and their sexual partners are two of the groups that continue to have high rates of newly diagnosed human immunodeficiency virus (HIV) infection. Tuberculosis rates continue to climb in the addicted population because of poor nutritional and immune-system status and exposure to the disease and the elements. Cellulitis is common in persons using needles to administer drugs, and pneumonia is common in heroin addicts who are motionless ("on the nod") for extended periods following intravenous heroin injection.

Sexually transmitted diseases are more frequent in the addicted population for two primary reasons. First, intoxication impairs judgment about having unpro-

tected sex. Persons who are otherwise careful become less so when intoxicated. Second, there is a high rate of prostitution among both male and female addicts. Sex is traded either directly for drugs or for money to purchase drugs.

A final element of the nursing assessment of the addicted patient should be an assessment of the patient's family. A genogram can be helpful in assessing

TABLE 31–3 DRUGS OF ABUSE AND SYMPTOMS

Drug Class	Symptoms
Depressants	
Narcotic-Analgesics	
Opium	Constricted pupils,
Heroin	respiratory depression,
Morphine	hypotension, bradycardia
Codeine	nausea, drowsiness,
Methadone	euphoria
Demerol	
Fentanyl	
Dilaudid	
Percodan	
Talwin	
Benzodiazepenes	
Valium	Slurred speech,
Ativan	disorientation,
Halcion	staggering, relief from
Xanax	anxiety
Dalmane	
Librium	
Alcohol	Slurred speech, disorientation, staggering
Barbiturates	
Seconal	Slurred speech,
Tuinal	disorientation,
Phenobarbital	staggering
Amytal	
Stimulants	
Cocaine	Hypervigilance,
Amphetamine	euphoria, excitation,
Desoxyn	insomnia, anorexia,
Dexedrine	hypertension, tachycardia
Biphetamine	
Ritalin	
Hallucinogens	Visual, tactile,
Lysergic acid diethylamide	auditory, or olfactory
Phencyclidine	hallucinations;
Psilocybin	delusions; labile
Mescaline	emotions

the transmission of addiction as well as other medical problems across generations. The simple act of genogram construction often has the effect of removing much of the guilt, blame, and shame from the addict as he or she realizes that addiction is a systemic rather than an isolated problem. In addition, the genogram permits potential support systems within the family to be identified.

STIMULANTS

Stimulant drugs are consumed by millions of people daily. Many people cannot imagine beginning the day without a cup (or three) of coffee or tea. Caffeine, while not meeting the criteria for causing tolerance, does produce withdrawal symptoms and can be considered addictive.

Nicotine is also addictive. Although the development of tolerance to nicotine is still being debated, there is no doubt that nicotine produces potent withdrawal symptoms and creates strong urges to relapse in its users. It has been called the single most addictive drug in America today, and is certainly directly responsible for the greatest number of drug-related deaths in America (Ray and Ksir, 1993). Although caffeine and nicotine create many health problems, discussion of addicting stimulant drugs in this chapter will be confined to the illegal drugs cocaine and amphetamine, since there is much information elsewhere on the dangers of caffeine and nicotine.

History

Cocaine has been used for centuries by Native Americans in the higher elevations of South America. Cocaine is consumed there orally by chewing the leaves of the coca plant. This serves to raise the pulse slightly and to increase the cardiac output in a high-altitude environment with lower oxygen concentrations. The chewed coca leaves do not, however, produce the "high" that cocaine is reputed to produce in its other ingested forms.

Cocaine was introduced into the United States in the late 19th century in patent medicines. The popular story that the soft drink Coca-Cola contained cocaine is indeed true. Coca-Cola was one of many over-the-counter tonics that one could purchase for the relief of fatigue. These patent medicines all became illegal to sell or purchase with the passage of the Harrison Act in 1914.

Cocaine in its current incarnation was introduced in the 1920s. Cocaine powder has been popular among the same population described as heroin users—"musicians, entertainers, (and) gangsters." This was generally true until the 1980s, when a generation of young, ambitious, middle class, and upwardly mobile people discovered that cocaine not only produced euphoria but also provided seemingly boundless energy for work and play. An entire generation found itself at risk for cocaine addiction.

The cocaine problem was compounded exponentially in the mid-1980s with the introduction of crack cocaine. Crack cocaine is made by blending powdered cocaine hydrochloride (an acid) with an equal amount of a chemical base and mixing the resulting compound with a volatile liquid to free the pure cocaine from the base and impurities. What is left is a clear to dark tan crystal chunk that is 95 to 99% pure cocaine. The crystal makes a cracking noise as it is heated, thus the name *crack*.

The processing of cocaine powder sounds as if it would be laborious and economically unsound. The reality is quite the opposite. Crack cocaine can be sold in very small amounts, and persons smoking this form of the drug develop an immediate euphoric "high" that lasts only 15 to 20 minutes. After this time a profound "crash" occurs, with immediate dysphoria. The person smoking the drug is strongly motivated to use it to an increasing degree, both to maintain the euphoria and prevent the subsequent crash. What began as a drug used by the wealthy or upwardly mobile became cheap and available for use by the poor.

Amphetamines, methamphetamines, and dexedrine, known for years as *speed*, also has a history of waxing and waning popularity. The Chinese have been using herbs containing ephedrine for centuries. Amphetamine was discovered in the 1920s; its effectiveness as a bronchodilator confirmed the Chinese use of the herb for respiratory problems.

Amphetamine was widely used by the militaries of most of the countries involved in the Second World War. Soldiers given dexedrine could march longer and stay more awake and alert while on guard. The use of dexedrine by persons needing to stay awake for long periods, such as long distance truck drivers, continued after the war.

The concomitant anorexic effects of amphetamine were noticed in a culture that was beginning an obsession with slenderness, as the United States was in the 1950s. Many drug companies began the manufacture of diet pills that were consumed by millions of people trying to lose weight. However, long-term weight loss was not maintained with the use these diet pills. In 1970, the U.S. Food and Drug Administration (FDA) restricted the use of amphetamines to attention deficit/hyperactivity disorder, short-term weight loss, and the treatment of narcolepsy.

The pills consumed for energy and weight loss were discovered by a generation experimenting with drugs in the 1960s. Amphetamine and methamphetamine were taken orally, nasally, and intravenously.

These drugs produced euphoria, high energy levels, and an attitude and affect of expansiveness and mastery of life. Unfortunately, at high doses, they may also produce severe paranoia.

In the mid-1980s, a production process was devised for methamphetamine that was similar to the process used for producing crack cocaine. At that time a smokable, crystalline form of methamphetamine, known as *ice*, was introduced into the United States. It has the same general effects of crack cocaine with one notable exception—instead of lasting 15 to 20 minutes, the effects of a single dose of ice may last for up to 14 hours. The use of ice has been somewhat limited in parts of the United States by the ready availability of crack cocaine.

Pharmacokinetics

Cocaine has the effect of blocking the re-uptake of norepinephrine, dopamine, and serotonin at their individual synapses. The resulting accumulations of these neurotransmitters stimulate the central nervous system, specifically the sympathetic nervous system. In addition to producing "fight or flight" physical reactivity, this stimulation produces a sense of well-being, energy, and euphoria, especially with the first use of cocaine. There is some evidence that a first dose of cocaine generates a permanent alteration of neurotransmitter function such that the same sense of well-being and euphoria is never quite replicated.

Cocaine is metabolized in the liver. Its half-life in the body is relatively short, lasting approximately 1 hour. Because of its short half-life, cocaine is measured in the body by testing for its metabolites, which have a half-life of approximately 8 hours. In general, even the heavy user of cocaine will test negatively for cocaine metabolites within a few days after the most recent use of the drug.

Assessment

The individual who is dependent on stimulant drugs is likely to present for treatment in poor physical condition. Energy levels may be extremely low. Fatigue and psychomotor retardation may be so great as to resemble clinical depression.

Assessment of the stimulant addict involves the same systemic overview of psychiatric/psychological and physical sequelae of drug use discussed in connection with alcohol and depressants. The stimulant addict in withdrawal presents with dysphoria and anhedonia, and is literally incapable of feeling pleasure at this time. Mood and affect may be difficult to assess in such an individual as a function of withdrawal because even after the last drug dose has been detoxified, neurotransmitter levels may be so unbalanced as to produce signs of clinical depression. The depression accompanying withdrawal may be severe enough to warrant hospitalization.

Physical effects of stimulant addiction include the sympathetic effects of tachycardia, hypertension, increased metabolic and respiratory rates, anorexia, restlessness, and pupillary constriction. With each new use of cocaine, particularly via inhalation, there is massive systemic vasoconstriction. This vasoconstriction is responsible for many of the untoward sequelae associated with cocaine use, which can include coronary artery spasm, and myocardial infarction, cerebral vascular constriction with a cerebral vascular accident, and uterine artery constriction with spontaneous abortion. Other potential health complications include epistaxis from repeated snorting of cocaine, and trauma from the occasionally violent life-style accompanying illegal drug use. With poor nutrition and rest habits, the stimulant addict is infection-prone. The previously discussed infectious complications of drug abuse (tuberculosis, sexually transmitted disease, and HIV with or without acquired immune deficiency system, and hepatitis) are also prevalent in the cocaine-addicted population. Careful assessment must be done for these diseases.

Malnutrition is very common in the cocaine addict as a result of marked anorexia, hyperactivity, and the use of money for drug acquisition rather than food. The addict usually presents with an emaciated appearance, or at the very least will report significant

E CASE EXAMPLE

Marty is a 36-year-old stockbroker referred by the employee assistance program at his company for treatment of cocaine addiction. He began snorting cocaine 2 years ago at a party and was astounded by the euphoria and energy it produced. Almost immediately, he began using it daily at work "to get more done." Initially, he was minimally more productive, but has now missed many days from work, and random urine testing has twice proved him positive for cocaine. He now must report for treatment or be fired.

weight loss during the time of greatest use of the drug. It is not unusual for the addict to be unable to recall the last meal eaten, especially if there has been recent major drug ingestion. Appetite may take some time to return, or the addict may crave foods of high sugar content.

The possibility of high levels of paranoia with stimulant use coupled with illegal and large sums of money exchanging hands in a group of people who are essentially strangers sets the stage for violence-related trauma. Persons who use illegal stimulants are at high risk for traumatic assault and injury.

Withdrawal from the stimulant drugs has a less dramatic presentation than the withdrawal syndromes associated with depressant drugs. The overwhelming symptom is fatigue. The individual addicted to stimulant drugs is likely to have a long-term history of sleep disruption and sleep deprivation. The addict withdrawing from stimulant drugs may spend hours "catching up" on sleep.

HALLUCINOGENS

The deliberate use of hallucinogens has its roots in religious practice. The Native American Church has as a practice the use of peyote buttons, a product of an indigenous cactus of the southwestern United States, for the production of visions. Marijuana was used in ancient India and mushrooms in pre-Christian Europe for the same effect.

Accidental ingestion of hallucinogens may also have a long history. Some of the witch-killing frenzy in France in the Middle Ages may have been sparked by the eating of bread made with moldy wheat and ergot—a precursor of lysergic acid diethylamide (LSD).

LSD has the effect of interfering with dopamine at the sensory synapses of the nervous system. Signals that are allowed across the synapse are altered in such a way as to markedly affect the individual's perception of reality. Visual, auditory, and tactile hallucinations are common. Pain and motor neurons are not affected by LSD.

The laboratory creation of LSD grew from accidental ingestion. In 1938, the creator of LSD, Dr. Albert Hoffman, spilled some of the fluid on his hand before realizing that it is absorbed through the skin. After experiencing hallucinations and an altered state of consciousness, Dr. Hoffman deliberately tested LSD by taking a dose of 0.25 mg (the usual dose 50 *micrograms*). He experienced aural and visual hallucinations and severe distortions of the sense of time.

LSD was tested by the United States military and intelligence agencies to evaluate its use against enemy soldiers. Psychiatrists tried using LSD to increase patient insights and shorten or facilitate treatment. When publicized by Dr. Timothy Leary in 1966, LSD spread to the general population as a recreational drug.

Phencyclidine (PCP) was developed by the Parke-Davis pharmaceutical company in 1956 for use as a general anesthetic. It proved to be an excellent anesthetic in that it produced anesthesia without concomitant decreases in blood pressure. When the patient began to awaken, however, the drug produced violent and frightening hallucinations that often resulted in injury to both the patient and recovery room personnel. The medication was subsequently removed from the market as a human anesthetic agent and released for use in the veterinary population.

At low doses, PCP produces euphoria. At higher doses, however, PCP affects dopamine at the synaptic clefts in a manner that produces hallucinations. In addition, the PCP user becomes delusional and experiences **peripheral anesthesia**. Most persons set limits on their physical behavior on parameters of the comfort and discomfort it evokes. With peripheral anesthesia, these constraints disappear. The popular media portrait of the drug user whom the police shoot several times without effect can apply to the user of large amounts of PCP. Such an individual can therefore be very dangerous to those around him.

There is no withdrawal from LSD or PCP. However, both drugs create another long-term potential health problem, in that when they are used to excess, they may be inefficiently metabolized. Since both of these drugs are highly fat-soluble, quantities that are not metabolized are stored in fat tissue and may be released into the circulation during times of fat metabolism, producing hallucinations. This may contribute to the "flashback" phenomenon encountered in users of LSD and PCP, in which hallucinations occur without the ingestion of drugs.

The individual using a hallucinogenic drug will display the following sympathomimetic signs: dilated pupils, salivation, hypertension, and hyperthermia. The half-life of LSD is 3 hours; within 6 hours most of the effects of the drug are gone. Assessment of the user should be deferred until effects of the drug have worn off. While there are fewer systemic health risks with LSD and PCP than with stimulant and depressant drugs, the user of a hallucinogenic drug is at risk for trauma because of the altered state of consciousness produced by the drug. This is exemplified in the following case:

■ DRUG TESTING

Many companies now require drug testing as a condition of employment. These tests can be done on samples of blood, urine, or hair, or with perspiration-collecting patches. Popular wisdom holds that drug testing results can be nullified by the drinking of large amounts of water or the use of herbal treatments (goldenseal) to cleanse the body. These tactics have had some limited success in confusing the results of blood and urine testing, but do not affect hair and perspiration testing.

A danger associated with drug testing is inaccuracy resulting in falsely positive or falsely negative results. False-positive results can be caused by the resemblance of metabolites of certain foods and legitimate drugs to the metabolites of illegal substances. Some of these foods and drugs include:

Test Positive For:	Caused By:
Alcohol	Cough syrup or any medication in tincture
Opiates	Poppy seeds (large quantities), ibuprofen
Amphetamines	Decongestants containing ephedrine or pseudoephedrine

■ CARE OF THE DRUG-ABUSING PATIENT

PLANNING

In planning care for the individual with an addiction, the nurse must first be very clear about his or her goals. If the addicted individual is presenting for treatment of the addiction, it is appropriate for the nurse to adopt long-term measures that include addiction management.

If, however, the addicted individual has presented for the treatment of appendicitis or bipolar disorder and is in denial about his or her addiction, the nurse is guaranteed increased frustration and an angry, noncompliant client when addressing the addiction. In this situation, the nurse and all other health-care providers should keep the addiction in mind when considering the patient's anxiety and pain levels and the doses of

TABLE 31–4 WITHDRAWAL AND OVERDOSE SYMPTOMS

Drug Category	Withdrawal	Overdose
Alcohol	Hypertension, tachycardia, tremors, nausea, anxiety, delirium, vomiting, seizures, death	Respiratory depression, bradycardia, hypotension.
Depressants		
Narcotics	Anorexia, nausea, vomiting, chills, diaphoresis, panic, muscle cramps, watery eyes, runny nose.	Shallow respirations, constricted pupils, shock, coma, death
Benzodiazepenes	Anxiety, nausea, seizures	Respiratory depression
Stimulants		
Cocaine	Depression, hypersomnia, apathy, anhedonia, irritability	Seizures, hyperthermia, agitation, hallucinations
Amphetamines	Depression, hypersomnia, apathy, anhedonia, irritability	Paranoia, hyperthermia, agitation, seizures
Hallucinogens	None	Psychosis

medication required to manage them. The nurse should also be aware of potential withdrawal symptoms (see Table 31–4). The addicted patient in denial should be offered educational information pamphlets and/or telephone numbers "just in case the drug use or drinking ever becomes a problem." In this way, the patient is given an opportunity to address his or her problem in a less ego-threatening way.

Planning for care of the addicted patient also requires a holistic approach that takes into account the stage of the patient's addiction or recovery. Popular wisdom dictates that a person cannot be treated effectively for addiction until he or she has "hit bottom" and lost

E CASE EXAMPLE

Joey is a 17-year-old white high-school student who has spent the past 2 days with a friend smoking marijuana soaked in phencyclidine. The initial euphoria has progressed to delusional and hallucinatory behavior. Joey believes that his friend is an agent of the Central Intelligence Agency and is trying to control his mind. He has been hearing voices telling him to get rid of the friend and protect himself. The noise of the resulting fight disturbs the neighbors, who call the police. Joey's friend is now unconscious from a head injury in the fight. The police surround the house and ordered Joey to come out. He charges out of the house and assaults two of the police officers, who shoot him several times. Joey is peripherally anesthetized and continues to fight until he loses enough blood from his wounds to cause hypotension and collapse. Even then, it requires four officers to put him in handcuffs.

everything. It is true that an addicted person must be strongly motivated to recover; addiction is a powerful force, and the motivation to change must be equally powerful. Regardless of the assessment made by members of the health-care staff, the individual's readiness, an addicted person requesting help must be offered assistance and information. Even if the addict relapses, the information received and the affirmative treatment experience serve as positive reinforcements to seek treatment again.

IMPLEMENTATION

The first treatment priority for the addict must be physiological stabilization and detoxification. As previously mentioned, withdrawal from some drugs can be life-threatening. Hospitalization may be necessary for some detoxifications; much of the time, however, detoxification can be accomplished on an outpatient basis or at a detoxification center. Nursing responsibilities in this phase include monitoring the addict for physiological stability, assuring adequate fluid and nutritional intake, and providing emotional support and education.

Following the period of detoxification, the addict requires ongoing treatment to prevent relapse. The treatment selected depends upon the theoretical framework used by the health care provider to define addiction, and on the resources available in the community. Treatment options are presented in the following sections according to the theoretical framework.

Medical Model

Several medications have been used in relapse prevention. Perhaps the most widely known is disulfiram (Antabuse). Disulfiram blocks the metabolism of alcohol at the stage of acetaldehyde formation. Acetaldehyde is toxic; at high levels it produces palpitations, nausea and vomiting, facial flushing, and diaphoresis. The person taking disulfiram is unable to metabolize alcohol and becomes ill when drinking. Disulfiram is effective as long as the alcoholic patient continues to take it. Because of the unpleasant effects it creates with alcohol ingestion and the strong urge to drink, many alcoholic individuals simply stop taking the medication. Moreover, the cardiac symptoms of disulfiram may be dangerous to the alcoholic individual who either relapses or has an accidental ingestion of alcohol (such as with medications that are tinctures) while taking disulfiram.

Another medication helpful in relapse prevention is naltrexone. Naltrexone is a long-acting narcotic antagonist that acts to block the craving for alcohol that is believed to arise from the pleasure center in the brain and is experienced strongly in the early stages of recovery. The primary drawback of naltrexone is that it blocks the action of narcotic and synthetic narcotic analgesics as well as blocking craving for alcohol. The alcoholic individual requiring analgesia must either use non-narcotic analgesics or stop taking naltrexone.

Medication therapy is also used in preventing relapse in opiate addiction. Methadone is a long-acting synthetic opiate that prevents the withdrawal symptoms associated with heroin addiction. Methadone may be used in two primary ways in the treatment of opiate addiction. The first is in a tapered withdrawal that is designed to prevent withdrawal symptoms while gradually decreasing the dose of methadone until it is discontinued. The second method of methadone administration is to simply give the addict a stable dose of methadone and leave him or her on it permanently. Ciritics of this method say that it simply changes the drug of addiction without changing the addict's behavior. While this criticism is certainly true, the treatment removes addict from an illegal drug–seeking lifestyle, and eliminates the potential for using contaminated intravenous needles, thus decreasing other health risks associated with opiate addiction.

Researchers continue to seek drugs that will prevent or mediate the craving associated with cocaine addiction. Thus far, research with amantadine and selegiline in reducing relapse in cocaine addicts has been inconclusive. Nursing responsibilities in programs using a medication for relapse prevention include medication education (effects and side effects), addiction education, and emotional support for the addict.

Also within the medical model of addiction are the 12 Step programs, such as those of Alcoholics Anonymous and Narcotics Anonymous. These programs consider addiction to be a disease of the body, mind, and spirit. Rather than treating addiction medically or psychiatrically, the 12-step programs are directed at self-help and generally aim to stop participants from seeking assistance from the medical community.

Alcoholics Anonymous is a world-wide, loosely organized system of self-help groups. It uses peer support to achieve total abstinence from drugs and alcohol. It is free to anyone wishing to attend its meetings. With a huge international membership, Alcoholics Anonymous has undoubtedly helped many people in their efforts to stop drinking and/or using drugs.

Begun in 1935 by two middle-class American men struggling with alcoholism, the Alcoholics Anonymous program uses daily meetings, peer support, assistance from a "sponsor" (a person who has achieved sobriety through the program), and rigid adherence to the goal of sobriety to help alcoholics and addicts in their recovery. While certainly meeting the needs of many people in this effort, Alcoholics Anonymous has sometimes been less successful for women and members of other ethnic groups. There is little in the way of controlled research either to support or to challenge the organization's methods.

E CASE EXAMPLE

Lynnette is a crack-addicted 32-year-old single black mother of five children, and is 6 months pregnant. The department of human services in her community has custody of her children. She says that her primary reason for being in drug treatment is to regain custody of her children, but despairs of doing so, since she has been unable to avoid drugs for more than 5 days. After telling the group about her most recent relapse, she says that she is thinking of giving up. The group points out to her that in spite of her continued use of crack, she has kept all of her prenatal appointments and has been able to pay her rent and stay in the same apartment for the past 8 months—a record unprecedented for the past 3 years of her addiction. The group also points out that her relapses are not lasting as long as they formerly did. This is interpreted as Lynnette's making better decisions and keeping better track of her responsibilities. She realizes that her attitude toward crack use has changed.

In practical terms, the meetings of Alcoholics Anonymous provide a place for the struggling addict or alcoholic individual to be with other people who are not using alcohol or drugs. They prevent isolation of the recovering individual and provide a sober social environment with recreational activities. The organization also provides a support system that is available 24 hours a day for the individual who may be in crisis at 3:00 A.M. Finally, Alcoholics Anonymous is free of charge and offers a wide variety of meeting times and places. Most clinical treatment programs advise recovering alcoholic individuals and addicts to attend a twelve-step program as additional support.

For patients needing support groups but who find Alcoholics Anonymous, Narcotics Anonymous, or Cocaine Anonymous unacceptable, alternatives do exist. Women for Sobriety is a program that acknowledges differences in the ways women and men experience addiction. Women for Sobriety achieves abstinence through building self-esteem rather than through spirituality. The group teaches new coping skills and ways of thinking through thirteen affirmations and increasing personal power rather than by admitting powerlessness.

A second and larger alternative to Alcoholics Anonymous is Rational Recovery. Rational Recovery also rejects spirituality and powerlessness. Members are encouraged to build on the strengths they have and to "think themselves sober." Personal responsibility, choice, and decision-making are emphasized with the eventual goal of independence from the drug or alcohol addiction and the Rational Recovery group itself. Nursing responsibilities for clients in self-help programs include education about available choices and additional emotional support.

Psychosocial Model

The psychosocial model for the treatment of alcoholism or addiction uses either cognitive therapy, behavior modification, or humanistic techniques to achieve changes in addictive behavior. Early research was done with aversion therapy, using electric shocks or nausea-producing medications coupled with drinking to make drinking a less desirable behavior. The nausea-producing medication worked better than the electric shocks, but neither was successful enough to be a basis for treatment.

Cognitive therapy has been more successful in altering the thinking and behaviors associated with alcoholism or drug addiction. In this therapy, both the cognitions and activities of the patient prior to drug and/or alcohol use are analyzed. Instead of perceiving

E CASE EXAMPLE

Mrs. J. has suffered from alcoholism for the past 15 years. After the death of her mother (also an alcoholic), and with her husband and children's support, she was motivated to attempt sobriety. After being hospitalized for 1 month she returned home to discover that family decisions were being made without her input or approval. When she pointed this out, her children became annoyed and her husband stated that it had certainly been easier to get things done when she was drunk. She relapsed within a week.

E CASE EXAMPLE

▶ THE CHEMICALLY-DEPENDENT PATIENT

Terry, a 27-year-old black woman with dependence on crack cocaine, alcohol, and nicotine, comes to the clinic to get help for her drug problem because she doesn't want to lose her children. She began smoking cigarettes at the age of 16 and has been smoking crack for the past 6 years, after her boyfriend introduced her to it; she discovered 4 years ago that drinking a 40-ounce container of beer after smoking crack "took the edge off" and made it possible to enjoy the crack. She denies using other drugs.

Terry is 3 months pregnant. She now leaves her six children with her mother for days at a time while she is smoking crack. None of her family or friends trust her to be alone in their homes because she has stolen from them repeatedly to obtain money with which to buy drugs. She is at risk for losing her apartment because she has not paid the rent for 2 months. The local department of human services is investigating her for possible removal of her children to foster care. Terry verbalizes fear, anger, and hopelessness when talking about losing her children.

Terry has two sisters and a mother. Both sisters use crack and her mother is a recovering alcoholic. Terry never knew her father, but believes that he was an alcoholic, on the basis of comments by her mother. She has never felt close to her family, stating "My mother was drunk all the time when I was little—I don't know what she wants from me now."

Terry graduated from high school but was pregnant at the time. Her plans to continue school were delayed by repeated pregnancies. She has no job skills and has never been employed in a full-time job outside the home.

Terry is receiving prenatal care. Her health history is negative except for a well-healed broken arm received in a fight while intoxicated. She is unaware of her HIV status and says that she doesn't want to know it.

She comes to the clinic for her initial interview 8 hours after her last use of crack and alcohol. She is tired and depressed, and emaciated in appearance, appearing to be about 30 pounds underweight. She has a fine tremor in her hands. Her pulse and blood pressure are elevated. Her temperature is 100 degrees Fahrenheit.

Her mental status reveals a flat affect with a depressed mood. She is casually and somewhat sloppily dressed. Her hair is uncombed. She has difficulty focusing on questions and displays psychomotor retardation. She verbalizes some suicidal ideation, but has no plan or means for acting on these ideas.

Diagnostic Impressions, *DSM-IV* Multiaxial Diagnoses:

Axis I:	Cocaine dependence
	Alcohol dependence
	Depression
Axis II:	No diagnosis
Axis III:	Alcohol withdrawal syndrome
	Malnutrition
	Sleep deprivation
Axis IV:	Potential loss of children
	Potential loss of home
	Lack of support system
	Economic instability
	Educational and occupational deficits
Axis V:	Global Assessment of Function = 25 (current and highest in previous year)

Diagnostic impressions, nursing diagnoses:

- Ineffective individual coping related to cocaine and alcohol dependence.
- Potential for sensory-perceptual alteration related to chemical withdrawal.
- Altered nutrition, less than body requirements.
- Altered sleep patterns.
- Impaired social interaction.

Nursing Diagnosis:

- Ineffective individual coping related to cocaine and alcohol dependence.

Short-term Goals:

- The patient will agree to stop using cocaine within 24 hours.
- The patient will assume responsibility for her behavior.

Long-term Goal:

- The patient will substitute healthy coping responses for substance-abusing behaviors.

Nursing Interventions:

- Assist the patient in identifying his or her substance-abuse problem.
- Aid the patient in identifying behaviors and activities leading to substance abuse.
- Involve the patient in identifying alternative responses to cues that prompt drug abuse.
- Provide constant support with affirmations that the patient is strong enough to stop abusing drugs.
- Re-frame previous patient behaviors to demonstrate client strength, resourcefulness, and problem-solving skills.
- Provide information about effects of drug use across physical, cognitive, emotional, and spiritual domains.
- Encourage patient's attendance at group education and group therapy sessions.

Outcome Criteria:

- The patient will abstain from using all mind-altering drugs.

Nursing Diagnosis:

- Potential for sensory-perceptual alteration related to chemical withdrawal.

Short-term Goals:

- The patient will have stable vital signs.
- The patient will remain free of the symptoms of increased autonomic reactivity.

Long-term Goal:

- The patient will regain a sense of pleasure.

Nursing Interventions:

- Monitor vital signs every 4 hours if stable, more frequently in the presence of tachycardia, hypertension, or hyperthermia.

E CASE EXAMPLE Continued

- Assess patient's orientation whenever vital signs are assessed.
- Observe patient for signs and symptoms of autonomic reactivity: irritability, agitation, tremors, confusion, nausea, diaphoresis, hallucinations.
- Offer sedation as needed in the presence of increased vital signs, tremors, and increasing irritability.
- Encourage fluid intake of 2,000 ml daily.
- Provide education about expected course of detoxification from alcohol and cocaine.
- Provide constant emotional support with information that withdrawal is time-limited and that patient is capable of enduring the withdrawal process.
- Provide information about longer-term effects of drug withdrawal, such as craving and anhedonia; assure patient that these are also time-limited.

Outcome Criteria:

- Patient completes withdrawal process safely.
- Patient verbalizes pleasure and sense of pride in accomplishment.

Nursing Diagnosis:

- Alteration in nutrition, less than body requirements.

Short-term Goals:

- Patient will gain at least 1 pound per week until reaching desired body weight.
- Patient will verbalize connection between loss of appetite and alcohol and cocaine ingestion.

Long-term Goal:

- Patient will demonstrate integration of nutritional principles into daily menu plans.

Nursing Interventions:

- Encourage intake of small, frequent feedings every 2 to 3 hours rather than three large meals daily.
- Monitor patient's use of vitamins and dietary supplements.
- Initiate consultation with dietitian to incorporate patient's preferences into a healthy diet.
- Begin teaching patient about healthy eating. Teach patient about conflicts that may arise between new dietary information and family loyalties.

Outcome Criterion:

- Patient balances caloric intake with body requirements to maintain a healthy weight.

Nursing Diagnosis:

- Altered sleep patterns.

Short-term Goal:

- Patient will be able to sleep 6 hours per night within 2 weeks.

Long-term Goal:

- Patient will report satisfaction with the quality of her sleep.

Nursing Interventions:

- Assess sleep patterns prior to chemical dependence.
- Provide information about sleep-disturbing effects of alcohol and cocaine.
- Assist patient in learning relaxation techniques.
- Encourage use of relaxation techniques at bedtime.
- Assist patient in establishing a bedtime routine that will be followed each night.
- Discourage use of chemical sleep aids other than warm milk.

Outcome Criterion:

- Patient sleeps 6 hours each night.

Nursing Diagnosis:

- Impaired social interaction related to drug-seeking and drug-using life-style.

Short-term Goal:

- Patient will attend group sessions on a regular basis.

Long-term Goal:

- Patient will establish a nurturing and satisfying support group for herself.

Nursing Interventions

- Establish a therapeutic nurse-patient relationship, using a contract format to enhance the patient's understanding of roles and responsibilities.
- Develop mutual goals with patient.
- Provide honest and supportive feedback to patient's verbalized concerns and behaviors.
- Maintain confidentiality.
- Provide patient with opportunities to assist others.
- Provide patient with opportunities to succeed in task accomplishment.
- Analyze and reframe situations perceived as negative.
- Encourage patient to attend a self-help support group; provide patient with choices of types and times of groups.
- Encourage patient to enlist assistance of sober family members and friends in her recovery.

Outcome Criterion:

- Patient will have in place a strong and satisfying support group of sober individuals.

themselves as being without skills, individuals are taught to view survival on the street and obtaining drugs as examples of complex problem-solving that can be adapted to other situations. In one cognitively based group, a client was helped to reframe her behaviors in the following way:

Behaviorism looks at specific drug-seeking or drug-using behaviors and teaches alternatives to them. The therapist will have the individual incorporate some substitute behavior rather than having a drink after work and before dinner, for example. This behavior may involve exercise, napping, or food preparation during these same hours. Eventually the individual will stop associating these time periods with drinking.

Another behavioral approach is to extinguish the conditioned response to the drug of choice. In one study, this involved repeated exposure to the drug of abuse and drug-delivery paraphernalia in a controlled laboratory environment, without use of the drug itself (Childress et al., 1995). On the basis of the classical conditioning model, it was correctly hypothesized that repeated exposure without the reinforcement of drug use would decrease physiological reactivity to withdrawal.

Humanistic therapy seeks to discover what motivates the addict to use the addict's drug of choice. Not all addicts or alcoholic individuals use drugs and alcohol for the same reasons: some use them to blunt feelings, while others use them to allow themselves to feel. The humanistic therapist helps the patient to understand his or her addiction, and then teaches the patient different ways of coping than drinking or drug use.

Nursing responsibilities in programs using psychosocial modalities of therapy for alcoholism or addiction may involve one-to-one therapy, group therapy, education, and emotional support. In in-patient settings the nurse may also be responsible for coordinating services for the patient.

Family-Systems Theory

Family-systems theory views addiction as a function of anxiety. When anxiety rises in a family, the addict uses his or her drug of choice in response to the anxiety. In this way the addict carries the family's symptoms of dysfunction so that the family itself may continue to function. Within this theoretical framework, it is less than useless to limit therapy to the addicted individual. An example illustrates this.

Using family-systems theory, the therapist works not only with the addicted individual but also with as many of the individual's family members as will come to treatment sessions. The family needs to understand repetitive patterns of behavior that it has practiced for generations in order to decrease some of its blaming of the addicted member as the source of its problem. The addict learns ways of dealing with problems other than drinking or drug use; the family learns to deal with the addict as a healthy individual rather than as one who is sick or defective. The family also learns new ways of dealing directly with anxiety-provoking situations. With subsequently lower levels of anxiety in the family, the addict has less need to use alcohol or drugs. AlAnon for adult family members and Alateen for adolescent family members are excellent resources for both support and teaching emotionally nonreactive ways to deal with the addict.

EVALUATION

The single most important indicator of the success of treatment for alcoholism or drug addiction is sobriety. Regardless of the therapeutic model that is chosen, the addict will need lifelong support to maintain sobriety. It is critical that the addict, the family, and the providers of health care realize that in times of great stress, relapse is possible (if not likely). Thus, it may be more appropriate to measure sober and intoxicated periods in the client's life and to consider treatment successful if intoxicated periods shorten and become increasingly rare while sober periods lengthen and become more productive.

The addict should be taught practical coping skills and have realistic expectations. The family and health-care providers must avoid rescue fantasies and emotional reactivity. Alcoholism and addiction are extremely serious threats to physical, cognitive, and emotional health; the addict can, with help, achieve sobriety.

O AN OVERVIEW

- Addiction is a process—usually comprising the five stages of experimentation, recreation, habituation, abuse, and dependence—in which use of a psychoactive substance leads to physical or emotional dependence on that substance.

- Medical, psychosocial, and family-systems models of substance abuse view it in terms of physical correlates, social learning and anxiety reduction, and the dynamics of tension within the family.

- A stimulator of the dopamine pathway, alcohol is metabolized differently by different individuals, produces tolerance in users, and has a potentially fatal withdrawal syndrome marked by increased autonomic reactivity.

- Depressant drugs—sedatives, hypnotics, and narcotic analgesics—depress the central nervous system or stimulate the parasympathetic nervous system by altering neurotransmitter levels. Withdrawal from opiates produces increased pain perception and anxiety as a consequence of low serotonin levels, whereas abrupt withdrawal from the benzodiazepene group of sedative-hypnotics can lower the seizure threshold.

- Cocaine, amphetamines, methamphetamines, and dexedrine are stimulant drugs that produce feelings of euphoria, a high level of energy, and mastery of life. Anorexia is common among chronic stimulant users, who may also present with tachycardia, hypertension, increased metabolic and respiratory rates, restlessness, and pupillary constriction.

- Hallucinogens such as LSD and PCP interfere with dopamine activity at the synapses, altering the transmission of sensory signals to produce hallucinations. Users of PCP also become delusional and peripherally anesthetized, and are potentially dangerous.

- The first goals of treatment for addicted patients are physiological stability and detoxification; long-term psychological and social support, such as the support provided by twelve-step groups, can then be initiated.

TD TERMS TO DEFINE

- addiction
- alcoholic hepatitis
- chemical dependence
- denial
- depressant drugs
- dual diagnosis
- hallucinogenic drugs
- hypnotic drugs
- impairment
- intoxication
- narcotic-analgesic
- peripheral anesthesia
- rationalization
- sedative drugs
- stimulant drugs
- substance abuse
- tolerance
- withdrawal

Q STUDY QUESTIONS

1. Which of the following is not a narcotic?
   a. Opium
   b. Cocaine
   c. Methadone
   d. Codeine

2. The addiction process begins with
   a. habituation.
   b. recreation.
   c. experimentation.
   d. abuse.

3. Withdrawal from narcotics
   a. produces symptoms similar to an exaggerated case of the flu.
   b. may be life-threatening.
   c. is likely to result in temporary paralysis.
   d. is typified by psychotic-like behavior.

4. Police sometimes have trouble subduing a heavy PCP user because
   a. the user is anesthetized and feels no pain.
   b. the user is at times very violent.
   c. the user's behavior is unpredictable.
   d. all of the above
   e. none of the above

5. Depressant drugs mimic or exaggerate which of the following?
   a. Sympathetic nervous system
   b. Parasympathetic nervous system
   c. Autonomic nervous system
   d. Central nervous system

6. Benzodiazepenes are not usually dangerous unless mixed with
   a. cocaine.
   b. methaqualone.
   c. alcohol.
   d. nicotine.

7. Believing that alcoholism is an illness reflects use of the
   a. psychosocial model.
   b. systems model.
   c. medical model.
   d. role model.

8. The medical model approach to addiction would take into consideration all of the following EXCEPT
   a. genetic markers.
   b. enzyme differences.
   c. personality type.
   d. medications to prevent craving of the drug.

9. The primary difference between drug abuse and drug dependence is
   a. the person who is drug dependent does not develop a tolerance to the drug.
   b. the person who abuses drugs shows only cognitive symptoms of withdrawal.
   c. the person who is drug dependent shows no sign of wanting to stop using drugs.
   d. the person who is drug dependent has signs and symptoms of emotional, cognitive, and physical withdrawal.

10. T F In the family-systems approach to addiction, the addicted person acts out the symptoms of anxiety for the whole family.

11. The best approach to take when looking for the cause of addiction is one that
    a. considers biology as the most important of the frameworks.
    b. is based on family systems theory
    c. takes into account psychosocial and cultural factors.
    d. is holistic.

Gawin FH, Ellinwood EH: Cocaine and other stimulants: actions, abuse, and treatment, *New England Journal of Medicine,* 1988; 318(18):1173–1181.

O'Brien CP: Drug dependence, in DiPalma JR, DiGregorio GJ, Barbieri EJ, Ferko AP (eds): *Basic Pharmacology in Medicine,* ed. 4, 1994.

O'Brien CP, Eckardt M, Linnoila M: *Neuropsychopharmacology.* New York, Raven Press, 1994.

Preble E, Casey JJ: Taking care of business—the heroin user's life on the streets. *Int J Addict,* 1969; 4(1):1.

Ray O, Ksir C: *Drugs, Society, and Human Behavior.* St. Louis, CV Mosby, 1993.

Rice DP: (1993). The economic cost of alcohol abuse and alcohol dependence: *Alcohol Health Res World* 1990; 17(1):10–11.

Stanton MD, Todd TC: *The Family Therapy of Drug Abuse and Addiction.* New York, Guilford Press, 1982.

U.S. Department of Health and Human Services, Public Health Service: *Healthy People 2000.* Boston, Jones and Bartlett, 1992.

Volpicelli J: Psychoactive substance use disorders, in Rosenhan DL, Seligman MEP (eds): *Abnormal Psychology.* New York, WW Norton, 1995.

Weil A, Rosen W: *From Chocolate to Morphine.* Boston, Houghton Mifflin, 1993.

Weinreib R, O'Brien CP: Persistent cognitive deficits attributed to substance abuse. *Neurologic Clinics,* 1993; Aug, 11(3):663–691.

■ REFERENCES

Childress AR, Ehrman R, Robbins S, Kung H, O'Brien CP: Using cue reactivity strategies to study the psychophysiological and neurochemical correlates of drug craving. Paper presented at the NIDA Technical Review on Clinical Neurobiology and Treatment of Drug Abuse and Dependence, May 20–21, 1992.

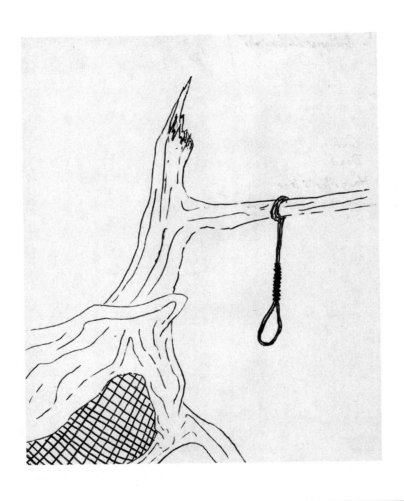

"... the sense of being accompanied by a second self—a wraithlike
observer who, not sharing the dementia of his double is able to watch
with dispassionate curiosity as his companion struggles against the
oncoming disaster, or decides to embrace it . . . I watched myself in
mingled terror and fascination as I began to make the necessary
preparation. . . ."

William Styron

Darkness Visible: A Memoir of Madness

(pp. 64–65) Random House, 1990

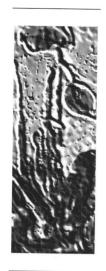

32
Management of Suicidal Patients

Sharon M. Valente

In the United States, a total of 384,262 suicides were recorded from 1980 to 1992 (Kachur et al., 1995). Suicide is the 9th leading cause of death, accounting for more than 30,000 deaths each year, or 1.4% of the total (Kachur et al., 1995). The incidence of suicide has increased significantly since the 1950s (5.2 per 100,000 population) to 12.4 per 100,000, despite advances in the treatment of mental illness. Rates of suicide have increased among those aged 10 to 19 years, young black males, and elderly males (Kachur et al., 1995). Increases in suicide rates are not limited to the United States but are also found in most other countries studied. Firearms "were disproportionately responsible for increases among the young and elderly" (Kachur et al., 1995, p. iii). Suicide is a self-inflicted mode of death that involves undue suffering; suicidal behavior is typically a cry for help. When possible, nurses should strive to relieve conditions that produce suffering and apply a broad range of suicide prevention measures.

Understanding suicide and the methods of screening, early intervention, and monitoring appropriate for suicidal individuals are important priorities for nurses in all settings. Preventing suicide is like preventing fires, in that the critical actions are to maintain vigilance at all times, sound an alarm at an early stage, reduce hazards or methods, detect risk, notify others of danger, and act immediately to ensure safety. Although the principles of suicide prevention remain constant, in-patient and out-patient settings may allow different approaches to risk detection, evaluation, and management of the suicidal patient. Successful management depends on accurate assessment, interdisciplinary collaboration, and examination of attitudes toward suicide.

This chapter examines definitions of suicidal behaviors; the nature, incidence, and epidemiology of suicide; and the application of empirical knowledge to estimating the severity of suicide risk. Suicide assessment and intervention guidelines and case examples are provided to guide practice for the professional nurse. To meet standards of practice, nurses need to detect and evaluate a patient's suicide risk, provide for adequate safety, inform the health-care team of the risk, and document ongoing assessments (ANA, 1994; Bongar et al., 1993; Maris et al., 1992).

■ IMPORTANCE OF ATTITUDES TOWARD SUICIDE

One of the most profound yet invisible influences on a patient's suicide risk is the professional's attitudes and assumptions about suicide (Fishbein and Ajzen, 1975; Valente, Saunders, and Grant, 1994). Attitudes are tendencies to behave in certain ways. The nurse needs to examine his or her personal beliefs and distinguish them from professional attitudes that have an impact on care. Consider the nurse who conveys the attitude that suicidal patients are wrong, immoral, or bad. When patients detect this attitude and feel devalued, they may hesitate to disclose suicidal inclinations or follow the nurse's prescriptions for safety. Favazza (1987) provides a worst-case scenario involving emergency departments in which staff attitudes implied that suicidal patients were not really sick and did not deserve treatment (e.g., in contrast with cardiac patients). Favazza found that suicidal, self-mutilating patients reported receiving negative and abusive treatment from emergency departments to an extent that made them lie about the cause of their self-inflicted injuries (Favazza 1987; Valente, 1993). Nurses need to separate their personal beliefs and religious values from their professional attitudes toward the suicidal patient, which should be therapeutic. Consulting with a colleague or an advanced-practice psychiatric nurse can help nurses monitor their attitudes about suicide.

Suicidal patients tend to elicit feelings of inadequacy, anxiety, and fear of failure from both novice and expert health-care professionals. In a national, random survey of over 400 nurses, respondents reported that their knowledge of, and personal experience with suicide, and the weight of their professional responsibilities, made caring for a suicidal patient difficult (Valente, Saunders, and Grant, 1994) (see Table 32-1). Nurses who consistently explore and understand their feelings about suicidal patients will develop their capacity for empathy and expertise.

■ DETAILED DESCRIPTION

Suicide may be defined as killing oneself on purpose by direct (e.g., by one's own hand) or indirect methods (Durkheim, 1951; Shneidman, 1981; see Table 32-2).

TABLE 32–1. NURSES' DIFFICULTIES IN RESPONDING TO SUICIDAL PATIENTS

Category	Nurses' Comments	Recommended Actions
Religious, spiritual, or other values about suicide	Religious beliefs are anti-suicide. Topic is taboo in society; my religious conviction (suicide is wrong, a mortal sin, a coward's way out).	Seek consultation to discuss your values/ feelings and provide unbiased care: find ways to evaluate risk and act. Distinguish personal values from professional duty.
Uncomfortable feelings and/or fears (e.g., failure to prevent suicide)	Fear of my failure. If the patient commits suicide, did I do enough? Fear of feeling helpless. Fear of my inadequate response. Fear of not being able to care for patients' needs that are not being met.	Seek consultation, recognize fear as a common response. As part of a team, your duty is to detect, evaluate, take action, get help, and notify health-care team. Do not let fears prevent assessment. Provide high-quality care but recognize that not every suicide will be prevented.
Inadequate skills, knowledge, experience	Don't want to say the wrong thing. Unsure of ability to help. Uncertainty of my own skill/knowledge to assess risk. Frustration with inability to convince patient they're needed and loved. Failure "I may not be able to fix things" I'm not a psychiatrist, don't have skills to deal with this. Don't know what to say. How can I impact one who is so troubled?	Recognize feelings. Do not avoid assessment. Improve knowledge and skills. Use consultation. Your task is not to "fix things" or be the expert. You need to say, "I care about your pain and distress and want to make sure you get treatment you need." We need to talk about this, make sure you are safe, and consult with our team of experts.
Personal experiences with a loved one's suicide	Due to a chronic illness, my parent committed suicide when I was young. My young brother impulsively committed suicide.	Seek consultation to help resolve painful loss. Detect risk and get support and consultation patient.
Weight of professional responsibility	Not wanting to get involved but knowing I already am; Fear of not having the best response: Feeling responsible for patient's actions. Tension in medical, legal, ethical duty.	Consultation or case consultation to discuss duties and plan for care. Clarify duty and roles. Nurse is not responsible for patient's action. Duty is to detect, assess, monitor risk, take action, and notify others.

Sources: Valente, Saunders & Grant, 1994 and Saunders, JM and Valente, SM. National survey of oncology nurses' attitudes and knowledge about suicide. *Unpublished data,* personal communication. Funded by Oncology Nursing Society and American Cancer Society.

Parasuicide includes all non-fatal suicidal thoughts, acts, attempts, or wishes. *Lethality* is the potential of an action to cause death.

Because clinicians lack consensus about terms and definitions relating to suicidal behavior, they must clearly describe such behavior in the individual patient. For instance, a nurse who learns that a patient is "suicidal" does not know how recent or lethal this behavior was. Recounting the behavior is essential (e.g., ideas of suicide with no actions; low-lethality attempts with two sleeping pills; a high-lethality attempt with a gun). The American Association of Suicidology discourages the use of commonly misunderstood terms such as "suicide gesture" (Bongar, 1992).

The following vignette illustrates the need to avoid confusing terms and to depict suicidal behavior clearly. During a team conference, the discharge of a young, suicidal man was planned. A new nurse asked for a suicide evaluation. Her concern was ignored, and she was told not to worry because the patient had "only made a suicide gesture." In fact, the patient had poured gasoline on himself and ignited it. The term suicide gesture masked the patient's high risk for suicide and the lethality of his act, and hindered necessary pre-discharge evaluation and safety precautions. Unless the behavior is described, the staff may miss serious clues, a patient's cry for help, and opportunities for preventing suicide.

■ EPIDEMIOLOGY

As previously noted, self-inflicted death claims approximately 30,000 individuals yearly in the United States and is the 9th leading cause of death overall. The age-adjusted suicide rate is 11.3 per 100,000 persons (see Table 32-3). Among elderly men, one in four suicide attempts ends in death. Increases in suicide among the young and high rates among older adults have evoked concern (Berman and Jobes, 1991; Kachur et al., 1995; Leenaars et al., 1992). One unique aspect of suicide among the young is its contagion, often referred to as "copycat suicide," which may be triggered by media events or other suicides (Phillips and Carstensen, 1986).

TABLE 32-2. DEFINITIONS OF SUICIDE TERMS

Term	Definition	Examples and Comments
Ambivalence	Presence of opposite feelings (e.g., love/hate) about the same object, outcome or situation.	Suicide note: Dear Mary: I hate you. Love, Tom. Suicidal comment, "I want to live; but I can't stand this misery."
Suicide	The act of taking one's own life intentionally and voluntarily; a mode of death that excludes homicide, accident, and natural causes of death. This does not differentiate (1) the level of intent, lethality, desired or actual outcome, or (2) persons who commit or attempt. Suicide (completed) should define one who has killed him/herself.	A 49-year-old man who had talked about suicide left the hospital on a pass, went home, and shot himself. A 58-year-old woman with cancer sent her family home. She had read a book on how to commit suicide. She drank gin, overdosed on her pain medications, and died.
Completed suicide	Intentional, self-inflicted, voluntary acts that end in death.	A woman was never tested but believed she had AIDS. She planned suicide on her anniversary, took barbiturates at 4:30 P.M., turned on the gas, fell asleep, and died.
Attempted suicide	Nonfatal, deliberate self destructive acts (e.g., wrist cutting, self poisoning) and include many degrees of intent, lethality, mitigating circumstances, and rescue plans. Lethality, initial or repeated attempts should be detailed.	A young nurse with depression drank a large amount of vodka, took a few antidepressants, and asked for a ride to the hospital, where her stomach was pumped. A young man tried to hang himself with his cloth belt but it broke.
Parasuicide (also called deliberate self injury)	Non-lethal, deliberate, self-inflicted behaviors that were not intended to cause death.	Sara, age 15, took two tranquilizers and hoped this would reverse her parents' pending divorce.
Suicidal ideas	All thoughts inferred or observed via behaviors that threaten the person's life. Separating ideas from behavior is complicated because mental rehearsal may overlap impending action.	
Suicide gesture	This concept and term is misleading because it implies that some suicidal behaviors are innocuous. The actor planned to communicate that the self destructive act was tentative, but not lethal and not intended to cause death.	For example, superficially cutting wrists.
Indirect self destructive behavior	Subtle, covert, indirect and perhaps unconscious methods that exist at all ages (e.g., smoking, alcohol/drug abuse or omission of life-sustaining activities such as neglecting prescribed treatment or refusing medications or nourishment needed for life).	In a national survey of nursing homes, patients' refusal of medications or food or fluids necessary to sustain life was counted as indirect suicide (Osgood, ref).
Lethality of method and plan	The level of danger or potential to cause death by an action.	Highly lethal suicide methods include guns, knives, hanging, jumping, and carbon monoxide.
Survivor-victims	Individuals who have had a loved one die by suicide. They survive bereavement and cope with painful memories of a suicidal death.	A woman whose father committed suicide thought that suicide was her destiny; she attempted suicide each year.
Psychological Autopsy	Method of investigating the details, motives, and mode of death, which involves interviewing family, friends, and significant others of the deceased to identify motives and dynamics. It determines mode of death.	A 35-year-old physician died of an overdose of illicit drugs; both suicide and accident were suspected. An autopsy labeled the death an accident because the dose of drug was not lethal.

■ PRESENTATIONS OF SUICIDE

Wide variations of suicidal ideas, behaviors, and attempts occur in diverse school, community, and hospital settings. The frequency, intensity, duration, and goals of these suicidal behaviors differ. Often, suicidal patients emphasize physical complaints and do not share their suicidal ideas unless asked about suicidal impulses. Some persons may have vague, fleeting suicidal thoughts while others have a chronic history of lethal attempts.

A person with suicidal behaviors may be:

- Covertly suicidal and complaining of symptom distress.
- Overtly suicidal and reporting suicidal thoughts.
- Denying suicide and brought by their loved ones for medical attention.

TABLE 32–3. SUICIDE FACTS

Completed suicides, U.S., 1992

- Suicide is the 9th leading cause of death in the United States, accounting for 1.4% of total deaths
- The 1992 age-adjusted rate was 11.1/100,000, or 0.0111%, down from 11.4/100,000 in 1990
  - Only 1.4% of total deaths were from suicide. By contrast, 33% were from diseases of the heart, 24% were from malignant neoplasms, and 6.6% from cerebrovascular disease, the three leading causes
- Suicide by firearms is the most common method for both men and women, being used in 60% of all suicides
- More men than women die by suicide
  - The gender ratio is over 4:1
  - 73% of all suicides are committed by white men
  - Nearly 80% of all firearm suicides are committed by white men
- The highest suicide rates are for persons over 65; however, it is not a leading cause of death in this age group
- The 1992 suicide rate for white men older than 85 was 67.6/100,000
- Suicide is the third leading cause of death among young people 15 to 24 years of age, following unintentional injuries and homicide. In this age group:
  - Suicide rates are lower than for any other group except children less than 14 years of age
  - The rate was 13.0/100,000 in 1992, down from 13.1/100,000 in 1991
  - The total number of deaths in 1992 was 4,693, compared with 30,484 for all ages
  - The gender ratio was over 6:1 (men:women)
- Among young people 15 to 19 years of age the suicide rate was 10.8/100,000 in 1992, down from 11.0/100,000 in 1991
  - The total number of deaths was 1,847, compared with 30,484 for all ages
  - Rates among both young women and young men in this age group have increased since 1979; rates for young men have increased at a greater rate than rates for young women
  - The gender ratio was over 5:1 (men:women)
- Among young people 20 to 24 years of age the suicide rate was 14.9/100,000 in 1992, unchanged from 1991
  - The total number of deaths was 2,846, compared with 30,484 for all ages
  - The rate among young women in this age group has steadily decreased since 1979; the rate among young men has remained relatively flat
  - The 1992 gender ratio was over 6.5:1 (men:women)

Agency for Health Care Policy and Research, 1993; Alcohol, Drug Abuse, and Mental Health Administration, 1989; Maris, 1992; National Center for Health Statistics, 1992.

- A suicide attempter.
- A suicidal patient whose risk is identified by other staff members.
- A terminally ill patient who requests assistance to die.
- Someone who has engaged in self mutilation.

The patient's loved ones and friends as well as different members of the health care staff, often provide important observations about suicidal behavior.

Although some forms of self-mutilation (e.g., ear piercing, flagellation) may be condoned by culture or religion, most patients who mutilate themselves by means of cuts, burns, or other forms of self-injury fear criticism or rejection. Intentional self-injury that destroys or alters body tissue occurs in an estimated 24 to 40% of psychiatric patients, who may also be suicidal (Favazza, 1982; see Table 32-4). Understanding the motives, history, and precipitants of self-injury is challenging. Severe mutilations usually accompany psychopathology such as major depression, mania, schizo-

phrenia, organic mental disorders, eating disorders, or multiple personality disorders, and often reflect religious or sexual themes (Favazza, 1987). Self-mutilation may become treatment-resistant, repetitious, and chronic, and be imitated by other patients. Chronic self-mutilators typically alienate staff members, who feel that their therapeutic efforts have been ineffective or wasted (Valente, 1993). Nurses must monitor suicide risk among self-mutilators.

TABLE 32-4. SELF-INJURY IN SELECTED DIAGNOSTIC GROUPS

Group	Percent
Prisoners with antisocial personality	24%
People with bulimia	40.5%
People with anorexia	35%
Patients with multiple personality disorder	34%

Putnam, 1986; Virkkunen, 1976.

E CASE EXAMPLE

Gerry, a 34-year-old man with schizophrenia, electrocuted his genitalia and attempted to cut off his genitalia with a razor blade. He explained that "God and my voices told me to purify myself and be with Him; I will die." Nurses discounted Gerry's suicide risk because of his non-lethal injuries and their belief that self-mutilating patients were not sui-cidal. Having failed to identify earlier clues to Gerry's potential for suicide, nurses did not foresee or prevent his jump to his death several months later. His suicide might have been prevented had the nurses evaluated his hallucinations, monitored suicidal clues in his behavior (see Table 32-5), and used suicide precautions.

■ THEORIES RELATED TO SUICIDE

To collaborate with colleagues in a patient's treatment, nurses need to understand the major psychological and sociological perspectives for evaluating and treating suicidal patients. Because a unified and integrated theory of suicide is lacking, nurses typically need many theories to understand and treat such patients. A synopsis of the common theories is presented here. Because suicide typically results from many factors, each theory emphasizes understanding and assessment of different elements in an individual's life history, from unconscious wishes to coping strategies, that influence suicide (Hatton and Valente, 1984) (see Table 32-6).

PSYCHOLOGICAL THEORIES

Psychological theorists suggest that suicide may arise from diverse intrapersonal, interpersonal, and develop-

TABLE 32-5. COMMON RISK FACTORS FOR SUICIDE

Risk Factor	Illustration	References
Psychiatric disorder,* depressive disorder, chemical dependency	Major depression (40-60%); chronic alcoholism (20%), schizophrenia (10%), phobias, post-traumatic stress disorders, borderline and narcissistic personality	Bongar, 1992; Maris et al., 1993
Age, race, sex, being an older white male.*	Male Gender (70%); young adult, adult and older age caucasians > other groups Black, hispanic men (high risk age 15-40)	Maris et al, 1992 Bongar, 1992
Physical illness.* Higher risk if unrelieved pain or symptoms, advanced disease, or depression.	AIDS, cancer (head and neck, gastrointestinal neoplasms), Huntington's chorea, temporal lobe epilepsy, multiple sclerosis, peptic ulcer disease, spinal cord injuries, anorexia nervosa, head injury, Cushing's disease and hemodialysis	Cote et al., 1992; Marzuk et al., 1988; Kizer et al., 1988; O'Dowd et al., 1993; Valente, 1993
Prior suicide attempts*	About 15% of nonfatal attempters die by suicide	Bongar, 1992
Suicide ideas, talk,* preparation	Verbal or written messages of suicide, "I want to die"; "I'd be better off dead"; jokes and diaries	Leenaars, 1992 Valente, 1994
Lethal suicide methods*	Firearms used by >60% males; hanging, poisoning by >40% females	Bongar, 1992 CDC, 1985
Isolated, lives alone, loss of support*	40-50% of suicides lived alone or had no close friends vs. 20% nonfatal attempters	Maris, 1981
Hopelessness	No alternatives to suicide, rigid (either/or) thinking, tunnel vision. "Suicide is the only thing I can do."	Weishaar and Beck, 1993
Modeling of suicide in the family* genetics	Suicides and depressive illnesses tend to run in families. Modeling or imitation predicts suicide among adolescents	Phillips and Carstensen, 1986
Marital problems, family pathology*	Divorced/widowed > married, early separation from parents, physical/sexual abuse	Stack, 1993
Aggression/anger*	Murderous revenge, dissatisfied with life	Maris et al., 1993
Problems at work or school	Unemployment, retirement, no productive activities	Maris, 1981 Valente, 199
Stress, life events*	Stress that erodes self-esteem and raises guilt, fear, interpersonal problems	Bongar, 1992

*Single-variable predictors of suicide that experts agree are present in most suicides (excluding problem of comorbidity or interactions).

TABLE 32-6. SYNOPSIS OF MAJOR PERSPECTIVES AND THEORIES OF SUICIDE

Type	Theory	Major Themes	Assessment Focus
Biological	Neurochemical-hormonal imbalance; serotonin abnormality	An imbalance in biochemistry leads to depression with sequelae of suicide. Research explores the link between suicide, blood cortisol, 5-HIAA, and other chemicals	When future research refines biochemical predictors, laboratory tests may provide markers for suicide risk. Currently used for research and not reliable clinically.
Sociological	Anomie, Alienation (Durkheim, 1951)	Suicide reflects disruptions between the individual and society (e.g., social ties, social status, alienation, or alliance with society's pro-suicide norms which advocate suicide)	Evaluate stigma, discrimination, alienation, relationship with social norms, ties and status.
Psychological			
	Psychodynamic (Lovett and Maltsberger, 1992)	Suicide is an intrapsychic phenomenon emerging from early childhood trauma, anger, or death wishes toward self or others. Suicidal wishes can be unconscious, preconscious or conscious. Defense mechanisms may keep suicidal impulses hidden from the patient's awareness.	Analyze defenses, feelings, death wishes, impulses and dynamics. Evaluations of suicide risk based only on mental status exam or patient's self-report or denial of suicide may be inaccurate. The decision to commit suicide rests at deeper, less conscious levels.
	Crisis (Bongar, 1992; Shneidman, 1981, 1985)	Suicide is a response to a crisis. A crisis is an acute, time-limited period of severe disorganization and disequilibrium with severe symptoms, painful feelings, and failure of coping mechanisms (Shneidman, 1981). The patient feels out of control and suicide appears to be one way to escape this distress.	For the suicidal crisis, determine the precipitants, hazard, crisis, feelings, symptoms, thoughts, coping strategies, significant others, resources, and help-seeking behaviors. Crisis intervention is one of the most common frameworks for suicide prevention.
	Interpersonal Family (Richman, 1986)	Suicide emerges from disrupted relationships with significant others. A dyad or family bond is broken (e.g., divorce, death, abandonment). Family messages may encourage self hatred and self-destructive behavior (Richman, 1986)	Evaluate impact of family and significant others and patient's perceptions of messages about self-worth and suicide.
	Cognitive (Beck et al., 1979)	Depression arises primarily from distorted processes of thinking, knowing and perceiving; people have a triad of beliefs that the self is worthless, the world is barren, and the future is bleak. Interventions help patients' reconsider their automatic negative perceptions (e.g., "I'm worthless and better off dead") and irrational beliefs.	Elicit collaboration. Closely monitor all suicidal thoughts, hopelessness, and depression. Regular use of screening tools such as Beck Depression Inventory. Evaluate thought processes, reasons for living and dying, problem solving, and negative thoughts (e.g., "I'm a burden; I've failed at life. I'll never get better")

mental sources, such as crisis, disrupted relationships (Shneidman, 1981), negative thinking patterns (Beck et al., 1979), vulnerability and failed coping strategies, and long-standing psychological distress. Crisis and cognitive theories, the most common and most useful ones for nursing, are summarized here.

Crisis Theory

A crisis is a normal, time-limited response to a distressing event that overwhelms one's coping strategies, resources, and social support. What is most important is the patient's perspective on the circumstances that precipitated the crisis. Clearly, an earthquake, death, di-

vorce, or disease could provoke a crisis for anyone, but the nurse needs to identify other hazards, such as money problems or a facial blemish, that overwhelm the client. Moving from a $500,000 home to a $200,000 home, finding ants in the kitchen, or having a pet duck die may all evoke suicidal crises. Nurses need to guard against any impulse to discount or belittle the patient's perception of the crisis.

Using crisis intervention, the nurse focuses the patient on the patient's current situation, evaluates the patient's distress, and takes action to reduce powerlessness and to improve the patient's safety, coping, and interaction with significant others. Suicidal risk and feelings are monitored carefully. Crisis intervention is particularly useful for an acute disruption, whereas chronically suicidal patients need more extensive treatment. Crisis intervention neglects to explain how to evaluate or manage the multiple or chronic suicidal crises that occur with psychiatric disorders.

Cognitive Theory

Cognitive theory posits that depression arises primarily from distortions in cognitive processes: thinking, knowing, and perceiving. Beck et al. (1979) describe a cognitive triad in depression:—that the self is worthless, the world is barren, and the future is bleak. Depressed persons often alienate others by rejecting help, asking to be alone, and behaving in an uncooperative manner. They then feel more isolated, alone, and worthless, but rarely recognize the impact of their negative and self-isolating behaviors on their mood or self esteem.

Cognitive distortions and irrational beliefs automatically guide thoughts and shape emotional responses, and these thinking patterns can be changed. Automatic beliefs become habitual even when they lead to a negative outcome such as depression. Examples of cognitive distortions include selective negative focusing in which an individual emphasizes bad news or catastrophes (e.g., sees the worst outcome possible for a situation). For example, the patient whose laboratory reports are normal except for a borderline low platelet count might respond, "I'm always the one with the worst laboratory results. My platelets are so low I'll bleed and get an infection."

The nurse intervenes by eliciting the patient's co-operation and increasing the patient's awareness of a negative focus and its influence on coping and depression. For example, the clinician can question automatic thoughts about an event. When the patient expresses negative thoughts, the clinician asks about the sequence of thoughts that led to this conclusion, examines how often the patient's conclusions result from a single fact, and clarifies the meaning and consequences of this pattern of thinking. Upon reflection, the patient may discover that the negative event that "always" happens has really only happened once.

The nurse also helps the patient to examine unrealistic goals, set practical goals, transform unrealistic goals into practical steps, and take pride in the effort to reach a goal. Failure to reach overly ambitious goals reinforces a negative self-image. Many patients also need help to change the rigid thinking and limited problem-solving approaches that are commonly associated with suicide. For instance, suicidal individuals often see the limited choices of either continuing with unabated suffering or committing suicide. Interventions include clarifying irrational beliefs (e.g., everyone must love me) and re-examining negative views of the future, the

self, and the world (Wright et al., 1993). Homework assignments can enable patients to identify pleasant or mastery experiences that they habitually discount or ignore. Suicide risk declines as negative thought patterns and depression decline and problem solving improves.

Psychodynamic Theory

Psychodynamic theories argue that suicide results from a person's ongoing responses to intolerable psychological distress, frustration, and unmet needs (Maltzberger, 1993; Richman, 1986; Shneidman, 1981). Suicidal impulses reflect long-standing self-destructive attitudes and a history of feeling ostracized or devalued (Farberow, 1981) as seen in the following example:

> I . . . tried to hang myself . . . with my bathrobe belt; it broke. I tried my belt . . . it didn't work; I gave up. I couldn't do it right. I want to be dead . . . to sleep and never wake up. I feel . . . discouraged; I'm getting worse and feel hopeless; I want relief from physical and emotional pressure; I fear I'll never be well. (Valente, 1994)

Suicidal persons talk of feeling hostile, ashamed, guilty, aggressive, vengeful, afraid, frustrated, unloving (Maltzberger, 1993; Richman, 1986), and ambivalent.

SOCIOLOGICAL THEORIES

Sociological theories indicate that alienation, broken relationships, social ties, and lost or poor status lead to suicide (Durkheim, 1951); this may explain suicide among vulnerable or minority groups (e.g., elderly people, gay men or lesbians, immigrants, homeless people, children) (Rofes, 1983). Stigma disrupts relationships, provokes rejection, and increases the social distance between clinicians and patients.

APPLICATION OF THEORY

The various theories for suicide help to explain its bases and to guide treatment for its prevention. In general, until an out-patient begins treatment, the nurse provides support, monitors suicide risk, and encourages follow up. For instance, crisis intervention might guide one's approach with a friend. Ali, who is not a patient but who suddenly says that "everything is falling apart; I cannot go on, and I'm a worthless failure or crazy." With crisis intervention, the focus is on the "here and now" and what happened recently to prompt the friend's distress (e.g., the triggers, resources, feelings, supports, and coping strategies). In this case, Ali's mother was diagnosed as having breast cancer about a month earlier, and since then Ali's symptoms (e.g., crying, inability to sleep or eat, slowed behaviors, anhedonia, fatigue, and fears of her mother's death) have intensified. Because she comes from a Middle-Eastern culture that expects calm, stoic behavior, Ali sits in her car and cries alone; no one discusses her mother's diagnosis. Her typical coping strategies have been useless. As a student, her worst worry is failing her final examinations because she cannot concentrate. Ali says that if she fails she will feel ashamed and wish for death. Currently she occasionally thinks of suicide but has no suicide plan or history, and her religion forbids suicide.

Crisis intervention guides her assessment (e.g., evaluate symptoms, risk, significant others, suicide plans, etc.) and therapeutic actions (e.g., estimate risk, provide safety, and enlist resources). Here, a depression or suicide screening inventory provides baseline data. Ali's Beck Depression Inventory score suggests depression, but she has a low score on the suicide items, which indicates that she is at low risk for suicide and that her suicide risk should be monitored. Consulting an advanced-practice colleague improves the comprehensiveness and accuracy of assessment and of interventions and referrals for her.

The next step is to summarize the precipitants and crisis intervention plan with Ali (e.g., seek treatment for her depression and improve her coping strategies and social support). Ali is told that anyone in her situation could feel depressed, but that effective treatment will improve her concentration and coping strategies. Sometimes, perspective on the situation, a plan for help, and a referral for treatment reduce distress. On the basis of a recommendation, Ali consults with a faculty member and seeks treatment for her depression. About a week after Ali begins her therapy and antidepressant medication (fluoxetine [Prozac]), her mood, behaviors, and concentration improve. With therapy and medications, she passes her final examinations and begins to cope with her mother's cancer.

■ CLINICAL ASSESSMENT

Assessment of the suicidal patient includes a comprehensive physical and neurobehavioral mental status examination to rule out treatable diagnoses (e.g., depression or chemical dependency), screening and determination of risk factors to identify persons at risk for suicide, and examining individual risk by observations and interviews of the patient. Gathering data from significant others and other members of the health-care team often yields useful data about suicide risk.

SCREENING

Patients in community as well as in-patient settings can complete simple, brief, self-report questionnaires that permit the rating of severity of depression and/or suicide potential, such as the Beck Depression Inventory (Wright et al., 1993) or Hamilton Depression scale for depression and suicide. Common screening tools for adults are summarized in Table 32-7. The 20-question Beck Depression Inventory takes adults about 5 to 10 minutes to complete and contains 21 items about cognitive, somatic, and behavioral symptoms of depression as well as items about suicide. Other screening tools are available for specific age groups. When patients have abnormal scores as defined by the authors of these screening tools, a suicide assessment interview should be conducted to determine the patient's risk status. For young children or non-verbal individuals, evaluations done through art and play therapy help to determine risk. Typically, standard criteria (*Diagnostic and Statistical Manual of Mental Disorders, Fourth Edition [DSM-IV]*, 1994) are used to diagnose depression.

EVALUATION OF RISK FACTORS

Although researchers have identified many clinical indicators of suicide risk, consensus on the key risk factors and pathognomonic predictors of suicide does not exist (Bongar, 1993; Simon, 1988). Determination of risk includes a systematic examination of group and individual risk factors (see Table 32-5). Recognizing risk factors for suicide is as important as detecting signs of infection or cardiovascular disease.

Both group (e.g., incest history, abuse, chemical dependence, schizophrenia, or depression) and individual (e.g., prior attempts or suicide messages) risk factors require evaluation (see Table 32-5). Groups with high suicide rates include those with disorders such as cancer, acquired immune deficiency syndrome (AIDS), or depression; those undergoing renal dialysis; and men with cardiorespiratory disorders and neurological diseases associated with depression (e.g., Huntington's disease, stroke, Parkinson's disease). Major depression, which occurs in 25% of chronically ill persons, often goes untreated. Failure to adapt to the multiple stressors of aging may increase suicide risk among elderly males who have no prior psychiatric history. These factors suggest that someone may belong to a high-risk groups; however, further evaluation of suicidal or hopeless feelings, behaviors, and attitudes is needed to determine an individual's risk.

ASSESSING INDIVIDUAL RISK

The next step in the evaluation of risk factors for suicide is to collect data about the individual patient. The nurse may begin an interview with observations such as "You sound discouraged, I wonder if you are feeling depressed or hopeless? Tell me more about these feelings.

TABLE 32-7. SCREENING INSTRUMENTS FOR ADULTS

Instrument	Characteristics	Scoring
Beck Depression Inventory (BDI)	Patients rate cognitive, affective, and somatic symptoms on a brief 21-item self report scale. Easily administered.	≤10 = normal Cognitive/affective items best indicators of depression in medically ill. Valuable measure for medically ill (Cavanaugh; Schwab)
Hamilton Rating Scale (HRS)	Interviewer-scored. Somatic symptoms = 52% of total score.	Gives more credit to somatic symptoms than BDI and can give false positives and low specificity. Measures different components of depression than BDI.
Hospital Anxiety and Depression (HADS) Scale	Easily administered self-report questionnaire. Reported the best measure of stable patients free of disease and effective for patients in treatment	Score ≥8 warrants psychiatric evaluation. Score ≥11 likely to have Anxiety or Depression (*DSM IV* criteria)
Hopelessness Scale (HS) (Beck, Weissman, Lester and Trexler, 1974)	A 20-item scale containing true-false self-report statements testing pessimism about the future. The scale differentiates threateners, attempters, and controls. It has three factors and internal consistency of .93 (Kuder Richardson); a 91% sensitivity for inpatients and 94% for outpatients. Some experts argue that HS is a better index of suicidality than depression scales.	One point is given for each item that the respondent marks in the direction of pessimism. The total score is an excellent indicator of suicidality among adults, but not among adolescent minority females.
Center for Epidemiological Studies Depression Scale (CES-D) (Radloff, 1977) for general populations	A 20-question, self-administered tool. The scale has high reliability and discriminant validity. It is unclear whether the scale measures depression or psychological distress.	Myers and Weissman (1980) suggest a cut-off score of 16 or above for major depression. Scale has a low false positive and a high false negative rate.

Beck A, Weissman A, Lester D, Trexler L: Classification of suicidal behaviors: II. Dimensions of suicidal intent. *Arch Gen Psychiatry* 1976; *33*, 835-837.
Corcoran K, Fischer J: *Measures for Clinical Practice: A Sourcebook.* New York, Free Press, 1987.
Radloff LS: The CES-D Scale. A self report depression scale for research in general populations. *Appl Psychol Measurement* 1977; *1*: 385-401.
Myers J, Weissman MM: Use of a self report symptom scale to detect depression in a community sample. *Am J Psychiatry* 1980; *137*.

TABLE 32-8. GUIDELINES FOR PRACTICE

Key Concepts

A. Suicide is the 8th leading cause of death in the United States; elderly Caucasian men are at highest risk for completed suicide; all males age 15 to 50 years are at high risk.

B. Establish rapport; and do not avoid or refuse to discuss suicide. Avoid being judgmental or asking why.

C. Take any reference to suicide seriously! Look for suicidal ideas behind defenses such as joking, anger, laughter, pretense, denial. Patients are ambivalent, wanting to disclose distress but also fearing discovery.

D. Confidentiality: A nurse's duty is to protect the patient's safety and to share information about suicide risk with the health-care team and often with guardians and significant others. It is most therapeutic if the patient agrees or at least knows in advance that suicide risk be shared.

E. Pick up clues and take therapeutic actions to decrease risk. Clinicians who communicate honest concern, detect and reduce risk, reduce symptom distress, and enhance support and resources can reduce risk and offer a life-line to survival. A suicidal patient's thinking typically narrows into "either-or" thinking (e.g., "Either I remove this pain or I'll die; no one can remove the pain, therefore I must commit suicide."), problem solving and coping strategies diminish, hope wanes, and help seems impossible.

F. Give a message of concern and hope: ("No one feels this way without a good reason; your health care team and I want to understand your distress and do whatever possible to improve the quality of your life.")

G. Use consultation and monitor risk. Seek consultation regarding management of patient and regarding any role conflict when a suicidal patient contradicts your religious, spiritual, or cultural values or beliefs; elicits grief or personal distress; or provokes ethical dilemmas. Plan support for yourself because suicidal patients can be stressful and also because professionals experience grief when a patient dies by suicide.

H. Refer to theories to improve assessment, understanding, and management.

I. Maintain ongoing documentation, inform others.

Detect risk by recognizing risk factors and clues: evaluation of suicide risk requires systematic inquiry about risk factors. Presence of risk factors implies that the nurse should suspect that the patient may have ideas of suicide. Examination of individual risk factors provides information about intensity of suicidal intent and suggests lethality.

A. Group Risk: Factors indicating individual is in a group at risk for suicide.

   1. Psychiatric Diagnosis: Depression, substance abuse, schizophrenia, post-traumatic stress disorder, organic brain syndrome, anxiety

   2. Medical Diagnosis: Cancer (head, neck, gastrointestinal tract), AIDS

   3. Demographics: age > 18 years, adult or older age, male, single (with no responsibility for children under age 18), unemployed, recent death of spouse. (Note: females have higher rates of attempted suicide; gay men and lesbians have had higher rates of attempted suicide)

    4. Personal or Family history of suicide and current risk
    5. Mood improvement among depressed patients often precedes suicide
    6. Prior suicide attempts (determine intent and pattern of attempts)
    7. Hospitalization

B. Individual Risk Factors

1.	Historical	Prior suicide attempts
2.	Communication	Verbal suicide messages, jokes, writings, diaries
3.	Behavioral	Changes in behavior, saying good-bye (e.g., making a will[1], giving away prized possessions)
4.	Mood	Depressed, hopeless, helpless, ambivalent
5.	Social	Social isolation
6.	Death Wishes	Themes in art, play, or conversation

Assess for individual risk of suicide and lethality

A. Determine acuity and lethality/conduct a thorough assessment
    1. Ask about, monitor, and continue to assess suicide risk
    2. Evaluate pattern, detail, and intensity of suicidal thoughts/behaviors
    3. Inquire about suicide plan, method, means and details
    4. Estimate immediate and long-term lethality
    5. Collect data from colleagues, family or friends

B. Acute management
    1. Crisis assessment
    2. Evaluate for possible injury, overdose, blood loss, extent of injury
    3. Provide a safe environment; remove access to pills, sharp objects, and/or provide close supervision when such objects are used (e.g., safety razors, blunt scissors).
    4. Provide safety by close or constant observation
    5. Monitor intensity of thoughts and risk
    6. Communicate patient's risk of suicide to all staff members; document.
    7. Arrange consultation when a second opinion is indicated or when health-care team lacks expertise in suicide management

C. Obtain complete, focused psychiatric and psychosocial history
    1. Past suicidal thoughts, behaviors, attempts
    2. Past psychiatric treatment, medications, therapies
    3. Psychosocial and cultural history (e.g., include drugs, caffeine, support systems and relationships, resources, coping strategies)

D. Neurobehavioral mental-status examination

E. Physical examination

F. Family history and patient's educational, social, and occupational history

G. Evaluate need for or review results of psychological testing

Management Strategies

A. Determine acuity of risk and take action to improve safety (e.g., remove method; increase supervision; consider hospital or alternatives)

B. Acute treatment for high lethality (immediate risk of suicide attempt)
    1. Complete psychiatric evaluation
    2. Hospitalization or close supervision if necessary:
        a. Consult as needed to move patient to secure environment or arrange close supervision
        b. Arrange consultation, inform primary physician
    3. Evaluate safety of environment; remove dangerous objects from patient; institute suicide precautions; monitor medications
    4. Consult regarding effectiveness of current treatment plan (goals: improve symptom management and treatment plan)
    5. Improve social support and resources
    6. Discuss no-suicide contract
    7. Ongoing monitoring and documentation of mood, behavior, suicidal ideas; notify others
    8. Plan for living

C. Short-Term and Long-Term Treatment
    1. Individual counseling (e.g., cognitive strategies, reduce helplessness)
    2. Treatment of depression
    3. Reduce symptom distress (e.g., enhance management of pain, depression PRN)
    4. Enhance social support (social services, chaplain, family, friends)
    5. Improve resources and coping (self-concept, self-esteem)

TABLE 32-9. A COMPARISON OF PATTERNS AND EXAMPLES OF COMPLETERS' AND ATTEMPTERS' MESSAGES

Pattern	Completers' Messages	Attempters' Messages
Unbearable Psychological Pain: flight from pain, other motives, emotional states. Suicide solves urgent problems or injustice.	"I'm depressed. I have a fear of the future; I feel down and will kill myself." "I want to be dead; sleep, never wake up. I want relief from physical and psychological pressure."	"I feel hopeless; feel like hurting someone. I'd be better off dead." "I feel defeated, hopeless, and I look for places to hang myself."
Interpersonal Relationships: Unresolved problems, needs and frustrations are obvious and overwhelming.	"I've seriously considered cutting off my hand to kill myself to make amends for causing my wife's abortion."	"I feel hopeless; wish I were dead; I set fire to my bed to burn and die; no one would care if I burned."
Inability to Adjust: sees self as weak, inferior unable to adapt.	"I want to end it all because I can no longer handle everyday problems."	"He (e.g., I) is homosexual and is going to kill himself because he can't deal with being me. Life is garbage; I'm a black cloud, at the bottom of the heap, a failure; undeserving. I feel dead already."
Cognitive Constriction: Evidence of adult wanting to kill self. Intoxicated by emotions, constricted logic and perceptions.	If you send me home, I'll kill myself "I'd be better off dead. I have plans to slit my wrists. I'm losing it; I feel high too much."	"I plan to overdose on heroin; I tried to slit my throat with a razor blade; I want to kill myself. I want to commit suicide. I thought I heard a voice say, find a way to kill yourself. If I left hospital, I'd probably OD on heroin."

Valente, 1994

Have you thought of doing anything to hurt yourself?" The nurse uses therapeutic communication skills to introduce the topic of suicide and asks direct questions about suicide. What are your thoughts about suicide? Do you have a plan for suicide? What is it? When will you act on your plan? What do you hope will happen (e.g., rescue or death)? How deadly are your plans? What prompted these suicidal thoughts now? All past and present suicidal behavior requires evaluation (see Table 32-8).

Essential to individual risk assessment is continuous observation and monitoring of suicidal communications, changes in behavior and mood (e.g., depression, anxiety, agitation, hopelessness, and ambivalence), increasing social isolation, and clues to suicide (e.g., giving away prized possessions or making final arrangements). Suicide messages may be overt (e.g., "I'm going to kill myself; I should be dead.") or less obvious comments that life isn't worthwhile or that "you won't have to worry about me any more." Persons who express suicidal thoughts often tentatively say that they may attempt suicide if things become worse, while those who complete the act say that suicide is the only option (see Table 32-9). Some persons signal their risk nonverbally by social withdrawal, self-mutilation, anxiety, depression, or a hopeless mood (Bongar, 1992; Maris et al., 1993). Nurses should assess suicidal themes in essays, diaries, art, or jokes. One hospitalized suicidal youth draped a hospital call bell cord around his neck and made seeming jokes about being dead. When staff members misinterpreted this as play, and failed to evaluate it as a cry for help, the youth tried to hang himself. Other clues to a patient's suicide risk may come from other patients and family members, friends, or loved ones. The nurse should continue to explore and document the patient's mood and behaviors, and notify the physician and other team members of any changes in the patient's behavior. Nurses often need not do all of this alone, and can benefit from collaborating with experienced colleagues. Once the risk of suicide is detected, evaluating the potential for lethality and providing safety for the patient are urgent goals.

EVALUATING LETHALITY

The evaluation of lethality involves making an estimate of the likelihood that an individual will die from a suicide attempt or plan (Bongar, 1992; Maris et al., 1993). A high lethality rating reflects a clear plan with a deadly method and means for suicide (e.g., a gun, knife, jumping from a height, drowning, or carbon monoxide poisoning). A moderate rating reflects a moderately lethal method (e.g., barbiturates) or an incomplete or imprecise plan; a low rating indicates a vague plan, a low-risk method (e.g., wrist cutting), and a low risk of death. In long-term-care facilities, patients have successfully committed suicide by refusing to take necessary medications (Osgood, Brant, and Lipman, 1988). A patient with an imminent, precise, and lethal suicide plan and the method and means for accomplishing it has a high short-term risk and requires immediate intervention and suicide-preventive measures. A team conference confirms the lethality of the patient's intent and permits the planning of therapeutic interventions to prevent it.

The nurse estimates short-term lethality and judges the capacity of the staff and setting to provide reasonable assurance of the patient's safety. In in-patient settings, the nurse and staff members arriving for duty need to ensure that the unit environment and staffing provide adequate safety for a suicidal patient. A serious nursing error is failure to monitor the patient and provide such safety. Based on an evaluation of suicide risk and lethality, the nurse collaborates with the health-care team, consults the physician, and recommends or institutes safety precautions (one-to-one supervision, transfer to a locked unit, close observation, removal of suicide methods).

EVALUATING RESOURCES AND SOCIAL SUPPORT

Assessment includes determining deficits in resources and social support that could increase the risk of suicide. Suicidal patients may doubt that significant others or staff members will provide support, and may negatively perceive supportive intent (e.g., "if they loved me, they would automatically know what I need; no one really cares about me"). Patients often neglect to ask for support and fail to use internal (e.g., sense of humor or coping strategies) and external resources as means of support. The patient's family or social network resources, their ability to provide support both need in-

vestigation (Richman, 1986). Ongoing assessment and strengthening of resources and support are important in monitoring the risk of suicide.

■ MANAGEMENT STRATEGIES

REDUCING LETHALITY

Nurses need to express concern for and establish an alliance with the patient, and formulate a plan to reduce the risk of suicide. Many nurses who wish to resolve all of the patient's problems fail to realize this as an unrealistic goal that often keeps nurses from intervening. Instead, the nurse should focus on surveillance, safety precautions, communication, documentation, and actions to reduce risk. One therapeutic response is "we are concerned about your distress and pain, we will help reduce your symptoms and to keep you safe." A concerned non-judgmental response, direct questions about suicide, action to reduce current distress, and/or provide referrals are important. A patient's request for confidentiality is often ambivalent, representing a test of the care team's responsiveness and a cry for help. If asked to keep suicide plans confidential, the nurse

TABLE 32-10. PLAN OF CARE FOR SUICIDAL PATIENT
DSM-IV DIAGNOSIS: MAJOR DEPRESSION
NURSING DIAGNOSIS: POTENTIAL FOR SELF-HARM DUE TO DEPRESSION, SUICIDAL THOUGHTS, LOW SELF-ESTEEM

Assessment	Outcomes/Goals	Nursing Actions
High risk for suicide due to: depression, alcoholism, isolation	Patient will not physically harm self during treatment or hospitalization.	Notify physician and team of risk. Assign one to one close nursing observation, suicide precautions, place on locked unit near nurse's station.
Concrete, immediate, lethal suicide plan; may have prior lethal attempts;	Patient will not elope from hospital unit or endanger self or others	Staff will: *Monitor mood *Remove harmful objects. *Assist patient with activities of daily living *Help patient ventilate feelings and use constructive physical outlets for anger
Inconsistent impulse control	Patient will inform staff promptly of thoughts/feelings of wanting to harm self	*Observe closely and ask patient to report any suicidal ideas/feelings *Advise and monitor participation in activities *Teach alternate coping strategies
Feels hopeless, helpless, ambivalent about life/death	Patient will identify constructive alternatives to self harm	*Encourage patient to begin forming or using social support system and to expand resources *Reassess and document *Set realistic goals
High risk due to being elderly, substance abuse, diagnosis of AIDS, and cancer		*Evaluate/improve pain or symptom management *Build self esteem *Evaluate goal of suicidal behavior and desired outcome *Evaluate plans for rescue
History: suicidal ideas/feelings, or acts, social isolation, anger or homicidal impulses		*Investigate how patient handles anger and frustration *Help patient establish relationship with nurse then others *Help patient begin to socialize

firmly asserts that anything related to the patient's safety must be shared with the health-care team. Based on the assessment, the professional nurse collaborates with colleagues and care-team members to design an effective plan of care (see Table 32-10).

SAFETY PRECAUTIONS: THE FIRST PRIORITY

Protecting patients from suicidal impulses is critical. Safety precautions for suicidal patients include hospitalization, close supervision, and the least restrictive but safe environment. Evidence of clear and immediate self-endangerment by the patient is one criterion for involuntary hospitalization for a high lethality patient. Management for patients with a low risk of lethality includes supervision, consultation, medications, and other actions to further reduce the risk (e.g., improving problem solving, involving significant others, helping the patient to mobilize internal and external resources and, harness coping mechanisms, and referral). Monitoring risk and helping patients to examine alternatives to suicide, reducing distress, monitoring treatment outcomes, and improving supports, resources and the patient's quality of life all help to reduce risk (Bongar, 1992; Maris et al., 1993).

The nurse may be the first person to detect lethal impulses and to initiate safety precautions. For example, the night or weekend nurse may discover a highly suicidal patient on an unlocked unit. Ideally, the nurses, supervisor, and physician discuss the safety precautions needed for any particular patient. Failing this, the nurse evaluates whether the existing staff and the patient's current environment can provide adequate safety. The nurse is often responsible for safeguarding a patient in the minutes or hours before physicians respond to a call for care. The greater the risk of the patient's self-lethality, the more critical are the nurse's observations and precautions. Depending upon the patient's needs, agency policy, and legal guidelines, a safe environment requires the removal of potential means for suicide (e.g., sharp objects, ropes, pills), and may involve close supervision in a locked hospital unit (Bongar et al., 1993). Suicidal in-patients should have a room close to the nurses' station, and should not have a private room. Nurses are typically responsible for regular environmental surveillance to eliminate the presence of any dangerous conditions (e.g., drapery cords or bathroom fixtures that could support a person's weight).

Nurses in all settings must remain vigilant and alert to the risk of suicide. In an orthopedic hospital, one young-adult patient intentionally overdosed on diazepam (Valium) from her purse. The nearly fatal overdose might have been prevented had the nurses removed all pills from the patient at the time of her

admission, and investigated her unexplained, excessive sleepiness and suicide clues a few days before her suicide attempt. Surveillance of suicidal in-patients includes ensuring that they do not swallow or hoard medications. Suicidal patients often communicate their fear of suicide and hope that nurses will take precautions to prevent it. One male out-patient disclosed a lethal plan to shoot himself within a day, and told the clinic nurse that he was not safe at home. The nurse correctly rated his suicide risk as high, had a gun removed from his home, and immediately sent the patient for psychiatric evaluation and admission to a locked unit.

Managing suicidal inpatients requires clinical judgment and an ongoing investigation of suicide risk before approving a patient's privileges, discharge, and treatment plan. Managing suicidal patients is a multidisciplinary activity because psychotherapy, psychopharmacology, milieu management, family counseling, education, and adjunctive therapy all make important contributions to monitoring and reducing their risk of suicide (Bongar et al., 1993). Nurses have a critical role in removing contraband when patients enter or return to the nursing unit, in monitoring visitors and non-professional staff personnel, and in safeguarding any cleaning solvents or dangerous equipment on a unit where potentially suicidal patients are housed.

To prevent the hoarding of pills by inpatients, nurses should carefully administer medications and check to make sure that patients swallow their pills. Before discharge or during an outpatient's evaluation, the astute nurse investigates whether the patient can safely administer antidepressants. When an outpatient is unreliable or may self-overdose with antidepressants, the physician should be notified and a reliable adult should administer the patient's medications. Often, although not responsible for prescribing medications, the nurse has a critical role in risk management by alerting the physician to the possibility of drug self-overdosing. Suicide risk often increases during the months after discharge, but carefully monitored prescription drug quantities and refills can reduce the potential for overdosing. Except for medicating pain such as cancer pain, clinicians are wise to prescribe non-lethal quantities of narcotic or antidepressant drugs for suicidal patients, and to allow refills only after seeing the patient. Particular caution is needed when patients take tricyclic antidepressants, which are common and potentially lethal agents of suicide (Kapur, Mieczkowski, and Mann, 1992).

OFFERING HOPE OR HELP

Suicide risk is often decreased by helping patients to develop realistic goals, believe that help is available, and hope for realistic outcomes. Patients need regular reminders and reliable evidence that nurses and the other health-care team members want to help them and believe that they can improve. Observing and praising patients' efforts to ask for help is useful.

INFORMING OTHERS AND SEEKING CONSULTATION

Bongar (1993) emphasizes the vital role of informing others and consulting routinely with suicidal patients. Nurses have an obligation to observe, document, and report the patient's response to therapies. Prompt investigation and reports of changes in the patient's condition and of changes in or effects of medications are particularly important. The nurse needs to notify other care-team personnel, physicians, and supervisors when poorly managed pain or depression result in increasing suicide risk.

Consultation with colleagues is critically important when dealing with any suicidal patient; it also helps staff members to manage chronic or high-risk suicidal patients and resolve counter-transference issues (Shneidman, 1981). However, in one national survey, oncology nurses caring for suicidal patients reported that they rarely sought consultation (Valente, Saunders, and Grant, 1994). Consultation helps nurses in planning care for any patient with a moderate to high risk of suicide, or who has made previous suicide attempts, or who has organic or psychotic symptoms (e.g., hallucinations, delusions, or dementia). Consultation can also renew nurses' hope about the treatment of manipulative patients, and provide renewed energy and encouragement, expanded perspectives, and better means for environmental safety and suicide prevention. Finally, a patient's suicide is a significant occupational hazard in psychiatry. Because psychiatric nurses providing direct care have a good chance of losing a patient to suicide, consultation helps nurses to cope with this occupational stress.

NO-SUICIDE CONTRACTS

A no-suicide contract is a time-limited verbal or written promise by a patient to not do anything self-destructive either accidentally or intentionally before informing the primary clinician. Patients are encouraged to clarify any circumstances that could limit their keeping the contract. However, contracts do not guarantee that suicidal impulses will be contained, and contracts are not substitutes for continued assessment or safety measures. Although no-suicide contracts are widely used, sparse and only empirical support for their value has led to debate about their usefulness (Davidson, Wagner, and Range, 1995). Such contracts are more effective when patients have reliable impulse control and a relationship with the nurse or clinician.

No-suicide contracts may be ineffective and provide false reassurance when entered into with manipulative or impulsive patients. These patients often learn that threatening suicide achieves hospitalization and that promising not to commit suicide will yield privileges or a pass. Nurses cannot take such promises at face value, but must instead validate the patient's words by investigating inconsistencies in the patient's dynamics and behaviors and comparing their assessment with that of other team members. Clinicians have viewed no-suicide contracts as more effective with adults and adolescents than with children or moderately suicidal patients (Davidson, Wagner, and Range, 1995).

REDUCING SYMPTOMATIC DISTRESS

The professional nurse is likely to care for patients with persistent pain, side effects of medication, fatigue, and symptom distress. These are among the most common reasons for requesting euthanasia or planning suicide (Breitbart, 1993), particularly among medically ill patients. Unless the nurse investigates the depressive effects of medications and alerts the physician to them, patients may fail to report them. Adequate pain and symptom management must be a priority in treating medically ill patients, particularly those with suicidal ideas (Breitbart, 1993; Valente, 1993).

Physical symptoms offer clues to the risk of suicide and must be carefully evaluated. For example, one hospitalized patient with major depression wrote several notes before he committed suicide. In one of these he wrote: "Dear Doctor and Nurses: "I've had these terrible headaches for over 15 years. Please do something about this pain; I can't live with it any longer" (Valente, 1994). His complaints of headaches had frequently been charted, but his nurses had not charted their evaluation or treatment of the headaches or the patient's response to treatment. Based on an evaluation of the patient's dynamics underlying somatic symptoms, the treatment team may encourage expression of feelings and discourage somatic complaints. Although it is unlikely that the patient's headaches alone led to his suicide, the nurses' failure to evaluate his symptoms and document their response to them could have put them in legal liability (Bongar et al., 1993).

IMPROVING PROBLEM-SOLVING AND COPING STRATEGIES

Suicidal persons tend to use narrow and negative thinking patterns and fail to consider alternatives to suicide. Helping such patients to consider options, prioritize problems, and plan constructive strategies can build hope in them and reduce their helplessness. Asking patients about their past coping strategies can help them to rediscover effective coping strategies such as help-

CASE EXAMPLE

Irena, a bereaved outpatient whose son had died, feared that her pattern of severe isolation, despair, and suicide attempts would increase during a period of upcoming holidays, but saw no options for herself. She was reluctant to remove a gun that she kept at her bedside, or to ask her friends for help. Because of her bereavement, depression, isolation, past suicide attempts and lethal planned method for suicide, Irena was at high risk. Initially, she told the clinic nurse and the advanced practice nurse that "Nobody wants me. I can't call and ask for a holiday invitation, I'd feel worse with people any-

way." Aiming to remove the means for Irena's planned suicide, decrease her isolation, explore options for her, and recommend psychiatric consultation, the advanced practice nurse helped Irena to call a supportive friend, ask for an invitation for the holidays, and ask the friend to keep the bullets for her gun. This plan decreased Irena's suicide risk. She had a safe, enjoyable holiday. Both nurses encouraged Irena's resolution of grief (see Table 32-11).

seeking, saying no, or focusing on their own needs, as seen in the following example.

INVOLVING SIGNIFICANT OTHERS AND MOBILIZING RESOURCES

Feelings of being worthless, unlovable, and alone through divorce, death, or other kinds of separation may intensify suicidal thoughts; increasing social isolation may signal increasing suicide risk. Depending on suicidal patients' level of social skill and independence, interventions include helping them to name supportive others and practice help in seeking skills. Recognition of their resources, skills, and help-seeking strategies can empower them. Suicidal patients often need to learn how to tell their loved ones about their feelings in ways that elicit understanding. Nurses can teach significant others to express their concern for the patient, enhance the patient's self esteem, decrease the patient's isolation, set realistic limits for achievement, and seek consultation in case of an increasing suicide risk. Patients can practice making friends in the hospital and at their church, temple, or support groups. Discharge planning includes making sure the patient has a list of more than two resources, such as a suicide hotline, psychiatric emergency room, or significant other person. Out-patient psychotherapy, group therapy, family ther-

TABLE 32-11.—DO'S AND DON'TS OF GRIEF SUPPORT

Helpful Responses: Do	Don't
Understand the survivor's perspective of this loss and its meaning.	Impose your meaning or values; avoid mentioning the decreased, or act as if nothing happened.
Use therapeutic communication: listen, accept emotions, invite sharing of thoughts and feelings; there are no right/wrong feelings.	Blame the bereaved survivor for the deceased's mental problems or suicide or criticize the family's actions or omissions.
Give permission to grieve; establish a safe environment. Encourage feelings, confusion, and questions (e.g., "Why did this happen?")	Insist the bereaved "get on with life", find a new love, have a stiff upper lip or stop brooding. Expect them to be the life of the party.
Educate clients about normal grief responses. Patterns of grief vary.	Imply that a "one size of grief fits all" (e.g., you *should* be . . . sad etc)
Encourage use of available support and resources (e.g., bereavement groups). Volunteer to offer support.	Expect the person to have the energy and skills to seek help and support when they fear rejection.
Monitor physical health, symptoms and coping (e.g., sleep, alcohol, suicide, exercise, diet). Advise safety and health (e.g., seat-belts)	Ignore potentially dangerous behaviors (e.g., excessive alcohol, pills or sexual behavior).
Invite talk of practical problems and solutions (e.g., how to tell children, should they attend the funeral, handling tough questions.)	Assume you know the best solutions (e.g., "tell everyone the truth about the suicide" or when to sort through the deceased's belongings.)
Respect the survivor's need for time to experience sad, angry, or other feelings. Expect some personal discomfort as you listen to painful, sad, guilty or angry feelings.	Diminish grief by a cheery, positive focus; justify the death as "God's will" or encourage replacement of the deceased (e.g., just have another child!)"

E CASE EXAMPLE

Mr. Hilt, a 40-year-old gay man, is admitted to an open unit in a small psychiatric hospital for detoxification from addiction to high doses of antianxiety medications. The patient has a past history of depression and risk of suicide. During almost every hour of the evening Mr. Hilt complains of increasing anxiety and symptoms of withdrawal. When the nurse reviews the patient's prescription for chlordiazepoxide (Librium), ordered during detoxification, she correctly determines that the dose of the drug is unusually low for detoxification. The nurse's duties include evaluating, monitoring, and docu-

menting the patient's suicide risk and notifying the physician of the patient's withdrawal symptoms and seemingly inadequate dose of librium, and providing safety through suicide precautions. In addition, the nurse must evaluate whether the open unit and its staff provide enough safety for the patient. If the open unit lacks adequate staffing for close supervision and suicide prevention, the nurse should consult the nursing supervisor and the on-call or treating clinician. If needed, the nurse should arrange for another staff member for to attend the patient or should transfer the patient to a closed, secure unit.

---

apy, and post-discharge groups are other useful resources.

Suicidal individuals typically feel powerless, helpless, weak, and unresourceful. Although they tend to discount their resources, helping them to recognize, develop, and expand these resources can decrease their risk of suicide. Such resources include humor, creativity, persistence, faith, skills, or knowledge, and external resources such as finances or employment. Reinforcing the patient's capacity for problem solving and using resources helps to decrease the sense of powerlessness.

DEVELOPING A PLAN FOR LIVING

Once a suicidal crisis is resolved and the patient can plan for the future, the nurse should select a time at which to encourage a plan for living that includes pleasurable activities and supportive relationships. The timing of this intervention is critical: if it begins during the suicidal crisis or before the patient is ready to plan ahead, the patient can easily feel overwhelmed and depressed.

The plan for living can include strategies to reduce automatic, negative thinking patterns. Questions such as, "What would make your life worthwhile today and help you feel better about yourself?" can help patients set realistic goals. As patients recognize their power to take small steps to improve the quality of their lives, their self-confidence grows. Many patients with vague suicidal ideas, no specific plan for suicide, and low-lethality methods can be managed on an outpatient basis with monitoring of their suicide risk. If suicidal ideas, behaviors, threats, or attempts increase, out-patient treatment should be re-evaluated. The patient's family, significant others, and social network can help monitor and evaluate the risk of suicide and offer support.

SEEKING CONSULTATION AND PSYCHIATRIC EVALUATION

Failure to recognize the risk of suicide, inform the health-care team of this risk, seek consultation, and take precautions to reduce the risk can be deadly. Nurses cannot discount a patient's suicide warnings or keep secrets about suicide. The nurse who discovers that a patient is at risk for suicide must notify the treating clinician and take action to ensure the patient's safety.

■ SUICIDE PREVENTION

To prevent suicide, nurses need to request, seek, or recommend consultation for patients with a high risk of suicide, when treatment fails to reduce the risk of suicide, when suicidal behaviors escalate, and when the treatment team lacks expertise in suicide prevention (see Table 32-12). When an advanced practice nurse is responsible for treating an outpatient and the patient attempts suicide, a psychiatric consultation is indicated because all treatment plans require evaluation, and the patient's need for safety and hospitalization must be considered. A good practice is to seek consultation for patients who make serious suicide attempts during hospitalization or who remain on suicide precautions for extended periods.

Effective primary prevention strategies include gun control, medication control (e.g., barbiturates), safety barriers (e.g., bridge railings), and educational campaigns. School-based prevention programs that identify and refer students at risk for suicide and provide grief counseling after a suicide are popular, but scant research has been done on their costs and benefits. A serious issue in suicide prevention is that media reports of suicides may increase suicide risk among some individuals (Philips and Carstensen, 1986).

TABLE 32-12. GUIDELINES FOR SUICIDE PREVENTION IN THE HOSPITAL

Identification

  At admission

    Inquire about current suicidal behavior

    Inquire about prior suicidal behavior

    (Two or more previous events indicate high risk)

    Record presence or absence of above (if present, obtain details of method, place, motivation)

  After admission

    Watch for suspect behavior

      Refusing food, medication

      Saving medication

      Asking about suicidal methods

      Talking of death, futility

      Giving away possessions

      Checking locks, windows, layout of the ward

      Loosening bolts, tearing sheets into strips

    Watch for suspect mood

      Hopelessness, helplessness, worthlessness

      Depression with agitation, restlessness

      Depression with apathy, withdrawal

      Unrelieved anxiety

      Excessive guilt and self-blame

      Severe frustration

      Bitter anger

    Observe personality characteristics

      Severe personal disorganization

      Dependent-satisfied behavior

      Dependent-dissatisfied behavior

      Diagnosis of schizophrenia

      Recent object loss

      Negative feelings about hospital

      Feeling of no future

Safeguards

  Environmental

    Install safety glass in windows

    Restrict window openings with stops

    Block off stair wells, access to roof

    Use breakaway shower curtain rods, breakaway clothes hooks in bathrooms and clothes lockers

    Cover exposed pipes

    Avoid grilles over ventilators, porch screens and railings

Procedure

  Remove from vicinity of suicidal patients all articles easily used in self-harm such as belt, suspenders, bathrobe cord, light cords, shoe laces, glass, ashtrays, vases, razor, pocketknife, nail file, nail clippers

  Be alert when suicidal patients are using sharp objects, such as scissors, needles, pins, bottle opener, can opener, dining room utensils, occupational therapy tools

  Be alert when suicidal patients are using the bathroom (to prevent hanging, jumping, cutting)

  Be alert when giving suicidal patients medication (patients may save or discard medicine)

  Observe acutely suicidal patients on a one-to-one basis

  Check suicidal patients at least every 15 minutes at night

  Be alert to whereabouts of suicidal patients during shift changes

  Room suicidal patients with others close to nurses' station; do not room alone if avoidable

  Warn visitors about bringing or leaving anything with lethal potential

  Apprise off-ward escort of suicide concern

  Keep suicidal patient in escorted group; examine anything patient picks up

  Define staff responsibility thoroughly

  Ensure continuous availability of help

Communication

  Document records completely to show that:

    Risk is recognized and evaluated

    Reasonable measures are ordered

    Orders are followed (if not, indicate why not)

  Ensure that all staff record pertinent observations

  Write orders specifically to show:

    Plan and rationale

    Specific restrictions

    Specific staff responsible for observation or escort

    Specific frequency of night observation

  Obtain frequent consultation

Attitudes

  Avoid preoccupation and fear

  Avoid harsh, repressive measures

  Use positive interest and build mutual trust

  Restore and strengthen hope

  Rebuild self-esteem to overcome helplessness

  Accept the reality that mistakes occur; aim for minimum

The Guidelines are reprinted by permission of Norman L. Farberow, Ph.D., and *HOSPITAL AND COMMUNITY PSYCHIATRY*. Dr. Farberow is clinical professor of psychiatry (psychology) at the University of Southern California School of Medicine, and principal investigator at the Central Research Unit of the Veteran's Administration Wadsworth Medical Center, Los Angeles, California. The Guidelines appeared as part of a copyrighted article on *Suicide Prevention in the Hospital*, published in HOSPITAL & COMMUNITY PSYCHIATRY, February, 1981 (Volume 32, Number 2).

An educational campaign for suicide prevention conducted by the mass media, and public policy aimed at preventing suicide among older adults and high risk individuals, could increase referrals and treatment at existing health-care facilities. A media public education campaign would include: (1) responses to depression and substance abuse; (2) the treatment of emotional problems and depression; (3) resources for psychiatric treatment; (4) friends' and relatives' roles in bringing an individual at risk for suicide to treatment; and (5) explanation that a quest for psychiatric help does not signify insanity. Such a campaign could help efforts to increase the accessibility of mental health care and to encourage primary practitioners' evaluation of mental-health needs. Such educational and policy efforts should be combined with process and outcome research.

Suicide is a significant and potentially preventable clinical problem. Nurses have an obligation to emphasize its primary prevention and the early detection and evaluation of patients with risk factors for suicide.

■ ETHICAL ISSUES

The current controversy about euthanasia, assisted dying, and AIDS is based not on facts but opposing ethical views (Coyle, 1992). Although patients have the right to fully understand their treatment choices and to refuse them, some experts equate refusing treatment with suicide (Valente and Saunders, 1933). In their suffering and vulnerability, many patients with serious or terminal physical illnesses ask a nurse to help them end their lives, and family members ask for an end to the lives of their seriously ill relatives. Nurses anguish over responses to these requests, and few guidelines exist for practice in this area. The values guiding clinical nursing practice have their roots in a tradition of preserving life, leaving clinicians to struggle with how to respond to requests that touch the heart of professional and personal values. Media reports of physician-assisted death, and the publication of "how-to" suicide books, are debated (Quill, 1993). Organizations such as the Hemlock Society, Choice in Dying, and Americans Against Human Suffering have sponsored initiatives for assisted suicide in California, Oregon, and Washington. Although many health-care professionals accept assisted suicide, the American Medical Association Council on Ethical and Judicial Affairs and the California Nurses Association oppose active euthanasia and assisted suicide (ANA, 1994; Lipman and Battin, 1996). Many supporters of assisted suicide in principle voice concern about inadequate safeguards for legislation regarding euthanasia.

Clinicians encounter conflicts between their duties to prevent suicide and to respect the patient's autonomy. Some argue that their duty is to respect a patient's right and free will to choose suicide instead of a life of disease with pain and unrelieved suffering. However, many patients who commit suicide may be unable to exercise autonomy because a severe psychiatric disorder, such as depression which undermines their ability to think clearly.

Slome et al. (1992) examined physicians' attitudes toward assisted suicide in the context of AIDS. They found that 23% of their sample in San Francisco would be likely to grant a patient's initial request for help in committing suicide. When physicians grant a request for suicide, they often overlook the need to treat depression, improve pain management, reduce symptoms, improve the quality of life, or evaluate whether the request for suicide is a cry for help or a rational consideration. If a moral conflict about suicide impairs one's ability to care for a suicidal patient, referrals should be considered.

Although many nurses believe they have a duty to sound the alarm at the first hint of suicide, they also feel a conflicting responsibility to protect the patient's confidentiality (Coyle, 1992; Lipman and Battin, 1996). Battin (1992) provides a way of evaluating a suicidal patient's rationality (see Table 32-13). For most suicidal patients, the concept of autonomy, taken naively, neglects the transforming effects of illness.

Rational suicide is a controversial issue. Terminally ill persons are prototypes for arguments favoring rational suicide. Although controversy exists about whether a person of sound mind can plan suicide, patients deserve the chance to discuss the rationality of their re-

---

TABLE 32-13. ASSESSMENT OF RATIONAL SUICIDE

1. The purpose and motives of the person considering suicide
   Is the person making a request for help?
   Why is the person consulting a health professional?
   Is the request for help in suicide a request for someone else to decide?
   Is the suicide plan financially motivated?
   What has kept the person from committing suicide so far?
   Does the person fear becoming a burden?

2. Stability of request
   How stable is the request?
   Has suicide been planned for a long time or is it a response to a recent event?

3. Is the request consistent with the person's basic values?

4. Are the medical and nonmedical facts cited in the request accurate?

5. Has the person considered the effects of suicide on others?

6. Suicide plan and options
   How far in the future would this take place?
   Has the person picked a method of suicide?
   Would the person be willing to tell others about his or her suicide plan?
   Does the person see suicide as the only way out?

7. What cultural influences are shaping a person's choices?

8. Are the person's affairs in order? Have arrangements been made for a funeral or durable power of attorney? In most states a health professional's relationship with a patient implies a legal and professional duty to refrain from assisting suicide. Terminally ill patients with suicide plans, however, deserve thoughtful evaluation of their rational and irrational requests and appropriate treatment options for their depression, pain, or symptom distress. Clinicians need to understand the ethical issues and criteria for evaluating rational suicide.

Adapted from Battin MP: Rational suicide: How can we respond to a request for help? *Crisis* 1991; 2:73-80.

E CASE EXAMPLES

▶ JOHN LIN

John Lin, a 65-year-old Caucasian, divorced attorney lives a fast-paced life and suffers from hypertension, obesity, insomnia, and a high blood cholesterol concentration. His hypertension has been treated with diuretics and antihypertensive medications. Because of his many cardiac risk factors, stress reduction, diet, and counseling have been recommended for him.

He complains of fatigue, poor appetite, difficulty in concentrating, and a loss of interest in work, sex, and sports. He reveals that he has purchased a gun and bullets, and reluctantly discloses that he does not know how much longer he can go on. He denies having hallucinations or delusions, and says that his sadness began a few weeks after he began taking hydrochlorothiazide and propranolol. He asks whether his blood pressure medications might have changed his outlook.

A clinical evaluation for depression and suicide risk indicate that John's severe depression followed the diagnosis and treatment of his hypertension. Because of his severe depression and symptoms, with a score of 28 on the Beck Depression Inventory, and the depressive side effects of propranolol and his diuretic, his antihypertensive medications are changed and antidepressants therapy is started. Psychiatric evaluation and psychotherapy are recommended because of his age, high depression score, and suicide risk. His suicide risk is closely monitored, and he agrees to enter into a no-suicide contract. Both exercise and joining a social sports group are recommended to him. Four months later, John is no longer suicidal and his depression is mild and resolving.

▶ SALLY HERNANDEZ

Sally Hernandez, a single, 19-year-old with asthmatic bronchitis, reports having felt sad and listless for 3 months since having had an abortion. She cries constantly and doesn't want to do anything. She expresses the wish that she had died during the abortion because her mate then left her and her parents are ashamed of her. Although Sally has no idea of how to kill herself, she thinks about it often. Although her religion teaches that suicide and abortion are sins, she says that she has sinned by killing her baby, and doubts that God meant her to live with this misery.

An evaluation shows that Sally is moderately depressed and has vague thoughts of suicide. She is begun on antidepressant medication and referred for psychotherapy, a bereavement support group, and pastoral counseling. She is willing to join a support group and talk with a pastoral counselor, but refuses psychotherapy and prefers to talk to her nurse-practitioner. She develops a good relationship with the nurse practitioner and promises not to do anything to harm herself without first calling for help. Helping her to improve her coping strategies and social support resources, and obtaining spiritual support from her priest, reduces her suicide risk. Her depression and suicidal thoughts are evaluated at every visit, and a Beck Depression Inventory indicates less depression and fewer suicidal thoughts after 4 weeks of antidepressants medication. By the 5th month of antidepressant therapy and other supportive measures, her Beck depression score reaches 10, which is normal.

▶ ALEXIS FORBES

Alexis Forbes, a 40-year-old gay man with a history of depression, recovery from alcohol addiction, social isolation, and anxiety, is admitted at dinner time to an open psychiatric unit for detoxification from high doses of anxiolytic agents. During his admission history, he confides that he fears growing old and alone, and doubts that he can successfully go through detoxification or live without his alprazolam (Xanax.) He tells three members of the psychiatric staff that he does not think life is any longer worth living; that he was a disappointment to his family and that no one loved him. Although he is given chlordiazepoxide (Librium) for detoxification, he complains several times during the evening of his admission about nausea and somatic symptoms. After telling Alexis to express his feelings instead of symptoms, the evening nurse records on his chart that his Librium did not control his withdrawal symptoms.

Alexis' complaints increase through the evening, and he repeats that he has little reason to live. However, the nurses on his unit do not document any suicide assessment, evaluate his need for safety, or notify the physician of his withdrawal symptoms or suicide risk. One nurse assigns an aide the responsibility for checking Alexis at 30-minute intervals. At about 2 A.M., when the charge nurse realizes that rounds have not yet been made, she sends the aide on rounds. When Alexis is not found in bed, the aide returns to the nurses station and asks the registered nurse to inspect the bathroom with her. When they enter the bathroom, they find Alexis cyanotic from asphyxiation. They call the paramedics, who try to resuscitate him, but he dies. His family sues the hospital, psychiatrists, and nursing staff for negligence. The negligence charged against the nurses; is the failure to have detected, evaluated for, and documented a suicide risk in a patient with this risk; failure to notify the psychiatrist of the patient's ongoing withdrawal symptoms and to request adequate symptom management; and failure to provide safe supervision or transfer the patient to a locked unit. Some nurses deny any responsibility for knowing the patient was suicidal because they routinely never read admission or chart records. At trial, an expert witnesses maintains that nurses are expected to review admission documents, noting any patient's suicidal feelings, comments, and risk factors; to have knowledge and competence to evaluate suicide risk; and to have provided ongoing supervision and a safe environment given this patient's suicide risk.

This case highlights the nurse's duty to review pertinent chart records, detect clues, evaluate suicide risk, act to provide a safe level of supervision, and notify the physician of suicidal risk and symptomatic distress. When staff personnel on an open unit do not provide adequate safety, the nurse is obligated to take reasonable action to improve the unit's safety (e.g., by arranging close supervision or transferring the patient to a locked psychiatric unit).

quest for suicide. Proponents of rational suicide recommend the following criteria for terminally ill adults who plan suicide: (1) a mental status examination showing clear mental processes without depression; (2) understandable motivation for suicide; (3) societal understanding of the patient's motives for suicide; and (4) evidence that all options have been thoroughly explored before suicide is selected (Siegel, 1986). One patient with AIDS planned to commit suicide when her pain was overwhelming, her quality of life unacceptable, and her life meaningless. She had psychotherapy, was given antidepressants for depression, and returned to clear thought processes about the nature, meaning, and consequences of her suicide plan and other options. Still she wanted suicide.

These criteria do not guide clinicians through complex situations. They also neglect the impact of suicide on loved ones, family, or friends.

When the pain of living is greater than the fear of dying, people may consider suicide an impulsive response to persistent pain, depression, dementia, or an unacceptable quality of life. When a patient in pain says "I would be better off dead," clinicians may believe the patient. Only a thorough assessment of a patient's suicidal intent will identify symptoms that require treatment, such as persistent pain, depression, or dementia. Nor can clinicians assume that the risk of suicide is absent when suicide is not mentioned, because many patients will not spontaneously mention suicide unless asked. Hence, nurses have a duty to routinely detect, monitor, and evaluate patients for their risk of suicide.

Patient quotes from a study funded by DHHS, PHS STC 1 A23 NU0024–01.

O AN OVERVIEW

- When a patient says that the pain of living seems worse than dying, the nurse needs to evaluate the risk of suicide, relieve suffering, and protect the patient from suicidal impulses.

- The nurse's non-judgmental attitudes can encourage the patient to disclose suicide plans.

- Several theories help explain the pathways to suicide, and persons in high-risk groups should be carefully evaluated for suicide risk.

- Clinical assessment begins with screening and the investigation of clues, warnings, and behaviors indicating suicidal intent.

- Interventions to reduce suicide risk include providing safety, removing means for suicide, monitoring suicidal behavior, increasing the patient's social support, resources, and coping mechanisms, and communicating suicide risk to the health-care team. Nurses also reduce patient distress and ensure that depression and other disorders are effectively treated.

- Management of suicidal patients is enhanced by consultation, collaboration, and referrals. The family and significant others can be helpful allies in treating the patient.

- Nurses have an important role in developing an agency's suicide prevention and treatment policies, improving social policy and access to care for high-risk groups.

- Ethical issues such as rational suicide, assisted suicide, and euthanasia are controversial; the nurse's role remains one of detecting, evaluating, monitoring, and preventing suicide, and abstaining from assisting in suicide.

TD TERMS TO DEFINE

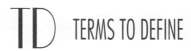

- ambivalence
- attempted suicide
- completed suicide
- crisis
- indirect self-destructive behavior
- lethality
- parasuicide
- suicidal ideas
- suicide
- suicide gesture

Q STUDY QUESTIONS

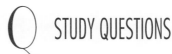

Case example: Jon Lima, a 35-year-old patient, is admitted to a psychiatric unit with low self-esteem and suicidal behavior. It is his third admission. He speaks negatively of himself and states that he would be better off dead. He is concerned about insomnia. Although he has been suicidal during past hospitalizations, he now denies suicidal ideas and is not put on suicide alert status. He is quiet and withdrawn, and responds slowly to all stimuli.

1. Mr. Lima seems less lethargic today, and agrees to participate in an occupational therapy program. To help make the session most successful, the nurse would do which of the following?

   a. Introduce him to wood carving; show or tell him how to use the carving and burning tools safely.
   b. Stay away from Mr. L. in occupational therapy so that he is free to express himself.
   c. Teach him to make a macramé belt from long rope, and encourage him to take it to his room and work on it later.
   d. Structure his session to help him complete one small task, such as painting a picture.

2. The possibility of suicide is a most important concern in the care of Mr. Lima. When is Mr. L. most likely to attempt suicide?

   a. When he is mute and unlikely to tell anyone about it.
   b. When he is ready to go home and afraid of leaving the hospital.
   c. When his family goes on vacation.
   d. When he begins to demonstrate improvement.

3. Mr. Lima begins to demonstrate an increased risk for suicide and his treatment orders include suicide precautions. Which of the following is not considered a suicide precaution?

   a. Searching personal effects for toxic agents (drugs, alcohol).
   b. Removing sharp instruments (razor blades, glass, knives).
   c. Removing clothes that could be made into straps (belts, suspenders),
   d. Asking the patient to focus on positive feelings

4. Mr. Lima is put under one-to-one observation and objects strongly to being "followed around and watched" and not trusted to behave like an adult. He screams when the nurse says that she must accompany him to the bathroom. The best response for the nurse would be:

   a. "I understand you are angry, but I must be able to see you at all times to make sure you are safe."
   b. "Stop yelling at me! I can't change the rules—anyway, what did you expect if you talk about suicide!"
   c. "Well, you are better; I'll wait outside the bathroom and you can close the door until you are finished."
   d. "You should stop being angry and uncooperative and focus on happy things."

5. Which of the following would NOT be an appropriate question for the nurse to ask when assessing Mr. Lima?

   a. "What are your expectations of yourself?"
   b. "How do you cope with anger?"
   c. "What kinds of things are pleasurable for you?"
   d. "Don't you think that it is morally wrong to think of suicide?"

6. The nurse selects a diagnosis of "ineffective individual coping related to feelings of anger, suicide, and hopelessness," and focuses on goals for the patient. Which is the most appropriate goal for this nursing diagnosis?

   a. The patient will deny feelings of hopelessness, anger and suicide.
   b. The patient will demonstrate joyful and cheerful mood.
   c. The patient will voice no complaints.
   d. The patient will share angry, suicidal feelings with the nurse.

7. Which would be the LEAST effective approach to assisting Mr. Lima to cope with painful feelings of anger and suicide?

   a. Encourage him to smile and be cheery.
   b. Encourage him to share his feelings
   c. Help him to keep busy.
   d. Provide reality orientation and encourage him to have realistic expectations of himself.

8. The nurse's highest priority for a patient with a high suicide risk is to

   a. administer tranquilizers so that the patient will be less suicidal.
   b. constantly monitor the patient's location and behavior.
   c. change the subject whenever the patient mentions suicide.
   d. keep the patient in isolation in order to prevent other patients from witnessing a possible suicide attempt.
   e. get the patient to talk about suicide to lower the risk of accomplishing it.

9. Patients with which diagnosis would be at LOWEST risk for suicide?

   a. Major depression
   b. Obsessive-compulsive disorder
   c. Schizophrenia
   d. Chemical dependency

10. Which population group is NOT in a high-risk group for suicide?

   a. Elderly
   b. Adolescents
   c. Drug/alcohol abusers
   d. Women in their 40s

Case example: Loyola Grim, a 53-year-old woman, is admitted to an intensive care unit. She is accompanied by her husband, who tells the nurse that he recently asked his wife for a divorce. He left the house yesterday to attend a 3-day business meeting in another state. Some of the meetings were canceled and he returned home on the morning of her admission to find his wife unconscious. An empty bottle of sleeping pills was at her bedside.

11. In assessing the seriousness of Mrs. Grim's suicide attempt, which of the following facts is the LEAST important?

   a. She is unconscious.
   b. She used a potentially lethal method.
   c. She planned the attempt for a time when she thought no rescue was possible.
   d. She did not leave a suicide note.

12. The following day, Mrs. Grim regains consciousness. She is in tears and tells the nurse. "I'm a failure at everything, as a woman, as a wife; I've even failed at killing myself." In interpreting this statement, which of the following is LEAST likely to be true?

   a. Mrs. Grim is depressed.
   b. Mrs. Grim is remorseful about her suicide attempt and therefore unlikely to make a second attempt.
   c. Mrs. Grim is feeling hopeless and the potential for another attempt is great.
   d. Mrs. Grim is ambivalent about whether to live or die.

■ REFERENCES

Position Paper on Assisted Suicide. Washington, DC, American Nursing Association, 1994.

Agency for Health Care Policy and Research: Clinical Practice Guidelines: *Depression In Primary Care* Vols. 1 and 2. AHCPR Publication no. 93–0 551. Rockville, Maryland, United States Department of Health and Human Services. Public Health Service, 1993. pp. 1–98;

Alcohol, Drug Abuse, and Mental Health Administration. (1989). Report of the Secretary's Task Force on Youth Suicide. Vol. 3. Publication No. (ADM)87–1623. United States Department of Health and Human Services Washington, DC, U.S. Government Printing Office.

Diagnostic and Statistical Manual of Mental Disorders, ed. 4. Washington, DC, American Psychiatric Association, 1994, pp. 128–131.

Battin MP: (1992) Rational suicide. *Crisis* 1992; 12:73–80.

Beck AT, Rush AJ, Shaw BF, Emery G: *Cognitive Therapy of Depression.* New York, Guilford, 1979.

Berman A. et al. Case consultation: Inpatient treatment planning. *Suicide Life Threat Behav* 1993; 23:162–169.

Berman AL, Jobes DA: *Adolescent Suicide Assessment and Intervention,* Washington DC, American Psychological Association, 1991, pp. 100–270.

Bongar B: Consultation and the suicidal patient. *Suicide Life Threat Behav* 1993; 23:299–306.

Bongar B: *Suicide.* Oxford, Oxford University Press, 1992.

Bongar B, Maris RW, Berman AL, Litman RE, Silverman MM: Inpatient standards of care and the suicidal patient. *Suicide Life Threat Behav* 1993; 23:245–262.

Breitbart W: Suicide risk and pain in cancer and AIDS patients, in Chapman CR, Foley KM (eds): *Current and Emerging Issues in Cancer Pain: Research and Practice.* New York, Raven Press, 1993.

Coyle N: The Euthanasia and physician-assisted suicide debate: Issues for Nursing. *Oncol Nurs Forum* 1992; 19(Suppl):41–47.

Cote T, Biggar R, Dannenberg A: Risk of suicide among persons with AIDS: A National Assessment. *JAMA* 1992; 268:2066–2068.

Davidson MW, Wagner WG, Range LM: Clinician's attitudes toward no-suicide agreements. *Suicide Life Threat Behav* 1995; 25:410–415.

Durkheim E: *Suicide: A Study in Sociology* (Spaulding JA, Simpson G, Trans.). Glencoe, IL, Free Press, 1951 (Original work published in 1897).

Farberow NL: Suicide prevention in the hospital. *Hosp Commun Psychiatry* 1981; 32:99–104.

Favazza AR: Why patients mutilate themselves. *Hosp Commun Psychiatry* 1982; 40:137–145.

Favazza AR: *Bodies Under Siege. Self-mutilation in Culture and Psychiatry.* Baltimore, Johns Hopkins University Press, 1987.

Fishbein M, Ajzen I: *Belief, Attitude, Intention and Behavior.* Reading, MA, Addison-Wesley, 1975.

Hatton CL, Valente SM: *Suicide: Assessment and Intervention,* ed. 2. Norwalk, CT, Appleton & Lange, 1984, pp. 61–148.

Hazell P, Lewin T: Postvention following adolescent suicide. *Suicide Life Threat Behav* 1993; 23:101–110.

Jamison S: AIDS and assisted suicide. *Hemlock Q* July 1992; 4–6.

Kachur SP, Potter LB, James SP, Powell KE: *Suicide in the United States 1980–1992.* Violence Surveillance Summary Series, No. 1. Atlanta, GA, National Center for Injury Prevention and Control, United States Department of Health and Human Services, 1995.

Kapur S, Mieczkowski T, Mann JJ: Antidepressant medications and the relative risk of suicide attempt and suicide. *JAMA* 1992; 268:3441–3445.

Kizer KW, Green MA, Perkins CI, Doebbert G, Hughes MS: AIDS and suicide in California. *JAMA* 1988; 260:1581.

Lipman A, Battin MP (eds): Position papers on euthanasia and assisted suicide. *J Pharmaceut Care Pain Symptom Control* 1996;

Litman RE: Suicide prevention in treatment settings. *Suicide Life Threat Behav* 1995; 25:134–142.

Lovett CG, Maltzberger T: in Bongar B. (ed): Psychodynamic factors in suicide. *Suicide.* Oxford, Oxford University Press, 1992, pp. 160–186.

Leenaars A, Maris R, McIntosh J, Richman J (eds): *Suicide and the Older Adult.* New York, Guilford, 1992.

Maltzberger JT. The psychodynamic formulation: an aid in assessing suicide risk, in Maris RW, Berman AL, Maltsberger JT, Yufit R (eds): *Assessment and Prediction of Suicide.* New York, Guilford, 1993, pp. 25–49.

Maris R: Overview of the study of suicide assessment and prediction, in Maris RW, Berman AL, Maltsberger JT, Yufit R. (eds): *Assessment and Prediction of Suicide* New York, Guilford, 1992, pp. 3–25.

Maris RW, Berman AL, Maltsberger, JT, Yufit R (eds): *Assessment and Prediction of Suicide* New York, Guilford, 1992, pp. 3–98.

Marzuk PM, Tierney H, Tardiff K: Increased risk of suicide in AIDS. *JAMA* 1988; 103:1333–1338.

Menninger WW: Patient suicide and its impact on the psychotherapist *Bull Menninger Clin* 1991; 55:216–227.

National Center for Health Statistics (NCHS), Vital Statistics. U.S. Public Health Service. Washington, DC, Government Printing Office. 1992.

O'Dowd M, Biderman D, McKegney F: Incidence of suicidality in AIDS and HIV+ patients attending a psychiatry outpatient program. *Psychosomatics* 1993; 34:33–40.

Osgood N, Brant BA, Lipman AA: Patterns of suicidal behavior in long term care facilities. *Omega* 1988; 19:69–77.

Phillips DP, Carstensen LL: Clustering of teenage suicides after television news stories about suicide. *N Engl J Med* 1986; 315:685–689.

Putnam FW, Guroff JJ, Silberman EK: The clinical phenomenology of multiple personality disorder. *J Clin Psychiatry* 1986; 47:285–293.

Quill T: Doctor, I want to die. Will you help me? *JAMA* 1993; 270:870–876.

Richman J: *Family Therapy for Suicidal People.* New York: Springer, 1986.

Saunders JM, Valente SM: Cancer and suicide. *Oncol Nurs Forum* 1988; 15:580–585.

Simon RI: *Concise Guide to Clinical Psychiatry and the Law.* Washington, DC, American Psychiatric Press, 1988, p. 89.

Rofes E: *I thought People Like That Killed Themselves.* San Francisco, Grey Fox Press, 1983.

Shneidman EH: Postvention: The care of the bereaved. *Suicide Life Threat Behav* 1981; 11:349–359.

Shneidman EH: *Definition of Suicide.* New York, Wiley, 1985.

Slaby A: Suicide as an indicium of biologically based brain disease *Arch Suicide Res* 1995; 1:59–74.

Slome L, Moulton J, Huffine et al. Physicians' attitudes toward assisted suicide in AIDS. *J AIDS* 1992; 5:712–718.

Valente SM, Saunders JM, Grant M: Oncology nurses' knowledge and misconceptions about suicide. *Cancer Pract* 1994; 2:209–216.

Valente SM: Suicide among medically ill patients *Nurse Pract* 1993;

Valente SM, Saunders JM: Suicide among the terminally ill: A case study. *Suicide Life Threat Behav* 1993; 23:76—82.

Valente SM: Messages of psychiatric patients who attempted or committed suicide. *Clin Nurs Res* 1994; 3:316–333.

Virkkunen M: Self-mutilation in anti-social personality disorder. *Acta Psychiatr Scand* 1976; 54:347–352.

Weishaar ME, Beck AT: Clinical and cognitive predictors of suicide, in Maris RW, Berman AL, Maltsberger JT, Yufit R (eds): *Assessment and Prediction of Suicide.* New York, Guilford, 1993; pp. 467–484.

Wright JG, Thase ME, Beck AT, Ludgate JW: *Cognitive Therapy with Inpatients.* New York, Guilford, 1993.

Zung WWK: Index of potential suicide, in Beck AT, Resnick HLP, Lettieri DJ (eds): *The Prediction of Suicide.* 1974, New York, Guilford, pp. 221–249.

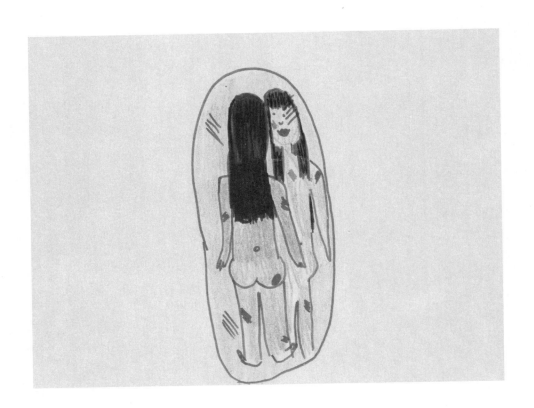

Anger is a weed.

St. Augustine (354–430)

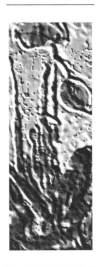

33
Managing Assaultive Patients

Burton Thelander / Denise Ribble

Interpersonal violence has been an important public health issue since 1985, when violent crime was declared a national public health emergency in the United States by Surgeon General C. Everett Koop. Between 1960 and 1987 the rate of violent crime in the U.S. increased by almost 400%. This increase is evident in general-hospital emergency rooms, psychiatric settings, and prisons.

Within inpatient psychiatric settings the occurrence and perception of aggression, violence, and assaultive behavior between patients and staff has also increased (Davis, 1991). Violent patients within hospital settings are managed by utilizing milieu and alternative interpersonal interventions, medications and less restrictive physical restraints, and seclusion. The focus of practice is to promote safer and more effective response patterns among patients, thereby helping to prevent aggressive behavior before it occurs. Patients who have shown such behavior should use this competence to recover and take better care of themselves in less restrictive environments outside the hospital. The inpatient practice paradigm must evolve from that of coercive management and control of behavior to humane, effective treatment that stresses learning, prevention of violence, rehabilitation, and promotion of health. This chapter outlines interviewing and management techniques for aggressive behavior.

■ AGGRESSIVE BEHAVIOR

Aggressive behavior is defined as an event of actual or threatened contact (hitting, striking, spitting, kicking, throwing objects) in which the target is a person or object in the environment. This definition includes verbal threats and/or physical acts.

THEORIES

The origins of aggressive or violent behavior are said to be multi-causal, including biological, interpersonal, family-system, socio-economic, cultural, and environmental factors (Barnes, 1989). The belief that mental illness predisposes a person to behave violently has also been explored, but without establishing a definitive causal relationship or correlation between such illness and violent behavior (Monahan, 1992).

Various theories have been proposed to explain aggression and violence. Four prominent theories attribute it to biological or psychological factors, frustration, and social learning (see Table 33–1). Each has a specific focus and direction for treatment (Morrison, 1996).

What is important to stress when working with violent patients, their families and significant others, and the nursing staff, supervisors, peers, and subordinates is that the patterns of violence are amenable to understanding, intervention, and ultimate reversal. Communicating, overtly or covertly, the belief that violent behavior is predetermined (with genetic, neurological, or biochemical origins) promotes a hopeless, helpless response by patients and health-care staff members that seriously impairs efforts to promote learning and recovery. Before they can effectively intervene, prevent violence, and promote recovery, nurses must confront myths, fear, anxiety, and stigma about interacting with people who display violence.

The multifaceted nature of aggressive behavior is reflected in the theories that attempt to explain it. This multifaceted characterization of human aggression is also reflected in the variable and diverse nosology of violent behavior contained in the *Diagnostic and Statistical Manual of Mental Disorders, Fourth Edition (DSM-IV)*. For example, an adolescent who demonstrates violent behavior might be given a diagnosis of conduct disorder. An adult who displays the same behavior might be categorized as having an impulsive disorder. In other examples, child abuse could be coded as a parent-child problem rather than a mental disorder of any kind. Violent behavior may also be considered a symptom of psychiatric disorders including dementia, schizophrenia, drug intoxication, depression, mania, personality disorders, mental retardation, or attention deficit disorder.

RESEARCH

Psychiatric clinicians are often required to assess the risk of violent behavior among persons with mental disorders. However, research is only beginning to address the potential for violence among such individuals. A study by McNiel and Binder (1994), consistent with previous research, found a higher level of hostile-suspiciousness at admission among assaultive patients with manic disorders, organic psychotic conditions, and other mental disorders than among non-assaultive patients with these same disorders. Among patients with schizophrenia, on the other hand, there were no significant differences in the level of hostile-suspiciousness between patients who later became assaultive and those who did not.

Lanza's pioneering nursing research on patient assault argues that assault on nurses is a much larger problem than has been recognized (Lanza, 1985). Nurses can experience intense physical and emotional

TABLE 33–1 THEORIES OF AGGRESSION AND VIOLENCE

Theory	Focus	Directions for Treatment
Neurobiological theory	Violence has a biological basis (i.e., genes, biochemistry)	Address the biological imbalance and control symptoms Pharmacologic therapy Seclusion and restraint
Psychodynamic theory	Aggression is the result of the effects of the unconscious; unresolved issues motivate behavior	Uncover patient's unconscious instincts through talking therapies Performance of expressive, non-destructive acts
Frustration–aggression hypothesis	Aggression is a result of the build-up of frustration (e.g., drive theory) External stimuli affect frustration level	Release of frustration through other activities (sports, punching bag, pillow fights, arts)
Social learning theory	Violence is learned through witness of violence; positive reinforcement (tangible rewards, social reward and approval); negative reinforcement); cycle of violence	Contingency management (alter the reward system) Emphasize verbal techniques (negotiation and conflict resolution) Problem-solving training

Source: Morrison, 1996. Personal communication.

reactions when they are victims of a patient assault. One reaction is role conflict, which may result when the nurse believes it is unprofessional to express his or her feelings about the assault.

Although there is a dearth of evidence that violence can be reliably predicted in community or hospital settings, factors that may be related to the risk of violence, and which suggest that an individual is at risk for violent behavior, include the following.

- A history of violent behavior (criminal, intrafamily, or with significant others or in other social systems, during previous or current hospitalizations).
- A history of childhood psychological, physical, or sexual abuse or the witnessing of family violence.
- Alcohol/substance abuse.
- Rigid, controlling, and/or exploitative family systems.

The expectation of non-violent behavior must be communicated to patients and their families. Violence inside or outside the hospital or home setting is unacceptable. The belief that everyone has the right to work and live in a safe and humane environment must be communicated by nursing and the other mental-health professions and enacted consistently within the treatment environment.

■ APPROACH TO AGGRESSIVE PATIENTS

A calm, systematic approach is critical in approaching an aggressive, violent, or acutely excited patient regardless of the treatment setting (see Figure 33-1). The patient's behavior is viewed as a symptom of an illness and should be taken very seriously. Potentially violent patients who are not immediately seen in the emergency room or other out-patient settings should not be kept waiting, since they may interpret the wait as a sign that they are not important or do not need immediate treatment. The nurse should act promptly, introduce her- or himself by name and title, and ask to begin talking with the patient.

Back-up help should be available for the management of patients who are overtly aggressive or psychotic. The environment should be free of objects that could be used as weapons. The treatment team should never turn their backs or let the patient come between them and the door; the door should be readily available to both the patient, nurse, and other members of the care team. If a violent patient escapes, security guards and/or police should be called immediately. Threatening calls or letters from patients should never be ignored, since doing so may escalate the potential for violence.

Some specific steps should be taken when interviewing a potentially violent patient. First, it is important to be aware of one's own anxiety and fear, and prevent that anxiety from overtly effecting the intervention. The nurse should maintain a distance adequate to permit avoiding or deflecting blows. No attempt should be made to deal with a violent patient without help. Be sure the patient has been checked for weapons. Talk in a calm and soothing voice. If talk does not de-escalate agitated behavior, restraints or medication may be necessary. If they are needed, they should be applied as gently as possible. An early show of authority and control may prevent injury and property damage (Goldman and Levy, 1995).

■ ASSESSMENT OF AGGRESSION

The following areas are important in assessing aggression, whether during a home visit, patient admission, or in the course of treatment.

ENVIRONMENTAL FACTORS

Assessing a potentially aggressive patient requires a quiet setting or room. There should be minimal noise and interruption by television, telephone, radio, and persons walking in and out. For patients who have a low impulse threshold for violence, use comfortable furniture that cannot be easily picked up and thrown. There should be an absence of objects (lamps, computer terminals, pens, pencils, staplers, etc.) that can be used as weapons. Decorations must be securely attached to walls in hospital units that treat aggressive patients.

Environmental factors may adversely affect patient behavior and staff response, yet they are often amenable to alteration. These factors include furniture that may be used as obstacles and objects that could be used as weapons or for defense, It is important to know the location of restraints, of exits, light switches, door locks and their opening direction, and the telephone, and other staff personnel; to have equipment in working condition; to keep patients from dangerous situations; to understand the importance of personal space for the patient; and to prevent the presence of hot beverages or food and lighted cigarettes.

A separate environment within a psychiatric unit that reduces distraction promotes the opportunity to attend to what the patient presents during the assessment process, and reinforces the importance of the effort to understand the patient's experience and develop alternative responses.

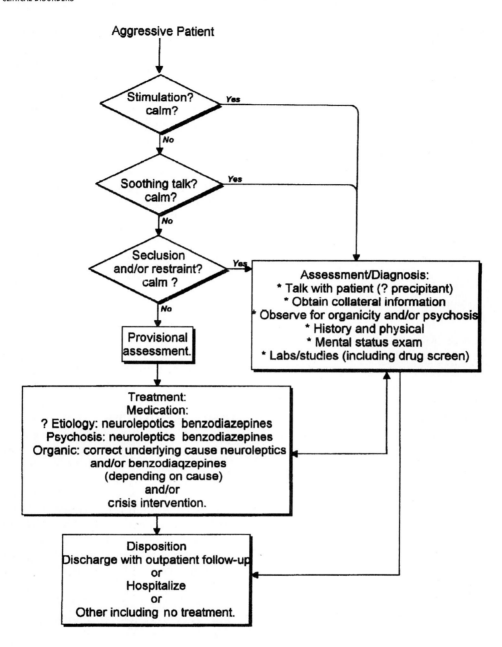

Adapted from: Goldman and Levy. In: Goldman H. *Review of General Psychiatry,* 4ed. Appleton & Lange, Stamford, CT; 1995, 514–515.

Figure 33–1: Interviewing the Aggressive Patient.

HISTORY OF AGGRESSION OR ABUSE

An essential component of the assessment process is obtaining a comprehensive history of criminal behavior resulting in arrest and/or conviction; physical, emotional, or sexual abuse; displays of violence toward the self or others; the context and precipitants of violence; the patient's response; and consequences of the patient's actions.

The importance of a comprehensive interview cannot be underestimated. The nurse must assess the seriousness of the patient's behavior and be able to ask questions that will promote descriptions of this behavior and a response to interventions. Questions to ask the patient include:

- Have you ever caused physical injury to another person?

- What is the closest you have come to being violent?
- Have you ever been harmed? How? When?
- Describe what occurred just before you were violent.
- Have you ever been arrested? What were the charges?
- Have you ever been in jail?
- When you get excited, what helps you to calm yourself?
- What do you believe causes you to be angry or aggressive?
- Do you worry about being violent?

Litwack (1994) discussed the need to differentiate between the **assessment of dangerousness** and the prediction of violence. The prediction of violence has been shown to be unreliable (McNiel and Binder, 1995), but the assessment of dangerousness may more accurately predict the potential for violence. Determining the patient's history of violence can assist this effort. Comparing and contrasting the patient's memory and perception with that of other sources (documents from other hospitals or treatment settings, staff descriptions, interviews with family members and significant others, and a criminal history) can provide further illumination. It is essential to assess whether the patient is vulnerable to violent behavior.

DETAILING AGGRESSION

Specific characteristics of violent behavior include its precipitants, social context, environment, and the patient's response, perception, and thought processes before, during, and after a violent episode.

PROMOTING NON-VIOLENCE

Assessment should focus on the capacity of the patient to employ non-violent strategies of behavior. If violent behavior has occurred, the nurse should explore with the patient those factors that worked to stop the violence. Questions directed at this include:

- How has the patient avoided being violent?
- What strengths, supports, or resources are available to the patient?
- How does the patient successfully get along with people?
- How has the patient been able to calm him- or herself?
- What medication has helped calm the patient?
- How does the patient perceive his or her violence?
- What ability does the patient have to learn?

Family members, significant others, and treatment staff personnel should be questioned in order to elicit information that will complement the review.

Measurement of behavior may be done with an assessment tool. The St. Lawrence Overt Aggression Scale (see Figure 33–2) can yield specific information about a patient's violent behavior patterns and response to treatment interventions. All treatment staff personnel working with the patient should have input into the recording of information about the patient's behavior. Accurate recording of information in conjunction with the patient, for specific periods of time, can be utilized in the treatment-planning process.

Behavioral Warning Signs

Specific **behavioral warning signs** can alert nurses to potential aggression and violence by a patient. Some of these signs include pacing, an angry demeanor or behavior, fearful looks, threatening actions, staring, extreme quietness, arguments, mumbling, threatening statements, clenched fists, a tense posture, refusal to talk with staff members, and changes in the patient's usual behavior.

Other factors that can alert nurses to potential patient aggression and violence include displaced anger, frustration, or guilt; rejection by others; bad news from home; projection of the patient's self concept; the desire to be punished; broken promises; threats to personal safety; loss of autonomy; lack of communication; a need to test limits and/or control the environment; a lack of choices; and unaddressed sexual needs.

A careful evaluation of variables that influence behavior in a given situation is important. This information can be utilized to provide specific feedback that may help the patient identify behavioral patterns and effects of which he or she is not aware, or may deny.

Nurses may need to consult with other specialists for further diagnostic or evaluative measures, such as psychological testing for cognitive and intellectual functioning. A neurological evaluation or laboratory tests may be indicated to assess other factors that may contribute to the occurrence of violence and/or influence treatment decisions. A neurological assessment can reveal seizure activity, organic brain disorders, or dementia; psychological testing may uncover mania, paranoia, or character disorders; a history of injury with subsequent behavioral changes may be discovered through imaging techniques. Diagnoses to consider include attention deficit with hyperactivity disorder in the patient's childhood or adolescence; alcohol or substance abuse; and developmental trauma and delays. Requesting consultations for such information will augment the nursing assessment.

Physiological Responses to Stress

Dealing with a potentially violent patient is stressful. Some physiological responses to stress in either the patient or staff member health-care professional include

OVERT AGGRESSION SCALE
ADULT SERVICES

PATIENT NAME:_____ **"C" NUMBER:**_____ **WARD:**_____

DIRECTIONS: Each shift notes degree of aggressive behavior and interventions used by marking the shift (M,D,E) in the box in column for that date.   (over...)

WEEK OF:_____

BEHAVIOR DATE →							
(12) Attacks others causing severe injury, fracture, laceration							
(11) Mutilates self through severe laceration, deep bites, fracture							
(10) Sets fires, throws objects in dangerous manner							
(9) Attacks others causing bruises, sprains, mild to moderate welts							
(8) Breaks objects, violently destroys property							
(7) Self inflicts cuts, bruises, minor burns (cigarette)							
(6) Punches objects or wall with minor or no injury; headbanging							
(5) Self inflicts scratches or minor injury							
(4) Destroys property or throws objects without breaking							
(3) Serious verbal threats to hurt others or self							
(2) Moderate verbal threats to hurt others or self							
(1) Makes loud, angry noises							
(0) No aggressive behavior							
INTERVENTIONS:							
(14) Injury to others requiring medical treatment							
(13) Injury to self requiring medical treatment							
(12) Restraint							
(11) Seclusion							
(10) 1:1's							
(9) Ward restrictions or observations							
(8) PRN medication, IM							
(7) PRN medication, oral							
(6) Holding patient							
(5) Relocation							
(4) Verbal limit setting							
(3) Verbal redirection							
(2) Verbal calming							
(1) Problem solving, counseling							
(0) None							

Figure 33–2. Front

OVERT AGGRESSION SCALE

DIRECTIONS

This sheet is to be filled out, documenting a single patient's behaviors and staff interventions addressing those behaviors, over the course of 1 week.

Please keep this sheet filed near the shift report book for easy documenting each shift.

A staff member on each shift (Midnights, Days, Evenings) will note the degree of aggressive behavior exhibited by the patient by marking the shift (M,D,E) in the corresponding box under behavior for that date.

The staff member will also note the corresponding staff intervention by marking the shift (M,D,E) in the corresponding box under interventions.

At the end of 1 week, a connecting line may be drawn through the most aggressive behaviors on each date in order to obtain a graphic profile of the severity of aggression and nature of staff interventions during that week.

for example:

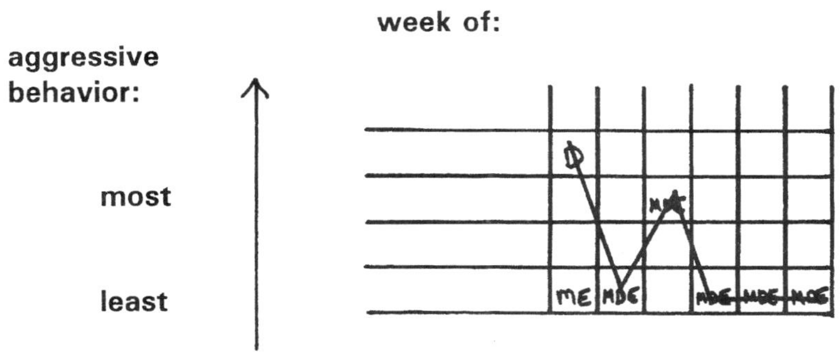

Weekly profiles may be grouped together to form a profile over a longer period of time.

Adapted from: Goldman and Levy. In Goldman H. *Review of General Psychiatry*, 4ed, Appleton & Lange Stamford CT; 1995, 514–515.

Figure 33–2. Back

an increased heart rate and respiration; elevated blood pressure; rapid, shallow mouth breathing; dryness of the mouth; palpitations; headaches; shaky knees; a need to urinate; diarrhea; anger; restlessness; weakness; a pounding pulse; a squeaky voice; confusion; nervousness; sweating; silliness; cold hands; and sweaty palms.

Staff assessment of their own emotional and intellectual response to violence is important. Answers to the following questions are helpful.

- What anxiety or fear do you experience?
- How do you cope with being anxious or afraid?
- How do you let your peers know about your response?
- Does your response interfere with effective treatment?
- What expectations do you have for the patient?
- Are they realistic?
- Do you believe the patient will recover?

Developing self awareness, exploring one's response with peers and supervisors, and determining how that response affects the patient's treatment are all recommended steps.

■ NURSING DIAGNOSIS

After assessment, the nurse participates with other treatment staff members and the patient in a case formulation that involves hypothesizing the intrapersonal, interpersonal, and systems dynamics that contribute to the patient's violence. Identifying the etiology, possible cause(s), and past and current patterns of behavioral responses to specific precipitants of violence will help in developing treatment strategies for promoting patient understanding and changes in behavior and outcomes.

A nursing diagnosis is a statement that represents a truly or potentially altered pattern of human functioning (in this case related to the occurrence of violence), and that describes defining characteristics (empirical indicators) and behavioral manifestations of this alteration (McFarland and Wash, 1986). The North American Nursing Diagnosis Association has established a list of approved nursing diagnoses. Some nursing diagnoses related to violence are:

- Defensive coping
- Denial, ineffective
- Fear
- Self esteem, situational low
- Thought processes altered
- Risk for violence: self-directed or directed at others

■ OUTCOME IDENTIFICATION

Once the nurse has formulated a nursing diagnosis and a case formulation that addresses the patient's violent behavior in conjunction with the patient and treatment staff, specific patient outcomes must be identified. The American Nurses Association (ANA, 1994) suggests that outcomes be individualized, measurable, realistic, and attainable. Outcome statements addressing violent behavior should define exactly what the patient is expected to display as he or she learns to change his or her response pattern. The patient's understanding of his or her behavior can be addressed. For example, the patient will describe:

- Precipitants prior to assaulting peers
- The emotion experienced prior to destroying property
- Two warning signs that have occurred during group sessions

The expectation that violent behavior will be reduced can be addressed:

- by having the patient ask staff members to permit him or her to use the quiet room when feeling the urge to strike peers.
- by having patient request PRN medication when he or she has the impulse to throw furniture.

Generic outcome statements such as "the patient will develop insight," unrealistic statements such as "hallucinations will be eliminated," or negative statements such as "will not be assaultive" should be avoided. The specific patterns of patient behavior and response to interventions identified during the assessment process should be integrated into the outcome statements. The patient should participate in this development process to foster specific understanding of what is expected of him or her in terms of behavioral change.

Behavior contracts can be effective with patients who have the intellectual and cognitive capacity to participate and agree to establish specific expectations about interventions and behavioral change. The patient should participate in the development of the contract and agree to specific response patterns and expected changes in behavior. The contract should describe staff interventions that evolve from least restrictive (counseling, feedback, suggestion of alternative behaviors/calming techniques) to more restrictive (identification of consequences, offer of medication, use of quiet area, physical interventions) according to the patient's response.

■ NURSING INTERVENTIONS

Various nursing interventions can assist in promoting an environment that discourages aggression and violence. These interventions may be undertaken in crisis situations or in less urgent situations. The trend toward the least possible restrictive environment for psychiatric patients is a positive step in mental-health care delivery. However, the issue of providing a safe and minimally restrictive environment for all patients while caring for an assaultive patients creates a serious dilemma for nurses; in addition to helping patients cope with their aggressive feelings and behavior, nurses must also deal with violence directed at themselves.

■ CRISIS MANAGEMENT OF AGGRESSION

When less restrictive interventions are unsuccessful in promoting patient learning, changing patient outcomes, and preventing violence, alternate and restrictive crisis interventions may be necessary to manage uncontrolled behavior. The purpose of crisis intervention techniques is to:

- Assess patients who are losing control of their behavior.

- Recognize the causes of violent behavior.
- Provide a co-ordinated team response to violent behavior.
- Teach the patient self-calming techniques.
- Reduce the use of restraint and seclusion.
- Reduce the number of patient and staff injuries.

The use of a team approach in which all staff members (physicians, psychiatric nurses, ancillary mental health workers, psychologists, and social workers) collaborate in sharing assessment ideas, and plan and implement coordinated and consistent interventions congruent with the patient's response, can be effective in preventing patient violence.

WHEN VIOLENCE PREVENTION FAILS

As with least restrictive interventions, it is important to cease negotiation when the patient begins to display patterns of behavior that may precede violence. Staff members should then set limits ("the expectation within this unit is that you not threaten to harm others; you are expected to stop immediately; what can we do with you so you can calm yourself?"), and define specific consequences for unacceptable behavior ("if you continue with your behavior [describe exactly] you will be asked to use the quiet room and take an available PRN medication", "if you are not able to stop threaten-

E CASE EXAMPLE

Joe Jones, a 29-year-old African-American male, is admitted to an inpatient psychiatric unit from an alcohol treatment center. He makes statements expressing the wish to kill himself. Two weeks ago his wife left him for another man. He threatened to stab himself with a knife. He is having difficulty sleeping and wants to harm his wife's new boyfriend.

Patient History

Joe is the second of three children; his siblings work in semi-professional positions. Joe describes a close, supportive relationship with his mother. His father deserted the family when Joe was a child. He had little subsequent contact with his father, who died of alcoholism and cirrhosis of the liver several years ago. Joe denies having been physically or sexually abused. He has a 7-year-old daughter who he has not seen since being estranged from her mother, and a 3-month-old son with the wife who recently left him. This stressor precipitated his recent episode of drug and alcohol abuse and suicidal ideation.

As a child, Joe was diagnosed as having attention deficit disorder. He did not take medication for it because of the objection of his mother. He has abused alcohol since the age of 13, and had used crack cocaine since his early twenties. He has been to a

detoxification center twice in the past 2 years, and has been admitted to rehabilitation programs at least twice, once just prior to his current psychiatric admission. He has a criminal history of robbery and armed robbery, with a 3-year incarceration 10 years ago. He has had one arrest related to drug possession

During his 6-week admission, Joe does not describe suicidal ideation or a plan to harm himself. He makes no effort to harm himself. He states that his suicidal thoughts were a symptom of his depression. Joe is alert and oriented, and participates in clear and goal-directed discussions with staff members of his unit. His activities of daily living skills are satisfactory; he is always neatly and casually dressed. On Wexler testing, he displays average intelligence (his test results are 92 on the full scale, 85 on the verbal scale, and 106 for performance), and describes a limited education (he completed 9th grade in special-education classes for hyperactive children, and acquired a general equivalency diploma [GED] in a correctional institution). He has established a positive therapeutic relationship with a female therapist, but does not trust other members of the treatment team. He believes that certain staff members are hostile toward him. He wished to return to the rehabilitation program to get help with his impulse control and anger.

Continued

E CASE EXAMPLE   Continued

Joe describes himself as being anxious. He fidgets and bounces his feet while seated, establishes eye contact for brief periods, and rises out of chairs and paces back and forth frequently during scheduled group and individual sessions, and during psychological testing sessions. He frequently asks that questions be repeated. When his requests for food, medication, or to make telephone calls are not immediately met, he threatens to harm staff members, intrudes physically upon personal space, and sometimes enters restricted office areas, having to be physically restrained and removed. He often misinterprets other's behavior and motives as being hostile, and at times describes himself as being paranoid and mistrustful. He also believes that he has a poor memory, which he attributes to his past use of crack cocaine. Among his statements are "I will kick your ass," and "I'm going to hurt you." He also threatens riots on the unit, and curses. He would push through doors and aggressively enter a morning staff meeting when his request for pain medication (tooth ache) was not acted upon immediately. Once, in the dining room, he threatened to assault staff when he was denied certain food he wanted for his insulin dependent diabetes mellitus. Several staff were required to restrain and physically return him to his unit. When restrained, he blames others for this. He rarely displays this behavior when he encounters social difficulties or frustration with peers.

Joe does not take medications prescribed to help reduce his anxiety and impulsive behavior. He initially agreed to take these medication, but then refuses, when they are offered at scheduled times. He also refuses to take offered PRN medications when displaying anxiety, anger, threatening staff members, or pacing, and says that he will not take medication after his discharge. He also does not comply with dietary recommendations to prevent complications of his insulin-dependent diabetes mellitus. He claims that he understands the need for dietary compliance and monitoring of his blood glucose concentration, but does not follow the schedule for his dietary, or eat at scheduled times. When provided the diet at scheduled meals he would threaten ("You better give me the right food at lunch or I'll throw my tray in your face, you stupid bitch! You're the only f——— one that does this to me, no one else restricts me!")—He would minimize the long-term effects of his noncompliance with medication and diet and its immediate effects on his behavior and mental health.

He attends scheduled unit programs, and had participated in several alcohol/substance abuse rehabilitation programs in the past, including having been detoxified 2 weeks prior to his admission. He says that rehabilitation programs were been helpful to him in the past.

Three aggressive episodes (one resulting in staff injury) result in his transfer to the hospital's secure unit. During one of these episodes he was in a designated smoking area with about 20 other patients and two staff members, and began to insist that he be allowed to make a telephone call and insisted that he wanted "to get the hell out of here." When told that he would be given an opportunity to use the telephone upon return to his unit, he suddenly stood up, threw several chairs, and ran out of the room yelling that he was leaving and going to "kick ass."

The unit staff members used defensive physical interventions to stop Joe's behavior. They said "We want to listen to you. What do you want? We are not going to hurt you or let you hurt anyone else. What do you need to calm yourself right now?" Joe

was directed to a hallway away from other patients and staff members. Although displaying agitation by pacing and speaking rapidly and clenching his fists, he was able to establish eye contact and listen to questions and answers to his questions. He was offered medication; he refused and stated he wanted to call his mother. Within ten minutes he was calm enough to be escorted to a room where he could use a telephone. He was then informed that he would be transferred to the secure unit.

Patient's Strengths

- Joe states that he wants to "get better," leave the hospital, and return to the rehabilitation program.
- He participates in goal-directed counseling, and is alert and oriented.
- He has excellent self-care skills (dressing, bathing, grooming).
- He has regular contact with his mother, and relies on her for emotional support.
- He displays effective social interpersonal skills.

Nursing Diagnosis

- Potential for violence (self directed) related to recent separation from wife/child.
- Hopelessness as evidenced by threats to harm self and statements that he wants to die.
- Potential for violence (directed at others) related to low frustration tolerance, difficulty in controlling impulses, a history of alcohol and controlled-substance abuse, and a history of violence as evidenced by assaults (resulting in injury) on staff members and peers, threats to harm or kill staff members, and inability to enact contractually established behaviors when feeling angry or anxious.
- Altered health maintenance related to denial of significance of diagnosis of insulin-dependent diabetes mellitus, non-compliance with prescribed diet, and health-learning deficits evidenced by extreme fluctuations in blood glucose levels and repeated refusal to comply with prescribed diet/insulin coverage.

Short-term goals

- Patient will continue to maintain daily blood glucose levels within normal limits while in the hospital.
- Patient will communicate daily without verbal threats or assaultive behavior.

Interventions

- Develop contract with patient to control behavior.
- Read and review daily unit rules.
- Have patient identify three precipitating events leading to his aggressive behavior.
- Have nursing staff provide immediate feedback to patient when changes in his behavior are noted; explain consequences of poor behavior; and provide least restrictive interventions to calm him.
- Have staff provide a consistent response by teaching patient, providing interpersonal counseling, and using environmental interventions. PRN medication and restraint will be used as needed. There will be debriefing with the patient.
- Health teaching about diet for blood glucose maintenance.

ing harm you will be escorted to the restraint room to remain until you calm yourself"), and reinforce their belief that the patient can calm him- or herself. It is also important to employ varied interventions that progress or recede as the patient's response changes. When an intervention is unsuccessful, and an alternate intervention that may have previously worked or may not have been attempted but is indicated on the basis of the etiology of the patient's violence, patterns of behavior, and the case formulation should be attempted.

When **de-escalation techniques** fail to prevent violent behavior, more restrictive interventions must be attempted to control a patient's behavior. Maintaining safety and security within the care setting is a primary responsibility for nursing. Members of the team responsible for the patient must collaborate when making decisions about how and when to intervene. Leadership should be exercised to reach a consensus quickly and provide direction for all interventions. Once the patient's behavior has become violent or violence is believed imminent, team action should take place without overt ambivalence. Further negotiation or failure to act will reduce the effect of efforts intended to change the patient's behavior, and may result in manipulation by the patient and staff splitting. Restrictive interventions indicated when violence is impending include:

- STAT medication (this requires physician evaluation of the patient, and is often given intramuscularly)
- Protective and restrictive physical measures.
- A code response to provide sufficient staff to respond to physical violence.
- The use of restraint devices or seclusion.

These interventions may increase the potential for injury to the patient and staff members. Struggling with a patient to provide intramuscular medication, utilizing take-down procedures to prevent further violence, escorting an unwilling patient out of an area, and putting a patient under restraint or seclusion are high-risk interventions. The need for competent, calm staff personnel, working cooperatively and effectively, is paramount in such situations. This can be accomplished through rapid, overt communication, assessment, and mutual planning prior to implementing all interventions.

Five **crisis-management** interventions emphasize behavior-control techniques directed at preventing a crisis or dealing with its escalation; they consist of the provision of a therapeutic environment, verbal communication with the patient, a team approach, and pharmacological and mechanical restraint.

PROVISION OF A THERAPEUTIC ENVIRONMENT

Factors within the therapeutic environment may constitute the precipitants for aggressive patient behavior. Thus, the environment should be structured to minimize the potential for such behavior. Attention should be given to the ambient temperature, noise control, lighting, furniture, and other factors, with the goal of establishing routines and attitudes that are conducive to peaceful conditions.

Christenfeld et al. (1989) have explored the effects of the physical environment on patients and staff personnel in psychiatric settings. Specific design features can have deleterious effects such as depersonalization, regimentation, and sensory deprivation. Careful design and configuration of the physical environment in an inpatient setting can promote social interaction, reduction of isolation, and privacy without impairing staff members' ability to observe patients without excessive intrusion. Waist-high partitions can be constructed in large living and common areas to promote small-group formation and allow staff members to observe patients. Nursing stations and offices should be accessible to patients in order to promote interaction. Quiet areas with low levels of stimulus should be available to patients upon request. Decorated, clean, and well maintained living areas with comfortable furniture should be provided. Seclusion rooms and private areas for the use of approved restraint devices must be prepared, available, and accessible. Bathrooms and sleeping areas should provide privacy while permitting unimpeded observation by staff members. Partitions with large, unbreakable windows can separate living and treatment areas to allow privacy and observation of patients and their interactions with other patients, family members, visitors, and staff personnel. Mirrors can permit observation around corners while minimizing intrusion. The seemingly conflicting needs of providing privacy while ensuring observation; security; and humane, comfortable, and non-restrictive living can be accomplished creatively. Physical space can be seen as nourishing and can connect the treatment milieu with practice concepts.

Nursing interventions can fail to prevent violence unless the physical structure of the treatment milieu supports the philosophy and implementation of treatment.

VERBAL INTERVENTION

Staff members' verbal intervention with patients should be based on knowledge and skills in psycho-social interaction, information processing, and levels of care and assertion, as well as methods for the stepwise prevention, intervention into, and resolution of various behavioral disorders.

When patients exhibit threatening behavior, staff members can provide immediate verbal feedback and ask the patient to stop. If the patient does not stop, the staff can provide the option of a time-out. This intervention includes the temporary separation of a patient from the unit milieu through movement to an isolated area. Its goal is to provide a setting in which a patient who has experienced a loss of self control can regain control.

If the patient refuses or the time-out proves ineffective, the staff may escort the patient to a quiet area and intervene verbally to calm the patient.

De-escalation techniques include verbal and nonverbal interventions, including environmental manipulation, designed to provide positive and corrective feedback to the patient and to define the consequences of unacceptable behavior.

TEAM APPROACH

When individual patients do not respond to individual verbal interventions or seclusion in a quiet room, it is important that team members show coordinated concern to the patient. Any show of concern should be non-threatening, and have a code name to alert the staff that it should assemble. Verbal threats should not be used. The strategy and goal of this team approach is to convey that the patient can control his or her impulses in a safe environment. It is critical to have the team prepared before the patient's behavior goes out of control. Once the team members arrive and are told the circumstances of the intervention, they are located physically in such a way that they are visible but non-threatening to the patient. Their presence acts as a means of security and conveys to the patient that physical action is inappropriate and will not be tolerated, and that self-control is of prime concern. However, the first team approach should be to verbally calm the patient, and this should take precedence over any form of physical contact.

PHARMACOLOGICAL INTERVENTION

When individual and team efforts are only partly effective or completely fail, and physical danger is imminent, rapid tranquilization of the patient is generally required. This intervention involves giving doses of antipsychotic medication that are titrated against the severity of the patient's symptoms. Oral medications can be as effective as intramuscular injections if the patient will cooperate. This approach is utilized after a physician trained in techniques of rapid tranquilization has evaluated the patient. If the patient does not comply with oral or intramuscular medication, the team upon the physician's order, should utilize additional techniques of behavioral control. The four-point personal-control tech-

nique is a suggested format. At no time should only one or two staff members try to make physical contact with a patient; rather, five staff members should be used, one for each limb and one to protect the patient's head.

The quiet room, scheduled or PRN medication, or defensive physical interventions such as maintaining distance and having trained staff members hold a patient's wrists or shoulders in a team approach has been shown to be effective in reducing patient aggression and staff injury (Martin, 1995).

MECHANICAL RESTRAINT

Mechanical restraint should be the last resort in seeking to control a patient who may be harmful to him- or herself or others, and should be used only in cases of noncompliance with the first four interventions described above. Patients should not be threatened with mechanical restraints, and when restraint is inevitable, only selected and approved devices should be used (e.g., well-padded wristlets and anklets).

A patient in mechanical restraints represents a psychiatric emergency and once restraint has been applied, a staff member must be constantly present with the patient in a one-to-one situation to monitor the patient's response and progress.

Restraint and seclusion (R/S) are safety interventions and not therapeutic techniques. Whereas therapeutic interventions are directed at increasing a patient's capacity for self-control, the use of restraint and seclusion indicates a failure of treatment. Imposing physical control on a patient does not provide a therapeutic opportunity to explore the patient's experience, promote learning and use competence and self-generated behavior to effect change. Definitions of restraint and seclusion follow:

- Seclusion is the placement of a patient in an area or room that the patient cannot leave at will
- Restraint is the placement of a patient in a device that interferes with the free movement of the body, and which the patient cannot easily remove, for the purpose of preventing imminent harm to the self or others. These devices include four-point ankle and wrist bindings, five-point (ankle, wrist, and chest strap), bindings, camisoles, restraint sheets, and preventive aggressive devices (a waist belt with wrist attachments to impede upper extremity movement).

Indications for restraint and seclusion may include:

- Assaultive or aggressive behavior (swinging of the arms at people, kicking, threats to harm, grabbing objects to use as weapons).

- A lack of response to verbal or non-verbal interventions.
- Refusal to consider such options as moving voluntarily to another area or to take medication.
- Behavior consistent with a past pattern of behavior that has resulted in violence or harm to the self or others.

Once a decision is made to put a patient in restraint and seclusion, evaluation and monitoring of the patient's emotional and physical status is of primary importance. Comfort and privacy must be provided for the duration of time the patient spends in restraint and seclusion. The nurse must continually evaluate the need for continued use of restraint and seclusion to reduce the potential for violence. The patient's vital

E CASE EXAMPLE

Henry Lee, a 47-year-old, white male, is admitted to a state psychiatric facility from a family-care home. He displays the following behaviors and problems:

- Poor sleep patterns and irritability.
- Setting small fires with cigarettes.
- Psychomotor agitation, pacing, and rubbing of his fingers.
- An increased rate and volume of speech.
- A report that his family plans to "sell the house."
- Withdrawal and aloofness.
- Minimum ability to complete activities of daily living and hygiene.
- Multiple stains/burns on his fingers/nails from cigarettes.
- Eating from the garbage.
- Defecating and urinating on himself and the floor, and attempting to drink his urine.
- Dermatitis of the buttocks.

Henry was first admitted to a psychiatric facility at age 25, following service in Viet Nam for 1½ years. At that time he believed that he was being injected with "needles" and that a magnetic signaling device had been implanted in his skin. He stated that others could monitor him and tell what he was doing. He responded well to psychotropics drugs (thiothixene; Navane), but failed to continue medications or after-care when discharged. His subsequent readmissions revealed further delusional thinking, including "bugs implanted in his buttocks by his father because he was bad as a child, and which accounted for noises in his ears." He had repeated psychiatric admissions and discharges for approximately a 10-year period. When out of the hospital, he engaged in excessive alcohol use, minor thefts of food and mail, and use of marijuana. He was unable to re-establish a relationship with his former wife and three children; his multiple threats and break-ins of their property had led to the involvement of a child protective services agency on the part of his family and an order of protection for them. He was able to recall events of his childhood, school, and family history. He was one of six children: three girls and three boys; he had left school in the 10th grade but had been awarded a general equivalency diploma while in the Army. He stated that his father was "bossy, opinionated, hard tempered, and difficult to get along with." He recalls having had difficulty making and keeping peer relationships because of his family's frequent moving. He has had no adult involvement in religion. In the past, he has threatened harm to his children and ex-wife, but cannot account for these actions.

Nursing Assessment

Henry smokes, carries a cup, and has episodic incontinence and rapid changes in clarity of thought, ranging from a short attention span to increasing confusion, and rapid changes in mental status, such as irritability and aggressive behavior. He has frequent abnormalities of his serum sodium. He drinks fluids excessively.

Presenting Problems

- Physically threatening behavior (i.e., spitting, assaulting, encroachment). He is verbally aggressive, yelling, swearing, and cursing.
- Hyponatremia, with excessive drinking of water, urinary incontinence, and a high level of irritability, as well as aggressive (physical and verbal) behavior that often revolves around fluids.
- Dermatitis due to enuresis, related to hyponatremia.

Course of hospitalization: For the 2 weeks after his most current admission, Henry does not wash himself, change his clothes, or brush his teeth unless directly supervised by staff personnel. He relates superficially with the staff, making eye contact, but remains aloof from peers. He paces continuously and raps on doors while laughing inappropriately and conversing without a partner. He denies bizarre, somatic, religious, persecutory, or grandiose delusions; auditory, visual, or sensory hallucinations; and suicidal or homicidal ideation or plans. He smokes safely during the supervised smoking program on the unit, but would otherwise burn his fingers and nails. His attention span and concentration last for approximately 20 minutes if the topic is of fair interest to him. He states he is not "bugged out" and does not need medications. He says he is residing in the facility "due to a need for housing."

As his hospitalization progresses, Henry demonstrates frequent periods of noncompliance with psychotropic medication and associated escalation of aggression, especially when approached about excessive cigarette smoking and with attempts at supervision and direction by staff members. He is often noted to be ingesting large amounts of fluids, with ensuing periods of irritability and threatening behavior. It is noted that when he consumes excess fluids, he exhibits increased psychomotor agitation, pacing, loudness, demandingness, and grandiose and threatening behavior both verbally and physically. Further, he shows no insight into the need for his hospitalization and treatment of his mental illness, or for his personal safety, but rather expresses feelings of being persecuted by legal authorities and by his ex-wife, and demands release on the grounds of his rights as a veteran. When given a psychotropic medication PRN in response to his increasingly threatening, aggressive behavior, he drinks fluids and has periods of exces-

Continued

E CASE EXAMPLE   Continued

sive fluid intake. One episode of fluid intoxication results in an extremely low blood sodium concentration, which is treated in an acute medical facility after he suffers grand mal seizures. When medically re-stabilized, he continues to show limited insight into the harmful effects of fluid intoxication, laughing inappropriately and stating that it produces a "high" for him. He also continues to berate peers, is reluctant to join leisure activities, and occasionally shouts demands, threatens staff members and peers, and refuses interactions unless they occur on his "terms."

Patient's Strengths:
- Is oriented to person, place, and time; has good recall of past events.
- Has a history of a favorable response to psychotropic medications.
- Has attained a general equivalency diploma; has completed 1½ years in the Army in Viet Nam.
- Communicates needs and feelings for short durations (15 to 20 minutes).
- Can minimally perform activities of daily living in an independent manner with verbal prompting and supervision.

DSM-IV Diagnosis: schizophrenia, paranoid type

Nursing diagnosis:
- Disordered water balance related to knowledge deficit about the effects of excessive fluid intake, as evidenced by poor impulse control (assaultive behavior) and fluid-seeking behavior.
- Alteration in thought processes related to inability to trust, as evidenced by delusional thinking, inappropriate social behavior, and inability to demonstrate interpersonal/social skills.
- Risk for infection related to compromised skin integrity caused by frequent, extended periods of exposure to urine, as evidenced by dermatitis.

Nursing interventions:

Acute Crisis Phase:
- Observe patient for increased thirst and fluid seeking behavior or psychotic behaviors.
- Teach patient to report an increase in thirst.
- Counsel patient to reduce fluid intake to prevent low sodium levels.
- Fluid restriction; control access to water, other fluids.
- Give electrolytes as ordered. Notify physician if serum sodium is below 130 mg/dL.
- Weigh patient twice daily. Inform physician if there is a 5% increase in body weight.
- Give hard, sugarless candy to stimulate saliva and prevent dry mouth.
- Give small amount of hyperosmotic beverage (Gatorade) with medications, instead of juice or water.
- May require 1:1 supervision when fluid intake is intensified.
- Reduce access to fluids immediately after patient smokes.
- Provide support to decrease acting-out and blaming when ward environment is restricted.

Continuing treatment phase:
- Monitor patient daily for excess fluid intake.

- Monitor patient for changes in mental status (i.e., headaches, gastrointestinal symptoms, nausea, vomiting, and diarrhea.)
- Monitor changes in medications including psychotropics drugs, lithium, and carbamazepine (Tegretol), which may cause symptoms of dry mouth and increased thirst.
- Monitor weight and electrolytes.
- Teach patient to report increased thirst or fluid consumption to staff.
- Contract with patient to maintain weight or serum sodium within agreed range.
- Patients who have a chronic condition should have highly structured activities that divert behavior such as that in this case.
- Reduce smoking; nicotine stimulates release of antidiuretic hormone (i.e., have patient enroll in smoking cessation program.)

Discharge planning:
- Health education about patient's hyponatremic condition. Nursing group therapy, focusing on the hyponatremia patient (fluid restriction, toileting, vital signs, weight).
- Encourage positive coping mechanisms on a 1:1 basis and in nursing group therapy to maintain controlled behavior and reduce aggressive behavior (verbal and physical).

Outcome:

Following the introduction of clozapine (Clozaril) 100 mg in A.M. and 225 mg at hour of sleep, Henry is more receptive to interventions, socialization, and participation in leisure activities. He agrees to thrice daily monitoring of his weight fluctuations and a daily fluid intake of 2000 to 3000 ml. If there is a 5% deviation in his weight (gain or loss), a physician is notified to evaluate his physical status and a STAT sodium level may be obtained. Further, there may be a change in his level of supervision, fluid intake, and monitoring of his vital signs. He is observed daily and asked to note any sudden changes in his behavior, which he does. There is significant correlation between his irritability, nicotine-seeking behavior, intrusiveness, excessive talkativeness, delusional and persecutory thoughts, psychomotor agitation and pacing, and withdrawn and aloof demeanor with increased fluid intake.

Henry has been able to attend nursing psycho-educational groups that focus on the harmful effects of excessive fluid intake. He has actively participated in identifying events in his life (past/current) that may result in his increased fluid intake. He shares his experiences and recovery strategy with others in a peer-support group. These interventions reinforce a contract to maintain a sodium level above 130 mg/dL, and recognize his efforts to manage his condition with the help of the nursing staff.

Clozaril therapy and nursing interventions have given Henry increased insight into his illness and self management of his fluid-seeking behavior. He can identify and use coping strategies such as keeping his mouth moist with sugarless hard candy or decreasing his level of physical exertion in warm weather. He has been able to join a vocational program that involves maintenance activities, completing his assignments in a thorough, motivated fashion.

signs, any injuries, hydration status, circulatory and respiratory status, and other physical features must be assessed continually. Changes in the patient's condition must be reported to a physician immediately. A primary purpose of the continuous evaluation is to release the patient from restraint and seclusion as soon as the potential for violence has diminished. Focused counseling about the patient's understanding and perception of the behavior that led to restraint and seclusion and questioning about the patient's immediate plans should be conducted. Once the decision to release the patient is made (in consultation with a physician and with assessment data from ancillary staff personnel), the patient should be given an opportunity to talk about the incident of violence and how his or her behavior can be changed. The patient's physical status on release from restraint and seclusion must be assessed.

■ PREVENTING VIOLENCE AND PROMOTING MENTAL HEALTH

Preventing violence and promoting mental health are critical goals in psychiatric mental-health nursing. These goals may be set in an in-patient setting through **milieu therapy.**

Milieu therapy is defined as the prevention, structuring, and maintenance of a therapeutic environment by the psychiatric nurse in collaboration with the patient and other health-care providers (ANA 1994). Hall (1995) refers to the interpersonal contact, structure, and control employed in the milieu, and the need to create a shared environment that preserves consensus and promotes wellness. What is essential to understand is that the milieu is much more than furniture, decorations, and a physical structure that provides (or eliminates) privacy and the opportunity for interpersonal accessibility and socialization. The nurse has the responsibility to promote humane interaction, communication, and structured socialization between the patient and the nursing staff. Safety and security can be established and maintained without relying solely on physical or environmental control and a coercive or directive management style.

Leadership can be defined as guidance or direction of the course of an effort. To successfully promote the creation and maintenance of a therapeutic milieu that prevents violence and provides the opportunity for patients to change their behavior, the nurse must exercise leadership. Articulating clear expectations for personal, peer, and subordinate performance, that are congruent with the hospital or unit philosophy, personally collaborating with other staff personnel, and engaging violent patients clinically are very important.

An essential intervention in milieu therapy is establishing unit rules and clearly defined expectations of patient behavior and responses. The importance of safety and security, and the right of all persons within the milieu to feel safe and not be intimidated or threatened, must be clearly articulated. The expectation that violence or aggression is unacceptable and will not be tolerated, and the ways in which this expectation will be implemented by patients and staff should be described in writing. Expression of strong feelings without resorting to threats, intrusion, aggression, or violence should be encouraged. The rule-development process should include meaningful participation by patients and all levels of staff personnel. Optimally this can take place during regularly occurring unit meetings. Patients and staff entering the milieu for the first time should be oriented to the rules. Regular review and evaluation of the rules by patients and staff can be used for their revision.

Unit rules established at the Middletown Psychiatric Center in New York State identify unacceptable behavior as including: physical violence in any form; verbal threats of physical violence; efforts to intimidate or coerce; unwelcome touching or invasions of personal space; sexual contact; and claims of ownership (e.g., my girlfriend, my chair, my table). The rules set forth security measures for patients and visitors that include methods of searching for contraband; visiting rules; standards for the care of personal belongings; shower schedules; and rules for sleeping and access to sleeping areas, the use of telephones, dining room behavior, television and radio use, smoking, and the use of laundry facilities.

PREVENTING AGGRESSION

Morrison (1990, 1993) presents a conceptual framework for nursing interventions that promotes social interaction within in-patient settings as a means of preventing (not managing or controlling) violence. The model focuses on contingency management, negotiation and conflict resolution, and the development of problem-solving skills. Violence is viewed as a social problem within a context rather than as an individual patient problem resulting from personal characteristics, or as an inevitable component of mental illness. Adverse characteristics of the in-patient environment (confusion, provocation by patients and staff, mistrust, and coercive patient and staff interactions) may promote rather than reduce violence. Staff members' behavior may actually reward or promote violence, such as by withdrawal from patients (perhaps through fear or the environmental structure), leading patients to behave violently in order to receive attention from staff personnel. Staff members may also reinforce the unacceptable expression of anger by not paying attention when anger is expressed appropriately (verbally and without physical intrusion, threats, or threatening gestures).

The philosophical basis for Morrison's model is that nurses and other treatment personnel must examine the context of patients' behavior, including factors that provoke various behaviors, the tactics and goals of patient aggression, and the consequences of such aggression. Contingency management can promote behavioral change by rewarding appropriate behavior and providing negative consequences and the loss of privileges for aggression. Patients wanting to be left alone may use violence to be removed from the environment. When practicing negotiation and teaching conflict resolution, staff members can listen to patients' requests and needs, explore options within the limits of the treatment milieu and patients' own responsibility to try to improve and define compromise solutions to problems for patients and staff members. Negotiation ceases and defined consequences are implemented when threats, intrusion, and violence occur.

PROBLEM SOLVING

When attempting to solve problems with a potentially violent patient, the nurse should focus on how to think, not on what to think. Staff members can teach the steps of the problem-solving process, which are:

- Stop and think: How do you problem solve? What is the problem? What are the different ways in which a particular problem can be solved? How have you been successful or unsuccessful in solving past problems?
- Evaluate the alternatives.
- Choose and implement one or more alternatives.
- Know the resources you will need.
- Plan to implement your chosen solution and implement it.
- Reinforce patients' efforts to learn by paying attention to them.

When the patient refuses to examine problem-solving techniques and resorts to threats or violence, verbal interaction stops. The effects and consequences of such behavior should be clearly defined for the patient. This interventional model can decrease the possibility of overt conflict between patients and staff members, and encourage patients to assume control over their lives. It is important for staff members to avoid participating in a patient's hostile behavior.

Peplau (O'Toole and Welt, 1989) describes the role of the psychiatric mental-health nurse as promoting, maintaining, and restoring patients' health. This interpersonal theory of nursing practice has relevance in the effort to prevent violence and assist changes in patients' behavior. As in the Morrison social-interaction model,

Peplau advocates the use of daily verbal interaction to transform brief, irritating interactions between patients and staff members into experiences that can be clarified, understood, and explored. Recognizing and exploring patients' anxiety and anger without avoidance or denial promotes learning and behavioral change. What impedes this process is the unwarranted use of controlling, coercive intervention (physical intervention, medication, physical restraint, or seclusion), which stifles patients' verbal responses and interaction; it is important to identify what occurs during uncomfortable situations and to establish trust between the patient and the staff. Nurses can avoid participating in dysfunctional interactions, and can utilize counseling, listening skills, and feedback to help patients clarify their thoughts and feelings so as to make more adaptive decisions. The purpose of verbal intervention is to transform the energy generated by an uncomfortable, anxious, or angry situation so as to make it available for exploring the precipitants of the situation, relating them to past experience, and determining what can be done differently.

Scheduled, predictable, and meaningful therapeutic and recreational group programming is an essential part of the effort to prevent violence. Anger management of anger and symptoms, behavior-modification programs, token economy behavior modification programs, communication and social skills training, community meetings, group counseling, and therapy complement the milieu and the interventions that have been described. Integrating group programming into the violence-prevention effort, and making the content of the programming congruent with individual patients' diagnosis (psychiatric and nursing) and sources of illness is important.

Within this interactive interpersonal model of nursing care, it is difficult to determine when a patient lacks the ability to control his or her behavior, especially impulsive and violent behavior that can compromise safety within the milieu. Decisions about when to cease counseling, use verbal interactions, and take other least-restrictive psychiatric nursing measures is a function of the nurse's experience and self-knowledge, the nurse's knowledge of the patient's prior patterns of response, awareness of available resources, and clinical skill.

The importance of an effective, competent staff development program in achieving the goals described above cannot be underestimated. Staff members must be educated about the use of verbal and non-verbal interventions, interpersonal communication techniques, de-escalation techniques, restrictive physical interventions, restraint, and seclusion, and the team approach for responding to violent patients. The training should be competency based, with the opportunity to practice, demonstrate and evaluate skills. The training should be updated regularly with a review of patient outcomes.

■ OUTCOME EVALUATION

Evaluation is a continuous process of appraising the effect of nursing interventions and treatment regimens on patients' health status and expected outcomes (ANA, 1994, p. 34). If it is to promote improvements in practice and individual and institutional outcomes, outcome evaluation with patients and staff must be systematic and ongoing. An effective evaluation process for preventing violence should include:

- Patient outcome evaluation.
- Staff outcome evaluation.
- Staff performance evaluation.
- Review of outcomes with senior clinical staff members.
- Patient-satisfaction surveys.

When exploring patient responses (debriefing), effective interpersonal skills are important in communicating the belief that the patient can understand and recover from his or her violent behavior. The nurse should provide privacy and confidentiality when debriefing the patient. Identifying unacceptable behavior while focusing on patient strengths, capacity, and competence can be difficult. An effective method of accomplishing this is to promote descriptions of violent behavior (after the extreme emotional and physical response has subsided), and to follow this with identification and evaluation of the thoughts and feelings that accompanied the behavior.

Exploration of staff members' intellectual, physical, and emotional response to violence is as important as evaluation of the patients' response. Debriefing of staff members should also occur after episodes of violence, at a time when their emotional responses are still available for review. The focal point should be the emotional response and overall staff response, a discussion of techniques that worked and did not work with the patient and care-team members, and recommendations for improving interventions. Staff members' denial of experiencing emotional reactions ("Its part of the job," "I expected to get hit.") and denying the potential for violence should be explored. Tension, anxiety, fear, hopelessness, and helplessness ("I don't know what we are going to do with this patient," "We tried everything.") are common staff reactions that must be overtly recognized. Staff withdrawal, distancing, and responding to problems by applying more rigid control are problems that must be identified in a supportive manner. This process should not be implemented solely on a supervisory basis, but rather as an effort to promote emotional accessibility among the staff and to provide staff members with support.

Regular review of practice and patient outcomes with senior clinical staff members is recommended as part of an effective outcome evaluation process. Daily staff meetings, including members of the direct-care staff, physicians, and nurses can provide an opportunity for education and clinical supervision in the prevention of violence. A comprehensive evaluation of team responses to patient behavior should take place at scheduled team meetings. Staff members on all shifts must have an opportunity to participate in or provide input into these sessions.

Assessing patient satisfaction (apart from the individual debriefing process, which focuses on violent episodes) through group meetings (community meetings, focus groups) and surveys can complement individual outcome evaluation. The effects of a milieu on its patients, satisfaction with the physical environment, perceptions about the responsiveness of staff to patient needs, and how to improve the environment and staff–patient interactions, should be explored in an open and supportive forum.

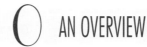

AN OVERVIEW

- Aggressive patient behavior can occur in all practice settings.
- An effective method for talking with aggressive patients is to project a calm, soothing manner.
- Nurses should use the least restrictive method for physically managing violent inpatients.
- Physical restraints are used for safety rather than for therapeutic reasons.

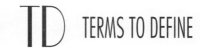

TERMS TO DEFINE

- acute crisis phase
- aggressive behavior
- assessment of dangerousness
- behavioral warning signs (of aggression)
- crisis management (of aggression)
- de-escalation techniques
- mechanical restraint
- milieu therapy

Q STUDY QUESTIONS

1. Which of the following factors may explain the origin and cause of violent/aggressive behavior?
   a. Family system interaction patterns
   b. Socioeconomic situation
   c. Major mental illness
   d. All of the above
   e. A and B only

2. When working with patients, family, and staff, it is important to stress that
   a. violent/aggressive behavior is best managed by strict behavioral controls, rigid unit rules, and medication.
   b. exploring the history of violence within a family is contraindicated.
   c. the nursing staff should not discuss with peers their feelings of fear and anxiety.
   d. violent/aggressive behavior is predetermined by genetic and biological factors.
   e. patients can understand the reasons for their behavior and change their response pattern.

3. When conducting an admission evaluation or an assessment of the patient within the unit for the potential for violent/aggressive behavior, it is important for the nurse to
   a. reassure the patient that everything will be all right, and staff will make sure that nothing untoward happens.
   b. reinforce that the patient is solely responsible for his or her own actions and will suffer the consequences of acting out.
   c. explain that violence is not acceptable and that staff will work with the patient to prevent aggressive behavior.
   d. All of the above
   e. A and B only

4. When interviewing a potentially violent/aggressive patient, which of the following environmental factors is most important?
   a. The interview should take place in a private area with the door closed to reduce external stimulation.
   b. Care should be taken to make sure that other staff do not interrupt.
   c. Restraint devices should be in full view of the patient to reinforce consequences for behavior.
   d. Plans should be made to have staff support immediately available if it is needed.
   e. Soothing music may be used to calm the patient.

5. Which of the following questions would NOT be appropriate to ask a patient while taking a comprehensive history to assess the patient's potential for violence/aggression?
   a. What is the closest you have come to being violent?
   b. Have you ever been arrested?
   c. When were you sexually or physically abused?
   d. Do you worry about being violent?
   e. How have you successfully avoided violence?

6. Which of the following information would be helpful when detailing the characteristics of individual patient violence?
   a. The behavioral warning signs identified by patient
   b. Specific patient behaviors measured using an assessment tool, such as OAS
   c. What patient peers express during a community meeting as the cause of violence in a specific patient
   d. All of the above
   e. A and B only

7. Each staff member should develop an awareness of his or her own response to violence/aggression because
   a. fear or anxiety must not be displayed with peers or patients.
   b. expectations for patient behavior can be more easily identified and clarified.
   c. that awareness will facilitate staff understanding of how their responses may help or hinder work with patients.
   d. B and C only
   e. All of the above

8. Which of the following expected patient-outcome statements is NOT realistic or CANNOT be accomplished?
   a. The patient's anxiety will be eliminated.
   b. The patient will identify precipitants to violence.
   c. The patient will not experience hallucinations.
   d. The patient will describe one alternate behavior he can use when he feels impulsive.
   e. A and C only

9. When responding to patients who display the potential for violence, the most restrictive intervention would be
   a. meeting in a quiet room to reduce stimulation.
   b. counseling to describe specific consequences for specific behavior.
   c. giving PRN medication.
   d. providing physical interventions, such as a two-person escort out of a program area.
   e. using restraints, such as a camisole or four-point restraint.

10. The most important intervention when patients demonstrate that they are not responding to less restrictive interventions and are rapidly escalating toward violence is

   a. cease negotiation with patient and implement plan of intervention to control patient and provide safety.

   b. bargain with patient to determine what can be done to prevent assaultive behavior.

   c. offer PRN medication.

   d. ask patient to move to a less stimulating, private area and spend some time alone.

■ REFERENCES

A Statement on Psychiatric-Mental Health Clinical Nursing Practice and Standards of Psychiatric Mental Health Clinical Nursing Practice. Washington, DC, American Nurses Association, 1994.

American Psychiatric Association, Diagnostic and Statistical Manual of Mental Disorders, Fourth Edition, 1992, Washington, D.C. Authors.

Barnes DM: The origins of violent behavior: what research strategies will emerge? *J NIH Res* 1989; 1:27–30.

Christenfeld R, Wagner J, Pastva G, and Acrish WP: How physical settings affect chronic mental patients. *Psychiatr Q* 1989; 60(3):253–264.

Davis S: Violence by psychiatric inpatient: A review. *Hosp Commun Psychiatry* 1991; 42:585–590.

Hall B: Use of milieu therapy: The context and environment as therapeutic practice for psychiatric-mental health nurses, *in* Anderson C (ed): *Psychiatric Nursing 1946 to 1994:*

A Report on the State of the Art, Columbus, Ohio, Ohio State University Press, 1995, pp. 46–56.

Goldman B, Levy R: Emergency psychiatry, *in* Goldman H. (ed.): *Review of General Psychiatry.* Stamford, CT, Appleton & Lange, 1995.

Lanza, M.L.: How nurses react to patient assault. *J of Psychosocial Nurs,* 1985; 23:6–11.

Littwack TR: Assessments of dangerousness: Legal, research and clinical developments. *Administr Policy Mental Health* 1994; 21:361–377.

Martin K: Improving Staff Safety Through an Aggression Management Program. *Arch Psychiatr Nurs* 1995; 9:211–215.

McFarland G, Wash R: *Nursing Diagnoses and Process in Psychiatric Mental Health Nursing.* Philadelphia, JB Lippincott, 1986.

McNiel D, Binder R: Correlates of accuracy in the assessment of psychiatric inpatients' risk of violence. *Am J Psychiatry* 1995; 152:901–906.

Monahan J: Mental disorder and violent behavior perceptions and evidence. *Am Psychologist* 1992; 47:511–521.

Morrison EF: The tradition of toughness: a study of non-professional nursing care in psychiatric settings. *Image* 1990; 22:32–38.

Morrison EF: Aggression and violence in psychiatric settings. Personal communication.

Morrison E: Toward a better understanding of violence in psychiatric settings: debunking the myths. *Arch Psychiatr Nurs* 1993; 7:328–335.

Morrison E: *Violence and the Mentally Ill: Theories, Treatment Approaches and Policy Recommendations.* Washington, DC, American Nurses Association. (in press).

O'Toole A, Rouslin Welt S: *Interpersonal Theory in Nursing Practice: Selected Works of Hildegard E. Peplau.* New York, Springer, 1989.

7

Level 7

Cataclysmic Crises

A cataclysmic crisis may be an interpersonal or external event.

An interpersonal event involves a Level 3 traumatic crisis and a Level 4, 5, or 6 crisis. It can occur in the aftermath of multiple traumatic crises, such as losing several family members in an airplane crash, or consist of a traumatic crisis and unresolved cumulative crises, such as following a diagnosis of HIV infection.

As an external event, a cataclysmic crisis may be a war; a natural disaster such as an earthquake or storm; or a technological disaster, such as uncontrolled seepage of radiation from an industrial site. These events are sudden and potent, and are likely to affect large numbers of people. Intervention is specific to the type of event. In interpersonal cataclysmic crises, supportive counseling and grief counseling are indicated. In external crises, community disaster teams are mobilized.

A condition representive of a Cataclysmic Crisis is discussed in the following chapter:

- *HIV Positive Persons and Their Families*

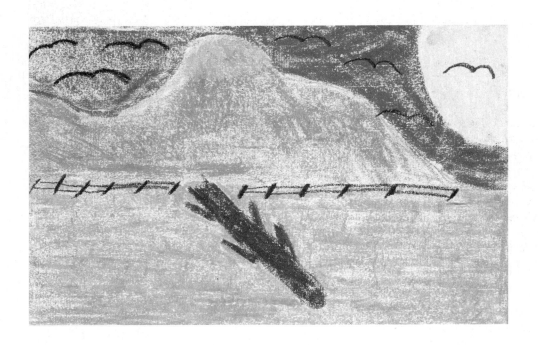

"*Patients in the initial crisis stage of AIDS typically have difficulty retaining information and may distort what they are told regarding their illness. Contact with support services such as crisis counseling. . . . and psychotherapy should begin as early as possible.*"

—John G. Bruhn, PhD
Vice President for Academic Affairs and Research
University of Texas at El Paso
(in *HIV Manual for Health Care Professionals*, Muma et al.)

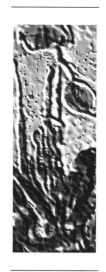

34

HIV Positive Persons and Their Families

Theresa M. Croushore

Caring for psychiatric patients with human immunodeficiency virus (HIV) infection or acquired immune deficiency syndrome (AIDS) demands knowledge, compassion, dedication, and tolerance, and can be emotionally exhausting. Nurses must be able to accept the limitations of what they can do for such patients and their families, while helping patients and families to accept and deal with the physical and emotional demands of these diseases.

The single most important component of nursing care for HIV-infected patients is optimism. Maintaining hope that not everyone infected with HIV will die and that new and promising therapies are being pursued helps nurses communicate optimism to the patients for whom they care. Coupled with respect for and acceptance of the patient, hope can help in restoring and maintaining a patient's self-esteem, often eroded by years of stigma and disapproval.

Nurses confront many legal, moral, and ethical issues in the course of assessing, planning, and implementing care for HIV-positive or AIDS patients. They feel the impact of obstacles and conflicts in the health care and social systems that undermine successful outcomes when dealing with the many physical and psychosocial needs of these patients.

In this work, nurses struggle with such topics as sex and sexuality, drugs and drug use, AIDS prevention and education, the right to privacy, the right to know, multiple losses, and issues of death and dying. After confronting these difficult subjects, however, the nurse emerges not only enlightened but also challenged to provide unconditional acceptance to every patient. Caring for the HIV-infected psychiatric patient truly encompasses every dimension of nursing.

■ HIV DISEASE

According to the Surgeon General of the United States, AIDS constitutes the greatest health threat of the 20th century. The World Health Organization (WHO) estimates that 18-million adults and 1.5-million children worldwide have been infected with HIV, which causes AIDS. More than 85% of adults infected with HIV live outside the Western industrialized world; more than 75% of cases of HIV infection in adults have been transmitted through heterosexual intercourse, and more than 45% of HIV-infected individuals are women. These WHO estimates herald future trends of HIV disease in the United States.

As of October 1995, only 4.5 million (or about 23%) of persons infected with HIV worldwide had been reported as progressing to AIDS. Just over 500,000 of these people are in the United States (Table 34–1); nearly half have been reported as having AIDS since 1993 (MMWR, 1995). Clearly, even if transmission of HIV were stopped, the number of persons manifesting signs of HIV infection and progression to AIDS would continue to grow.

In 1993, the Centers for Disease Control and Prevention amended the definition of AIDS to include the following:

- Persons with less than 200 T helper cells
- HIV positive persons with any form of tuberculosis
- Persons with recurrent bacterial pneumonia
- Infected women who develop cancer of the cervix.

This expanded definition does not change current understanding of the course of the infection or disease, but it does help to explain both the recent increase in reported cases of AIDS in women and the explosion of reported cases of AIDS in the United States.

The continuum of **HIV disease**—the term used to describe all diseases resulting from infection with the human immunodeficiency virus—is divided into three stages. Each stage is associated with distinct physical changes; there are also common psychosocial issues for the patient, the patient's significant others, and caregivers, whether they are health-care professionals, family members, or friends.

EXPOSURE

The first stage of HIV disease is acute infection, generally lasting from 6 to 12 months. It begins with **exposure** to HIV-infected body fluids through high-risk sex, perinatal transmission or the use of contaminated hypodermic needles or transfusion equipment. Each type of exposure entails a different risk and leads to a different course of disease; for example, recipients of contaminated transfusions almost always become infected (Lang, 1993), but their course of disease is typically longer than that of persons infected in other ways (DiMarzo, 1993). In contrast, only about 30 to 50% of infants born to HIV-infected mothers become infected (Lang, 1993), but those that are infected rarely survive for more than 5 years.

Infection occurs when HIV successfully enters the body and incorporates itself into deoxyribonucleic acid—the genetic material in the hosts cells. Sometimes the infection is accompanied by an influenza-like illness with fever, muscle aches, a rash, swollen lymph nodes, sore throat, and headache occurring within a few weeks

Rebecca Leibowitz, RN, BSN, assisted in the development of the case studies and case examples presented in this chapter.

TABLE 34–1 NUMBER AND PERCENTAGE OF PERSONS WITH AIDS, UNITED STATES, 1981–OCT. 1995

	Cumulative	
Characteristic	No.	(%)
Sex		
Male	428,480	(85.8)
Female	72,828	(14.5)
Age group (years)		
0–4	5,432	(1.1)
5–12	1,385	(0.3)
13–19	2,300	(0.5)
20–29	91,054	(18.2)
30–39	227,754	(45.4)
40–49	122,569	(24.4)
50–59	36,640	(7.3)
>60	14,176	(2.8)
Race/Ethnicity		
White, non-Hispanic	238,171	(47.5)
Black, non-Hispanic	170,271	(34.0)
Hispanic	87,387	(17.4)
Asian/Pacific Islander	3,457	(0.7)
American Indian/		
Alaskan Native	1,283	(0.3)
HIV-exposure category		
Men who have sex with men	254,437	(50.8)
Injecting-drug use	125,440	(25.0)
Men who have sex with men		
and inject drugs	32,429	(6.5)
Hemophilia	4,258	(0.8)
Heterosexual contact	38,541	(7.7)
Transfusion recipients	7,700	(1.6)
Perinatal transmission	6,124	(1.2)
No risk reported	32,381	(6.4)
Region		
Northeast	156,595	(31.2)
Midwest	49,036	(9.8)
South	165,348	(33.0)
West	113,954	(22.7)
U.S. territories	15,971	(3.2)
Vital status		
Living	189,929	(37.9)
Deceased	311,381	(62.1)
Total	501,310	(100.0)

Adapted from Morbidity and Mortality Weekly Reports (MMWR), Center for Disease Control, Atlanta, Ga, Nov. 24, 1995.

after exposure. The virus multiplies rapidly and spreads throughout the body, crossing the blood-brain and placental barriers. The host's immune system develops antibodies, but they are not effective against the virus for more than a few months. The immune system gradually weakens and the number of T-helper lymphocytes (the major target cells of HIV, which are highly important to the body in combating infection), falls below its normal range of 800 to 1,200 per cubic millimeter, to 650 cells/pmm^3. At this point the decline in immunologic capacity becomes less rapid, indicating some successful functioning of the body's immune system. One physical manifestation of this immune response is widely scattered swelling of the lymph nodes, persisting for long periods and marking the end of the first stage of HIV disease. Often, however, no physical symptoms are evident; awareness of infection follows a positive antibody test or occurs even later in the course of HIV disease, when associated serious illnesses occur.

LATENT INFECTION

In the second stage of HIV disease, known as **latent infection,** most infected individuals feel well and have few indications of infection. The most common physical complaints during this stage of the disease are swollen lymph nodes and fatigue. Antibodies to HIV are still present, and the number of T-helper lymphocytes continues to slowly but progressively decline. This stage of HIV infection usually lasts from 3 to 5 years, although it has in many cases lasted for 10 years or longer. For reasons not clearly understood, this stage of HIV infection is accompanied by greater psychological distress than any other stage.

CLINICAL DISEASE

The third, **clinical disease** stage of HIV infection occurs when the number of T-helper lymphocytes falls below 200/mm^3 and the immune system can no longer fight off certain diseases. "Opportunistic infections," such as caused by *Pneumocystis carinii* pneumonia (PCP) or certain cancers (e.g., Kaposi's sarcoma), have come to be associated with this stage of HIV infection; however, a host of other illnesses can occur during this third stage. Some (including oily skin rashes) directly affect a patient's body image and self esteem, while others sap the patient's energy and compromise supportive interactions with others. Neuropsychiatric complications of HIV infection are sometimes misdiagnosed as mental illnesses and, as a result, are mistreated.

During the third stage of HIV infection illnesses may develop and resolve over periods of months to several years. Approximately 80% of persons infected for more than 10 years progress to this stage of the infection, and once it has begun, death typically occurs within 18 to 36 months. Researchers believe that anyone infected with HIV will progress to the clinical disease stage of the infection and succumb to an associated illness. The unfavorable natural history of HIV disease presents many challenges in caring for those it affects.

■ IDENTIFICATION OF PATIENTS AT RISK

Psychiatric nurses are in a key position to identify patients with risk factors associated with HIV infection, particularly factors related to a patient's mental illness, as well as to identify patients already infected with the virus. In the mental-health setting, this requires knowledge of the signs and symptoms of HIV infection, **AIDS-related complex (ARC),** and AIDS (see Figure 34–1). The nurse must also be able to complete a physical assessment and mental-status examination, including the taking of a sexual history of the patient and assessment for drug use. Nurses are called on to collect data that can specifically identify patients exhibiting psychosocial distress related to HIV, those whose HIV status has ex-

acerbated a pre-existing psychiatric diagnosis, and those whose symptoms are a direct result of HIV infection. This can become extremely difficult, since the patient can easily fall into all three categories. Therefore, every psychiatric patient must be assessed for the risk factors associated with HIV infection, as well as for the signs and symptoms of the infection itself.

Risk factors for exposure to HIV include homosexuality, (men who have sex with men), intravenous drug use, hemophilia, heterosexual contact with an infected partner, transfusion, and perinatal transmission. Rape victims and children who have been sexually abused are at risk. Adult survivors of childhood sexual abuse are often repeatedly victimized and/or engage in sexually promiscuous, impulsive, and dangerous behaviors as sequelae of their abuse. Their risk of contracting HIV infection is high (Brady and Carmen, 1990).

A 5-year study of psychiatric patients infected with HIV found that one-third had a psychiatric history before becoming HIV infected, one-half had a history of

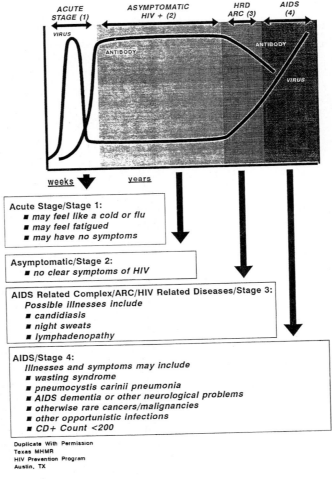

Figure 34–1. Signs and Symptoms of HIV Infections, ARC, and AIDS

drug and/or alcohol abuse; and one-fourth had a family history of psychiatric illness or problems with drugs and/or alcohol (Wiener et al., 1994). Clearly, psychiatric patients are at increased risk for becoming HIV positive.

The chronically mentally ill are a neglected high-risk population for HIV infection. Although the stereotype of the mentally ill population as being asexual is pervasive, patients with severe psychiatric disorders may be more likely than the general public to engage in HIV-related risk behaviors (Brady and Carmen, 1990). The majority of such patients are sexually active and engage in unprotected sex with multiple partners, often meeting these partners in psychiatric clinics. One-third have sexually transmitted infections, and many exchange sex for money or drugs (Kalichman et al., 1994). Poor judgment, hypersexuality, and impulsivity are associated with many chronic psychiatric illnesses (Brady and Carmen, 1990).

The incidence of homosexuality or bisexuality has been reported to be 51% among patients with borderline personality disorders and 14% among patients with mania. Another group at high risk for exposure to HIV are patients with personality disorders, who commonly engage in impulsive and self destructive behaviors and characteristically have transient and unstable relationships (Perkins, 1993). They meet more sex partners in psychiatric outpatient clinics or bars than patients with other psychiatric diagnoses, and are more likely to be forced to have sex.

A large number of patients with affective disorders are intravenous drug users. Kalichman and associates (1994) report that psychiatric patients with dual diagnoses often have inaccurate information about HIV transmission and may be unaware of the degree to which their behavior puts them at risk for HIV infection.

■ ASSESSMENT OF THE PATIENT WITH HIV DISEASE

Although a full review of physical assessment is beyond the scope of this chapter, the nurse must observe the general physical condition of the patient when conducting a mental-status examination. A nurse who takes time to establish a trusting rapport with a psychiatric patient is much more apt to elicit meaningful information than one who proceeds immediately to questions, expecting honest answers. The psychiatric patient, especially one who practices risky behaviors, is already conditioned to expect judgmental, non-accepting attitudes from others (Kalichman et al., 1994).

The patient's history should include sexual preference and drug and alcohol use (see Chapter 31, Substance Abuse, for discussion of drug and alcohol assessment). The nurse should also focus on behaviors and the patient's mental status. Because HIV disease presents the patient and family with many stressors, the interview must also include an evaluation of the patient's adjustment and coping skills, the patient's personal way of dealing with the disease, and psychosocial and environmental problems.

Assessment of the patient's capacity for judgment includes the patient's ability to organize thoughts and make decisions: Are the patient's decisions logical? Can the patient describe his or her thinking in coming to a decision? To determine whether the patient's thinking is organized, the nurse should listen for tangential conversation, illogical conclusions, or obviously scattered thinking. The patient with difficulties in thought organization due to HIV infection may be able to draw but not write clearly.

Orientation and memory may fluctuate in the patient with HIV disease, but can usually be regained with

E CASE EXAMPLE

Jessie is a 24-year-old woman admitted to a psychiatric unit with a diagnosis of major depression. She complains of fatigue, headaches, blurred vision, increased sleep, and weight loss. She has recently stopped attending her college classes, stating that she was unable to keep up with the work. Prior to her admission she refused outpatient care and retreated to her apartment. During the course of her admission interview she admits to having had multiple sexual partners and is afraid that she may be pregnant. Her expectation of her admission is to identify why she is unable to keep a boyfriend; she believes that she will then be less depressed.

During the course of her treatment, it is revealed that Jessie was sexually abused by her uncle while she was a teenager. Although her depression is easing, she continues to be tired and to complain of headaches and other neurological symptoms. When it was learned that the uncle was HIV positive, Jessie was tested and determined to be HIV positive also.

visual or verbal prompting. Patients may be easily distracted and lose track of what they were doing or saying.

The affect, or emotional expression, of patients with HIV infection may be blank or apathetic; however, it is important not to conclude too quickly that the patient is depressed. Early neurological signs of HIV infection can be confused with typical signs and symptoms of depression. In the absence of other vegetative or dysphoric signs of depression, the HIV patient's blank, uninterested look may have an organic basis.

At the other extreme of emotion, the HIV patient with an organic mental syndrome may be very labile, displaying the range of emotions characteristic of mania. It is necessary to clarify with patients and/or their friends whether this emotional response is typical for the patient or is of recent onset.

The most common defining characteristic of the organically impaired patient with HIV disease is cognitive slowing, which may be apparent in conversation or may manifest itself as easy distractibility. The patient may be able to count backward from 100 by 7s, but will need time to do so. By proceeding too quickly in an assessment, the nurse may falsely conclude that the patient is cognitively impaired.

Similar slowing can be observed in HIV-infected patients' motor skills, such as picking up a cup or climbing stairs. The patient seems to have to think in order to perform these automatic movements. Many HIV-infected patients describe themselves as feeling "stoned," though they have no history of recent drug use (Singer, 1990).

A sexual history should be taken to determine the patient's risk for contracting HIV infection, knowledge of AIDS, and awareness of risk-related personal behaviors (see Figure 34–2). These data must be incorporated into the patient's treatment plan so that all members of the treatment team can actively work to reduce any risk-related behaviors.

Many HIV-infected patients may resist answering "personal" questions, but usually cooperate when offered a simple, straightforward reason for such questions. Nurses must make sure that their questions are understood by asking the patient if he or she understands and that their verbal and nonverbal communication is non-judgmental. Remember that the purpose of information gathering is not to make a judgement but to make a nursing diagnosis. Does the patient have the potential for self injury or injury to others in relation to risky sexual behavior? Does the patient lack knowledge of the means of transmission of HIV?

The process of gathering information and assessing risk is itself an opportunity for educating the patient. When a patient comments that he and his male lover do not use condoms because both are seropositive, the nurse can point out that HIV mutates quickly and that the partners may be cross-infecting each other, increasing the likelihood of disease progression.

■ PSYCHOSOCIAL IMPACT OF HIV INFECTION

The psychosocial impact of HIV infection begins long before the affected individual learns that he or she has a positive HIV antibody test or experiences symptoms of HIV infection. It begins as soon as the individual begins to consider how the AIDS epidemic affects him or her.

Recent research has found that different groups of infected individuals show a similar degree of psychological distress both before and after learning of positive results of HIV testing. Moreover, similar frequency of psychological distress among persons who are told of HIV-negative results and those who are told of HIV-positive results has led many persons to conclude that this distress stems from factors other than knowledge of HIV infection status (Perry, et al., 1993). Thirty percent of the subjects studied by Perry and colleagues (1993) were found to have suicidal thoughts both before and after testing, despite the results.

Daniolos and Holmes (1995) report that the emotional and behavioral responses to news of HIV infection are not necessarily like those seen with reports of other chronic or infectious illnesses. When informed that an HIV antibody test is positive, patients sometimes appear to be relieved, perhaps because their situation is clarified. When patients confront a certain and perhaps even imminent death, other issues and problems, which had previously seemed intolerable, lose much of their urgency. It is important to assess how each patient and the patient's family and friends react to the diagnosis and progression of HIV disease. The generalization that only positive test results for HIV produce intense adverse emotional consequences can lead to further stigmatization, implying that HIV-positive adults are distraught, depressed, and dysfunctional. The patient may respond to such cues with increased hopelessness, helplessness, and depression.

Knowledge of HIV seropositivity often results in some behavioral risk reduction among homosexual men; conversely, a negative test for anti-HIV antibodies can lead to an increase in high-risk activity, which is probably caused by feelings of invulnerability (Daniolos and Holmes, 1995). A patient who tests positively for HIV may also experience a post-traumatic stress disorder–like reaction, including severe anxiety, intrusive ruminative thoughts about failing health and death, and hypervigilance for signs of physical deterioration, as well as insomnia, depression, and guilt. HIV-infected women may especially feel isolated and try to cope alone because of the general lack of social support

Name: _____   Date: _____

Sexually active with others?   Yes ( )   No ( )
Last sexual contact within the
Last week ( )   Last month ( )   Last 6 months ( )   Last year ( )
1+ year ( )
Frequency of sexual contact _____
Number of partners?
   One partner   ( )   How long same? _____
   Multiple   ( )   How many? _____
Kind of partners?
   Same sex ( )   Other sex ( )   Both ( )   Mostly which? _____
   Known to you?   Always ( )   Sometimes ( )   Never ( )
   Bisexual partners ( )   IVDU partners ( )

Use of IV drugs?   No ( )   Yes ( )   Frequency/type _____
If yes, needle sharing?   No ( )   Yes ( )   Frequency _____
Extent of alcohol, other drugs?   Specify _____
_____

Females: LMP _____   G _____   P _____   Ab _____
Physical abuse in childhood/adulthood/at present/never (circle all that apply).
Sexual abuse in childhood/adulthood/at present/never (circle all that apply).

Currently homeless?   No ( )   Yes ( )

Condom use?   Always ( )   Mostly ( )   Sometimes ( )   Never ( )
Other contraceptives?   Specify which _____

History of sexually transmitted diseases?   Yes ( )   No ( )
   GC/syphilis ( ) Treatment _____
   herpes ( ) Treatment _____
   other ( ) Specify/Tx _____
ARC/AIDS ( ) Treatment _____

Ever tested for HIV antibodies/"AIDS test"?
   Yes ( )   No ( )   Results _____   Year _____
Worried about HIV/AIDS infection? Yes ( )   No ( )   If yes, why? _____
_____
_____

Knowledge about AIDS (check which)
   What it is ( )   Transmission ( )   Prevention ( )   None ( )
HIV teaching: Sex ed ( )   Contraception ( )
Transmission/prevention ( )   Condom distribution ( )   HIV ( )
Referral _____

Clinician _____

(Brady and Carmen, 1990)

Figure 34–2. Sexual history/HIV risk assessment

for women who have the infection (Daniolos and Holmes, 1995).

The loss of physical and cognitive abilities, friends, and even certain freedoms contributes to the demoralization and grieving that is common in the HIV-infected population. These and other issues can be identified in a patient's life story, in which patient writes or tells of the meaning of disease to him- or herself. This effective therapeutic tool not only helps in the continuing assessment of the patient's psychological status, but also offers an opportunity to review the patient's life and identify "unfinished business." The nurse can help the patient begin to deal with these issues by listening, offering support and encouragement, and teaching. The patient's life story can be updated whenever the patient is readmitted or attends out-patient support groups.

■ NEUROPSYCHIATRIC COMPLICATIONS OF HIV DISEASE

It is estimated that 30 to 40% of patients with AIDS have neuropsychiatric manifestations of this disease. These manifestations range from myelopathy and peripheral neuropathy to **AIDS dementia complex.** Patients with a history of aseptic meningitis as the initial response to HIV infection are at high risk of developing AIDS dementia complex (Bartlett et al., 1993).

AIDS dementia complex is caused by direct HIV infection of the brain's glial cells, targeting deep structures such as the thalamus, basal ganglia, and white matter. The complex is often the first clear sign of AIDS, preceding systemic involvement in more than 10 to 20% of patients (Scherer, 1990). Bornstein and associates (1992) reported a 65 to 70% prevalence of AIDS dementia complex in patients with AIDS related complex or AIDS.

AIDS dementia complex is a subcortical dementia that primarily affects mood and motor activity. A typical early presentation includes cognitive, motor, and behavioral symptoms. Cognitively, there may be mental slowing (slowing of thought, reduced verbal ability, loss of spontaneity), memory loss, a poor concentration and attention span, forgetfulness, confusion about time and place, and visual–spatial disorientation. Motor symptoms include an unsteady gait, leg weakness, tremor, spasticity, hyperreflexia, and loss of coordination. Among the behavioral symptoms of AIDS dementia complex are apathy, withdrawal, agitated psychosis (occasionally mania), social isolation, and changes in personality characterized by irritability (Price, 1995; Singer, 1990).

The patient with AIDS dementia complex may experience organic denial, a condition in which there is unawareness of cognitive deficits (Bocceleri and Zeifert, 1994), and may, for example, insist on driving a car when unable to do so. The patient with organic denial cannot accept realistic limitations, thus requiring the nurse to calmly assert authority and redirect the patient to unit areas (or topics) of less stimulation. This is frequently helpful in helping the patient to regain equilibrium.

The phenomenon of **organic denial,** coupled with the sudden and intense mood changes and irritability typical of AIDS dementia complex, may make it difficult to care for the patient with this condition. Support systems may diminish as the patient's inconsistent interactions and prolonged withdrawal drive friends and family away.

Because AIDS dementia complex shows considerable variability in presentation, its symptoms can be confused with those of depression, anxiety, or psychotic disorders. Depression does not appear to account for the neuropsychological deficits observed in many HIV-infected patients (Bornstein et al., 1992); however, increased frequencies of suicide and fire setting have been reported among patients with AIDS dementia complex, including those not considered to be depressed (Alfonso and Cohen, 1994).

Opportunistic infections of the central nervous system (CNS) can easily be mistaken for AIDS dementia complex. Lumbar puncture is important to exclude opportunistic infection in patients suspected of having the complex. It is also important to rule out metabolic derangement caused by hypoxia or sepsis.

As dementia progresses, new learning and memory deteriorate, further slowing of mental processes occurs, and language impairment becomes more obvious. Because the patient becomes unable to adapt to changes, the environment must be adapted to the patient's needs for safety, orientation, and consistency (Bocceleri and Zeifert, 1994). Eventually, the patient becomes unable to walk without assistance. Slowing and clumsiness of the arms also develop. The terminal phase of AIDS dementia complex is characterized by global impairment with severe psychomotor retardation and mutism (Price, 1995).

Disability brought on by neuropsychiatric and neurological pathology compounds the psychosocial problems of patients with AIDS dementia complex and their families at a time of physical, emotional, and social crisis. Eventually, friends and family may be asked to make important decisions. Early discussions of the patient's preferences with regard to experimental treatment protocols, care options, the use of heroic measures, and estate planning make these decisions less stressful. It is recommended that the patient get legal advice before AIDS dementia complex progresses; many local AIDS organizations help arrange for free legal services for patients (Scherer, 1990).

■ HIV-ASSOCIATED PSYCHOSIS

Psychosis is an uncommon but serious complication of infection with HIV. The presence of psychotic symptoms in patients with AIDS contributes to difficulties in providing these patients with medical care, arranging aftercare, and finding placement for them. The etiology of such psychosis remains undetermined, but the psychosis may be related to substance abuse, adverse reactions to antiretroviral drug therapy such as with azidothymidine (AZT), neoplasms of the central nervous system, premorbid psychiatric conditions, or the HIV infection itself (HIV encephalopathy). Acute psychotic episodes can also result from drug interactions, such as between isoniazid given for antimycobacterial therapy and disulfiram for treating alcoholism.

Patients at greatest risk for HIV-associated psychosis have a higher lifetime prevalence of stimulant and sedative/hypnotic abuse or dependence than do others; they also tend to have more global neurological impairment as a result of HIV infection and a higher mortality rate than other HIV-infected patients (Sewell et al., 1994). Often, the psychosis appears very early in the disease, even in the absence of other signs of AIDS. Therefore, any adult with a first presentation of psychosis should be carefully evaluated for the presence of HIV. The same advice holds for patients with depression of new onset.

■ AIDS ANXIETY SYNDROME

It is reasonable to assume that anyone dealing with HIV infection experiences significant anxiety. This includes not only persons infected or fearful of infection, but also family members, friends, and care-givers. However, the term **AIDS anxiety syndrome** applies only to those whose coping is ineffective, leading to a range of destructive and debilitating symptoms.

Persons needing help with AIDS-associated anxiety report symptoms ranging from panic attacks and morbid obsessions to persistent hypochondria and self-absorption. Their symptoms are disruptive to normal routines, including work, school, and social activities. They usually exhibit one extreme or the other of withdrawal from the outside world or morbid interest in any report about AIDS. Extremely anxious patients have been known to convince themselves and others that they have AIDS. Interestingly, the most severe anxiety symptoms in infected persons occur early in the course of the illness (Tartaglia, 1993).

A factor that appears to be significant in extreme AIDS-associated anxiety in many homosexual men is the strong tendency to identify themselves primarily in terms of their sexual orientation. This phenomenon also occurs, although to a lesser extent, in substance abusers. This emphasis on sexual orientation or substance abuse serves as a constant, relentless reminder of life-threatening risk. Any guilt or ambivalence about sexual orientation compounds the anxiety and produces persistent and serious loss of self-esteem. Social withdrawal typically follows; men with these problems move away from their families of origin and known support systems. A cycle of depression, obsession, hypochondria, frustration, and anger consumes the patient. HIV-negative adults who engage in high-risk behaviors face the possibility of future changes in their status and are often dealing with bereavement and the continuous challenge of modifying behaviors associated with HIV risk (Perry et al., 1993). These challenges add to the patient's stress and anxiety.

Approaches to caring for the patient with AIDS-associated anxiety are aimed at restoring self-esteem and identifying multiple aspects of the patient's personality. Helping the patient to understand that the origin of his or her anxiety involves more than dealing with the threat of AIDS.

It is important to show the patient acceptance without endorsement of his or her behavior. For example, some nurses attempt to assure the male homosexual patient that his sexual orientation is "normal and healthy" for him; in doing so, they may shut out unexpressed feelings of ambivalence, guilt, or other negative emotion on the part of the patient. Instead, showing neutrality and acceptance without judgment is crucial to building trusting therapeutic relationships in the face of controversial subjects (Tartaglia, 1993).

■ DEPRESSION

Many studies indicate a higher incidence of depression in HIV-infected patients than in other comparably ill patients following the diagnosis of illness. Manifestations of this depression can range from mild, transient symptoms to mood disturbances or organic mood disorder. The diagnosis can be difficult because the HIV-infected patient may have physical signs such as anorexia, fatigue, and weight loss. It is important to consider the cause of symptoms: toxoplasmosis of the central nervous system, for example, may be reversible, whereas a neurodegenerative process such as AIDS dementia complex is not.

About one-third of both asymptomatic HIV-infected and uninfected homosexual men have a lifetime history of major depression, suggesting that a significant proportion of HIV-infected homosexual men may be at high risk for major depression (Perkins et al., 1994). In theory, HIV may directly or indirectly cause an organic mood disorder in some infected individuals. A depressed mood may be a symptom of HIV-related impairment of the central nervous system.

Many health-care professionals have proposed that HIV-infected individuals are at high risk for attempted or completed suicide, while many others dispute these assertions. It is documented that substance abuse correlates positively with both suicide risk and HIV infection, and HIV substance-abusing patients are much more likely to be admitted to psychiatric facilities for suicidal thoughts and suicide attempts (Wiener et al., 1994). Heterosexual sex partnerships with intravenous drug users are also linked with suicidality (O'Dowd et al., 1993).

Some authors have suggested that AIDS-related complex, with its accompanying sense of impending doom in an uncertain time frame, may be psychologically the most difficult stage for infected patients. Perhaps suicidality and overall distress diminish in AIDS patients because of the greater certainty about the future progression of their disease, their having had more time to accept their fate, or their progressing organicity and accompanying denial (O'Dowd et al., 1993).

In order to increase recognition of the potentially depressed or suicidal patient, it is necessary to identify the subset of AIDS and HIV-infected patients who are substance abusers or substance dependent. HIV-infected substance abusers may be less prone to seek the benefits of rehabilitation when pessimism about HIV infection dominates their thoughts. Addressing this pessimistic outlook is an important step toward providing the rationale for referral to alcohol- and drug-rehabilitation services (Wiener et al., 1994).

Among the benefits of hospitalization in the treatment of depression is empathy on the part of the inpatient staff. Baer and colleagues (1993) noted that patients with AIDS and AIDS-related complex can experience marked changes in hope and hopelessness over brief periods. An empathetic attitude is recommended; an attitude that is "too understanding" might suggest that depression is an inevitable consequence of HIV rather than a treatable disease (Beckett and Rutan, 1990).

■ PERSONALITY DISORDERS

Personality disorders occur when personality traits are "inflexible, maladaptive, and cause either significant functional impairment or subjective distress." Thirty-three percent of HIV-infected individuals were diagnosed with personality disorder in studies done by Perkins and associates (1993). This compares with 5 to 15% in the general population.

Personality disorder is common in the HIV-positive population. Impulsiveness, overdramatization, poor recognition of future consequences of current behavior, and inability to tolerate discomfort or delay all contribute to the risk of HIV infection.

Compared with other HIV-infected patients, those with a personality disorder may experience greater dysphoria and be more likely to cope with AIDS in a dysfunctional way. In Perkins and associates' study, individuals with personality disorder showed significantly greater use of denial and **helpless coping** styles than other HIV-infected patients. Denial is exemplified by the following beliefs: "I refuse to believe it has happened; I pretend it hasn't really happened." People who use helpless coping styles endorse such statements as "I feel that there is nothing I can do to help myself; I am unable to handle the stress of AIDS" (Perkins et al., 1993).

These coping strategies may hinder patients from accepting and dealing with their HIV infection. Alternatively, the greater dysphoria experienced by individuals with personality disorders may affect their coping ability. Denial and helpless coping may potentially affect the relationship between the patient and the medical-care provider and, ultimately, compliance with treatment.

Patients with personality disorder report significantly more social conflict than those without the disorder. There is no difference between these patients and others in the number of their social supports or the satisfaction with these supports. To work successfully with the HIV-infected patient with personality disorder, the entire treatment team needs to be involved so as to prevent splitting, to identify target symptoms and behaviors, and to set firm limits with fixed consequences that are collectively planned in advance.

■ MEDICATING THE HIV-INFECTED PATIENT

The nurse must be aware of some special circumstances when medicating the patient with HIV infection. Knowledge of the way in which a particular psychotropic medication works and affects the body of the HIV-infected patient is imperative to assure accurate assessment of new or concurrent manifestations of HIV and to prevent serious side effects of medication. In addition, the side effects of antiviral medications and other agents commonly used to treat HIV-associated infections can mimic or exaggerate psychiatric symptoms or syndromes. Many drugs affect the nervous system, and their effects can be mistaken for HIV-related conditions. A thorough record of the patient's medication use and drug history is necessary and should include over-the-counter drugs, nutritional supplements, and animal and plant extracts.

Unlike depressed patients with cancer or chronic renal failure, HIV-infected patients have a high rate of response to psychotropic medications. However, the dosage must coincide with the patient's potential reaction to the medication. For example, tricyclic antidepressants are usually begun at lower doses than usual (only 10 to 25 mg at bed-time) and are gradually increased by 10 to 25 mg every 2 days, because of patients' extreme sensitivity to anticholinergic affects. The adage "start low and go slow" is important when medicating HIV-infected patients. Cognitive difficulties are aggravated, and in some cases antidepressant drugs can precipitate delirium in HIV-infected patients. In addition, anticholinergic agents can cause excessive drying of the mucous membranes, which can contribute to the development of candidiasis.

Lithium is usually avoided except to augment other psychotropic medications, because it is generally too toxic at the levels needed to be effective. Carbamazepine and valproic acid are avoided because they pose a significant risk of myelosuppression in immunocompromised patients already taking agents such as AZT.

The risk of seizures in the neurologically compromised HIV-infected patient is increased with psychotropic medications that lower the seizure threshold. Additionally, the HIV-infected patient is extremely susceptible to developing neuroleptic malignant syndrome. Frequent measurements of creatinine phosphokinase should be made until the patient is stabilized on a neuroleptic medication.

As previously noted, many HIV-infected patients receive antiviral therapy. The use of zidovudine (AZT) has been associated with acute mania as well as major depression. Patients receiving AZT should be monitored closely for major mood changes. If such changes occur, and other neurological causes for them are not identified, it is probable that the AZT is their cause. Both mania and depressive symptoms linked to AZT respond well to lithium and other psychotropic agents, even when AZT is continued.

Sedative, hypnotic, and antidepressant drugs, as well as many other groups of medications, enter the central nervous system and have the potential to cause neurological symptoms. AZT can cause headaches, depression, malaise, and somnolence—symptoms that can be confused with early AIDS depression complex or encephalitis. Amphotericin B, vincristine (Oncovin), and pyrimethamine can cause seizures, as can some opportunistic infections and lymphoma. Systemic fluocytosine can cause confusion, hallucinations, and drowsiness, and ganciclovir produces headaches, disorientation, and hallucinations—which are also symptoms of encephalitis (Scherer, 1990). Drug combinations can cause effects that may not be seen when each drug is used alone. Zidovudine plus lorazepam (Ativan) may slow mental and physical responses, producing an effect that resembles Parkinson's disease.

The psychiatric nurse can help the HIV-infected patient avoid the use of medications that may lead to tolerance and abuse, such as benzodiazepines. Use of tranquilizing medications can not only be harmful but also may prevent the patient from dealing with long-term distress. Teaching relaxation techniques and imaging, rather than reliance on medication, is prudent. The most common method of attempted suicide in HIV-infected patients is drug overdose (Wiener et al., 1994). An ongoing assessment of the patient's compliance with medication and risk of self-harm is necessary.

■ PAIN MANAGEMENT IN THE HIV-INFECTED PATIENT

More than 50% of patients hospitalized with HIV disease require treatment for pain. Pain is second only to fever as the most frequent presenting complaint among persons with AIDS. It is important to remember both that pain has a profound impact on levels of emotional distress and that psychological factors, such as anxiety and depression, intensify pain. Studies show an increased frequency of anxiety, depression, and confusion in patients with pain, particularly in the late stages of an illness (Breibart, 1990). Uncontrolled pain has been implicated as a major factor in suicide among patients with cancer and those infected with HIV (Hendin, 1991).

Barriers to pain control are many. Assessment of pain is difficult for any patient, but when the patient has communication difficulties because of an organic mental disorder, or has a limited expectation of pain relief, the true degree of pain may not be expressed. The physician may be afraid that the patient will become addicted or abusive with a pain-controlling medication, or the physician may fear respiratory depression from such a drug. In any case, consultation with nurses experienced with pain control, such as those working in hospice settings, may be helpful.

The effective treatment of pain often decreases psychiatric problems and occasionally eliminates a perceived psychiatric disorder. Measures that diminish anxiety and mood disturbances can also reduce pain. Many non-pharmacological approaches to pain control are available; either alone or in conjunction with medication, they can be quite effective. Cognitive and behavioral techniques for pain control, including relaxation, imagery, hypnosis, and biofeedback, are beneficial in patients with HIV disease, who may have an increased sensitivity to the side effects of medications. These techniques build on the elements of relaxation and distraction, and give patients a sense of increased control over their pain and their bodies (Breitbart, 1990).

The use of medications to control pain in HIV-infected patients is controversial, especially in those with histories of substance abuse. Studies show, however, that intravenous drug abusers neither complain of greater pain nor require more analgesics for relief than do other patients (Lebovits and Lefkowitz, 1990).

Psychiatric disorders, such as AIDS dementia, can complicate pain management. Medications such as opiates, which are typically used to control pain, may worsen dementia or cause excessive sedation, confusion, or hallucinations in neurologically impaired patients. The use of psychostimulants to diminish sedation and neuroleptics to clear analgesic-related confusion can be helpful, but monitoring the effects of myriad medications is difficult. Relief is best achieved when analgesics are given on a fixed-time, fixed-dose schedule, rather than PRN. This approach establishes a steady blood level of such drugs and helps diminish the patient's memory and expectation of pain (Lebovits and Lefkowitz, 1990).

Newer, non-tricyclic antidepressants, such as trazodone and fluoxetine, have potent analgesic properties and are widely used to treat chronic pain syndromes. They are most beneficial in the treatment of peripheral neuropathies, which are commonly seen in persons with HIV infection (Breitbart, 1990).

■ TEACHING HIV-INFECTED PATIENTS AND THEIR FAMILIES

Interventions that focus on teaching about AIDS provide risk sensitization and allow the practice of risk-reducing skills have great value for psychiatric populations. In particular, role playing activities can assist patients in identifying risky situations and developing strategies for avoiding HIV risk (Kalichman et al., 1994).

Barriers to learning about HIV infection include a perceived risk of such infection; patient values, attitudes and beliefs; prejudice; and stigma. Almost everyone has the capacity to learn, provided the information is conveyed in such a way that the patient can clearly see its significance to him- or herself. The nurse must personalize the information and teach it in a comfortable setting. Usually, same-sex groups are ideal settings for HIV/AIDS education.

In long-term psychiatric settings, safe-sex education and distribution of condoms are being incorporated into policies and practices, recognizing that patients with "grounds privileges" or who leave the facility on short passes often engage in sexual activity. Indeed, consenting sex may to occur between patients while in the hospital, especially among those hospitalized for long periods.

All teaching begins with an assessment of the patient's, family's, or caregivers' learning needs, as well as their capacity and willingness to learn. Nurses must also be aware of the personal attitudes that they have concerning the learning needs of the psychiatrically compromised AIDS patient. For example, if the nurse experiences the same helpless coping felt by many patients, the nurse may be conveying the thought that extensive teaching need not be pursued to help the patient and family cope, because the outcome is evident. A great difference, however, can be made in the remainder of the patient's and caregivers' lives, by the nurse helping them to have some control over their experience.

PLANNING FOR THE FUTURE

First, the nurse should establish the reasonableness of having goals and plans for the future. Explore the pa-

tient's belief system concerning the value of his or her life and its impact on others. Remember, the purpose of all teaching is to facilitate living at the highest possible level of independence, interacting with others, and experiencing happiness.

EXPLORING OBSTACLES

Next explore the obstacles with both the patient and family. Obstacles to living with both a psychiatric illness and HIV disease frequently involve conflicts within the health care environment (for example, insurance coverage, access to care) and the social support systems. Often referral to medical social workers who are skilled in navigating the myriad social agencies is required. The nurse should ensure that contact is made early in the course of the illness so that a rapport can be established and relied on throughout the course of the disease.

INTERDISCIPLINARY PLANNING

Throughout the course of dealing with the psychological impact of AIDS and the pre-exisiting or comorbid factors, teaching and learning in therapeutic settings must occur in concert with the multidisciplinary treatment plan. The nurse may teach about relaxation techniques, self-awareness and esteem building, risk reduction, sex and sexuality, drug use and abuse, medication teaching and compliance. This is often accomplished in scheduled programs that include patients with differing problems, and then during individualized "one to one" meetings with the patient and family. Frequently, the individualized teaching can only occur after a patient is discharged and involved in outpatient care. Nursing teaching, therefore, must focus on the patient's compliance with continued treatment and contact with helping professionals.

FAMILY AND CAREGIVER NEEDS

Families and caregivers benefit when teaching is targeted to support the many stresses they feel. Often caregivers wish to do everything possible for the patient and neglect their own needs. They need permission to take care of themselves, and the nurse can stress the importance of self-care. In addition, the nurse must reinforce the need for caregivers to share their feelings and fears, develop support systems separate from the patient's, and continue activities and interests of their own.

The nurse may help by preparing the family and caregiver for potential hurdles, without communicating that they are inevitable. For example, conflict between the patient's family of origin and family of choice is common, especially as the disease progresses. Early efforts should be made to solidify communication between these two important parts of the patient's life.

Ongoing teaching is necessary about the symptoms of disease progression and how to deal with them. Advice about dealing with the patient experiencing organic denial, for example, should be concrete and related to specific events. "If he does this, then you try this approach . . ." Information about the effects of new medications and treatments should be included, and follow-up provided by home health nurses, whenever possible.

Sometimes, families and caregivers have many questions about infection control. Straightforward answers can be given; however, don't miss the unasked questions and concerns. Use the opportunity to quickly review the risks of infection, the disease course, and its prevention. Also, allow the caregiver to talk about his or her fears. Everyone sees the AIDS epidemic from a personal perspective.

O AN OVERVIEW

- HIV disease, which encompasses all diseases resulting from infection with the human immunodeficiency virus, is a three-stage continuum that begins with exposure to HIV and acute infection, progresses to latent infection, and culminates in clinical disease (AIDS).

- Because of the high correlation between psychiatric illness and substance abuse, hypersexuality, and impulsivity, psychiatric patients are at increased risk for HIV infection. Patients with severe psychiatric disorders may be more likely than the general public to engage in HIV-related risk behaviors.

- A careful patient history that includes information about sexual behavior and drug and alcohol use is important in identifying risk factors for HIV infection, since the latter may produce signs and symptoms similar to those of depression or other psychiatric disorders.

- Similar levels of psychological distress may occur both before and after HIV testing and with positive as well as negative HIV test results. AIDS anxiety syndrome may develop in individuals whose inability to cope with their distress leads to destructive and debilitating symptoms.

- AIDS dementia complex, caused by direct HIV infection of the brain, is a neuropsychiatric complication of AIDS that can produce cognitive slowing, memory loss, concentration and attention deficits, and disorientation.

- HIV-associated psychosis, depression, and personality disorder require careful assessment by the nurse to determine the relative contribution of psychological and organic-disease factors to their manifestations.

- Medication and pain management in patients with HIV disease require attention to drug interactions and to physical changes caused by the disease that may affect drug activity.

TD TERMS TO DEFINE

- acquired immune deficiency syndrome (AIDS)
- human immunodeficiency virus (HIV)
- HIV disease
- AIDS-related complex (ARC)
- AIDS dementia complex (ADC)
- organic denial
- AIDS anxiety syndrome
- helpless coping

Q STUDY QUESTIONS

1. Do you feel that hospitals and physicians are obligated to report AIDS cases to local and state health agencies? Is an AIDS patient's consent necessary before the disease is reported to the CDC?

2. Present an argument for and against a health care insurer refusing or cancelling coverage for an AIDS patient.

3. Do you believe that a health care provider has the right to refuse to care for an AIDS patient?

4. Does a health care professional have a greater obligation to protect an AIDS patient's privacy or to inform the individual's sexual partner(s) of the risk of infection?

■ REFERENCES

Alfonso CA, Cohen MA: HIV dementia and suicide. *Gen Hosp Psychiatry,* 1994; 16:45–46.

Baer JW, Hall JM, Holm K, Koehler SL: Treatment of people with AIDS on an inpatient psychiatric unit, in Dilley JW, Pies C, Helquist M (eds): *Face to Face: A Guide to AIDS Counseling.* San Francisco, AIDS Health Project, 1993.

Bartlett JA, Gallis HA, Shipp KW, Nabors KL: Diagnosis and treatment of patients with HIV infection, in Bartlett JA (ed): *Care and Management of Patients with HIV.* North Carolina, Glaxo, 1993.

Beckett A, Rutan JS: Treating persons with ARC & AIDS in group psychotherapy. *Int J Group Psychother* 1990; 40:19–29.

Bocceleri A, Zeifert P: Management of the neurobehavioral impairment in HIV-1 infection. *Nurs Clin North Am* 1994; 17:183–203.

Bornstein RA, Nasrallah HA, Para MF, Whitacre CC, Rosenberger P, Fass RJ, Rice R: Neuropsychological performance in asymptomatic HIV infection. *J Neuropsychiatry Clin Neurosci,* 1992; 4:386–394.

Brady SM, Carmen E: AIDS risk in the chronically mentally ill: Clinical strategies for prevention, in Goldfinger SM (ed): *Psychiatric Aspects of AIDS and HIV Infection.* San Francisco, Jossey-Bass, 1990.

Breitbart W: Psychiatric aspects of pain and HIV disease. *FOCUS: A Guide to AIDS Research and Counseling,* 1990; 5:1–2.

Daniolos PT, Holmes VF: HIV public policy and psychiatry: An examination of ethical issues and professional guidelines. *Psychosomatics* 1995; 36:12–21.

DiMarzo D. John: A man with hemophilia, in Dilley JW, Pies C, Helquist M (eds): *Face to Face: A Guide to AIDS Counseling.* San Francisco, AIDS Health Project, 1993.

Hendin H: The psychodynamics of suicide. *Am J Psychiatry* 1991; 148:1150–1158.

Lang W: Natural history of HIV disease, in Dilley JW, Pies C, Helquist M (eds): *Face to Face: A Guide to AIDS Counseling.* San Francisco, AIDS Health Project, 1993.

Lebovits AH, Lefkowitz M: Pain Management in People with HIV Disease. *FOCUS: A Guide to AIDS Research and Counseling,* 1990; 5:3.

Kalichman SC, Kelly JA, Johnson JR, Bulto M: Factors associated with risk for HIV infection among chronic mentally ill adults. *Am J Psychiatry* 1994; 151:221–227.

O'Dowd MA, Biderman BA, McKegney FP: Incidence of suicidality in AIDS and HIV-positive patients attending a psychiatry outpatient program. *Psychosomatics* 1993; 34:4595.

Perkins DO, Davidson EJ, Leserman J, Liao D, Evans DL: Personality disorder in patients infected with HIV: A controlled study with implications for clinical care. *Am J Psychiatry* 1993; 150:309–315.

Perkins DO, Stern RA, Golden RN, Murphy C, Naftolowitz D, Evans DL: Mood disorders in HIV infection: Prevalence and risk factors in a nonepicenter of the AIDS epidemic. *Am J Psychiatry,* 1994, 151(2):233–236.

Perry SW: Organic mental disorders caused by HIV: Update on early diagnosis and treatment. *Am J Psych* 1990:147:696–710.

Perry S, Jacobsberg L, Card CAL, Ashman T, Frances A, Fishman B: Severity of psychiatric symptoms after HIV testing. *Am J Psychiatry* 1993; 150:775–779.

Price N: The role of the consultation-liaison nurse. *J Psychosoc Nurs* 1995; 33:31–34.

Sacks M, Silberstein C, Weiler P, Perry S: HIV-related risk factors in acute psychiatric inpatients. *Hosp Commun Psychiatry* 1990; 41:449–452.

Scherer P: How AIDS attacks the brain. *Am J Nurs* 1990; 90:44–52.

Sewell DD, Jeste DV, Atkinson JH, Heaton RK, Hesslink JR, Wiley C, Thal L, Chandler JL, Grant I: HIV-associated psychosis. *Am J Psychiatry* 1994; 151:237–242.

Singer EJ: Management of the patient with AIDS dementia complex. *AIDS Med Rep* 1990; 3:131–136.

Tartaglia CR: AIDS anxiety syndromes, in Dilley JW, Pies C, Helquist M (eds): *Face to Face: A Guide to AIDS Counseling.* San Francisco, AIDS Health Project, 1993.

Wiener PK, Schwartz MA, O'Connell RA: Characteristics of HIV-infected patients in an inpatient psychiatric setting. *Psychosomatics* 1994; 35:5965.

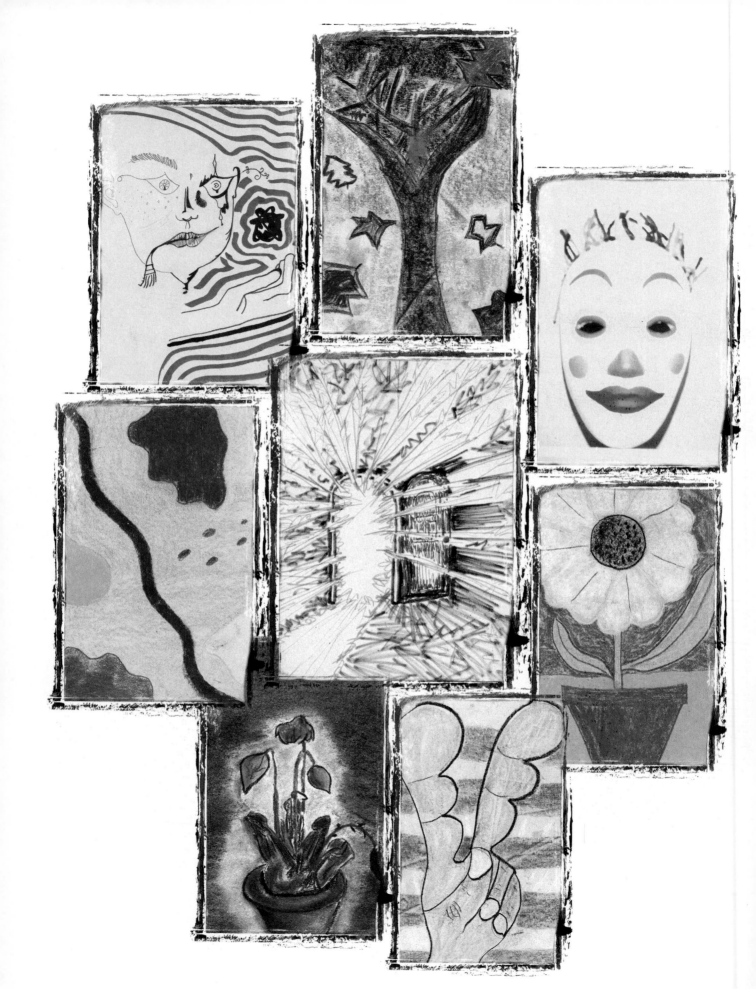

IV

PSYCHIATRIC NURSING PRACTICE

Nursing practice is based on conceptual frameworks that provide a rationale and direction for the nursing process as it is exercised in inpatient and community settings. The core content of psychiatric nursing addressed in the final section of this text includes developing a therapeutic nurse–patient relationship, learning the skills necessary for clinical assessment and nursing diagnosis, and identifying critical pathways for the planning of care. The generalist practicing in in-patient psychiatric settings needs to know the principles of the therapeutic milieu, pharmacotherapy, crisis intervention, treatment modalities, and management of therapeutic groups. Additional core content for community practice includes the skills of case management and psychiatric home care.

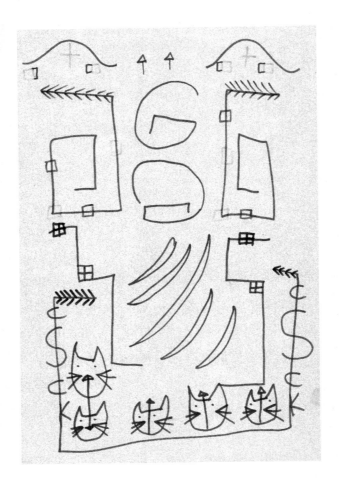

. . . Questions that occupied nurse scholars in the past were related to creating models as overall frameworks for nursing and its practice. Other questions followed related to the utility of these models in research, practice, teaching, and administration. To articulate future directions and agendas for knowledge development in nursing, existing knowledge needs to be articulated and integrated.

Afaf Ibrahim Meleis, R.N., Ph.D., Dr.Ps. (Hon)

Dept. of Mental Health, Community and Admin. Nursing, UC, San Francisco

The Neuman Systems Model, Foreword, 1995, Appleton & Lange

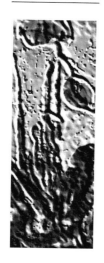

35
Conceptual Models as Guides for Psychiatric Nursing Practice

Jacqueline Fawcett

Conceptual models have existed since human beings began to think about themselves, their family members and friends, and their surroundings. Conceptual models now exist in all areas of life and in all fields of study and practice. Indeed, everything that people see, hear, read, and experience in their lives is perceived and understood through conceptual frames of reference (Lachman, 1993).

The terms conceptual model, conceptual framework, conceptual system, paradigm, and disciplinary matrix are used interchangeably and have the same definition: a set of abstract and general concepts and statements that describe or link those concepts. Each conceptual model presents a particular perspective about the phenomena of interest to a particular discipline, such as nursing. Conceptual models of nursing, for example, present diverse perspectives on the recipient of nursing, which can be an individual, a family, or a community; the recipient's environment and the environment in which nursing occurs; the health state of the recipient; the definition and goals of nursing; as well as the nursing process used to assess, label, plan, intervene, and evaluate.

■ CONCEPTUAL MODELS OF NURSING

The works of several nurse scholars are recognized as conceptual models (Table 35–1). Among the best known are Johnson's Behavioral System Model, King's General Systems Framework, Levine's Conservation Model, Neuman's Systems Model, Orem's Self-Care Framework, Rogers' Science of Unitary Human Beings, and Roy's Adaptation Model (Johnson, 1990; King, 1990; Levine, 1991; Neuman, 1995; Orem, 1995; Rogers, 1990; Roy and Andrews, 1991).

VOCABULARIES OF CONCEPTUAL MODELS

Each conceptual model is stated in a distinctive vocabulary that should not be considered jargon. Rather, the terminology is the result of considerable thought about how to convey the meaning of that particular perspective (Biley, 1990). Furthermore, as Akinsanya (1989) pointed out,

> Every science has its own peculiar terms, concepts and principles which are essential for the development of its knowledge base. In nursing, as in other sciences, an understanding of these is a prerequisite to a critical examination of their contribution to the development of knowledge and its application to practice. (p. ii)

Indeed, the differences in the vocabularies of the various models described in Table 35–1 are the same as the differences in the vocabularies of the diverse psychiatric modalities used by physicians, clinical psychologists, or family therapists, such as psychoanalytic theory, interpersonal theory, self theory, and family systems theory (Burton, 1974; Drapela, 1995; Hall and Lindzey, 1957).

FUNCTIONS OF CONCEPTUAL MODELS OF NURSING

Vocabulary reflects one function of any conceptual model, which is to provide a distinctive frame of reference and "a coherent, internally unified way of thinking about . . . events and processes" (Frank, 1968, p. 45). A conceptual model helps nurses to know how to observe and interpret the phenomena of interest to their particular practice specialty, such as psychiatric mental health nursing. Each conceptual model, then, presents a unique focus that has a profound influence on a nurse's way of thinking about patients and their environments, as well as on health-related events and situations.

Another function of a conceptual model of nursing is to identify a particular "philosophical and pragmatic orientation to the service nurses provide patients—a service which only nurses can provide—a service which pro-

vides a dimension to total care different from that provided by any other health professional" (Johnson, 1987, p. 195). Conceptual models of nursing provide explicit orientations not only for nurses but also for the general public. The models identify the purpose and scope of nursing and provide frameworks for objective records of the effects of nursing assessments and interventions. Johnson (1987) explained, "Conceptual models specify for nurses and society the mission and boundaries of the profession. They clarify the realm of nursing responsibility and accountability, and they allow the practitioner and/or the profession to document services and outcomes" (pp. 196–197).

The most tangible benefit of using a conceptual model of nursing is its delineation of goals for nursing practice (Table 35–1). Another tangible benefit is the articulation of a nursing process format that encompasses parameters for assessment, labels for patient/client problems, a strategy for planning nursing care, a set of nursing interventions, and criteria for the evaluation of the outcomes of nursing practice (see Tables 35–2, 35–3, and 35–4).

The particular philosophic and pragmatic orientations provided by three conceptual models of nursing are described below. Although any one of the conceptual models listed in Table 35–1 could be used to guide psychiatric mental health nursing practice, the discussion here is limited to Johnson's Behavioral System Model, Neuman's Systems Model, and Roy's Adaptation Model. These three models, more than the others, focus on phenomena that are of particular interest to psychiatric mental health nurses. Furthermore, all three models reflect the systems approach that has proven to be so effective in psychiatric mental health nursing practice.

JOHNSON'S BEHAVIORAL SYSTEM MODEL

Dorothy Johnson began to develop the Behavioral System Model in the early 1940s, when she first taught in a baccalaureate nursing program. She explained that the model was developed to clarify nursing's social mission from the perspective of a scientifically sound view of the person served by nursing and to identify the nature of the body of knowledge needed to attain the goal of nursing (Johnson, 1990).

Philosophic Orientation

The Behavioral System Model is based on Johnson's interpretation of the philosophic values of the nursing profession, as well as those of the individual nurse. Johnson (1990) values a focus on the person's behavior and views it as a manifestation of the momentary condition of the whole behavioral system, as well as the sub-

TABLE 35–1. OVERVIEW OF SEVEN CONCEPTUAL MODELS OF NURSING

Conceptual Model	Recipient of Nursing	Environment	Health	Nursing
Johnson's Behavioral System Model	A behavioral system with seven subsystems: attachment, dependency, ingestion, elimination, sexual, aggression, and achievement.	Internal External	Behavioral system balance and stability. Efficient and effective behavioral functioning. Purposeful, orderly, and predictable behavior.	*Definition:* A service that is complementary to that of medicine and other health professions, but which makes its own distinctive contribution to the health and well-being of people. *Goal:* Restore, maintain, or attain behavioral system balance and stability. *Actions:* Impose external regulatory or control mechanisms. Alter set or add choices for behavior. Provide protection, nurturance, or stimulation.
King's General Systems Framework	*Personal system:* Focus on perception, self, growth and development, body image, time, space, learning. *Interpersonal system:* Focus on interaction, communication, transaction, role, stress, coping. *Social system:* Focus on organization, authority, power, status, decision making, control.	Internal External	Dynamic life experiences of a human being. Ability to function in social roles.	*Definition:* Perceiving, thinking, relating, judging, and acting vis-a-vis the behavior of individuals who come to a nursing situation. *Goal:* Help individuals maintain their health so they can function in their roles. *Actions:* A process of action, reaction, interaction, and transaction directed toward establishment of goals and goal attainment.
Levine's Conservation Model	A holistic being, a system of systems. Organismic responses are fight or flight, stress, basic orienting system, visual system, auditory system, haptic system, taste-smell system.	Operational Perceptual Conceptual	Health and disease are patterns of adaptive change	*Definition:* A human interaction. *Goal:* Promotion of wholeness for people, sick or well. *Actions:* Conservation of energy, structural integrity, social integrity, and personal integrity.
Neuman's Systems Model	A patient system composed of five variables: physiological, psychological, sociocultural, developmental, and spiritual. Central core surrounded by flexible and normal lines of defense and lines of resistance	Internal External Created	Client system stability	*Definition:* A unique profession that is concerned with all the variables affecting an individual's response to stressors. *Goal:* To facilitate optimal wellness through retention, attainment, or maintenance of client system stability. *Actions:* Primary prevention, secondary prevention, and tertiary prevention.
Orem's Self-Care Framework	Self-care agent Therapeutic self-care demand made up of universal self-care requisites, developmental self-care requisites, and health deviation self-care requisites.	The person's external surroundings	Soundness or wholeness of developed human structures and of bodily and mental functioning	*Definition:* A helping service, a creative effort to help people. *Goal:* Help people to meet their own therapeutic self-care demands. *Actions:* Wholly compensatory, partly compensatory, and supportive-educative nursing systems. Assist by acting for or doing, guiding, providing physical and/or psychological support, providing a developmental environment, and teaching.
Rogers' Science of Unitary Human Beings	A unitary human being, a patterned, open, pandimensional energy field.	A patterned, open, pandi-mensional energy field	An expression of the life process	*Definition:* A learned profession that is both a science and an art. *Goal:* Help people achieve maximum well-being. *Actions:* Deliberative mutual patterning that involves environmental patterning to promote helicy, integrality, and resonancy.
Roy's Adaptation Model	An adaptive system with four response modes: physiological, self-concept, role function, and interdependence. Regulator and cognator coping mechanisms.	Focal stimuli Contextual stimuli Residual stimuli	Being and becoming an integrated and whole person	*Definition:* A theoretical system of knowledge that prescribes a process of analysis and action related to care of the ill or potentially ill person. *Goal:* Promotion of adaptation. *Actions:* Management of environmental stimuli, including increasing, decreasing, maintaining, removing, altering, or changing.

systems. She also values nursing intervention before, during, and following illness. Moreover, she values patients' contributions to their care, as indicated by her recommendation that contracts for nursing intervention be established between nurses and patients. Johnson (1990) believes that nursing views the person as a behavioral system, whereas medicine views the person as a biological system.

Pragmatic Orientation

Johnson's Behavioral System Model focuses on the degree to which seven interrelated behavioral subsystems and the entire behavioral system function efficiently and effectively. Each behavioral subsystem has a special function, which reflects a basic drive or goal of human behavior.

The function of the *attachment* or *affiliative subsystem* is attainment of the security needed for survival, as well as social inclusion, intimacy, and the formation and maintenance of social bonds. The function of the *dependency subsystem* is succoring behavior that calls for a response of nurturance, as well as approval, attention, or recognition, and physical assistance. The function of the *ingestive subsystem* is appetite satisfaction, with regard to when, how, what, how much, and under what conditions the individual eats, which is governed by social and psychological considerations, as well as biological requirements for food and fluids. The function of the *eliminative subsystem* is the appropriate disposal of bodily waste products, with regard to when, how, and under what conditions the individual eliminates wastes. The functions of the *sexual subsystem* are procreation and gratification, with regard to behaviors dependent on the individual's biological sex and gender role identity, including, but not limited to, courting and mating. The functions of the *aggressive subsystem* are protection and preservation of self and society. The function of the *achievement subsystem* is mastery or control of some aspect of self or environment, with regard to intellectual, physical, creative, mechanical, social, and caretaking skills (of children, spouse, and home), and as measured against some standard of excellence.

The functions of the behavioral subsystems reflect their respective *drive* or *goal,* which is one structural element of each subsystem. The other structural elements of each are set, choice, and action or behavior. *Set* refers to the person's predisposition to act in a certain consistent way to fulfill the function of each subsystem. *Choice* refers to the person's total behavior repertoire for fulfilling subsystem functions and achieving particular goals. *Action* refers to the actual organized and patterned behavior in a situation and is the only structural component that can be directly observed; the others must be inferred from the observed behavior.

The ability of the behavioral subsystems to fulfill their functions depends on three requirements that are met by the person or through outside assistance from a nurse:

- *Protection* from noxious influences with which the subsystem cannot cope.
- *Nurturance* through the input of appropriate supplies from the environment.
- *Stimulation* to enhance growth and prevent stagnation.

The goal of nursing action is "to restore, maintain, or attain behavioral system balance and dynamic stability at the highest possible level for the [person]" (Johnson, 1990, p. 29). The nursing process that is used with Johnson's Behavioral System Model is outlined in Table 35–2.

Using Johnson's Model in Psychiatric Mental Health Nursing

Johnson's Behavioral System Model (JBSM) has been used to guide psychiatric mental health nursing practice for many years. Dee (1990) presented a detailed description of the use of the model at the UCLA Neuropsychiatric Institute and Hospital in Los Angeles. She explained that JBSM is implemented in the child and adult psychiatric in-patient services with patients ranging from 2 years to older than 90 years. Clinical settings include a child and an adolescent psychiatric unit, a child and an adolescent developmental disabilities unit, general adult psychiatric units, and a geropsychiatry unit.

The Patient Classification Instrument (PCI) used at the Neuropsychiatric Institute is directly derived from JBSM (Auger and Dee, 1983; Dee and Auger, 1983). The PCI operationalizes each behavioral subsystem as a list of critical behaviors. The overall level of behavior for each patient is categorized as adaptive, in the process of being learned and/or minimally maladaptive, or maladaptive. Specific nursing interventions are linked to specific behaviors and are categorized according to the particular level of nursing care required.

In category I, patient behaviors that are appropriate to the patient's developmental stage and adaptive to the environment are linked with nursing interventions that provide general supervision, maintain and support healthy, developmentally appropriate behaviors, and reinforce independent behaviors.

In category II, patient behaviors that are inconsistent, in the process of being learned, or maladaptive to the environment, along with behaviors that may or may not be appropriate to the patient's developmental stage, are linked with nursing interventions that provide moderate or periodic supervision, modify mal-

TABLE 35–2. THE NURSING PROCESS FOR JOHNSON'S BEHAVIORAL SYSTEM MODEL

I. Determination of the existence of a problem
  A. Obtain past and present family and individual behavioral system histories
  B. Specify condition of the subsystem structural components
    1. Determine drive strength, direction, and value
    2. Determine the solidity and specificity of the set
    3. Identify the range of behavior patterns available to the individual
    4. Identify the usual behavior in a given situation
    5. Assess and compare behavior with indices of behavioral system balance and stability
      a. Determine whether the behavior is succeeding or failing to achieve the consequences sought
      b. Determine whether more effective motor, expressive, or social skills are needed
      c. Determine whether or not the behavior is purposeful, that is, whether or not actions are goal-directed, reveal a plan, cease at an identifiable point, and are economical in sequence
      d. Determine whether or not the behavior is orderly, that is, whether or not actions are methodical, systematic, build sequentially toward a goal, and form a recognizable pattern
      e. Determine whether or not the behavior is predictable, that is, whether or not actions are repetitive under particular circumstances
      f. Determine whether or not the amount of energy expended to achieve desired goals is acceptable
      g. Determine whether or not behavior reflects appropriate choices
        (1) Determine whether or not actions are compatible with survival imperatives
        (2) Determine whether or not actions are congruent with the social situation
      h. Determine whether or not the individual is sufficiently satisfied with the behavior
    6. Determine the organization, interaction, and integration of the subsystems
II. Diagnostic classification of problems
  A. Internal subsystem problems
    1. Functional requirements not met
    2. Inconsistency or disharmony among structural components of subsystems
    3. Behavior inappropriate in the ambient culture
  B. Intersystem problems
    1. Domination of entire system by one or two subsystems
    2. Conflict between two or more subsystems

III. Management of nursing problems
  A. General goal of action
    1. Restore, maintain, or attain the patient's behavioral system balance and stability
    2. Help the patient achieve a more optimum level of balance and functioning when this is possible and desired
  B. Determine what nursing is to accomplish on behalf of the behavioral system
    1. Determine what level of behavioral system balance and stability is acceptable
    2. Determine who makes the judgment regarding acceptable level of behavioral system balance and stability
      a. Identify value system of nursing profession
      b. Identify own explicit value system
  C. Select a type of treatment
    1. Fulfill functional requirements of the subsystems
      a. Protect patient from overwhelming noxious influences
      b. Supply adequate nurturance through an appropriate input of essential supplies
      c. Provide stimulation to enhance growth and to inhibit stagnation
    2. Temporarily impose external regulatory or control measures
      a. Set limits for behavior by either permissive or inhibitory means
      b. Inhibit ineffective behavioral responses
      c. Assist patient to acquire new responses
      d. Reinforce appropriate behaviors
    3. Repair damaged structural elements in desirable direction
      a. Reduce drive strength by changing attitudes
      b. Redirect goal by changing attitudes
      c. Alter set by instruction or counseling
      d. Add choices by teaching new skills
  D. Negotiate treatment modality with patient
    1. Establish a contract with the patient
    2. Help patient understand meaning of nursing diagnosis and proposed treatment
    3. If diagnosis and/or proposed treatment are rejected, continue to negotiate with the patient until agreement is reached
IV. Compare behavior after treatment to indices of behavioral system balance and stability (c.f. I.B.5.a-h)

Reprinted from Fawcett J. *Analysis and Evaluation of Conceptual Models of Nursing.* 3rd ed. Philadelphia: Davis; 1995:82–83, with permission.

adaptive behaviors and maintain newly adaptive ones, and structure the environment to provide limits on behavior. The interventions are carried out in group settings and include implementation of the medical treatment regimen.

In category III, patient behaviors that are severely maladaptive to the environment and are not appropriate to the patient's developmental stage are linked with nursing interventions that provide direct supervision, modify maladaptive behaviors, teach new behaviors, reinforce adaptive behaviors, structure the environment to provide limits on behavior, and include implementation of the medical treatment regimen.

In category IV, patient behaviors from category III that are of acute intensity, duration, and/or frequency, as well as behaviors that represent self-destructive acts or aggression toward others, are linked with nursing interventions that provide one-to-one supervision and are directed toward the reduction of the intensity, frequency, and/or duration of the maladaptive behaviors and the protection of the patient. It is noteworthy that the PCI encompasses all behavioral subsystems and the entire nursing process, from problem determination (assessment) to evaluation of post-treatment behaviors (see Table 35–2).

Poster (1989) reported the results of a study on the use of the PCI. She stated that 90% of the 38 adolescent psychiatric in-patients studied had an adaptive change in at least one behavioral category after 1 week of Behavioral System Model–based nursing care.

A JBSM-based nursing diagnostic system also was developed for use at the UCLA Neuropsychiatric Institute and Hospital. Randell (1991) and Lewis and Randell (1991) described the development of the diagnostic system and documented its advantages over the North American Nursing Diagnosis Association (NANDA) system. Randell (1991) explained that JBSM-based nursing diagnoses "reflect the nature of the ineffective behavior and its relationship to the regulators in the environment" (p. 154). She went on to point out that JBSM "helps distinguish what counts as a problem and what counts as etiology, calling into question existing [NANDA] labels" (p. 159).

NEUMAN'S SYSTEMS MODEL

Betty Neuman developed the Neuman Systems Model in 1970, when she was teaching students in a community mental health master's degree program. She explained that the development of the model was motivated by her desire to respond to the expressed needs of her students for course content that would present the breadth of nursing problems prior to content that emphasized specific nursing problem areas (Neuman, 1995).

Philosophic Orientation

Neuman's (1995) approach to health care reflects her assumption that systems thinking is a comprehensive way of viewing clients and their environments. Neuman also values intervention prior to manifestations of variances from wellness, as well as after they occur. She emphasizes the need to consider both the client's and care-giver's perceptions of stressors, and assumes that nursing goals are effectively established when negotiated with the client. Furthermore, Neuman focuses on the extent of the client system's wellness rather than illness. Moreover, although Neuman believes that nursing is a unique profession, she considers her conceptual model appropriate for all health care disciplines.

Pragmatic Orientation

Neuman's Systems Model regards the person as a client system that must defend its central core from the invasion of environmental stressors. The client system, which can be an individual, a family or other group, or a community, is a composite of five interrelated variables. *Physiological variables* encompass bodily structures and functions; *psychological variables* include mental processes and relationships; *sociocultural variables* encompass social and cultural functions; *developmental variables* include the developmental processes of the life cycle; and *spiritual variables* include aspects of spirituality on a continuum from complete unawareness or denial to a consciously developed high level of spiritual understanding.

E CASE EXAMPLE

Jed Stewart is a 16-year-old male who was admitted to an inpatient psychiatric unit after attempting suicide. Jed's suicidal behavior indicates an imbalance in the aggressive subsystem. The underlying cause of this imbalance was revealed through interviews with Jed and his parents. Jed stated that he thought that he was a "total failure" in school, varsity sports, and even in committing suicide, which indicates an imbalance in the achievement subsystem. Both Jed and his parents stated that he had "no friends" and "couldn't get dates with girls," which indicates an imbalance in the attachment subsystem. Because of his suicide attempt, Jed is initially placed in the PCI category that mandates nursing interventions on a one-to-one basis for his protection.

One goal of nursing intervention will be to help Jed to attain balance and stability in the achievement subsystem by contracting with him to use more effective study habits and to explore various options to varsity sports. Another goal will be to help Jed attain balance and stability in the attachment subsystem by initially providing regular intensive one-to-one interactions to help him understand the components of effective interpersonal relationships and then contracting with him to use more effective communication skills with the staff and other patients. All of these nursing interventions are directed toward repairing damaged structural elements by altering set and adding choices (see Table 35–2).

TABLE 35–3. THE NURSING PROCESS FOR NEUMAN'S SYSTEMS MODEL

I. Nursing diagnosis
  A. Establish data base that includes the simultaneous consideration of the dynamic interactions of physiological, psychological, sociocultural, developmental, and spiritual variables
    1. Identify client/client system's perceptions
      a. Assess condition and strength of basic structure factors and energy resources
      b. Assess characteristics of the flexible and normal lines of defense, lines of resistance, degree of potential or actual reaction, and potential for reconstitution following a reaction
      c. Assess internal and external environmental stressors that threaten the stability of the client/client system
        (1) Identify, classify, and evaluate potential or actual intrapersonal, interpersonal, and extrapersonal stressors that threaten the stability of the client/client system through deprivation, excess, change, intolerance, etc.
        (2) Identify, classify, and evaluate potential and/or actual intrapersonal, interpersonal, and extrapersonal interactions between the client/client system and the environment, considering all five variables
      d. Assess and discover the nature of client/client system's created-environment
        (1) Assess client/client system's perception of stressors
        (2) Determine degree of protection provided
        (3) Identify the cause and effect relationship between the created environment and client/client system in terms of bound versus available energy
      e. Evaluate influence of past, present, and possible future life processes and coping patterns on client/client system stability
      f. Identify and evaluate actual and potential internal and external resources for optimal state of wellness
    2. Identify care-giver's perceptions (repeat 1 a, b, c, d, e, and f from care-giver's perspective)
    3. Compare client/client system's and care-giver's perceptions
      a. Identify similarities and differences in perceptions
      b. Facilitate client awareness of major perceptual distortions
      c. Resolve perceptual differences
  B. Variances from wellness
    1. Synthesize client data base with relevant theories from nursing and adjunctive disciplines
    2. State a comprehensive nursing diagnosis
    3. Prioritize goals
      a. Consider client/client system wellness level
      b. Consider system stability needs
      c. Consider total available resources
    4. Postulate outcome goals and interventions that will facilitate the highest possible level of client/client system stability or wellness (i.e., maintain the normal line of defense and retain the flexible line of defense)

II. Nursing goals
  A. Negotiate desired prescriptive change or outcome goals to correct variances from wellness with the client/client system
    1. Consider needs identified in I.B.3.b.
    2. Consider resources identified in I.B.3.c.
  B. Negotiate prevention as intervention modalities and actions with client/client system

III. Nursing outcomes
  A. Implement nursing interventions through use of one or more of the three prevention as intervention modalities
    1. Primary prevention as intervention nursing actions to retain system stability
      a. Prevent stressor invasion
      b. Provide resources to retain or strengthen existing client/client system strengths
      c. Support positive coping and functioning
      d. Desensitize existing or possible noxious stressors
      e. Motivate toward wellness
      f. Coordinate and integrate interdisciplinary theories and epidemiologic input
      g. Educate or re-educate
      h. Use stress as a positive intervention strategy
    2. Secondary prevention as intervention nursing actions to attain system stability
      a. Protect basic structure
      b. Mobilize and optimize internal/external resources to attain stability and energy conservation
      c. Facilitate purposeful manipulation of stressors and reactions to stressors
      d. Motivate, educate, and involve client/client system in mutual establishment of health care goals
      e. Facilitate appropriate treatment and intervention measures
      f. Support positive factors toward wellness
      g. Promote advocacy by coordination and integration
      h. Provide primary preventive intervention as required
    3. Tertiary prevention as intervention nursing actions to maintain system stability
      a. Attain and maintain highest possible level of wellness and stability during reconstitution
      b. Educate, re-educate, and/or reorient as needed
      c. Support client/client system toward appropriate goals
      d. Coordinate and integrate client system health resources
      e. Provide primary and/or secondary preventive intervention as required
  B. Evaluate outcome goals
    1. Confirm attainment of outcome goals
    2. Reformulate goals
  C. Set intermediate and long-range goals for subsequent nursing action that are structured in relation to short-term goal outcomes

Reprinted from Fawcett J. *Analysis and Evaluation of Conceptual Models of Nursing.* 3rd ed. Philadelphia: Davis; 1995:234–235, with permission.

The client system is depicted as a central core, which is a basic structure of survival factors common to the species, surrounded by three types of concentric rings. The **flexible line of defense** is the outermost ring, which is a protective buffer for the client's normal or stable state; it prevents invasion of stressors, keeping the client system free from stressor reactions or symptomatology. The **normal line of defense** lies between the flexible line of defense and the lines of resistance; it represents the client system's normal or usual wellness state. The **lines of resistance** are the innermost concentric rings; they are involuntarily activated when a stressor invades the normal line of defense, and they attempt to stabilize the client system and foster a return to the normal line of defense. If the lines of resistance are effective, the system can reconstitute; if ineffective, death may ensue.

Environment encompasses all internal and external influences surrounding the client system. The **internal environment** consists of all forces or interactive influences internal to or contained within the boundaries of the defined client system; it is the source of **intrapersonal stressors**. The **external environment** is all forces or influences external to or existing outside the defined client system; it is the source of **interpersonal** and **extrapersonal stressors.**

The **created-environment** is subconsciously developed by the client as a symbolic expression of system wholeness and supersedes and encompasses the internal and external environments. It functions as a subjective safety mechanism that may block the true reality of the environment and the health experience.

The goal of nursing is to facilitate optimal wellness through retention, attainment, or maintenance of client system stability. The nursing process for Neuman's Systems Model is outlined in Table 35–3.

Using Neuman's Model in Psychiatric Mental Health Nursing

Neuman's Systems Model (NSM) has been used to guide psychiatric mental health nursing practice in various settings. Scicchitani and colleagues (1995) presented a detailed description of the process used to select and implement NSM at Friends Hospital in Philadelphia. Among the many beneficial outcomes cited were "a fairly dramatic increase in the attention focused on client perceptions"; the nurses' "commitment to assessment of all five variables [physiological, psychological, sociocultural, developmental, and spiritual], even in the face of pressure to focus on the 'most significant reason' for hospitalization"; and "an increase in the scope of [client system] teaching and in the creativity with which it is accomplished" (pp. 392–393).

A project to implement NSM-based nursing practice at the Whitby Psychiatric Hospital in Ontario, Canada, was described by Craig and Morris-Coulter (1995). In addition, community psychiatric nursing practice projects in Wales and in the Netherlands were outlined by Davies (1989) and Verberk (1995), respectively.

Baker (1982) described a NSM-based continuing education program for nurses in a psychiatric mental health hospital that could be used as part of a project for implementing the model. The content of the program seminars was organized according to the psychological, physiological, and sociocultural variables; the stressors and lines of defense relevant to each variable area; and the nurse–client relationship in primary, secondary, and tertiary prevention interventions.

Turning to practice with individual clients, Stuart and Wright (1995) pointed out that NSM leads to a comprehensive psychiatric nursing assessment. They noted that comprehensive assessment includes

> the individual's basic structure or predisposing factors; precipitating and possible stressors; the flexible line of defense, characterized by the client's appraisal of the stressor and coping resources; and the individual's lines of resistance, or coping mechanisms. (p. 268)

Stuart and Wright (1995) went on to explain that NSM-based psychiatric nursing diagnoses "identify problems that may be overt, covert, existing, or potential . . . [and] that nursing diagnoses complement [DSM] diagnoses; they are not contingent upon them" (pp. 268–269). Finally, they underscored the NSM-based emphasis on a continuum of nursing intervention modalities (rather than nursing intervention focused on episodic symptom relief), that is, primary, secondary, and tertiary prevention.

Clark (1982) explained how NSM can be used to guide comprehensive care of depressed clients in community settings. She described the development of a Depression Assessment Guide and a Depression Symptom Checklist that focus attention on the stressors and variables of NSM, rather than only on the symptom of depression.

Herrick and associates (1991) described the use of the NSM as a guide for a continuum of care for children who require psychiatric services. They identified the use of primary and secondary prevention interventions for children requiring out-patient services or partial hospitalization, and tertiary prevention interventions for children who require residential treatment or treatment in an acute care setting.

Moore and Munro (1990) explained how NSM can be applied to the mental health nursing of older adults. They emphasized the unique role of nursing intervention within an interdisciplinary approach by outlining the use of primary, secondary, and tertiary prevention with an elderly woman who has assumed total care of her husband who has dementia.

Beitler and co-workers (1980) identified common stressors experienced by clients with personality disorders, including denial of anxiety and needs for help, broken relationships, manipulative behavior, and use of rationalization. They went on to identify primary, secondary, and tertiary prevention interventions to deal with each stressor.

The effectiveness of NSM-based practice is documented by a study conducted by Waddell and Demi (1993). They reported that post-test fear of fear, severity of psychological impairment, and general emotional distress scores were lower than pretest scores among a sample of 32 participants in a 5-week partial psychiatric hospitalization program based on NSM.

Neuman's Systems Model is equally effective with individual psychiatric nursing clients and troubled families. Herrick and Goodykoontz (1989) described a NSM-based framework to guide the assessment and intervention of a dysfunctional family. Moreover, Goldblum-Graff and Graff (1982) adapted NSM to family therapy by linking it with contextual family therapy.

ROY'S ADAPTATION MODEL

Sister Callista Roy began to develop the Adaptation Model in 1964, while she was a graduate student studying with Dorothy Johnson at the University of California, Los Angeles, School of Nursing. She explained that the model was developed as a way to articulate a body of scientific nursing knowledge that can be taught in nursing programs and can be used to guide nursing practice.

Philosophic Orientation

The Adaptation Model is based on Roy's assumption that people are integrated wholes capable of action. More specifically, the model is based on Roy's belief in the general principles of humanism and veritivity. Humanism refers to "a broad movement in philosophy and psychology that recognizes the person and subjective dimensions of human experience as central to knowing and valuing" (Roy, 1988, p. 29). Veritivity is a philosophical premise that asserts that "there is an absolute truth" (p. 29) and "a common purposefulness of human existence" (p. 30).

Roy values the active participation of persons in their nursing care. She noted that, although participation may not always be possible, as in the case of infants and unconscious or suicidal patients, the nurse "is constantly aware of the active responsibility of the patient to participate in his own care when he is able to do so" (Roy and Roberts, 1981, p. 47). Furthermore, Roy believes that medicine focuses on biological systems and the person's disease, whereas nursing focuses on the person as a total being who responds to internal and external environmental stimuli.

Pragmatic Orientation

Roy's Adaptation Model focuses on the responses of the person, as a human adaptive system, to a constantly changing environment. Adaptation is the central feature of the model. Problems in adaptation arise when the adaptive system is unable to cope with or respond to constantly changing stimuli from the internal and external environments in a manner that maintains the integrity of the system.

E CASE EXAMPLE

Dorothy Foster, who is 85, and her husband, Joseph, who is 90, live alone in their own home. They have been receiving home care since Dorothy was discharged from an inpatient rehabilitation unit following successful surgery for a fractured hip. A comprehensive NSM-based nursing assessment revealed several stressors. Dorothy's intrapersonal stressors include urinary incontinence and mobility limited to ambulation with a walker. Joseph's major intrapersonal stressor is impaired vision due to bilateral cataracts. The major interpersonal stressor is Dorothy and Joseph's continuing disagreement about where they should live—Joseph would prefer to move to a retirement community and Dorothy insists on remaining in their own home. One major extrapersonal stressor is a lack of stimulation—Dorothy and Joseph have become increasingly reclusive since

Joseph retired 25 years ago. Another major extrapersonal stressor is the couple's reliance on neighbors to shop for groceries. Dorothy states that she does not want to go out because she is afraid of "accidents," but also has refused to participate in a urinary incontinence training program. Joseph states that he is afraid to leave Dorothy alone. The psychiatric nurse at the home health care agency discusses a variety of possible secondary and tertiary prevention interventions with Dorothy and Joseph, including employment of a housekeeper/companion and use of community resources, such as "Meals on Wheels." In addition, the nurse encourages Dorothy and Joseph to discuss their feelings about their current lifestyle and their vision of the future to facilitate primary prevention.

There are three types of environmental stimuli.

1. **Focal stimulus:** the one most immediately confronting the person.
2. **Contextual stimuli:** all other stimuli that contribute directly to adaptation.
3. **Residual stimuli:** all other unknown factors that may influence the situation.

When the factors making up residual stimuli become known, they are considered focal or contextual stimuli.

Adaptation to changing environmental stimuli occurs through two types of coping mechanisms. The **regulator mechanism** receives input from the internal and external environment and processes it through neural-chemical-endocrine channels to produce responses. The **cognator mechanism** also receives input from external and internal stimuli and processes it through cognitive/emotive pathways, including perceptual/information processing, learning, judgment, and emotion.

Responses to environmental stimuli take place in four modes: physiological, self-concept, role function, and interdependence. The **physiological mode** is concerned with basic needs requisite to maintaining the physical and physiological integrity of the human system, including oxygenation, nutrition, elimination, activity and rest, protection, the senses, fluids and electrolytes, neurological functions, and endocrine functions. The **self-concept mode** deals with the person's conceptions of the physical self, including body sensation and body image, and the personal self, including self-consistency, self-ideal, and the moral-ethical-spiritual self. The **role function mode** is concerned with the person's performance of roles on the basis of his or her position within society. The **interdependence mode** involves the person's willingness and ability to love, respect, and value others and the ability to accept and respond to love, respect, and value given by others. This mode focuses primarily on relationships with significant others and social support systems. The four response modes are interrelated, such that responses in any one mode may have an effect on or act as a stimulus to one or all of the other modes.

Responses in each mode are judged as either **adaptive responses,** which promote the integrity of the person in terms of the goals of the human adaptive system, including survival, growth, reproduction, and mastery; or **ineffective responses,** which do not contribute to these goals.

The goal of nursing is the "promotion of adaptation in each of the four [response] modes, thereby contributing to the person's health, quality of life, and dying with dignity" (Roy and Andrews, 1991, p. 20). Roy's Adaptation Model's nursing process is outlined in Table 35–4.

Using Roy's Model in Psychiatric Mental Health Nursing

Robitaille-Tremblay (1984; personal communication, August 4, 1982) reported that Roy's Adaptation Model (RAM) is used as the basis for nursing practice with psychiatric patients at Centre Hospitalier Pierre Janet in Hull, Quebec, Canada. She explained that a nursing history tool that is organized according to the four response modes of Roy's model enhanced the patients' satisfaction with their nursing care, quoting them as saying, "It is the first time a professional has evaluated me so fully," "I realize that most of my problems interrelate," and "I have learned to know myself better than I have during any previous hospitalization" (1984, p. 28).

Use of the tool also increased the nurses' satisfaction with practice by helping them to

> . . . get to know the patient more fully and to broaden their perspective in establishing priorities on the basis of identified stimuli. Some felt closer to the patient with whom the tool was used. One nurse stated, "I have acquired more confidence in my independent role and I'm proud, very proud." (Robitaille-Tremblay, 1984, p. 28)

In addition, use of the nursing history tool led to more comprehensive assessments and nursing care plans, which in turn led to more comprehensive treatment and increased the patients' length of stay in the hospital; however, as Robitaille-Tremblay speculated (personal communication, August 4, 1982), the more comprehensive treatment would most likely reduce the rate of rehospitalization.

Miller (1991), a student nurse, reported that RAM guided the comprehensive nursing practice with a 22-year-old man who was in a "special hospital" for patients with dangerous, violent, or criminal behavior located in England. She pointed out that the locked units and other environmental constraints required for security represented detrimental contextual stimuli that prevented complete negotiation of goals and interventions. Furthermore, commenting on the detrimental effects of the contextual stimuli, Miller stated:

> As [these] detrimental contextual stimuli could not be removed, the only other option for intervention using Roy's model was to increase the patient's level of adaptation. This identified a great flaw in the special hospital system: patients who adapt well to their environment may be considered institutionalized. Should we discourage this because the behavior needed to adapt to a special hospital could be considered [ineffective] outside its confines? When and how are we to expect patients to re-adapt their roles to prepare them for discharge and what plans do we have to aid them? (p. 32)

TABLE 35–4. THE NURSING PROCESS FOR ROY'S ADAPTATION MODEL

I. Assessment of behaviors
  A. Methods used to collect data
    1. Observation
      a. Sight
      b. Sound
      c. Touch
      d. Taste
      e. Smell
    2. Objective measurement
      a. Paper and pencil instruments
      b. Measures of physiological parameters
    3. Interviews
  B. Behaviors to assess
    1. Physiological mode
      a. Oxygenation
      b. Nutrition
      c. Elimination
      d. Activity and rest
      e. Protection
      f. Senses
      g. Fluid and electrolytes
      h. Neurological functions
      i. Endocrine functions
    2. Self-concept mode
      a. Physical self
        (1) Body image
        (2) Body sensation
      b. Personal self
        (1) Self-consistency
        (2) Self-ideal
        (3) Moral-ethical-spiritual self
    3. Role function
      a. Primary role
        (1) Instrumental component(s)
        (2) Expressive component(s)
      b. Secondary roles
        (1) Instrumental component(s)
        (2) Expressive component(s)
      c. Tertiary roles
        (1) Instrumental component(s)
        (2) Expressive component(s)
    4. Interdependence mode
      a. Significant others
        (1) Contributive behavior
        (2) Receptive behavior
      b. Social support
        (1) Contributive behavior
        (2) Receptive behavior
  C. Judgment of behaviors
    1. Adaptive or ineffective responses
      a. Nurse's judgment
      b. Person's perception

    2. Criteria for judgment
      a. Person's individualized goals
      b. Comparison of behavior with norms signifying adaptation
      c. Regulator mechanism activity
      d. Cognator mechanism effectiveness
II. Assessment of stimuli
  A. Criteria for priorities for further assessment of the person's behaviors
    1. Behaviors that threaten the survival of the individual, family, group, or community
    2. Behaviors that affect the growth of the individual, family, group, or community
    3. Behaviors that affect the continuation of the human race or of society
    4. Behaviors that affect the attainment of full potential for the individual or group
  B. Methods used to determine influence of stimuli
    1. Observation
    2. Objective measurement
    3. Interview
    4. Validate hunch about relevant stimuli with the person
  C. Stimuli
    1. Focal stimulus
    2. Contextual stimuli
      a. Culture
        (1) Socioeconomic status
        (2) Ethnicity
        (3) Belief system
      b. Family structure and tasks
      c. Developmental stage
        (1) Age
        (2) Sex
        (3) Tasks
        (4) Heredity
        (5) Genetic factors
      d. Integrity of response modes
        (1) Physiological mode and disease pathology
        (2) Self-concept
        (3) Role function
        (4) Interdependence
      e. Cognator effectiveness
        (1) Perception
        (2) Knowledge
        (3) Skill
      f. Environmental considerations
        (1) Change in internal or external environment
        (2) Medical management
        (3) Use of drugs, alcohol, and/or tobacco

    3. Residual stimuli
      a. Beliefs
      b. Attitudes
      c. Traits
      d. Cultural determinants
III. Nursing diagnosis
  A. Three approaches
    1. State behaviors within each response mode and with their most relevant influencing stimuli
    2. Provide a summary label for behaviors in each response mode with relevant stimuli
    3. Provide a label that summarizes a behavioral pattern across response modes that is affected by the same stimuli
  B. Arrange diagnoses in order of priority using criteria in II.A
IV. Goal setting
  A. Statement of behavioral outcomes of nursing intervention
  B. Determine that the person agrees with goal
V. Nursing intervention
  A. Management of stimuli
    1. Alter stimuli
    2. Increase stimuli
    3. Decrease stimuli
    4. Remove stimuli
    5. Maintain stimuli
  B. Priorities
    1. Manage focal stimulus first if possible
    2. Manage contextual stimuli next
  C. Selection of nursing intervention approach
    1. List possible approaches
    2. Outline consequences of management of each stimulus
    3. Determine probability for each consequence
    4. Judge value of outcomes of each approach
    5. Share options with the person
    6. Select approach with highest probability of reaching valued goal
VI. Evaluation
  A. Methods used
    1. Observation
    2. Objective measurement
    3. Interview
  B. Criteria for judgment of effectiveness of nursing intervention
    1. Goal attained or not attained
    2. Person does or does not manifest behavior stated in goal

Reprinted from Fawcett J. *Analysis and Evaluation of Conceptual Models of Nursing.* 3rd ed. Philadelphia: Davis; 1995: 462–464, with permission.

Leonard (1975) discussed the links between RAM and the findings from her study of psychiatric patients' attitudes toward nursing interventions. She noted that nursing interventions should be directed toward the management of contextual stimuli, such as changes in the administrative structure of a psychiatric unit to enhance patient adaptation.

Roy's Adaptation Model has been used to guide nursing practice with patients who have various psychiatric symptoms. For example, Schmidt (1981) presented two case studies of RAM-based, individualized nursing practice. Both cases were adult patients who suffered from schizophrenia and exhibited withdrawn behavior. Schmidt managed both focal and contextual stimuli to promote the long-term nursing goal of decreasing withdrawn behavior through short-term goals, such as establishing one-to-one relationships, increasing participation in ward recreational activities, and increasing interaction with others.

Furthermore, Coleman (1993) explained the influence of biological and social factors on the development of depression during menopause within the context of RAM. She noted that the use of the model to guide nursing intervention results in holistic care for menopausal women who suffer from depression. In addition, Frederickson (1993) described the beneficial effects of using RAM to help patients to deal with the symptom of anxiety.

Roy's Adaptation Model also has been linked to particular types of therapy. Hamer (1991) used RAM as the basis for the application of music therapy for patients diagnosed with organic brain damage, mild to moderate mental retardation, and schizoaffective disorder. Although the effects of the music therapy could not be clearly distinguished from other therapies, improvements were noted in the patients' ego strength, socialization, activity levels, and psychotic symptoms.

Moreover, Kurek-Ovshinsky (1991) described RAM-based group therapy for patients on a 15-bed acute in-patient psychiatric unit located in a metropolitan trauma center. She explained narcissism within the context of the self-concept and interdependence response modes and discussed the effects of the patients' narcissistic behavior on their participation in group therapy.

■ SELECTING A CONCEPTUAL MODEL FOR PSYCHIATRIC MENTAL HEALTH NURSING PRACTICE

The process of selecting the conceptual model for psychiatric mental health nursing may be facilitated by the six steps that follow.

1. State your philosophy of nursing in the form of beliefs and values about the nursing recipient, the environment, health, and nursing goals.
2. Identify the particular patient population with which you wish to practice.
3. Thoroughly analyze and evaluate several conceptual models of nursing, with emphasis on philosophic claims and utility for psychiatric mental health nursing practice.
4. Compare your philosophy of nursing with the philosophical claims upon which each conceptual model is based.
5. Determine which conceptual models are appropriate to use with the patient population of interest.

E CASE EXAMPLE

Ellen Cooper is a 25-year-old married primipara who delivered a healthy, full-term infant son 3 weeks ago. Now Ellen's husband, Dan, brings her to the emergency room at their community hospital. Ellen says, "I'm afraid I will hurt the baby because he cries so much, and I am so tired." Initial nursing assessment indicates that Ellen is exhibiting ineffective behaviors in all four response modes. More specifically, assessment of the physiological mode responses reveals that she has not been eating regular meals and feels "listless and very, very tired." Assessment of the self-concept mode responses indicates that Ellen feels like a failure because the baby was born by cesarean section due to a breech presentation. Assessment of the role function mode responses reveals that

Ellen had no prior experience with infant care and feels "overwhelmed by motherhood." Assessment of the interdependence mode responses indicates that Ellen and Dan have had no time to spend alone and that they regard the changes in their relationship negatively. After discussing appropriate options with the Coopers, the emergency room nurse, who has a background in both psychiatric and maternity nursing, recommends that Dan immediately arrange for a relative or friend to help Ellen with the baby while he is at work. The nurse also recommends that Ellen make an appointment at the local mental health clinic to talk to a nurse about her feelings.

6. Select the conceptual model that most closely matches your philosophy of nursing and patient population of interest.

FIRST STEP

In the first step, answering the following questions will help you to identify your particular beliefs and values.

- Are all people, regardless of health state or psychiatric diagnosis, potential recipients of psychiatric mental health nursing?
- Or, are only people with documented psychiatric illnesses legitimate recipients of psychiatric mental health nursing?
- Who are the significant people in the recipient's environment?
- What are the significant objects in the recipient's environment?
- In what settings can psychiatric nursing practice take place?
- What is health? What is mental health?
- What are the appropriate goals of psychiatric mental health nursing practice?
- What part do recipients of psychiatric mental health nursing play in determining nursing goals and identifying interventions used to attain those goals?

SECOND STEP

The patient population that one identifies to work with (the second step in selecting a model) may be based on a specific psychiatric diagnosis, such as schizophrenia or bipolar disorder; an age group, such as children, adolescents, or the elderly; a type of psychiatric illness, such as an acute crisis or chronic illness; or a particular symptom, such as anxiety or depression.

THIRD STEP

To carry out the third step in the process of conceptual model selection—the systematic analysis and evaluation of several models—the book *Analysis and Evaluation of Conceptual Models of Nursing* (Fawcett, 1995) should be consulted. The text includes comprehensive analyses and evaluations of seven nursing models; they are summarized in Table 35–1.

FOURTH AND FIFTH STEPS

Regarding the fourth step (comparing the philosophic claims of a conceptual model with one's own beliefs and values), the philosophic claims are identified during the analysis described in step 3. Similarly, identify-ing the appropriate models for nursing with a particular patient population (step 5) may be accomplished during step 3.

SIXTH STEP

After a model is selected (step 6), it is used to guide practice with several patients. If it is found that the model is not useful, another model is selected and its utility determined.

Initially, using a conceptual nursing model may seem forced or awkward. Adopting a model requires using a new vocabulary and restructuring how one thinks about nursing situations. Repeated use of the model, however, should lead to more systematic and organized applications. Broncatello's (1980) comments are encouraging for those starting to use a conceptual model for psychiatric mental health nursing practice. She stated:

> The nurse's consistent use of any model for the interpretation of observable [patient] data is most definitely not an easy task. Much like the development of any habitual behavior, it initially requires thought, discipline and the gradual evolvement of a mind set of what is important to observe within the guidelines of the model. As is true of most habits, however, it makes decision making less complicated. (p. 23)

O AN OVERVIEW

- Three conceptual models that are particularly useful for psychiatric mental health nursing practice are Johnson's Behavioral System Model, Neuman's Systems Model, and Roy's Adaptation Model.

- Each conceptual model presents a unique focus that has a profound influence on a nurse's way of thinking about patients, their environments, and health-related events and situations.

- The distinctive vocabulary of every conceptual model has been carefully selected to convey the meaning of that particular perspective.

- The most tangible benefit of using a conceptual model of nursing is its delineation of goals for nursing practice.

- Although initially using a conceptual model of nursing may seem forced or awkward, repeated use should lead to more systematic and organized applications of the model.

TD TERMS TO DEFINE

- conceptual model
- Johnson's Behavioral System Model
    - achievement subsystem
    - aggressive subsystem
    - attachment subsystem
    - dependency subsystem
    - eliminative subsystem
    - ingestive subsystem
    - sexual subsystem
    - action
    - choice
    - drive or goal
    - Patient Classification Instrument (PCI)
    - set
- Neuman's Systems Model
    - client system
    - flexible line of defense
    - created environment
    - external environment
    - internal environment
    - interpersonal and extrapersonal stressors
    - intrapersonal stressors
    - lines of resistance
    - normal line of defense
- Roy's Adaptation Model
    - humanism
    - veritivity
    - mechanisms
        - cognator
        - regulator
    - response modes
        - interdependence
        - physiological
        - role function
        - self-concept
    - responses
        - adaptive
        - ineffective
    - stimuli
        - contextual
        - residual
        - focal

Q STUDY QUESTIONS

Johnson's Behavioral System Model

1. According to Johnson, system and subsystem balance and stability are equivalent to
    a. high level system function.
    b. structural alignment of elements.
    c. orderliness.
    d. efficient and effective behavior.

2. In Johnson's model, the only structural element that is directly observable is
    a. drive or goal.
    b. set.
    c. choice.
    d. behavior or action.

3. The onset of puberty may create an imbalance in which behavioral subsystem?
    a. Dependency
    b. Sexual
    c. Achievement
    d. Attachment

4. Eating disorders represent an imbalance in which behavioral subsystem?
    a. Sexual
    b. Eliminative
    c. Ingestive
    d. Achievement

5. Bob Scott is a 16-year-old patient on the psychiatric unit. He has expressed suicidal thoughts to several people. The nursing care plan, which requires a nurse to be with Bob at all times, reflects application of which functional requirement?
    a. Nurturance
    b. Protection
    c. Stimulation
    d. Choice

Neuman's Systems Model

6. Neda Zelana is a 40-year-old secretary who works in a large corporate office. During her visit to the office clinic nurse, she states that she rarely gets up from her desk and that her back hurts by noon almost every day. Work demands that require prolonged sitting are which kind of stressor?
    a. Intrapersonal
    b. Interpersonal
    c. Extrapersonal

7. When asked by the office clinic nurse how things are going at home, Ms. Zelana (question 1) mentions that she and her 16-year-old daughter have frequent arguments. The arguments are which kind of stressor?

    a. Intrapersonal
    b. Interpersonal
    c. Extrapersonal

8. Paul Solomon is a 65-year-old widower who lives with his daughter, son-in-law, and two teenaged grandsons. He has been especially quiet recently and acts depressed. Depression represents instability in which type of variable?

    a. Physiological
    b. Psychological
    c. Sociocultural
    d. Developmental
    e. Spiritual

9. Mr. Solomon's daughter brings him to the local mental health clinic. The initial plan of nursing care for Mr. Solomon would emphasize which kind of intervention?

    a. Primary prevention
    b. Secondary prevention
    c. Tertiary prevention

10. This morning, Allison Banks left her husband, who has been verbally abusive to her for several years. She and her 3-year-old son have just come to the women's shelter in their suburban community. As the "shelter nurse," your assessment of Allison includes which of the following numbered variables?

    1. Physiological
    2. Psychological
    3. Sociocultural
    4. Developmental
    5. Spiritual

    a. 2,3
    b. 1,4
    c. 2,5
    d. 1,2,3,4,5

Roy's Adaptation Model

Questions 11 and 12 pertain to the following statement: Breast cancer support groups are based on the proposition that increased social support facilitates adaptation.

11. When viewed from the perspective of the Roy Adaptation Model, increased social support could be regarded as the management of which type of stimulus?

    a. Focal
    b. Contextual
    c. Residual

12. When viewed from the perspective of the Roy Adaptation Model, the age and family situation of each support group participant could be regarded as which kind of stimuli?

    a. Focal
    b. Contextual
    c. Residual

13. Rod Longstreet, who is 17 years old, is brought to the emergency room at a major trauma center with a gun shot wound to the abdomen. Which response mode should be assessed first?

    a. Physiological
    b. Self-concept
    c. Role function
    d. Interdependence

14. During his recovery, Rod (question 3) tells you that he has been "dealing drugs," but has decided to go back to school and "get away from the drugs." Rod's decision reflects a change in which response mode?

    a. Physiological
    b. Self-concept
    c. Role function
    d. Interdependence

15. A comprehensive nursing assessment reveals that Rod (questions 3 and 4) requires help making sound judgments and solving problems. The results of the assessment indicate the ineffectiveness of which coping mechanism?

    a. Regulator
    b. Cognator

Essay Questions

16. Select one conceptual model of nursing. List the model's concepts that describe the person. Select one of those concepts and describe how you would assess a patient with the psychiatric diagnosis of bipolar disorder.

17. Select one conceptual model of nursing. Outline the interventions that are consistent with that model. Discuss the application of one intervention with a patient with the psychiatric diagnosis of post-traumatic stress disorder.

■ REFERENCES

Akinsanya JA. Introduction. *Recent Adv Nurs* 1989; 24:i–ii.

Auger JR, Dee V. A patient classification system based on the behavioral system model of nursing: Part I. *J Nurs Admin* 1983; 13(4):38–43.

Baker NA. The Neuman systems model as a conceptual framework for continuing education in the work place. In: Neuman B. *The Neuman Systems Model: Application to Nursing Education and Practice.* Norwalk, Conn: Appleton-Century-Crofts; 1982:260–264.

Beitler B, Tkachuck B, Aamodt D. The Neuman model applied to mental health, community health, and medical-surgical nursing. In: Riehl JP, Roy C, eds. *Conceptual Models for Nursing Practice*. 2nd ed. New York: Appleton-Century-Crofts; 1980:170–178.

Biley F. Wordly wise. *Nursing (London)* 1990; 4(24):37.

Broncatello KF. Auger in action: Application of the model. *Adv Nurs Science* 1980; 2(2):13–23.

Burton A, ed. *Operational Theories of Personality*. New York: Brunner/Mazel; 1974.

Clark J. Development of models and theories on the concept of nursing. *J Adv Nurs* 1982; 7:129–134.

Coleman PM. Depression during the female climacteric period. *J Adv Nurs* 1993; 18:1540–1546.

Craig DM, Morris-Coulter C. Neuman implementation in a Canadian psychiatric facility. In: Neuman B. *The Neuman Systems Model*. 3rd ed. Norwalk, Conn: Appleton and Lange; 1995:397–406.

Davies P. In Wales: Use of the Neuman systems model by community psychiatric nurses. In: Neuman B. *The Neuman Systems Model*. 2nd ed. Norwalk, Conn: Appleton and Lange; 1989:375–384.

Dee V. Implementation of the Johnson model: One hospital's experience. In: Parker ME, ed. *Nursing Theories in Practice*. New York: National League for Nursing; 1990:33–44.

Dee V, Auger JA. A patient classification system based on the behavioral system model of nursing: Part 2. *J Nurs Admin* 1983; 13(5):18–23.

Drapela VJ. *A Review of Personality Theories*. 2nd ed. Springfield, Ill: Thomas; 1995.

Fawcett J. *Analysis and Evaluation of Conceptual Models of Nursing*. 3rd ed. Philadelphia: Davis; 1995.

Frank LK. Science as a communication process. *Main Curr Mod Thought* 1968; 25:45–50.

Frederickson K. Using a nursing model to manage symptoms: Anxiety and the Roy adaptation model. *Holistic Nurs Pract* 1993; 7(2):36–43.

Goldblum-Graff D, Graff H. The Neuman model adapted to family therapy. In: Neuman B. *The Neuman Systems Model: Application to Nursing Education and Practice*. Norwalk, Conn: Appleton-Century-Crofts; 1982:217–222.

Hall CS, Lindzey G. *Theories of Personality*. New York: John Wiley & Sons; 1957.

Hamer BA. Music therapy: Harmony for change. *J Psychosocial Nurs Mental Health Services* 1991; 29(12):5–7.

Herrick CA, Goodykoontz L. Neuman's systems model for nursing practice as a conceptual framework for a family assessment. *J Child Adolescent Psychiatric Mental Health Nurs* 1989; 2:61–67.

Herrick CA, Goodykoontz L, Herrick RH, Hackett B. Planning a continuum of care in child psychiatric nursing: A collaborative effort. *J Child Adolescent Psychiatric Mental Health Nurs* 1991;4:41–48.

Johnson DE. Guest editorial: Evaluating conceptual models for use in critical care nursing practice. *Dimen Crit Care Nurs* 1987;6:195–197.

Johnson DE. The behavioral system model for nursing. In: Parker ME, ed. *Nursing Theories in Practice*. New York: National League for Nursing; 1990:23–32.

King IM. King's conceptual framework and theory of goal attainment. In: Parker ME, ed. *Nursing Theories in Practice*. New York: National League for Nursing; 1990:73–84.

Kurek-Ovshinsky C. Group psychotherapy in an acute inpatient setting: Techniques that nourish self-esteem. *Iss Mental Health Nurs* 1991; 12:81–88.

Lachman VD. *Communication Skills for Effective Interpersonal Relations*. Concurrent ses-

sion presented at the American Nephrology Nurses Association 24th National Symposium. Orlando, Fla; 1993, June.

Leonard, C. (1975). Patient attitudes toward nursing interventions. *Nursing Research, 24*, 335–339.

Levine ME. The conservation principles: A model for health. In: Schaefer KM, Pond JB, eds. *Levine's Conservation Model: A Framework for Nursing Practice*. Philadelphia: Davis; 1991:1–11.

Lewis C, Randell BP. Alteration in self-care: An instance of ineffective coping in the geriatric patient. In: Carroll-Johnson RM, ed. *Classification of Nursing Diagnoses: Proceedings of the Ninth Conference: North American Nursing Diagnosis Association*. Philadelphia: Lippincott; 1991:264–265.

Miller, F. (1991). Using Roy's model in a special hospital. *Nursing Standard, 5*(27):29–32.

Moore SL, Munro MF. The Neuman systems model applied to mental health nursing of older adults. *J Adv Nurs* 1990; 15:293–299.

Neuman B. *The Neuman Systems Model*. 3rd ed. Norwalk, Conn: Appleton and Lange; 1995.

Orem DE. *Nursing: Concepts of Practice*. 5th ed. St. Louis: Mosby Year Book; 1995.

Poster EC. Behavioral category ratings of adolescents on an inpatient psychiatric unit: The use of the Johnson behavioral system model [Abstract]. In: Brackston A, Cooper-Pagé L, Edwards S, Light M, Cardinal S, Du Gas B, Hinds C, McNamara M, eds. *Proceedings: Putting it All Together*. Ottawa, Ontario, Canada: University of Ottawa; 1989:99.

Randell BP. NANDA versus the Johnson behavioral systems model: Is there a diagnostic difference? In: Carroll-Johnson RM, ed. *Classification of Nursing Diagnoses: Proceedings of the Ninth Conference: North American Nursing Diagnosis Association*. Philadelphia: Lippincott; 1991:154–160.

Robitaille-Tremblay M. A data collection tool for the psychiatric nurse. *The Canadian Nurse* 1984; 80(7):26–28.

Rogers ME. Nursing: Science of unitary, irreducible, human beings: Update 1990. In: Barrett EAM, ed. *Visions of Rogers' Science-based Nursing*. New York: National League for Nursing; 1990:5–11.

Roy C. An explication of the philosophical assumptions of the Roy adaptation model. *Nursing Science Quarterly* 1988; 1:26–34.

Roy C, Andrews HA. *The Roy adaptation model: The definitive statement*. Norwalk, Conn: Appleton and Lange; 1991.

Roy C, Roberts SL. *Theory Construction in Nursing: An Adaptation Model*. Englewood Cliffs, NJ: Prentice-Hall; 1981.

Schmidt CS. Withdrawal behavior of schizophrenics: Application of Roy's model. *J Psychosocial Nurs Mental Health Services* 1981; 19(11):26–33.

Scicchitani B, Cox JG, Heyduk LJ, Maglicco PA, Sargent NA. Implementing the Neuman model in a psychiatric hospital. In: Neuman B. *The Neuman Systems Model*. 3rd ed. Norwalk, Conn: Appleton and Lange; 1995:387–395.

Stuart GW, Wright LK. Applying the Neuman systems model to psychiatric nursing practice. In: Neuman B. *The Neuman Systems Model*. 3rd ed. Norwalk, Conn: Appleton and Lange; 1995:263–273.

Verberk F. In Holland: Application of the Neuman model in psychiatric nursing. In: Neuman B. *The Neuman Systems Model*. 3rd ed. Norwalk, Conn: Appleton and Lange; 1995:629–636.

Waddell KL, Demi AS. Effectiveness of an intensive partial hospitalization program for treatment of anxiety disorders. *Arch Psych Nurs* 1993;7:2–10.

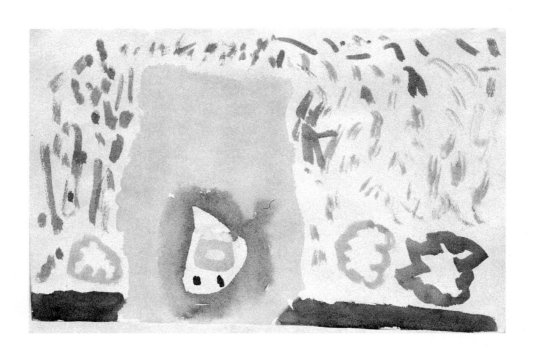

There never were in the world two opinions alike, no more than two hairs or two grains; the most universal quality is diversity.

Michel Eyquem de Montaigne (1533–1592)

Essays, book III

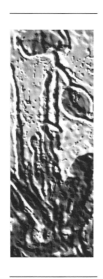

36
Therapeutic Nurse–Patient Relationship

Margaret P. Shepard

Psychiatric nursing involves the therapeutic use of self in the care of individuals experiencing distress. Use of self therapeutically requires knowledge of self, as well as a mastery of the therapeutic relationship (Armstrong and Kelly, 1993; Holden, 1991). Therapeutic use of self is the process by which the nurse draws on his or her unique interpersonal skills in a thoughtful fashion to assist the patient to achieve health. The therapeutic relationship is based on the assumption that each person has an innate drive toward health. It is the process that uses the nurse to motivate the patient to desire healing and healthy behaviors. In the context of the therapeutic relationship, the nurse provides information, empathy, nondirective listening, respect, and feedback as an actual treatment modality (Peplau, 1952). The patient, in turn, experiences the therapeutic relationship as an opportunity to address and redress the sources of his or her distress.

The mutual drive toward health is exemplified within the therapeutic relationship by the case example of a psychiatric nurse, Michelle, and a patient, Simon, who was recently admitted into the day hospital program. Simon has had a long-standing pattern of depression and suicidal ideation related to his history of abuse and abandonment as a child. He describes himself as "unworthy, unlovable, stupid trash." In the context of their therapeutic relationship, Michelle and Simon identify low self-esteem as a problem. To address this problem, Michelle helps Simon see his strengths as she and others see them: his wry sense of humor, the way he expresses concern for his peers, his attention to detail, and his respect for others. Simon's ability to recognize his strengths initiated the process that allowed him to change his self-concept.

The therapeutic nurse-patient relationship also includes sanctions for professional nursing care, a philosophy of nursing, and the context for patient growth. Professional nursing care embodies thoughtful, deliberate goals, as well as attitudes and actions of concern for individuals and groups to support their well-being. In psychiatric nursing, care is further distinguished by acceptance of the person as he or she is, focusing on the here and now, remaining nonjudgmental, and recognizing the person's uniqueness and potential for growth and self-actualization (Hosking, 1993). The therapeutic relationship provides the framework for nursing care. It is a dynamic process in which the patient and nurse become oriented toward one another. With the help of the nurse, the patient learns to identify problems, exploit resources, and resolve distress. Hildegard Peplau first described the nurse-patient therapeutic relationship in 1952. She described four phases: orientation, identification, exploitation, and resolution. Each phase is characterized by overlapping purposes for the nurse and patient. This landmark nursing theory is as applicable in the twenty-first century as it was in the middle of the twentieth century.

■ ORIENTATION

The orientation phase of the nurse–patient relationship is the beginning phase of the process in which the patient and nurse engage with each other to form their ongoing relationship. It is during this phase that the patients learn what to expect from the nurse, as well as what is expected of them. This phase may be as short as one meeting or may never be completed depending on the patient's previous experience with health care professionals and his or her ability to trust and collaborate. The goal of orientation is for the nurse and patient to become acquainted with one another and assist the patient to identify seeking help as a learning process. Viewing the stage of seeking help as a dynamic learning experience can lead to personal and social growth for both the patient and nurse. Patients may initially view their illness, and the need for help, as a failure of self due to a character deficit or weakness. It is for this reason that it is essential for the patient to acquire the perception of their illness and the need for help as a learning process. When the need for help is viewed in this mode, the patient can actively pursue the appropriate knowledge in the learning process. The problem becomes one of a knowledge deficit rather than a personal or characterological deficit. For example, the patient experiencing difficulty coping with numerous stressors will view their experience as a need to learn about alternate coping strategies, rather than as a personal failure in coping. The orientation phase begins when the patient seeks assistance on the basis of a felt need in relation to a health crisis.

The individual may be aware of changes in his or her mental health. This person will be in a position to plan for and choose mental health services. Alternatively, the patient may be experiencing a major mental illness crisis or a psychiatric emergency. This person may be aware of the need for assistance but, in all likelihood, will not have the capacity to seek assistance independently. He or she may seek assistance through the support of a family member, a friend, or the police. Expressed needs should be interpreted as educative needs. What does the patient need to know about the present situation in order to resolve the crisis and to develop adaptive or productive ways of coping with present and future situations? Often the patient provides clues to how he or she visualizes needs. For example, a patient with bulimia might view the problem as being unable to stop the habit of binging and purging. Such clues provide opportunities for the nurse to recognize gaps in information and understanding. The nurse, in turn, may be able to assist the patient to learn about the function of the bulimic symptoms in relation to the patient's coping, perception of self, and family relationships.

FROM INITIAL CONTACT

The nurse enters the orientation phase of the therapeutic relationship at the point of contact with the patient. Into this encounter, the nurse brings all of his or her prior knowledge, previous experiences, attitudes, and feelings. How the nurse feels about helping others can make a great difference in the outcome for the patient. Nurses may have many different feelings about giving help, and many different factors arising from the situation, the patient, or the nurse may influence those feelings. For example, some people believe that a person with mental illness became that way because of laziness, lack of discipline, or an unwillingness to help themselves. Such beliefs would certainly influence a nurse's ability to effectively care for patients with mental illness. Similarly, the patient with poor self-care skills may present with a strong body odor, and the nurse may form a negative opinion about the patient based on his or her physical presentation.

On the other hand, some patients may have had negative or unpleasant encounters with helping professionals in the past, and this patient may have difficulty engaging in a relationship with a nurse based on past experiences. The learning process can be enhanced for the nurse as well when he or she takes the time to reflect on those feelings, prior to engaging a patient, during the relationship, and at the resolution of the relationship. During orientation and throughout the relationship, four interlocking nursing functions may operate. The nurse may function in the role of resource person, counselor, technical expert, and surrogate.

A Resource Person

Helping the patient to identify needs and the resources available to meet those needs is a paramount function in the orientation phase. First, the patient needs to feel safe in the environment, whether it is in an in-patient hospital setting, a clinic, or a day hospital program. The nurse facilitates the patient's efforts to feel safe by orienting them to the environment. Specifically, the patient needs to know about where he or she is, the rules and routine of the setting, and the rights and responsibilities of the patient role. Further, the patient needs to know, well in advance, about any procedures, tests, or meetings in which the patient is expected to participate. This is essential to gain the patient's informed consent.

Second, the patient needs to recognize and understand the crisis he or she is experiencing and the extent of his or her need for help. Helping the patient to become oriented to his or her identified problem can be a challenging experience for the nurse. The nurse serves as a resource person by conveying specific information about how the patient is functioning and by helping the patient to see relations to symptoms that accompany the illness. The nurse engages the patient as an active partner in identifying and assessing the presenting problems.

Counselor

Often, during the phase of orientation, the patient is not completely ready to disclose difficult underlying issues related to the current crisis. For example, a patient with a history of sexual abuse is not likely to discuss this information until he or she is confident of the trust in the context of the therapeutic relationship. The nurse who responds unconditionally, while assisting the patient to focus on the problem, permits the patient to express his or her feelings and develop increased awareness about what those feelings are. Often, in the orientation phase, the nurse may feel compelled to want to say something to make the patient feel better. It is important for the nurse to remember that the focus is on encouraging the patient to identify and express his or her feelings. "Advice, reassurance, suggestion, persuasion are of little value when offered in connection with feelings" (Peplau, 1952, p. 28). The focus, for the nurse and patient, in this stage of the relationship is to gain an understanding of the situation as it is seen by the patient. Enhanced understanding of the situation as it is seen by the patient will lead to the possibility of voluntary control and effective nursing actions.

Technical Expert

The role of the nurse as a technical expert is somewhat different in psychiatric nursing than it is in other nursing settings. The psychiatric nurse generally uses fewer pieces of technical equipment in the care of patients. Nonetheless, the role of technical expert is still an essential component of psychiatric caring, especially in relation to increased understanding of the biological correlates of mental illness. During the orientation phase, the nurse may function as a technical expert in relation to diagnostic testing, preparing the patient for an electroencephalogram, a magnetic resonance imaging scan, or other diagnostic procedures. Technical procedures may also be involved in treatments, such as electroconvulsive therapy. The role of technical expert will include the need to educate the patient about other aspects of treatment, including medications, changes in diet related to medication, stress management techniques, or helping the patient to resume activities of daily living.

Surrogate

The role of surrogate is often enacted through the unconscious dynamic processes of **transference** and **countertransference.** Transference occurs when the patient projects onto the nurse feelings, thoughts, or wishes held about another person, such as a family member or another person in authority. Projected feelings may involve past or current relationships. The feelings involved in the process of transference are often intense and can be either positive or negative.

Countertransference is an unconscious response on the part of the nurse to projected content from the patient. In the example below, if Martha were to respond to James in a motherly fashion, these actions would represent countertransference. On the other hand, in her interactions with James, Martha could have acted out some of the negative feelings she holds about substance abusers because of her own experience of growing up in an alcoholic family. Countertransference also includes all of the feelings, both positive and negative, the nurse may hold in relation to the patient.

Transference and countertransference are naturally occurring processes. They can, however, seriously impede the development of the therapeutic relationship. Recall that psychiatric nursing care requires that the nurse focus on the here and now, remain nonjudg-

E CASE EXAMPLE

James, who is 28 years old, had a close and loving relationship with his mother until she died when he was 8 years old. Recently, he was admitted to a day hospital program for treatment of schizophrenia. In this program, the patients usually interact with many different staff members throughout the day. James, however, begins to show a marked preference for Martha, a nurse 20 years his senior. He chooses to speak exclusively with her, begins writing her "private" notes, and offers her small gifts. On Martha's days off, James prefers not to speak with any of the other staff members. The staff is aware of James' family history and soon recognizes that he has transferred the feelings he once held for his mother onto the nurse Martha.

mental, and recognize the uniqueness of each person. Enacting past relationships, whether consciously or unconsciously, takes the therapeutic relationship out of the present tense; it denies the unique quality of the patient, and may invoke judgments that are not appropriate in the therapeutic context.

A WORKING UNDERSTANDING

Toward the end of the orientation phase, the patient and nurse will have developed a working understanding of the presenting concerns. The level of understanding will be reflected in the nursing diagnoses and the interdisciplinary treatment plan. In addition, the patient will have some knowledge about what the treatment situation can offer to help him or her learn more about the illness and related needs. This phase may be very brief, or it may linger for months, especially for patients experiencing transference issues or for those having difficulty trusting due to the nature of their illnesses. (See Research Highlight.)

■ IDENTIFICATION

Following successful orientation to the illness experience and the treatment process, the patient may indicate that he or she feels stronger and less helpless. The patient will begin to selectively respond to persons who offer help. Peplau (1952) labeled this phase "identification" because of the unconscious process of identification that occurs between the patient and nurse. Identification is considered an ego defense mechanism wherein one person assumes the attitudes and behaviors of an authority or parent figure. In the close nurse–patient therapeutic relationship, the patient may aspire to the strengths and healthy traits of the nurse. As the nurse role models effective problem solving or expression of feeling, the patient identifies with those traits. The patient will, in turn, demonstrate more effective problem solving and expression of feelings.

The process of identification is natural and reasonable; however, it may evoke some unsettling feelings for the nurse to know that his or her behavior is being so closely examined and incorporated into the actions of another. In any treatment setting, professional nursing can be emotionally complicated. It requires the nurse to be meaningfully related to the patient, yet separate enough to distinguish one's own feelings and needs. It is essential for the nurse to preserve self while caring for others. Preservation of self occurs when the nurse is able to maintain well-defined boundaries between the nurse and patient. Boundaries refer to where self leaves off and the other person begins (Barnsteiner and Gillis-Donavan, 1990; Jerome, 1992). They help give nurses a

RESEARCH HIGHLIGHT

In American and Canadian surveys, Peplau's theory has been identified by at least half of the psychiatric nursing samples as the theory that guides their practice. Although, Peplau's theory has been widely used in practice, it has not been empirically tested through research. The purpose of this nursing investigation (Forchuk, 1994) was to test Peplau's theory regarding influences during the orientation phase of the nurse–patient relationship.

Previous research has indicated that the initial phase of the nurse–patient relationship significantly influences treatment outcomes for patients with severe and persistent mental illness. Difficulty in establishing therapeutic relationships has been related to poor treatment outcomes. When a good alliance was not established in the first 6 months of treatment, it was unlikely to develop at all. The length of the orientation phase has been linked to the patient's previous hospitalization pattern. Severely and persistently mentally ill patients who took longer in the orientation phase also tended to have longer hospitalizations. Thus, the orientation phase is a clinically significant phase of treatment for the patient with chronic mental illness. Information about nurse and patient contributions to the orientation phase may ultimately lead to improved patient outcomes.

This study focused on nurse and patient variables measured at the beginning of the relationship that were expected to be related to the development of the therapeutic relationship. Independent variables in this study included nurse preconceptions of the patient, patient preconceptions of the nurse, characteristics of nurse and patient interpersonal relationships with others, and patient and nurse levels of anxiety. Dependent variables in this study included the relationship form (a measure of nurse and patient behaviors at each phase of the relationship) and the Working Alliance Inventory (a measure of the nurse's and the patient's perceptions of the bonds, goals, and tasks within the evolving therapeutic relationship).

The research sample consisted of 124 newly formed nurse–patient pairs. Pairs were interviewed at the beginning of the study and at 3 months and 6 months into the nurse–patient relationship.

Results of this research provided support for the importance of the role of the nurse and the role of the patient for the evolving therapeutic relationship. Preconceptions of both the nurse and the patient were most strongly related to the development of the therapeutic relationship. Patient's other interpersonal relationships contributed to the working alliance. Neither nurse nor patient levels of anxiety were related to progress in the relationship. The finding that both the nurse's and the patient's preconceptions were significant is supportive of an interpersonal approach. Peplau's theory recognizes that the nurse must use awareness of self and self-reflection as vigilantly as assessment of the patient situation.

sense of who they are and promote the patient's control over the illness experience. For example, the nurse demonstrates effective boundaries when she or he recognizes at the end of the shift that it is time to go home and attend to personal needs. Ineffective boundaries are demonstrated when the nurse stays with the patient beyond the shift, serving the patient's needs rather than the needs of the nurse or the treatment setting.

The nurse maintains well-defined boundaries through periodic review of the therapeutic relationship, both with the patient and with the interdisciplinary treatment team. The nurse should observe and ask the patient about preconceptions of nurses and nursing. This will facilitate the patient's ability to make use of the therapeutic relationship as each comes to know and respect the other as persons who have likes and differences of opinions. Similarly, interdisciplinary treatment team reviews provide opportunities to assess progress toward established goals. The team may also provide feedback that the nurse is making use of professional education and skills in aiding the patient to achieve health.

Patients in the phase of identification will begin to experience some clarity about their needs and perceptions. With increased comfort in the treatment setting, some patients may identify and explore some feelings of which their culture does not ordinarily approve. A patient may express some powerful feelings, such as anger, helplessness, dependency, self-centeredness, and grief. Although these feelings may be distressing for all who experience them, the role of the nurse in this phase of identification is to permit the patient to express what he or she feels and still receive caring professional attention. The nurse's acceptance of the patient's expression of feelings will promote the patient's acceptance of self as he or she learns about those feelings and eventually learns how to manage them effectively. In the role of counselor or surrogate, the nurse quietly listens and facilitates the expression of feeling. As a resource person or technical expert, the nurse can aid the patient to identify means for managing those feelings. For example, when the patient expresses intense feelings of anger, the nurse might suggest writing in a journal, hitting a punching bag, or talking to a supportive friend as a means to master the anger. Once the patient is able to trust the experience of the nurse–patient relationship, the patient will be able to challenge other negative feelings and perceptions of self.

DIFFICULTIES WITH IDENTIFICATION

Some patients will have more difficulty moving into the phase of identification in the therapeutic relationship. This may be due to symptoms of the illness or to earlier traumatic relationship experiences. Patients may not feel worthy of care and may isolate themselves, resisting nursing efforts toward engagement in the therapeutic relationship. Most resistances represent the patients' defenses against their feelings of discomfort (Shea, 1988). When the patient fears a loss of control, he or she may show discomfort in the form of angry resistance. Patients demonstrate resistance in many unique ways. Some examples include coming to meetings late, not completing tasks that were previously negotiated, or challenging the professional role of the nurse.

Some patients will guard against identification by maintaining an angry negative facade. The threatened patient will not sit easily with the nurse in a one-to-one conversation. The nurse, however, can creatively facilitate the therapeutic relationship with the resistant patient by engaging the patient in routine care. The nurse might assist the patient with activities of daily living or

E CASE EXAMPLE

Natasha, a 15-year-old girl, is being treated on an in-patient adolescent unit for a 2-year history of bulimia and substance abuse. She is making good progress in her treatment, learning to identify and manage her feelings without the numbing effects of marijuana and without binging and vomiting. One evening she is anticipating a visit from her parents; however, they do not arrive at the anticipated time. Forty-five minutes after their expected arrival, her primary nurse finds Natasha vomiting in the bathroom. Rather than talking about her anxiety and disappointment over her parents' lateness, Natasha resorts to an earlier coping behavior—vomiting. Although the nurse can readily interpret Natasha's actions, she recognizes that telling Natasha what she has done will not help Natasha learn from this situation. Instead, they find a quiet room and sit down and talk. The nurse, through her gentle questioning and the trust they established in the context of their therapeutic relationship, helps Natasha to identify the feelings that led to her vomiting. Eventually, Natasha is able to identify that many of her bulimic episodes are preceded by feelings similar to the ones she experienced that evening. Natasha and the nurse work out a plan for Natasha to talk to one of the nurses rather than vomiting when she feels anxious or despondent.

participate with the patient in diversional activities. Accompanying a patient to a diagnostic procedure can do a lot toward facilitating trust in the relationship. Patients identify with nurses on the basis of services that are recognized as useful. Identification is noted when the patient responds selectively to persons who offer the help that he or she needs, and the professional nurse may offer help in many different forms. The focus of the help, however, is always to assist the patient in developing feelings of being related to others in ways that allow expression of underlying needs and wishes (Peplau, 1952).

Some patients will identify with the nurse, not on the basis of the present helping behavior, but rather on the basis of the patient's past experiences. In such cases, the presentation, actions, and gestures of the nurse will be evaluated in terms of a symbolic past relationship. Identification on the basis of past relationships reinforces the patient's fixed repertoire of coping responses and allows for little learning or growth. Ultimately, it undermines the success of the therapeutic relationship. In order for the patient to effectively learn about his or her illness experience, he or she must be able to identify and focus on the events in the current treatment situation. Moreover, the patient must be able to identify treatment issues through his or her own efforts and eventually to develop responses to them independently of the nurse. The nurse facilitates this process by assessing the patient's responses and gently providing feedback about them.

■ EXPLOITATION

The phase of exploitation is considered the true working phase of the relationship. Once the patient and nurse have sufficiently learned about the other as unique individuals in a therapeutic relationship, the patient is ready to make full use of the available resources. Peplau called this phase "exploitation" because the patient takes advantage of all of the goods and services available. Exploitation occurs on the basis of self-interest and need as the patient explores all of the possibilities of the changing situation.

The phase of exploitation can be noted in terms of the nursing process when the patient begins to demonstrate goal-oriented behavior. For example, the goal for Mr. Jones was to spend 10 minutes each day talking to his primary nurse about treatment-related issues. For the first several days of treatment, the nurse needed to seek out Mr. Jones to facilitate his achieving the treatment goal. Soon Mr. Jones came to identify with his primary nurse as one whom he could trust, and he started to seek her out for their daily meetings. Mr. Jones' self-

directed, goal-oriented behavior indicated that the phase of exploitation had been reached in the therapeutic relationship.

The quality of the exploitation phase of the relationship will depend on features of the nurse and patient, as well as the goals and setting of treatment. Some patients with greater interpersonal strengths, or less severe illness, will exercise more independence in the phase of exploitation than other patients with more enduring crises. The independent patient may pursue treatment goals, identify new and related issues, and acknowledge progress toward goals with few cues or urgings from the nurse. This patient may occasionally check in with the nurse to inform him or her about progress made. Some patients may need more guidance and feedback from the nurse in order to pursue treatment goals. Dynamics of the interaction between the nurse and patient should be a negotiated component of the treatment plan. It is helpful for the nurse to discuss candidly with the patient how they can best work together. The nurse can offer feedback to the patient about how he or she seems to use treatment resources most effectively. Part of the learning process for the patient includes identifying issues and how to ask for assistance.

The quality of the work that takes place in the exploitation phase also depends on the work that has occurred in the previous stages of the relationship. Exploitation, or making use of treatment resources, also takes place during the orientation and identification phases. Similarly, exploitation continues through the phase of resolution and after treatment has ended. Exploitive behavior is characterized by an intermingling of needs and testing of new behaviors. The role for the nurse, in this phase of the relationship, is to facilitate exploitive learning whenever possible. The illness experience provides cues for exploitive learning. The nurse might encourage the patient to try new problem-solving skills, or the nurse might assist the patient to identify alternative resources that might be helpful. An additional function of the nurse during the phase of exploitation is to encourage the patient to develop insight into past behaviors through the application of newly learned skills. In the case example of Natasha, the nurse helped the patient to apply a new behavior (talking) in the current situation, and she helped Natasha see that many of her past binging episodes were precipitated by similar feelings of despondency and anxiety.

Peplau (1952) likened this phase of the relationship to the phase of adolescent development in which a need for some dependence remains but the individual is exercising new skills of independence. Just as for the parent of the adolescent, the challenge for the nurse is to assist the patient to balance the opposing needs safely and effectively. In the role of counselor, the nurse can talk with the patient about the opposing needs demonstrated by the patient. Together, the nurse and patient can explore the meaning of these needs and develop a plan of action in response to the expressed needs.

The phase of exploitation may also stir some opposing feelings and needs for the nurse. The nurse may experience intense pride as the patient successfully exercises increased independence. Occasionally, the nurse may also experience feelings of ambivalence. Conflicting feelings may arise from loss of role clarity as the patient's need for support from the nurse diminishes. They may also arise from the desire to protect the patient from anxiety and potential harm. It is helpful for the nurse to acknowledge these feelings as natural and identify their meaning both personally and in the context of the therapeutic relationship. Nurses do experience many conflicting feelings in relation to their patients but acting on them would only impede the progress of the therapeutic relationship. When the feelings persist, it is helpful to discuss them with a trusted colleague.

■ RESOLUTION

The final phase of the therapeutic relationship is called resolution. The hallmark of this phase is termination of the relationship between the nurse and patient. It is signaled by the patient's imminent discharge from the treatment program or the meeting of the patient's goals. Termination of treatment is initiated at the start of treatment because it is something that is planned by the interdisciplinary team. The length of a hospital stay or a course of out-patient treatment is contingent on achievement of therapeutic goals. When treatment is initiated, it usually involves some specific planning about the duration of treatment. As such, resolution of the therapeutic relationship should be anticipated from the moment of orientation.

Resolution occurs on several levels for the patient. The acute crisis of the illness is resolved and gradually has become integrated into the patient's life experience. The nurse and patient can reflect on what they have learned from the patient's experience with the illness. On a very practical level, treatment is resolved and the patient prepares for life after treatment: planning for out-patient follow-up; medication; returning to home, work, or school; and planning to implement newly learned coping skills.

Resolution also occurs on a psychological level. "The stage of resolution implies the gradual freeing from identification with helping persons and the generation and strengthening of ability to stand more or less

alone" (Peplau, 1952). Freedom from identification is the outcome of unconditional acceptance when the emphasis in the therapeutic relationship has been on learning and growth.

The focus in this phase, for both the nurse and patient is often on saying good-bye and the physical preparation necessary for discharge from treatment. A measure of the patient's increased independence should include participation in planning for discharge. For example, the patient can make phone calls for follow-up treatment and returning to work. It is not unusual for some patients to experience increased anxiety in the phase of resolution. Anxiety may be related to the patient's lack of confidence in themselves and what they have learned about their illness. It may be manifest by the return of symptoms and increased reliance on the nursing staff. Return of symptoms can be disheartening and frightening for both the nurse and patient. When it occurs in this phase of the relationship, however, it is usually related to issues about discharge from treatment. It may be helpful to anticipate increased anxiety in this phase of the relationship and to encourage the patient to exercise new coping behaviors to manage anxiety. Success in this phase can serve to strengthen the patient's confidence in preparation for discharge.

Saying good-bye at the end of the therapeutic relationship can be an awkward and difficult time for both the nurse and patient. As such, it should not be left for the last moment. The nurse and patient should plan for enough time and a comfortable space to terminate their relationship. This is a time to review, synthesize, and consolidate all that has been learned about the individual patient's illness experience. The nurse might ask the patient "what has your experience with your illness taught you about yourself?" The patient should be encouraged to review perceived weaknesses, as well as new skills and insights. In turn, the nurse may choose to share what he or she has learned from the patient, possibly about such topics as perseverance, human spirit, or growth potential.

The patient may wish to express gratitude. Occasionally, patients will offer a gift or money in expression of gratitude. This should be discouraged. It is natural to want to offer something as an expression of gratitude but a concrete or monetary gift infers a burden of indebtedness that is not appropriate in a professional relationship. The patient should be encouraged to verbalize or write about their feelings, just as he or she did throughout the relationship. Similarly, the patient may ask to keep in touch with the nurse after the relationship has terminated. It may be tempting for the nurse to want to maintain contact with the patient as well. Some nurses will be anxious to hear about the patient's success. After working so intensely with the patient throughout the illness experience, some nurses may want to be available to support the patient if difficulties arise. Maintaining contact with the patient after termination conveys a subtle message of lack of confidence in the patient's independence. A nurse–patient relationship, after treatment has ended, is outside of the therapeutic context, and it is usually without the support of the interdisciplinary team. Finally, most treatment settings have a policy against such contact after discharge from treatment. Resolution is not achieved for either the nurse or the patient when contact is prolonged after treatment has ended. Peplau (1952) asked the following thought provoking questions about nursing actions in the phase of resolution.

What courses of action are required by nurses who wish patients to free themselves from dependency on others when crises have been met? Can a patient free himself when a nurse fixes all courses of action and evaluates attainment in these terms? Can a patient learn to free himself if every move has been managed by someone else? (p. 41)

■ THE ROLE OF THE NURSE IN THE THERAPEUTIC RELATIONSHIP

The role of the nurse, in relation to the patient experiencing a mental health crisis, reflects a dynamic balance between knowledge of the patient and knowledge of self. It incorporates sound therapeutic skills and creative use of self. Skills that specifically facilitate the therapeutic relationship include empathy and unconditional positive regard.

"Empathy is the ability to accurately recognize the immediate emotional perspective of another person while maintaining one's own perspective" (Shea, 1988, p. 14). That is, empathy involves the experience of the other's feelings without losing the experience of self. Carl Rogers (1974) first developed the concept of empathy in the context of the counseling relationship. Rogers distinguished empathy from the process of identification with the patient. When the therapeutic professional identifies with the patient, the professional not only recognizes the emotional state of the other but also feels the emotions of the other as if they were their own. Experiencing the patient's feelings at this level can lead to such therapeutic obstacles as burn out and unrecognized countertransference.

Empathy on the other hand, helps the nurse to understand the patient's needs without the loss of professional boundaries or skill. Empathy develops over the course of the therapeutic relationship. During the phase of orientation, the nurse may not have adequate knowledge of the patient to fully understand and empathize with his or her experience. As the nurse learns more about the patient as a unique individual, empathy is also likely to increase. Empathy facilitates the therapeutic relationship in that it conveys the additional message to the patient that his or her feelings are understood and accepted by a helping professional. The patient's trust in the nurse is likely to increase when there is empathetic understanding.

Unconditional positive regard is another skill that advances the therapeutic relationship. This involves relating to and accepting the patient with deep and genuine caring and without attaching conditions. Attached conditions might include moral judgments, relating from a position of power, or withholding care contingent on some behaviors of the patient. In many cases, patients who seek help bring with them some evocative issues, such as violence, rape, abortion, incest, different religious or sexual preferences, substance use, or legal entanglements. In the context of the therapeutic relationship, however, it is essential for the nurse to relate to the patient as another person deserving of care. Also, in the relationship, the nurse can explore with the patient the meaning of these issues in connection to his or her history and the current crisis.

Unconditional positive regard is essentially an attitude about participating in a therapeutic relationship. It is reflected in each of the actions made by the nurse on behalf of the patient. In order to relate from the position of genuine caring, it is important for the nurse periodically to identify and assess potentially disturbing responses to the patient's feelings and issues.

The case example of Melissa on page 656 demonstrates that a healthy knowledge of self is important for obtaining a therapeutic relationship (Jerome and Ferraro-McDuffie, 1992). Each individual comes into nursing with personal motivations, values, beliefs, and unresolved relational issues that can have repercussions for the therapeutic relationship. In addition, our self-concepts contribute to the ways in which a nurse and patient relate to one another (Hosking, 1993).

Self-concept develops as a result of interaction with the environment, society, and significant others. Self-concept, for all nurses, is to some degree defined by our role as nurses—as helping caring professionals. Although the neediness of patients is easily recognized in the health care setting, the need of nurses to be needed is often overlooked. When the patient responds well to the care provided by a nurse, the nurse will feel a sense of satisfaction. This kind of interaction contributes to a positive self-concept. On the other hand, when the patient does not respond to the care offered, it is important for the nurse to examine his or her need to be needed in the context of the therapeutic relationship. The nurse's need to be needed can unwittingly offset the balance in the relationship, resulting in amplification of the neediness and helplessness of the patient

E CASE EXAMPLE

Melissa has been working on an inpatient general psychiatric unit for 4 years. Her colleagues always regard her as a thoughtful and caring professional, and her patients usually respond well to her warm and accepting demeanor. Recently, Melissa was selected as the primary nurse to care for Richard, a 28-year-old gay man with a history of IV substance abuse. Richard was admitted for major depression following his recent diagnosis as HIV positive. Although Melissa thought she could care for Richard, just as she had her previous patients, she finds herself avoiding her daily contacts with him, making excuses, and finding reasons to be off the unit when they are scheduled to talk. Melissa recognizes her behavior but is not aware of the reason for it, so she asks to discuss it with the advanced practice nurse on the unit. Together, they are able to identify that Melissa blames Richard for his condition because of his lifestyle and high-risk behavior. Eventually, Melissa is able to recognize that Richard also blames himself for his condition and that this is probably contributing to his current depression. Melissa is then able to empathize with Richard; she recognizes the pain and the self-blame he is experiencing. From this position, she is able to care genuinely and deeply for her patient.

(Barnsteiner and Gillis-Donavan, 1990). The therapeutic relationship requires the nurse to be meaningfully related to the patient, yet separate enough to distinguish one's own feelings and needs.

Actions and feelings on the part of the nurse can inhibit or enhance the formation of a therapeutic relationship. When the nurse becomes aware that he or she is acting or thinking in ways that inhibit the relationship, the nurse needs to complete a self-assessment, taking stock of feelings and thoughts in relation to the patient. Does the patient remind the nurse of someone from the past? Does the patient remind the nurse of a previous patient who did not respond well to the nurse's effort to care? Does the patient remind the nurse of someone from his or her family of origin? It is always helpful for the nurse to examine the original feelings and to manage them effectively outside of the context of the therapeutic relationship. When the nurse identifies feelings that can inhibit the progress of the therapeutic relationship, the nurse should consult with peers or others for supervision in managing the feelings.

■ NURSING FACTORS THAT INHIBIT DEVELOPMENT OF THE THERAPEUTIC RELATIONSHIP

Many factors can inhibit the formation of a therapeutic relationship (Morse, 1991). Some factors are related to the nurse's thoughts and feelings. Some are a by-product of the treatment delivery system. In most cases, inhibiting factors can be regarded as a signal that the nurse consciously or unconsciously wishes to maintain some emotional distance in the therapeutic relationship. Often they occur because of tension or anxiety on the part of the nurse. Perhaps the nurse fears he or she cannot help the patient who presents with severe mental illness. Perhaps the nurse fears that the patient will respond with hostility to any caring efforts. Such signals can function as cues to implement remedial action.

DEPERSONALIZATION OF THE PATIENT

Depersonalization of the patient occurs when the patient is regarded as a diagnosis, a bed number, or a quirk of the illness. For example, one nurse referred to a patient with a fixed delusion that he was an alien space traveler as "Captain Kirk." Depersonalization can also occur when the nurse refuses to chat, does not make eye contact, or uses unnecessarily formal terms of address.

MAINTAINING AN EFFICIENT ATTITUDE

Maintaining an efficient attitude can occur when the nurse attempts to convey a professional aura. This can happen when the nurse has some doubts about the adequacy of her or his skill to care for the patient. Many patients will balk at such pseudoprofessionalism, preferring a nurse who interacts with gentle responsiveness (Shea, 1988). A flexible style for interacting with patients should include an honest presentation, a well-timed sense of humor, and a nondefensive attitude toward questions asked by the patient.

FAILURE TO TRUST/SUSPICION OF ULTERIOR MOTIVES

Failure to trust the patient or suspicion of ulterior motives can occur when the nurse believes he or she has been manipulated by a patient. Sometimes, when a patient is not yet ready to trust the nurse, the patient will test or manipulate the nurse to have his or her needs met. For example, a patient may feign a headache to get both attention and medication rather than directly expressing the need for support about a particular stressor or event. An experience of being manipulated can make the nurse wary that it might happen again. Rather than recognizing the manipulations as a symptom that requires therapeutic intervention, the nurse may guard against further events by consciously or unconsciously deciding not to trust patients again.

ETHNOCENTRIC BELIEFS ABOUT ILLNESS BEHAVIOR

Ethnocentric beliefs about illness behavior may hinder the development of the therapeutic relationship. When the nurse and patient do not share the same cultural beliefs, the nurse, fearing the unknown, may cling to known and understood beliefs. Inclusion of the patient's belief system in the interdisciplinary treatment plan will facilitate the therapeutic relationship. Murphy and Clark (1993) found that spending time with the patient, using nonverbal communication, and being patient were particularly helpful in building a relationship with ethnic minority patients who did not speak the language of the nurse.

MULTIPLE CAREGIVERS

The issue of multiple caregivers is a treatment system issue that can inhibit the formation of the therapeutic relationship. Rotating shifts and days off may be perceived by the patient as a lack of caring, particularly when the nurse has been working closely with the patient. The nurse should explain changes in scheduling and prepare the patient in advance when he or she is planning to be off for some time.

CHARTING CONFIDENTIAL MATERIAL

Charting material considered confidential by the patient may inhibit the patient from trust and further disclosure. Patients may wish to keep some information between themselves and one nurse. This situation may pose a serious dilemma for the nurse; on the one hand, the nurse wants to respect the patient's wishes, and on the other hand, the nurse feels compelled to share pertinent information with the treatment team. In situations like these, the nurse needs to explain to the patient that the whole team cares about the patient and will maintain the patient's dignity and confidentiality. For the safety of the nurse and patient, pertinent information must be shared with the treatment team.

TIME

Time is essential to the development of the therapeutic relationship, yet treatment programs are becoming shorter and more intensive than they were a few years ago. Patients occasionally express a feeling that the health care delivery system only cares as long as the insurance company is paying. In light of shorter hospital stays and the brief psychotherapy programs prevalent in out-patient settings, it is essential to accurately prioritize the patient's needs effectively. It is helpful to involve the patient in planning treatment goals to be accomplished within the usual length of treatment. Faster and increasingly cost-effective service also can limit the time available for nurses to have the opportunity to develop the self-awareness fundamental to the therapeutic relationship (Hoskings, 1993). Some nurses have found it helpful to participate in a peer group that focuses on enhancing therapeutic skills through the development of self.

■ SPECIAL CONSIDERATIONS FOR THE STUDENT NURSE IN THE THERAPEUTIC RELATIONSHIP

Students often express concern about their ability to function in the therapeutic relationship. They may wonder "why should the patient trust me when there are so many experienced professionals around," or "how can I help my patient when I have so little experience?" Many students express concern about saying the wrong thing to the patient and the consequences that may follow. These are genuine concerns of the student's professional learning to use new skills with a new patient population in a new clinical setting. Recall that the therapeutic relationship is to be viewed, by the patient, as a learning experience about the illness and self. Armstrong and Kelly (1993) found it helpful for the student to use the phases of the therapeutic relationship in learning about the work of the therapeutic relationship. Thus, the student goes through the phases of orientation, identification, exploitation, and resolution in relation to learning about the role and self.

At the beginning of the psychiatric nursing experience, the student must be oriented to role responsibilities, boundaries, and available resources. In the **orientation phase,** the student is likely to ask many questions, seek help frequently, and test new boundaries. The student may feel the need to meet frequently with clinical faculty. This should be encouraged as part of the phase of orientation. Once the student becomes more familiar with the role and concomitant expectations, the student is ready to identify learning needs.

Identification involves articulation of learning needs. Perhaps the student has observed an experienced nurse conduct a patient interview with what appeared to be ease. The student may identify that he or she would like to experience greater confidence in the clinical interview. After the learning need is identified,

RESEARCH HIGHLIGHT

The nursing student must be aware of personal attitudes and self-awareness in relations with others when establishing the therapeutic relationship. Increased awareness of thoughts and behaviors may help the nursing student become more therapeutic in the nurse–patient relationship. Specific techniques to assist students in developing positive attitudes and self-awareness toward psychiatric patients, however, have not been identified or tested.

The purpose of this study (Landeen, et al., 1992) was to evaluate the use of keeping a journal to assist students in examining their attitudes and self-awareness in their relations with others within the context of the clinical experience. The study examined the effects of keeping journals by comparing three groups of third year baccalaureate nursing students pre- and post-clinical experience on their attitudes toward the mentally ill, awareness of interpersonal relations, and comfort in working with psychiatric patients. The study group included students in psychiatric clinical placements who were instructed to keep a journal. The control groups included students in their psychiatric and students in medical-surgical placements who did not keep journals. A total of 35 students participated in the study.

Journals are similar to diaries in that they contain a description of an event, but different in that there is also a reflective component included. Students were instructed to write in their journals at the end of each clinical day for a maximum of 20 minutes. They were asked to describe the most significant event of the day. In addition, the students were asked to reflect on the impact of the event in terms of understanding a patient situation, their own attitudes in the situation, and future learning needs as a result of the event.

The researchers measured the effect of keeping journals on a scale assessing the students' attitudes toward mental illness pre- and post-clinical experience. Attitude domains included authoritarianism, benevolence, mental hygiene ideology, social restrictiveness, and interpersonal etiology. The effect of journal keeping was also tested on a scale measuring students' self-awareness in relationships with others. Dimensions of self-awareness measured by the scale included inclusion, control, and affection.

Results of this study indicated that the journal group did have statistically significant changes in their attitudes toward the mentally ill on the subscales of authoritarianism and interpersonal etiology. The direction of changes in the students' attitudes indicated that the journal group viewed psychiatric patients in a less authoritarian manner and viewed mental illness as caused less by interpersonal experience in childhood by the end of their experience. There were no statistically significant changes among the groups of nursing students over time on any of the subscales measuring self-awareness in relationships with others. The authors speculated that perhaps changes in self-awareness occur over a longer period than the 13-week clinical rotation. Findings from this study support the use of journals to assist students in exploring and changing their attitudes but not necessarily in changing their interpersonal style.

the student then considers options and resources to meet the need.

In the **exploitation phase,** the student is ready to make use of the resources available to expand professional knowledge. With increasing independence, the student is able to exploit faculty, staff, and literature to meet learning needs. In this phase, the student is also likely to identify new learning objectives. As the student learns more, the student realizes what he or she wants to learn.

Finally, **resolution** occurs when the learning needs have been met, and the student identifies the level of competency that has developed. The student is able to recognize the skills that have been acquired.

Part of the learning process also involves learning about self. The student is likely to learn more about his or her identity as a helping professional. The student is also likely to learn more about personal strengths and weaknesses in relation to others. In the psychiatric mental health setting, students are likely to be confronted by personal attitudes and preconceptions about mental illness and human vulnerability. As in any nursing setting, the student is also likely to experience some frustrations. These are all key issues of which the nursing student should become increasingly aware when establishing a therapeutic relationship. Research supports the use of journals to assist students in exploring and changing their attitudes toward patients with mental illness. (See Research Highlight.) Clinical conferences with faculty and peers also provide an arena for students to develop increased awareness about self in the therapeutic relationship.

■ ROLE OF THE PATIENT IN THE THERAPEUTIC RELATIONSHIP

Each patient will function uniquely in the therapeutic relationship depending on the crisis they are experiencing, parameters of the illness, and personal strengths and limitations. In general, however, all patients will present with the following three needs.

1. The patient needs to recognize and understand the current situation and the extent of his or her need for help.
2. The patient needs to recognize and collaborate in developing and implementing a plan of care.
3. Each patient needs to focus their energy positively to define, understand, and meet the problem at hand (Peplau, 1952).

It is tempting to think that all patients will present for treatment with knowledge of the above needs and with the skill to address those needs readily. In many cases, however, the patient will need assistance and support from the nurse in order to recognize and work on addressing these needs. Some patients may not acknowledge their need for help. Others may not be aware of, or be ready to use, the resources available through the nurse and the treatment setting. Still others may be experiencing aspects of their illness, such as acute anxiety or psychosis, that deters them from fully participating in the therapeutic relationship.

PATIENT RECOGNITION OF THE NEED FOR HELP

Patient orientation to the presenting problem can be a complex task. This usually involves developing an awareness of the relationship between symptoms and the accompanying illness.

The nurse can assist the patient to recognize the need for help by gently asking questions and probing the patient's understanding of his or her situation. For Bill, in the case example below, the nurse might ask him to describe his drinking behavior, when, where, and why he thinks he drinks. The nurse would ask about how his mood changes and how he sees others responding to him when he is drinking alcohol. Part of Bill's treatment would include helping him to develop a better self-concept so he no longer feels the need to drink. Bill, however, will not be motivated to work on his self-concept if he does not see the relation between his symptoms and his illness. Once the patient develops some recognition and understanding of the situation, the patient is also likely to grasp the extent of the need for help. The patient will be ready to collaborate in developing a plan of care.

PATIENT COLLABORATION IN THE TREATMENT PLAN

To encourage the patient to participate in treatment is to engage him or her as an active partner in an enterprise of great concern to the patient (Peplau, 1952). In order to ensure full participation in treatment, the patient must have an understanding of their situation, and he or she must be informed of treatment options.

This is a dynamic process. While the nurse helps the patient to learn about treatment options, the patient, in turn, helps the nurse learn about ways in which the patient feels he or she can best use the treatment options available. For example, one of the treatment options available to Bill was to participate in group psychotherapy; however, Bill did not feel ready to share his issues in a group context. He chose instead to work one-to-one with the nurse and other members of the treatment team. Later in the course of treatment, as his self-confidence improved, Bill was ready to participate in group psychotherapy.

Collaborative participation in treatment is dependent on the patient's needs, consent and understanding of the prevailing problems, related reality factors, and existing conditions for all participants. The patient, when aided in identifying and understanding facets of the problem, can recognize what is involved and can base consent and subsequent actions on known data. The key factor in eliciting collaborative participation is the patient's identification and understanding of the problem. Some patients may be experiencing such severe illness at the time treatment is initiated that they will not be able to cognitively comprehend the presenting problem. The patient may be experiencing auditory hallucinations, symptoms of substance abuse withdrawal, severe anxiety, or the depths of a depressive illness, all of which will interfere with the patient's ability to hear and understand the situation. In these situations, the nurse can augment the patient's deficits by periodically assessing the patient's level of understanding and by repeating information about treatment at regular intervals. Usually, with the passage of time and implementation of appropriate medical management, the patient's understanding will improve, and he or she will be able to collaborate in treatment planning.

PATIENT FOCUS ON TREATMENT

The patient's perception of self, including strengths and limitations, will influence how he or she perceives

E CASE EXAMPLE

Bill, a 46-year-old sales representative, has started a 6-week out-patient program for treatment of alcohol abuse. His chief complaint is, "I'm going to lose my job if I don't get this drinking under control." Bill needs to develop an awareness of the consequences of the illness for *himself* before he can focus his energy on changing his behav-

ior. Moreover, Bill needs to identify some of the underlying issues related to his drinking; his poor self concept and lack of confidence. Bill thinks he is funnier and has more confidence when he is under the influence of alcohol, so he frequently drinks to excess when he is entertaining customers.

the treatment process. For example, the patient with a negative view of self will have a negative view of hospitalization. It may also affect the person's ability to solve problems and learn (Morse, 1991). This patient may say "nothing is going to help me" or "spend your time with another person who is going to get better." The patient is hopeless about his or her situation and is consequently hopeless about treatment outcomes. The nurse will be challenged to assist this patient to obtain a more optimistic view of treatment and elicit the patient's participation in treatment. It is helpful to spend time with the patient, perhaps engaging in diversional activities together. The goal is to help the patient develop a more positive view of self and available treatment options.

To encourage the patient's participation in the treatment process is to engage the patient in the therapeutic relationship. Recall that the therapeutic relationship is the process that uses the nurse to motivate the patient to desire healing and healthy behaviors. It is the context in which the patient has the opportunity to address and redress the sources of his or her distress, the outcome of which is for the patient to have gained a better understanding of self. How the patient best learns about self and to desire healing is largely dependent on the many unique features of the individual. In what context does the patient function optimally? Can the patient express needs better verbally or in writing? Does the patient become anxious with one-to-one encounters or does the patient need a less threatening approach? The nurse can facilitate the patient's ability and desire to participate in treatment by maximizing situations for learning and growth.

■ PATIENT FACTORS THAT INHIBIT DEVELOPMENT OF THE THERAPEUTIC RELATIONSHIP

Many patient-related factors can inhibit the development of the therapeutic relationship (Morse, 1991). Some inhibiting factors are a consequence of the illness, while others can be regarded as an indication that the patient has not yet experienced the therapeutic situation as one that he or she can trust. Just as for the nurse, inhibiting factors can function as a signal for remedial action.

PSYCHOSIS

When an individual is experiencing alterations in thought processes, he or she may not be able to focus adequately on the actions or efforts of the nurse to evaluate the nurse's trustworthiness. Patients may not be able to focus on treatment goals because they are confused and overwhelmed by the psychotic processes they are experiencing. The nurse should first respond to the patient's symptoms. Once the symptoms are under control, the nurse can again attempt to orient the patient to the therapeutic relationship.

LACK OF TRUST

Lack of trust is usually evidenced by strategies to keep the nurse at a distance including avoiding eye contact, looking into space, fidgeting, sharing less, talking less about self, or keeping the conversation focused on mundane issues. When there is lack of trust, the therapeutic relationship cannot proceed. The nurse can help the patient to verbalize the lack of trust by asking questions, such as, "It seems like you feel uneasy talking to me. Is there something we can do together to help you feel more comfortable?" Very often, it is simply that the patient needs time to trust. If the patient is unwilling to accept the nurse, the nurse can demonstrate continued willingness to engage in a therapeutic relationship by persevering and continuing to provide routine care (Morse, 1991).

PATIENT BEHAVIORS

Patient behaviors can signal inhibition in the therapeutic relationship. Behaviors such as withdrawing from contact with the nurse, attempting to elope, focusing on symptoms, or demanding coercive or manipulative interactions can all be indications that the patient feels inhibited in the therapeutic context. When any of these behaviors become apparent after the nurse and patient have established a therapeutic relationship, the patient may be inhibited about current treatment issues. The behaviors can be taken as clues to the patient's response to treatment.

IMPAIRED COMMUNICATION

Impaired communication can present a barrier to the formation of the therapeutic relationship. Nurses identified greater difficulty in forming a good relationship with the patient when the nurse and patient did not have a common language (Murphy and Clark, 1993). Impaired communication may also be the result of cognitive deficits. Since communication is an essential component of the therapeutic relationship, it is important to assure the availability of interpreters or to implement other forms of communication, such as writing, the use of pictures, and nonverbal messages of care and support. Extra effort on the part of the nurse to communicate with a patient when there is a communication barrier can also enhance trust.

PRECONCEPTIONS ABOUT TREATMENT

Preconceptions about treatment can be an inhibiting factor for either the nurse or patient (e.g., whether the nurse or patient are capable of viewing the illness experiences as a learning process). One study found that preconceptions of both the patient and nurse were related to the development of the therapeutic relationship (Forchuk, 1994). Both patient and nurse perceptions developed early in the relationship and underwent almost no change over a 6-month period. These research findings emphasize how influential preconceptions can be to the outcome of the therapeutic relationship. Part of the function of the orientation phase is for the patient and nurse to become aquainted with one another and to assess the other's understanding of the mutual roles in the relationship. This can help to combat the inhibiting influence of preconceptions of the relationship for both the patient and nurse.

■ TYPES OF MUTUAL NURSE–PATIENT RELATIONSHIPS

From qualitative research of nurse–patient relationships, Morse (1991) identified an explanatory model for describing the relationship types that occur. Four types of mutual relationships were identified: clinical, therapeutic, connected, and over involved. In this model, nurse–patient relationships are negotiated until a mutually satisfying relationship is reached. The type of relationship that is achieved is dependent on the duration of contact between the nurse and patient, the needs and desires of the patient, the commitment of the nurse, and the patient's inclination to trust the nurse.

CLINICAL RELATIONSHIP

The **clinical relationship** is one where the duration of contact is relatively brief. Usually the patient has sought treatment for a minor concern, such as medication evaluation or diagnostic procedures. Interaction between the nurse and patient is courteous and superficial. The clinical relationship is not a therapeutic relationship as defined by Peplau (1952). The patient and nurse may spend a brief time becoming oriented to one another; however, they will not go through the phases of identification, exploitation, and resolution.

THERAPEUTIC RELATIONSHIP

The **therapeutic relationship** identified by Morse (1991) is usually of short duration. The patient's needs are not great, and care is given quickly and effectively. Treatment interventions are not serious or life threatening. This level of relationship might develop when the patient has a reasonable support system but is temporarily unable to care for self, for example, during the post-operative period. Although this type of relationship is also called therapeutic, the nurse and patient do not experience the phases of the therapeutic relationship as defined by Peplau (1952).

CONNECTED RELATIONSHIP

The **connected relationship** is one where the patient chooses to trust the nurse and the nurse chooses to enter the relationship to meet the patient's needs. Trust evolves in the connected relationship either due to sufficient duration or to the patient's presentation of extreme need. In addition, the nurse is able to maintain a professional perspective while having empathy for the patient. The connected relationship most closely resembles Peplau's therapeutic relationship. Both relationships share the fundamental ingredients of time, trust, empathy, and caring. There is also a collaborative component to the connected relationship: The patient consults with the nurse about the treatment plan, and the nurse serves as the patient advocate. Like Peplau's therapeutic relationship, the connected relationship is likely to develop in many psychiatric or mental health settings.

OVER-INVOLVED RELATIONSHIP

The **over-involved relationship** resembles a very close personal relationship. It develops when caring between the nurse and patient exceeds professional boundaries. The nurse's commitment to the patient becomes the paramount concern and is no longer balanced by a professional commitment to the treatment goals, the interdisciplinary treatment team, and the institution. In many cases, the over involved relationship involves the reciprocal processes of transference and countertransference. As such, it is not a therapeutic relationship as described by Peplau since it is usually not focused on the here and now, nor is it based on the nurse's unconditional positive regard for the patient. When the nurse chooses to overfunction, a reciprocal underfunctioning results on the part of the patient (Barnsteiner and Gillis-Donavan, 1990). Overfunctioning on the part of the nurse fosters dependence on the part of the patient. Certainly the goal of any treatment plan is to move the patient toward maximum independence. This requires thoughtful and competent functioning from the nurse and patient.

The issue of duration is important in distinguishing the above relationships. If the duration of contact is to be relatively brief, there may not be sufficient time to develop a connected relationship. Given the realities of shortened lengths of treatment, both in-patient and out-patient, the nurse, as a member of the interdisciplinary team, should participate in treatment planning that is consistent with the patient's needs and projected length of treatment. Even in the context of reduced contact with the patient, when the nurse conveys empathy and unconditional positive regard, the patient will respond with trust in the therapeutic nurse–patient relationship. The type of relationship that develops is negotiated and planned by the nurse and patient. The intensity of negotiations depends on the patient's perception of the seriousness of the situation and his or her feelings of vulnerability and dependence (Morse, 1991).

O AN OVERVIEW

- The therapeutic relationship is the context in which the nurse and patient work to assist the patient to desire healing and health.
- Four phases, which overlap and interlock, are identified in the therapeutic relationship: orientation, identification, exploitation, and resolution.
- The nurse and patient fulfill identifiable roles in the therapeutic relationship.
- Empathy and unconditional positive regard are the specific nursing skills that facilitate development of the therapeutic relationship.
- In general, the patient needs to learn about the current situation and how to collaborate in meeting identified needs.
- When development of the therapeutic relationship is inhibited by the nurse or patient, the inhibiting factors can be viewed as signals that the therapeutic relationship cannot proceed and remedial action is needed.
- In addition to the therapeutic relationship phases described by Peplau, four types of mutual nurse–patient relationships have been identified: clinical, therapeutic, connected, and over involved.
- An established relationship is the result of nurse–patient negotiations and is dependent on duration of contact, needs of the patient, and commitment of the nurse.

TD TERMS TO DEFINE

- countertransference
- clinical relationship
- connected relationship
- exploitation
- identification
- orientation
- over-involved relationship
- resolution
- therapeutic relationship
- transference

Q STUDY QUESTIONS

Multiple Choice Questions

1. Four phases of the therapeutic relationship include
   a. orientation, identification, exploitation, and resolution.
   b. introduction, development, modification, and closure.
   c. orientation, problem identification, working, and resolution.
   d. introduction, orientation, reflection, and closure.

2. The goal of orientation is
   a. for the patient to become oriented to the treatment setting.
   b. for the nurse to become oriented to the patient's problems.
   c. for the nurse and patient to become acquainted with one another.
   d. for the nurse and patient to become oriented to the treatment process.

3. To assist the patient to express his or her own feelings and to develop increased awareness about what those feelings are, the nurse should respond
   a. with reassurance.
   b. authoritatively.
   c. unconditionally.
   d. emphatically.

4. When the patient projects onto the nurse feelings, thoughts, or wishes held about another person, such as a family member or other person in authority, this process is called
   a. psychosis.
   b. countertransference.
   c. transference.
   d. projection.

5. In the therapeutic relationship, the nurse is encouraged to maintain well-defined boundaries between the self and the patient. Boundaries help the nurse to

   a. effect limit setting with a demanding patient.
   b. avoid the pitfalls of countertransference.
   c. evaluate progress toward established goals.
   d. maintain a sense of self and promote the patient's control over the illness experience.

Essay Questions

6. Discuss journal keeping as an educational strategy described in the study by Landeen and collegues (1992).

7. Discuss several ways the nurse can facilitate the therapeutic relationship with a resistant patient.

8. Discuss the role of the nurse in each of the phases of the therapeutic nurse–patient relationship.

9. Discuss the role of the patient in each of the phases of the therapeutic nurse–patient relationship.

10. Discuss some of nurse and patient factors that can inhibit the formation of the therapeutic relationship.

Barnsteiner JH, Gillis-Donovan J. Being related and separate: A standard for therapeutic relationships. *MCN; Am J Mat Child Nurs* 1990; 15:223–224,226–228.

Forchuk C. The orientation phase of the nurse–client relationship: Testing Peplau's theory. *J Adv Nurs* 1994; 20:532–537.

Holden RJ. In defense of Cartesian dualism and the hermeneutic horizon. *J Adv Nurs* 1991; 16:1375–1381.

Hosking P. Utilizing Roger's theory of self concept in mental health nursing. *J Adv Nurs* 1993; 18:980–984.

Jerome AM, Ferraro-McDuffie AR. Nursing self awareness in therapeutic relationships. *Pediatr Nurs* 1992; 18:153–156.

Landeen J, Byrne C, Brown B. Journal keeping as an educational strategy in teaching psychiatric nursing. *J Adv Nurs* 1992; 17:347–355.

Morse JM. Negotiating commitment and involvement in the nurse–patient relationship. *J Adv Nurs* 1991; 16:455–468.

Murphy K, Clark JM. Nurses' experiences of caring for ethnic-minority clients. *J Adv Nurs* 1993; 18:442–450.

Peplau HE. *Interpersonal Relations in Nursing.* New York: JP Putnam; 1952.

Rogers CR. In retrospect: Forty-six years. *Am Psychol* 1974; 29:115–123.

Shea SC. *Psychiatric Interviewing: The Art of Understanding. A Practical Guide for Psychiatrists, Psychologists, Social Workers, Nurses, Counselors, and Other Mental Health Professionals.* Philadelphia: Saunders; 1988.

■ REFERENCES

Armstrong MA, Kelly AE. Enhancing staff nurses' interpersonal skills: Theory to practice. *Clin Nurse Special* 1993; 7:313–317.

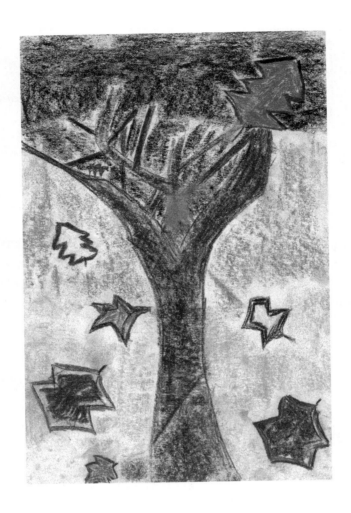

Healing is a matter of time, but it is sometimes also a matter of opportunity.

Hippocrates (460–400 B.C.)

Precepts, ch. 1

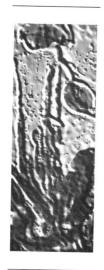

37
Therapeutic Milieu Management

Doris Vallone

Milieu is the general psychosocial context within which care takes place. Health care reform and managed care incentives that mandate mental health services be provided in the least restrictive or intensive setting have created the need for a more dynamic formulation of milieu than the carefully planned environment previously provided in in-patient psychiatric settings (LeCuyer, 1992). The term "milieu management" is appropriate today in that it implies that the environmental factors in any setting can be assessed and managed on a continual basis. In this chapter, "therapeutic milieu management" refers to the efforts taken to release an environment's therapeutic potential.

Discussions of the evolution of milieu in psychiatric care generally involves four models: moral treatment, custodial, therapeutic community, and therapeutic milieu. Each reflects the attitudes of people from various historical periods toward mentally ill people.

■ MORAL TREATMENT

The advent of the deliberately planned milieu occurred at the end of the eighteenth century with the institution in Europe and America of what was termed "moral treatment" (Bockoven, 1963). Moral treatment provided a supportive, attractive environment that emphasized fresh air, rest, and recreation. These "retreats" were located in aesthetically pleasing locations. Moral treatment was not a particular technique but a comprehensive approach to patient care based on Christianity, enlightenment, and reason (Maxmen, et al., 1974). The rationale for this treatment was that psychological stressors had robbed the "lunatics" of their reason and the physical setting and social influences were curative agents (Bockoven, 1963). The new treatment brought claims of high cure rates (although unsubstantiated) and an era of optimism for the mentally ill.

Championing the cause for improved facilities for the mentally ill was Dorothea Dix, a reform advocate who exposed the poor conditions in the almshouses and asylums and lobbied across the United States to build institutions that would provide moral treatment. Dix was successful in persuading legislators to provide funds for large hospitals, which were inundated with large numbers of chronic cases transferred from almshouses, jails, and private homes. Immigrants entering the country in increasing numbers were labeled as insane and admitted to these asylums. The state hospitals quickly became overcrowded and understaffed. The leaders of the moral treatment movement failed to train successors, and the administrators of the state institutions were politically and economically motivated (Maxmen, et al., 1974).

■ CUSTODIAL MODELS

By the end of the nineteenth century, a new view of the physiological origins of mental illness replaced the belief that mental illness was the result of moral stress (Almond, 1974). Darwin's *Origin of the Species* was used as the rationale for the inhumane treatment of the mentally unfit. Successful treatment was viewed as impossible, and institutions provided only shelter and safety. The mentally ill were socially isolated, often for years. Albert Deutsch (1948) exposed the conditions of state hospitals in his book *The Shame of the States*. The segregation of the patients and staff became a breeding ground for the "total institution" described by Goffman (1961), as social organizations in which all elements of human life occurred in the same place and under the same authority. All activities were organized to meet the institution's goals rather than the goals of the resident or inmate. Residents were induced to conform through a complex organization of privileges and punishments.

■ THERAPEUTIC COMMUNITY MODELS

Talbott (1978) cited several factors relating to World War II as influencing the change from custodial asylums to more therapeutic models. First, the many draftees who revealed mental illness upon induction increased people's sensitization to psychiatric disorders. Second, combat neurosis appeared in increasing numbers, resulting in the development of new methods for short-term treatment that were employed on the battlefield. Third, about 3,000 conscientious objectors performing alternative service in mental hospitals reported the deplorable conditions they found there. The federal government responded by appropriating monies to develop for the mental institutions the treatments that were used during the war. Similar efforts were occurring in Great Britain. Most notable of these was the pioneering work of psychiatrist Maxwell Jones who publicized his efforts at creating a therapeutic community in 1953.

MAXWELL JONES' THERAPEUTIC COMMUNITY

This was a very specific treatment approach developed by Jones (1953) shortly after World War II. Jones (1953, 1968) viewed the psychiatric hospital as a small society and believed in the patient's right to participate in treatment. An underlying premise is that all relationships and activities in the hospital can have therapeutic value. Jones focused on social and group interaction, living–learning opportunities, and "shared responsibilities" among patient and staff. The shared responsibility was the most basic to Jones' model, and he used the term to imply that treatment is a concern of not only the trained staff, but of all community members. The democratic process was used to mediate problems during several daily forums. Privileges, such as off-grounds trips, were granted by the community as a whole. The therapeutic community requires several preconditions: sanction by the administration, a willingness to examine conflicts, and a stable patient population (Kernberg, 1981). It was impractical in its pure form, but many of the principles were applied to the newly evolving therapeutic milieu model.

■ THERAPEUTIC MILIEU MODEL

Any therapeutic milieu normally retains some of the elements of the therapeutic community (Gunderson,

1978), including the distribution of responsibility and decision-making power; clarity of treatment programs, roles, and leadership; and a high level of staff–patient interaction. Elements that differ include the maintenance of a medical hierarchy and the retention of staff control in decision making.

These principles of the therapeutic community were applied to many in-patient settings during the 1960s and 1970s, and the concept of the therapeutic milieu evolved. Almond (1974) wrote extensively about the Yale-New Haven Unit called Thompkins I, which he called a "healing community." He attributed the healing power to *communitas,* or a sense of support and belonging shared by all staff and patients, and to the healing charisma or expanded therapeutic roles and abilities of the unit staff.

During the 1980s, the advancement of somatic and medical treatments de-emphasized the value of psychosocial treatments. Currently, the negative effects of some medications coupled with renewed interested in psychosocial models has renewed interest in the milieu management principles.

THE NURSING ROLE IN THE EVOLUTION OF THE THERAPEUTIC MILIEU

Sills (1975) detailed the participation of nurses in therapeutic milieus during several time periods. Therapeutic milieu models fostered collaboration among the disciplines of nursing, medicine, social work, and social science and helped to solidify psychiatric nursing as a clinical specialty. A concrete symbol of the distinction of psychiatric nursing from other nursing specialties was the adoption of street clothes by the psychiatric nurse (Hurteau, 1963).

Nurses delivered much of the care within the context of the milieu and described models of group and individual methods. The role of the nurse as "sociotherapist" was outlined by Hays (1962), who traced the evolution of the nursing role through the custodial, somatic, and rehabilitative phases of psychiatric care in the United States. In in-patient settings, the nurse's 24-hour presence was fundamental to the nurse's centrality in the milieu. Nurses developed many treatment methods within the milieu and contributed to theory building and research.

THERAPEUTIC PROCESSES IN THE MILIEU

As a treatment context, the milieu itself provides certain functions that can enhance any therapeutic intervention. In order to identify common threads in all milieus, Gunderson (1978) described five therapeutic processes in the milieu that form this treatment context. These processes are containment, support, struc-

ture, involvement, and validation. They serve as a focus for the assessment and management of the milieu. While all milieus contain these processes, it is the degree to which they are shaped and managed that characterize the individuality of the each milieu. The atmosphere of the milieu is influenced by the attitudes and beliefs of the setting's leaders and treatment team.

MILIEU PROCESSES

Containment

Containment represents that which sustains the physical well-being of patients and prevents assaults, homicides, suicides, and physical deterioration or accidents in those who lack judgment (Gunderson, 1978). Additionally, the effect of containment is a reinforcement of the internal controls of the patient. Gunderson added that too much of an emphasis on containment suppresses initiative and reinforces isolation. Emphasis on containment was a characteristic of large state hospitals and Goffman's (1961) "total institutions." Puskar and associates (1990) adopted Gunderson's model to design nursing interventions for medication-free psychotic inpatients. Their examples of containment included the use of seclusion, cold wet packs, and suicidal observation as nursing interventions based on the concept. LeCuyer (1992) identified milieu concepts as having a richness of impact on treatment. She described containment as facilitating the patients' feelings of safety because their illness would not overwhelm the staff or treatment facility. Kahn and White (1989) identified safety as one of five essential environmental elements necessary for an adequate treatment environment for acute schizophrenics. They stated that the concepts formed a hierarchy of needs for the patient who is hospitalized in crisis. To establish safety, Kahn and White (1989) stated that the staff must create expectations for conduct and develop a hierarchy of interventions, such as suicide precautions, time-out, seclusion, and restraints to deal with potential dangers.

Support

Gunderson (1978) stated that the function of support is to assist patients to feel comfortable and secure. There is a readiness to see patients as having needs that staff can fulfill. Support can be given as concrete provisions, such as food and clothing, or as direction, advice, and education. Keltner's (1986) concept of balance between encouraging independence while meeting patients' dependency needs is similar to the concept of support. Both Gunderson (1978) and LeCuyer (1992) pointed out that too much support may confirm a sense of inadequacy and dependence thereby fostering the feeling that the patient is unable to cope on his or her own. LeCuyer (1992) further stated that withholding support is a nursing intervention sometimes needed to prevent regression. Puskar and colleagues (1990) identified interventions based on support as including patient education on topics such as coping skills, medications, stress, and symptom management. Gunderson (1983) stated that support was the underlying concept of the moral treatment era.

Structure

Structure is all aspects of the milieu that provide a predictable organization of time, place, and person (Gunderson, 1978). Structure includes all regulation, hierarchy, and role definitions. Keltner (1986) included in his concept of unit structure environmental modification, community meetings, and other activities. Puskar and co-workers (1990) related all formal aspects of the milieu to unit structure. They included such nursing interventions as open reports, community meetings (see Table 37-1 for the elements of community meetings), nursing rounds, and education groups as being derived from structure. Gunderson (1983) identified structure as a later development in milieu evolution.

Involvement

Involvement refers to those processes that cause patients to attend actively to their social environment and interact with it (Gunderson, 1978). Interventions that facilitate interaction derive from involvement. Kahn and White (1989) used the term socialization as one of their essential milieu elements. In Keltner's (1986) model, structure consists of both structure and involvement and includes group therapy and formal and informal discussion groups. Keltner also discussed the therapeutic nurse–patient relationship within the context of the milieu. This therapeutic relationship is distinguished from therapy as the provision of a consistent adult relationship in an atmosphere in which the patient can try out new interpersonal skills. This relationship connects the patient to the environment. In a classic study, Tudor (1952) systematically investigated the involvement aspect of the milieu by observing the interactions between staff and a specific patient in a state hospital. She observed that the patient and staff gradually withdrew from each other if staff responses were not planned to interrupt the withdrawal process. She found that the symptomatic behavior of the patient provoked anxiety in the staff, who resorted to providing only basic physical and custodial needs. Interaction with the patient on a consistent basis was necessary to retard the withdrawal pattern. This required a plan for structured interaction by a relief staff member if the as-

signed staff member was absent. Tudor's case study demonstrated the value of consistent and planned social interaction within the context of the milieu.

Validation

Validation refers to the ward processes that affirm a patient's individuality (Gunderson, 1978). This is characterized by respect and honor for the individual. Validation affirms the patient's worth (Puskar, et al., 1990) and is thought to overlap and permeate all other milieu functions. Kahn and White's (1989) concept of self-understanding is analogous to the concept of validation. Keltner's (1986) concept of norms relate to validation and help to build a climate of universality and shared experience. They are the values that underlie what is and is not acceptable and tolerated behavior. Gunderson (1978) identified wards with a high focus on validation as tolerant of regression and expression of symptoms. This function underscores the uniqueness of individuals and the exploration of capacities. Calnen (1972) expressed the spirit of the concept of validation when he advocated that nurses take a noncoercive role in the therapeutic community. He observed that the value of the milieu is the power of the group, but that the individual's needs must not be subordinated to the group by coercion or a demand for behavior socially defined by the group. Sills (1975) also cites Calnen (1972) as the lone nurse critic of milieu interventions. Validation ensures that treatment remains patient focused.

TABLE 37–1. ELEMENTS OF COMMUNITY MEETING

Preparation
  Community members designated to prepare room.
  Community leaders and staff meet to review agenda.

Meeting order
  Chairperson calls meeting to order.
  Roll is called and missing members are accounted for.
  Minutes are read.
  Agenda is followed.
  Meeting is terminated on time with supportive ending (i.e., thought for the day).

Typical agenda
  New members introduced and welcomed.
  Members who are leaving say good-bye and where they are going.
  Community jobs are filled if applicable.
  Old business is discussed.
  New business is discussed.
  Committee and treasurer reports (if applicable).
  Daily schedule is read and reviewed.
  Meeting ends on time.

Post-meeting process
  Staff meet with community leaders to provide support and give feedback.

■ THE CHANGING NATURE OF INPATIENT HOSPITALIZATION

The changing nature of the inpatient psychiatric unit has rendered some of the ideals of the therapeutic milieu difficult to operationalize (Warner, 1993).

These changes include:

- Decreased length of stay
- Higher acuity
- Heterogeneity of patients
- Increased physical complications and medical complexity
- Decreased or inconsistent staff
- Devaluation of psychosocial methods by biologically oriented psychiatrists (Watson, 1992)

The function of inpatient units has evolved from "storing the mentally ill" to "dispatching the mentally ill" according to Wilson (1982). Because the deinstitutionalization movement and managed care cost containment incentives greatly decreased length of stay, the gathering of diagnostic and assessment information and transfer to a suitable nonacute setting dominates the activities of the staff on many inpatient units.

THE IMPACT OF MANAGED CARE

Managed care is the delivery of health care that influences utilization, monitors cost of services, and measures performance. The goal is to provide access to quality, cost-effective health care. Managed care refers to the administration and organization of a health care delivery system. In order to effectively manage care, a company has to control, direct, maneuver, and oversee all aspects of treatment delivery and operation (Selan, 1995).

Managed care providers serve as gatekeepers for third party reimbursement for services. These organizations have endeavored to ensure that treatment in high-intensity settings is medically necessary. To fill in the gaps in the care systems, managed care companies have created incentives for health care providers to develop several levels of care, which decrease in both cost and intensity. This has resulted in the development of vertically integrated systems that offer crisis intervention, inpatient treatment, partial hospitalization, assisted living assistance, out-patient services, and home care. Several of these settings are amenable to milieu interventions. Home care is a growing psychiatric specialty. Home care mental health nurses can incorporate milieu principles in their patient and family education programs.

PARTIAL HOSPITALIZATION PROGRAMS

Partial hospitalization programs consist of day, evening, or weekend programs that provide structured activities, medication monitoring, and living skills. Patients live at home or in structured residential facilities and arrive at the program either by car, public transportation, or program sponsored vans. Patients usually attend three to five times per week. These programs provide opportunities for socialization, positive reinforcement of strengths, and a connection with a consistent therapist. Most programs include activities based on the patient's culture and community, as well as living skills, such as shopping, banking, and cooking. These programs have become diverse and flexible and, in addition to supportive services, offer therapeutic interventions for a variety of disturbances. These programs are for subacute patients who are assessed for suicide and violence potential prior to admission to these settings.

ASSISTED LIVING

Patients who have become socially isolated from their families and need continual supervision and monitoring may be placed in assisted living or personal care homes. These settings vary in quality, but most provide cooked meals, laundry services, safety screening, and medication monitoring. Resident supervisors manage the home, and patients participate in the upkeep and chores. Many of the patients attend day hospital programs for structure. Some of these homes have on-site programs and activities. Milieu management techniques are being explored for application to these settings with excellent results. Murray and Baer (1993) discussed the application of milieu techniques to a transitional residential program.

■ THERAPEUTIC MILIEU PROCESSES APPLIED ACROSS SETTINGS

The therapeutic milieu processes are applied in Table 37–2 to a crisis intervention center, an inpatient unit, a partial hospital program, and assisted living.

CONTAINMENT

Crisis intervention centers, inpatient psychiatric hospitals, and maximum security units provide the most concrete examples of containment. Involuntary commitments, locked doors, and barred windows are forms of containment. The use of physical restraints and locked seclusion are intensive care measures regulated by law and hospital policies because of past misuse and are used only when the patient is a danger to others or self.

Another form of containment is staff observation. For patients who are at risk of hurting themselves, one-to-one observation by a staff member who is at arm's length may be necessary. This may be provided around

TABLE 37–2. THERAPEUTIC MILIEU PROCESSES APPLIED ACROSS SETTINGS

Milieu Function	Crisis Intervention Center	Inpatient Unit

Containment	Intensive care procedures:
	  Restraints
	  Sedatives
	  One-to-one staff
	  Quiet rooms
	  Staff trained in behavior management
		Intensive procedures
		  Restraints
		  Medication
		  One-to-one staff
		  Quiet rooms
		Level or privilege system
		Belongings restriction
		Access monitoring and restriction

Support	Nourishment if needed Clean clothes if needed Facilities for hygiene Medical screening Minimal bureaucracy for access to services	Clean attractive unit Availability of supplies Nutritious meals and snacks
Structure	Explanations of all procedures Introduction and role of all who contact patient	Clear hierarchy of staff Written expectations Opportunity to participate in a staff–patient forum Schedule of activities Predictable routines Patient handbook
Involvement	One-to-one contact with crisis worker	Opportunities to participate in unit planning Group activities and therapies Consistent therapist/RN Participation in treatment plan Family groups and meetings
Validation	Maintenance of privacy and confidentiality	Privacy Alternative track if needed Opportunities for growth and leadership

	Partial Hospital Program	Assisted Living
Containment	Plan for management of aggression and suicide Hot line for after hours Mechanism for admission to an in-patient unit, if necessary Clear behavioral expectations	Plan for management of aggression and suicide Hot line for after hours Therapist on call House rules Assistance with controlling drug and alcohol abuse
Support	Transportation to the center Assistance with budgeting Assistance with obtaining medication and prescriptions	Supervised ADLs if needed Assistance with meals Assistance with obtaining health care Medication self-administration program
Structure	Defined schedule Assistance with time management	Each member has a flexible schedule Assistance with time management Participation in the larger community through a job, school, or sheltered workshop
Involvement	Participation in program planning Community meetings Social as well as therapeutic activities Group excursions	Planned social activities Social skills education Celebration of important events, such as holidays and birthdays Facilitated family interventions
Validation	Opportunities for growth and leadership Education regarding the patient's specific illness Facilitation of completion of GED or college Opportunity for paid work	Access to patient advocate Ritualized acknowledgement of strengths and successes Focused education Tolerance of occasional regression

the clock and maintained during hygiene and elimination. Decreasing levels of observation include observations at 15 minute, 30 minute, or 1 hour intervals.

Most inpatient units also have policies requiring a search of belongings on admission. Commonly restricted items include smoking materials, glass items, medications, and appliances with cords. Certain items of clothing may also be restricted. Nurses must be careful to explain the reasons for restrictions to patients and families and emphasize safety rather than punishment. The restriction of smoking and smoking materials continues to be debated by psychiatric nurses.

A decrease in restrictions can be facilitated through a level or privilege system where clients may participate in off-unit activities, visit public areas of the hospital, or receive passes to go home for a period of several hours. Elaborate privilege systems are no longer practical in inpatient settings where the length of stay has decreased to 5 to 7 days. Patients needing reduced restriction may be transferred to less intensive settings that have minimal containment.

Most partial programs, residential programs, and intensive outpatient settings have a plan for emergency management in the event of a patient losing impulse control. By their very nature, these settings have a minimal degree of containment.

Nurses must be able to assess patients and provide for their safety by monitoring the degree of restriction necessary. Patients who perceive the environment as too restrictive may act out by using substances, engaging in sexual behavior, physically acting out, or eloping (running away) from the institution.

SUPPORT

Support provides for the fulfillment of basic needs and decreases anxiety and stress. In an inpatient setting, food, clothing, linens, social services, information, and medications are provided to the patient. Acutely ill patients depend on staff to assist them to meet basic needs until they reintegrate and attain stability. Staff then facilitate the patient's independence and withdraw support. Another form of support is the affective support given by staff members. Staff will encourage patients to develop coping skills and to recognize and draw on their inner strengths. Hospitals in the past often provided too much support and created dependency on the institution and staff. Too much support can retard patient growth and promote further dysfunction.

Partial settings and assisted living programs provide support to the patient to maintain independence by facilitating negotiation with social agencies, assisting with job placement, and improving life skills.

RESEARCH HIGHLIGHT

The Patient Staff Community Meeting: Intervention or Tea Party with the Mad Hatter?

In his article on the application of therapeutic community principles to short term units, P. H. Klein observed many difficulties that occurred in trying to apply the formula of the therapeutic community to an acute inpatient setting without modifying the techniques to the unique environment. Klein criticized the "faddish and uncritical application to all forms of mental illness" (p. 206). Klein gave examples of boundary problems which occurred from a lack of determining the purpose of holding community meetings and the lack of structure in its implementation. Some observations made on a specific ward included:

Task boundary problems—Staff created a rigid agenda avoiding emotionally charged issues and patients became disruptive to bring up topics. Staff issued open-ended invitations to bring up any topic resulting in rapidly shifting personal subjects and increased anxiety, confusion, and vulnerability experienced by the patients.

Membership boundary problems—*Attendance:* It was not clear who should attend the meeting. Both staff and patients were inconsistent in attendance. Staff rounded up patients or announced meeting over loudspeaker. Sometimes patients attended on time and all staff were late. *Participant roles:* It was unclear who should initiate discussions. Staff did not raise critical issues because they said the patients ought to initiate discussion. Different levels of staff, visiting staff, and new staff were not given guidelines on meeting participation and then were censured for inappropriate behavior.

Leadership boundary problems: Patients sometimes led the meeting with or without staff assistance. When staff led the meetings most members were silent. When senior staff attended, everyone waited to hear from them.

Time boundary problems: Agreed upon beginning and ending points were not maintained.

The problems observed by Klein can still be seen in community meetings on short-term inpatient units. E. M. Kahn discussed techniques and more importantly, principles that can result in the community meeting being a useful tool on these units.

Kahn recommended Gunderson's framework as a guide for developing a meeting which is valuable and has a therapeutic effect. Kahn advised against concretely following a rigid formula as the need for safety and structure could be met, but that there would be no cohesion and sense of belonging and giving. He suggested providing an extensive structure while promoting interaction and involvement (p. 24). The steps include 1) Planning ahead: leaders are designated and meet briefly before the meeting; 2) Operating procedures: rules and norms are reviewed at the beginning of every meeting, time structures are reviewed and maintained; 3) Get everyone involved: a structured exercise can be used such as each member saying something about the workings of the unit; 4) Infuse energy: use humor and creativity, make the meeting interesting; 5) Choose relevant topics: keep the discussion simple, don't avoid difficult issues; 6) Address unit processes: use unit issues for teaching and problem-solving.

STRUCTURE

A world without structure is frightening. Structure gives the qualities of order, consistency, and predictability to the patient's life. Structure decreases the chaos of the patient's environment and provides a matrix within which healthy functioning can be regained. In an in-patient setting, staff provide boundaries and limits. Structure is found in a program's schedule of activities. Most in-patient programs are highly structured to maximize the benefits of short stays. Nurses choose from the available activities to develop schedules with the patient based on individual desires and abilities. Sometimes reluctant patients are urged to participate to combat a tendency toward inertia and inactivity. Depressed patients, in particular, often benefit from staff encouragement.

Other examples of structure include bulletin boards and schedules that are current, patient handbooks, and community meetings where schedules are reviewed and reinforced. Community meetings will be discussed in more detail in the section on involvement.

In other settings, patients learn to structure their time and make choices among alternatives. The patient's schedule needs to be individualized and realistic. Tools, such as appointment books, calendars, and buddy systems, may be provided as part of the program. Depending on the setting, staff members facilitate structured activities, such as shopping, meal preparation, and recreational excursions. In assisted living settings, a case worker will facilitate planning sessions with the house members to assist them to structure activities. Psychiatric home care nurses may assist patients and their families with time structuring.

INVOLVEMENT

In all communal settings, participation and socialization play an important role in treatment. Patients engage in group activities, participate in the setting's operation as they are able, and develop social and therapeutic alliances. The possibilities for group activities are limited only by staff and patient creativity, skills, and inventiveness. Even mundane household tasks can become fun activities. Any member of the community can have an opportunity to develop leadership skills. Group activities reflect the interests, culture, and age group of the patients.

A powerful technique that originated in the therapeutic community is the community meeting. While the original community meetings encouraged patients to express intrapersonal and interpersonal conflicts, the community meeting in current practice is more structured and focused on community living issues. The unfocused community meeting has been maligned and compared to "a tea party with the mad hatter" (Klein, 1981; see Research Highlight on previous page). The community meeting can be conducted in any setting, and certain elements can be modified depending on the setting and the population. Table 37-2 describes these elements.

Most frequently, community meetings are held with the chairs in a circle, but an additional row of chairs may be added for more disorganized patients (Russakoff and Oldham, 1982). Patients are not forced to attend the meeting, but the importance accorded the meeting by leaders and community members provides encouragement. It is important to provide an alternative structure for those patients who are too ill to attend.

Patients take the responsibility to gather members for the meeting. The community leader with the support of a staff member, if needed, reviews the agenda and then calls the meeting to order. All community members are acknowledged, whether or not they are present at the meeting. This reduces anxiety and fantasies about missing staff and patients. Any new patients, visitors, and students are introduced. This may decrease the sense of invasion of personal space by strangers that is common in many psychiatric settings and respects the right of the patients to know who is attending their groups and activities. Patients who are leaving the community are given an opportunity to make closure, and if they have a community responsibility or job it can be filled.

Once introductions and separations are completed, the agenda of business continues. Appropriate topics include unit or house order and cleanliness, management of community funds, programming, meal planning, and other issues of living or sharing a community space. The leaders provide modeling and set limits on inappropriate topics by referring them to a more appropriate forum. Administrative problems and concerns can be clarified, and appropriate guests can be invited. The setting structure and rules can be reviewed, and community values can be reinforced. The meeting needs to be time limited and is rarely extended.

Another important function of a community meeting is the potential for assessment of a patient's level of functioning. Patients who participate and maintain a role in the meeting demonstrate strengths not readily observable in other activities. Patients who demonstrate problematic or regressed behaviors may be supported by staff or removed from the meeting to an alternative situation.

Community meetings can be held once or twice daily or as often as is optimal for the setting. Patients who are accustomed to the format will respond to an emergency meeting held during or following a crisis, such as a suicide, fire, death, or violence. This creates an opportunity for assessment and rapid intervention.

VALIDATION

Validation acknowledges and affirms the patient as an individual. All patients are entitled to treatment that maintains their dignity and uniqueness. Individual treatment plans within the milieu include creative strategies to assist the patient to maintain optimal functioning. Patients participate in activities that are appropriate to their age, culture, and developmental level. Staff maintain a nonjudgmental attitude and curiosity about each patient's uniqueness. An example of validation is a staff who treats patients in the same manner they would treat a family member. Patients are not labeled or dehumanized in any way. Any contribution by a patient is valued and acknowledged. Staff continually search for strengths and competencies and offer opportunities for expression. In some community programs, such as partial hospitalization programs, community run businesses offer patients the opportunity for paid work as part of the treatment program. Patients develop job skills and are given the opportunity to demonstrate responsibility.

Even with the best treatment, patients sometimes regress. Regressed behavior, while not encouraged, is accepted and tolerated. Patients are not coerced into attending activities, and modifications to the routine affirm the individuality of the patient.

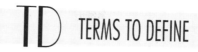

TERMS TO DEFINE

- containment
- custodial model
- involvement
- managed care
- milieu
- milieu management
- moral treatment
- structure
- support
- therapeutic community
- therapeutic milieu
- validation

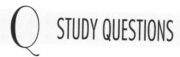

AN OVERVIEW

- Early forms of institutionalized psychiatric care were often inhumane and cruel. Mentally ill persons were thought to be subhuman and not bothered by harsh conditions.

- The moral treatment model was the first significant step in humane care for the mentally ill. Attempts to establish moral treatment in the United States on a large scale failed due to political and demographic shifts.

- Following World War II, therapeutic community models were developed to treat large numbers of returning mentally ill soldiers.

- Therapeutic milieu principles evolved from therapeutic community models. Gunderson (1978) described these principles as containment, support, structure, involvement, and validation.

- These principles can be applied to many settings, including inpatient, partial hospitalization, and assisted living.

STUDY QUESTIONS

1. Prior to the 18th century, a person who was mentally ill received
   a. moral treatment.
   b. harsh physical treatment.
   c. chemical treatment.

2. Each of the following individuals is associated with moral treatment EXCEPT
   a. Pierre Janet.
   b. William Tuke.
   c. Phillip Pinel.

3. The primary concern of Dorothea Dix in her crusade for the mentally ill was
   a. the nature of treatment in hospitals.
   b. the classification and causes of mental illness.
   c. the improvement of staff education in mental hospitals.

4. Which of the following interventions best illustrates the milieu function of structure?
   a. Individualized care plans
   b. Daily community meetings
   c. Nutritious snacks

5. Which of the following illustrates application of the milieu function of support?
   a. Having clothing available if the client has none
   b. Providing group therapy
   c. Instituting a smoking policy

6. Which of the following concepts differentiates therapeutic community (pioneered by Maxwell Jones) from therapeutic milieu?
   a. Living–learning experiences
   b. Emphasis on social interactions
   c. Highly democratic governance

7. Tudor studied nurse–patient interaction in the therapeutic milieu and observed a phenomenon of nurses and patients growing distant from each other. What name did Tudor give to the phenomenon?
   a. Termination
   b. Mutual withdrawal
   c. Therapeutic distance

8. Respecting a client's religious beliefs and cultural background is an example of the milieu function of
   a. containment.
   b. validation.
   c. involvement.

■ REFERENCES

Almond, R. *The healing community.* New York: Jason Aronson, 1974.

Bockoven, J.S. *Moral treatment in American psychiatry.* New York: Springer, 1963.

Calnen, T. Whose agent? A re-evaluation of the role of the psychiatric nurse in the therapeutic community. *Perspectives in Psychiatric Care, 1972;* 10(5), 211–219.

Deutsch, A. *The shame of the states.* New York: Harcourt, Brace, 1948.

Goffman E. *Asylums.* New York: Anchor Books, 1961.

Gunderson JG. Defining the therapeutic processes in psychiatric milieus. *Psychiatry* 1978;41:327–335.

Gunderson JG. An overview of modern milieu therapy. In: Gunderson JG, Will OA, Mosher L, eds. *Principles and Practice of Milieu Therapy.* New York: Jason Aronson, 1983.

Hays, J.S. The psychiatric nurse as sociotherapist. *American Journal of Nursing,* 1962; 62(6): 64–67.

Hurteau, P. Street clothes or uniform for psychiatric nursing personnel? *Nursing Outlook,* 1963; 11: 359–360.

Jones M. *The Therapeutic Community.* New York: Basic Books, 1953.

Jones N. *Beyond the Therapeutic Community.* New Haven, Conn; Yale University Press, 1968.

Kahn, EM. The patient-staff community meeting: Old tools, new rules. *J Psych Nurs:* 1994; 32(8), 24–26.

Kahn EM, White EM. Adapting milieu approaches to acute inpatient care for schizophrenic patients. *Hosp Commun Psych* 1989; 40(6):609–614.

Keltner N. Psychotherapeutic management: A model for nursing. *Perspect Psychiat Care* 1986; 23:414–418.

Kernberg, O.F. The therapeutic community: A re-evaluation. *National Association of Private Psychiatric Hospitals Journal,* 1981;12(2): 46–55.

Klein PH. The patient-staff community meeting: A tea party with the mad hatter. *Internat J Group Psychotherapy* 1981; 31:205–221.

LeCuyer EA. Milieu therapy for short stay units: A transformed practice theory. *Arch Psychiat Nurs* 1992; 6(2):108–116.

Maxmen JS. Tucker GJ, & LeBow MD. *Rational Hospital Psychiatry: The Reactive Environment.* New York: Brunner/Mazel, Inc., 1974.

Murray RB, & Baier M. Use of therapeutic milieu in a community setting. *Journal of Psychosocial Nursing and Mental Health Services* 1993; 31(10): 11–6; 36–7.

Puskar KR, McAdam D, Burkhart-Morgan CE, et al. Psychiatric nursing management of medication-free psychotic patients. *Arch Psychiat Nurs* 1990; 4(2):78–86.

Russakoff M, Oldham J. The structure and technique of community meetings: The short-term unit. *Psychiatry* 1982; 45:38–44.

Selan E. *Managed Care in Mental Health.* Presentation at Medical College of Pennsylvania Psychiatric Nursing Update '95. Philadelphia; 1995.

Sills GM. Use of milieu therapy. In: Huey FL. *Psychiatric Nursing 1946–1974: A Report on the State of the Art.* New York: American Journal of Nursing Company; 1975:23–35.

Talbott JA. *The Death of the Asylum.* New York: Grune & Stratton, 1978.

Tudor G. A sociopsychiatric nursing approach to intervention in a problem of mutual withdrawal on a mental hospital ward. *Psychiatry,* 1952; 15: 193–217.

Warner S. The milieu enhancement model: A nursing practice model, Part I, *Arch Psychiat Nurs* 1993; 7:53–60.

Watson J. Maintenance of therapeutic community principles in an age of biopharmacology and economic restraints. *Arch Psychiat Nurs* 1992; 7: 183–188.

Wilson H.S. Limiting intrusion: Social control of outsiders in a healing community. *Nursing Research* 1977; 26: 103–107.

Wilson HS. *Deinstitutionalized Residential Care for the Mentally Disordered: The Soteria House Approach.* New York: Grune & Stratton; 1982.

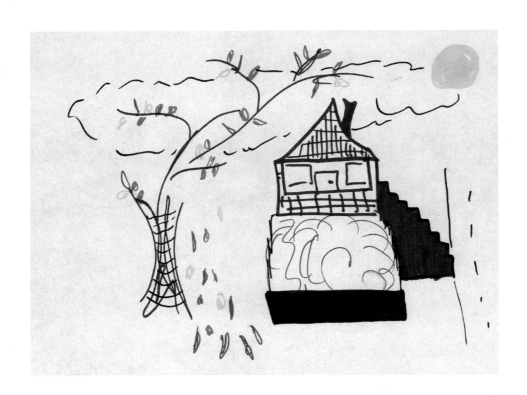

Nursing diagnosis is a clinical judgment about individual, family, or community responses to actual or potential health problems/life processes. Nursing diagnoses provide the basis for selection of nursing interventions to achieve outcomes for which the nurse is accountable.

North American Nursing Diagnosis Association (NANDA), 1990

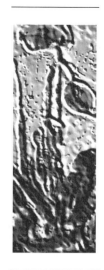

38
Clinical Assessment and Nursing Diagnosis

Denise J. Ribble / Regina Gavlick / Burton Thelander

The psychiatric nursing assessment guides the entire nursing process and is the basis for interactions between the nurse and the person receiving the psychiatric nursing services. Assessment is also basic to interactions the nurse has with others in the behavioral health system while coordinating and managing care. It is the critical step that leads to developing nursing diagnoses that direct the planning of patient care.

A holistic approach to psychiatric nursing assessment includes the use of conventional nursing strategies. In looking beyond the medical model of disease and cure, symptoms and psychosis, the holistic approach to assessment looks at the connections between mind-body-spirit and environment for their impact on the person's well-being, self-advocacy, rehabilitation, and recovery.

The Japanese concepts of shiki shin funi and esho funi describe the relationship of mind-body-spirit and self and environment as "two but not two." An analogy would be the head and tail of a nickel: These characteristic parts are viewed separately but are integral to the nickel. It is at the fundamental level of "but not two" that recovery is thought to occur.

Recovery may be defined as an act, process, or instance of recovering, to get back, to regain, or to save from loss and restore to usefulness. Nursing care in *behavioral health includes education, health promotion, support of self-controlled lifestyle modifications, advocacy, empowerment, primary care, prophylaxis, and a high degree of assessment and interaction directed toward supporting the person's goal of recovery. A holistic approach to the nursing process promotes mental, emotional, motivational, environmental, spiritual, systems, and biological outcomes. This is particularly useful in behavioral health because a medical cure is elusive and pharmacological interventions are unable to address all of the issues, concerns, and desired outcomes involved in providing care and in recovery. This holistic nursing response to promote recovery begins with the first nursing interactions and assessment.*

■ NURSING ASSESSMENT AND EMPOWERMENT

In a holistic model of behavioral health, empowerment is one of the conceptual outgrowths of facilitating well-being (quality of life) and recovery. Providing opportunities for empowerment to people who receive mental health services in contemporary behavioral health systems is a specific, challenging area for nurses, particularly as managed cost, access, resource, and outcome factors increasingly dominate.

Empowerment is a process by which people are supported and valued as they learn about themselves, make decisions, mobilize resources, and accept power, control, and direction of their lives. In assuming that the empowerment process begins with assessment and is related to the nursing process, several self-assessment concerns emerge.

SELF-AWARENESS

Is the nurse personally prepared to advocate for the diversity of people who may seek services? The Oracle of Delphi said, "Know thyself," and self-awareness of beliefs, values, and attitudes is essential to the professional, ethical, and therapeutic conduct of the psychiatric mental health nurse. Mental illness is tremendously stigmatizing. Issues of racism, classism, able-ism, religion, ethnicity, language, sexism, ageism, culture, homophobia, addictophobia, and xenophobia in society and in the nurse may make assessment more difficult. Stigmatizing attitudes could inhibit the assessment process and fail to obtain adequate data for the nursing plan.

NONLABELING ASSESSMENT

Patients with mental illness are people, not symptoms or psychiatric labels. Labeling and pathologizing are two mechanisms of professional distancing that usually relate to fear, a sense of superiority, or a sense of inadequacy and powerlessness on the part of the practitioner. Self-assessment is indicated when labeling and pathologizing are used in describing the patient rather than classifying a mental disorder. Such patient labeling practices have implications for providing substandard nursing care.

THERAPEUTIC USE OF SELF

The practice of psychiatric nursing is largely carried out by the therapeutic use of self, not by the application of highly mechanical apparatus or techniques. Self-awareness develops into a higher level of knowledge and skill in identifying transference, countertransference, and defense mechanisms.

When psychological processes are unconscious, as in transference, countertransference, and defense mechanisms, they affect assessments and interactions, usually in a nonproductive way. When the nurse has

Standard 1. Assessment

The psychiatric–mental health nurse collects patient health data.
Rationale: The assessment interview, which requires linguistically and culturally effective communication skills, interviewing, behavioral observation, database record review, and comprehensive assessment of the patient and relevant systems, enables the psychiatric–mental health nurse to make sound clinical judgments and plan appropriate interventions with the patient.

Standard II. Diagnosis

The psychiatric–mental health nurse analyzes the assessment data in determining diagnoses.
Rationale: The basis for providing psychiatric–mental health nursing care is the recognition and identification of patterns of response to actual or potential psychiatric illnesses and mental health problems.

Standard III. Outcome Identification

The psychiatric–mental health nurse identifies expected outcomes individualized to the patient.
Rationale: Within the context of providing nursing care, the ultimate goal is to influence health outcomes and improve the patient's health status.

Standard IV. Planning

The psychiatric–mental health nurse develops a plan of care that prescribes interventions to attain expected outcomes.
Rationale: A plan of care is used to guide therapeutic intervention systematically and achieve the expected patient outcomes.

Standard V. Implementation

The psychiatric–mental health nurse implements the interventions identified in the plan of care.
Rationale: In implementing the plan of care, psychiatric–mental health nurses use a wide range of interventions designed to prevent mental and physical illness, and promote, maintain, and restore mental and physical health. Psychiatric–mental health nurses select interventions according to their level of practice.

Note: V.a to V.g are basic level interventions. V.h to V.j are advanced practice interventions.

Standard V.a. Counseling

The psychiatric–mental health nurse uses counseling interventions to assist patients in improving or regaining their previous coping abilities, fostering mental health, and preventing mental illness and disability.

Standard V.b. Milieu Therapy

The psychiatric–mental health nurse provides, structures, and maintains a therapeutic environment in collaboration with the patient and other health care providers.

Standard V.c. Self-Care Activities

The psychiatric–mental health nurse structures interventions around the patient's activities of daily living to foster self-care and mental and physical well-being.

Standard V.d. Psychobiological Interventions

The psychiatric–mental health nurse uses knowledge of psychobiological interventions and applies clinical skills to restore the patient's health and prevent further disability.

Standard V.e. Health Teaching

The psychiatric–mental health nurse, through health teaching, assists patients in achieving satisfying, productive, and healthy patterns of living.

Standard V.f. Case Management

The psychiatric–mental health nurse provides case management to coordinate comprehensive health services and ensure continuity of care.

Standard V.g. Health Promotion and Health Maintenance

The psychiatric–mental health nurse employs strategies and interventions to promote and maintain mental health and prevent mental illness.

Standard V.h. Psychotherapy

The certified specialist in psychiatric–mental health nursing uses individual, group, and family psychotherapy, child psychotherapy, and other therapeutic treatments to assist patients in fostering mental health, preventing mental illness and disability, and improving or regaining previous health status and functional abilities.

Standard V.i. Prescription of Pharmacologic Agents

The certified specialist uses prescription of pharmacologic agents, in accordance with the state nursing practice act, to treat symptoms of psychiatric illness and improve functional health status.

Standard V.j. Consultation

The certified specialist provides consultation to health care providers and others to influence the plans of care for patients, and to enhance the abilities of others to provide psychiatric and mental health care and effect change in systems.

Standard VI. Evaluation

The psychiatric–mental health nurse evaluates the patient's progress in attaining patient's expected outcomes.
Rationale: Nursing care is a dynamic process involving change in the patient's health status over time, giving rise to the need for new data, different diagnoses, and modifications in the plan of care. Therefore, evaluation is a continuous process of appraising the effect of nursing interventions and the treatment regimen on the patient's health status and expected health outcomes.

Figure 38–1. Standards of Care: 1994 ANA Standards of Psychiatric Mental Health Clinical Nursing Practice.

E CASE EXAMPLES

A nurse is involved in assessing two women who both answered "yes" to the question, Do you hear voices? The first woman describes her experience as one of hearing voices that are sometimes pleasant and at other times derogatory. She states, "There is another person who goes everywhere with me. She is a real friend and has been giving me advice for years. But now she tells me what to do and say all the time. She tells me if I don't do and say what she wants she'll go away or she'll hurt me." She also describes that the voices just "pop into her head." They never occurred when she was around people before, but now they do. They mostly occur when she is alone.

The second women describes her experience as one of hearing voices that always repeat the same message: "It's your fault," "You're bad," and "Don't tell anybody." The woman states the voices are episodic and usually occur during or after stressful interpersonal situations. This woman also reports recurring nightmares and disturbing "pieces of dreams." She states she has no clear memories of events in her life from the age of 3 to the age of 23.

As these examples illustrate, both women responded affirmatively regarding hearing voices. As the nurse encourages them to describe their experiences (to do a more thorough assessment), it is clear that the two women have arrived at hearing voices differently. The nurse who stops assessing at "yes" would probably develop the same interventions for both women; however, the interpersonal interventions for the first woman, probably diagnosed with altered perceptions and schizophrenia, would be unlikely to benefit the second woman, who probably has flashbacks and post-traumatic stress disorder.

---

self-awareness, obtained through the self-inventory (see Chapter 1), the processes can become conscious. Self-awareness, validating feelings, and exploring intuitive reactions can be used as a mechanism for assessing transference and the therapeutic use of transference and countertransference.

■ NURSE–PATIENT INTERACTION

There are a number of ways to view the interaction in the relationship between the nurse and patient. The nursing problem is different from the nurse's problem or the patient's problem, although there may be a unique way that the nurse and patient work together on the patient's problem. The elements in psychiatric nursing situations are the nurse, patient, and whatever happens between them that can be characterized either as a nursing problem, a patient's problem, or a theme of the relationship. To recognize and validate themes in nursing situations is difficult.

■ ASSESSMENT AND THE NURSING PROCESS

The *Statement on Psychiatric–Mental Health Clinical Nursing Practice* (1994) includes "Standards of Care" (see Figure 38–1). These standards relate to the direct clinical care a patient receives as demonstrated through the nursing process. The six standards include the assessment of the patient's health data, the nursing diagnosis, identification of expected outcomes individualized to the patient, development of a plan of care that prescribes interventions to attain expected outcomes, implementation of interventions identified in the plan of care, and evaluation of the patient's progress in attaining expected outcomes. For optimal care, these six sequential steps are used concurrently and recurrently in nursing practice.

ASSESSMENT

Assessment begins the nursing process and is the systematic ordering of the steps that provide the organizational structure for psychiatric nursing practice. The Standards cite two important rules of the assessment process. First, the nurse has a responsibility to inform the patient of their mutual roles and responsibilities in regard to the data collecting interview. The nurse needs to inform the patient who she or he is, why she or he wishes to interview the patient, and what the goal of the meeting entails. Concurrently, the patient needs to inform the nurse regarding his or her intent to cooperate, as well as discuss the meaning of the interview. Second, the nurse uses clinical judgments to determine what information is needed. As a nurse gains proficiency in conducting admission interviews, the amount of time needed to ask specific questions is reduced.

Assessment and Data Collection

In the first step of the nursing process (assessment), data are collected on functional areas and the behavioral and mental status of the patient in order to formulate nursing diagnoses of the health concerns and problems. The psychiatric nurse uses such skills as observing, encouraging the patient to talk, listening, and keeping the interview focused on collecting essential data.

E CASE EXAMPLES

A pediatric nursing teacher was commenting to a supervisor about how she missed opportunities to see children because her administrative activities kept her away from clinical contact. "I love to see the children's faces light up for me," she said quite innocently. "I go around and hug them every chance I get." At about the same time a male nurse commented to the same supervisor, "I have a patient on my ward, and he is giving me a hard time. He is constantly complaining of feeling nervous and begging for medication. How can I keep him out of my hair?" Each nurse had failed to observe what was going on in the nurse–patient relationship. Their recitations were like dreams told glibly and easily, events for which each of these two nurses took no responsibility. Their participant roles with the patients were not noticed. The needs of one nurse to give love and of the other nurse to be free of the complaints of patients seem self-evident, yet they did not notice them. The pediatric nurse was not aware of the way in which children served as a potential audience for her and the male nurse did not see the implication that he was seeking a more reliable management technique, as if he thought the patient perpetrated complaints merely to annoy the nurse. The needs of these two nurses, to have a love object and to have patients who would not make demands, were important elements in their interpersonal contacts and integration with patients.

In another example, a nursing student walked into a patient's room one day and observed that the patient looked worried. Immediately, the patient commented to the nurse, "My, what lovely hair you have." The student did indeed have very attractive, neatly groomed red hair. The student replied, "Do you think so? I am glad you like it."

Then the patient continued, "It is so lovely, how do you take care of it?" Whereupon the student discussed how she cared for her hair: what shampoo she used, her shampooing technique and setting procedure were all discussed at length while she bathed the patient. The patient seemed interested. Afterward, the student thought she had done a good job of health teaching with reference to care of the hair. At some point a nursing arts instructor had given out a list of subjects to be taught to patients, and care of the hair was on that list.

Some months later when this student was asked to describe a health teaching situation in which satisfaction had been experienced, she described the foregoing event. She was asked, "What happened to the patient's worries?" The student blushed and mumbled hastily, "I never thought of that." What had happened was not a great crime, in this instance, but it is one step in a long series of steps in nursing education by which nurses fail to notice more and more of what goes on in a situation that is significant. It was obvious that the student, months later, was noticing for the first time how her own needs interfered with serving the needs of the patient, how the patient had been permitted to operate as an audience for the nurse, and how the needs of the patient went unnoticed and unattended.

All three situations were reduced by the nurses to a deceptively simple level. Consequently, important interpersonal events went unnoticed. What took precedence was the need of one nurse to show love, another to have an orderly quiet situation, or to talk about herself.

The key elements in formulating a nursing diagnosis for people with emotional problems or distress are their patterns of interaction, methods of coping, emotional status, and general lifestyle. In order for psychiatric nurses to develop appropriate interventions, the careful collection of this information is critical. Throughout the assessment process, which may vary from one to several interviews, the main task of the nurse gathering the data is to remain in touch with how the patient is feeling. The therapeutic intent is to diminish or lessen the distress symptoms of the patient as well as to obtain the necessary information for a nursing diagnosis.

The goal of collecting data is to assess for patterns defined as a sequence of behavior over time. Sequences of behavior, rather than isolated events, are the data used in clinical inference and judgment.

Beginning the Assessment Interview

The nursing assessment interview provides a way for the nurse and patient to become oriented to each other while the nurse elicits information preliminary to arriving at nursing diagnoses supporting positive mental health.

The nurse introduces him- or herself and orients the newly admitted patient to the unit. The nurse then sits down and says, "I would like to do a nursing assessment, the first part of which deals with your being here at the (hospital, clinic, etc.). The second part of the interview deals with your understanding of how your past experiences have influenced your being here now."

This initial part of the interview includes observing the patient, how the patient makes initial contact with the therapist, and the gathering of essential identifying demographic information (i.e., name, address, type of work, names of family members). Questions may include some of the following:

- What problem brings you here?
- When did you first note it?
- What do you believe is causing or contributing to it?
- What, if anything, alters or relieves the problem?

- What do you believe has to be done? and by whom?
- How will you be if the problem has been solved?
- What resources are available to you at this point in time?

The patient's ability to provide answers to the above questions rests on the skill of the nurse in establishing a therapeutic alliance as described in Chapter 36, whereby the patient feels safe and that he or she can trust the nurse. The answers provide the nurse with an overall view of how the patient comes for assistance at this particular point in time.

Assessment does not stop with the interactions between the nurse and the person receiving services. As the coordinator of care, the RN is responsible for using the nursing assessment to prescribe nursing interventions that impact on the patient's continued stay in one setting (or movement within or between settings). This involves assessment by the nurse of resources available and their management, supervision of subordinate staff and assessment of their care delivery, and cost considerations. As each person moves through the service delivery system, the nurse assesses the system for cross-functional integration and areas for system or process improvement.

Integral to assessment is eliciting accurate information and transmitting it correctly and efficiently to the person receiving services, their support network, peers, and colleagues, as well as to individuals or groups who are responsible for systems processes. In order to collaborate, communicate, and coordinate, it is essential that the nurse also accurately assess the interpersonal relationships, responsibility or authority hierarchy, and continuum of care. This can be likened to case managing the system. Finally, the nurse needs to assess if the person receiving services is satisfied. Do they feel they have received value for the money, time, and effort spent? Have the services, in their perception, improved their quality of life?

A common example of this multilevel process is the nurse's assessment of a person's response to medications.

- Is it the right medicine?
- Is the desired response occurring?
- Who is defining the desired response? (The desired response is not blind compliance but a true assessment of benefit by all partners in recovery.)
- What does the person understand about the condition and symptoms the medication treats, and the benefits, risks, and side effects of the medication?
- Is the prescriber receptive to input about the medication and its outcomes from the nurse? The person prescribed for?

- If the person finds the medications helpful, can they self-administer medications? Fill a prescription? Afford their medications?
- Does the person's family, culture, or both support or sabotage the use of medication?

■ ASSESSMENT AND EMPOWERMENT

The standards of care and practice for psychiatric mental health nurses describe an inclusive and empowering process. Standards of care delineate what the patient can expect to receive, and standards of practice delineate what the nurse is expected to provide. Sample standards of care and standards of practice for assessment appear in Figure 38–1. Sample tasks and standards used for performance evaluation of the entry level RN appear in Figure 38–2.

Assessment involves skills in both the science and art of nursing. Knowledge about major mental illnesses, personality disorders, mental status evaluation, organic syndromes, and substance abuse, or ready access to symptomatology and diagnosis is essential. There is an entire body of knowledge regarding laboratory values, medications, psychological evaluation, and so on with which the nurse needs to be conversant. These are areas of dependent and interdependent practice.

The science of nursing is integrated with the art of nursing. For the student, mastery begins with the synthesis of holistic, professional, and scientific principles:

- To interview and attend.
- To hear and listen.
- To observe and see.
- To analyze and understand.
- To treat and help.

The Narrative Nursing Assessment form (Figure 38–3) includes general assessment categories with space to detail patient information. A second Nursing Assessment form (Figure 38–4) is filled out for a patient.

Category I, Feeling, in Figure 38–4, assesses anxiety, a condition that has both psychic and somatic components. The psychic manifestation is the sensation of apprehension, which is a critical perception of discomfort or actual pain. It is perceived by the conscious aspect of the personality. The somatic manifestations are the result of physiological responses of the various bodily systems. For example:

- *Cardiovascular response* may be tachycardia or palpitation.
- *Gastrointestinal response* may be anorexia, nausea, vomiting, cramps, or diarrhea.
- *Respiratory response* may be rapid or slow respiration.

Directions

The following is a competency based description of tasks and standards consistent with the Nurse I position at Middletown Psychiatric Center. This description is consistent with ANA Standards of Adult Psychiatric and Mental Health Nursing Practice.

Upon hire or assignment change or annually, the nursing supervisor with the Nurse I will review the tasks/standards, *check* those that are applicable to nurse's current assignment, taking into consideration employer expectations and the nurse's abilities. For the Nurse I position, it is expected that the nurse will be learning to perform many of these tasks and standards throughout the evaluation period and that these areas will be identified as training needs at the beginning of the evaluation period. Areas that are not applicable to the Nurse I position (i.e., acting as relief Nurse Administrator I) should be marked as nonapplicable. Additional tasks/standards may be added as necessary in the blank spaces.

At the beginning of the evaluation period, the nurse will be asked to use this form to do a self-assessment of competency for each task/standard that is checked. Using the left margin, the nurse will assess each task and write in a **C,** indicating *competent* to perform this task or a **T,** indicating that the nurse identifies they have a *training need* in this task. This initiates the nurse's performance program and provides practice guidelines for the nurse in his or her current assignment. The nurse receives a copy of their performance program at this time.

As directed, the Nurse I demonstrates applicable skills and competencies with the supervision, training, and guidance of the Nurse Administrator I and Registered Nurse II, according to this performance program. Throughout the year, the nurse may be involved in training/cross-training, continuing education and performance improvement programs, supervisory sessions for commendation or counseling and quality assurance/improvement activities under the direction of their supervisor. At the end of the evaluation period, supervisory staff will use this individualized performance program to provide a competency based evaluation of the nurse's performance. This evaluation will be used to generate the performance rating.

Both employee and supervisor must sign and date the performance program. At the beginning and end of the evaluation period a copy of the completed evaluation is given to the employee, supervisor, and Director of Nursing. The original completed evaluation is sent to Personnel at the end of the performance period.

Standards and Tasks

The nurse uses critical thinking and selective use of theory that is scientifically sound as a basis for guiding understanding of the phenomena of the patient's response, application of the nursing process, and decisions regarding nursing practice.

Duties may include

Use of the nursing process

1. *Assessment:* The Registered Nurse systematically collects patient health data in order to make sound nursing judgments and develop nursing recommendations.

Assessment:

_____ Collects data about the mental and physical health status of the patient, beginning with the admissions process. Pertinent information is gathered through interviewing the patient, the family/significant others, review of historical documents, records, and reports, and observational skills.

Assessment
_____ interview observed
S or **U**

_____ Documents on an ongoing basis the observed behavior, the results of staff/patient interactions, changes in the patient's conditions or status. Reviews and analyzes documents on a regular basis, adding and/or revising data as indicated.

_____ Identifies patient health problems, needs, and strengths through the review and analysis of the patient's:

_____ Review of quality assurance follow-up
S or **U**

- Central complaint, symptoms, or focus of concern.
- Biophysical, psychosocial, emotional, behavioral status, and life/developmental stages.
- Health history, including previous treatment.
- Diagnostic test results.
- Presenting signs/symptoms.
- Bodily responses to the disease process, including co-morbidity of mental and physical illness.
- Family, social, cultural, and community systems.
- Activities of daily living abilities and capacities.
- Daily activity, interaction, and coping patterns.
- Safety needs.
- Strengths and weaknesses in achieving goals.
- Patient's expectations for interacting with the health care provider and health care system.
- Strengths and competencies that can be used to promote health.
- Spiritual, religious, or philosophical beliefs.
- Economic, environmental, legal, and political factors affecting patient's health.
- Personally significant support systems, as well as unused but available support systems.
- Knowledge, perception, and satisfaction change motivation regarding current health status and illness.
- Knowledge of advanced health care directive.
- Contributing data from family, significant others, health care team, and support systems in the community.

_____ Records data on the nursing assessment form Part I and II as per facility standards

- Completes Part I of the nursing assessment within 24 hours.
- Completes Part II, of the nursing assessment update within 11 days of the admission.
- Uses clinical judgments to determine what information is relevant to patient care.
- Reassesses patient status on routine basis and as indicated for any significant change in condition.

_____ Nursing assessment reviewed for quality and timeliness
S or **U**

_____ Note additional assessment skills for adult specialty areas (e.g., subacute admissions, MICA, psychiatric rehabilitation, extended care, disordered water balance, secure care). *Circle assigned specialty area.*

_____ Cross-training/continuing education completed (attach)
S or **U**

_____

_____

_____

Identified training needs/learning activities with time frames

_____

_____

_____

Employee/Supervisor Comments

_____

_____

_____

Figure 38–2. Tasks and standards for the adult psychiatric nurse, Nurse I position, Middletown Psychiatric Center, Middletown, NY.

```
┌─────────────────────────────────────────────────────┐
│ PATIENT'S NAME ____ DATE ____ ADM. TIME ____ CHART NO. ____ │
│                                                       │
│ AGE ___ SEX ___ S: ___ M: ___ DIV: ___ SEP: ___ WID: ___ │
│ REFERRAL SOURCE _____          │
│                                                       │
│ PERSONS INTERVIEWED: PATIENT ___ SPOUSE ___ OTHER (list) ___ │
│                                                       │
│ COMMITMENT STATUS: 201 ___ 302 ___ 303 ___ 304 ___ OTHER ___ │
│                                        PSYCHIATRIC HISTORY │
│                                                       │
│ CHIEF COMPLAINT                                       │
│ What necessitated admission            _____ │
│                                                       │
│ PRESENTING PROBLEMS                                   │
│ Psychiatric signs, symptoms, duration  _____ │
│ Substance abuse                        _____ │
│ Problems (if applicable)               _____ │
│ Previous treatment                     _____ │
│                                                       │
│ PRECIPITATING FACTORS                                 │
│ Stressors                              _____ │
│ Stop medication/treatment              _____ │
│                                                       │
│ FAMILY/SOCIAL HISTORY                                 │
│ Parents, siblings                      _____ │
│ Family problems, deaths, family illness history, living _____ │
│ arrangement, education, employment, legal problems _____ │
│                                                       │
│ PHYSICAL APPEARANCE                                   │
│ Dress, grooming, eye contact           _____ │
│                                                       │
│ INTERVIEW BEHAVIOR                                    │
│ Cooperative, hostile, anxious, withdrawn _____ │
│                                                       │
│ MENTAL FUNCTIONS                                      │
│ Orientation                            _____ │
│ Memory                                 _____ │
│ Concentration                          _____ │
│ Suicidality                            _____ │
│ Hallucinations                         _____ │
│ Delusions                              _____ │
│ Phobias                                _____ │
│ Obsessions                             _____ │
│                                                       │
│ AFFECT                                                │
│ Depressed, labile, euphoric            _____ │
│                                                       │
│ SPEECH                                                │
│ Tone, pattern, rate                    _____ │
│                                                       │
│ STRENGTHS                              _____ │
│                                                       │
│ GOALS OF TREATMENT                     _____ │
│                                                       │
│ DISCHARGE                              _____ │
│ PLANNING                               _____ │
└─────────────────────────────────────────────────────┘
```

Figure 38–3. Narrative nursing assessment.

- *Genitourinary response* may be urgency or frequency of urination.
- *Musculoskeletal response* may be various muscular aches or joint symptoms.

During the admission interview and subsequent interactions, the psychiatric nurse and the patient will assess the problem that resulted in admission, attend to and analyze responses, and assess expectations and capacity. The nurse and patient enter into an interactive

role with the health care system, other providers, and the family in order to collect and present information and formulate interventions. It is important to remember that the patient's experience is the bedrock that creates his or her behaviors. Therefore, it is essential that the nurse be attentive to the experiences. The patient's understanding of his or her experience forms the basis of recovery.

Most hospitals, clinics, and agencies have their own form or outline that provides a structure for interviewing and documenting information. It is critical that nurses use the patient's own words in writing narrative comments rather than relying on their own interpretation or language.

■ FUNCTIONAL BEHAVIOR STATUS

A third type of nursing assessment is functional behavior status. An interview is structured with an organized set of questions and dialogue (Figure 38–5) that may be carried out during the admission process and either read by the nurse to the patient or completed by the patient himself. The patient responds to each of the 84 items in one of four ratings: I do this independently, I do this with reminders, I need some assistance with this, and I cannot do this. The areas assessed include assertiveness/self-advocacy training, community integration and resource development, rehabilitation counseling, daily living skills, health services, medication management and training, skill development services, socialization skills, substance abuse services, symptoms management, and parent training.

■ MENTAL STATUS ASSESSMENT

The purpose of the mental status assessment is objectively to determine and record observable aspects of the patient's psychological functioning. This contrasts with the history, which is based on recollections. The mental status assessment has several major functions:

- It is a method of organizing clinical observations.
- It provides a clinical baseline for a patient's psychological state.
- It provides specific information that assists in establishing certain diagnoses, for example, organic brain disease.

The mental status assessment generally includes the following five categories: presentation and appearance, motor activity and behavior, cognitive status, content of thought, and mood and affect (Figure 38–6).

NURSING ASSESSMENT

Form 444 MED (MPC 5/93)

Patient	Last Name	First Name	M.I.

INSTRUCTIONS: (this form must be completed by a Registered Nurse)
- Part I must be completed within 24 hours of admission to the extent possible
- Part II must be completed within 11 days of admission.
- Update annually thereafter.

C#		DOB
		__ / __ /70

Unit/Ward	Sex
	☐ Male ☒ Female

Part I - Initial Assessment

1. IDENTIFYING DATA

A. Physical Characteristics:

Height __5'0"__   Eye Color __brown__

Weight __150 lbs__   Hair Color __brown__

Race/Ethnicity __Caucasian__

Physical Disability __none noted__

Scars/Birthmarks/Tatoos __see skin integrity__

B. Vital Signs:

Blood Pressure __130/78__

Temperature __98__

Pulse __100__

Respirations __22__

C. Language:

Primary __English__   Secondary __--__

D. Religion:

Religion __Catholic - states no__
Practice __longer believes in God__

E. Cultural Issues:

Cultural Identification __Caucasian__
Practice ____

F. For Women:

Pregnant	Menopause	Last Menstrual Period	Last Pap Smear	Last Breast Exam	Last Mammogram
☐ Yes ☒ No	☐ Yes ☒ No	1992	1995	1995	n/a

2. ALERTS

List risk factors including danger to self/others, elopement risk, fire setting risk, allergies, compromised gag reflex, h/o violence or suicide, h/o drug/etoh use, etc. Ms. _____ reports that she has been hospitalized since age 10. She describes several suicide attempts and multiple episodes of self-inflicted violence. Denies allergies. Denies drug and alcohol use.

States suicide attempts were by "drinking bleach" and O.D. Self-inflicted violence includes cutting and self-induced vomiting (using "little girl voice" here).

3. PATTERNS

The following classification represents an arrangement of human responses into categories or patterns based on their relationships. Note 'P' = Past, 'C' = Current, 'NA' = Information Not Available.

A. Exchanging: *(Human responses involving mutual giving and receiving between systems)*

• Circulation *(Include edema, chest pain, hypo/hypertension, tachycardia, bradycardia, cyanosis, pacemaker)* _____
States past and current "low blood pressure" and "palpitations"

• Elimination *(Include incontinence, fluid intoxication/hyponatremia/DWB, constipation, diarrhea, urination problems, ostomy device)*
Past and current constipation - "from meds" and from not eating.

• Nutrition *(Include food allergies, dentures, special diet, altered appetite, abnormal weight gain/loss, eating disorder, underweight, obesity)*
Vegetarian; states she has had periods in past where she has refused to eat and was fed through a "tube in my nose"; current - self-induced vomiting.
Reports she takes "Tagamint" (Tagamet) for "an ulcer in the stomach."
Reports weight gain in last year. Overweight.

Figure 38-4 A. Nursing Assessment.

Reproduced with permission of the Middletown Psychiatric Center, Middletown, NY.

Middletown Psychiatric Center
Form 444 MED (MPC 5/93)

| Page 2 | Patient | Last Name | First Name | M.I. | C# | NURSING ASSESSMENT Part I - Initial Assessment |

A. Exchanging: *(Continued)*

• **Oxygenation** *(Include cough, difficulty breathing, respiratory problems, pattern of smoking)* Smokes two packs
 per day. Sometimes at night feels like being "smothered."

• **Skin integrity** *(Include bruises, lacerations, rashes, pale/flushed skin)* Multiple scars on both arms -
 mid-biceps to wrist; all perpendicular to veins and arteries. About 50
 1/2" x 1/4" scars on each arm. Superficial scars "on top of" scars
 described above.

• **Potential for infection** *(Include HIV, TB, Hepatitis B, sexually transmitted disease; note HIV testing)* States no risk
 "can't have sex when you're locked up."   "They can't get in" - "don't want to
 have sex with anybody."   (Marked change in appearance from pleasant to
 defiant/angry)

B. Communicating: *(Human responses related to sending and receiving messages)*
 Listens and responds to questions; marked changes in body language and affect
 during interview.

C. Relating: *(Human responses relating to establishing bonds with others)*

• **Support Systems** *(Include whether family is involved, visitors are expected, socially isolated, comfortable with groups*
 Father, foster mother, and paternal grandmother in area. States does not want
 visits - does not want family to know she is "still in hospital."

• **Sexuality** *(Indicate whether sexually active outside the hospital, sexual orientation, sexual acting out, knowledge of safe sex practices,*
use of contraceptives) States she is celibate, heterosexual, "innocent but not a virgin."
 Has a Norplant, placed 2 years ago, was sexually active with men "by choice"
 since 15.

• **Trauma** *(Include history of child abuse/neglect as victim/abuser, rape, spouse abuse, sexual abuse)*
 "I don't remember anything about my childhood. I was in foster care."
 (head down, face averted, eyes closed)

D. Valuing: *(Human responses related to selecting and implementing alternatives)*

• **Spiritual Concerns** States she used to believe in God, but God doesn't help her.
 "Hates" God now.

E: Choosing: *(Human responses related to selecting and implementing alternatives)*

• **Adjustment to Hospitalization** Would like to get help but "no one can help me."
 "You should just let me die."   "I desire to die."

Figure 38–4 B.

Middletown Psychiatric Center   Form 444 MED (MPC 5/93)

Page 3	Patient	Last Name	First Name	M.I.	C#	NURSING ASSESSMENT Part I - Initial Assessment

F. Moving: *(Human responses related to activity)*

• **Mobility** *(Indicate whether ambulatory, needs ambulatory aides, needs safety devices, needs staff assistance)* _____
Ambulatory

• **ADL** *(Indicate whether well-groomed, dresses appropriately, bathes independently, toilets self)* Well-groomed, clean,
light makeup, slightly provocatively dressed. Can bathe and toilet self.
Demands privacy in showering/bathroom.

• **Sleep Patterns** *(Describe and note any changes)* States she has nightmares and difficulty
falling and staying asleep nightly. States she has had this for years
(at least 10 years that she can remember)

G. Perceiving: *(Human responses relating to sending and receiving/integrating information)*

• **Hallucinations** *(Describe)* States she hears voices - always male, always say the
same things - "you're bad," "it's your fault," "don't tell anybody," "drink
the bleach/cut yourself - you should die." Describes feelings of being
touched at night, but nobody there.

• **Self-esteem** *(Include coping/dysfunctional coping, problems expressing anger, self-destructive behavior, h/o or current drug/etoh
use, psychological response to physical/mental illness)* _____
Multiple episodes of self-destructive behavior

H. Knowing: *(Human responses related to cognitive functioning)*

• **Thought Content** *(Include delusions, obsessions, preoccupations; describe)* _____
Reports many rituals around bathing and eating, induced vomiting and cutting
and blood.

• **Altered Thought Processes** *(Describe)* Limited insight into behaviors, large memory
gaps

• **Orientation** *(Person, place, time)* Oriented x 3

• **Educational Needs** *(Consider medication, symptom management, coping skills, safe sex, health, HIV counselling, discharge planning)*
Psychoeducation to decrease self-harm; individual therapy; symptoms management

I: Feeling: *(Human responses related to subjective awareness)*

• **Mood** Showed euphoria to depression during interview

• **Affect** Marked changes

• **Physical Pain** Stomach ache

Figure 38–4 C.

						Form 444 MED (MPC 5/93)
Page 4	Patient	Last Name	First Name	M.I.	C#	**NURSING ASSESSMENT** Part I - Initial Assessment

SUMMARY AND TREATMENT RECOMMENDATIONS *Identify and prioritize nursing diagnoses/patient needs. Include strengths/assets relevant to nursing interventions and recommended interventions.*

Assessment of Strengths/Needs *(Psychiatric)* Intelligent, would like help, young. Needs to reduce harm to self behaviors and explore effect of past events in present situation

Nursing Diagnosis *(Psychiatric)* Unresolved post-traumatic response related to altered memory, altered perceptions, spiritual distress, altered sleep and altered self-concept as evidenced by self-mutilation, reports "voices," nightmares, insomnia, no early memories, "I deserve to die," suicide attempts, rituals.

Nursing Interventions (1) Assessment of lifetime history of traumatic events. (2) "No harm" contract to maintain her safety. (3) Psychoeducational interventions to manage distress during flashbacks/memory recovery - keeping log, create a safe space, ice for hands for orientation. (4) Careful evaluation of any psychotropic medications for effectiveness and side-effects. (5) Individual counselling or psychotherapy.

Assessment of Strengths/Needs *(Medical/Other ie: MICA, DWB, functional, etc.)* _____

Nursing Diagnosis *(Medical/Other ie: MICA, DWB, functional, etc.)* Altered nutritional processes related to altered eating, reported gastric ulcer, and obesity as evidenced by self-induced vomiting, taking Tagamet, many rituals with mood, obesity, vegetarian.

Nursing Interventions (1) Ask for dietary consult/monitor labs/weight. (2) Supervise meals to prevent vomiting. (3) Administer Tagamet. (4) Observe rituals around food and document.

RN Signature	Title	Date

Figure 38–4 D.

Name: _____   C: _____

MPC MR6020 (3/94)

Name: _____

MIDDLETOWN PSYCHIATRIC CENTER

C : _____

STATE OPERATED COMMUNITY RESIDENCE

Sex: _____ DOB: _____

FUNCTIONAL BEHAVIOR ASSESSMENT

Date Completed: _____

Date of Next Review: _____

INSTRUCTIONS: Resident completes assessment upon day of admission. (If a question does not apply, enter N/A for non-applicable in the "I DO THIS INDEPENDENTLY" column.) Primary counselor completes staff ratio as Ste &a. prior to the service plan. When a staff rating disagrees with resident's assessment, a comment will be entered. The assessment is to be reviewed every three months by the resident and staff during the service plan review on the continuation sheet.

RATINGS: (1) Agrees   (2) Disagrees   (3) Unable to assess (Comment)

ASSERTIVENESS/ SELF-ADVOCACY TRAINING	I DO THIS INDEPENDENTLY	I DO THIS WITH REMINDERS	I NEED SOME ASSISTANCE WITH THIS	I CANNOT DO THIS	RATING
1. Are you able to resolve conflicts with others?					
2. Are you able to assert yourself without becoming angry, agitated, or verbally/physically abusive to self/others?					
3. Are you able to respond to medical, safety, and other personal issues?					
4. Are you able to differentiate between your values and the values of others?					
5. Are you able to identify when you need assistance with problems?					
6. Are you able to communicate with others in a socially acceptable manner?					

COMMENTS:

COMMUNITY INTEGRATION RESEARCH DEVELOPMENT	I DO THIS INDEPENDENTLY	I DO THIS WITH REMINDERS	I NEED SOME ASSISTANCE WITH THIS	I CANNOT DO THIS	RATING
7. Do you get up on time and allow enough time for morning routine?					
8. Do you keep scheduled appointments?					
9. Do you notify program/work when unable to attend?					
10. Do you attend individual meetings with your primary counselor?					
11. Do you utilize the public transportation system regularly or as needed?					
12. Do you use other support systems when needed (social clubs, self-help groups, etc.)?					

COMMENTS:

Figure 38–5A. Nursing assessment form.

Reproduced with permission of the Middletown Psychiatric Center, Middletown, NY.

Name: _____   C: _____

REHABILITATION COUNSELING	I DO THIS INDEPENDENTLY	I DO THIS WITH REMINDERS	I NEED SOME ASSISTANCE WITH THIS	I CANNOT DO THIS	RATING
13. Do you utilize your therapist and psychiatrist to deal with therapy issues?					
14. Do you use what you learn in therapy in your life?					
15. Are you able to identify your future goals?					
16. Do you participate in goal planning?					
17. Are you able to identify stressful situations and behaviors that will prevent you from reaching your goals?					

COMMENTS:

DAILY LIVING SKILLS	I DO THIS INDEPENDENTLY	I DO THIS WITH REMINDERS	I NEED SOME ASSISTANCE WITH THIS	I CANNOT DO THIS	RATING
18. Do you shower at least five (5) out of seven (7) days per week?					
19. Do you wash your hair between one (1) and three (3) times weekly?					
20. Do you prepare balanced, nutritious meals?					
21. Do you brush your teeth at least once daily?					
22. Do you maintain your living area?					
23. Do you complete household chores?					
24. Do you complete laundry tasks (clothing and bed linens)?					
25. Do you budget your money (rent, earnings, bank accounts)?					
26. Do you obtain and maintain items needed for personal hygiene?					

Figure 38-5 B.

Name: _____   C: _____

HEALTH SERVICES	I DO THIS INDEPENDENTLY	I DO THIS WITH REMINDERS	I NEED SOME ASSISTANCE WITH THIS	I CANNOT DO THIS	RATING
27. Do you make and keep medical/dental appointments?					
28. Do you eat two (2) to three (3) meals per day?					
29. Do you cook a variety of different meals and follow nutritional guidelines?					
30. Can you follow recommended special diets?					
31. Do you follow through on aftercare recommendations?					
32. Do you seek medical attention when ill?					
33. Do you go to a medical doctor at least once a year?					
34. Do you go to a dentist at least once a year?					
35. Do you use the proper precautions following the Universal Infectious Disease Guidelines (HIV/AIDS Guidelines)?					
36. Do you have and use basic first aid?					

COMMENTS:

MEDICATION MANAGEMENT AND TRAINING	I DO THIS INDEPENDENTLY	I DO THIS WITH REMINDERS	I NEED SOME ASSISTANCE WITH THIS	I CANNOT DO THIS	RATING
37. Do you take your medication on time as prescribed by your physician?					
38. Do you fill and refill your prescriptions as needed, and make them available to staff for recording?					
39. Do you store your medication properly in a locked box if on self-medications?					
40. Do you hand in doctor's orders and notifications to staff?					
41. Do you speak to your psychiatrist when you have problems with your medications and are you aware of your med changes?					
42. Do you understand what symptoms your medication treats and what side effects may occur?					
43. If you receive an injection, do you know when your appointments for the injection are scheduled?					
44. Are you aware of changes in your behavior before and after the injection?					
45. If you receive PRNs, are you aware of what symptoms they treat and when you need one?					

COMMENTS:

Figure 38-5 C.

Name: _____   C: _____

SKILL DEVELOPMENT SERVICES	I DO THIS INDEPENDENTLY	I DO THIS WITH REMINDERS	I NEED SOME ASSISTANCE WITH THIS	I CANNOT DO THIS	RATING
46. Are you interested in furthering your education?					
47. Are you interested in work or job training?					
48. Do you attend scheduled daily activities/programs?					
49. Are you aware of and able to apply for vocational and educational programs (i.e., VESID, IPRT, BOCES, MHA)?					
50. Do you have a job history and can you prepare/update a resume?					
51. Are you aware of job opportunities in your area for which you may qualify?					
52. Are you able to fill out a job application?					
53. Do you possess appropriate interviewing skills?					
54. Are you able to maintain employment for a significant period of time?					
55. Do you know how to dress appropriately for interviews or work?					
56. Are you able to recognize when you become stressed, need assistance, or need time off?					
57. Are you able to relate to a boss/co-workers effectively?					
58. Are you able to recognize and manage your symptoms at work?					
59. Are you able to identify stressors at a job and identify solutions?					

COMMENTS:

SOCIALIZATION SERVICES	I DO THIS INDEPENDENTLY	I DO THIS WITH REMINDERS	I NEED SOME ASSISTANCE WITH THIS	I CANNOT DO THIS	RATING
60. Do you participate in leisure activities with others at least once weekly?					
61. Are you willing to participate in recreational activities offered by the program?					
62. Can you identify when you become withdrawn or isolated and seek assistance?					
63. Are you comfortable and able to handle yourself on social outings?					
64. Are you aware of social activities in your community?					
65. Are you open to redirection by staff if needed while on an activity?					

COMMENTS:

Figure 38-5 D.

Name: _____ C : _____

SUBSTANCE ABUSE SERVICES	I DO THIS INDEPENDENTLY	I DO THIS WITH REMINDERS	I NEED SOME ASSISTANCE WITH THIS	I CANNOT DO THIS	RATING
66. Are you able to recognize and seek treatment when you abuse alcohol or drugs?					
67. Are you aware of support services/rehabilitation programs in your community?					
68. Are you able to get to and participate in such support groups (AA, NA, OA, etc.)?					
69. Are you able to recognize when you feel like you will have a relapse and notify the appropriate people?					
70. Can you identify techniques, strategies, therapeutic approaches that help prevent relapses?					
71. Are you able to recognize your triggers to relapse?					

COMMENTS:

SYMPTOMS MANAGEMENT	I DO THIS INDEPENDENTLY	I DO THIS WITH REMINDERS	I NEED SOME ASSISTANCE WITH THIS	I CANNOT DO THIS	RATING
72. Are you aware of crisis services available in your community?					
73. Can you identify your symptoms of mental illness?					
74. Can you identify techniques that help you manage your symptoms?					
75. Can you develop/use coping strategies to help you manage your symptoms?					
76. Can you identify stressors (internal and external) that increase your symptoms?					
77. Are you able to alert the appropriate people when your symptoms increase?					

COMMENTS:

PARENT TRAINING	I DO THIS INDEPENDENTLY	I DO THIS WITH REMINDERS	I NEED SOME ASSISTANCE WITH THIS	I CANNOT DO THIS	RATING
78. Are you aware of support groups to foster effective parenting skills or to address single parenting issues?					
79. Do you know how to link your child up with children's services if necessary?					
80. Do you know how to enroll in programs/classes for parenting skills?					
81. Are you able to obtain additional services/funding for your child (food stamps, WIC, etc.)?					
82. Can you identify how/when your symptoms may affect your child and where to get help?					
83. Are you aware of appropriate housing options available to families?					
84. Do you know what child care, education, and/or services are available in your community?					

COMMENTS:

Figure 38-5 E.

Name: _____   C : _____

SUMMARY

Resident Comments: _____
_____
_____
_____
_____

Staff Comments: _____
_____
_____

RESIDENT SIGNATURE: _____
STAFF SIGNATURE: _____
QUALIFIED MENTAL HEALTH STAFF: _____
DATE: _____

Figure 38- 5 F.

PRESENTATION AND APPEARANCE

In assessing the general appearance of the patient, special attention needs to be paid to grooming, dress, facial expression, posture, gait, and hygiene.

General Appearance

Is the patient taking care of his or her appearance? What is the appearance of the teeth, hair, nails, and body? Is there any body odor? If a woman patient uses cosmetic makeup, is it done appropriately for the situation? For example, a 60-year-old patient enters the emergency room with her face made-up in a clownlike manner.

Dress

Is the dress appropriate for the season and situation? For example, a young college man arrives at the walk-in psychiatric service in mid-July dressed in boots and a long winter coat. Is the appearance neat or unkempt? Is the dress meticulous, slovenly, eccentric, or seductive?

Facial Expression

What is the patient's facial expression? Sad, expressionless, hostile, worried, or avoids gaze? Does the patient look around the room, stare down, or into space?

MOTOR ACTIVITY AND BEHAVIOR

The nurse should assess for posture, gait, tics, tremors, posturing, grimaces, and other abnormal bodily movements. The speed of these movements is important to note. Is there a general slowness of movement? Does much effort appear to be expended to talk, walk, or gesture? Or do the movements appear to be intense and rapid? Behaviors, including nail biting, wringing of the hands, tapping of the foot, and chewing movements, may be clues to the individual's anxiety, and an increase or decrease of these behaviors can be noted as the interview progresses and deals with emotionally charged material.

Posture and Gait

How does the patient sit in the chair? Erect, slumped down, on the edge of the chair, leaning forward, backward, or on his elbows? When the patient walks, does he move quickly, slowly, with hesitation or a limp, or with the head erect or hung down?

A number of abnormal motor behaviors are frequently related to specific mental disorders. Echopraxia (the pathological repetition by imitation of the movements of another person) and cerea flexibilitas (waxy flexibility) are often seen in catatonic schizophrenia in which a person can hold his body in one position for a long period of time. Catalepsy (a generalized condition of diminished responsiveness) often is characterized by trancelike states and immobility and can occur in organic and psychological disorders. Cataplexy is temporary loss of muscle tone and may be precipitated by surprise, laughter, or anger and is seen in schizophrenics.

CHECK NUMBER FOR MOST APPROPRIATE DESCRIPTION: 1, MILD; 2, MODERATE; 3, SEVERE.

Presentation/appearance

Normal

Unkempt	1	2	3
Body habits	1	2	3
Facial expression:			
Sad	1	2	3
Expressionless	1	2	3
Hostile	1	2	3
Worried	1	2	3
Avoids gaze	1	2	3
Dress	1	2	3
Meticulous	1	2	3
Slovenly	1	2	3
Eccentric	1	2	3
Seductive	1	2	3

Motor activity + behavior

Normal

Increased amount	1	2	3
Decreased amount	1	2	3
Agitation	1	2	3
Tics	1	2	3
Tremor	1	2	3
Peculiar posturing	1	2	3
Unusual gait	1	2	3
Repetitive acts	1	2	3

Cognitive/intellect

Normal

Above normal	1	2	3
Below normal	1	2	3
Paucity of knowledge	1	2	3
Vocabulary weak	1	2	3
Mathematical deficit	1	2	3
Unable to abstract	1	2	3

Content of thought

Normal

Suicidal thoughts	1	2	3
Suicidal plans	1	2	3
Assaultive ideas	1	2	3
Homicidal thoughts	1	2	3
Homicidal plans	1	2	3
Antisocial attitudes	1	2	3
Suspiciousness	1	2	3
Poverty of content	1	2	3
Phobias	1	2	3
Obsessions—			
compulsions	1	2	3
Feelings of unreality	1	2	3
Feels persecuted	1	2	3

Thoughts of running away

Thoughts of running away	1	2	3
Somatic complaints	1	2	3
Ideas of guilt	1	2	3
Ideas of hopelessness	1	2	3
Ideas of worthlessness	1	2	3
Excessive religiosity	1	2	3
Sexual preoccupation	1	2	3
Blames others	1	2	3

Illusions

Present	1	2	3

Hallucinations

Auditory	1	2	3
Visual	1	2	3
Other	1	2	3

Delusions

Of persecution	1	2	3
Of grandeur	1	2	3
Of reference	1	2	3
Of influence	1	2	3
Somatic	1	2	3
Other	1	2	3
Are systematized	1	2	3

Interview behavior

Normal

Angry outbursts	1	2	3
Irritable	1	2	3
Impulsive	1	2	3
Hostile	1	2	3
Silly	1	2	3
Sensitive	1	2	3
Apathetic	1	2	3
Withdrawn	1	2	3
Evasive	1	2	3
Passive	1	2	3
Aggressive	1	2	3
Naive	1	2	3
Overly dramatic	1	2	3
Manipulative	1	2	3
Dependent	1	2	3
Uncooperative	1	2	3
Demanding	1	2	3
Negativistic	1	2	3
Callous	1	2	3

Cognitive/flow of thought

Normal

Blocking	1	2	3
Circumstantial	1	2	3
Tangential	1	2	3
Perseveration	1	2	3
Flight of ideas	1	2	3
Loose association	1	2	3
Indecisive	1	2	3

Speech

Normal

Excessive amount	1	2	3
Reduced amount	1	2	3
Rush of speech	1	2	3
Slowed	1	2	3
Loud	1	2	3
Soft	1	2	3
Mute	1	2	3
Slurred	1	2	3
Stuttering	1	2	3

Sensorium

Normal

Orientation impaired	1	2	3
Time	1	2	3
Place	1	2	3
Person	1	2	3
Memory:			
Clouding of			
consciousness	1	2	3
Inability to concentrate	1	2	3
Amnesia	1	2	3
Memory impaired			
Recent memory	1	2	3
Remote memory	1	2	3
Confabulation	1	2	3

Insight and judgment

Normal

Insight lacking	1	2	3
Faulty judgment	1	2	3
Unrealistic regarding			
degree of illness	1	2	3
Doesn't know why			
he is here	1	2	3
Unmotivated for			
treatment	1	2	3

Mood and affect

	1	2	3
Normal	1	2	3
Anxious	1	2	3
Inappropriate affect	1	2	3
Flat affect	1	2	3
Elevated mood	1	2	3
Depressed mood	1	2	3
Labile mood	1	2	3

DSM IV-R MULTIAXIAL DIAGNOSIS

AXIS I: _____

AXIS II: _____

AXIS III: _____

AXIS: IV: _____

AXIS V: Global Assessment of Functioning Scale: Current GAF ____ Highest GAF Past Year ____

Case formulation: _____

NURSING DIAGNOSIS

1: _____

2: _____

3: _____

4: _____

Figure 38–6. Mental status checklist.

COGNITIVE OR INTELLECT

The nurse can assess an individual's general intellectual capacity by listening to his or her history. The patient's level of knowledge can be measured against the years of formal education and family and cultural background. Does the patient appear average, above, or below normal in intellect? Is there a paucity of knowledge? Is the vocabulary weak or strong? Is there a mathematical deficit? Is the patient able to abstract?

Content of Thought

The nurse can assess thought content by listening carefully to the patient's preoccupations, ambitions, and dreams. By assessing the major themes and issues discussed by the patient, the nurse can identify the dominant themes the patient is expressing. For example, does the patient relate most of what he or she considers his or her difficulty to a sense of failure, fear of harm, loss of an important person, phobias, fear of losing impulse control, or certain ritualistic compulsive behaviors?

A compulsion is an insistent, repetitive, intrusive, and unwanted urge to act contrary to one's usual wishes or standards. The suffix mania is used with Greek terms to indicate a preoccupation with certain kinds of activities or a compulsive need to behave abnormally. Examples are egomania (the pathological preoccupation with self), erotomania (the pathological preoccupation with erotic fantasies or activities), kleptomania (the compulsion to steal), megalomania (the pathological preoccupation with delusions of power or wealth), necromania (the pathological preoccupation with dead bodies), and pyromania (the morbid compulsion to set fires).

An important area for the nurse to assess is the suicidal and homicidal ideation. The patient should be asked if he or she has had any thoughts about hurting her- or himself or others. If the answer to either of these questions is "yes," the following data must be obtained:

- Does the thought only occur infrequently or is there a serious plan?
- When did the thought start and how often does it occur?
- Does the patient have the means to implement the thought or plan?
- Has the patient told anyone else about these thoughts or plans?

Thought Process

As the nurse attends to the content of the patient's speech, observations may be made regarding disturbances in the thought processes, the structure and rate of association, and the flow of ideas. Among the areas to be considered are form, disorders of perception, delusions, and phobias.

Form. Does the patient's thinking and communication proceed in a relatively clear, understandable manner? The following list describes thought disorder abnormalities.

- Circumstantiality: The person digresses into unnecessary detail and unusual thoughts before saying the central idea (often seen in patients who are schizophrenic).
- Incoherence: Difficult to follow or understand the patient because of an impairment in the manner of speech.
- Blocking: Sudden stopping in middle of sentence with no understanding of why.
- Loose association: Lack of logical order in content.
- Neologisms: New words or condensations of words (often seen in psychotic disorders).
- Word salad: An incoherent mixture of words (often seen in schizophrenia).
- Preservation: Repetition of the same response to different questions (often indicates organic involvement).
- Echolalia: The pathological repetition of words used by one person.
- Condensation: One symbol stands for a number of others and results in the fusion of various ideas into one.
- Flight of ideas: Describes a succession of thoughts without logical connections.
- Retardation: The slowing down of thought processes.

Disorders of Perception. Perception is the capacity to be aware of objects and to discriminate between them. The nurse can assess the patient's perception of reality during the interview and determine if any of the three major perception disorders, illusion, hallucination, or depersonalization, are present. Illusion is the misinterpretation of some real external sensory experience. For example, the patient looks out the window and sees the shadow of a tree as a real person and hears the wind calling his or her name.

Hallucinations are sensory perceptions without external sources. Hallucinations may have different origins, such as psychosis, brain tumor, drug reaction, drug overdose, alcohol overdose, sleep deprivation, and hepatic failure. They may be vague sounds, flashes of light, or recognizable voices, faces, insects, or odors. There may be one or more of the following types: visual, hallucinations of sight; auditory, hallucinations of sound; olfactory, hallucinations of smell; tactile, hallucinations of touch; gustatory, hallucinations of taste; or visceral, hallucinations of sensation. Auditory hallucinations are the most common. In evaluating them one should ask the patient if he or she can identify the voice and sex of the person. Also, is the voice friendly or threatening? What is the voice saying to the patient? (This is important to assess the directive of the hallucination.)

Depersonalization is a feeling that one is outside of one's body. This often is accompanied by a derealization in which the person feels a kind of strangeness about his or her immediate surroundings. They almost feel like they are in a dream.

Delusions. Delusions are a process by which a person adheres to a false or unreasonable idea from which no logic or experience can dissuade him or her. The patient's views, opinions, or ideas differ greatly from those generally accepted. There are five types of delusions: (1) persecutory, in which the person believes there is an organized conspiracy to hurt or harm the patient in some way; (2) somatic, in which the person is certain that his or her body is deteriorating from within or that someone is in the brain; (3) grandeur, in which the person believes that he or she is a famous or an important person (i.e., God, Clark Gable, or Queen Elizabeth); (4) guilt, in which the person believes that his or her bad thoughts have the power to affect or influence others; and (5) influence, in which the person believes his or her thoughts are being controlled by outside objects or persons.

Phobias. Phobias are a persistent, unrealistic, obsessive fear or dread of an object or situation. Four major phobias are acrophobia, a fear of heights; agoraphobia, a fear of open places; claustrophobia, a fear of closed spaces; and panphobia, a fear of everything.

Speech

The nurse can assess several aspects of the patient's form of speech. When assessing volume the following things must be considered: How loudly or softly does the patient speak? Does the examiner have to adjust his or her position to hear? When assessing what the speed of the patient's speech is or how rapid a person speaks and whether they use few pauses or long pauses between words, the nurse assesses the rate of speech. When assessing tone the nurse checks to see if there is a wide range in the pitch of the voice sounds or if the sound of the voice is strong, tedious, or monotonous. When productivity is assessed, the nurse checks to see if the questions are answered in one-word responses, for

example, yes or no; if any details are offered or if the questions are expanded; or if simple questions yield complex or overly detailed responses.

When assessing goal direction the following must be considered: Do the answers follow a logical sequence? Do the answers make sense? Does the focus remain clear?

Sensorium

Several factors are included in examination of the sensorium. They are the patient's level of attention and consciousness or how alert the patient is. The nurse also examines the person, for example, does the patient know who he is (i.e., name and age); time, that is does the patient know the day of the week, month, and year; and place, which examines whether the patient knows where he is and lives, and how he got to where he presently is.

Memory

This can be divided into recent and remote memory. Recent memory is whether the patient can remember the events of last week, what was eaten for breakfast, or the name of the examiner. Anterograde amnesia is the absence of memory of recent events. Remote memory is whether simple facts (e.g., who was last governor of the state, who is the current president, and who was the president before him) are recalled. Retrograde amnesia is the absence of memory for past events. (A test for immediate memory is to name three objects and ask the patient to recall them in 5 minutes, 10 minutes, etc.)

Concentration

The focus of the responses (Does patient have difficulty in focusing his answers? Is the patient easily distracted?) is one form of concentration. Simple calculation (Can the patient perform simple math additions, subtractions, and so on?) is another. The following is a sample exercise to test a person's level of concentration.

1. Add any two small whole numbers.
2. Multiply any two small whole numbers or spell the word "world" backward or state the number of nickels in $1.35.
3. Name the days of the week backward or perform a "serial threes" test; that is, subtract 3 from 100, then an additional 3 from the result, and so on until zero is reached. (The normal standard is fewer than two errors in 120 seconds or less.)
4. Name the months of the year backward, or perform a "serial sevens" test; that is, subtract 7 from 100, then an additional 7 from the result, and so on until zero is reached. (The normal

standard is fewer than four errors in 90 seconds or less.)

5. Repeat a random series of numbers forward, beginning with a series of three numbers, then increasing the series by one number at a time. (The normal standard is a forward series of five to eight numbers.)

6. Repeat a random series of numbers backward, beginning with a series of three numbers, then increasing the series by one number at a time. (The normal standard is a backward series of four to six numbers.)

Ability to Abstract

Can the patient see any pattern to his or her life? Is the patient able to interpret a proverb in a less literal, personal manner? Or is his or her interpretation very concrete and personal? One exercise to test a person's capacity of abstraction is to ask the patient to state the meaning of two proverbs (see following list for examples) and describe their application to his or her own present circumstances. Proverbs need to be used with caution, as people, especially young people and those from other cultures may not be familiar with the point that is expressed.

- Don't cry over spilled milk.
- People who live in glass houses shouldn't throw stones.
- Birds of a feather flock together.
- A stitch in time saves nine.
- The tongue is the enemy of the neck.
- Don't count your chickens before they hatch.
- The proof of the pudding is in the eating.
- A rolling stone gathers no moss.
- The squeaky wheel gets the grease.

Also ask the patient to describe the similarity between the objects in each of these pairs: an apple and an orange, a chair and a table, a fly and a tree, and a child and a dwarf.

Insight

Does the patient realize that he or she is having emotional or mental problems? What is his or her level of motivation to work on the difficulties? Is he or she aware of how the difficulties affect his or her life in general?

Judgment

The nurse assesses the patient's judgment by observing his or her ability to make and carry out plans, take the initiative, discriminate accurately, and behave according to accepted practice.

A person's judgment may be considered impaired if his or her thoughts and actions are inconsistent with reality. To test for such a process, the nurse can ask questions, such as, "What would you do if you found a stamped envelope in the street?" "Explain why criminals are put in prison." "Describe what you would do if stopped for speeding."

Attitude

The attitude of the patient may be assessed by observing if he or she is cooperative, evasive, arrogant, ingratiating, spontaneous, assertive, or withdrawn. What is the patient's attitude about coming to the clinic or hospital? Toward the interview? These observations provide clues regarding patterns of relating to people as well as clues to the patient's defense mechanisms.

MOOD AND AFFECT

The term "affect" refers to what the individual is feeling at the moment, including the emotional state and the outward appearance. Several areas can be noted when assessing affect. One is range, which can be limited or narrow and means only a few emotions are expressed. A wide or labile range means the patient has frequent shifts between very different emotions. For example, a 39-year-old depressed woman vacillates between crying and laughing about her current experiences. The quality of emotion expressed is the intensity. Intensity can be flat, with little energy, or exaggerated, with great energy. Mood and affect also involve types, or different categories of emotions, such as fearful, happy, angry, elated, and so on. It also means the appropriateness of what is expressed must be assessed (Does the expressed affect fit the content being expressed?). For example, an appropriate affect is when a young woman is crying and fearful as she describes an attempted rape, but an inappropriate affect is when a 40-year-old man smiles when describing how angry he is at his father.

The individual's subjective description of his or her feeling is mood. Ask the patient to describe his or her mood. Have there been any mood changes noted? If so, were these changes in mood rapid, cyclic, or situational? Assess the patient's dominant mood during the interview (i.e., depressed, anxious, or angry).

CONCLUDING THE ASSESSMENT INTERVIEW

As a conclusion to the nursing assessment interview, a series of questions and discussions can ensure that closure is brought to the interview and to help the nurse in the formulation of current and continuing care for the patient. These questions elicit information that help the nurse know something about the person in a straightforward manner and impart that the nurse is interested in a whole sphere of experience. The interaction between the nurse and patient may be recorded in narrative format.

- What are your expectations of being here?
- What is your expectation of the staff?
- What have you noticed that helps you feel better, think better, or behave better than you are presently?
- What do you believe to be your greatest assets both personally and interpersonally?
- What areas do you find that are problematic for you personally, interpersonally, and achievement-wise?

The time orientation of a patient is important to assess. Questions related to time orientation include

- What do you find yourself thinking about the most: things in the past, present, or future?
- When you think of the past, what kind of thoughts come to mind; when you think of the present what kind of thoughts come to mind? When you think of the future what kind of thoughts come to mind?
- When you think about time, where would you most like to be: in the past, present, or future?
- Are there special things you regret? Are there special things that you are afraid of? Are there special things that you want to do or achieve in the future?

Other concluding questions to close the interview include

- Are there any questions you wish to ask?
- When comparing yourself today to when you felt the best about yourself and the world, what differences do you note in how you feel, think, and behave?
- Of all the ideas we have talked about, what are some you think are important in relation to what is presently concerning you?

■ CASE FORMULATION, DIAGNOSIS, PLAN, AND EVALUATION

Nursing is a holistic science that treats the totality of the patient. Primary prevention intervention is aimed at maintaining a state of wellness, and secondary prevention minimizes the patient's negative response to an acute physical or mental health state. Tertiary prevention assists the patient to maintain an optimal functioning despite a long-term illness or chronic mental health disability. How can the data that have been collected be assembled to formulate preliminary nursing diagnoses and a plan care and evaluation? How can preventive measures be instituted?

The next step is to sit with the patient and formulate the plan of care. The patient and nurse together will recognize behaviors that are manifested, determine which need to be improved or changed, which strengths are available to bring to bear on the process, and what resources are needed.

The summary of information collected during the assessment process is called the case formulation. This is not analogous to selecting five symptoms from a list or referencing psychiatric diagnosis. For example, ineffective individual coping related to schizophrenia as evidenced by poor coping skills is neither a formulation or a nursing diagnosis. The intent of formulation is to generate understanding about the dynamics of what brings the person to the in-patient setting and to develop agreement on how to proceed. It is brought about by the process of engagement and trust and is started during the assessment.

CASE FORMULATION

The nursing diagnosis comes after the information collected in assessment has been summarized holistically as the nurse and patient prioritize the specific areas on which to work. Formulation of relevant nursing diagnoses have the purpose of expressing the needs and goals of the patient and interfacing with other care providers.

Standard II, diagnosis, states that, in addition to psychiatric mental health nurses analyzing assessment data, they must provide nursing care that recognizes and identifies patterns of response to actual or potential psychiatric illnesses and mental health problems. Diagnoses conform to the accepted classification systems, such as the North American Nursing Diagnosis Association (NANDA) Nursing Diagnosis Classification and the Diagnostic and Statistical Manual of Mental Disorders (APA, 1994).

The diagnoses are organized into nine human response patterns as they appear in Section 3 of the MPC Nursing Assessment Form (Figure 38–4).

1. Exchanging: mutual giving and receiving.
2. Communicating: sending and receiving messages.
3. Relating: establishing bonds with others.
4. Valuing: assigning relative worth.
5. Choosing: selecting alternatives.
6. Moving: activity.
7. Perceiving: receiving information.
8. Knowing: meaning of information.
9. Feeling: subjective awareness of information.

Components

A nursing diagnosis is the conceptualization of the patient's health problems identified from the assessment process. They are abstractions proposed by clinicians in their attempts to make sense out of what has been observed and recorded.

DETERMINING NURSING DIAGNOSIS

When nurses complete the patient assessment, they review the NANDA list of nursing diagnoses. Once the nursing diagnosis is developed and agreed on, nursing interventions to effect change or improvement in that area can be formulated. Diagnoses are hypotheses. Based on the nursing diagnosis, implementing the intervention plan with proposed interventions regarding what treatment services combined with what patient strengths will promote the desired outcome in a cost-effective and satisfactory way (see case example of Henry Lear below).

Outcome Identification

Standard of Care III is outcome identification. In this standard of care, the psychiatric–mental health nurse identifies expected outcomes individualized to the patient. Within the context of providing nursing care, the ultimate goal is to influence health outcomes and improve the patient's health status.

PLANNING CARE

Standard of Care IV is planning care. The psychiatric–mental health nurse develops a plan of care that prescribes interventions to attain expected outcomes. A plan of care is used to guide therapeutic intervention systematically and achieve the expected patient outcomes.

Nursing diagnoses must be identified and prioritized with patient needs. The strengths and assets relevant to nursing interventions must be included and interventions recommended.

IMPLEMENTATION

Standard of Care V is implementation of the nursing care plan. The psychiatric–mental health nurse implements the interventions identified in the plan of care.

E CASE EXAMPLE

HISTORY/PAST EXPERIENCES

Patient Henry Lear (a 47-year-old white male) was admitted to a state psychiatric facility from a family care home displaying the following behaviors/problems:

- Poor sleep patterns, irritability.
- Setting small fires from cigarettes.
- Psychomotor agitation, pacing, repeated patterns of rubbing fingers.
- Increased rate and volume of speech.
- Report that family care provider is relocating him as there are plans to "sell the house."
- Withdrawn and aloof.
- Poor ADLs and hygiene.
- Multiple stains/burns on fingers/nails from cigarettes.
- Eating from the garbage.
- Defecating/urinating on self and floor.
- Dermatitis of buttocks.

The patient shared information about his childhood, family history, interpersonal relations, alcohol and drug use, spiritual beliefs and practice, education, employment, military history, and physical and mental health. He was first admitted to a psychiatric facility at age 25, following service in Vietnam for 1½ years. At that time he believed that he was being injected with needles and that a magnetic device, like radar, was implanted in his skin. He made statements of "they can see you and what you are doing." He responded well to psychotropics (Navane) but failed to continue medications

or aftercare when discharged. His subsequent readmissions revealed further delusional thinking: bugs implanted in his buttocks by his father because he was bad as a child, which accounted for the noises in his ears. He had repeated admissions and discharges for approximately a 10-year period. When out of the hospital, Mr. Lear engaged in excessive alcohol use, minor thefts of food and mail, and used marijuana. He was unable to re-establish a relationship with his former wife and three children; the multiple threats and break-ins of their property resulted in the involvement of Child Protective Services and an order of protection. He was able to recall events of childhood, school, and family composition. He was one of six children; three girls and three boys. He had quit school in the tenth grade but was awarded his GED while in the army. He stated that his father was "bossy, opinionated, hard tempered, and difficult to get along with." He recalls having difficulty making and keeping peer relationships due to his family moving frequently. He has no adult involvement in religion. In the past, he has threatened harm to his children and ex-wife but cannot account for these actions.

NURSING ASSESSMENT ON THE WARD

- He smokes.
- He carries a cup frequently.
- He has episodic incontinence.
- He has rapid changes in clarity of thought from short attention span to increasing confusion.
- He has frequent electrolyte abnormalities of serum sodium.

- He drinks excessively.
- He has rapid changes in mental status, such as mood irritability and aggressive behavior.
- He may urinate in clothes, on floor, or in cup/shoes and attempt to drink urine.

PRESENTING PROBLEMS

Problem one: Physically threatening behavior (i.e., spitting, assaulting, encroachment). He is verbally aggressive (yelling, swearing, and cursing).
Problem two: Hyponatremia (excessive water drinking, urinary incontinence, increased irritability). Aggressive (physical and verbal) behavior that often revolves around fluids.
Problem three: Dermatitis due to enuresis, related to hyponatremia.

COURSE OF HOSPITALIZATION

For the 2 weeks following his most current admission, Mr. Lear did not wash himself, change his clothes, or brush his teeth unless directly supervised by staff. He related superficially with staff, made eye contact, but remained aloof from peers. He paced continuously and rapped on doors accompanied by inappropriate laugher and conversation without the presence of a person. He denied bizarre, somatic, religious, persecutory, or grandiose delusions, auditory/visual/sensory hallucinations, and suicidal/homicidal ideations or plans. He smoked safely during the supervised smoking program on the unit, otherwise he would burn his fingers and nails. His attention span and concentration lasted for approximately 20 minutes if the topic was of fair interest to him. He stated he was not "bugged out" and did not need medications. He stated he is residing in the facility "due to a need for housing."

As 6 months of hospitalization progressed, the patient demonstrated frequent periods of noncompliance to psychotropic medication and associated escalation of aggression, especially when approached regarding excessive cigarette smoking and supervision and direction from staff. He was frequently noted to be ingesting large amounts of fluids followed by periods of irritability and threatening behavior.

It was noted that when he consumed excess fluids, he would exhibit increased psychomotor agitation, pacing, becoming loud, demanding, grandiose, and threatening verbally and physically. Further, he demonstrated no insight into the need of his hospitalization and treatment of his mental illness or personal safety, but rather expressed feelings of being persecuted, victimized by legal authorities and his ex-wife, and demanded release on the grounds of his rights as a veteran. When provided a psychotropic P.R.N. medication in response to the increasingly threatening, aggressive behavior, he would seek fluid and have periods of excessive urination. Mr. Lear later would relate this behavior as an effort to dilute the medication and wash it from his body. One episode of fluid intoxication resulted in an extremely low sodium (Na 114 to 117), and he was treated in an acute medical facility following grand mal seizures. Once medically stable, he continued to demonstrate limited insight into the harmful effects of fluid intoxication, laughing inappropriately and stating that it produced a high for him. He continued to berate peers, was reluctant to join leisure activities, and occasionally shouted demands, threatened staff and peers, and refused interactions unless on his terms.

STRENGTHS

- Oriented to person, place, and time.
- History of favorable response to psychotropics.
- Recall of past events.
- Attained GED.
- Completed 1½ years in army/Vietnam.
- Ability to verbally communicate needs and feelings for short duration (15 to 20 minutes) and remain with topic.
- Ability to minimally perform ADLs in an independent manner with verbal prompts and supervision.

NEEDS

- Poor insight judgment reporting personal health and safety as demonstrated by excessive fluid intake resulting in hyponatremia and unsafe cigarette smoking resulting in fire setting.
- Difficulty trusting, making and keeping peer relationships, and demonstrating appropriate socialization skills.
- May become physically threatening, pace, become irritable, excited if perception of environment is threatening.
- Difficulty coping, identifying stressors or support systems.
- History of noncompliance to medication and aftercare program.
- History of disrupted sleep patterns.
- Presenting inguinal hernia.
- Poor orientation to situation, or stressor precipitating admission.

NURSING DIAGNOSIS

Disordered water balance related to knowledge deficit regarding the effects of excessive fluid intake on the total person as evidenced by poor impulse control (assaultive behavior) and fluid seeking behavior.

Alteration in thought processes related to inability to trust as evidenced by delusional thinking, inappropriate social behavior, and inability to demonstrate interpersonal and social skills.

Potential for infection related to compromised skin integrity caused by frequent, extended periods of exposure to urine as evidenced by dermatitis.

NURSING INTERVENTIONS

Acute phase

- Observe patient for increased thirst and water seeking or psychotic behaviors.
- Teach patient to report an increase in thirst.
- Counsel patient to reduce fluid intake to prevent low sodium levels.
- Fluid restriction; control access to water and/or fluid.
- Electrolytes as ordered. Notify physician if serum sodium is below 130.

E CASE EXAMPLE   Continued

- Weigh patient twice per day. Inform physician if there is a 5% increase in body weight.
- Give hard sugarless candy to stimulate saliva and prevent dry mouth.
- Give small amount of hyperosmotic beverage (Gatorade) with medications instead of juice or water.
- Patient may require one-to-one supervision at the time when fluid drinking is intensified.
- Reduce access to fluids immediately after smoking.
- Provide support for patient and peers to decrease acting out and blaming when ward environment is restricted.

Chronic phase
- Monitor patient daily for excess fluid intake.
- Monitor for mental status changes (i.e., headaches, gastrointestinal symptoms, nausea, vomiting, and diarrhea).
- Monitor changes in medications, including psychotropics (Lithium and Tegretol), that may cause symptoms of dry mouth or increased thirst.
- Weight and electrolytes to be monitored.
- Teach patient to report increased thirst or fluid consumption to staff.
- Contract with patient to maintain weight or serum sodium within agreed upon range.
- Patient, because of his chronic condition, should have highly structured activities that divert this behavior.
- Reduce smoking consumption (nicotine stimulates ADH release) that is, smoking cessation program.

NURSING IMPACT ON DISCHARGE PLAN

Give health education regarding hyponatremic condition, such as nursing group therapy, focusing on the hyponatremia patient (fluid restriction, toileting, vital signs, weight) (see attached review sheet and hyponatremia group outline for protocol).

Encourage positive coping mechanisms on a one-to-one basis and in nursing group therapy to maintain control over behavior and reduce aggressive behavior (verbal and physical).

OUTCOME

At present, following the introduction of Clozaril 100 mg AM and 225 mg H.S., Mr. Lear is more receptive to interventions, socialization, and participation in leisure activities. He agrees to monitoring of weight fluctuations t.i.d. and a daily fluid intake of 2000 to 3000 cc. If there is a 5% deviation in weight (gain or loss), a physician is notified to evaluate his physical status, and a STAT Na level may be obtained. Further, there may be a change in his level of supervision, fluid intake, and monitoring of vital signs. He is observed daily and asked to self-report to note any sudden changes in behavior, which he does with this person. There is significant correlation in irritability, nicotine seeking behavior, intrusiveness, hypertalkativeness, delusional or persecutory thoughts, psychomotor agitation or pacing, and withdrawn or aloof demeanor with increased fluid intake.

The patient has been able to attend nursing psychoeducational groups that focus on the harmful effects of excessive fluid intake. He has actively participated in identifying triggers or events in his life (past and current) that may result in increased fluid intake. He shares his experiences and recovery strategy with others in a peer support group. These interventions reinforce a contract to maintain a Na level above 130 and recognize his efforts to manage the condition with the help of nursing staff.

Clozaril therapy and nursing interventions have allowed this patient to have increased insight into his illness and to self-manage his fluid seeking behavior. He can identify and use coping strategies, such as keeping his mouth moist with sugarless hard candy or decreasing physical exertion in warm weather. He has been able to join a vocational program that involves maintenance activities, completing his assignments in a thorough, motivated fashion.

When implementing the plan of care, psychiatric–mental health nurses use a wide range of interventions designed to prevent mental and physical illness, and promote, maintain, and restore mental and physical health. Psychiatric–mental health nurses select interventions according to their level of practice.

Discharge plans are included in any plan of care. Although the nurse is assessing the patient for his or her current condition, the future is also a consideration, and thus, the following questions will be useful for the patient's continuing care.

- Describe your current living condition.
- Does your current living situation meet your needs?

- What help do you think you will need after discharge?
- Who will be available to help?
- Have you ever had follow-up care after a hospitalization?

EVALUATION

Standard of Care VI is evaluation. As with any hypothesis or intervention, continued evaluation and reassessment to determine if the desired effects are occurring is essential.

O AN OVERVIEW

- Psychiatric nursing assessment guides the entire nursing process and is the basis for interactions between the nurse and patient and between the nurse and other members of the health care team.

- A holistic approach to the nursing process promotes mental, emotional, motivational, environmental, spiritual, systems, and biological outcomes.

- The Standards of Psychiatric Mental Health Clinical Nursing Practice relate to the direct clinical care a patient receives as demonstrated through the nursing process.

- Assessment includes collecting data concerning the patient's functional areas and behavioral and mental status.

- The key elements in formulating a nursing diagnosis for people with emotional problems or distress include their patterns of interaction, methods of coping, emotional status, and general lifestyle.

- The nursing assessment interview provides a way for the nurse and patient to become oriented to each other, while the nurse elicits information preliminary to arriving at nursing diagnoses.

- Information elicited is transmitted correctly and efficiently to the patient, the patient's support network, the nurse's peers and colleagues, and individuals or groups who are responsible for systems processes.

- The summary of information collected during the assessment process is called case formulation; its intent is to generate understanding about the dynamics of what brings the person to the in-patient setting and develop agreement on intervention.

TD TERMS TO DEFINE

- case formulation
- data collection
- empowerment
- functional behavior status
- holistic psychiatric assessment

- human response patterns
- mental status assessment
- nursing diagnosis
- primary prevention
- secondary prevention
- Standards of Psychiatric Mental Health Clinical Nursing Practice
- tertiary prevention

Q STUDY QUESTIONS

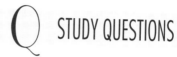

1. Describe and analyze a situation that you have experienced or observed in which a nurse allows his or her own needs to take precedence over interpersonal events with the patient. How could the nurse have handled the situation differently?

2. Complete a functional assessment of yourself or a colleague. How would you integrate this information into a nursing diagnosis? Case formulation? Interventions?

3. Complete a mental status examination of yourself or a colleague. Explain the implications of "mental status" for both psycho-educational interventions and interpersonal interventions.

■ REFERENCES

American Nurses Association. *Standards of Psychiatric Mental Health Clinical Nursing Practice.* Washington, DC: Author; 1994.

American Psychiatric Association. *Diagnostic and Statistical Manual of Mental Disorders,* ed 4, Washington, D.C. 1994, The Association.

Macrae JC. Nightingale's spiritual philosophy and its significance for modern nursing image. *J Nurs Scholarship* 1995; 27(1):8–10.

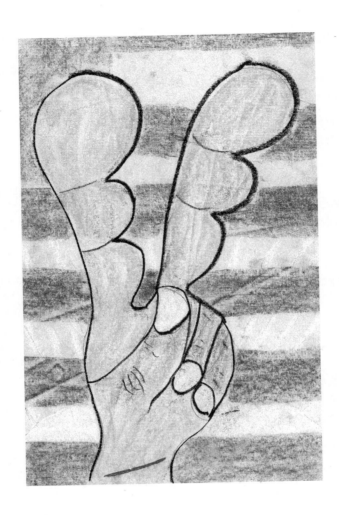

Most people live, whether physically, intellectually or morally, in a very restricted circle of their potential being. They make use of a very small portion of their possible consciousness, and of their soul's resources in general. . . . Great emergencies and crises show us how much greater our vital resources are than we had supposed.

William James (1842–1910)
Letter to W. Lutoslawski (May 6, 1906)

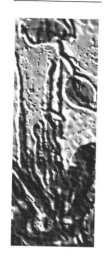

39
Crisis Intervention

Albert R. Roberts / Ann Wolbert Burgess

Nurses are in daily contact with patients who are under stress, experiencing anxiety, or having difficulty coping and managing their lives (Hoff, 1995). When the stress or stressors overwhelm individuals, a crisis situation may develop. This chapter continues the discussion of stress, coping, and anxiety and focuses on crisis theory and techniques to assess and intervene with people in crisis. The theory is based on a biopsychosocial perspective.

A crisis is a period of psychological disequilibrium, which is experienced as a result of a hazardous event or situation that constitutes a significant problem that cannot be remedied by using familiar coping strategies.

A crisis occurs when a person faces an obstacle to important life goals that generally seems insurmountable through the use of customary habits and coping patterns. The goal of crisis intervention is to resolve the most pressing problems within 1 to 12 weeks through focused, directed intervention aimed at helping the patient develop new adaptive coping methods.

Crisis reaction refers to the acute stage, which usually occurs soon after the hazardous event (i.e., death of a loved one, battering, suicide attempt, or serious diagnosis). During this phase, the person's acute reaction may take various forms, including helplessness, confusion, anger, anxiety, shock, or *disbelief. Low self-esteem and serious depression are often produced by the crisis state. The person in crisis may appear to be incoherent, disorganized, agitated, and volatile or they may be calm, subdued, withdrawn, and apathetic. It is during this crisis reaction period that the individual is often most willing to seek help, and crisis intervention is usually more effective at this time.*

■ THEORETICAL DEVELOPMENT

As long ago as 400 BC, physicians have stressed the significance of crisis as a hazardous life event. Hippocrates himself defined a crisis as a sudden state that gravely endangers life. The development of a cohesive theory of crisis, however, and approaches to crisis management had to wait until the twentieth century.

Although the movement to help people in crisis began in 1906 with the establishment in New York City of the first suicide prevention center (National Save-A-Life League), contemporary crisis intervention theory and practice were not formally elaborated until the 1940s. Erich Lindemann and Gerald Caplan were primarily responsible for introducing crisis intervention theory.

ERICH LINDEMANN

Lindemann and associates at Massachusetts General Hospital introduced the concepts of crisis intervention and time-limited treatment in 1943 in the aftermath of Boston's worst nightclub fire, at the Coconut Grove, in which 493 people perished. Lindemann (1944) and colleagues based the crisis theory they developed on their observations of the acute and delayed reactions of survivors and grief-stricken relatives of victims. Their clinical work focused on the psychological symptoms of the survivors and on preventing unresolved grief among relatives of the persons who had died. They found that many individuals experiencing acute grief often had five related reactions: somatic distress, preoccupation with the image of the deceased, guilt, hostile reactions, and loss of patterns of conduct.

Furthermore, Lindemann and colleagues concluded that the duration of a grief reaction appears to be dependent on the success with which the bereaved person does his or her mourning and "grief work." In general, this grief work refers to achieving emancipation from the deceased, readjusting to the changes in the environment from which the loved one is missing, and developing new relationships. People need to be encouraged to permit themselves to have a period of mourning and eventual acceptance of the loss and adjustment to life without the deceased. By delaying the normal process of grieving, negative outcomes of crises will develop.

GERALD CAPLAN

Gerald Caplan (1961), who was affiliated with Massachusetts General Hospital and the Harvard School of Public Health, expanded on Lindemann's work with the fire survivors. He studied various developmental crisis reactions, as in premature birth, infancy, childhood, and adolescence, and accidental crises, such as illness and death. Caplan (1964) defined crisis as psychological disequilibrium when a person confronts a hazardous circumstance that he or she can for the time being neither escape nor solve with customary problem-solving resources.

Caplan also described four stages of a crisis reaction:

1. The initial rise of tension that comes from the emotionally hazardous, crisis-precipitating event.
2. An increased level of tension and disruption to daily living because the individual is unable to resolve the crisis quickly.
3. As the individual attempts and fails to resolve the crisis by emergency problem-solving mechanisms, tension increases to such an intense level that the individual may go into a depression.
4. The person may experience either a mental collapse or breakdown, or they may partly resolve the crisis by new coping methods.

CRISIS THEORY

Crisis theory is based on the concept of homeostatic balance and the relationship of coping processes to stable psychological functioning. The principle of homeostasis is borrowed from physiology and, in that context, is defined by the need to preserve stable chemical or electrolyte balances within the body necessary to sustain life. When these balances are upset, self-regulatory mechanisms are triggered that help restore these balances to healthy levels. Crisis theory applies this principle to psychological functioning.

For each individual, a reasonably consistent balance exists between affective and cognitive experience. This homeostatic balance, however, may vary considerably from person to person. The primary characteristic of this balance is its stability for that individual. The stability is "normal" for that person and becomes a frame of reference against which to evaluate changes in psychological functioning. A healthy homeostatic balance requires stable psychological functioning with a minimum of dysphoric affect, the maintenance of reasonable cognitive perspective on experience, and the retention of problem-solving skills.

When there is an imbalance, coping processes or psychological self-regulatory mechanisms facilitate a return to homeostatic balance. Through development and experience, individuals learn a repertoire of coping behaviors that are used in various types of stressful situations. The coping mechanisms are designed to reduce, control, or avoid unpleasant emotions in order to re-establish homeostatic balance, facilitating the person's return to normal functioning. Coping behaviors occur at various levels of the individual's awareness, and the behaviors at different levels may be used simultaneously as responses to stressful situations.

Most adults have developed a range of coping behaviors; some are adaptive, others less than adaptive. Maladaptive coping responses are typically used in situations where the individual feels vulnerable. At best, coping is the process of mastering a particular problematic situation. At worst, coping behaviors serve primarily to protect a vulnerable sense of self without mastery of the situation. Coping behaviors cannot be dichotomized into categories of adaptive or maladaptive but should be viewed as a continuum, with behaviors manifesting various levels of adaptiveness depending on the person and the situation. When an individual encounters a situation in which there is a significant psychological threat and great personal vulnerability, coping behaviors are more likely to be self-protective than oriented toward mastery.

Baldwin (1978) identified four distinct phases in the life cycle of an emotional crisis.

Phase 1 THE EMOTIONALLY HAZARDOUS SITUATION

- A rise of uncomfortable affect signals disruption of homeostatic balance.
- Unpleasant affect produces motivation to reduce it and return to a normal state of psychological homeostasis.
- Previously learned and used coping behaviors are brought to bear on the situation in attempts to reduce unpleasant affect.
- In most instances, learned coping behaviors succeed in returning the individual to homeostatic balance in a short period of time.

Phase 2 THE EMOTIONAL CRISIS

- Previously learned coping behaviors are tried but are inadequate or ineffective responses to the crisis situation.
- Unpleasant and uncomfortable affect intensifies, and cognitive disorganization increases over time.
- The individual is motivated to attempt new and/or novel coping behaviors or problem-solving techniques.
- The individual seeks out others for support in resolving the crisis.

Phase 3 CRISIS RESOLUTION
Adaptive Resolution

- With help, the individual defines issues, deals with feelings, makes decisions, or learns new problem-solving or coping behaviors.
- Underlying conflicts represented in the crisis situation or reactivated by it are identified and at least partially resolved.
- Internal and external sources of support are mobilized, and the individual's resources for resolving the crisis are defined.
- Unpleasant or uncomfortable affect is reduced, and the individual returns to at least a precrisis level of functioning.

Maladaptive Resolution

- The individual does not seek or find adequate help to define issues, deal with feelings, make constructive decisions, or learn new problem-solving or coping behaviors.
- Underlying conflicts represented in the crisis situation or reactivated by it remain unidentified and unresolved.

- Internal and external sources of support for the individual are not mobilized and needed resources remain unavailable.
- Unpleasant and uncomfortable affect is reduced somewhat, thereby defusing the immediate crisis situation; the individual returns to a less adaptive level of functioning than in the precrisis period.

Phase 4 POSTCRISIS ADAPTATION
Adaptive Resolution

- The individual becomes less vulnerable in a particular problematic situation because underlying conflicts have been resolved and will not be reactivated in similar situations.
- The individual has learned new and more adaptive coping behaviors or problem-solving skills that can be used as responses to future stressful situations.
- The individual's general level of functioning may have improved, and personal growth and maturation have occurred.
- The likelihood is reduced that future emotionally hazardous situations of a particular type will develop into an emotional crisis.

Maladaptive Resolution

- The individual remains vulnerable or becomes more vulnerable in particular problematic situations because underlying conflicts have not been resolved and will be reactivated in future, similar situations.
- The individual has learned maladaptive, self-defeating mechanisms to cope with stressful situations.
- The individual's general level of functioning may be reduced to a less adaptive level than that of the precrisis period.
- The likelihood is enhanced that future emotionally hazardous situations of a particular type will develop into an emotional crisis.

TRANSITIONAL SITUATIONS

J. S. Tyhurst (1957) studied transition states (i.e., migration and retirement) in the lives of persons experiencing sudden change during civilian disaster. Based on his field studies on individual patterns of responses to community disaster, Tyhurst identified three overlapping phases, each with its own manifestations of stress and attempts to reduce it: a period of impact, a period of recoil, and a post-traumatic period of recovery. Tyhurst recommended stage-specific interventions. He con-

cluded that persons in transitional crisis states should not be removed from their life situations, and intervention should focus on bolstering the network of relationships.

LYDIA RAPOPORT

Lydia Rapoport built on the pioneering work of Lindemann and Caplan. In her first article on crisis theory (Rapoport, 1962), Rapoport defined a crisis as an "upset steady state" that places the individual in a hazardous condition. Rapoport pointed out that a crisis situation results in a problem that can be perceived as a threat, loss, or challenge. She stated that usually three interrelated factors create a state of crisis:

- A hazardous event.
- A threat to life goals.
- An inability to respond with adequate coping mechanisms.

In their early works, Lindemann and Caplan briefly mentioned that a hazardous event produces a crisis; however, Rapoport (1967, 1970) most thoroughly described the nature of this crisis-precipitating event. Rapoport clearly conceptualized the content of crisis intervention practice, particularly the initial or study phase (assessment), pointing out that in order to help persons in crisis, it is necessary that the patient have rapid access to the crisis worker. She stated, "A little help, rationally directed and purposefully focused at a strategic time, is more effective than more extensive help given at a period of less emotional accessibility" (Rapoport, 1967, p. 38).

This was echoed by Naomi Golan (1978) who concluded that during the state of active crisis, when the usual coping methods have proven inadequate and the individual and his or her family are suffering pain and discomfort, a person is frequently more amenable to suggestions and change. Clearly, intensive, brief, appropriately focused treatment during a period when the patient is motivated can produce more effective change than long-term treatment during periods when motivation and emotional accessibility are lacking.

Rapoport (1967) asserted that during the initial interview, the first task of the practitioner is to develop a preliminary diagnosis of the presenting problem. It is most critical during this first interview that the crisis therapist convey a sense of hope and optimism to the patient concerning successful crisis resolution. Rapoport suggested that this sense of hope and enthusiasm can be properly conveyed when the interview focuses on mutual exploration and problem solving, along with clearly delineated goals and tasks. The underlying message is that patient and therapist will be working together to resolve the crisis.

■ SEEKING HELP

What motivates people in crisis to seek help? Ripple and colleagues (1964) suggest that a balance of discomfort and hope is necessary to motivate a distressed person to seek help. Hope, defined by Stotland (1969), is the perceived possibility of attaining a goal. The pressure to act comes from a sufficient amount of both discomfort and hope for the individual in crisis to make a concerted effort to seek help.

The crisis nurse knows that coping patterns differ for each individual. The crisis nurse also knows that for an individual to suffer and survive a crisis (such as losing a loved one, living through an earthquake or a tornado, attempting suicide, or being sexually assaulted) that person must have a conscious purpose to live and grow. Each individual in crisis must define his or her own purpose. Each needs to ventilate, be accepted, and receive support, assistance, and encouragement to discover the paths to crisis resolution.

It is useful for the patient to understand the specific personal meaning of the event and how it conflicts with his or her expectations, life goals, and belief system. Thoughts, feelings, and beliefs usually flow freely when a patient in crisis talks. The crisis nurse should listen carefully and note any cognitive errors or distortions (i.e., overgeneralizing, catastrophizing) or irrational beliefs. The nurse should avoid prematurely stating rational beliefs or reality-based cognitions for the patient, and instead, the nurse should help the patient to recognize discrepancies, distortions, and irrational beliefs. This is best accomplished through carefully worded questions, such as, "How do you view yourself now that you realize everyone with less than 5 years seniority got laid off?" or "Have you ever asked your doctor whether he thinks you will die from cancer at a young age or what your actual risk is of having cancer?"

Experiencing an unwanted pregnancy, a divorce, or a broken engagement, being the victim of a domestic assault, and being a close relative of a person killed in an automobile or plane crash are all highly stressful events. The persons involved may use denial and express anger and fear, grief and loss, but they can all survive. Crisis intervention can reduce immediate danger and fear, as well as provide support, hope, and alternative ways of coping and growing.

■ CRISIS INTERVENTION MODELS

Several models have been developed to guide practitioners who work with patients in crisis. The most widely known models are Caplan's (1964) four-stage model, Rapoport's (1967) three-stage model, Baldwin's (1978, 1980) four-stage model—all defined earlier in this chapter—and Golan's (1978) three-phase model. Roberts, expanding on the previously developed systems, has devised a seven-step model that offers an integrated problem-solving approach to crisis resolution. Before discussing that model, Golan's model, the most useful of the earlier ones, will be described.

GOLAN'S MODEL

Naomi Golan's (1978) model is very useful for clinicians because it provides the crisis nurse with examples of selective empathetic statements and questions to ask patients during each phase of treatment—the beginning (first interview), middle (first to fourth interviews), and end (the last one or two interviews). More specifically, during the first interview, Golan directs the crisis nurse to begin with the "here and now" by focusing on the precipitating event, including "scope, persons involved, outcome, severity of effect, and the time the event occurred" (p. 84). The triggering factor is the event or incident that prompted the individual to contact the crisis center.

After allowing the patient to verbalize what happened, he or she should be encouraged to ventilate by expressing such feelings as frustration, anger, or guilt. The crisis nurse is encouraged to elicit from the patient subjective reactions about the event, while trying to obtain his or her affective responses to the recent past and to the part the patient played in it. Among Golan's prompting statements for the crisis workers to use are

- You must have felt terrible about it.
- No wonder you sound so upset.
- Can you put your finger on what started this?
- Things really began to change after you came to college.
- I suppose in the beginning you were in a state of shock.
- You're in a real dilemma; I guess the most important thing is to come to a decision as to whether to leave your husband.

ROBERTS AND BURGESS MODEL

The Roberts and Burgess seven-stage model (Table 39–1) can be applied to specific patients in crisis and can promote effective early crisis resolution. This model is an expansion and adaptation of Roberts (1991) and Baldwin (1978) models. The order of stages 1 and 2 can be reversed, depending on the type of crisis. It is essential that the nurse immediately assess the lethality of the situation. If the patient is not in any immediate distress, establishing rapport is the first step.

TABLE 39–1. ROBERTS AND BURGESS SEVEN STAGE CRISIS INTERVENTION MODEL

Stage	Intervention
1	Assess danger and safety
	Are patient and family in danger or safe from others?
	Is patient safe to him or herself?
2	Establish therapeutic alliance
	Contract for meeting
	Active listening
	Provide support
3	Identify the precipitating event
	Time and place of precipitating event
	Interpersonal dimensions of the event
	Physical and emotional response to event
	Psychodynamic issue of the crisis
	Processing the precipitating event
4	Meaning of the crisis
	Effect of crisis on present and future
	Changes to life plan or goals
5	Explore coping alternatives
	Past and present coping
	Adaptive and maladaptive coping
6	Develop action plan
	Short-term approach for the crisis
	Long-term approach for mastery
7	Follow-up
	Evaluation of crisis resolution
	Referral

Assess Lethality and Safety Needs

Determine the person's degree of risk for serious injury or death from self-destructive acts or from the violent acts of another person. On the telephone, it is necessary to assess the level and seriousness of threats to the caller's safety. Roberts and Roberts (1990) studied the crisis intervention techniques used by telephone hotlines and emergency shelters for battered women. The shelters indicated that their first priority is to ensure the safety of the women and their children. Examples of the questions crisis workers ask are

- Are you or your children in danger now?
- Is the abuser there now?
- Do you want me to call the police?
- Do you want to leave, and can you do so safely?
- Do you or your children need medical attention?

If the patient is a battered woman, she should be encouraged to call the police, go to the emergency room of the nearest hospital if medical care is needed, or take refuge at the local battered women's shelter if emergency housing is needed. To detect and assess bat-

tery systematically, adult abuse protocols have been developed at large city hospitals, including Boston, Chicago, Indianapolis, Philadelphia, and Seattle. The first and most comprehensive protocol was developed by Karil Klingbeil and Vicky Boyd at Harborview Seattle (Roberts, 1984). Although the adult abuse protocols were developed for use in emergency wards, they have been adapted for use by crisis units in community settings and for use in private practice and prenatal clinics.

Establish Rapport and Communication—the Therapeutic Alliance

Initial rapport can be established when the nurse lets the patient know that he or she has done the right thing by contacting a crisis unit. The nurse should also convey a willingness and ability to help, which is accomplished by active listening in an accepting, concerned, patient, and helpful manner.

People experiencing stress of crisis proportions often feel frightened and vulnerable. Part of establishing a therapeutic alliance is to help the individual feel safe and secure, and that he or she will be listened to respectfully. The nurse directly provides appropriate support for the patient or helps mobilize it. In addition, the nurse helps the patient restore a realistic perspective of the crisis situation and to define viable options or courses of action. The personal resources of the patient are assessed and identified as essential to the development of an adaptive response to the crisis.

Identify the Precipitating Event

It is useful to explore with the patient the immediate past and the present. The immediate past refers to the "last straw," the precipitating factor (i.e., a violent assault, rejection, or an extremely humiliating event) that led the patient to seek help at this time. Nurses also find it useful to determine how the patient was functioning just prior to the crisis. Many patients present with multiple problems, including those of other people, such as a spouse or a sibling. The clinician should help the patient to focus on his or her own problems, not those of a third party. Efforts should center on helping the patient to rank, order, and prioritize the problems, with the goal of attending to the immediate and major problem. In general, it is usually much more productive to isolate the precipitating event or problem that led the patient to seek help and to focus first on that central concern.

Crisis theory is based on the interaction of an individual and a stressful situation. Understanding in detail the precipitant event that resulted in a failure to cope and an emotional crisis is necessary in crisis assessment.

This information helps to structure and focus intervention. It cannot be assumed that the patient is aware of or understands the relationship of the precipitating event to the emotional crisis, and creating this understanding may be an important aspect of helping the patient organize the crisis experience. Several aspects of the precipitating event warrant closer scrutiny and exploration by the nurse.

Time and Place of the Precipitating Event.

Sometimes patients easily define the time and place of the event that precipitated the crisis. This, however, is not always the case. In many instances, the patient has not defined the event that evolved into the crisis nor its emotional meaning. Defining the event and placing it into the framework of the patient's recent experience is important. Sometimes the event is quite subtle and difficult to detect, even by a skilled therapist. Yet, the crisis always has a situational trigger that, when conceptualized, is helpful to both patient and therapist in understanding the crisis.

Patients with little or no psychological-mindedness or capacity for insight may have difficulty defining the time and place of the precipitating event. With such patients, examining emotional cause-and-effect relationships can be very helpful and often is part of the psychological education that becomes part of the crisis assessment process. At other times, the precipitating event will not be evident even with close scrutiny of the patient's recent past. Then the course of crisis intervention is initiated on the basis of available information; it is not uncommon that the precipitating event becomes clearer during the course of crisis resolution.

Interpersonal Dimensions of the Problem Situation.

It is extremely important for the nurse to assess not only the time and place of the precipitating event, but also the interpersonal parameters of the situation. Sometimes significant others from the past are involved in the present crisis because conflicts or traumas associated with them are reactivated by a current situation. The interpersonal dimension of a crisis often represents an actual loss or potential loss to the patient. It is the defending against such losses, or attempting to replace them, that determines many maladaptive coping responses to problem situations and precipitates the crisis.

Affective Response to the Precipitating Event.

Reacting to the precipitating event, the patient experiences disruption of homeostatic balance. This disruption is characterized by a rise of unpleasant or dysphoric affect that intensifies with time because no effective coping responses are available to reduce it. The longer this situation (the crisis) continues, the more intense this disruptive affect becomes and the more incapable the patient becomes of retaining perspective of the situation, defining viable courses of action, and mobilizing problem-solving or coping skills. It is frequently very helpful early in the crisis assessment process to encourage the patient to express such affect and thereby defuse (at least temporarily) some of the intensity of the crisis.

The nature of the dysphoria experienced by a patient is also important in crisis assessment. It helps to determine whether or not any emergency measures must be taken to ensure patient welfare. The patient may be experiencing guilt, anger, anxiety, or depression, or may have already decompensated and be overwhelmed. The nature of patient stress is diagnostic and often reflects a particular type of vulnerability that has been instrumental in producing the crisis. The nurse needs to elicit a description of the affective experience of the crisis in the patient's own words for future reflection during the crisis work.

Psychodynamic Issues in the Crisis.

Many emotional crises are determined, at least in part, by unresolved conflicts or traumas that occurred in the past and are again brought to awareness by a particular event. The psychodynamic component of the crisis, the precipitant, is frequently instrumental in producing a failure to cope and impedes adaptive crisis resolution unless addressed as part of the crisis intervention process.

Although not all crises have psychodynamic determinants, most do involve antecedent factors reactivated by the precipitating event. When this is the case, the patient experiences an emotional overreaction that is often surprising in its intensity. The precipitating event has activated a dormant vulnerability of the patient, and the intensity of the affect produced is often overwhelming and confusing. When this occurs, usual coping behaviors become inoperable, and the patient may use coping responses that are orientated more toward ego protection than mastery of the situation.

It is the task of the nurse, when a precipitant is detected, to help the patient respond adaptively to the current situation, using the situation to simultaneously address and work through the reactivated conflicts and traumas from the past.

Detecting and Working Through the Precipitant.

Perhaps the most challenging aspect of crisis intervention is identifying and addressing the precipitant. The precipitant may be activated in two basic ways: by an experience that is somehow directly analogous to a past conflict or trauma, or by an event that activates anticipatory fear of experiencing a past trauma again. When the latter is the case, coping responses are mobilized to avoid anticipated pain and to protect the self.

The nurse may explore the crisis situation for clues to the precipitant in a number of ways. Some strategies follow.

- Define similarities between current patient affect and affect recalled from past painful experiences (When have you felt this way before?).
- Explore situational similarities between the present experience and past experiences that remain painful and unresolved (When has this type of experience happened before?).
- Detect specific types of interactions that remind the patient of past pain (Who are you reminded of in this situation?).
- Determine whether or not the time of onset of the crisis is an anniversary reaction (Is this time of the year reminiscent of a past stressful experience?).
- Determine the worst possible outcome of the present situation and relate it to past experiences (What would be the worst outcome now and has such an outcome happened before?).
- Link the patient's present coping behavior for possible secondary gain and compare it to past unresolved issues (How is your current response helping you and has that helped in the past?).
- Review past maladaptive coping behaviors (Have you had prior difficulty dealing with stress?).
- Examine the present problem within the context of the patient's fear of being similar to a significant person with whom there is an ambivalent relationship (Who have you known that reacts like this to stress and are you like that person?).
- Explore dream and/or nightmare material that occurred in close proximity to the precipitating event for significant links of past to present (What have you been dreaming about at night?).
- Inquire whether recent memories, feelings, or thoughts have emerged unexplained into consciousness (What types of thoughts have popped into your mind recently?).

Understanding the precipitant is important in crisis assessment, and inquiry is essential. When the precipitant cannot be defined during assessment, using the basic strategy of crisis intervention by helping to modify responses to a present stressor often reveals the precipitant.

Processing the Meaning of the Crisis

After identifying the triggering, or precipitating, event and the person's level of functioning prior to the crisis, the nurse should focus on the person's current feelings (affect). Also important is the impact of the crisis on relationships with family members and friends, on daily living and routines (work, exercise, and entertainment), and on the person's physical health (somatic symptoms). In addition, what is the cognitive impact, including fantasies and daydreams, intrusive thoughts, fears and phobic reactions, and dreams and nightmares?

This stage involves active listening and communicating through empathetic statements. The nurse should encourage the patient to express the intense feelings around the crisis. With patients who are used to expressing their feelings, empathic statements may be all that is necessary. Other patients will need to be informed about feelings and given permission to express themselves verbally. Fear, anxiety, sadness, and guilt are normal reactions to crisis, and patients often must be reassured that they are not "crazy." Catharsis of feelings is often very productive.

Finally, nurses should listen for and note cognitive distortions (overgeneralizations, catastrophizing), misconceptions, and irrational belief statements, but not confront the patient with the cognitive errors prematurely. Instead, the nurse should use questions and clarifying statements, such as, "What do you think of yourself now that he has walked out?" "Do you really have that view of yourself?" "Should we trust Anthony's insulting judgments? Anthony has insulted you again and again for years! Can you trust his opinion of you?" "You feel very sad and angry that a person like that doesn't love you? Why should Lisa's problem be reflected in your self-image?" Most experienced clinicians concur that cognitive crisis treatment has a better chance of success when the patient discovers cognitive errors and distortions independently.

The stages of the therapeutic tasks are discussed next.

Explore the Crisis Event. The crisis event is explored in detail and in terms of the patient's thoughts, feelings, and actions. The patient is encouraged to acknowledge and express feelings generated by the crisis situation, and the therapist helps the patient restore a realistic perspective of the crisis situation and define viable options or available courses of action.

Conceptualize Dynamic Meaning of the Crisis. It is important to define the emotional meaning of the precipitating event that produced the crisis. The patient is helped to conceptualize the precipitant or the psychodynamic meaning of the crisis situation that links present to past (if this is a component of a crisis). The therapist obtains an agreement from the patient on a concise statement of the core conflict or problem that has produced the crisis.

Unlink the Sensory and Perceptual Crisis Components. Limited relevant background information is obtained from the patient to help understand the crisis situation more fully. The patient is helped to develop an awareness of those feelings that impair or prevent use of adaptive coping behaviors and to work through feelings that support maladaptive coping responses (e.g., resistance) and thereby prevent adaptive crisis resolution.

Process the Cognitive Component of the Crisis. The therapist and patient agree on a tentative therapeutic strategy or plan to attain the goals necessary for crisis resolution. The therapist defines and directly supports the patient's strengths and adaptive responses to the crisis situation. The patient is supported and helped to respond directly and appropriately to the crisis situation in terms of both issues and feelings (i.e., direct communication involving significant others is encouraged).

Store the Crisis Event in Past Memory. Part of crisis resolution is "therapeutic forgetting." For this task, the therapist directly teaches or helps the patient develop new or more adaptive coping responses or problem-solving skills that will assist in moving the thoughts of the crisis to past memory. The therapist prevents diffusion of the therapeutic process away from the focal problem and the goals defined for crisis resolution.

In addition to facilitating patient movement through these stages of crisis work, the therapist must also accept goals for crisis intervention that are different from those of longer term psychotherapy. It is not the task of the nurse to effect major changes in the patient, deal with all the patient's problems, restructure personality, or restore deep-seated conflicts or chronic problems. A single general goal for crisis intervention becomes the sole criterion for success in this form of therapy: to facilitate return of the patient in crisis to at least a precrisis level of functioning as quickly as possible, even though that level of functioning may not be optimal for the individual. Any gains made by the patient beyond restoration of precrisis levels of functioning is a therapeutic bonus that will be helpful in preventing future crises.

Explore Coping Alternatives

Exploring alternatives involves examining past adaptive and maladaptive coping methods. One of the key components of crisis intervention is identifying and modifying the patient's coping patterns at both the preconscious and conscious levels. It is useful for the nurse to attempt to bring the patient's coping behavior that is operating just below the surface (at the preconscious

level) to the conscious level and then to inform the patient about methods of modifying maladaptive coping responses.

Nurses, in an effort to counteract a person's feelings of helplessness and despair, should encourage alternative ideas, coping methods, and solutions. The nurse can suggest other solutions, including potential obstacles. Solutions must be thoroughly discussed to help the individual recognize possible pitfalls.

DEVELOP AN ACTION PLAN

In addition to the general goal of crisis intervention, several subgoals are part of successful crisis resolution:

- The individual in crisis is prevented from using or learning maladaptive coping responses and/or regressing, thereby avoiding maladaptive crisis resolution.
- The individual in crisis is helped to learn new, more adaptive coping responses that will result in reintegration at a more mature and stable level of functioning in the postcrisis period.
- The individual in crisis is helped to use the experience to become aware of and resolve underlying conflicts and/or ambivalence that is manifest in and that determines the crisis.
- The individual in crisis is helped to integrate changes resulting from adaptive crisis resolution at both cognitive and affective levels to expand his or her repertoire of coping skills.

FOLLOW UP

As part of terminating the crisis intervention process, the therapist evaluates the patient's goal attainment or nonattainment. Anticipatory guidance will help integrate adaptive change and help prepare the patient to meet future similar situations more adequately. The patient is given information about additional services or community resources. A direct referral to continue therapy is made when appropriate.

O AN OVERVIEW

- Every crisis involves an individual responding to a stressor within a particular psychosocial context.
- Crisis assessment that emphasizes the individual in a stressful situation focuses on the interaction of that person's coping responses with the situation stressor.

- The emphasis in crisis work is on the "here and now" problem, not past difficulties, although the psychodynamic implications of the crisis situation are not neglected.

- In crisis therapy the question is not whether an emotional crisis will be resolved; rather, it will be resolved within a reasonably short period, usually 4 to 6 weeks.

- A crisis should be resolved in an adaptive fashion that results in enhanced maturity and stable functioning.

- Maladaptive resolution of a crisis increases a patient's vulnerability to future crises.

- When using the crisis model, nursing intervention is begun with less than complete information about the patient.

TD TERMS TO DEFINE

- affect
- crisis
- crisis reaction
- crisis theory
- hazardous event
- homeostasis
- maladaptive coping responses
- precipitating event
- therapeutic alliance
- transition states

Q STUDY QUESTIONS

1. T F The goal of crisis intervention is to resolve the most pressing problems within a 1- to 4-week period.

2. Which of the following statements is NOT true about the acute phase of a crisis reaction?
   a. The acute phase generally occurs soon after some hazardous event.
   b. The individual is least willing to seek out help during the acute phase.
   c. The reaction is varied as it ranges from feelings of helplessness, anger, shock, and disbelief.
   d. Crisis intervention is most effective during the acute phase.

3. Which of the following statements is NOT true about the concept of homeostatic balance as it relates to crisis theory?
   a. Homeostatic balance is a physiological, not psychological, principle involving the need to preserve stable chemical or electrolyte balances within the body.
   b. Homeostatic balance varies from one person to the next.
   c. A homeostatic imbalance triggers coping mechanisms that have been attained through development and experiencing stressful situations.
   d. The primary characteristic of homeostatic balance is its stability for the individual.

4. T F Maladaptive coping behaviors should not be viewed as negative. They are behaviors that primarily protect a vulnerable sense of self without mastery of the situation.

5. Which of the following statements about the Roberts and Burgess crisis intervention model is NOT true?
   a. It is the only model that first identifies the person's degree of danger and need for safety.
   b. The model involves seven distinct stages to crisis resolution.
   c. The model focuses on identifying the precipitating event to aid in crisis assessment.
   d. The model should only be applied when the patient is in imminent danger.

6. A crisis includes all of the following EXCEPT
   a. psychological disequilibrium.
   b. hazardous event.
   c. psychotic thinking.
   d. lack of coping.

7. The goal of crisis intervention includes all of the following EXCEPT
   a. resolving the most pressing problems.
   b. helping the patient develop insight.
   c. helping the patient develop coping skills.
   d. working within a 12-week time period.

8. Maladaptive crisis resolution involves all of the following EXCEPT
   a. lack of professional help.
   b. unresolved issue(s).
   c. patient guilt feelings.
   d. unavailable resources.

9. T F Golan's crisis intervention model emphasizes eliciting the patient's subjective and affective responses.

10. T F Developing the therapeutic alliance requires establishing communication and rapport.

11. Give two examples of Golan's prompting statements.

12. The first step in the Burgess and Roberts crisis intervention model is to
    a. calm the patient.
    b. assess for safety and danger.
    c. determine the type of crisis.
    d. assess for suicide risk.

13. The "last straw" refers to the
    a. crisis.
    b. precipitant.
    c. stressor.

14. List three strategies to explore the crisis precipitant.

15. Describe how goals for crisis intervention differ from the goals of psychotherapy.

■ REFERENCES

Baldwin BA. A paradigm for the classification of emotional crises: Implications for crisis intervention. *Am J Orthopsychiatry* 1978; 48:538–551.

Baldwin BA. Styles of crisis intervention: Toward a convergent model. *J Prof Psych* 1980; 11:113–120.

Caplan G. *An Approach to Community Mental Health.* New York: Grune & Stratton,1961.

Caplan G. *Principles of Preventive Psychiatry.* New York: Basic Books, 1964.

Golan N. *Treatment in Crisis Situations.* New York: Free Press, 1978.

Hoff LA. *People in Crisis: Understanding and Helping.* 4th ed. San Francisco: Jossey-Bass, 1995.

Lindemann E. Symptomotology and management of acute grief. *Am J Psychiatry* 1944; 101:141–148.

Rapoport L. Crisis-oriented short-term case work, *Soc Service Rev ,* 1967; 41:31–43.

Rapoport L. Crisis intervention as a mode of brief treatment. In Roberts RW and Nee, RH (eds) *Theories of Social Case Work,* 1970; 265–312.

Rapoport L. The state of crisis: Some theoretical considerations. *Soc Service Rev* 1962; 36:211–217.

Ripple L, Alexander E, Polemis B. *Motivation, Capacity, and Opportunity,* Chicago: Univ of Chicago Press, 1964.

Roberts AR. *Battered Women and Their Families.* New York: Springer; 1984.

Roberts AR, Roberts BS. A comprehensive model for crisis intervention for women and their children. In: Roberts AR, ed. *Helping Crime Victims and Witnesses: Policy, Practice, and Research.* Newbury Park, Calif: Sage, 1990; 186–205.

Roberts AR (ed). *Contemporary Perspectives on Crisis Intervention and Prevention.* Englewood Cliffs, N.J.; Prentice Hall, 1991.

Stotland E. *The Psychology of Hope,* San Francisco; Jossey-Bass, 1969.

Tyhurst JS. The role of transition states—including disasters—in mental illness. In *Symposium on Social and Preventive Psychiatry.* Washington, DC: Walter Reed Army Institute of Research, 1957.

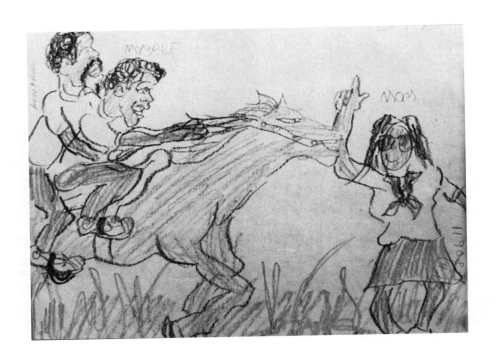

We never know how high we are
Till we are called to rise
And then, if we are true to plan
Our statures touch the skies.

Emily Dickinson (Letter, 1870)

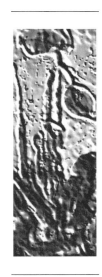

40

Treatment Modalities—Crisis, Behavioral, Relationship, and Insight

Carol R. Hartman

Patient assessment and diagnosis give direction to the selection of the therapeutic focus. The context wherein the treatment will occur can be an inpatient unit or clinic; it can be a community-based clinical agency, such as a homeless shelter; or it can be an institutional setting, such as a prison. The context also will define the resources available. In an inpatient setting, the milieu and group activities are available; in a clinic, referrals can be made; in a home, social network support is available; and in a prison, educational and athletic facilities may be present.

This chapter examines four major therapeutic modalities: crisis management, behavioral change, relationship therapy, and insight therapy. For each modality, the principal tasks, strategies, and techniques are identified. Many case examples illustrate the challenges of treatment.

■ CRISIS MANAGEMENT

Crisis management tasks can be classified by what the person experiencing crisis needs at the point of professional contact. The task is to provide support for the person, while the strategy is to modify and stabilize acute symptoms, control impulsive behaviors, and fos-ter the person's rational problem solving. Techniques are active guidance, stress reduction, medications, environmental manipulation, self-control procedures, and focused problem solving. Through the use of community and social support resources, the goal of crisis management is to reduce the patient's sense of being overwhelmed and strengthen the patient's coping capacity.

E CASE EXAMPLE

Mrs. Rosenberg appears at the clinic unkempt, agitated, and weeping. She reports that her daughter sent her because of her weight loss, insomnia, social isolation, uncontrolled crying over her husband's recent death, and her inability to complete daily activities. If we focus on Mrs. Rosenberg's inability to follow the advice of her daughter, or if we attempted a program of reinforcing her positive rather than sad thoughts, or if we focused on her early upbringing and her sense of dependency, we could be employing treatment strategies that had little or nothing to do with the immediate therapeutic tasks. While giving her sleeping medication may help her sleep through the night (attending to an immediate symptom), there is every indication that this too would miss the point of her present needs.

Mrs. Rosenberg is emotionally overwhelmed. She is symptomatic, in that she is not sleeping, eating, or taking care of herself. The context of this reaction appears to be most immediately connected with the death of her husband. Her daughter expressed expectations of the mother's response to the death that do not match her mother's current behavior, thus setting up a pattern of tension. Nevertheless, the mother did come to the clinic. An assessment tells us that Mrs. Rosenberg is in an acute state of grief, there is daughter–mother tension and confusion; and a crisis because the daughter also feels incapable of carrying on. Stabilization is necessary for the mother and the daughter. A basic active intervention is one of psychoeducational strategies that aim at reframing the response to a normal, yet overwhelming, event: the loss of a loved one. Helping both mother and daughter connect symptoms to the loss and the process of grieving, will often reduce the level of anxiety and allow for more self-directing processes to take over.

■ BEHAVIORAL CHANGE

Behavioral change targets behavior that is excessive, lacking, or inappropriate. The task is to change behaviors that are connected with symptoms, unwanted consequences, or antisocial behaviors. Possible strategies are **classical conditioning,** operant techniques, modeling, and self-regulating procedures, such as biofeedback.

Behavioral change identifies internal and external triggers, which start and sustain a particular behavior pattern, and consequential factors, which support the continuation of the behavior pattern. In cognitive behavioral approaches, the reinforcing capacity of self-thought processes are the focus of behavior change, as well as internal and external triggering events. For example, a fear of flying may be approached primarily from exposure to airplanes and flying in airplanes while in a deep state of relaxation. The thoughts, ideas, and imagined experiences of flying and the self-talk become a focus of intervention (these are viewed as behaviors with their own reinforcing capacities), as well as the exposure to the flying experience.

■ RELATIONSHIP THERAPY

Relationship therapy aims at changing interpersonal expectations, reducing debilitating social behaviors, and fostering affectionate and trusting relationships.

E CASE EXAMPLE

▶ BEHAVIORAL CHANGE

George, a freshman in college, comes to the counselor saying he is failing two courses. As he continues talking, part of the reason he is failing becomes obvious: he is partying every night and drinking beer. He does not really like beer, but he is finding it difficult to refuse going out for a beer; further, when he is studying, he feels he is getting nowhere with his efforts. Thus, he begins to think more and more about drinking and getting drunk. George thinks he is an alcoholic because he has just heard that his father is an alcoholic. He believes he needs help to not drink alcohol.

George has identified a specific behavior that needs to be addressed. The behavior is drinking alcohol. While there are many routes that could be taken, the important issue is the drinking pattern must be interrupted. At this point in his life, certain situations and perceptions are suggested as being linked with his drinking behavior. These will be the focus of the intervention techniques to be employed.

E CASE EXAMPLE

▶ RELATIONSHIP THERAPY

Jill seeks counseling because she is constantly fighting with the head nurses at the hospital units where she works. She is upset because her nursing career is threatened, and she has been told to seek counseling. As luck would have it, the counselor assigned to her is a nurse. Jill is uncomfortable as she reveals her reasons for coming. When the nurse counselor inquires as to what is the difficulty, Jill states that she wonders in part about seeing a nurse since she has so much conflict with head nurses on the unit. The

nurse asks if she has had difficulty with other work situations, and Jill reflects on the variety of jobs she had in high school, some of them with women where there was no difficulty and some with women where she did find herself fighting. When asked about male bosses and relationships, Jill feels that while she got along better with men, she often felt inferior to them. Jill and the nurse agree that examining Jill's reactions and behaviors with authority figures might be an important point of therapy and provide clues as to her handling work relationships better.

The therapeutic task is a corrective emotional experience. The strategy most relied on is the therapy relationship. The goal is to improve positive attachments, reduce distortions from past experiences with people in current and new relationships, and enhance a positive sense of self.

Relationship therapy questions what factors move a patient toward one or away from another and whether this is done in an aggressive or passive way. Questions also asked regard tolerance levels for closeness, self-differentiation, trust of self, and others. The case example of Jill illustrates issues in relationship therapy.

■ INSIGHT THERAPY

Insight therapy is for patients who experience little or no dysfunctional patterns. Rather, they have subtle problems in relationships revealing interpersonal

deficits, defensive avoidance of feelings, or both. The therapeutic task is self-awareness and insight. The strategies used are methods to increase verbalization and insight and methods that focus and direct emotional experiences and behavioral–emotional change and analyses of the therapeutic relationship. The goal is to reduce defensive behaviors and increase self-awareness and self-control without defensive patterns.

Insight therapy questions repetition of dysfunctional patterns that connect past persons and experiences to the present. Questions address the patient's capacity for self-observation and differentiation, patterns of expectation and defensive patterns, and the ability to use insight to change internal and external behaviors. The case example of Jeff illustrates insight therapy.

All case examples presented in this chapter highlight general theoretical positions and their principal therapeutic task and focus; however, in each case, some strategies and the form of therapy can overlap. For example, techniques that help persons observe and evalu-

E CASE EXAMPLE

▶ INSIGHT THERAPY

Jeff came to the therapist because he does not feel satisfied with his life. He is a handsome and successful business man, an excellent amateur golfer, has friends and dates, but it is unclear as to what prevents him from making a marriage commitment. He has been repeatedly involved with women only to break off with them when close to becoming engaged. In addition to this pattern, Jeff is not comfortable with who he is and

where he is going. He is perplexed by this since he feels that he had a privileged upbringing, though there was an early loss. Jeff's mother died of heart disease when he was younger, and his father, a caring man, was often called on extended business activities out of the country. Jeff remained home with his father's sister and family but looked forward to his father's return. In adult life, they continue to have a caring relationship, though separated by each one's busy schedules.

ate their response to whatever bothers them could be used with all of the patients described, regardless of the theoretical orientation of the therapists. Herein lies the important differentiation: therapeutic task and outcome is facilitated by the use of therapeutic techniques.

■ THERAPEUTIC TECHNIQUES

Techniques are like colored pens and pencils, typewriters and computers. They are basic tools organized by a theoretical orientation to the therapeutic task.

LINKING TECHNIQUE TO TASK

The following analogy involving the game of golf illustrates the link of technique to task. Each golf course represents the therapeutic task. The process is playing the course. The techniques are represented by a variety of clubs. The importance of clubs is that they basically operate in a similar manner, that is, they impact on the ball. The impact on the ball depends on the correct choice, control, management, and use of the club by the golfer, the lie of the ball, and the condition of the course.

Beginning golfers find that they often hit the same distance regardless of the club. Further, they struggle with control, that is, they get the distance, but it goes right or left rather than straight. As the beginning golfer gains more insight and practice, the clubs become more specific in their use, each demanding practice to learn how to use it best. Corrections are needed. The terrains of different courses present different experiences. The golfer may use past experience, judgment, and insight, and sometimes observe others to make corrections to accommodate the situation.

The technique of communication is the common denominator in therapeutic modalities. The golf club, the grip, and the swing are analogous to communication. The selection of clubs and the corrections and alterations are the refinement of technique, which comes about when the knowledge of what the technique has to accomplish is understood at a basic level. Therapeutic techniques seek to accomplish one or more of the following: separating, combing, changing, sorting patterns for positive or negative, changing criteria to alter priorities, and rehearsing something new.

To return to the golf analogy: If the process requires that the ball be driven a long distance, the golfer will select the club that gives the most distance. If the same strength is used by both hands and arms swinging the club, the golfer may lose control of the ball to the right or left rather than straight ahead. Thus, the correction requires that the left hand (in the case of the right-handed golfer) be the stronger dominant hand and arm and the right hand and arm gently guide the left. They must be separate in function.

If patients believe that they wish to die because they think suicide is a relief of pain, they need to attend to the fact that the two thoughts do not go together. Suicide as a means of relieving pain is one assumption. Wanting to die is another. The patient is not saying, "I want to die," rather he or she wants to be relieved of pain.

Patients who say they want to die because their life holds nothing present another fundamental assumption. Here there is an assumption that life in general, and/or their life in particular, holds nothing for them. What would it take for their life to have something for them? It might be, "If my husband would stop the divorce." The dilemma is that the only criterion being used by the patient to place value on her life is that her husband not divorce her. Would she say the same thing if he died in an automobile accident? Would she think and feel the same thing if she wanted to leave him? These questions prompt not only the need to separate cause and effect, but also to challenge and examine the criteria of thoughts and beliefs and their connection to emotional states. The strategies demonstrated by these examples are the use of questions and engaging the patient in comparing and contrasting and observing the reactions and responses of oneself to different emotional states associated with different thoughts and perceptions. So a basic strategy used in therapies is to ask questions; however, it has been demonstrated that questions have to be understood by the type of information they elicit. The theoretical orientation often becomes the framework for the interpretation of the information that comes forward.

The four therapy orientations, their tasks, and the use of techniques, such as questions, to achieve subgoals that lead to the major therapy outcomes are examined in the following sections.

CRISIS MANAGEMENT

Support is the overall therapeutic task. Some strategies are talking, diversion, medication, focusing on reality, interrupting negative fantasies and emotions, protection and safety, removal of stressful circumstances, environmental manipulation, scheduling, direct supervision and protection, mobilizing logical thought patterns, evaluation of coping strategies and unhealthy behaviors, and mobilizing social support. Briefly, the strategy is to reduce negative reactions and to foster, create, and reestablish self-maintaining behaviors. Crisis management may be done within a few hours, days, weeks, or months. The steps are evelation, stabilization, and protection.

Evaluation

Evaluation examines how severe the crisis is; what the personal intellectual, emotional, and interpersonal resources are, including the hope structure and motivation of the person and what the risk factors are.

To ask what is overwhelming a patient at a particular point in time can be helpful if the patient can tolerate the issue. While the goal is to help the patient regain control, it is important to understand where the patient locates the source of the crisis, externally or internally.

Patient answers should be evaluated for the amount of anxiety that is increased or reduced and the regaining of personal control. How, what, when, and where questions and attributions regarding the crisis help sort events, both external and internal, thus establishing parameters to the crisis reaction. It is from this information that an assessment of personal resources are made. This includes an assessment of the degree of hope or hopelessness of the patient, his or her energy and motivation to engage in self-enhancing activities, and the potential risk factors that need to be considered to move on to the process of stabilization.

Evaluation of a patient's intellectual resources provides a basis for determining the amount and level of questions, explanations, and directives that can be absorbed by the patient. It also indicates how one prepares the patient to be as self-sufficient as possible. The patient's ability to respond interpersonally gives an indication of the patient's capacity to attach and relate to others, as well as whether the engagement is dependent, hostile, rejecting, or simply absent with no connecting. This capacity gives some indication as to whether the patient is at all comforted by the presence of another and whether separation is tolerated. Emotional control and impassivity are assessed not only for the safety capacities of the patient but to understand to what extent the patient can control her- or himself and alter upsetting waves of emotion. If the patient cannot tolerate intense emotion, he or she may be prone to impulsive acts. Is the patient able to handle strong, aggressive, and angry emotions without acting aggressively? The ability to foresee a positive future despite the crisis may be the critical factor in stabilizing strategies (i.e., management of suicidal potential). Assessing patient motivation and energy to help oneself is a difficult area to assess, but it is important to the extent that the patient will follow through on positive activities as opposed to self-defeating behaviors.

Stabilization

Stabilization strategies are derived from the assessment. First, does the contact with the nurse have a calming ef-

fect? If so, in what way? Does it reduce a sense of being alone? Does the person feel heard? Is it a relief to just tell someone else how miserable one feels? Is the contact a disappointment? In this latter situation, further evaluation of patient expectations is needed. Does talking, both by the therapist and the patient, help the patient calm down?

The nurse may need to consistently repeat comments that ground the patient in the safety of the here and now. If they are overwhelmed by terrible images and thoughts of what has happened (e.g., witnessing a shooting) or by unexplainable shifts in his or her thinking processes, the patient is at risk. Here the nurse assumes an active part in directing the patient, while at the same time helps the patient gain perspective on processes that are contributing to the sense of being overwhelmed. Directing patients to note what they are thinking, feeling, and experiencing and relaxing their body, supports the self-observing capacity. The calm, reassuring voice and presence of the nurse assist the person to regain a sense of self-observation and control. Engaging the patient in appropriate diverting activities and demonstrating to the patient that he or she can gain relief reinforce a sense of control. Even immediately after a crisis situation, taking time out to have a drink of water or something to eat brings a patient back to a reality beyond the crisis.

Sometimes it is necessary to use medication. This is best done with the cooperation and understanding of the patient. Focusing on reality and concrete events helps divert the patient from upsetting fantasies of what might be or should have been. This process introduces patients to the power of their own thoughts over their emotional states and that by diversion and focusing on what is reasonable, they can do much to control their emotional state. As patients gain mastery over this step of stabilization, they build upon resources that move them to a more problem-oriented solution to the distress and prepares them for learning what they have to do to achieve what they need.

Protection

Protection of the patient moves from a variety of very restrictive to least restrictive strategies. Assessment gives the nurse insight into how restrictive the strategies should be. If hospitalization is decided on, the extent to which the patient participated in making the decision, will reflect the patient's conflict over his or her loss of control or the fantasy that others are in charge and controlling what happens. The following are straightforward actions that can be taken to protect the patient: remove the patient from the stressful circumstances; manipulate of the stressful circumstances or stressors,

E CASE EXAMPLE

In the earlier case example of Mrs. Rosenberg, assessment reveals an overwhelmed woman who is able to relate to others and willing to try to cooperate. She has a tendency to be dependent on others for direction. The more her daughter interprets her situation as disastrous, the more upset Mrs. Rosenberg becomes. Stabilization, in part, is effected by having her daughter participate in the educational efforts regarding loss and grieving.

---

for example, limit contact with a stressor, such as a job situation or a person; or select a roommate if patient is fearful of being alone. Behavioral prescriptions and scheduling can also be strategies to protect the person. For example, in preparing the patient to be at home (make sure someone is in the house), teach the patient to do relaxation exercises before retiring at night, make plans to counteract insomnia, prepare a morning routine, and schedule phone calls.

Once evaluation, stabilization, and protection have been established, supportive efforts are directed at restoring logical thought and inner controls by improving and developing coping behaviors. This technique requires a review of how the person is trying, and has tried, to cope and defend him- or herself and an evaluation of what changes are needed. Again, in line with the tenets of supportive therapy, the strategies used are aimed at containing anxiety, not intensifying it as one might do with the tenets of relationship or insight oriented therapy. An effort is made to increase emotional awareness through reflection and reframing.

The first task is analyzing sources of stress and establishing inner controls. The person should attend to the stressors and the self-talk that moves the individual away from logical considerations and toward distressing emotions. The process of detailing the events in an objective manner often assists the person to clarify responsibility for events and gives balance to perceptions.

The process and experience of re-establishing inner controls moves the person and the therapeutic efforts to a basic analysis and understanding of coping behaviors. Problem-solving strategies become the focus: taking time to make decisions rather than acting on impulse, consideration of options, and possible outcomes. The patient's finding of new ways to cope is fostered by direct advice, suggestion, modeling, and encouragment in independent discovery through a variety of sources, such as books or other people.

New coping behaviors are implemented through rehearsal and setting up the environment to reduce stress and promote healing and health. Taking new behaviors and imaging and using them in new and potentially stressful future situations will help solidify the gains made.

Mrs. Rosenberg, discussed in the case example, had gained emotional control over her reactions to her husband's death and the images that confronted her from the last hours of his life. As this control was estab-

E CASE EXAMPLE

As Mrs. Rosenberg begins to detail the loss of her husband, sources of stress become more apparent to her, and she can shift her thinking and patterns of reasoning around the events. For example, a particularly distressing aspect of her husband's death is the fact that he had a heart attack at the kitchen table. He fell to the floor and struggled to the door of the apartment. When she realized that he was in distress, she ran from the apartment to get help from a neighbor. In the process, the apartment door closed and locked. The image of her husband lying inside a locked apartment keeps coming to her mind and in the image she believes her husband was terrified that he was left alone.

This provokes great distress in her and much self-blame. The fact that she really does not know what her husband was experiencing has to be emphasized, as well as the possibility of another scenario in which her husband lay quietly, knowing his wife had gone for help (reframing). Mrs. Rosenberg can then remind herself when the distressing thoughts and images come to mind that there is an alternative scenario, and she has a choice. Gradually, she learns that by attending and noting the illogical premises of internal images and thoughts, she can contain and modulate her internal reactions. This increases her sense of control.

lished, more self-focused concerns occurred that produced distress and anxiety. They were associated with the steps she needed to take to care for herself and to deal with being alone. Handling relationships with former friends and family and meeting new people became areas of stress, needing clarification of both external and internal tasks and concerns. Moving into a new life without her husband required anticipatory preparation for a variety of events. This was done in part through role playing, writing concerns, and meeting with other people going through the same transition she was confronting.

Now that the patient is moving from the past to the present and future with more agility and awareness, preparation for termination is the final step in supportive therapy. Termination and follow-up are accomplished through a gradual decrease in therapeutic contact, refinement of coping skills, and anticipation of and preparation for future stresses, both of a positive or negative type.

BEHAVIORAL CHANGE

Behaviorism developed in the laboratories of psychology departments. The major thesis of behaviorism is that learning is at the core of every behavior and if we know the principles of learning, we can change the behavior. There is a rather defined history to the evolution of behaviorism, starting with Pavlov's 1927 classical conditioning theory, whereby he investigated the means by which a neutral stimulus, such as a tone, comes to elicit a reflexive response, such as salivation. Thorndike's (1911) work on rewards and punishment are the basis of **operant conditioning,** which emphasizes associative learning. Skinner, Kelley, and Cautela's (1973) contributions have led to the investigation of learning and change being directed to behavioral self-control and the cognitive learning therapies of Ellis (1970) and Beck (1976).

Assessment in behavioral approaches emphasizes measurement. In most instances, the strategies used are derived from learning theories and principles. Issues of psychopathology and its origins, personality theory, and defenses are not the organizing framework for the behaviorally oriented therapist, rather the symptom or problem is the focus. The treatment efforts would most likely proceed as follows:

1. Identification of frequency and intensity of symptoms and problem behaviors.
2. Evaluation of the conditions, both internal and external, under which these symptoms and problematic behaviors occur. Conditions refer to environmental and **internal stimuli,** such as thoughts and emotional reactions.
3. Development of hypotheses about the functional relationship between the symptoms and behavioral problems and the conditions that elicit them.
4. Testing hypotheses by using specific treatment methods derived from the functional analysis of the interaction and measuring their effect on the problem behaviors.
5. Revise treatment approaches depending on the basis of the measured effect.

Other nonspecific factors in the learning process of patients are external pressures that motivate them to continue in therapy and the rewards experienced or anticipated by the patient. The therapy setting and sessions themselves become an incentive to participate and change. The praise and encouragement of the therapist or simply the therapist's presence can be important factors in behavior change and learning.

As can be seen in behavioral therapies, there has been movement from the simple model of classical conditioning. Of particular note is the exposure of patients to prior traumatic event information under controlled conditions with enhanced relaxation. The risk of this approach is that the individual may be retraumatized if the exposure is too great and the countering relaxing elements are missing from the patient's capacities.

In the area of severe mental illness, efforts to design a community that rewards the patient for nonpsychotic behavior (token economy) have been useful. We see that the principles and strategies can be applied to individuals, as well as groups. A process of arranging reinforcers, strengthening the capacities and skills basic to coping, and refraining self-defeating thought patterns can aid, not only in change, but in solidifying the retention of therapeutic effects.

RELATIONSHIP THERAPY

The central therapeutic task of relationship therapy is providing a corrective emotional experience. This therapeutic approach draws on a broad area of information regarding therapy. Attachment theory attends to the deep fears patients have regarding affection from others and fear of interpersonal hurt. Cognitive theories deal with the perceptual schema that need to be addressed so that the negative expectation of others and the overgeneralization of negative expectations can be altered. Psychodynamic theory gives attention to the defensive nature of behavior and gives direction to the need to keep others and oneself at a distance. The object of this therapy stance is to give way to more positive behaviors and insights that reduce inner stress and move the person to more fulfilling relationships. Humanistic theories also play a role in the thinking and

E CASE EXAMPLE

In the second case example in this chapter, George, a freshman at college, is concerned with his drinking. If one takes the position that his drinking is his sole and primary concern, the use of the drug Antabuse might be the treatment of choice. With this drug, if George lapses into drinking he, having taken the drug, will become violently ill. The association of drinking liquor to the illness response is the conditioning. This noxious condition would result in a withdrawal from the use of alcohol.

Another behavioral therapist might look at the behavior somewhat differently and assume that George loses self-control and, therefore, needs to develop skills to exert self-control. His first step will be to learn to self-monitor. This is fundamental to the process of operant conditioning in human conditions where there is an excess of an unwanted behavior. The self-monitoring involves self-recording, which brings into awareness the frequency and intensity of the unwanted behavior. George may note that when he is with his friends he wants to be a part of the group; therefore, he finds it difficult not to order beer. He can regulate the stimulus to drink by avoiding friends who drink and when he wishes to be with someone, he can go to the gym and play basketball. George may combine this with going out with his drinking friends and when time comes to order, ordering a soft drink instead. As reward for this, he not only praises himself, but his girlfriend praises him, and they spend the night together. By the same token, he may avoid a date with his girlfriend if he breaks his commitment not to drink. George may also associate his drinking with tension. When this occurs, he may profit from a form of biofeedback where he monitors his state of tension and the emerging desire to drink by learning to relax, noting the reduction in tension and the urge to drink. One or all of these methods for developing self-control may be used.

Covert conditioning may be employed with George. In this situation, the imaginable and ideational processes generated in George will be used to reduce the drinking behavior. One method of sensitization that can be used is similar to the noxious association of Antabuse. In this situation, George is trained to associate his urge to drink with a noxious image of the consequence of drinking. He is encouraged to imagine vomiting or wetting his trousers with losing control and the urge to drink. An aversion to the thought of drinking is thus set up.

Another approach may be to have George create a hierarchy of events, both internal and external, that ultimately are associated with the urge to drink. He is then taught a type of deep relaxation associated with a state of calm rather than a desire to drink. He is then taught how to identify alternative thoughts that reduce the desire to drink, and he reinforces them by relaxing deeply himself. He may be taught "thought stopping," wherein he yells "Stop!" to himself when the drinking thoughts enter his awareness.

George may also be a candidate for cognitive learning strategies. He notes that in his studies he feels he does not know where he is going with his life, he thinks that he has problems in setting up an adequate study schedule, and he fears that he is doomed to be an alcoholic like his father. **Cognitive restructuring** strategies focus on the detailing of thoughts and their underlying premises that are associated with the conclusion that his life is going nowhere and his fear of becoming an alcoholic like his father. Problem-solving strategies would be used to assist him in overcoming the obstacles that prevent him from setting up a study schedule.

George may be concerned about how he is perceived by other people and feel awkward in social situations, and observational learning and rehearsal can help him with this. Bandura and Rosenthal (1978) have summarized the principal factors of effective therapeutic aspects of observational learning. There is capturing the patient's attention and a downloading of the information for retention. Then information, practice, and corrective feedback assists George to rehearse and correct his behavior. Approaching new groups of people and talking to them can be demonstrated by the therapist with George observing and then practicing. This may involve a mix of some of the aforementioned strategies. For example, a therapist may demonstrate the self-talk that pulls one away from engaging others and how this may be countered by the person, and dealing with comments that are potentially upsetting, all of which can be shown to George and practiced by him. It is obvious that this would require that George be motivated to participate in these activities, and the motivation would be linked to incentives, that is, George would have to have some reason or purpose for his participation in the learning process.

---

strategies developed in this type of therapy. Alienation, denial of inner experience, and fear of existential stress that stunt the discovery and development of goals, a purpose, and a positive social feeling also give direction to this type of therapy.

Many sources teach that life and people can be problematic. Early childhood abuse; shocking and sudden, if not frequent, losses through death; and failure all contribute to individuals pulling away from others and themselves. Patients come with a clear picture of the events and issues that drive them away from others. While a nurse can be sympathetic to the power of these

events, one has to learn that the patterns of often obnoxious behaviors guarantee that the patient will not have a positive relationship with other people. More often than not patients come not expecting that they have to change nor, for that matter, are they willing to change. Their deep distrust of others is understandable. In some cases, the degree of alienation can be so great that patients do not wish to make contact. For others, contact is painful because negative emotions are stimulated that are distressful; their strongest desire is to get away so that they might have peace. Closeness is associated with tension. Consequently, there is risk in making contact with unmotivated patients and patients who become extremely angry and destructive toward others and themselves when in a close relationship. Their deep anger and resentments can become a dominant factor in the relationship to the therapist.

Stages in the therapy process involve dealing with issues of motivation and resistance and suspiciousness; preventing premature closure with the therapist; maintaining a commitment to the patient; managing testing and heightened anxiety (defusing, confronting, and focusing); giving verbal emotional support; responding to patient's attachment and dependency; assisting the patient in self-observation, self-discovery, and self-evaluation; trying actively to change the patient's perceptions, expectations, and behaviors; encouraging and monitoring new relationships; and decreasing the therapeutic intensity and therapeutic relationship.

The initial stage of therapy is making contact with the patient. Suspiciousness, lack of motivation, and distrust of the therapist are the primary features of this stage. The therapeutic process and the use of the relationship for therapy are spelled out at this time. Contracting for emergencies and premature ruptures in the relationship are also anticipated, and the procedures for dealing with these events are detailed.

Once the patient is coming to therapy, a testing period ensues. It must be remembered that the testing period reflects mostly the thinking that the patient is conscious of regarding why there are good reasons not to get close to others. Furthermore, this testing is not always on a conscious level. Efforts can be made on an interpersonal level to get the nurse to agree to patterns of participation with the patient that cannot be fulfilled: for example, no hospitalization, no medications, no contact with relevant people in the patient's life, to always be available, and not to report injurious behavior to the self or others, to name a few. Efforts at anxiety containment are made during this time by increasing emotional awareness through reframing and reflection. In the face of emotional escalation, interpretation and confronting are used specifically in terms of the prior patterns of interpersonal disappointment and hurt that are now carried over to the nurse.

As the initial level of defensiveness weakens, the patient is supported in the heightened anxiety and anger that comes to the surface. This is done within the therapy sessions, and the patient is contracted with again not to act on these feelings with others or themselves. The point is that the relationship now holds the behavior. The initial contracting is reviewed.

As the stage of increased closeness evolves in the context of the supportive relationship, there is increased self-awareness on the part of the patient; however, with the closeness comes increased potential for

E CASE EXAMPLE

In the third case example presented in this chapter, Jill initially agrees to start a therapy that focuses on relationships. She is told that the therapeutic relationship becomes a focus of this exploration. Despite this orientation, Jill re-enacts her basic distrust of authority within the therapy sessions. J.=Jill; T.=therapist

J. "I didn't want to come today—" (looks away from therapist with wrinkled brow).

T. "When did the desire and the thoughts not to come start?"

J. "I don't think therapy is working I—"

T. "Go on . . ."

J. "There is nothing to say. You just keep asking questions!"

T. "When you say that, I get the feeling you think I am hiding behind the questions."

J. "Yeah, it isn't fair—I have to be here because of my crazy family—you just sit and judge me!"

T. "I must have done something that makes you feel that way. Was it something I said last session?"

J. "I don't think you believe me when I tell you how miserable my older sister was to grow up with! So what if she was only 3 years older than me. She bit me when I was a baby, and it continued. My parents did nothing, nothing."

T. "I guess it was like I took sides with your sister when you told me these things, and I only asked how old she was when these events occurred."

J. "I feel this way with you and with other people, no one will take my side. Everyone else can do what they want, but not me!"

The nurse asks Jill to share, if she can, more of her concerns regarding what she believes the nurse therapist thinks about her. Jill reveals a lengthy list of concerns of being judged by the nurse, and eventually reveals that she believes the nurse thinks she should not be in nursing. The nurse gently points out how Jill thinks these thoughts as if she is sure she knows what the nurse is thinking. She suggests this could be a habit that makes it difficult for her to deal with other people as well as with the nurse. She commends Jill on revealing these thoughts and encourages her to continue bringing them forward, no matter how strongly she feels.

E CASE EXAMPLE

J. "I was so angry, they ganged up on me—the head nurse and the nursing supervisor. They resent me for running for the union office. It all started when I thought that a patient had too much pain medication—not an hour and a half had lapsed from her last dose. She complained to the head nurse, and the head nurse went to the supervisor. They called me in without any warning. I was furious! Then I got depressed. I don't know. Can you come and meet with them and tell them to lay off. I am getting more depressed."

T. "Jill, what makes you think you need me to intercede for you?"

J. "It is two against one."

T. "You feel outnumbered, ganged up on?"

J. "It is the same old shit!"

T. "Explain what you mean."

J. "It's the family battles. I am alone against them all."

T. "Is the work situation and the family situation really the same?"

J. "It feels that way."

T. "It feels that way, but is it the same? Take time to think about it."

J. "Well, I did say to the head nurse that she acted without checking with me. They did ask me what had gone on, and I told them that I had given the medication only an hour and a half before. They did go over with me how I might approach the patient, but I just feel they have it in for me!"

T. "If they do, how might you handle this?"

J. "I don't know." Silence. "I guess that is why I want you to come, like I am a kid, not effective, but I really don't know what to do."

This brings the nurse and Jill to a point of discussing the combined efforts of exploring and learning possible ways of dealing with difficult situations. Expectations regarding the ability to change others are explored along with the realization that the person who has the most potential for change in these situations is Jill.

---

crisis, as anxiety is stimulated by the depth of the emotion and sensations. Shifts are made in using strategies to either contain the anxiety or to heighten it. Strategies used are focusing and questioning. They challenge irrational thinking and prompt the patient to seek alternatives.

As Jill approached reflecting on her own behavior, the nurse had to work with her through crises associated with guilt and low self-esteem. Time was needed to help Jill separate her behavior from her sense of self (self-regard). Accompanying these therapeutic activities, Jill was encouraged to develop outside activities, such as taking classes and eventually meeting new people.

Next, the patient's emotional commitment and attachment to the nurse emerges with a drop in the anxious hostile responses. During this stage the nurse assists the patient in self-discovery and self-evaluation. Through the relationship, the patient's capacity to view him- or herself and her or his behavior loosens the defensive posturing that was present at the beginning of the relationship.

During this period, Jill began to work on evaluating her work situation and whether it was time to seek a job elsewhere. This was done. Jill was able to spend much more of the therapy sessions evaluating her own behavior without feeling judged, guilty, or less of a person. This freed her, and she set new goals for herself.

With the resolution of the ambivalence toward close relationships via the reciprocal emotional commitment, a working stage emerges. During this stage, the

---

E CASE EXAMPLE

Jill continues to have conflicts at work. There is a week of getting along and then another with some sort of crisis. This brings forward a great deal of anger toward the nurse, followed by increasing anger toward her parents. This anger is met with fear that the nurse is turning her against her parents. At this point, it is important for the nurse to help Jill experience that no judgments are being leveled against her parents, but rather,

Jill is getting familiar with strong emotions that are hard to express in relationships. Jill becomes less anxious and worried about her emotional outbursts toward the nurse or her parents. She then shifts to her frustration with being raised in a family that continues to dominate her relationships with others. She expresses resentment over the fact that she has to work at changing her behavior.

patient actively engages in changing his or hers behavior with others, re-evaluating goals, and setting new goals. During this time, strategies that enhance self-monitoring, such as setting priorities, exposing oneself to anxiety provoking situations, and learning how to control and express anger, are part of the therapeutic work. Gradually this moves the patient to the stage of implementation of the goals in interpersonal situations. There is a shift in the attachment from the therapist to outside relationships.

Jill began to date. She also joined a group dealing with self-assertion. Later, she became active in a martial arts program. All of this expanded her contacts with both men and women. There was less pressure in the work setting, in part because it was not as central to her life as it had been. The final stage of therapy is marked by decreased contact with the therapist with only occasional communication.

As can be seen through the various stages, many of the behavioral strategies will be used in modified forms. The failure in relating is the primary focus of this therapy, and until the deep emotions are expressed in the context of a safe relationship and the patient makes an emotional commitment to the therapist, the patient is not open to learning.

INSIGHT THERAPY

Insight therapy has two broad areas of therapeutic work: (1) self-exploration and insight and (2) commitment to and enactment of behavior change. An overview of the process is as follows:

- Learning to identify and analyze repetitive patterns of behavior.
- Orientation to internal patterns of thinking.
- Evaluation of these patterns.
- Identifying defensive behavior and emotional presentations.
- Demonstrating application to ongoing threatening emotional awareness.
- Analysis of origins of emotional conflicts and defensive mechanisms.
- Development of areas of behavioral change, a move to make changes, extinction of old behaviors, and development of new behaviors.
- Solidifying changes.
- Preparing for termination and enhancing independence from therapy and commitment to changes.

Stages can help organize the treatment tasks and types of strategies. Initial self-exploration and insight deals with the process on an intellectual level rather than a deeper experiential level. It is necessary first to

build the abilities to handle the self-exploration and insights on a more emotionally charged level.

An initial therapy contract covers the provision of information and the structure of the therapy process. There is an early orientation of the patient to internal processes, in particular to the defenses of denial, projection, displacement, reaction formation, and protective aspects of repression. Expectations of what therapy can and cannot do are carefully evaluated and clearly stated.

Beginning self-exploration is fostered by having the patient focus on repetitive problem behaviors, which includes emotions, images, and so on; however, the anxiety level of the patient is managed by the therapist. Techniques, such as free association and interpretation, are used but are primarily guided by the ability of the patient to handle the anxiety associated with underlying themes of earlier relationships and events in the patient's life. In addition to the patient's organizing abilities, the therapist pays close attention to the patient's response to the therapist.

The next stage of analysis focuses on the dynamics of the patient's behavior. Here the defensive style and operations of the patient are analyzed. Interpretation is more along the lines of the protective use, as well as the dominant use, of defenses in certain situations, such as defensive styles with authority, intimate relationships, and so on. Questions both raise awareness and anxiety and focus and relieve anxiety.

After repetitive behaviors have been described and defensive behaviors identified and experienced, a deeper analysis of the historical roots of experiences are analyzed. Particular attention is paid to how behaviors and roots are brought out in the relationship with the therapist. From these experiences, the patient becomes aware of behavioral and emotional changes to be attempted. There is a renewal of the contract and the behavioral–emotional change stage begins to take place.

Instruction on change may come from the therapist. Much work is done on behavioral changes in the therapy setting in the relationship of the patient to the therapist. From this the patient is supported in carrying these changes outside of the therapy to relationships and life activities. Through self-awareness and insight, there is an increased expansion of self-control. As this occurs, preparation for the termination of therapy begins.

Termination can be done on a gradual, fading out of therapy, or it can incorporate another level of analysis related to separation and individuation that may not have been fully explored during the stage of self-exploration and analysis of historical roots.

A variety of techniques are used in self-exploration. Intellectual analysis is fostered by reflection and nondi-

E CASE EXAMPLE

Jeff comes to his session complaining that his days have been "gray." He is irritable.
J.=Jeff; T.=therapist

T. "What is on your mind today?"

J. "I don't know. My boss bothers me. I have been the most productive worker. I come on time, I stay late, I bring in the money—for what!"

T. Silent.

J. "What the hell, I might as well be working for a machine—just nothing!"

T. Silent.

J. "Aren't you going to say something?"

T. "About your boss or me not saying anything?"

J. "God, therapy is a crazy process. I feel foolish. In these past years, I have been a self-starter. I am surprised at my reaction—to my boss, to you."

The therapist and Jeff have an opportunity to evaluate the contract of therapy, the boundaries that exist between therapist and patient, and also how spontaneous presentation of thoughts and feelings facilitate the process. Surprise and other issues of expectations are reviewed.

Jeff at another session.

J. "It was a beautiful weekend. I just stayed in my apartment—again, this gnawing, gray feeling took up the whole weekend. I was so glad to get back to work."

T. "The gnawing, gray feeling—"

J. "I feel anxious when you say those words back to me . . ."

T. (Silence.)

J. "Oh," Deep sigh, "gray makes me think my life is going to be gray, nothing exciting, maybe with the exception of work. I feel stuck."

T. "Anxious and stuck?"

J. Laughs. "No, the stuck feeling blocks the anxious feeling . . . hum, gray . . . guess I don't want to deal with gray and gnawing . . . makes me anxious. I think it has to do with when I was a kid," intellectualizing, "Probably related to when my folks were not around for the weekend. Yeah, something like that, don't you think?"

T. "What do you think?"

J. Laughs. "Hell, I don't know. It makes a kinda sense. Oh, that contract I was working on came through."

Jeff has grasped some of the process of self-exploration. Being bright, he also anticipates what might be the answer. More importantly, he attempts to engage the therapist in a rather passive manner. He is not, on the surface, offended by the therapist asking him to reflect on his ideas, rather, he moves on to another area—work and accomplishment. Note that the therapist limits interpretation to the most obvious levels of the transactions. Jeff's implication of earlier roots is intellectualizing, suggesting that the anxiety associated with these earlier events is not yet ready to be faced and endured. The therapist does not prematurely interpret, thus managing the anxiety level within the defensive framework of the patient. During this stage, the patient can feel excited by what he is learning and discovering; however, he can become discouraged because he does not seem to be changing.

And, another session.

J. "I came today, thinking I wanted to tell you it was the last session . . ." Silence. Held back, choking sound. "It is like I am not making progress. I have been depressed. It doesn't make sense. Work is going well. Maybe, I don't know."

T. "Wanted this to be the last session and you feel depressed. When did you first note these thoughts and feelings?"

J. "After our last session . . . uhm . . . that night, my cousin phoned. My aunt passed away. She was like a second mother to me." Obviously holding back emotion.

T. "Go on."

J. "I'm just thinking, when you went out of town last week, I was depressed." Quietly crying. "I remember her dying in bed . . . She—" Sob. "Had heart trouble. She was beautiful. Oh, how I loved her. I would sit by her bed when dad was working late. It's like she is dying all over again." Sobbing hard.

This was the first time Jeff connected his deep feelings to the illness and death of his mother. He was at first overwhelmed by the intensity of his feelings and sobbed for 20 minutes. In the next session, he talked at length about the grief his father went through and his lack of availability to Jeff. Jeff recounted how he thought it was his job to work hard around the house and perform well in school, submerging his feelings. He linked this to his fear of getting close to anyone, women in particular. He also linked his anger toward the therapist as being connected to his father's absence. He was again very emotional, confessing how he longed for the tender attentions of the therapist. The grayness in his life lifted, and he had more energy and desire to participate in activities outside of work.

---

rective leads into areas not immediately within the awareness of the patient, open-ended questions, requests to logically analyze what has happened, dream analysis, review and summarization of patterns, and the interpretation of motives and feelings. Patients are moved into more direct experiencing by free associa-

tion, guided fantasy, role playing, interpretation, and confrontation of defenses. Other features of the therapy that keep the focus on the individual are the anonymity of the therapist, focusing on childhood relations, frequency of session, and the interpretation of transactions in the therapist–patient relationship.

O AN OVERVIEW

- Crisis management, behavioral change, relationship therapy, and insight therapy are four major therapeutic modalities. Each encompasses tasks, strategies, and techniques appropriate to it.

- In crisis management, the task is to provide support; the strategy is to modify and stabilize acute symptoms, control impulsiveness, and foster rational problem solving; and the techniques include stress reduction, environmental interventions, and medication.

- The task in effecting behavioral change is to alter behaviors that are connected with symptoms, unwanted consequences, or antisocial activity. Strategies and techniques derive from behaviorism (e.g., classical and operant conditioning) and learning theory.

- In relationship therapy, the task is to provide a corrective emotional experience that enables the individual to reduce debilitating social expectations and behaviors. The interaction between the individual and therapist is central to this approach.

- Achievement of self-awareness and insight is the task of insight therapy, which relies on verbalization and analysis of experience. This modality is effective with patients who have few or no dysfunctional patterns.

- Although therapeutic tasks can be discussed in terms of stages, it must be remembered that people are complex and that stages are merely an organizing effort to attend to tasks in a logical manner. Obviously, a crisis is a crisis no matter when it occurs in therapy.

- Therapeutic modalities have economic implications. We live in a cost-conscious society regarding therapies and need to learn how to be efficient.

- Each therapeutic modality acknowledges that therapy depends on the relationship context. When the relationship compromises the empowerment of the patient or when the relationship becomes a system of demand on the part of the patient to be totally cared for by the therapist, movement in therapy is jeopardized.

- Each orientation acknowledges techniques, verbal and action-oriented, that can help in modifying behavior.

- Each orientation relies on the development of a capacity for self-observation and evaluation.

- Each orientation acknowledges a point where patients need to be clear in their commitment to change their behavior. This acknowledgment is fostered when the individual does not have his or her core sense of value diminished. Effort needs to be directed to strengthening the ability to soothe the self, maintain one's self-esteem, and develop a sense of continuity and belonging before the evaluation of self and change can take place.

- To a lesser or greater degree, each orientation uses verbal and action strategies that are similar, though the understanding of how important they are to change varies. In behavioral therapy, the strategies dominate the causal links to change. In crisis management, the establishment of cognitive functioning regulates the recovery. In the relationship and self-exploration models, the analysis of re-enactment of childhood experiences is at the core of change.

TD TERMS TO DEFINE

- behavioral change
- classical conditioning
- cognitive restructuring
- covert conditioning
- crisis management
- insight therapy
- internal stimuli
- operant conditioning
- relationship therapy

Q STUDY QUESTIONS

1. What are the major therapeutic tasks of the following treatment modalities: supportive therapy, behavioral therapy, relationship therapy, insight therapy?

2. How is the nurse–patient relationship shaped for the four modalities? Give the similarities and differences.

3. Give examples of therapeutic strategies used to foster change in the thinking and behaving patterns of patients. Explain how the strategy changes the thinking/behaving.

4. From your clinical experiences and observations of case history characteristics, develop your rationale for choosing a particular modality.

5. Select two research articles that examine the effectiveness of a treatment modality.

■ REFERENCES

Bandura A. *Aggression: A Social Learning Analysis.* Englewood Cliffs, NJ: Prentice Hall, 1973.

Beck AT. *Cognitive Therapy and the Emotional Disorders.* New York: International Universities Press, 1976.

Bergin AE, Strupp HH. New directions in psychotherapy research. *J Ab Psych,* 1970; 175: 13–26.

Cautela JR. Covert processes and behavior modification. *Journal of Nervous and Mental Disease,* 1973; 157: 27–36.

Ellis A. *The Essence of Rational Psychotherapy: A Comprehensive Approach to Treatment.* New York: Institute for Rational Living, 1970.

Garfield SL, Bergin, AE (eds). *Handbook of Psychotherapy and Behavioral Change: An Empirical Analysis* (2nd. ed). New York: John Wiley & Sons, 1978.

Kelly GA. *The Psychology of Personal Constructs* (vol 1&2). New York: Norton, 1955.

Maris R, Connor HE, Jr. Do crisis services work: a follow-up of a psychiatric outpatient sample. *J Health and Soc Behav* 1973; 14:311–322.

Pavlov IP. *Conditioned Reflex.* New York: Dover, 1960.

Rogers CR. *Client Center Therapy.* Boston: Houghton Mifflin, 1951.

Rosenthal T, Bandura A. Psychological modeling: theory and practice, in Garfield SL and Bergin AE (eds) *Handbook of Psychotherapy and Behavior Change: An Empirical Analysis* (2nd ed.). New York: John Wiley & Sons, 1978.

Skinner BF. *Science and Human Behavior.* New York: Macmillan, 1953.

Thorndike EL. *Animal Intelligence.* New York: Macmillan, 1911.

Wolberg LR. *The Technique Psychotherapy* (2nd. ed). New York: Grune and Stratton, 1967.

Wolpe, J *Psychotherapy by Reciprocal Inhibition.* Stanford: Stanford University Press, 1958.

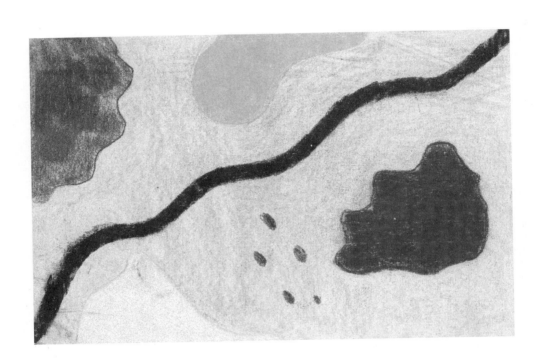

By the crowd they have been broken; by the crowd they shall be healed.

—L. Cody Marsh, psychiatrist

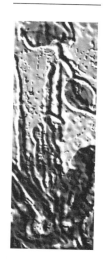

41
Therapeutic Groups

Ann Wolbert Burgess

"Tapping the motivational forces inherent in cohesive groups for therapeutic purposes," writes Scheidlinger (1993), *"is as old as human history."* Religious and tribal leaders used social aggregates to assist in healing and behavior change long before mental health therapists. Group therapy as a professionally guided, planned enterprise to treat psychological distress is an American invention of the twentieth century; however, the concept has been greatly expanded in the past decade.

The early pioneering efforts in group psychotherapy represented a psychoeducational approach. Group leaders incorporated a holistic body-mind concept that was coined *"collective counselling"* (Ettin, 1992).

■ EARLY TWENTIETH CENTURY

PRATT

Joseph Pratt, a Boston internist, first introduced therapy with a group in a medical setting in 1905. Pratt met once or twice a week with 20 to 30 patients, all of whom had tuberculosis. He lectured about the disease and the method of cure, and he was generally supportive and encouraging about the prognosis. Patients who had re-sponded successfully told the group how they had been helped. The positive therapeutic results were transferred to other groups of patients.

MARSH

L. Cody Marsh used his famous motto, "By the crowd they have been broken; by the crowd they shall be healed" as his inspirational approach to group therapy (Scheidlinger, 1994 p. 2).

L. Cody Marsh, both a minister and psychiatrist familiar with Pratt's work, used the group method of treatment with institutionalized mental patients. At weekly meetings, Marsh lectured on topics pertaining to mental illness. Marsh also arranged discussion groups with all hospital personnel who came into contact with patients (e.g., nurses, doctors, social workers, and attendants). He was one of the first psychiatrists to recognize that every encounter a patient had within the hospital setting had therapeutic potential. In this sense, he was a pioneer in the concept of the hospital as a therapeutic community.

LAZELL

Concurrent with Marsh's work, another psychiatrist, E. W. Lazell was gathering schizophrenic patients into groups and lecturing to them about schizophrenia. He concluded that the patients improved because, in part, their fears were reduced as a result of education. He also believed that the socialization process, defined most simply as patients getting to know one another, accounted for the positive changes he observed.

MORENO

In 1925, Jacob L. Moreno, a psychiatrist, introduced the technique of psychodrama. He encouraged the acting out of problem situations in a group setting to achieve a heightened awareness of the patient's actual conflict and its possible resolution.

FREUD

Although Sigmund Freud never ran therapeutic groups in his practice, he recognized the curative value of group participation, saying that where powerful impetus has been given to group formation, neurosis may diminish (Ettin, 1992). His Wednesday evening meetings of the Viennese Circle (1901 to 1907) have been likened to the first long-term psychoanalytic group.

In 1921, Freud published *Group Psychology and Analysis of the Ego*. He differentiated the leaderless group (a mob capable of great excesses) from the leader-centered group (a potential vehicle capable of diminishing anxiety). In the psychotherapy group, which has a leader, members identify with one another and have a common bond to the central figure, who is seen as a parental surrogate. Members react to each other as siblings within the family, and as a result, they have mutualities of both love and hate.

LEWIN

Kurt Lewin focused on "group dynamics" (a term he coined in 1939) in the same way that Freud focused on individual dynamics. To Lewin, acts of the individual cannot be explained on the basis of an individual's psychodynamics but must be explained on the basis of the nature of the social forces, the field to which the person is exposed. Lewin defined the concept of *group pressure,* whereby influence is brought to bear on a particular member of the group to the extent that the member's behavior can be altered. In turn, the individual member influences the group, and together they form a *gestalt* or whole. While the group includes individual members, it functions as a unit.

POST WORLD WAR II

During World War II, group therapy had its first growth spurt. Large numbers of psychiatric causalities and civilians were treated in the United States and England using this cost-effective and successful modality.

In the 1950s, the psychodynamic group model was the characteristic approach. Theoreticians, such as Freud, Sullivan, Horney, and Rogers, explored the applications of their conceptual frameworks to group therapy, theory, and practice.

A similar growth spurt occurred in the 1960s with the community mental health movement and the Vietnam War. New types of groups, such as encounter groups and Transcendental Meditation, functioned outside the traditional mental health establishment. These movements in the history of group therapy shed light on the need for short-term group models to replace the long-term intrapyschic techniques.

■ TYPES OF GROUP WORK

Three types of **group work** have been designed: traditional interpersonal group therapy, psychoeducational groups, and self-help groups. Both group therapy as a traditional interpersonal psychiatric treatment intervention and new contemporary methods of **psychoeducational group work** are being credited as therapeutic and responsive to the sociocultural needs of people. Self-help groups, designed from the 12-step Alcohol Anonymous model, have been useful as a single therapeutic method and in conjunction with professional intervention.

Group therapy is defined as a form of intervention in which carefully selected persons are placed in a group that is guided by a trained therapist for the purpose of changing the maladaptive behavior of the individual members.

Traditional group therapy is predicated on the assumption that people are consistent in their stylistic manner of behavior whether they are in a formal setting, such as in a group, or in an everyday, informal setting, such as a family scene. Because people behave in characteristic styles, a formal gathering is one mechanism whereby people can be helped to become more aware of their interaction and coping patterns, including their strengths and weaknesses. One of the roles of the nurse in group therapy is to help patients understand their characteristic manner of relating by examining their interactions with the leader and other group members.

THE INTERPERSONAL MODEL OF GROUP THERAPY

Beginning with the contributions of Harry Stack Sullivan to interpersonal theory and the ongoing growth of the model by Yalom (1995), the **interpersonal model of group psychotherapy** is used widely in both inpatient and outpatient settings. Members must be both affectively and cognitively engaged in the process of interpersonal learning (Brabender, 1993). Interpersonal learning is a two-stage process. In the first stage, members are plunged into a richly affective expression of their immediate reactions to one another. The second stage involves the analysis of the affective expressions. This learning, according to Yalom (1995), is more powerful than the exploration of early familial factors.

Goals of Treatment

A central goal of the model as derived from Sullivan is to foster members' development of effective social behavior that will enable them to achieve more intimate, gratifying interpersonal relationships.

Another goal on the inpatient unit is that the patient will overcome the feeling of isolation that is so common during hospitalization. There is evidence that hospitalized patients see their relationships to other patients on the unit as some of the most helpful experiences of their hospitalization (Yalom, 1983).

Role of the Interpersonal Group Leader

The leader assumes a highly active position, which is necessary to maintain the group in the here and now. It is also required to effect the appropriate balance between affect and cognition, a fundamental technique of the interpersonal approach (Table 41–1) (Yalom, 1995).

The therapist must cultivate an interactive style that is strong and authoritative, yet egalitarian. An egalitarian approach is important, as the group is responsible for self-disclosure. Self-disclosure on the part of the leader must be judicious, consonant with the goals of the group, and almost always concerns the therapist's reaction to some aspect of group process (Brabender, 1993).

The handling of conflict in the hospital group differs, depending on the setting and therapist. The practitioner must determine if more harm than benefit is derived from the exploration of anger and of members' hostility to one another. Most interpersonal group therapists would agree that neither the total squelching nor the full evocation of conflict is desirable (Brabender, 1993).

Use of the Here and Now

The use of the concept of the here and now is the central focus in applying the interpersonal model. According to the theories of Yalom (1995) most forms of psychopathology have an interpersonal aspect that can be explored within the immediacy of a relationship or, in the case of a group, a set of relationships. The use of the here and now is dualistic. Stage one is the activating phase, and stage two is the illumination phase, which performs a reflective loop to examine what just happened (Yalom, 1995).

The Agenda and Focus Groups

Two types of inpatient groups described by Yalom (1983) are the **agenda group** and the **focus group.** Both are highly structured in terms of session formats.

The agenda group, for the higher functioning patient, is designed to foster a positive attitude toward therapy, to enable the members to appreciate that talking is helpful, to isolate problems that can be addressed in long-term therapy, and to relieve iatrogenic anxiety (Brabender, 1993).

The focus group, which is suited to the lower functioning patient, holds to the same goals as the agenda group, but it also stresses the need for members to socialize in a nonthreatening manner and increase their reality orientation (Brabender, 1993).

Patient Preparation

In group therapy, the patient is prepared for the group experience during a preparatory session. During the preparation, the leader explains the processes to which the patient will be exposed, emphasizes the need to be open and honest with other patients, and alerts the patient to the possibility that he or she may not like all of the other group members, or that others might not like the patient. It is explained that by examining the interaction that evolves self-knowledge will increase, and in the process, more adaptive ways of thinking, feeling, and behaving will develop.

Patients who attend a preparatory session are more likely to develop positive feelings about being in a group, have a lower dropout rate, communicate more,

TABLE 41–1. THE LEADER'S ROLE IN EDUCATIONAL AND INTERPERSONAL PSYCHOTHERAPY

Educational	Interpersonal
Uses contract to set limits	Encourages discussion of contract violations
Contract renegotiable	Contract renegotiable
Focuses on external reality outside the therapeutic hour	Focuses on interpersonal issues within the group
Encourages dependence on the leader as an authority	Encourages self-reliance
Actively directs sessions	Actively directs sessions
May use formal agenda	Follows patients' agenda
Explains symptoms, feelings, behavior	Explores symptoms, feelings, behavior
Teaches	Provides interpersonal feedback
Stimulates positive transference	Allows negative transference
Explains away negative feelings	Explores negative feelings
Stimulates use of secondary process	Stimulates use of secondary process
Helps patients explain what they mean	Helps patients say what they mean
Helps patients use words, instead of behavior	Helps patients use words, instead of behavior
Provides structure to sessions	Less structured than educational therapy
Focuses on real-life issues	Focuses on relationships in group
Urges asking questions, instead of making assumptions	Urges asking questions, instead of making assumptions
Urges thinking before acting	May promote spontaneity
Accepts members' inability to tolerate emotional tension	Challenges members' attempts to avoid emotional tension
Avoids or explains intense feelings	Explores subjects that stimulate intense feelings
Emphasizes finding means to control symptoms	Relates symptoms to interpersonal events
Accepts members' defects in self-observation	Uses interpersonal feedback to promote self-awareness
Observations concern effective coping strategies	Leader has members observe and reflect back to each other
Maladaptive behaviors that occur in the group are redirected or reshaped	Maladaptive behaviors that occur in group members are considered in terms of their effects on others
Accepts defensive operations	Challenges maladaptive interpersonal defenses
Members' use of projection, denial, etc., is not confronted	Members' use of projection, denial, etc., is noted openly
Defensive operations used to gauge progress	Defensive operations used to gauge progress
Encourages accurate perception of reality	Encourages accurate perception of reality
Distracts from distorted ideation	Confronts distorted view of group members
Accepts real external problems	Examines members' roles in creating real problems
Encourages members to see themselves as ill	Encourages members to see themselves as having interpersonal problems
Develops ego by teaching and modeling coping skills	Develops ego by interpersonal learning
Fosters identification with healthier group members	Fosters identification with healthier group members
Helps patients see that they can function despite illness	Emphasizes use of will to overcome symptoms

Weiner MF. Role of the leader in group therapy. In Kaplan HI and Sadoch BJ (eds) *Comprehensive Group Psychotherapy* Baltimore, Williams & Wilkins, 1993, p. 89. Used by permission.

and have a greater sense of cohesiveness than those who are not prepared.

Patient Selection

Careful selection of patients and careful group organization are essential clinical responsibilities. Group psychotherapy cannot be applied as a psychiatric treatment for all types of emotional disorders, although a great variety of patient populations have been exposed to the method. To determine a patient's suitability for group psychotherapy, the therapist needs to gather a great deal of information in an individual session.

Key dynamic factors are assessed in selecting a patient for group therapy. The dynamics of the patient in current and past relationships with peers and authority figures, including commonly used defense mechanisms, are assessed and discussed.

Authority Anxiety

Patients whose primary difficulties center on their relationship to authority and who are very anxious in the presence of authority figures often do better in the group setting than in the didactic or one-to-one setting. Patients with authority anxiety may be blocked, anxious, resistant, and unwilling to verbalize thoughts and feelings in the individual setting, generally for fear of censure or disapproval from the therapist. They often welcome the suggestion of group psychotherapy to avoid the scrutiny of the dyadic situation. These patients gain support from the peer group and are, thus, aided in dealing with the therapist more realistically.

Adolescents often manifest authority anxiety, and for that reason, are often viewed as good candidates for group therapy. For the adolescent who has not had a peer group experience, which is a normal stage of adolescent development, such a choice is especially apt; therefore, the screening interview should include a careful history of attitudes toward parents, teachers, and other adults, but equally important, of the adolescent's participation in clubs and gangs. A clear indication for group therapy is the adolescent who gives a history of isolation, withdrawal, and no exposure to peers.

Peer Anxiety

The patients who have destructive relationships with their peer group or who have been extremely isolated from peer group contact generally react negatively or with increased anxiety when placed in a group setting. For example, some patients whose early development was characterized by sibling rivalry and whose hostilities toward or from their siblings were overwhelmingly intense may be unable to tolerate a group and may leave it. For those patients whose nuclear problem is rooted in the sibling relationship, the group can provide the corrective emotional experience necessary for relationship improvement; however, the group leader needs to evaluate the patient's ability to tolerate the degree of anxiety and discomfort that will be produced. The reality of having other patients with whom they can interact often leads to greater insight than does a verbal reconstruction in individual psychotherapy.

For the child who was raised without siblings, the group may provoke anxiety because the patient's central position is jeopardized—perhaps for the first time if the adult lifestyle is organized so that the patient remains the center of attention. Within the group, these patients demand to have their narcissistic needs gratified by the therapist, but the group setting demands that sharing occur, and such a setting may represent the first time the only child has been in such a position, one that may be very stressful. On the other hand, the only child may see the group as providing the sibling experience that was always denied. In either case (the only child who is unwilling to share or the only child who longs to share), the group setting rather quickly causes these dynamics to unfold and be subject to examination and ultimately resolution.

THE THERAPEUTIC PROCESS IN GROUP WORK

A discussion of the factors that assist in the therapeutic process of group work (therapeutic change) may be separated into the following three categories (Kaplan and Sadoch, 1993):

- Actional factors, consisting of reality testing, ventilation, catharsis, abreaction, and group pressure.
- Emotional factors, consisting of cohesion and transference.
- Cognitive factors, consisting of universalization, intellectualization, and spectator therapy (imitation and identification).

ACTIONAL FACTORS

Reality Testing

The group setting provides a reality testing forum for the objective evaluation of oneself and the world. Any transaction between two people contains three potential interactions:

- What each person wants the other to think the person is.
- What each thinks him- or herself to be.
- What each is in actuality.

In a group of eight people, these complexities may seem difficult to resolve, but through the process of consensual validation, the group defines the beliefs and actualities for each of its participants. When one member's perception of another is distorted, others in the group are able to bring their own observations to bear on the misperception. As a result, a constant assessment of reality takes place.

Honest and open communication within the group, which is encouraged by the therapist, helps the group maintain that assessment of reality. Some theoretical frameworks suggest therapists be open about themselves, thus acting as models for that standard. Those who hold a more traditional view of leadership suggest that therapists remain sufficiently apart from the group to maintain objectivity. That does not mean that they may not use examples from their own lives to illustrate certain points, but they must be constantly aware of the impact of such revelations on particular group members.

The group re-creates the family setting for many patients and may produce a revival of previous familial tensions and conflicts. Accordingly, it is common for patients to see other members as surrogate fathers, mothers, and siblings. Those reactions may be elicited because the surrogate figure actually may resemble the original family member, either physically or behaviorally. In successful reality testing, the patient is able to separate reactions that are appropriate to current stimuli from those that are carryovers from past conflicts. The therapist may attempt to elicit the association from the individual or make the interpretation directly in an effort to bring such associations to consciousness. For example, patient A may relate to patient B as his or her competitive sister.

Ventilation and Catharsis

Ventilation is the open expression of one's innermost thoughts and secrets. Catharsis is the evocation of feeling tones and affects that may be attached to the ventilated thought or secret. Ventilation allows for the amelioration of guilt feelings and anxiety through confession and provides the group with important information about the person's thoughts, feelings, and problems. It also stimulates in other members associations that may bring to awareness repressed material.

Each group develops its own mix of ventilatory and cathartic processes, with the mix depending on the composition of the group, leadership style, and theoretical framework.

Abreaction

Similar to catharsis, abreaction is the reliving of past events and the emotions associated with them; it is a more heightened process than catharsis in that the discharge of affect is greater. Moreover, it is associated with increased insight, because the patient is able to recognize the link between current irrational attitudes and previous emotional states. Abreaction also brings about an awareness, often for the first time, of degrees of emotion previously blocked from consciousness. While it is often a highly therapeutic experience, it may produce an unavoidable sense of distress in all concerned as the process unfolds.

Motor abreaction is the experiencing of an unconscious impulse through physical activity. It is known that emotional states may manifest themselves in physical ways. Hysterical paralysis, psychosomatic illness, and anxiety states are some examples.

EMOTIONAL FACTORS

Cohesion

Working groups are marked by some sense of cohesion. Members feel a "wellness" or a sense of belonging. They value the group, which engenders loyalty and friendliness. They are willing to work together and take responsibility for one another in achieving their common goals. They are also willing to experience a certain degree of frustration to maintain the group's integrity. A cohesive group is one in which members are accepting and supportive and have meaningful relationships with one another.

Individual evaluation of group members is often done using the measure of cohesion. The cohesive member is willing to take on responsibility for effective group functioning by participating actively in the meeting, by working hard to achieve difficult goals, by attending meetings regularly, and by remaining within the group for a long period of time. The cohesive member is willing to attempt to influence others and to listen to differences of opinion. Also, that member is willing to adhere to the standards of the group and to encourage others to do the same. It stands to reason that the more effectively the therapist can increase a member's cohesion in the group, the more probable is a successful outcome for the patient.

Transference

As an unconscious process, transference refers to when feelings, attitudes, and wishes, originally linked with a significant figure in one's early life, are projected onto new persons in the individual's life. When this happens in group therapy between an individual member and the leader, other group members will often help the individual member recall earlier treatment by a parent or significant other that was similar to the experience in group. Through this process, the patient is assisted in seeing the distortion and experiencing reality.

COGNITIVE FACTORS

Universalization

In the group, members recognize that they are not alone in having emotional problems and that others may be struggling with the same or similar problems. This process of universalization is a major therapeutic aspect of group work. The simple sharing of experiences fills an important human need.

As group members sense that they are important in the lives of one another, they seek to be of help to each other. This process, called altruism by some and support by others, is characterized by the sacrificing of personal interests to the group. In so doing, the sacrificing member receives help in return, for heightened self-esteem is gained by offering advice, attempting to guide, or otherwise influencing a fellow member to a greater awareness of psychological functioning. Supportive members also strengthen their own identities as they separate their problems from those of others and learn to share themselves realistically.

The mechanism of universality and its derivatives (altruism, support, advice giving, and reassurance) are processes that continue throughout the life of the group.

Intellectualization

This process implies a cognitive awareness of oneself, others, and the various life experiences, both good and bad, that account for current functioning. Not only does it connote more than a knowledge of personal history, it also implies that patients understand how they relate in the here and now. Feedback, in which each member confronts the others with immediate responses to events as they occur, is a learning experience. Confrontation groups, as used in drug rehabilitation groups, rely on the feedback mechanism extensively.

Interpretation

A derivative of intellectualization, interpretation also provides group members with a cognitive framework within which they can understand themselves better, whether that interpretation comes from the therapist or other group members.

Intellectualization does not necessarily lead to change because experiential factors must be added if effective learning is to take place. The concept of the corrective emotional experience, first formulated by Franz Alexander, combines both the intellectual and the experiential factors into a functional theoretical framework (Alexander and French, 1946). The corrective process unfolds as the patient experiences the therapist or a fellow group member in a distorted manner with the painful or pleasurable effects associated with that experience and as the patient later recognizes, through the transference phenomena, that the person acts in a manner different from what was expected (e.g., reality testing).

Identification

For the personality to be able to move in a health-functioning pattern, a person must be able to model him- or herself on a person with sound psychological makeup. Many psychiatric patients have identified with faulty models. During individual therapy, many patients attempt to learn new modes of adaptation by taking on the qualities of the therapist. In the group setting, a variety of other models are available and patients identify with certain qualities of these other members. The process of identification may occur either consciously by simple imitation or unconsciously and outside of awareness.

Other group mechanisms can be understood within the framework of identifications that take place among members. The sense of alienation is lost as patients develop feelings toward one another and toward the group as a whole. The group provides a sense of security, and a feeling of belonging develops. The mechanism of acceptance is therapeutic in that members realize that there is an appropriate place for differences of opinion. Arguments, the expression of hostility, and negativity do not disrupt the positive forces that link members of the group. For example, the group member exposed to parental arguments that led to dissolution of the family can find this mechanism of acceptance most beneficial.

■ CO-THERAPY

Co-therapy is a unique practice of psychotherapy in which two or more professionals treat an individual or a group (Crowthers, 1991). This therapeutic process may be performed by using an individual, couple, family, or group approach. Several benefits of co-therapy have been found (Bernard, Drob and Lifshutz, 1987; Crowthers, 1991; Roller and Nelson, 1991).

First, co-therapy presents professionals with an opportunity to discuss and learn through a collaborative process. Two professionals may agree to work together because they share a similar theoretical orientation or because they have a different theoretical orientation and hope to learn different techniques. It is important for each therapist to meet with the prospective partner before the beginning of a group. It has been recommended that each therapist fills out a questionnaire that addresses a number of clinical areas and compares it to the partner's questionnaire. This is recommended because it will allow the two therapists to see differences in their individual approaches that could cause tension in the group setting.

Co-therapy also allows for a wider or different perspective of a situation. Having a different perspective may initiate implementing different interventions, which one therapist alone might not have considered.

In addition, co-therapy allows for the possibility of a broader transference between patient and therapist. This is an area that the therapists should discuss. If therapists do not want to foster transference as a treatment goal, they need to identify what kind of bond they are trying to form.

Moreover, co-therapy is an opportunity for patients to expand their learning. They can accomplish this because they have two therapists working in collaboration to assist and direct them.

Finally, in co-therapy the therapists can check their behavior. This can result in less conflict in the therapeutic process and demonstrate appropriate interaction methods between two people through modeling.

CHOOSING A CO-THERAPIST

The ability of individual co-therapists to communicate openly is one of the most important qualities in choosing a co-therapist. Communication involves discussing the group, formulating a treatment plan, addressing areas of agreement and disagreement, freely discussing the co-therapist relationship, and being willing to disclose themselves in a group as persons.

According to Roller and Nelson (1991) the majority of co-therapists prefer to work with opposite-sex partners. The therapists in their survey stated that this partnership allowed for parental transference and the modeling of male–female communication.

SUCCESS OF A CO-THERAPY TEAM

Success of a co-therapy team means a balance of the therapists' abilities. One therapist may take a directive and confrontational role while the other therapist takes on a more passive role, letting the individuals of the group work through the issue at their own pace.

Theoretical compatibility is also essential. This refers to the framework from which each therapist functions during treatment. Differences in theoretical beliefs do not hinder the treatment process, if they are acknowledged by the therapists outside of treatment and are not addressed in the group.

An openness to communicate is another need for the partnership. This refers to the countertransference process. For example, the individual therapist who is struggling with a strong emotional response to a patient needs to share that with the co-therapist. It is also important for the co-therapist to address these feelings if detected in another therapist because the other therapist may not consciously be aware of them.

Equal participation among therapists is important. This refers to being actively engaged and sharing the leadership authority and responsibility of decision making. Partners do not have to perform in a 50–50 fashion; it is better to divide the responsibilities based on individual strengths.

Mutual respect and affinity for each other is not always necessary. If a therapist decides to work with a co-therapist to learn a skill, the therapist's desire to learn will transcend the desire or need to like the co-therapist.

DYSFUNCTION OF THE TEAM

Co-therapy becomes dysfunctional when the therapists fail to perform as a treatment team, communicate as peers, or a combination of the two. A dysfunctional team is oblivious to mistakes and fails to recognize or address its errors. It is similar to a dysfunctional family. It is recommended that the co-therapists have some form of supervision to help avoid these pitfalls. Five factors can contribute to a dysfunctional group.

Competition

Although competition can be a healthy aspect of a co-therapist team when acknowledged, it can also become detrimental to the process. When one or more therapists are competing to be "the best," it can lead to a battle for territory. This can signify an underlying insecurity in the therapist.

Countertransference

Countertransference, an aspect of any psychotherapeutic process, becomes detrimental to the treatment process when the therapists do not identify it or when one of the therapists recognizes it but does not address it.

Confusion and Lack of Communication

Confusion and lack of communication also occur in any treatment process at some point. Co-therapists need to maintain communication about the therapeutic process. If they do not, their patients will sense the confusion and it will become harmful to the process.

Incongruence Between Therapists

Co-therapists must agree on the treatment of their patients, otherwise, they run the risk of placing their patients in a double bind position. If each therapist has a differing opinion about a patient, their approach to that patient will send confusing messages to that patient. For example, one therapist viewed a patient as a borderline personality and the other therapist viewed him as nonpathological but imaginative. The patient finally confronted the therapists requesting their opinion regarding the state of his mental health. They presented him with both views. He dropped out of treatment 3 weeks later and was arrested by the police for his behavior.

Co-dependency Between Co-therapists

Becoming dependent on a co-therapist inhibits the growth process both professionally and individually.

■ USING GROUPS

Groups have a key role in the organizational structure of a society. The importance of the group process for

TABLE 41–2. CONTENT AND SEQUENCE FOR PSYCHOEDUCATIONAL GROUP MEETINGS

Meeting No.	Topic	Content
1	Depression	Do get-acquainted exercises; provide overview of the sessions; state group objectives and ground rules; discuss the holistic approach to depression; give information about depression (i.e., nature of depression, symptoms of depression, causes of depression, differences in depression in women and men, and social factors related to depression in women); and give information about medication for depression (ie, benefits and side effects, limitations of medications, and how to talk with the physician or nurse about medications).
2	Relationship of Thoughts to Depression	Discuss the role of thoughts in feelings, particularly depression, discuss irrational beliefs and steps in changing cognitive patterns; identify personal negative self-statements and irrational beliefs; and discuss the theory of learned helplessness.
3	Role of Social Factors in Depression	Discuss how current social expectations of women influence feelings; discuss realistic and unrealistic expectations women have of themselves; discuss the concept of multiple roles and identify number of roles each woman has; discuss expectations others have for women; identify factors in society that are oppressive for women and discuss how they affect their lives; identify which factors can be changed; and discuss marital and parenting relationships.
4	Goal Setting	Share importance of goal setting and steps in goal setting; share steps to take in setting goals; and discuss types of goals.
5	Self-Esteem	Share goals set over previous week; teach information related to self-esteem, including the nature of self-esteem, factors in development of self-esteem, and self-ideal, and share techniques for improving self-esteem based on awareness of self and self-messages, affirmations to substitute positive messages, and action to change behaviors (Gordon, 1991).
6	Understanding Family of Origin	Discuss family structures and messages received during childhood, and kinds of relationships between family members; discuss how childhood messages continue to influence adult life; discuss how to give up old messages and old hurts; discuss verbal, physical, and sexual abuse in the family; and discuss consequences and methods of handling abuse (Gordon, 1991).
7	Assertiveness	Give information about characteristics of assertive, passive, and aggressive behaviors; identify and discuss basic rights; and discuss and practice skills for accepting and giving criticism, communicating needs, and saying no.
8	Stress Management	Provide information about stress and its role in depression; discuss physiologic and psychologic responses to stress; and teach stress management strategies.
9	Caring for the Body	Teach the importance of diet, exercise, rest, and other preventive health practices; give information about such practices as breast self-examination; and discuss relationship of health practices to depression.
10–12	Review and Terminate	Teach role of social support and methods to increase social networks; discuss what each woman has gained from the meetings; discuss long-term goals and share positive feelings and experiences.

Maynard, C. A Psychoeducational Approach to Depression in Women, *Journal of Psychosocial Nursing and Mental Health Services* 1993, 31, p. 13. Used by permission.

coping and adapting in our society has heightened the need for nurses to develop skills in group approaches to patient care. The group method of intervention is increasingly used because it is effective and appeals to both patients and practitioners, it can be combined with individual therapy, and the same number of therapists can treat more people. Second, group intervention replaces individual therapy for selected patients and may be equally or more effective than individual therapy in many instances. It also may be the preferred intervention. Third, with the waning of natural social groups, such as the extended family, and the increase of single parent homes, the need for small group networks has emerged to counter social isolation. And fourth, there is an increasing need to educate patients about medications and various aspects of

their illnesses. Patient education has become highly valued both in psychiatric circles and the primary health care setting.

Table 41–1 on page 734 compares the leader's role in educational and interpersonal psychotherapy.

PSYCHOEDUCATIONAL GROUPS

Nursing's interest in psychoeducational groups has increased in the past several decades. Nurses are designing psychoeducational group programs to provide a more comprehensive intervention framework. The following Table 41–2 illustrates one such group that was designed as an intervention for depression in women. It includes the topic and content over 12 meeting times.

ETHNICITY AND GROUP

Many groups are multiethnic in composition due to the diverse cultural populations of American society. The group dynamics and culture that develops in a group with members from various ethnic backgrounds will be quite different than a group whose members all share the same ethnic heritage. The **multiethnic groups** do have unique dynamics and need appropriate cultural interventions.

The purpose of multiethnic groups can be viewed as offering an opportunity for members to address their reactions to cultural diversity, recognize their internalized bias and prejudice through exploration of cross-cultural issues, as well as to develop problem-solving skills to handle their individual life concerns (Bilides, 1991; Brown, 1984; Davis, 1980; Hurdle, 1991; Lee, Juan and Hom, 1984; Martinez, 1981).

DEFINITION OF ETHNIC

The term "ethnic" pertains to the characteristics of people who share either a common national origin, race, language, or religion. They may also share the consciousness of a common historical past, lifestyle, class, and value system and have aspirations for a common future. From a clinical point of view, ethnicity is more than a distinctiveness defined by these characteristics, it involves conscious and unconscious processes that fulfill a deep psychological need for an individual's secure identity in a group.

ETHNICITY FACTORS INFLUENCING THE GROUP

Ethnicity-bound values influence a group. Ethnicity may be transmitted through an ethnic message. The identifying specific ethnic message may be the key to distinguishing differences between ethnic groups. These traditions may be elements working against group cohesiveness, candor, and open expression of feelings, and they may affect group process and shape group culture.

Language

Language can be a major subissue of an ethnic group. Speaking a certain language is an expression of identity and is used in groups to form alliances with some members and to exclude or communicate covertly. Members may shift into their native language, especially when the group is working on an emotionally important issue. In addition, even when English is a common language, slang expressions might mean different things to group members and might result in a misunderstanding.

Physical Appearance

Skin color and other physical characteristics might attribute to subgroup factors and obstruct biculturalism. Subgrouping may be noted in initial sessions when the members subgroup by race in selecting seats. Paradoxically, it can also link culturally different members who bond on the basis of their color status.

Race-Linked Conversational Differences

The communication styles that result from cultural based differences may result in misperceived verbal messages and nonverbal cues, which may lead to an estrangement among group members. Examples include eye contact, physical contact, use of titles and surnames, and use of an indirect manner.

SPECIFIC GROUP DYNAMICS OF MULTIETHNIC GROUPS

Power Struggle in Groups

In general, the groups become microcosms of struggle and prejudices played out in larger social contexts. Group members often have values and opinions about the person's status who comes from a certain ethnic group. Power struggles commonly begin with racial motifs. It may be in a racial relationship to the leader that members begin breaking anti-bicultural patterns, either by unwittingly being against the leader or through experiencing emotional conflicts between personal feelings and long held stereotypes. Confrontation can be misinterpreted as racially based and a form of discrimination. Stereotyping, scapegoating, and polarization can easily occur.

Recapitulation of Family of Origin

When people participate in a group, their relationships with the leader and other group members will be based on their unique family of origin experience in their ethnic group. Explicit discussion of ethnic background, family of origin dynamics, and the connection to present group experience may be a method of addressing this concern. Awareness of these cultural family patterns also helps the leader to understand patients' behavior within the context of their ethnic heritage.

Cohesion

Group cohesion serves several psychological functions for a person, including adequate self-perception, individual security, and feelings of personal continuity. The cohesion of the group may be dependent on what issue is working within the group. Group issues are frequently framed in terms of race in a multiethnic group. Membership definition or exclusion becomes racially based when outsiders are involved. It is not uncommon for the same concerns to connect different ethnic groups.

Group Attendance

Attendance is another indicator of the ethnic effects. If a long-time ethnic group representative drops out of the group, inquiry should quickly be made as to the reason. Support systems are needed for minority ethnic group members. This support can come from the leader or through careful selection of members.

Silence

Silence may be the initial presentation in multiethnic groups, especially among the ethnic group members. Some ethnic group members remain quiet and withdrawn even when language proficiency is not the issue. For example, open sharing of problems in a group situation is intolerable for some Asian-Americans. Free participation and the exchange of views in treatment groups appears to be in conflict with Asian values of humility and modesty. Alternatively, the Asian members may become extraordinarily verbose. Verbosity is the Asian's way of struggling with the more verbal, active majority to gain control over the group process. It is a valiant attempt by the Asian member to define the group experience in a way that is comprehensible from that member's cultural vantage point and allows participation in the group.

Racial Balance in Group Work

The degree of intimacy in the group-proposed activity is influenced by the size of the group. Context of cross-racial contact and the numbers of those involved can potentially influence group interaction. The group member's preferences pose a critical problem for those trying to compose a group to the satisfaction of both populations. The goal of biracial groups should be to sustain intergroup contact until both parties are able to readjust themselves to what may be for them an atypical racial configuration. Another important task is to provide an atmosphere of trust in which the issue of race can be discussed openly.

Sterotypes of Other Ethnic Groups

Members typecast other racial groups on the basis of their most familiar context—cultural assumptions. It is important not to overlook their unique life experience. The focus should be on the individual in order to avoid stereotyping. A norm must be established in which diversity is valued rather than shunned.

Cultural Awareness of the Group Leader

The group leader needs to develop layers of bicultural awareness and understanding through personal examinations of ethnic background, values, race, color, class, and power. It is important for leaders to examine their own biases toward certain racial or ethnic groups before beginning to work with a new group. Leaders need to anticipate their own reactions and those areas of bias that might contaminate their responses. Such preparations will diminish potential areas of difficulty and allow construction of appropriate interventions.

Modeling

Group leaders are role models and must be willing to work through cross-racial tensions and issues with group members. Leaders should create an environment that is safe and accepting enough to allow members of different races, colors, ethnicities, and classes to interact in new and positive ways.

CLINICAL CONSIDERATION

Preparing the Group

Due to their cultural heritage and family structure, some ethnic patients will experience therapeutic groups differently than members of the dominant cultures. Other ethnic patients are frequently confused and anxious when faced with these expectations. Therapists have to develop culturally appropriate intervention responses, elicit comments from group members about their perceptions of group therapy, and discuss the group process and expectations.

Elicit Bias and Prejudice of Ethnicity Group

The process of identifying conscious and unconscious feelings and thoughts of race or ethnicity can stimulate major resistance, which can engender difficulties in maintaining a working alliance. Working through these feelings and thoughts, however, may have a catalytic effect and lead to a more rapid unfolding of the ethnic psychodynamic issue. To facilitate a positive multicultural environment, explicit discussion of feelings of bias and prejudice is necessary. Moreover, in a society that devalues cultural difference, ethnic and minority group members often internalize a negative sense of self. Building a positive cultural identity is an important part of transcultural therapeutic work.

Keep Neutral Status

Group leaders should become neither overprotective of other ethnic patients nor overly confronted. Unnecessary protection of a patient can arise from the leaders' projection of their own vulnerability or reactivation of their stereotype of certain ethnic groups, for instance, believing a stereotype that Asian patients are a fragile, inarticulate population. Such behavior also encourages other members to treat the overprotected patients in the same manner or ignore and devalue them. Excessive confrontation can result when the group leader becomes anxious, frustrated, or unable to draw the patient into the group or establish any meaningful participation.

STRATEGIES AND INTERVENTIONS

Confront the Issue

Confrontation is necessary especially when the group dynamics threaten to replicate the day-to-day oppression experienced by members. When these issues, such as color, race, and ethnicity, are discussed openly, the group becomes a safer place where bicultural interaction and learning can occur more easily.

Deal With Problematic Behavior

When a group member's behavior becomes problematic, for example, too silent, too withdrawn, or too argumentative, group leaders can facilitate the group's endeavors to understand, interpret, and confront the phenomenon. Group leaders also could encourage other group members who belong to the same ethnic group to reflect on the role of cultural difference in their behavior and make sure they know what a part unique personal issues play in the presentation.

Use Group Rules

Most groups have rules about respecting other members, such as no put-downs. When members use racial or ethnic slurs, it is important to explore the nature of the particular insult as one would deal with any other verbal insult. Exploring the meaning of these words and language begins to break down the walls created by racial subgroups' isolationism and ethnic divisiveness, thereby enhancing biculturalism.

Discuss Stereotypes at All Levels

One way of dealing with stereotypes is to point out how specific comments can become generalizations about an entire population. Another way to handle stereotypes might be to discuss how members learn them. It is useful to move from family and peers to societal means of indoctrination, such as media images.

Point Out Commonalities

Although group members may come from different backgrounds, they are still alike in many ways and dealing with the same issues of that life stage. When these linkages are explored, bicultural pathways are opened up.

Language Choice

Group leaders should be sensitive to language shifts and choices as they might relate to the content of the group session, and to state language preferences apart from fluency. In some of the monolingual groups, like Spanish, the members speak Spanish, or Spanish with many English words thrown in. This can be a problem for members who speak only Spanish. One method for handling the situation might be that the group leader speak only Spanish.

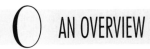

AN OVERVIEW

- Therapeutic groups are a cost-effective intervention.

- The two types of in-patient groups, agenda and focus, are designed to foster a positive attitude toward therapy, enable members to appreciate that talking is helpful, isolate problems that can be addressed in long-term therapy, and relieve iatrogenic anxiety. The focus group, suited to lower functioning patients, also stresses the need for members to socialize in a nonthreatening manner and to increase their reality orientation.

- Psychoeducational groups can teach patients specific content and increase social interaction.

- Co-therapy, in which two or more professionals treat an individual or group, is successful when communication is open and respectful and the therapists' abilities are balanced (e.g., one therapist may be confrontational within the group, the other more passive).

- Multiethnic groups are an opportunity for members to address their reactions to cultural diversity, recognize their internalized biases and prejudices through exploration of cross-cultural issues, and develop problem-solving skills to handle their individual life concerns.

TERMS TO DEFINE

- agenda group
- authority anxiety
- co-therapy
- focus group

- group work
- multiethnic group work
- peer anxiety
- psychoeducational group work
- interpersonal model of group psychotherapy

Q STUDY QUESTIONS

1. The first types of group therapy were
   a. psychoanalytic
   b. behavioral
   c. educational
   d. supportive

2. Match the group therapist with his or her major contribution
   a. Yalom   _____ group dynamics
   b. Marsh   _____ lectured on schizophrenia
   c. Freud   _____ psychodrama
   d. Moreno   _____ interpersonal psychotherapy
   e. Lewin   _____ first identified group therapist
   f. Lazell   _____ "let the crowd heal them"
   g. Pratt   _____ group psychology and analysis of ego
   h. Sullivan   _____ identified therapeutic group factors

3. Which of the following is NOT a benefit of co-therapy?
   a. Learning occurs through a collaborative process.
   b. Transference reactions are restricted.
   c. Different perspectives are provided.
   d. Therapists can check their own behavior.

4. Which of the following is NOT a benefit of group therapy?
   a. It can be combined with individual therapy.
   b. The therapist can treat more patients.
   c. It counters social isolation.
   d. It is economical for the patient.

5. T F Ethnicity does not affect group cohesiveness.

6. T F Language is part of ethnicity.

7. T F The group leader should avoid talking about a group member's race.

8. T F Group size affects the degree of group intimacy.

9. T F Group leaders should specifically protect a minority group member.

10. T F Depression is an effective topic for a psychoeducation group.

■ REFERENCES

Alexander F and French T. *Psychoanalytic Therapy: Principles and Application.* Univ. of Nebraska Press, Lincoln, 1946.

Bernard HS, Drob SL & Lifshutz H. Compatibility between co-therapists: an empirical report. *Psychotherapy.* 1987; 24(1):96–104.

Bilides DG. Race, color, ethnicity, and class: issues of bi-culturalism in school-based adolescent counseling groups. *Social Work with Groups.* 1991; 13(4):43–58.

Brabender V. Inpatient group psychotherapy. In Kaplan HI and Sadock BJ (eds). *Comprehensive Group Psychotherapy,* 3rd ed., Baltimore: Williams & Wilkens, 1993.

Brown AJ. Group work with low-income black youths. *Social Work with Groups.* 1984; 7(3):111–124.

Crowthers D. Co-therapists: learning to work together. *Perspectives in Psychiatric Care.* 1991; 27(4):18–25.

Davis LE. Racial balance—a psychological issue. A note to group workers. *Social Work with Groups.* 1980; 3(2):75–85.

Ettin MF. *Foundations and Applications of Group Psychotherapy.* Boston: Allyn & Bacon, 1992.

Gordon V, Tobin M. *Facilitator's Manual.* Minneapolis: Univ. of Minnesota School of Nursing, 1991.

Hurdle DE. The ethnic group experience. *Social Work with Groups.* 1991; 13(4):59–69.

Kaplan HI, Sadock BJ. (Eds.) 3rd ed. *Comprehensive Group Psychotherapy.* Baltimore, MD: Williams & Wilkins, 1993.

Lee PC, Juan G, Hom AB. Group work practice with Asian clients, a social cultural approach. *Int J Group Psychother* 1984; 37–48.

Martinez C. Group process and the Chicano: clinical issues. *Int J Group Psychother* 1981; 225–235.

Maynard C. Psychoeducational approach to depression in women, *J Psychosoc Nurs* 31, 1993; 13.

Roller B, Nelson V. *The Art of Co-Therapy.* Guilford Press: New York, 1991.

Scheidlinger S. History of group psychotherapy. In Kaplan HI and Sadock BJ (eds). *Comprehensive Group Psychotherapy.* Baltimore: Williams & Wilkens, 1993.

Storm CL, York CD, Sheehy, PT. Supervision of co-therapists: co-therapy liaisons and the shaping of supervision. *J Fam Psychother.* 1990; 1:65–74.

Weiner MF. Role of the leader in group psychotherapy. In Kaplan HI and Sadock BJ (eds). *Comp Group Psych.* Baltimore, Williams & Wilkens, 1993.

Yalom ID. *Inpatient Group Psychotherapy.* New York, Basic Books, 1983.

Yalom ID. *The Theory and Practice of Group Psychotherapy.* 4th ed., New York, Basic Books, 1995.

Yalom VG and Yalom ID. Brief interactive group psychotherapy, *Psy An.* 1990; 20:362.

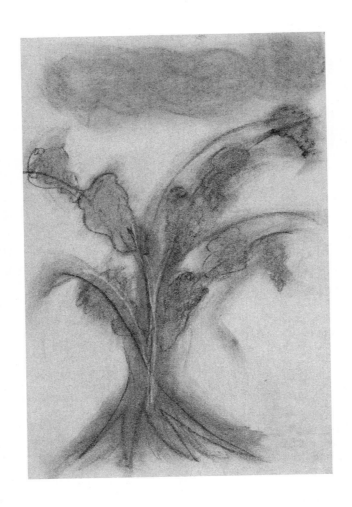

".   .   . a drug which takes away grief and passion and brings
forgetfulness to all ills."

—*The Odyssey*, bk.IV
Homer (9th–8 [?] century)

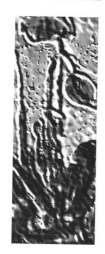

42

Pharmacotherapy

Carol R. Hartman / Margaret Knight / Carol A. Glod

The use of somatic or biological interventions is an important aspect of the nurse's work with the patient. Although the responsibility for prescribing drugs resides traditionally with the physician, the clinical nurse specialist's role has expanded to include prescriptive authority in many states. As of this writing, more than 35 states allow advanced practice nurses (nurse practitioners, clinical nurse specialists, certified nurse midwives, and nurse anesthetists) to prescribe medications in some capacity. The nursing role at both the specialist and generalist levels is most essential in pharmacotherapy and goes beyond the dispensing of drugs. In the mental health field, nurses are often the primary evaluator of behavior and have great influence over patients who receive drugs.

Before 1950, the availability of psychotropic medications was limited primarily to sedative agents and amphetamines, which had limited uses and carried the potential for addiction. Over the past 45 years, the development of psychopharmacology has expanded to include widespread use of antipsychotic, antidepressant, antianxiety, and mood stabilizing medications. Research into how these drugs work has provided an understanding of the etiology of major psychiatric disorders. With the development of newer techniques (e.g., magnetic resonance imaging and positron emission tomography), the evaluation of the effects of medications on brain structure and functioning are possible. Furthermore, sophisticated molecular biological methods have elucidated the probability of identifying genetic markers for psychiatric disorders and, in the future, may help with medication selection and efficacy.

Because the heart of psychopharmacotherapeutics relates in general to the regulatory functions of the brain and, in particular, to neuroregulation, the nurse must be knowledgeable about the actions and side effects of drugs. This knowledge is particularly important because it is the nurse who will have the most frequent contact with the individual receiving the drug. Teaching individuals and their families about drugs is an extremely important responsibility of the nurse. In settings where the nurse will work with other professionals and paraprofessionals (nonmedical), the nurse's knowledge of drugs is essential in helping these professionals carry out their work with patients.

In addition to the very helpful aspects of drugs, there are serious issues in their use. Informed consent is imperative. Drug therapy carries with it a degree of risk, as do other therapies. These risks must be known by nurses and must be conveyed to patients and their families in an appropriate manner (i.e., by the physician, advanced practice nurse, or by protocol). The nurse is in an important position to contribute to clinical information that confirms or refutes the efficacy of certain drugs. Furthermore, preliminary observations and distinguishing between the treatment-emergent side effects and worsening symptoms of disorders are key to the patient's overall treatment plan. Direct observation and reporting or systematic study may be done. Although somatic interventions place the nurse in close collaboration with the physician, the nurse is not relieved of independent responsibility regarding drug therapy. Assessment and reassessment of patient behavior are key tasks.

■ THE NURSE'S ROLE

Pharmacotherapy as a biological intervention that blends the specifics of medical diagnosis with nursing diagnoses demands critical assessment of the patient. This appraisal needs to include the sociocultural and psychological as well as the physiological contexts in which the behavior is manifested. The nurse has three tasks at this level of assessment: obtaining a baseline of patient behavior, monitoring the response pattern within the context of the drug regimen, and educating the patient and family about the medications.

BASELINE ASSESSMENT AND MONITORING OF BEHAVIOR

It is essential that the nurse have a baseline of patient behavior before drug treatment is instituted. The functional status assessment protocol and the mental status examination assist the nurse to assess with the patient his or her past responses to drug therapy, as well as his or her total drug history.

The functional health history includes the patient's beliefs and expectations regarding drugs, his or her willingness to participate in their use, myths and fears about taking drugs, and understanding the risks and potential side effects in the use of psychotropic drugs. Direct questions, as well as probing questions, encourage elaboration of these themes. Behavior and thought patterns that interfere with or limit these understandings must be fully noted by the nurse. Often, this part of the assessment strengthens the therapeutic alliance because of the thoughts shared by the patient and the decisions that the patient must make. This empowerment of the patient can prevent regression. Personal commitment to taking drugs through knowledge and negotiation counteracts fears of dependency, control by drugs, and other concerns of the patient.

The mental status examination provides information about behavioral movement patterns, such as spasms, flexibility, myoclonic movements, tremors, states of restlessness, rates and patterns of speech, and states of excitement. The examination assesses psychological processes, such as perception, memory, thought content and organization, sense of self, distorted perceptions, such as hallucinations (visual or auditory), and illusions, as well as self-care domains, such as grooming, appropriateness of dress, and interpersonal patterns.

In addition to the mental status exam, several valid and reliable rating scales are available for use in clinical practice. These scales rate specific symptoms and several areas of patient function. The use of popular rating scales, such as the Brief Psychiatric Rating Scale (Overall and Gorham, 1962; Overall, 1988) and the Global Assessment Scale (Endicott et al., 1976) at the point of drug initiation and at specified points throughout treatment assist in evaluating improvement, deterioration, or lack of change in behavior or symptoms. These scales are reproduced in Tables 42–1 and 42–2.

In addition to monitoring changes in the patient's behavior while on a drug regimen, ongoing assessment for the presence of side effects needs to be monitored carefully. The information obtained during the initial and subsequent assessments incorporates nursing observations, as well as self-appraisal by the patient, and assists in eliminating or reducing the untoward effects of drug intervention.

Initial nursing evaluation schemes are enhanced if they include questions and criteria that allow for observation and interview data for a patient status report. When this information is included with basic physiological assessment indices, such as weight, blood pressure, temperature, and a present history of the patient's health state and habits, nursing conclusions can be made regarding the patient's response to an instituted drug regimen.

DRUG EDUCATION

The psychoeducational needs of patients make clear the nurse's role in the variety of drug regimens used in psychiatric nursing practice. The nurse's knowledge of drugs becomes important not only for the monitoring of intervention programs but for the ultimate enhancement of the patient's independence and self-reliance.

An educational paradigm for drug taking that emphasizes the chemical imbalances that, when left uncorrected, influence thinking, perceptions, and interpretation of information, counteracts negative assumptions by the patient. Most negative assumptions by patients focus on drugs as a sign of their total incompetence, as being out of control, or "crazy." The use of drugs aims to restore balance to the body's chemical information–transmitting system when it is out of balance. The patient has to do the work to improve problem-solving skills, but the drugs will assist in that thinking process. Parallels can be drawn with other physiological conditions, such as the use of insulin to process sugar in the body or medication that "thins" the blood by reducing blood clots. Nurses need to be prepared for reluctance and challenges by the patient who feels compromised by the need to take a drug.

For patients who have been on drug therapy for some time and are stable, the converse may be true. They often need to understand that they can take the risk to reduce the dosage of the drug. In order for drug therapy to be effective, patients must feel they are included in the decision-making regarding their drug intervention program. Patients must learn self-monitoring procedures and communicate and negotiate drug increases and decreases in their drugs.

TABLE 42–1. BRIEF PSYCHIATRIC RATING SCALE

	Not Present	Very Mild	Mild	Moderate	Mod. Severe	Severe	Extremely Severe
Somatic concern: Preoccupation with physical health, fear of physical illness, hypochondriasis.	☐	☐	☐	☐	☐	☐	☐
Anxiety: Worry, fear, overconcern for present or future, uneasiness.	☐	☐	☐	☐	☐	☐	☐
Emotional withdrawal: Lack of spontaneous interaction, isolation deficiency in relating to others.	☐	☐	☐	☐	☐	☐	☐
Conceptual disorganization: Thought processes confused, disconnected, disorganized, disrupted.	☐	☐	☐	☐	☐	☐	☐
Guilt feelings: Self-blame, shame, remorse for past behavior.	☐	☐	☐	☐	☐	☐	☐
Tension: Physical and motor manifestations of nervousness, overactivation.	☐	☐	☐	☐	☐	☐	☐
Mannerisms and posturing: Peculiar, bizarre unnatural motor behavior (not including tic).	☐	☐	☐	☐	☐	☐	☐
Grandiosity: Exaggerated self-opinion, arrogance, conviction of unusual power or abilities.	☐	☐	☐	☐	☐	☐	☐
Depressive mood: Sorrow, sadness, despondency, pessimism.	☐	☐	☐	☐	☐	☐	☐
Hostility: Animosity, contempt, belligerence, disdain for others.	☐	☐	☐	☐	☐	☐	☐
Suspiciousness: Mistrust, belief others harbor malicious or discriminatory intent.	☐	☐	☐	☐	☐	☐	☐
Hallucinatory behavior: Perceptions without normal external stimulus correspondence.	☐	☐	☐	☐	☐	☐	☐
Motor retardation: Slowed weakened movements or speech, reduced body tone.	☐	☐	☐	☐	☐	☐	☐
Uncooperativeness: Resistance, guardedness, rejection of authority.	☐	☐	☐	☐	☐	☐	☐
Unusual thought content: Unusual, odd, strange, bizarre thought content.	☐	☐	☐	☐	☐	☐	☐
Blunted affect: Reduced emotional tone, reduction in formal intensity of feelings, flatness.	☐	☐	☐	☐	☐	☐	☐
Excitement: Heightened emotional tone, agitation, increased reactivity.	☐	☐	☐	☐	☐	☐	☐
Disorientation: Confusion or lack of proper association for person, place, or time.	☐	☐	☐	☐	☐	☐	☐

Adapted from Overall and Gorham (1962) and Overall (1988).

Given this overview of the nurse's role in the use and management of psychotropic drugs and the following descriptions of drug action within the body, the chapter will focus on three major units of antipsychotic drugs: mood-stabilizing agents, antidepressant drugs, and antianxiety drugs. The chapter focus will be on the general principles of these drugs, their specific actions, and the nursing management of the patient and drug.

■ KEY BIOLOGICAL ASSUMPTIONS IN PSYCHOPHARMACOTHERAPY

Psychopharmacotherapy is based on the study of drug action and interaction within the human being. Origi-
nal studies of drug effect, efficacy, lethality, dosage, and interaction are carried out with animals. Much knowledge is derived from animal models about the actions of endogenous signal substances and how drugs mediate and modulate behavior. The ultimate goal is to identify and understand these signal molecules (neurotransmitters, receptors, signal transducing proteins, and second messengers) as they relate to psychopharmacological mechanisms. These mechanisms are the molecular means by which exogenous and endogenous chemicals travel biochemical pathways. The primary functions of the pathways are to alter cellular activity, information flow, and ultimately behavior. Drug therapy is aimed at maintaining functional pathways.

TABLE 42–2. GLOBAL ASSESSMENT SCALE

Rate the subject's lowest level of functioning in the last week by selecting the lowest range that describes his or her functioning on a hypothetical continuum of mental health–illness. For example, a subject whose "behavior is considerably influenced by delusions" (range 21 to 30) should be given a rating in that range even though he or she has "major impairment in several areas" (range 31 to 40). Use intermediary levels when appropriate (e.g., 35, 58, 63). Rate actual functioning independent of whether or not subject is receiving and may be helped by medication or some other form of treatment.

Points	Functioning
100	No symptoms, superior functioning in a wide range of activities, life's problems never seem to get out of hand, is sought out by others because of his or her warmth.
90 to 81	Transient symptoms may occur, but good functioning in all areas, interested and involved in a wide range of activities, socially effective, generally satisfied with life. "Everyday" worries that occasionally get out of hand.
80 to 71	Minimal symptoms may be present but no more than slight impairment in functioning. Varying degrees of "everyday" worries and problems that sometimes get out of hand.
70 to 61	Some mild symptoms (e.g., depressive mood and mild insomnia) OR some difficulties in several areas of functioning, but generally functions pretty well, has some meaningful interpersonal relationships and most untrained people would not consider him sick.
60 to 51	Moderate symptoms OR generally functioning with some difficulty (e.g., few friends and flat affect, depressed mood and pathological self-doubt, euphoric mood and pressured speech, moderately severe antisocial behavior).
50 to 41	Any serious symptomology or impairment in functioning that most clinicians would think requires treatment or attention (e.g., suicidal preoccupation or gesture, severe obsessional rituals, frequent anxiety attacks, serious antisocial behavior, compulsive drinking).
40 to 31	Major impairment in several areas, such as work, family relations, judgment, thinking or mood (e.g., depressed woman avoids friends, neglects family, unable to do housework) OR some impairment in reality testing or communication (e.g., speech is at times obscure, illogical, or irrelevant) OR single serious suicide attempt.
30 to 21	Unable to function in almost all areas (e.g., stays in bed all day) OR behavior is considerably influenced by either delusions or hallucinations, OR serious impairment in communication (e.g., sometimes incoherent or unresponsive) or judgment (e.g., acts grossly inappropriately).
20 to 11	Needs some supervision to prevent hurting self or others or to maintain minimal personal hygiene (e.g., repeated suicide attempts, frequently violent, manic excitement, smears feces) OR gross impairment in communication (e.g., largely incoherent or mute).
10 to 1	Needs constant supervision for several days to prevent hurting self or others, or makes no attempt to maintain minimal personal hygiene.

Adapted from Endicott et al., 1976.

THE BRAIN AND NEURONAL FUNCTIONING

Neurochemical dysfunctions related to major mental illnesses appear to involve various subcortical structures of the brain: the limbic system, basal ganglia, reticular system, and brain stem. Their complex interconnection is vital to mediate primary affective states, biological rhythms and drives (sleep, sex, hunger, etc.), as well as memory and thinking. Irregularities in chemical transmission of information by neurotransmitters or hormones, as well as structural lesions and abnormalities, can upset the smooth relationship of these areas to one another and manifest this disruption in mental disorders. Mental illness is not associated with any one dysfunction or pathology in a brain structure or neurotransmission. Certain neuroanatomical areas, however, have been implicated in the distribution of neurotransmitters and associated with certain mental disorders. Examples of such neurotransmitters are norepinephrine (NE) in depression and anxiety, dopamine in schizophrenia and certain depressions, and serotonin in depression, particularly that associated with post-traumatic stress disorder, and in obsessive compulsive

disorders. Table 42–3 is a list of known and postulated neurotransmitters.

Every region of the brain is both activated and controlled by millions of neurons. These interconnecting neurons orchestrate the complex interactions necessary to carry out a host of functions, from reflex reaction and life support functions, such as the regulation of blood pressure, to highly developed abilities, such as abstract thought. When this neuronal functioning becomes derailed by damage to brain tissue from toxins, drugs, trauma, or disease or when the neuronal firing malfunctions because of basic disruption within the nerve cell, normal behavior and functioning are upset. Of particular concern in psychopharmacology is neurotransmission, the influence of drugs, and sites of malfunction.

In psychopharmacology, a two-compartment model describes neuronal processing (Greenblatt, 1995). The assumption of this model is that drugs administered intravenously enter directly into a central compartment, which consists of circulating blood as well as other flow tissues, such as brain, heart, lung, liver, and endocrine organs. Irreversible drug elimina-

TABLE 42–3. KNOWN AND POSTULATED NEUROTRANSMITTERS

Name	Group	Distribution in CNS
Adrenaline	Catecholamine/Monoamine	Subcortical
Noradrenaline	Catecholamine/Monoamine	Everywhere
Dopamine	Catecholamine/Monoamine	Everywhere
GABA	Amino acid	Supraspinal interneurons
Glycine	Amino acid	Spinal interneurons
Glutamic acid	Amino acid	Interneurons generally
Enkephalines	Neuropeptide	In numerous CNS regions
Substance P	Neuropeptide	In numerous CNS regions
Vasopressin	Neuropeptide	Sometimes together with
Angiotensin	Neuropeptide	other neurotransmitters
Somatostatin	Neuropeptide	
Serotonin	no specific group	Everywhere
Acetylcoline	no specific group	Everywhere

Adapted from Spiegle R. *An Introduction to Pharmacology*. 2nd ed. New York: Wiley; 1990.

tion occurs within the central compartment by hepaticbiotransformation, or renal excretion. Reversible distribution of the drug occurs between the peripheral and central compartments and usually requires a finite time for distribution and equilibrium to return (30 to 60 minutes after intravenous injection). The peripheral component (e.g., intracellular processes, neuromembrane processes, synaptic processes, and neuronetworks) is usually considered not accessible to direct measurement and study nor are the sites of drug elimination. These two component parts are amenable to mathematical formulation (and complexity) and provide the basis for understanding both pharmacodynamics (the drug's effect on the body) and pharmacokinetics (the body's effect on the drug).

Pharmacokinetics

Pharmacokinetics involves four factors: absorption, distribution, biotransformation, and excretion.

Absorption. Drugs taken orally are usually absorbed in the stomach or small intestines. Many factors influence the absorption of the drug. Whether medication is taken with or without food is an absorption characteristic of the drug itself and a host of biological barriers. What is central is knowing the bioavailability of the drug. The **bioavailability** of a drug can be decreased by what is called a "first-pass effect," in which a significant amount of the drug is metabolized before reaching the bloodstream. Many drugs, such as tricyclics and some antipsychotic drugs, demonstrate ranges of bioavailability from 30 to 60% (Hollister, 1992). Bioavailability is

the benchmark measurement for determining bioequivalence between brand name and generic drugs. Different clinical responses to the same drug—one the generic and the other a brand name—can be related to the compounding of the drug, the individual's reaction to the compounding difference, and the difference in the bioavailability of the drug under compounding differences. Additional concerns about the absorption of psychopharmacological agents are their ability to penetrate the blood–brain barrier of the central nervous system (CNS). The CNS has numerous mechanisms to protect it from the invasion of toxins, though the CNS is not totally impenetrable.

Distribution. Distribution follows when the drug has entered the bloodstream. The drug is then distributed to various organs or sites of action throughout the body. Drugs are also stored in tissues of organs, such as fatty tissues and muscle tissue. At times the reservoir of drugs stored in tissues is in excess of the drugs in the bloodstream, therefore, blood levels are not always an accurate estimate of the amount of drugs in an individual's body. For example, in psychiatry, tricyclic antidepressants and antipsychotic medications are stored in fat and muscle, in addition to drugs that are in the bloodstream.

In the two-compartment model, when a drug is distributed equally to all parts of the body, equilibrium is established. When drug distribution is completed and the flow of the drug between compartments is relatively stable, the body as a whole is considered a single compartment, and the distribution pattern is called a single-compartment model. In this case of equal distribution of the drug throughout the body, serum levels of the drug are equal to the concentration of drug in the organs and tissues.

The two-compartment model is demonstrated with some psychiatric drugs when equilibrium is reached more slowly because of the significant amount of drug that moves into muscle and fatty tissues or is bound by various proteins in the plasma. Only unbound drug is a free molecule and able to cross cell membranes and reach an eventual site of action; thus, bound drug is inactive and is a reservoir source of drug that is not easily accounted for in estimating the amount of drug with a potential for activation within an individual. Laboratory monitoring results typically indicate a total concentration that includes both bound and unbound drug (Greenblatt, 1994; Preston et al., 1994).

Individual physiological patterns of drug distribution vary greatly. Thus, there is great variability in how quickly each person reaches a therapeutic dosage and how much drug is in reserve. When patients do not take their drug correctly, stop taking it on their own, or implement a planned reduction of drug, there is great variability in how rapidly the drug will be eliminated from the system.

Biotransformation.

Biotransformation, or metabolism, is one way the body reacts to rid itself of a drug. The other way is excretion.

The metabolism of a drug occurs primarily in the liver, via specific action of enzymes that change the original chemical into compounds that are more easily excreted by the kidneys. The process of biotransformation is extremely complicated. The altered chemicals of a drug are called metabolites; some produce desired effects, and others produce side effects as they affect bodily tissues and processes. When metabolism is impaired, toxicity is a danger. Thus, impaired liver functioning can alter the metabolism of a medication and lead to side effects and toxicity, or in the case of increased liver enzymatic functions, a drug can be too quickly metabolized, resulting in a decreased drug level and an inadequate response to treatment.

Excretion.

The process of excretion (elimination) of drugs occurs primarily via the kidneys, although other routes include the gastrointestinal tract, respiratory system, sweat, saliva, and breast milk. Consequently impaired renal function can lead to a toxic buildup of drugs. Clinically and pharmacologically, a balance is needed between the ingestion of a drug and its elimination; one measure of this is a biological assessment to determine if a steady state has been achieved. This now moves to focus not only on the body's reaction to the drug but to the composition of the drug itself and its effects on various sites and the body.

Drug Effect

To understand the time required for a drug to reach a steady state, the drug's half-life is measured. Half-life is the time required for the serum concentration to be reduced by 50% (Benet et al., 1990). The half-life is used to determine dose amounts and the intervals between doses. When a concentration of a drug in the bloodstream reaches a plateau so that the amount administered is equal to the amount being eliminated, a steady state is attained. Steady state does not always correspond to the therapeutic effect (clinical improvement in key symptoms). With antidepressants, a steady state is often reached long before there is therapeutic effect. These effects of drugs are the pharmacodynamics.

Pharmacodynamics

Medication effects refer to the chemical reorganization of various metabolites and the desirable or undesirable effects of the resulting compounds. Preston and colleagues (1994) have organized the discussion of medication effects into five effects.

A pharmacological effect is the therapeutic effect. It is achieved when, for example, depressive symptoms, such as unremitting dysphoria are reduced, or hallucinations in schizophrenia are reduced.

Side effects are extensions of the pharmacological properties of a drug, such as dry mouth, blurry vision, or constipation. Sometimes the side effects can be useful to patients, like certain antipsychotic drugs that not only reduce hallucinations but also help the patient sleep.

Idiosyncratic effects are extremely rare, adverse effects. Prediction is difficult and often they represent the complex aspects of an individual's reaction to a drug or certain groups of people who share common genetic or biological features.

Allergic reactions are drug effects resulting from an individual's immune response to the drug, its metabolites, or both. The effects can range from a skin rash or hypersensitivity to severe, life-threatening allergic reactions, such as anaphylaxis.

Discontinuance syndrome results from the effects of stopping or interrupting a medication treatment. Examples are narcotic withdrawal or "cholingergic rebound" when tricyclic antidepressants or antipsychotic drugs are stopped.

Therefore principles of pharmacodynamics must also apply to drug interaction as well as drug action. The co-administration of other drugs with a primary psychotherapeutic medication must recognize the potential effect of these drugs on the kinetic properties of absorption, distribution, biotransformation, and excretion. Interaction effects can be realized immediately or over time. Symptoms that occur sometime after medications have been started can be a result of drug interactions over time. Because neuronal transmission of information is the central aspect of psychopharmacology, a review of the neurobiology relevant to psychopharmacology will follow.

The Neurobiological Basis of Psychopharmacology

The neurobiology basis includes neurotransmitters, receptor binding, signal transduction, and second messengers activation. In Chapter 4, the importance of neurons and their organization to behavior is detailed. This section highlights key points as they relate to a basic understanding of drug action and the pharmacokinetics of a drug. The capacity of the neuron to communicate specific neurotransmitters and hormones is key to understanding drug action and the interaction of a drug within an individual's body.

- Chemically, a substance necessary for the synthesis of the transmitter is present (e.g.,

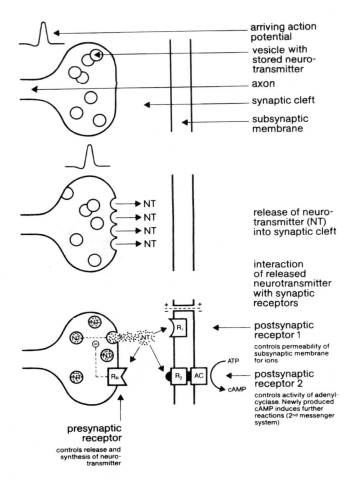

FIGURE 42–1. Processes occurring at the chemical synapse. Upper third represents action potential arriving at synapse nerve ending, which releases the neurotransmitter (NT) stored within the vesicles, which then travels to the synaptic cleft (middle third). A number of effects occur; 1 postsynaptic receptor 1 regulates the ion permeability of subsynaptic membrane. This activity prepares for further transmission of the electric signal in downstream neuron. Post-synaptic receptor 2 is linked to an enzyme system of subsequent nerve cells. Creates glucose metabolism and phosporylation reactions. The pre-synaptic receptors regulate further synthesis and release of the neurotransmitters. This is the principle of negative feedback.
(Adapted from Spiegle, 1990.)

tryptophan–serotonin, tyrosine hydroxylase, and aromatic amino acid decarboxylase–dopamine).

- Physiologically, pathways of neurotransmission can be identified as operant on certain areas of the brain.
- Pharmacologically, certain drugs have been demonstrated to act on certain sites of action, with the corresponding behavior altered in predictable ways from stimulating or lesioning tracts assumed to contain the neurotransmitter in the brain (Wilcox and Gonzales, 1995).

Most neurons are selective and release only one neurotransmitter. Neurotransmitters either activate or inhibit. Identified neurotransmitters within the brain associated with mental illness and drug therapy are dopamine, serotonin (5-HT), acetylcholine, norepinephrine, glycine, gamma-aminobutyric acid (GABA), enkephalins, substance P, and glutamic acid. Neurotransmitters are continually being discovered.

Nerve cells not only transmit information, they also have the capacity to synthesize, store, and metabolize neurotransmitters from biological precursors, as well as to re-use them following their re-uptake from the synaptic cleft. State of health, biological rhythms, fatigue states, and broader circadian and other functional demands at a specific point in time regulate and influence neurotransmission.

Receptor Binding. In early efforts to understand neurotransmission, receptors (coiled proteins that have on their exterior surface areas that bind to specific neurotransmitters) were classified by their ability to interact with specific drugs, a powerful addition has the ability to determine the amino acid sequence of a receptor. This has lead to an understanding of their signal molecules, their locations, and the interaction of classes of signal molecules with one another. Pathways are now understood for their open systems, linear transmission and close system, and cascading and redundant feedback pathways. Signal molecules have the capacity to excite or inhibit neural processing. In turn, neuronetworking results in complex systems of behavioral activation and inhibition.

Signal Transduction. Information via signal molecules (neurotransmitters, receptors, signal transducing proteins, and second messengers) are transmitted via the structures of the neuron (dendrites, cell body, axon, and terminal bouton). They continue transmission out of the bouton via the space (synapse) between the bouton and the next dendrite. The receptors act as complex cellular chemical gatekeepers demonstrating either an affinity for the neurotransmitter to bind it sufficiently to send it on or to store it (bind) and not release it or a lack of affinity or ability to receive the neurotransmitter. These latter functions occur intracellularly and on the surface membrane of the cell.

Second Messengers. Complex processes regulating signal molecules and their relationship with one another occurs within the neuron itself and on the suffice membrane of the neuron. Signal transduction (ion-based signaling and G-protein-linked signaling [see Chapter 4 for details]) and processes of second messengers derived from cellular metabolism ([cytosolic adenylate cyclase converts ATP to cAMP in the presence of magnesium ion] cAMP and adenylate cyclase) and from membrane pospholipids (inositol lipid-based second messengers and arachidonic acid). Second messengers are identified by the production of enzymes that ultimately lead to the regulation of cellular enzymatic functions and gene expression within the DNA of certain genes. In addition, second messengers regulate transmitter responsiveness so as to yield predictable change in cellular content of the substance to be transmitted, and they also demonstrate mimicry potentiation, whereby cellular actions mimic those of the transmitter. And lastly, the second messenger is identified by a specific molecular outcome (Wilcox and Gonzales, 1994).

Receptors can be on the nerve terminal (axon terminal autoreceptors, because they respond to the neuron's own transmitter) or on the nontransmitter cell (post-synaptic heteroceptors, because these neurons do not secrete the neurotransmitter or hormone being transmitted). Receptors have both the capacity to bind and release (conduction and transmission) or to inhibit (bind), acting as a break on nerve firing and reducing the sensitivity of the nerve cell (make it less likely to fire). In certain conditions, the number of inhibitory receptors may actually increase a process called up-regulation, which acts to decrease neuronal excitability. Conversely, in other conditions, down-regulation can occur when the number of inhibitory receptors results in increased neural sensitivity.

In essence, information flows from the dendrite, along the axon to the cell body, to and through the cell membrane to the synapse, from the synapse to the receptor with transmission to the dendrite of the receiving cell. Complementing this neuron conduction and transmission are molecular signaling processes within the receptor and membrane in cells that interact with neurotransmitter activity and regulate it, as well as restore the neuron to a resting state.

Transduction and integration occurs with every cell in the body (signal transduction molecules represent the conversion of incoming information to a transmittable molecular form), and special enzymes emitted from both the cell body and cell membrane result in second messengers (molecular signalers) that fine tune the flow of neurotransmitters and the restoration of neurons to their resting state. These second messengers not only allow for a brief period of simulated production of neurotransmitters, they also allow for an alteration in gene expression of certain molecular signals to either increase or inhibit the manifestation of neurotransmitters and hormones (Chin et al., 1995). This up- and down-regulation of transmission of information between neurons and receptors serves the adaptation of the organism to various levels of activation.

These processes can also become altered to the extent that specific forms of psychopathology occur. An example is in the current understanding of post-traumatic stress disorder (Yehuda and McFarlane, 1995; also see

Chapter 6 for detailed discussion of the neurobiology of stress and adaptation). In post-traumatic stress disorder, the chronic symptoms are seen to reflect neurobiological changes that are a consequence of the biologically overriding effects of a traumatic event (Yehuda and McFarlane, 1995).

A method of comprehending these complex processes is to think of the relationships between four complex biochemical factories as well as their internal processes. The first and major factory (the neuron) delivers a critical neurotransmitter. A second factory (the membrane of cells that make up neurons and receptors) facilitates its movement and prepares the product for delivery by a system that releases and adjusts the neuron to balance the flow. This mechanism returns unused neurotransmitters, making the neuron return to a resting state, so as to be prepared for reactivation. A third factory resides in the receptors (autoreceptors and post-synaptic receptors). It, too (the receptor), has to be kept in balance in its acceptance and further transmission of the neurotransmitter. This is done via the activity within its cells and their membranes. These intradepartmental relationships are highly complex and exacting to both the commitment of the transfer of the neurotransmitter and the level and duration of transmission. In concert with the other two factories, it determines whether the action needs to be of short duration or longer, depending on the demands on the organism (gene expresion).

Part of this critical information is determined by a variety of different neurotransmitters and hormones that are involved contemporaneously with the focused neurotransmitter, that is, each of these factories is responsive to the context of other supporting factors. This sets up a system of linking numerous chemical factories. Some transmit and mediate while others modulate. Modulation of fine tuning and balancing keeps balance or makes critical adaptations to preserve the organism. At times, neurotransmitters function not only as mediating signal molecules but as modulating signal molecules along with the other signal transduction systems and second messenger systems. The brain not only regulates both endogenous events and reactions, it responds to exogenous events. The brain regulates these actions by maintaining pathways for transferring and interpreting information and adapting and altering (gene expression) pathways for both short-term, extended-term and long-term actions.

Neuronal Malfunctioning

All of this is possible because of neuronal functions. If there is a neuronal malfunction and this leads to a neuronal misfiring, we have the basis for understanding what underlies major mental illnesses. Preston and associates (1994) outline some of the processes leading to a malfunction in neuronal firing.

- The first and most obvious issue is that there is not enough neurotransmitter. This can be a function of or a failure in the initial synthesis and production of the neurotransmitter.
- Diminished amounts or excesses of neurotransmitters at the pre-synaptic bouton can be caused by certain biological disorders and drugs.
- The process of recycling neurotransmitters by reabsorption (re-uptake) can be overstimulated or retarded by physiological malfunctions, medications, or both.
- The receptors on the membrane of cells that act as breaks to the firing of the neurotransmitter can, under certain conditions, increase (upregulation), thus resulting in the overinhibition and decrease of neuronal excitability, or there can be a decrease in receptors with a downregulation that results in increased neuronal sensitivity.
- Excesses of enzymatic activity may abnormally deplete neurotransmitters. An example of this is in certain types of depression where the intracellular enzyme monoamine oxidase (MAO) can cause significant inactivation of necessary neurotransmitters.

■ GENERAL CLASSIFICATION OF PSYCHOTROPIC DRUGS

Psychotropic drugs include antipsychotic, or neuroleptic, agents, mood-stabilizing agents, antidepressant agents, and antianxiety agents. In addition, anti-Parkinsonian agents are used in the treatment of certain side effects, and amphetamine-like stimulants are used in the treatment of attention deficit disorder. Antipsychotic drugs were first referred to as tranquilizers—a term that was not useful in distinguishing the drugs and their actions.

The logic of drug classification is, to a great extent, based on chemical structure and drug action. As discussed earlier, many psychotropic drugs were discovered by making slight molecular changes and studying the effect of these changes on behavior.

These initial changes were made at the R10, S, and R2 areas of the phenothiazine triple ring. These changes—aliphatics, piperidines, and piperazines—were made to alter side effects and potency. The variations of the effects of these manipulations are graphically represented in Table 42–4.

Not all psychotropic drugs follow from these chemical structures; however, those that do can be expected to generally manifest similar clinical characteristics

TABLE 42–4. SEVERITY OF ADVERSE EFFECTS OF ANTIPSYCHOTIC DRUGS

Drugs	EPS	NMS	Anticholinergic	Hypotension	Sedation
Thorazine	++	++	+++	++	+++
Mellaril	+	+	+++	+++	+++
Stelazine	++	++	++	+	+++
Trilafon	++	+	++	++	++
Prolixin	+++	+++	+	–––	+
Haldol	+++	+++	–––	–––	+
Moban	++	++	++	+	+
Loxitane	+++	+++	++	++	++
Clozaril	–––	–––	+++	+++	+++
Risperdal	+	–––	+	+	+

EPS, extra pyramidal symptoms; NMS, neuroleptic malignant syndrome; mild, +; moderate, ++; severe, +++; no information, –––.

based on their structural grouping. Milligram potency, dosage range, sedative actions, psychomotor inhibition, autonomic reactions, stimulating actions, and extrapyramidal reactions can be related to structure not only for antipsychotic drugs, but also for antidepressant drugs.

Drugs are generally broadly classified according to the symptoms that they primarily treat. Antipsychotic drugs are used to treat disorders of thought and perception. Antianxiety agents reduce anxiety and are, therefore, often used in crisis situations, major problems of adjustment, and as a short-term adjunctive treatment for many major mental disorders. Antidepressants are primarily used to treat major depression, though their success in the management of other disorders, such as eating disorders and obsessive compulsive disorders, has expanded over the last several years. Mood-stabilizing agents refer to drugs, such as lithium carbonate and certain anticonvulsant drugs, that have proven effective in the treatment of affective disorders.

■ ANTIPSYCHOTIC DRUGS

IDENTIFYING SYMPTOMS OF PSYCHOSIS

Prior to the initiation of antipsychotic agents, a clear history of the onset of the problem or illness and an accurate assessment of the patient's symptoms are critical. The data provide necessary information regarding the possible etiology of the symptoms and an initial direction for the overall pharmacologic plan. Prior to the treatment of psychotic symptoms with antipsychotic drugs, individuals often appear anxious and agitated. Information collected during the initial patient contact help to differentiate these multiple symptom clusters. This differentiation is essential because anxiety in and of itself ought not to be treated with antipsychotic drugs and psychotic states ought not to be treated with antianxiety agents. For the most up-to-date considerations of the classification of behavioral symptoms, physical status, personality structure, life stressors, and coping behaviors, the reader is referred to the DSM-IV (American Psychiatric Association, 1994).

Target symptoms most affected by antipsychotic drugs are delusions, hallucinations, change in the flow of ideas, changes in the structure and rate of associations, ideas of reference, suspicious behavior, incoherence, and marked illogical thinking. Agitation, which generally accompanies psychotic symptoms, also responds well to antipsychotic agents. Improvements in other symptoms, such as withdrawal, anorexia, and self-neglect presumably respond secondarily to the use of these drugs and follow the decreasing psychotic features (Hirsch, 1986).

Using a target symptom approach for the ongoing assessment of drug response maintains the focus on general areas of expected behavioral improvement. Personality structure and interpersonal communication styles remain unchanged as a result of medication administration. Therefore, changes in these areas should not be expected despite any contribution to maladaptation.

A listing of antipsychotic drugs and anti-Parkinsonian drugs used to treat target symptoms is in Table 42–5.

ANTIPSYCHOTIC DRUG ACTION

Antipsychotics are extremely effective and generally safe drugs, although their action is not well understood. Antipsychotic drugs, with the exception of the atypical antipsychotics, are often referred to as neuroleptics because of their many neurologic side effects. It is generally accepted that antipsychotics or neuroleptics alter the kinds and amounts of amines present at the synapse. These drugs block post-synaptic (D2) dopamine receptors (Seeman, 1993; Schatzberg and Cole, 1991; Baldessarini, 1985) particularly in the basal ganglia, hypothalmus, and limbic portions of the brain. Each of these systems has major integrating functions within the brain and nervous system. There is currently no proof that this selective action alone is responsible for their antipsychotic effect (Baldessarini, 1985). This action, however, is believed to be critical in selectively changing the transmission of information along dopamine pathways.

In addition to dopamine blockade, many of the neuroleptics have alpha adrenergic blocking effects, particularly the lower potency neuroleptics. This alpha adrenergic blocking action generally results in lowered

TABLE 42–5. ANTIPSYCHOTIC DRUGS AND ANTI-PARKINSONIAN DRUGS

Brand Name	Generic Name	Daily Dose Range (mg)
I. Antipsychotic agents		
A. Phenothiazine derivatives		
1. Aliphatics		
a. Thorazine	Chlorpromazine	100 to 1,000
b. Vesprin	Triflupromazine	20 to 150
2. Piperidines		
a. Mellaril	Thioridazine	30 to 800
b. Serentil	Mesoridazine	50 to 400
3. Piperazines		
a. Stelazine	Trifluoperazine	2 to 30
b. Trilafon	Perphenazine	2 to 64
c. Prolixin, Permitil	Fluphenazine	0.5 to 20
d. Prolixin enanthate or decanoate	(long-acting injectable)	4 cc (½ to 4 cc every 2 or 3 weeks)
B. Thioxanthene derivatives		
1. Navane (piperazine)	Thiothixene	6 to 60
C. Butyrophenone derivative		
1. Haldol	Haloperidol	1 to 100
2. Haldol Decanoate	Haloperidol	
D. Dihydroindolone derivative		
1. Moban	Molindone	20 to 225
E. Dibenzoxazepine derivative		
1. Loxitane	Loxapine	20 to 250
F. Diphenylbutylpiperidines		
1. Orap	Pimozide	0.3 to 0.5
II. Atypical antipsychotic agents		
A. Dibenzodiazepines		
1. Clozaril	Clozapine	200 to 450
B. Benzioxazols		
1. Risperdal	Risperidone	4 to 10
III. Antipsychotics under study		
A. Amperozide		
B. Seroquel/ICI204.636 Zeneca		
IV. Anti-Parkinsonian Agents (Drugs used in the control of side effects. They also have anticholinergic properties that can lead to toxic reactions.)		
A. Artane	Trihexyphenidyl	1 to 10
B. Benadryl	Diphenhydramine	25 to 200
C. Cogentin	Benztropine mesylate	1 to 6
D. Symmetrel	Amantadine	100 to 300

blood pressure, decreased pulse, and sedation. Sedation often contributes significantly to an individual's overall improvement and recovery from a psychotic episode. Sedation is particularly useful for manic or agitated states in which danger to oneself or others may be a concern.

In addition to relatively weak D2 and substantial alpha adrenergic blocking effects, clozapine has powerful D4 blocking effects. Clozapine also exerts strong effects at serotoninergic receptor sites (5-HT3) (Kane, 1993). Risperidone, another atypical and newer antipsychotic drug, also has a high affinity for serotoninergic (5-HT2), alpha adrenergic, and dopamine (D2) receptor sites (Kane, 1993). What this actually means regarding the etiology of the psychotic disorders is not known; however, it is clear that both of these drugs offer alternatives for individuals who do not tolerate standard antipsychotic treatment well.

Antipsychotic drugs are extremely useful in treating acute psychotic states and managing individuals with chronic psychotic symptoms (Bernstein, 1988). Not all chronically psychotic patients require large doses of medication for maintenance; many other therapies exist that provide essential adjunctive treatment to this group of individuals. The risk of the prolonged use of antipsychotic drugs must be evaluated against the benefits, and every patient deserves the opportunity to be medication-free whenever possible. The major serious consequence of prolonged use of antipsychotic drugs is tardive dyskinesia, for which there is no known corrective treatment. (See Side Effects below).

Dosage Considerations

Neuroleptic prescription practices have changed dramatically since the 1950s. Early on, it was not uncommon to observe patients taking 1 or 2 g of chlorpromazine per day for the treatment of acute psychosis or chronic schizophrenia. Perhaps initially it was believed that higher doses were needed to control acute and stubborn psychotic symptoms. In the late 1970s and early 1980s, the results of clinical studies changed prescription practices, and clinicians were directed to use lower doses in patient populations. In addition to determining that lower doses than expected were effective in managing psychotic illness, it was found that toxicity actually resulted from doses previously considered safe (Teicher and Baldessarini, 1985).

The dosage schedules vary according to the potency of the drug and the individual's differences. Drugs are available to minimize the unwanted pharmacologic effects of sedation, adrenergic blocking activity, and extrapyramidal effects (see Table 42–5). Because the antipsychotic drugs are long-acting, once a dose

level to control symptoms has been achieved, a single dose can be given at bedtime. This diminishes the problem of daytime sedation. In addition, for long-term treatment, high potency neuroleptics should be considered because they produce less autonomic nervous system effects (Bernstein, 1988).

In acute psychotic episodes, treatment with antipsychotic drugs may be brief, but in newly treated chronic patients, it might require 3 to 6 months of treatment before a change in medication is warranted. In schizophrenia, maintenance doses should be as low as possible while retaining therapeutic gains.

Pharmacokinetics

Antipsychotic drugs are metabolized in the liver and may cause hepatic toxicity. They are excreted via the kidney. Adults respond within a wide therapeutic margin. Most fatalities from overdoses have occurred with children or when the drugs are mixed with other drugs, which results in dangerous interaction effects.

Side Effects

Side effects and toxicity are not infrequent with antipsychotic drugs, yet as a group of drugs they are relatively safe (Bernstein, 1988). The side effects associated with antipsychotic drugs range from mild to extremely severe, including the potentially life-threatening neuroleptic malignant syndrome. Although some side effects are quite rare, consistent and ongoing assessment of patients on antipsychotics is critical for safe and effective practice. In general, most side effects are correlated with dosage (Baldessarini, 1985). The higher the dose, the greater the risk of side effects. In addition, low potency antipsychotics tend to produce a different side effect profile than high potency antipsychotics. Table 42–5 illustrates important differences.

As mentioned previously, because standard antipsychotic drugs often cause significant neurologic side effects, the term neuroleptic was introduced. With the exception of clozapine, most other antipsychotic drugs either cause or have the potential to cause serious **extrapyramidal symptoms (EPS).** Common EPS are dystonia, dyskinesia, akathisia, Parkinsonism syndrome, tardive dyskinesia, and choreathetoid movements. With the exception of tardive dyskinesia, the symptoms occur and disappear within the first several weeks of drug treatment.

Serious extrapyramidal effects occur as a result of the drugs blocking dopamine receptors at extrapyramidal and limbic sites. Clozapine, which does not cause EPS, seems to have a selective action against dopamine receptors only at limbic sites (Ereshefsky et al., 1989).

Risperidone is noted to cause fewer EPS when compared with haldol, although when the dose approached 10 mg/day, EPS increased (Kane, 1993). Mellaril, or thioridazine, a more standard neuroleptic, is also noted for having a relatively low incidence of EPS (see Table 42–4).

Tardive Dyskinesia.

Tardive Dyskinesia. Tardive dyskinesia is a syndrome that usually occurs later in the use of antipsychotic drugs. It is more often associated with the higher potency drugs. It cannot be predicted who will develop tardive dyskinesia or when. Data suggest, however, that of individuals on long-term antipsychotic maintainence, 2 to 4% per year develop tardive dyskinesia over the first 7 years of exposure. Therefore, within a 7-year period, one could predict that 14 to 28% of patients who have been on antipsychotics for this time period will develop dyskinesia. Further, in chronically institutionalized patients, 50 to 60% have developed tardive dyskinesia over years of treatment (Schatzberg and Cole, 1991). Prominent features of tardive dyskinesia consist of slow, sometimes stereotyped movements of the nose, tongue, mouth, and face (Bernstein, 1988). Chewing, smacking and licking of the lips (Marsden et al., 1986), sucking, tongue protrusions, tongue tremor with open mouth, wormlike movements on the surface of the tongue, blinking, and facial distortions are also common (Munetz and Benjamin, 1988). Choreic movements of the limbs and rhythmic dystonic contractions of the axilla muscles, giving rise to torticollis and pelvic thrusting, may also occur (Marsden et al., 1986). The movement is constant, though it may increase with emotional arousal and may decrease with relaxation or volitional effort. The movements are entirely absent during sleep (Kane and Lieberman, 1992). It is usually preceded by the **Parkinsonism syndrome.** Anti-Parkinsonian drugs, however, make the condition worse because of their anticholinergic actions.

Decreasing the antipsychotic drug or discontinuing it immediately following diagnosis of tardive dyskinesia reduces the symptoms; however, the dosage would soon need to be increased to control the symptoms. Substituting another antipsychotic drug would also result in the re-emergence of symptoms. Sudden withdrawal of an antipsychotic drug may reveal the latent syndrome.

Early detection of the disorder is most important to reduce its seriousness. For example, movements of the big toe can be so constant that the shoe top is worn through. In extreme conditions and with some young patients, despair has been so great they have committed suicide. Although many drugs have been studied as a potential treatment for tardive dyskinesia, none have proved efficacious. The only known treatment at this time is discontinuance of the drug.

Clozapine, however, represents a viable option for individuals with severe and persistent mental disorders. Due to the absence of tardive dyskinesia associated with clozapine use, this drug may offer an alternative for individuals who have developed tardive dyskinesia with traditional neuroleptics. To date, studies on the drug risperidone also indicate that it, too, may be another alternative drug with a lower incidence of tardive dyskinesia than observed with the use of traditional antipsychotics.

Dystonias and Dyskinesias.

Dystonias and Dyskinesias. Dystonic reactions are involuntary, irregular clonic contortions of the muscles of the trunk and extremities. Initially, patients complain of a thick tongue and the inability to hold their neck straight. Other early symptoms include cogwheeling (sudden, brief interruptions in breathing) and difficulty speaking and swallowing. Trismus (lockjaw) may develop. (Symptoms appear chiefly while walking, at which time the contortions twist the body forward and sideways (tortipelvis) in a grotesque fashion. Sometimes the dystonia can be quite dramatic, resulting in oculogyric crises (rolling back of the eyes in the head) and opisthotonus (extreme arching of the back with the head thrown back). This extreme reaction occurs mostly in young men and early in treatment.

Higher potency drugs are more often associated with acute dystonias. Anti-Parkinsonian drugs, such as benzotropine mesylate (Cogentin) or with diphenhydramine hydrochloride (Benadryl) are used for treatment.

Dyskinesia is impairment of the power of voluntary movement, resulting in fragmentary or incomplete movements.

Akathisia.

Akathisia. Akathisia is an extreme inability to sit still. The body is in constant movement. There is pacing and constant movement of the feet. It is difficult to concentrate, read, and do simple tasks. If movement in the trunk is stopped, the person's pelvis and feet will move. This side effect is frequently mislabeled as agitation or severe anxiety, often resulting in an increase of problems. Patients describe feeling as though they are "jumping out of their skin" or that their extremities will not stay still.

Parkinsonism Syndrome.

Parkinsonism Syndrome. Parkinsonism syndrome usually occurs after the first week but before the second month of treatment. The symptoms resemble Parkinson's disease, which has the following symptoms: akinesia (lack of interest, fatigue, slowness, heaviness, lack of drive or ambition, vague bodily discomforts), muscular rigidity, masklike faces, shuffling gait, loss of associated movements, hypersalivation, drooling, alterations in posture, tremor, and pill-rolling movements.

Agranulocytosis. Agranulocytosis is a serious and life-threatening blood dyscrasia associated specifically with clozapine use. This serious side effect led the drug company Sandoz to withdraw the drug from the market in the mid-1970s. It did not become available in this country again until 1990 when a distribution system was developed with the purpose of monitoring the white blood counts of individuals taking clozapine. Prescriptions are then filled only if white blood counts are within the designated range. Agranulocytosis is initially recognized by a sore throat, fever, and general malaise. Although agranulocytosis is rarely associated with other neuroleptics, it can occur and periodic blood counts are recommended.

Neuroleptic Malignant Syndrome. Neuroleptic malignant syndrome (NMS) is a rare side effect that has been referred to as an extrapyramidal crisis. The symptoms of this condition include labile blood pressure, elevated pulse and temperature, anxiety, dyspnea, profuse perspiration, cyanosis, and seizures. The best treatment is discontinuance of the neuroleptic agent. Often, patients must be admitted to the hospital for a symptomatic treatment of this disorder, such as ice blankets, hydration, and control of blood pressure.

Neuroleptic malignant syndrome usually develops over a 24 to 72 hour period and can occur hours or months after initial drug exposure. Its suggested incidence is 0.5 to 1% of patients on standard neuroleptics. Long-acting, high potency neuroleptics seem to be more responsible for the onset of NMS. Exhaustion and dehydration may place individuals at greater risk (Meuller, 1985; Birkhimer and De Vane, 1984). Neuroleptic malignant syndrome affects all ages and both sexes, but young adult men predominate the reported cases. They are affected twice as often as women. Why young men are more susceptible is unclear. In 80% of reported cases persons are under age 40, and the mortality rate for these individuals is 20% (Caroff, 1980; Meuller, 1985; Birkhimer and De Vane, 1984). Predisposing conditions include physical exhaustion, dehydration, and an infectious process in a compromised organic state (Caroff, 1980; Meuller, 1985).

Due to the potential emergent medical complications occurring in individuals with NMS, treatment on an acute medical unit may be necessary until stabilization occurs.

Progressive Obstructive Jaundice. Progressive obstructive jaundice is another rare and serious reaction. Increased

yellowing of the skin and sclera of the eyes are the most notable signs. The drug must be stopped. The patient can be changed to another drug because cross-sensitivity is rare. The usual intervention for the liver disruption is bed rest and a high-protein, high-carbohydrate, low-fat diet.

Seizures. Seizures may result from a lowered convulsive threshold. Seizures are particularly associated with clozapine use. This factor may limit the clinician's ability to reach therapeutic dosage. In addition, anticonvulsant drugs may be prescribed to prevent seizures in patients receiving relatively high doses of clozapine. In general, when seizures occur, the drugs should be stopped or decreased and anticonvulsant therapy initiated.

Hematologic System Symptoms. With the noted exception of clozapine causing agranulocytosis, other hematologic effects are rare. When they do occur, however, they are generally in the form of leukopenia or thrombocytopenia, and the drug must be stopped immediately and supportive measures instituted. Periodic blood counts may assist in detecting abnormalities.

Common Side Effects of Antipsychotic Drugs

Antipsychotic agents may impair physical and mental abilities, especially during the first few days of therapy. Other milder, more common side effects of antipsychotic drugs are described next.

Psychiatric Symptoms. Drowsiness and akathisia are often perceived as depression and anxiety, and therefore, these reported symptoms need to be assessed carefully. Akathisia is also often mistaken for psychotic agitation leading to potential increases in psychotropic medication, which will worsen the condition. Apparent exacerbation of psychosis is generally related to excessive anticholinergic activity of select antipsychotic drugs. A decrease in the dosage results in the correction of the problem.

Anticholinergic Effects. Anticholinergic effects these include blurred vision, flushing, pallor, and dry mouth. Reassurance usually helps. Urologic symptoms are less common, but there may be retention of urine, particularly with thioridazine (Mellaril). Also, there may be retarded ejaculation and painful urination. These symptoms can be handled by reducing the dosage, if possible, and if not, a cholinergic drug (bethanechol chloride [Urecholinel]) may be used.

Although rare, excessive anticholinergic activity can result in an anticholinergic psychosis. This generally occurs as a toxic reaction in individuals with extreme sensitivity to the pharmacologic agent, or alternatively, in individuals who are simultaneously taking other drugs with anticholinergic properties, such as cogentin or tricyclic antidepressants.

Other Central Nervous System Symptoms.
Central nervous system symptoms include drowsiness and ataxia, which may limit the clinician's ability to reach therapeutic doses quickly. Mild forms of dystonia, dyskinesia, and akathisia may all be treated by anti-Parkinsonian drugs. Severe reactions have already been discussed. Impaired motor function must be dealt with by warning the patient and having him or her not participate in dangerous activities. Fatigue, lethargy, and weakness are mild and usually subside when the patient becomes active and moves around. Any problems in breathing are best handled by stopping the drug or reducing the dose.

Cardiovascular System Symptoms (in Mild Form).
These symptoms include syncope and electrocardiogram changes and as not as common as ventricular tachycardia (usually associated with thioridazine) and coronary thrombosis (which has been suspected with imipramine hydrochloride), peripheral edema, and hypotensive crises. The heart rate changes may be handled by reducing the dose, if possible, and other cardiovascular complications must be weighed clinically against the benefits when considering stopping the drug.

Hypersalivation.
Hypersalivation is a common side effect associated with clozapine use. This side effect is poorly understood due to the anticholinergic properties of the drug (Lieberman et al., 1989). Hypersalivation, however, often restricts the clinician in increasing the dosage to therapeutic levels.

Dermatologic Side Effects.
The most common dermatologic side effect is photosensitivity, usually with chlorpromazine (Thorazine) and thioridazine (Mellaril). Staying out of the sun and wearing protective clothing are the best methods of dealing with this problem. Less common effects are skin rashes with edema on face, feet, or hands. Diphenhydramine chloride (Benadryl) may be used. A rarer effect, deep pigmentation of the skin, may occur with Thorazine.

Endocrine System Symptoms.
Common symptoms are obesity, menstrual irregularity, edema, abnormal lactation, and decreased sex drive for men and increased sex drive for women. These symptoms are usually handled by reassurance or trying another class of drugs.

Ophthalmologic System Symptoms.
Patients may manifest a mild disturbance in accommodation, in which the eye is not able to focus on an object, and miosis (small pupil). An ophthalmologist should assess the eye's ability to accommodate. Rare and serious side effects are glaucoma or aggravation of glaucoma, ulceration of the cornea, pigmentation of the retina (tissue darkening or discoloration in the eye ground), and fine reticular corneal opacities. The most important treatment for eye involvement is early detection and consultation with an ophthalmologist.

Gastrointestinal System Symptoms.
Gastrointestinal symptoms include fecal impaction, constipation, and diarrhea. The symptoms are easily managed by dietary supplements or other mild medications as needed. More severe symptoms requiring cessation of the drug are paralytic ileus and perforating ulcer, for which hospitalization is necessary.

■ NURSING MANAGEMENT OF EXTRAPYRAMIDAL SYMPTOMS

MANAGEMENT OF NEUROLEPTIC MALIGNANT SYNDROME

Neuroleptic malignant syndrome (NMS) is an underdiagnosed, potentially lethal complication of treatment with major antipsychotic drugs (Henderson and Wooten, 1981).

Nurses play a critical role in the important early assessments of patients who exhibit signs of NMS (Caroff, 1980). The four cardinal signs of NMS that nurses can observe are muscular "lead pipe" rigidity, hyperthermia, disturbance of consciousness, and autonomic dysfunction (Smego and Durack, 1982).

In a review of the cases of 53 patients reported in the literature who experienced NMS, Levenson (1985) noted that 89% had experienced lead pipe rigidity. Rigidity is often first observed as a dystonic reaction and commonly precedes an elevation in temperature (Gratz et al., 1992); however, there are generally several early accompanying symptoms that aid in the differential diagnosis of the syndrome. Hyperthermia characterized by temperatures in excess of 101°F is not uncommon, with most cases in the range of 101 to 104°F. Fluctuating changes in consciousness range from agitation and alert mutism to stupor and deep coma (Gratz et al., 1992). Blood pressure is generally elevated, but hypotension and labile blood pressure have also been reported. In Levenson's review, fever, tachycardia, rigidity, altered consciousness, abnormal blood pressure, tachypnia, and diaphoresis each occurred in more than two thirds of the patients. Also reported were dysarthria, dysphagia, and grand mal seizures.

TABLE 42–6. ABNORMAL INVOLUNTARY MOVEMENT SCALE (AIMS)

Observe patient unobtrusively while at rest.	Ask patient to open mouth. Observe tongue (twice).
Use a firm chair without arms to conduct examination.	Ask patient to protrude tongue. Observe (twice).
Ask patient whether there is anything in mouth. Remove gum or hard candy.	Ask patient to tap thumb with each finger rapidly for 10 or 15 seconds, both hands.
Ask patient about current condition of teeth. Dentures? Do they fit properly?	Observe facial and leg movements during above exercise.
Does the patient notice movements in mouth, face, hands, or feet?	Flex and extend patient's left and right arms. Note rigidity (may interfere with diagnosis).
Have patient describe movements and extent to which they interfere with activities.	Ask patient to stand. Note movements.
Have patient sit in chair with legs apart, feet on floor, observe for movements.	Ask patient to extend both arms in front. Note trunk, legs, and mouth.
Have patient sit with hands hanging, unsupported, between legs, observe movements.	Have patient walk a few paces back and forth. Observe hands and gait.

Modified AIMS Exam

	Instructions	Code
	Complete above examination procedure before making ratings. For movement ratings, rate highest severity observed. After completion, record results.	0 = none 1 = minimal, may be extreme normal 2 = mild 3 = moderate 4 = severe
Facial and oral movements	1. Muscles of facial expression (movement of forehead, eyebrows, periorbital area—include frowning, blinking, grimacing of upper face).	0 1 2 3 4
	2. Lips and perioral area (puckering, pouting, smacking).	0 1 2 3 4
	3. Jaw (biting, clenching, chewing, mouth opening, lateral movement).	0 1 2 3 4
	4. Tongue (rate only increased movement both in and out of mouth, NOT inability to sustain movement).	0 1 2 3 4
Extremity movements	5. Upper (arms, wrists, hands, fingers), include choreic movements (rapid objectively purposeless, irregular, spontaneous) and athetoid movements (slow, irregular, complex, serpentine). Do not include tremor (repetitive, rhythmic, regular).	0 1 2 3 4
	6. Lower (legs, knees, ankles, toes). Lateral knee movements, foot tapping, heel dropping, foot squirming, inversion and eversion of foot.	0 1 2 3 4
Trunk movements	7. Neck, shoulders, hips (rocking, twisting, squirming, pelvic gyrations). Include diaphramatic movements.	0 1 2 3 4
Global judgment	8. Severity of abnormal movements. Score based on highest single score on items 1 to 7 above.	None, normal: 0 Minimal: 1 Mild: 2 Moderate: 3 Severe: 4
	9. Incapacitation due to abnormal movements.	None, normal: 0 Minimal: 1 Mild: 2 Moderate: 3 Severe: 4
	10. Patient's awareness of abnormal movements.	No Awareness: 0 Aware, no distress: 1 Aware, mild distress: 2 Aware, moderate distress: 3 Aware, severe distress: 4
Dental status	11. Current problems with teeth and/or dentures.	No 0 Yes 1
	12. Does patient usually wear dentures?	No 0 Yes 1

Adapted from Munetz and Benjamin, 1988.

It is critical for the professional nurse to recognize potential symptoms of NMS early in their development. All observations and reports of muscle rigidity, elevated temperature, and changes in vital signs and levels of consciousness must be assessed and reported promptly to appropriate individuals. Further doses of medication must be held, and supportive measures instituted.

Elevated serum phosphokinase levels generally confirm the diagnosis. Anticholinergic agents, dantrolene sodium, and bromocriptine mesylate have been administered with varying success (Kahn et al., 1985; Zulbenko and Pope, 1983). These drugs act to decrease central dopaminergic blockade, believed to be one of the possible etiologies of the syndrome (Levenson, 1985).

Nursing interventions and comfort measures are essential in the ongoing management of these individuals. In addition to closely monitoring changes in the patient's status, cooling blankets to reduce body temperature, intravenous fluids to prevent dehydration and potential renal complications, and measures to assure safety are indicated. Furthermore, education and support of the individual, family, and significant others is a necessary aspect of the plan of care to decrease anxiety and fear throughout this medical and psychiatric emergency.

MANAGEMENT OF PARKINSONISM SYNDROME

The akinesia associated with Parkinsonism syndrome is often misinterpreted as depression or negativism. The weakness and lack of interest should be evaluated from the standpoint of muscle weakness. Usually, there is a lack of muscle strength in the individual's grip. In addition, increased muteness or comments about feeling slowed down, heavy, in slow motion, or under water are further subjective signs of akinesia.

The lack of facial expression or flatness of the face is often mistaken for signs of chronic schizophrenia or depression. The difference is that despite the facial expression, the person uses language to express variations of emotional reactions in contrast to schizophrenic or depressed patients.

Body rigidity is often mistaken for anxiety, again a misdiagnosis that can lead to more medication rather than treating this as the Parkinsonism syndrome. Rigidity is tested for by holding the patient's elbow in the palm of the nurse's hand with the nurse's thumb positioned over the flexor tendons, extending and flexing the patient's arm while asking him or her to relax. If there is a consistent resistance or lead pipe rigidity, or a ratchet-like phenomenon known as cogwheel rigidity, this is evidence of drug-induced rigidity. It usually starts 2 to 3 days or 2 weeks after drug therapy is begun.

The stooped posture and the lack of associative movements, such as the moving of arms while walking, are often mistaken for depression. If the person was not like this prior to drug treatment, chances are that such changes in posture and movement are connected with the drug.

Tremor, particularly in the hands, will be noted. The amount of tremor is usually more than in Parkinson's disease. The hand tremor interferes with fine motor coordination. Patients may try and hide the tremor, feeling embarrassed or attributing it to their emotional state.

The muteness and alterations in posture are often mistaken for worsening schizophrenic syndrome. Unfortunately, any increase in medication increases the symptoms. If left unchecked, incontinence, fever, and coma can ensue.

Improvement of these symptoms usually occurs slowly with the reduction of the dose of the drug and by the addition of an anticholinergic drug. Sometimes switching a patient to a different antipsychotic drug removes the symptoms. After 2 to 3 months, the symptoms will usually disappear. It is important to recognize this because anti-Parkinsonian drugs have powerful anticholinergic effects, and it is important to remove the patient from them as soon as possible.

MANAGEMENT OF PATIENTS WITH DYSKINESIAS AND DYSTONIAS

Dystonic reactions, acute dyskinesias and oculogyric crises typically occur during the early hours or days following an increase in the dosage of antipsychotic drugs. The symptoms of involuntary contractions, more common in men, are episodic and recurrent, lasting from minutes to hours. The importance in recognizing that these rather frightening symptoms are drug-related is that they can be misdiagnosed in an emergency situation. Consider the following example: A mental health worker reported that her daughter was about to have a tracheotomy performed in an emergency room when she came in with oculogyric crisis, torticollis, protrusion of her tongue, and opisthotonus. Fortunately, the mother informed the physician that her daughter was on an antipsychotic drug, and he administered diphenhydramine (Benadryl) intravenously, and the tracheotomy was avoided.

The symptoms of dystonias are painful and frightening. They can be acute or milder. Once they occur, the dosage of the medication should be lowered to avoid further episodes. Because the patient may complain of his or her eyes rolling up in the head or suspect peculiar things going on with his or her jaw, a nurse might wrongly assume the patient is delusional rather than having a drug-related response.

MANAGEMENT OF PATIENTS WITH AKATHISIA

Akathisia, with the most common effects of feeling restless and agitated (the "walkies and talkies") can be mistaken for anxiety and agitation. These symptoms are most uncomfortable, and patients often refuse to take antipsychotic medications because of them. The way of differentiating akathisia from anxiety is to note whether it gets worse when the drug is increased or if the subjective experience of the patient is different. The patient usually experiences the restlessness as something different. He or she also will report feeling better walking around and will identify an internal sense of restlessness that was not experienced before. The incidence peaks within 6 to 10 weeks with a decline in 12 to 16 weeks. Anti-Parkinsonian drugs and the shorter acting benzodiazapines will reduce the symptoms and demonstrate to the patient that the effects of akathisia are time-limited.

MANAGEMENT OF PATIENTS WITH TARDIVE DYSKINESIA

Patients on antipsychotic drug therapy, and in particular on long-term therapy, must be screened every 3 months for tardive dyskinesia. The earliest signs are excessive blinking and fine, vermiform movements of the tongue, and subtle spasmodic movements, particularly of the arms. The symptoms then progress with a fluctuating course until, finally, they interfere with activities of daily living, such as bathing, dressing, or eating. The symptoms can be suppressed only by intense, voluntary effort. During sleep they are absent. Patients are embarrassed by the symptoms.

As mentioned previously, both clozapine and risperidone are viable alternatives for patients who experience the onset of tardive dyskinesia. In those rare instances when either option does not seem appropriate, the lowest dose possible to maintain optimal mental status should be the rule, accompanied by drug holidays whenever feasible.

When tardive dyskinesia is identified, drugs used to treat extrapyramidal reactions should not be used, as they may exacerbate the condition. Increasing the antipsychotic drugs is contraindicated because it masks the symptoms and can lead to toxicity.

MANAGEMENT OF OTHER SIDE EFFECTS

Postural hypotension is an example of an *adrenolytic* side effect occurring frequently and, therefore, of particular concern in the nurse's, patient's, and family's daily evaluations of the patient. The effect may be precipitated by any antipsychotic drug but is triggered in particular by thioridazine and chlorpromazine. This problem is evaluated with the patient having the blood pressure taken in sitting and lying positions, both before and after the drug is administered. It is important to instruct the patient to take his or her time when getting up and to be careful when stooping in order to avoid fainting. If the patient is working with machinery, it is important that time away from the machines be taken after drug ingestion to avoid accidents. Drowsiness is another feature that can inhibit daily activities. This side effect is usually controlled by taking the medication at night. Nasal stuffiness is another manifestation of adrenolytic side effects.

For men, impotence and inhibition of ejaculation or retrograde ejaculation occur, especially with the use of thioridazine and mesoridazine. This can be extremely distressing for individuals and may lead to noncompliance. It is important to make sure that the sexual problems are not related to factors other than the drug.

Another important side effect is the reversal or blocking of administered epinephrine. This is most important for patients who need epinephrine for emergency reasons. Knowing that the patient is on antipsychotic drugs can alert the medical staff to use norepinephrine to counteract the blocking and potential paradoxical reactions.

Anticholinergic side effects include dry mouth, which can be helped with sugarless gum or gum drops or saliva substitutes. Constipation is best dealt with through the use of stool softeners. Cardiac changes, particularly rate problems, such as tachycardia, are best attended to by periodically checking the pulse and doing ECGs. Vision can be blurred because of interference with the accommodation processes. If this symptom interferes with the patient's life, it is usually treated with physostigmine.

A potentially serious problem for men, and in particular men with benign prostatic hypertrophy, is urinary retention. Intake and output records are important in establishing urinary retention.

A most confusing state is the induction of atropine-like psychosis marked by confusion, incoherence, visual hallucinations, disorientation, and impaired concentration. This can be differentiated from the psychotic disorder under treatment if the nurse has become familiar with the most anxious state of the patient. This becomes a baseline measurement for the nurse by which to assess behavior change. The marked confusion and acuteness of the symptoms, plus the vivid visual hallucinations are different from the psychotic episodes of schizophrenia, which usually do not manifest the same degree of confusion and disorientation. Symptoms are reduced by the use of physostigmine and withdrawal of the antipsychotic medication. Any onset of a psychotic episode needs to be fully evaluated by a physician with a review of drug therapy.

Hypothalamic side effects, such as disturbances of menstruation, temperature deregulation, fever, and appetite change, can all be addressed by having a daily program of evaluation and reporting. Risperidone increases prolactin levels, which are associated with galactorrhoea, disruption of the ovulatory cycle, and amenorrhea (Kane, 1993).

Lowering of the seizure threshold and the production of seizures are usually associated with clozapine and chlorpromazine and are dose related. Being prepared is facilitated by screening for a history of seizure problems with the patient or family members.

Phototoxicity is another important potential side effect that is best avoided by protective clothing and staying out of the sun. When sun exposure cannot be avoided, sun screening agents should be applied liberally.

■ NURSING MANAGEMENT OF OVERDOSE WITH ANTIPSYCHOTIC DRUGS

Although it is rare for a patient to overdose with antipsychotic drugs, it does occur. Many times the problems of overdose have to do with drugs other than antipsychotics. Nevertheless, it is important to remember that antipsychotic drugs last in human tissue for a long period of time. Phenothiazines are detoxified in the liver, and where there is hepatic dysfunction, coma may be prolonged.

Hypotension is usually the most serious symptom, and it responds to blood volume expansion. Treatment is very difficult because of the beta-adrenergic blockade. No epinephrine or isoproterenol are given to raise blood pressure because these drugs have beta-adrenergic activity. Instead, ephedrine or norepinephrine (Levophed) should be used (Arana and Hyman, 1991). Other serious complications of overdose are hypertension and hyperthermia, urinary tract infection with oliguria and renal failure, cardiac arrhythmias, skin lesions, and clinical relapse.

Treatment of overdose is best approached symptomatically. Gastric lavage, if initiated early postingestion, is useful to decrease absorption of the ingested drug. Maintenance of an adequate airway is also imperative. Induction of emesis is not advised because a dystonic reaction could ensue, which would cause aspiration of vomitus.

The use of stimulants should be avoided because convulsions may be initiated as a result of a reduced convulsion threshold. Extrapyramidal symptoms may be treated with anti-Parkinsonian agents, barbiturates, or diphenhydramine.

O AN OVERVIEW

Antipsychotic Drugs

- A clear history of illness and accurate assessment of symptoms is critical before initiating antipsychotic agents.

- Target symptoms most affected by antipsychotic drugs are delusions, hallucinations, change in the flow of ideas, changes in the structure and rate of associations, ideas of reference, suspicious behavior, incoherence, and marked illogical thinking.

- Antipsychotic drugs, often referred to as neuroleptics because of their many neurologic side effects, alter the kinds and amounts of amines at the synapse.

- Drugs are extremely useful in treating psychotic states and managing chronic psychotic symptoms.

- Extrapyramidal symptoms (EPS), which may be caused by most antipsychotic drugs, include dystonia, dyskinesia, akathisia, Parkinsonism syndrome, tardive dyskinesia, and choreathetoid movements.

- Nurses have a critical role in the assessment of patients with extrapyramidal symptoms and in interventions to treat patients.

■ THERAPY WITH ANTI-PARKINSONIAN AGENTS

Therapy with anti-Parkinsonian agents is directed at correcting a neurotransmitter imbalance (dopamine deficiency and acetylcholine excess in the corpus striatum). The use of levodopa or amantadine enhances dopaminergic action. Centrally active **anticholinergic agents** are useful in inhibiting acetylcholine (Table 42–3). Anti-Parkinsonian agents reduce the incidence and severity of akinesia, rigidity, and tremor. In addition to suppressing cholinergic activity, these agents may also inhibit the re-uptake and storage of dopamine, thereby prolonging the action of dopamine.

Peripheral anticholinergic side effects (e.g., urinary retention or tachycardia), frequently limit the dosages that can be instituted in therapy. Figure 42–2 shows the relative time range for the onset of a variety of side effects.

In spite of somewhat limited efficacy, anticholinergic anti-Parkinsonian agents are widely used in the therapy of drug-induced EPS. Once anticholinergic treatment is instituted, some clinicians argue the necessity to continue with prophylactic use while others suggest discontinuance whenever possible. This is generally a matter of personal preference. The patient, however, requires continued observation for the presence of side effects whether the anticholinergic drugs are continued or not.

Most important is the recognition of the toxic effects or the anticholinergic effects of these drugs when used with antipsychotic drugs, as detailed in the next two sections.

ANTICHOLINERGIC SYNDROME AS A CONSEQUENCE OF ANTI-PARKINSONIAN AGENTS AND ANTIPSYCHOTIC DRUGS

Acute overdose or excessive prescription of medications with antimuscarinic properties, especially when anti-Parkinsonian agents are combined with tricyclic antidepressants, other anti-Parkinsonian agents, some antipsychotics (especially thioridazine), many proprietary sedative–hypnotic drugs, many antispasmodic preparations, several plants, Jimson weed, and some mushrooms.

Signs of Toxicity

Neuropsychiatric signs include anxiety, agitation, restlessness, purposeless overactivity, delirium, disorientation, impairment of immediate and recent memory, dysarthria, hallucinations, and myoclonic seizures.

Systemic Signs

These include tachycardia and arrhythmias; large, sluggish pupils; scleral injection; flushed, warm, dry skin; increased temperature; decreased mucosal secretions; urinary retention; and reduced bowel motility.

Treatment

For both adults and children physostigmine salicylate (neostigmine, pyridostigmine, etc.) is used. The treatment may itself engender another imbalance; this time it would be a cholinergic excess. Familiarity with this syndrome is important.

PHYSOSTIGMINE-INDUCED CHOLINERGIC EXCESS

Neuropsychiatric Signs

The neuropsychiatric signs include confusion, seizures, nausea and vomiting, myoclonus, and hallucinations, often after a period of initial CNS improvement when physostigmine is given to treat the anticholinergic syndrome.

Systemic Signs

Systemic signs of physostigmine-induced cholinergic excess include bradycardia, miosis, increased mucosal secretions, copious bronchial secretions, dyspnea, tears,

sweating, diarrhea, abdominal colic, biliary colic, and urinary frequency or urgency.

Treatment and Prevention

For treatment and prevention atropine sulfate (CNS and systemic action) 0.5 mg/1.0 mg physostigmine, intramuscularly or subcutaneously; methscopolamine bromide (Pamine); and glycopyrrolate (Robinul) is used (Baldessarini, 1985).

THE EFFECT OF ANTI-PARKINSONIAN AGENTS ON DISEASE STATES

Although the anti-Parkinsonian agents are not contraindicated for patients with chronic liver or kidney disorders, these patients should be closely observed. Incipient glaucoma may be precipitated by these agents. When used to treat EPS caused by phenothiazine therapy, anti-Parkinsonian agents may exacerbate psychotic symptoms and precipitate a toxic psychosis. The possibility exists that the anti-Parkinsonian agents may mask the development of persistent EPS with prolonged phenothiazine therapy. These agents may impair mental or physical abilities required for the performance of potentially hazardous tasks.

OVERDOSE SYMPTOMS AND MANAGEMENT

Symptoms of overdose are similar in extent to those of antihistamine overdose, including dryness of mucous membrane; dilation of pupils; hot, dry skin; tachycardia; glaucoma; constipation; nausea and vomiting; mental confusion; convulsions; and circulatory and respiratory collapse. Severe CNS depression is followed or preceded by stimulation. (See description of anticholinergic syndrome.)

Overdose management consists of gastric lavage or emesis. Treatment should be symptomatic. Use of physostigmine salicylate will reverse the abovementioned symptom of anticholinergic intoxication. Artificial respiration and oxygen therapy should be instituted if respiratory depression is present. Maintain normovolemic state with intravenous supplement and vasopressor agents.

O AN OVERVIEW

Anti-Parkinsonian Drug Therapy

● Anti-Parkinsonian drugs are generally not started before the occurrence of side effects. Anti-Parkinsonian drugs have anticholinergic effects also and can compound the anticholinergic effects of the antipsychotic drugs.

- Anti-Parkinsonian drugs usually do not need to be given more than 3 months beyond the starting of antipsychotic agents and the occurrence of EPS. By 3 months, most side effects abate.

- Acute or increased agitation must be evaluated as a possible toxic side effect of anti-Parkinsonian agents. In this case, the drugs must be stopped and the anticholinergic effects treated medically.

- Tardive dyskinesia increases with anti-Parkinsonian drugs. When this side effect occurs, do not give anti-Parkinsonian drugs. Do not increase antipsychotic drugs. They mask the syndrome.

■ DRUG INTERACTIONS WITH ANTIPSYCHOTIC DRUGS

Highlights of important drug interactions of antipsychotic drugs are summarized in Table 42–9.

One of the most critical drug interactions involving antipsychotic drugs is the synergistic and cumulative effects that occur when combined with other CNS depressant agents. In addition, antidiarrheals and antacids reduce absorption of phenothiazines, antipsychotic agents may inhibit guanethidine, and chlorpromazine inhibits metabolism of propranolol. Another important consideration is that haloperidol (Haldol) and methyldopa may cause disorientation, aggressiveness, and assaultiveness.

ANTACIDS

Studies indicate that the concurrent administration of chlorpromazine and alum or magnesium gel-type antacids results in significantly lower serum levels of chlorpromazine.

HALOPERIDOL

When given in combination with anticoagulants, haloperidol reduces the prothrombin time, causing an enhanced anticoagulant effect.

DIBENZODIAZEPINES, PHENOTHIAZINES, AND THIOXANTHENES

The seizure threshold in some patients is lowered by dibenzodiazepines, phenothiazines, and thioxanthenes, thereby necessitating an increase in seizure-controlling medications.

ANTI-PARKINSONIAN DRUGS

Anti-Parkinsonian drugs usually decrease the extrapyramidal side effects of the antipsychotic agents. If the anti-Parkinsonian agent is prematurely withdrawn, a precipitation of EPS may occur.

ANTIPSYCHOTIC AGENTS AND CENTRAL NERVOUS SYSTEM DEPRESSANTS

Together antipsychotic agents and CNS depressants cause additive CNS depression. Also, because barbiturates affect liver function, an increased level of antipsychotic agents may be needed.

MONOAMINE OXIDASE INHIBITORS

Used with antipsychotic agents, monamine oxidase inhibitors may cause an additive hypotensive effect.

TRICYCLIC ANTIDEPRESSANTS

Concurrent administration of tricyclic antidepressants and phenothiazines increase anticholinergic effects and may lead to a toxic psychosis.

EPINEPHRINE

Epinephrine will have a paradoxical effect on blood pressure (i.e., lowering) in the presence of antipsychotic agents. Use ephedrine or norepinephrine.

PROPRANOLOL

Chlorpromazine inhibits metabolism of propranolol, resulting in increased hypotension.

■ IMPACT OF OTHER DISEASE OR ALTERED PHYSIOLOGICAL STATES AND NURSING MANAGEMENT

In view of the previously mentioned side effects of antipsychotic drugs, it is useful for the nurse to concentrate holistically on other ongoing disease processes unique to the patient. Patients suffering from pulmonary insufficiency should be watched for signs of bronchopneumonia. It has been postulated that lethargy and a decreased sense of thirst resulting from central inhibition may lead to dehydration, reduced pulmonary ventilation, and hemoconcentration.

■ PRINCIPALS OF PSYCHIATRIC NURSING PRACTICE REGARDING ANTIPSYCHOTIC DRUGS

Because antipsychotic drugs impact practically every organ system in the body, it is important for the nurse to understand the major objective of drug intervention. Side effects must be distinguished from the targeted symptoms. An early nursing assessment combined with the basic medical assessment provides a baseline of information for the nurse to monitor behavioral changes. This major principle is relevant to all drug therapy. In addition to the behavioral assessment, the use of laboratory tests, such as blood levels, to monitor toxicity and check on compliance, as well as a broad spectrum of laboratory tests to measure the impact of the drug on organ functions of the liver, kidney, heart, and the hematopoietic system are available and can be used to monitor the patient's clinical status.

Many severely and chronically disturbed patients are in service systems, both in-patient and community, that are medically underserved; that is, there are limited numbers of physicians and nurses. Therefore, it is imperative that the nurse take the initiative, when necessary, to establish adequate protocols for the health surveillance of patients taking drugs. In addition, the nurse may also be the one to initiate drug education for the patient, family, and auxiliary mental health personnel.

Dosage ranges are wide and related to the high therapeutic index of this drug class. Usually the patient is given a small test dose of the drug to rule out severe hypotension, oversedation, or severe allergic responses. These effects occur early in drug treatment. Chlorpromazine 50 mg or its equivalent of other antipsychotic drugs is used as a test dose. If the patient has no untoward reaction, he or she is usually started on a schedule of small, daily, divided doses leading to a total daily dosage in the range of 100 to 800 mg of chlorpromazine or its equivalent. Doses are gradually increased, observing for the onset of side effects. The dosage is maintained at a level where minimal side effects are present, and symptom improvement continues.

Within 5 to 10 days, symptoms are usually in control, and the patient has developed a tolerance to the acute side effects. Dosage schedules can then be rearranged. Most patients prefer fewer doses per day or one dose at bedtime. This allows the patient to carry out his or her daily regimen, and if there are mild, short-term side effects, they will occur during sleep.

Positive drug response should occur within 3 to 6 weeks. If there has been no improvement, and noncompliance is not an issue, the patient may require a drug from a different class or just a different drug. Variability of response is primarily a function of the individual. Approximately 10 to 12% of those diagnosed as schizophrenic do not respond to drug treatment.

RAPID NEUROLEPTIZATION

In the acute treatment phase of psychosis, some physicians use extremely large doses of antipsychotic drugs early in treatment. This approach is called rapid neuroleptization or digitalizing treatment. Although the purpose is to achieve rapid remission of psychotic states and early discharge from the hospital, studies do not support the efficacy of this approach over the standard regimen of gradually increasing drug dosage to effect. Furthermore, the rapid approach is associated with an increase in untoward reactions.

High potency drugs are preferable if the rapid neuroleptization regimen is adopted. The usual reason for using this approach is that a patient is highly excited or dangerous before administration. (Bassuk et al., 1983). In this case, the nurse must be prepared to monitor the administration of drugs and the patient's response. The locations of emergency supplies and their use in case of drug reactions and side effects must be known. While high potency drugs are preferred, as they are less likely to produce hypotension and seizures, chances of extrapyramidal side effects are increased. Rapid neuroleptization requires the close coordination of nursing and medical efforts. Clearly, a risk–benefit analysis is necessary prior to using this strategy.

After the cessation of the acute phase, the dose of a drug can be slowly lowered to a maintenance dose that is often one half to one fifth of the highest dose needed to control symptoms.

DURATION OF TREATMENT

Patients often ask how long they have to be on drugs. Usually, with people who have had an acute psychotic episode, there is a strong possibility that once they have gotten over the acute phase and stabilized, they can be slowly removed from drug therapy. When people have had recurrent psychotic episodes, long-term intermittent maintenance may be required. Children and adults who are maintained on long-term maintenance therapy risk tardive dyskinesia.

Whenever a patient is taken off a drug, it is usually necessary to remove the drug gradually. In addition, time must be taken between the administration of a new drug or somatic therapeutic intervention because these drugs tend to have a prolonged effect in the body due to breakdown or their mode of storage in the body. Only severe side effects warrant rapid removal of the drug, and this is best done under the direction of the physician. At these times, the management of the side effects as well as the impact of drug withdrawal requires medical management.

In many states, patients can refuse drug treatment even though they are hospitalized. Patients in the community, for a variety of reasons, may become annoyed or disenchanted with drug therapy and attempt to discontinue it. It is imperative that the nurse make it clear to these patients that they have a right to refuse treatment, but once a regimen is begun, they must work closely with the nursing and medical staff if they wish to discontinue drug therapy. All patients must be adequately informed as to the risks and gains assumed by drug intervention, and they must give their permission for therapy.

E CASE EXAMPLE

Carol, a 17-year-old black woman, is brought to the emergency room via ambulance, accompanied by her mother. The mother reports that the patient has not slept for 2 days and has refused to eat or drink for 24 hours. The patient's abrupt behavioral change also includes suspiciousness, complete withdrawal, hallucinations, and persecutory delusions. Carol's behaviors indicate an acute psychotic episode. She is admitted that night to the adolescent psychiatric unit for a complete psychiatric evaluation. All presenting features continue, and the patient remains awake the night of admission. On day one, she becomes physically combative during the routine medical workup and continues to refuse anything by mouth. The patient is begun on haloperidol (Haldol) 2.5 mg tid and receives the first two doses intramuscularly that evening. The following day the patient appears stiff and subdued, though not sedated. She makes a few vague complaints of general malaise. Later in the evening, the patient develops tachypnea and a temperature of 38.8°C; the patient is also tachycardic (heart rate: 140). Level of consciousness is strikingly altered with fluctuations of alertness. Subsequent dosages of medication are held, while an acute medical treatment and workup is begun. This includes IV therapy, blood gases and cultures, lumbar puncture, CT scan, x-ray, and consults from neurology and infectious disease. All test results are within normal limits with the exception of an elevated creatinine phosphokinase (CPK) (consistent with NMS).

In the early stages of recovery, respiratory, renal, and cardiovascular functions are monitored constantly for signs of decompensation. Level of consciousness is continuously assessed for degrees of unresponsiveness and alertness. Autonomic instability causes frequent episodes of tachycardia, diaphoresis, hyperpyrexia, and labile hypertension. Vital signs are monitored every 4 hours. The patient receives IV therapy for the first 72 hours for dehydration and absence of gag reflex. Hypertonic involvement of pharyngeal muscles results in intermittent dysphagia with inconsistent intake of fluids and food an ongoing problem. This necessitates strict I & O with close monitoring. Temperature and electrolyte balance are also followed closely. Due to minimal responsiveness initially, frequent position changes, elevation of extremities, and assisting the patient to ambulate are effective interventions in reducing associated health problems.

To respond to the psychological needs of the patient, nursing staff communicate with Carol in a way that assumes comprehension despite her changeable level of alertness. All medical procedures are carefully explained to her before implementation, and staff remain with her to provide support. A core group of staff is formed for consistency of care and to establish a safe and trusting environment for the patient. The use of touch becomes a therapeutic tool in diminishing feelings of isolation, fear, agitation, and helplessness. Family members are encouraged to become active participants in the patient's recovery and care.

Maintaining people on a useful dose of medication while they remain in the community requires educational programs for the patients, families, and community support providers. Employers of patients who are on medication can also be helpful. Group methods are useful in monitoring dosage effectiveness and side effects. Some drugs, such as fluphenazine (Prolixin) and haloperidol (Haldol) are prepared in suspensions, which when injected, can last 1 to 2 weeks, eliminating the need for daily medication.

The relationship between the medical team and the patient must be positive in preparing the patient to reduce or withdraw from antipsychotic drugs. There may be an exacerbation of symptoms after removal of the drug, which would necessitate a return to the drug. This return can be very demoralizing, and a supportive relationship is necessary to mitigate the patient's emotional response to remaining on drugs.

The patient, nurse, physician, patient's family, and, where appropriate, the work setting, must work together. Written information for patients, families, and employers; group presentations for family and patients; teaching what the objectives of drug intervention are and how to self-monitor; and group monitoring programs all aid in effective and successful drug intervention.

O AN OVERVIEW

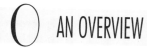

Nursing Implications

- Nurses must continually study and discern how to distinguish side effects from the disordered state.

- Nurses are responsible for collaborating with the patient, physician, and family on various levels of education regarding drug intervention and the establishment of policies and procedures.

- Nurses are responsible for assessing the psychological and cultural meanings associated with drug therapy for the patient and family. (For example, a large dose of drug does not necessarily indicate that a patient has a chronic problem or will need to be on drugs the rest of his or her life. This is the type of misconception that can interfere with the patient's recovery and his or her family relationships and, if the patient works, with the employer.)

- Nurses and physicians are responsible for making sure the patient and family are sufficiently informed of the risks and benefits expected from drug therapy.

■ MOOD STABILIZERS

IDENTIFYING MOOD DISORDERS

Affective disorders are characterized by a disturbance in mood. Mood is a prolonged emotion that affects the individual's social, affective, and behavioral experiences. Mood refers to the pattern presentation of depression or euphoria; disorders of mood include mania and depression, as well as cyclothymic and dysthymic disorders (Chapter 20). Often the terms bipolar disorder and unipolar disorder are used. A diagnosis of bipolar affective disorder is made when the individual has experienced at least one manic episode. This individual may also have suffered many major depressive episodes. A diagnosis of unipolar disorder describes an individual who has had depressive episodes but has never experienced a manic episode.

Clyclothymic disorder is characterized by alternating affective states of euphoria and depression, but they are not of sufficient intensity, severity, and duration to meet the criteria for major depressive or manic episodes. In dysthymic disorder, the symptoms are not of sufficient severity and duration for a major depressive episode, and there have been no hypomanic periods.

Two types of medication are currently being used to treat mood disorders: lithium preparations and anticonvulsants.

LITHIUM AS A TREATMENT FOR MOOD INSTABILITY

Lithium is widely recognized and used as a major treatment for affective disorders. Initially, it was believed that lithium's action was specific to mania, and while the best response to lithium occurs in manic individuals, lithium has also been used for the treatment of depression, cyclothymic, and dysthymic disorders. Varying results from treatment with lithium are reported in cyclothymic disorders. Individuals suffering from rapid cycling affective disorders seem to respond poorly to lithium, and while lithium is often used as an adjunctive treatment in depressive disorders, the most efficacious treatment for major depression is an antidepressant agent (Arana and Hyman, 1991). Lithium has been used to treat many states where mood is the prominent feature, including impulse disorders and personality disorders.

When lithium is used to treat mania, the person may be aware of a slowing of thought processes and actions. Lithium is often preferred over antipsychotics in the treatment of mania, as improvement is achieved without the sedating effect noted when antipsychotic drugs are used. Lithium takes 7 to 10 days at therapeutic blood levels to have any effect. Therefore, in severe manic states, antipsychotic agents may be used to bring about more immediate sedation and control of manic symptoms.

Lithium is used for maintenance therapy to prevent the recurrence of an affective disorder (Bernstein, 1988). Prophylactic use of lithium for both manias and depressions has been successful. In addition, lithium has been used to augment the antidepressant effect of tricyclics in the treatment of depression.

Lithium Absorption and Action

Lithium is readily absorbed through the gastrointestinal system and is distributed throughout body tissues. Peak blood levels occur within a few hours, with the exception of the longer acting lithium where peak levels occur after 4 to 5 hours. Lithium is eliminated almost entirely by renal excretion. Sodium diuresis and sodium deficiency tend to increase the retention of lithium, potentially leading to toxicity.

The mechanism of action is not yet clear. Some speculations deal with the electrolyte balance across membranes including neurons. Other hypotheses deal with the alteration of cellular processes due to the presence of lithium, changing calcium availability within the cell. Finally, lithium is known to have effects on the neurotransmitter serotonin, ultimately resulting in a stabilizing activity in the neurons. Whether this effect is related to improvement in symptoms or not is unclear, though serotonin has been indirectly linked to affective disorders (Arana and Hyman, 1991).

Dosage

Unlike most drugs, the dosage range of lithium is not indicative of its clinical effect (Table 42–7). When beginning treatment with lithium, the dosage must be

TABLE 42–7. LITHIUM DOSAGE

Preparation	Adult Dosage	Lethal Dose
Lithium carbonate (Eskalith, Lithonate, Lithotabs)	Initial: 300 to 600 mg (1,200 to 1,800 mg/day) until lithium blood level is reached (0.8 to 1.2 for therapeutic effect.	Toxicity results in blood levels > 2.0 mEq/L. Lethality generally occurs at levels greater than 3.0.
Lithium citrate Syrup (Cibalith)	Same as above.	
Lithium carbonate–Slow release (Lithobid, Eskalith CR).	Initial: 450 mg. Increase dosage to reach serum levels 0.8 to 1.2 mEq/L for therapeutic effect.	

adjusted carefully and slowly while monitoring blood levels. Generally speaking, blood levels should be checked with any change in dose, followed by weekly level checks to assure stability. Once the patient's blood level has stabilized, monthly levels surface. Any significant change in the patient's level of physical activity should be followed by lithium level monitoring. Significant changes in activity level may lead to increased sodium diuresis and, therefore, increased lithium retention. This is also a concern during the summer months for the same reason. Lithium is currently available in many preparations, including capsules, citrates, tablets, and slow release preparations. Lithium is usually administered in 150 to 300 mg increments in divided dosages in order to reach serum levels of 0.7 to 1.2. It must be understood that some individuals will require lower blood levels for a therapeutic response while some will necessitate higher levels.

Lithium Toxicity

Therapeutic levels of lithium closely approximate toxic levels, and the margin of safety is quite low. Prolonged blood levels greater than 1.5 usually result in toxicity. Blood concentrations of lithium greater than 2.0 mEq/L can result in lethal situations requiring immediate intervention. Therefore, careful nursing assessments accompanied by careful education of the patient regarding early symptoms of toxicity is critical.

Early symptoms of toxicity include nausea, vomiting, diarrhea, abdominal pain, and general malaise. Many patients experience mild toxicity associated with peak blood levels, but the symptoms are mild and are not prolonged.

Severe symptoms associated with serious toxicity include somnolence, confusion, motor restlessness, disturbed behavior, ataxia, incoordination, dysarthria, stupor, and coma. Incontinence of urine and feces and seizures may also occur. In addition to neurologic effects, individuals may experience an irregular pulse, decreased blood pressure, ECG changes, and peripheral circulatory failure, which ultimately results in circulatory collapse. Table 42–8 delineates symptoms of toxicity.

Management of Toxicity.
Early symptoms of toxicity are recognized readily and withdrawing lithium accompanied by replacing fluid and restoring the electrolyte balance is generally all that is required. Lithium serum levels fall rapidly once the drug is discontinued. With mild toxicity, changing to a slow-release lithium preparation generally resolves the problem. Serious symptoms of toxicity indicates a life-threatening event requiring immediate medical intervention. Dialysis and intravenous fluid replacement may be necessary; however, lithium toxicity rarely progresses to this state.

TABLE 42–8. LITHIUM TOXICITY AND SIDE EFFECTS

Lithium Concentrate (mEq/L)	Signs of Lithium Toxicity at Different Serum Levels
< 1.5	Nausea, vomiting, diarrhea, thirst, polyuria, lethargy, slurred speech, muscle weakness, fine hand tremor.
< 2.0	Persistent GI upset, coarse hand tremor, mental confusion, hyperirritability of muscles, ECG changes (moderate), drowsiness, incoordination.
> 2	Ataxia, giddiness, large output of dilute urine, serious ECG changes, tinnitus, blurred vision, clonic movements, seizures, stupor, severe hypotension, coma. (At this concentration, fatalities are secondary to pulmonary complications.)
> 3.0	Beginning of breakdown of many organ systems in the body.

Note: Treatment of toxicity: gastric lavage, hemodialysis (rapidly effective).

As already mentioned, changes in activity level, particularly during the hot weather increases sodium diuresis leading to higher serum levels of lithium, therefore, a change in daily dosage may be indicated.

Side Effects of Lithium

Kidney. Chronic ingestion of lithium may lead to a diabetes insipidus-like syndrome, evidenced by the inability to concentrate urine. Although this occurs commonly, it rarely causes long-term kidney damage when the individual's lithium level is maintained within the therapeutic range. Polyuria is another common renal side effect of lithium. There is evidence to indicate that individuals who take on a lower maintenance dose and individuals who take only a single daily dose have fewer reports of polyuria (Jefferson, 1992). The major problems associated with polyuria include inconvenience and the excessive liquid calories to replace lost fluid. Polyuria results from lithium's antagonistic effect with antidiuretic hormone (ADH) at the distal tubules. Therefore, while enough ADH may be circulating in the blood, it is unable to reserve fluid through its usual mechanism. This problem is easily managed by the addition of a thiazide diuretic.

Perhaps the most troubling effects of lithium on renal function were reported in 1977 (Hestbech et al., 1977). Morphologic changes associated with chronic interstitial nephritis were major concerns in the treatment of individuals with lithium carbonate. Fortunately, careful longitudinal studies have failed to confirm this fear (Arana and Hymen, 1991). Blood creatinine levels drawn at regular intervals are recommended, however.

Thyroid. A small percentage of patients taking lithium develop thyroid disturbances due to lithium's ability to interfere with the production of thyroid hormones. These disturbances sometimes result in the development of a goiter but do not require the discontinuation of lithium. The goiter may be present without abnormally low levels of T3 and T4. Therefore, depending on the presence of a clinical syndrome of hypothyroidism, decreased levels of T3 and T4, or both, treatment for the syndrome may be instituted. This involves the replacement of T4 with a synthetic form (synthroid). Elevated levels of thyroid stimulating hormone (TSH) have also been noted. While the importance of this finding in the absence of changes in T3 and T4 is unclear, it is prudent to follow TSH levels throughout lithium treatment (Arana and Hyman, 1991).

Tremor. Tremor may occur in individuals receiving lithium treatment. The tremor is characteristically a fine motor tremor that may be exacerbated with anxiety or when individuals are performing tasks that require fine motor control. Some individuals experience a worsening of the tremor with rising blood level 1 to 2 hours after the dose has been taken.

Other Side Effects. Some individuals complain of feeling unexcitable and disconnected from their effect. Many complain of weight gain as a result of lithium therapy, therefore, education regarding proper diet and exercise is indicated. Many also express concern about dermatologic problems, such as excessively dry skin, that may progress to more serious problems, such as psoriasis and severe acne. When appropriate, these conditions should be addressed seriously by referral to a dermatologist to prevent further complications.

Drug Interactions With Lithium

All these drugs increase renal clearance of lithium: sodium bicarbonate, acetazolamide, urea, mannitol, and aminophylline.

These drugs decrease renal clearance of lithium and may lead to lithium toxicity: thiazide diuretics, furosemide, and ethacrynic acid.

The drug indomethacin as well as other non-steroid anti-inflammatory agents can increase plasma levels of lithium by 30 to 60%, which may lead to toxicity.

The following drugs increase the CNS toxicity of lithium: mazindol, phenytoin, methyldopa, thioridazine, and carbamazepine.

An encephalopathic syndrome with irreversible brain damage has occurred in a few patients treated with lithium and haloperidol.

Lithium may lower chlorpromazine levels in blood and brain.

Nursing Responsibilities

Monitoring lithium blood levels necessitated by the drug's very narrow therapeutic index and the consequences of its buildup as a result of its patterns of excretion and binding. The dosage level of lithium does not determine its clinical effect; rather, the blood level does. Frequent assessment of blood levels is required until stability is reached, then monthly evaluation is sufficient.

Many people will experience side effects, even several hours after the first administration of the drug. Nausea, resting tremor of the hands, and slight abdominal discomfort are early symptoms. When antipsychotic drugs are used in conjunction with lithium, they are apt to mask side effects and signs of lithium toxicity because of their antinausea property. Even with frequent blood level assessment, there is great personal variation as to when the side effect or signs of toxicity will occur. Any attempt to equate symptoms with blood levels must be understood as a general position; each patient must be evaluated as an individual.

Mild side effects and signs of toxicity are usually registered with levels below 1.5 mEq/L. These are muscular weakness or fatigue, polyuria, polydipsia, nausea, diarrhea or loose stools, fine hand tremor while resting, and a metallic taste in the mouth. These symptoms often occur with rising blood lithium levels approximately 1 hour after receiving the medication. This can frequently be prevented by taking lithium with food or with meals. In this way, lithium absorption from the gastrointestinal tract is slowed, and blood lithium levels rise at a rate the individual can tolerate better.

Moderate symptoms are shown with levels between 1.5 and 2.5 mEq/L. These are severe nausea, vomiting, diarrhea, mild to moderate ataxia, incoordination, dizziness, sluggishness, giddiness, vertigo, slurred speech, tinnitus, blurred vision, increasing tremor, muscle irritability or twitching, asymmetrical deep tendon reflexes, and increased muscle tone. Some people show even more toxic effects at these levels. The clinical picture is usually more important than the blood level.

Severe and toxic symptoms are shown with levels of 2.5 to 7.0 mEq/L. These are coarse tremor, dysarthia, nystagmus, fasciculations, visual or tactile hallucinations, oliguria, anuria, confusion, impaired consciousness, dyskinesia, grand mal convulsions, coma, and death.

The best intervention is prevention. Lithium has an average serum half-life of 24 hours; the serum will gradually clear if no more lithium is given. Supportive measures need to be taken in severe and toxic states. Unfortunately, when serum levels are greater than 5.0 mEq/L and the individual survives the toxic reactions, there is apt to be a permanent aftereffect, such as dementia or cerebral ataxia.

Most side effects are reversible with a decreased dose and an increase in the time from onset of treatment. If the side effects do impede the patient, however, other measures may be necessary. For example, nausea can be offset by giving the drug with meals. Fine motor coordination may require the use of another drug, such as propranolol (Inderal).

Toxicity can occur for many reasons. Aside from overdosing, either through error or intention, dehydration caused by excessive heat, fever, or exercise, can cause a buildup of lithium through the loss of sodium. The other extremely important cause of lithium buildup and toxicity is renal disease. The kidneys are a prime source of excretion of the drug. The importance of these latter points cannot be sufficiently underscored. The need for patient and family cooperation and for thorough drug education is illustrated in the case of a young woman who was started on lithium without clear instructions. Her mother received no information regarding the drug. The girl developed the flu, and although she was vomiting and having diarrhea, she continued with the drug, only to develop a toxic condition and go into renal failure and tragically die.

Severe toxicity is a medical emergency. Some physicians believe that at 3.0 mEq/L or more, patients should be started on hemodialysis or peritoneal dialysis when the former is not available. Some attempts have been made to induce osmotic diuresis with mannitol, urea, or theophylline.

Gaining the patient's cooperation for the blood level assessment is challenging. Blood must be drawn between 10 and 14 hours after the last dose of lithium for accurate measurement. This requires that the patient remember not to take the lithium and not to come in and have blood drawn before the 10-hour limit. This is the only way to avoid false readings. It also points out that it is difficult to get an immediate lithium level that reflects accurate buildup levels; thus, the importance of clinical symptoms in making an initial decision.

When these nursing points are combined with the preceding information regarding drug interactions and the interplay of lithium with other disease states, such as thyroid problems, heart problems, and the drugs used to treat them, safe and very rewarding results can be derived for patients who have affective disorders.

◯ AN OVERVIEW

Mood Disorder and Lithium

- Disorders of mood include mania and depression, as well as cyclothymic and systhymic disorders.

- A diagnosis of bipolar affective disorder is made when an individual has had at least one manic episode; a diagnosis of unipolar disorder is made when an individual has had depressive episodes but never a manic episode.

- Two types of medication are currently being used to treat mood disorders: lithium preparations and anticonvulsants.

- Lithium is often preferred over antipsychotics to treat mania because improvement is achieved without the sedating effect noted with antipsychotic drugs.

- Because lithium takes 7 to 10 days at therapeutic blood levels to have any effect, antipsychotic agents may be used for severe manic states to bring about more immediate sedation and the control of symptoms.

- The dosage of lithium must be adjusted carefully and slowly when treatment is begun, and any significant change in a patient's level of activity should be followed by lithium level monitoring.

- Early symptoms of lithium toxicity include nausea, vomiting, diarrhea, abdominal pain, and general malaise. Among the severe symptoms of serious toxicity are somnolence, confusion, motor restlessness, disturbed behavior, ataxia, incoordination, dysarthria, stupor, and coma.

- Side effects of lithium may occur in the kidney and thyroid gland; tremors, weight gain, and dermatologic problems may also be seen.

- Because lithium has a very narrow therapeutic index and due to the consequences of its buildup, a major nursing responsibility is monitoring lithium blood levels; dosage levels of lithium do not determine its clinical effect.

ANTICONVULSANTS AS A TREATMENT FOR MOOD INSTABILITY

Since the early 1980s, anticonvulsants have been used in the treatment of affective disorders. Though not all of the anticonvulsants have been found to be efficacious, carbamazepine (Tegretol) and valproic acid (Depakene) have shown significant results. These drugs had previously been used primarily in the treatment of neuropsychiatric disorders, especially temporal lobe epilepsy (TLE), in which a large component of the illness manifests itself in behavior problems (Ballenger and Post, 1980).

More frequently, anticonvulsants are being used to treat affective disorders either as a single treatment or in conjunction with lithium. Studies have shown a 50% success rate in treating individuals whose illness appears to be refractory to lithium (Dalby, 1986). The literature that addresses the use of the anticonvulsants in the treatment of affective disorders does not indicate that these patients had electroencephalographic (EEG) abnormalities, although in some patients, nonspecific wave abnormalities were noted. Both manic and depressive symptoms have improved with therapeutic levels of carbamazepine. Valproic acid has been used primarily in the treatment of mania. These drugs represent a primary drug treatment for affective disorder, and they are often given in conjunction with lithium, neuroleptics, or both.

Action

The neurophysiologic action of these drugs is not known. As a result of their use in TLE and what seems to be behavioral improvement in all patients who have taken these medications, however, it is believed that the drugs induce alterations in the limbic system, which is responsible for thought and perception.

Early investigations into the action of carbamazepine focused on its ability to inhibit the kindling effect. Kindling is a process in which convulsive episodes occur in response to repeated stimulation. The ability of carbamazepine to inhibit this effect is thought to be related to its therapeutic effect (Bernstein, 1988; Post et al., 1982). Valproic acid is believed to increase levels of gamma aminobutyric acid, (GABA), blocking convulsive effects of the GABA antagonists (Arana and Hyman, 1991).

Dosage

Like lithium, the dosage of carbamazepine and valproic acid are based on blood level. The therapeutic range for carbamazepine is 4 to 12 μg/mL and valproic acid 50 to 100 μg/mL.

Of note is that with carbamazepine, when given in conjunction with antipsychotic drugs, increased metabolism occurs. The individual may experience a resurgence of psychotic symptoms. This is due to the fact that anticonvulsants induce liver metabolism; hence, both drugs (neuroleptic and anticonvulsant) are metabolized and excreted more rapidly, leading to a decline in blood levels of the antipsychotic, as well as the anticonvulsant drug.

Side Effects

Common side effects include nausea, vomiting, dizziness, ataxia, clumsiness, drowsiness, slurred speech, and diplopia. They frequently occur early in treatment. Once the liver has begun metabolizing the drug, the symptoms usually disappear. If they continue, a blood level evaluation should be obtained, and the dosage should be lowered, followed by a slower increase in

dosage if indicated. These effects have been noted both with carbamazepine and valproic acid.

Other more serious effects have been noted with the administration of both drugs. Incidents of heart block have been noted during treatment with carbamazepine, therefore, baseline ECGs should be taken. Routine white blood counts (WBC) should be drawn throughout treatment with carbamazepine because decreased WBC in all indices have been noted. Pruritus and exfoliative dermatitis have also been reported. These extreme side effects are not common. Hepatotoxicity has been noted with valproic acid, usually early on in treatment and with high doses. Lower dosages are indicated if these symptoms occur. Finally, valproic acid rarely causes platelet problems resulting in decreases in bleeding time.

Nursing Management of Patients Taking Anticonvulsant Drugs

Table 42–9 (on pages 774–775) indicates various drug interactions with anticonvulsants. In general, baseline complete blood counts with differential, ECG, and a careful history regarding hepatic and renal function should be completed before beginning a trial of carbamazepine or valproic acid. Levels should be adjusted upward carefully to avoid initial side effects. Patients should be observed carefully for colds, fevers, and flu-like symptoms due to potential hematologic effects. These drugs should not be administered to individuals within 2 weeks of receiving MAO inhibitors.

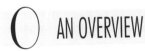 **AN OVERVIEW**

Anticonvulsants

- Although anticonvulsants are not a first choice for the treatment of affective disorders, they should be seriously considered for patients whose illness is refractory to lithium treatment or patients who previously required long-term prophylaxis with neuroleptics.

- Current literature indicates treatment with carbamazepine and valproic acid can be extremely fruitful when patients are monitored carefully.

- Clonazepam, which is a benzodiazepine, has been used recently to treat manic disorders. The results have varied, but at doses of 0.5 to 4.0 mg/day, control of manic symptoms has been achieved.

- Clonazepam is most often used as an adjunctive treatment during acute episodes.

- Clonazepam is tolerance producing and has the potential for addiction. It should not be the drug of choice in managing acute manic symptoms or in the long-term management of bipolar disorder.

■ ANTIDEPRESSANT DRUGS

IDENTIFYING DEPRESSION

It is important that the nurse be familiar with the symptoms of depression (Chapter 20) in order to evaluate the appropriate drug treatment. As a mood disorder, depressive states can be classified under many different headings: (1) bipolar disorder, depressed, (2) major depressive disorders, (3) dysthymic disorders, (4) bereavement and adjustment disorders with depressed mood, and (5) mood disorder due to a general medical condition or secondary to substance abuse.

BIPOLAR DISORDER, DEPRESSED

Bipolar affective disorders are those depressive states that are associated with a prior history of mania or clear hypomania. Bipolar disorders are discussed in connection with the use of lithium and other mood stabilizers earlier in this chapter. Here, the important distinction is that bipolar depression is treated with antidepressants and a mood stabilizer (e.g., with imipramine and lithium). The similarities are that the depressive symptoms observed in bipolar depression are similar to those seen in unipolar depression, although classic atypical symptoms tend to predominate (e.g., excess sleep, increased appetite, and fatigue). Also, like major depression, bipolar disorder is recurrent, with mood cycles of mania, depression, or mixed states. While treatment of bipolar affective disorders with antidepressants is often effective, the potential exists for the development of mania secondary to pharmacotherapy.

MAJOR DEPRESSIVE DISORDERS

The depressive disorders are divided into major depressive states (single-episode or chronic), and all antidepressants have been shown to be equally effective. Research is presently being conducted on milder forms of depression, such as dysthymia, and chronic depressive states. While a previous set of studies has demonstrated some effectiveness for the tricyclics in the treatment of dysthymia, recent case reports and popular books have suggested that the serotonin re-uptake inhibitors (e.g., fluoxetine [Prozac]) may have some utility. Studies on the long-term use of antidepressants in the maintenance of remission and prevention of future depressive states have found that, particularly in those with more treatment-resistant forms of major depression, long-term treatment is generally more successful (Schatzberg and Nemeroff, 1995).

Episodes of major depressive or unipolar states are marked by a dysphoric mood or loss of interest or plea-

sure in all or almost all usual activities and pastimes (DSM-IV, 1994). There is sleep- and appetite-pattern disruption along with symptoms of loss of energy, fatigability, and tiredness. There can be psychomotor retardation or agitation, decrease in sexual drive, feelings of self-reproach, difficulty in concentrating, and suicidal ideation. A person suffering from these symptoms for at least 2 weeks will be diagnosed with major depression and is likely to receive an antidepressant trial. Although no laboratory tests exist to diagnose the presence of major depression, abnormalities in sleep and neuroendocrine changes have been associated with the development of major depression.

For some, the depressive symptoms will have remained moderate to severe and persisted for years. Chronic major depressions are those episodes that meet the criteria for major depression, yet the person continues to suffer from symptoms for years without relief. Treatment-resistant depressions are those chronic depressions that persist long term, despite several adequate treatment trials, including several pharmacologic agents. Persons with treatment-resistant depressions generally will go on to be treated with less commonly prescribed medications (MAO inhibitors, stimulant medications), electroconvulsive therapy, or various augmentation strategies (e.g., thyroid, lithium, or combinations of antidepressants), to attempt to resolve the symptoms of depression.

Major depressive episodes may frequently coexist with many other psychiatric or medical disorders. Previously, persons with personality disorders were thought to suffer from characterological depressions. A characterological manifestation of depression is chronic and includes unhappiness, dissatisfaction, weeping, preoccupation with losses or unpleasantness, and feeling short-changed. They may evidence dramatic attention-seeking behavior; avoid personal blame; act in a manner that is demanding, complaining, clinging, irritable, and anxious; and be full of self-pity. These behaviors are not restricted to a particular personality profile, and in and of themselves may be responsive to various pharmacological treatment. Nonetheless, someone with a personality disorder may also be diagnosed with major depression and receive appropriate pharmacotherapy for depressive symptoms.

Similarly, persons with anxiety disorders (including post-traumatic stress disorder), substance or medical conditions, or other major psychiatric disorders (including schizophrenia) may also develop a major depression. In general, substantial comorbidity often exists with people who have major psychiatric disorders. For example, schizophrenia is not a protection against depression, and, at times, antidepressants combined with antipsychotic drugs can be helpful. In the early stages of schizophrenia, depression may occur. In this

TABLE 42–9. INTERACTIONS BETWEEN PSYCHOTROPIC AND OTHER DRUGS

Drug	Clinically Significant Interactions With	Clinical Effect of Interaction	Drug	Clinically Significant Interactions With	Clinical Effect of Interaction
Neuroleptics	Anticholinergics	Increased anticholinergic effect (particularly clozapine)		Quinidine	Cardiac conduction prolonged
	Antacids	Oral absorption delayed		Procainamide	
	Lithium	May increase CNS toxicity		Coumarin anticoagulants	Increased bleeding
	Phenytoin	May increase phenytoin toxicity		Neuroleptics	Increased tricyclic levels
		Decreased plasma levels and effect of neuroleptics		Anticonvulsants	Induces hepatic metabolism, decreasing clinical effect of antidepressants
	Tobacco	Lowered neuroleptic levels		CNS depressants	Additive cardiotoxicity possible
	Narcotics	Increased sedation		Anticholinergic drugs	Increased anticholinergic toxicity
		Analgesia augmented		Thyroid supplements	Tachycardia, arrhythmia
		Hypotension augmented		Lithium	Potentiation of antidepressant effect
		Respiratory depression augmented		Epinephrine	Hypotension augmented
		Anticholinergic effects augmented by mepenidine		Benzodiazepines	Increased CNS sedation, increased confusion, decreased motor functions
	Benzodiazepines	Increased CNS sedation		Neuroleptics	Increased sedation
		Possible severe orthostatic hypotension			Increased hypotension
	Cyclic antidepressants	Increased sedation			Increased anticholinergic effect
		Increased hypotension			Possible increased risk of seizures
		Increased anticholinergic effect		L-dopa	Delayed or decreased absorption of L-dopa
		Possible increased risk of seizures		Alcohol	Increased sedation
	L-dopa	May exacerbate psychosis		Tobacco	Increased metabolism of tricyclics
		Decreased anti-Parkinsonian effect of L-dopa	MAO inhibitors	Amphetamines	Increased blood pressure
	Amphetamines	May exacerbate psychosis		Ephedrine	
	CNS active drugs	Additive effects on CNS		Metaraminol	
	Isoniazid	Hepatic toxicity and encephalopathy		Levarterenol	
		Decreased neuroleptic effect		Methylphenidate	
	Antihypertensives	Increased hypotensive effect		Phenylephrine	
		May decrease antihypertensive effect		Pseudoephedrine	
	Anticonvulsants	Decreased antipsychotic effect		L-dopa	
		Increased clozapine levels (Valproate)		Methyldopa	
		Agranulocytosis on clozapine		Benzodiazepines	
	Bromocriptine	Decreased efficacy of phenothiazines		Dopamine	
	Methyldopa	Increased sedation		Novacain (dissolved in epinephrine)	
		Increased psychiatric symptoms		Tricyclic antidepressants	May have enhanced clinical effect
	Epinephrine	Hypotensive augmented			Conflicting reports on toxicity hyperpyrexia, excitability, muscle rigidity, convulsions, coma. Use with caution
	Alcohol	Sedation			Weight gain
Tricyclic Antidepressants	Cimetidine	Increased tricyclic levels, toxicity		Serotonin re-uptake inhibitors (scrotonergic agents)	Serotonin syndrome (ataxia, nystagmus, confusion, fever, tremor)
	Methylphenidate			Buspirone	
	Acetaminophen			Meperidine	Excitation, sweating, hypotension. Use other narcotics; can be life threatening
	Oral contraceptives				
	Chloramphenicol				
	MAO inhibitors			Succinylcholine	Phenelzine may prolong apnea with ECT
	Disulfiram	Inhibits metabolism, increasing blood levels of antidepressants		General anesthetics	May enhance CNS depression
		Possible induction of psychosis and confusional state		Insulin	Increased hypoglycemic effect
	Guanethidme	Decreased antihypertensive effect		Thiazide diuretics	Increased hypotension
	Clonidine	Decreased antihypertensive and antidepressant effect			
	Thiazide diuretics	Hypotension augmented			

Drug	Clinically Significant Interactions With	Clinical Effect of Interaction
	Guanethidine	Decreased antihypertensive effect
	Alcohol	Decreased MAO inhibition
		CNS system depression (wine and beer may cause hypertensive reactions)
Serotonergic antidepressants (SSRIs)	MAO inhibitors	Serotonergic syndrome, hypertensive crisis
	Tricyclic antidepressants	Increased tricyclic levels, tricyclic toxicity
	Carbamazepine	Increased carbamazepine levels
	Neuroleptics	Increased neuroleptic levels
	CNS active drugs	Interactions not established. Use with caution
		Cumulative effects
	Lithium	Increased lithium levels
		Partial serotonergic syndrome
	Buspirone	Partial serotonergic syndrome
	Alcohol	Possible potentiation
	Digoxin	Possible decrease in digoxin levels (paroxetine)
	Cimetidine	Increased SSRI concentration
	Warfarin	Tendency for increased bleeding
	Diazepam	Increased diazepam concentrations
	Alprazolarn	Increased levels with nefazodone
	Halcion	
	Terfenazine	
Lithium	Indomethacin	Increased lithium effect and toxicity
	Piroxicam	
	Ibuprofen	
	Phenylbutazone	
	Naproxen	
	Thiazide diuretics	Increased lithium effect and toxicity
	Spironolactone	
	Triamterene	
	Amiloride	
	Neuroleptics	Decreased nausea and vomiting from lithium
		Increased neurotoxicity (may be severe)
	Phenytoin drugs	May increase neurotoxicity of both
	Theophylline	Increased renal excretion of lithium, decreasing its effect
	Acetazolamide	
	Aminophylline	
	Succinylcholine	Prolonged apnea with ECT
	Sodium bicarbonate	Increased renal excretion of lithium, decreasing its effect
	Sodium chloride	
	Urea	
	Mannitol	
	Antiarrythmics	May potentiate cardiac conduction effects
	Calcium channel blockers	May raise or lower lithium levels

Drug	Clinically Significant Interactions With	Clinical Effect of Interaction
	Tetracycline	Increased lithium effect and toxicity due to decreased renal lithium clearance
	Spectinomycin	
	Carbamazepine	Increased neurotoxicity
	Digitalis	May cause cardiac arrhythmia by depleting intracellular potassium
Anticonvulsants (carbamazepine, CBZ; valproate, VA)	Lithium	Neurotoxicity with carbamazepine
	Neuroleptics	May decrease levels of both CBZ and neuroleptic
	Cimetidine	Increased CBZ and VA levels
	Fluoxetine	Increased carbamazepine levels, possibly to toxic levels
	Verapamil	
	Propoxyphene	
	Erythromycin and other antibiotics	
	Other anticonvulsants	Decreased levels of both drugs
	Quinidine	Decreased levels of drugs by CBZ
	Warfarin	
	Propranolol	
	Clonazepam	
	Anticoagulants	
	Oral contraceptives	
	Theophylline	
	Isoniazid	Increased effects of CBZ
	Benzodiazepines	Increased levels and effects by VA
	Tricyclic antidepressants	Serum levels increased by VA and decreased by CBZ
	Salicylates	Increased VA levels
	MAO inhibitors	Increased MAOI effects by VA
Benzodiazepines	CNS depressants	CNS depression
	Alcohol	
	Neuroleptics	
	Antihistamines	
	Anticholinergics	
	Cimetidine	Increased benzodiazepine levels
	Disulfiram	
	Isoniazid	
	Valproate acid	Increased effects of diazepam and decreased effects of alprazolam
	Amitriptyline	Potentiation of CNS effects
	Phenytoin	Increased phenytoin serum levels, risk of toxicity
	Antacids	Delay in oral absorption
	Digoxin	Increased digoxin levels
	L-dopa	Possible decreased effect of L-dopa
	Tobacco, caffeine	Decreased benzodiazepine effects
	Neuromuscular blocking agents	Increased respiratory depression
	Nefazodone	Increased levels of some benzodiazepines

775

case, treatment with antidepressants alone is usually not helpful and, in some instances, may precipitate or aggravate psychotic symptoms.

MOOD DISORDERS SECONDARY TO MEDICAL CONDITIONS OR SUBSTANCE ABUSE

If the depressed mood is thought to be a direct consequence of a major medical problem, then the most appropriate diagnosis is mood disorder due to a general medical condition. The health and medical assessment is the clinician's main tool for making and distinguishing this diagnosis from major depression. In contrast, if the depression is thought to be a psychological sequela from the medical condition, then the diagnosis made is major depression. Antidepressant treatment would then generally be considered in the latter condition, but the underlying medical problem should be corrected in the former to resolve the depressive symptoms.

In persons who abuse drugs or alcohol, the presence of depressed or anxious mood is often evident. Determining when the onset of mood and other vegetative symptoms occurred (e.g., prior to, concurrently, or upon withdrawal), is often difficult to assess. If possible, when the substance is thought to be the reason for the symptoms (e.g., alcohol withdrawal), then the diagnosis shifts to substance-induced mood disorder. Conversely, if the history and evaluation reveal clear present and past depressive symptoms, then a major depressive episode is diagnosed (DSM IV, 1994).

Dysthymia

In chronic depressive disorders, the individual has at least a 2-year history of a depressive syndrome, although the degree is not sufficient to call it severe. Once called depressive neurosis, dysthymia is relatively common and rarely leads to hospitalization. The ongoing quality of the person's life and ability to live to their full potential, however, is impaired. During this 2-year span, persons with dysthymia have at least two symptoms of depression, including appetite or sleep disruption, poor energy, low self-esteem, hopelessness, and difficulty with concentration. When the person has more symptoms of depression, they generally are diagnosed with major depression, and with chronic major depression, if they have been in a long-standing, more severe state. For dysthymia, antidepressants are increasingly being used to treat these depressive, mild symptoms, in part to prevent worsening and to help people improve their overall social and occupational functioning and level of happiness.

Situational Depressive States

Situational depressive states are marked by a clear precipitant. Classified as adjustment reactions with depressed mood, the individual manifests signs of depression and sadness. This is generally in response to a clear psychosocial stressor (job loss, divorce, etc.). Adjustment disorder with depressed mood may include some of the symptoms of major depression, but the person's symptoms fail to meet full criteria for the major depression. When these states are grief reactions associated with the death of an important person, they are classified as bereavement reactions, even though all of the criteria for major depression may be met. In both states, symptoms can include tearfulness, brooding, preoccupation with the loss, feelings of tension, inability to shift one's thoughts from the loss or situation, loss of appetite, and insomnia. Usually depressions of this type are self-limiting, but on occasion they can become symptomatic of a major depression and require more intensive treatment with antidepressants as one strategy. Psychotherapy and self-help groups are usually the main treatment to help the person through the immediate crisis or loss and to develop new or strengthen existing coping mechanisms.

Theoretical views of the etiology of depression include the following models:

- Loss and lowered self-esteem.
- Early deprivation.
- Psychoanalytic deficit.
- Cognitive set, disordered thinking.
- Learned behaviors: modeling, or gain-reinforcement.
- Biochemical amine.

Whatever the possible etiology of depression, the outstanding characteristic in depressive states is a lowering of self-esteem. This lowered self-esteem may be understood by a person as depression, or it may be experienced as simply not feeling oneself, being tired and irritable, or as not being functional in work or play with family or friends. Sometimes, particularly in the elderly, the person may simply complain of feeling physically ill.

ANTIDEPRESSANT DRUG ACTION

Antidepressant medications (Table 42–10) are traditionally used for the treatment of depression and related disorders, although recent advances have documented their actual or potential efficacy in anxiety, eating, and personality disorders, along with certain medical disorders (i.e., chronic pain, migraine headaches, or fibromyalgia). Antidepressants are indicated for the treatment of major depression, bipolar depression, dysthymic disorder, and depression associated with organic conditions, alcoholism, schizophrenia, or mental retardation. Emerging uses for these medications include panic disorder, obsessive-compulsive disorder, eating disorders, borderline personality disorder, and post-traumatic stress disorder.

TABLE 42–10. ANTIDEPRESSANT DRUGS

Class	Generic (Trade) Names	Daily Dosage
Tricyclic antidepressants (TCAs)	Amitriptyline (Elavil)	75 to 300 mg
	Clomipramine (Anafranil)	100 to 250 mg[a]
	Desipramine (Norpramin)	75 to 300 mg
	Doxepin (Sinequan)	50 to 300 mg
	Imipramine (Tofranil)	75 to 300 mg
	Nortriptyline (Pamelor)	75 to 150 mg
	Protriptyline (Vivactil)	15 to 60 mg
	Trimipramine (Surmontil)	75 to 300 mg
Monoamine oxidase inhibitors (MAOIs)	Isocarboxazid (Marplan)	20 to 40 mg
	Phenelzine (Nardil)	30 to 90 mg
	Tranylcypromine (Parnate)	10 to 60 mg
Serotonin re-uptake inhibitors (SSRIs)	Fluvoxamine (Luvox)	50 to 200 mg[a]
	Fluoxetine (Prozac)	10 to 80 mg
	Sertraline (Zoloft)	50 to 200 mg
	Paroxetine (Paxil)	10 to 50 mg
Miscellaneous antidepressants	Trazodone (Desyrel)	50 to 450 mg
	Bupropion (Wellbutrin)	150 to 450 mg[b]
	Venlafaxine (Effexor)	75 to 375 mg
	Nefazodone (Serzone)	200 to 600 mg
	Lithium carbonate (Lithane, Eskalith)	750 to 2,500 mg

a. Currently approved only for obsessive-compulsive disorder.
b. No single dose may exceed 150 mg.
Reproduced from Schatzberg and Nemeroff, 1995.

These medications increase the concentration of certain neurotransmitters acutely (within hours to days), primarily norepinephrine and serotonin. This is accomplished by blocking the re-uptake of these chemicals in the brain at the nerve synapse. One exception are the MAOIs (see below). The development of newer antidepressants has generally been to target certain chemicals selectively (e.g., serotonin). Although these effects are important, it appears that as a result of increased neurotransmitter levels, various other adaptive changes occur in the brain at pre- and post-synaptic parts of the neuron. In the end, it is unclear whether the neuron is actually "seeing" more or less of the neurotransmitter.

Monoamine Oxidase Inhibitors (MAOIs)

The MAO inhibitors have both peripheral and central neuronal action. The inhibition of MAO within the cell reduces the metabolism of endogenous amines (e.g., norepinephrine) and exogenous monoamines, thus increasing their concentration. Monoamine oxidase inhibitors also interact with amphetamine-like compounds, sympathomimetic amines, used in the treatment of allergies, and anticholinergic agents, used in the treatment of Parkinson's disease. Monoamine oxidase inhibitors may cause hypotension, as well as pro-

vide some relief from angina pectoris. They can also antagonize some of the pharmacological and biochemical effects of reserpine, used to treat hypertension. When used in conjunction with food containing tyramine or other restricted substances, they can cause severe hypertension and stroke.

Hypertensive Crisis. A hypertensive crisis, a severe and potentially life-threatening reaction, is characterized by a marked increase in blood pressure and is often accompanied by one or more of the following: severe occipital headache, neck pain or discomfort, sweating, and nausea and vomiting. The consequences may include stroke, coma, or death. Monoamine oxidase inhibitors have significant adrenergic effects, and MAO is responsible for destroying many substances within the body. When MAO is blocked, there is a buildup of these properties. This is why food intake becomes most important with these drugs. Foods that encourage the release of epinephrine and norepinephrine and foods that contain tyramine should be avoided, as well as sympathomimetic drugs. Foods high in tyramine content include aged cheeses, red wine, sherry or beer, fermented foods, smoked fish, preserved sausages, pickled herring, overripe fruits, and large amounts of soy sauce, yogurt, or caffeine. Many over-the-counter medications (e.g., cold preparations or diet pills) and prescribed drugs (Demerol, epinephrine, SSRIs) are contraindicated.

Selective Serotonin Re-uptake Inhibitors

For decades, the tricyclic antidepressants and MAO inhibitors were the only agents available for the treatment of depression. More recent development of medications has focused on the discovery of drugs that target one particular neurotransmitter; serotonin. Named the selective serotonin re-uptake inhibitors (SSRIs), these drugs primarily act at the nerve synapse acutely to block the process that allows the endogenous amine to be absorbed into the pre-synaptic neuron. The development of these and other, newer antidepressants has also moved away from the traditional uncomfortable side effects, such as the anticholinergic, sedating, and cardiac effects associated with the older agents. Thus, the SSRIs and newer medications fail to possess effects on those receptors associated with these potentially intolerable side effects (muscarinic, histaminic, and alpha-adrenergic receptors).

Other New Antidepressants

Another set of antidepressants are newer agents that do not comprise any one subgroup. These include trazodone, bupropion, venlafaxine, and nefazodone. They have varied effects on the pre- and post-synaptic norepinephrine and serotonin receptors, and they have little effect on cholinergic, histaminergic, and alpha-adrenergic receptors. As with any agent in this class, their efficacy in treating the symptoms of major depression remains equal to any other agent. Thus, while the SSRIs and newer agents may be more tolerable to many patients, no one medication is more effective than another.

A careful medical work-up is essential in the treatment of a depressed patient, as in all psychiatric states. This health baseline is necessary because of the possibility of pre-existing organic or metabolic reasons for the symptoms and because of the potential for side effects and adverse reactions. Once physical illness is ruled out, as are other possible toxic reactions, a decision can be made to use antidepressants. Special consideration must be given to how severe the depression is and how serious the suicidal threat is. A baseline of behavioral information is needed before a selection of a drug is made (e.g., symptom presentation and comorbidity). Although antidepressants do not differ in clinical efficacy, they do differ in their ability to cause side effects. Furthermore, if the person is suffering from a psychotic depression, which is a major depression with some paranoia, delusions, or hallucinations, both an antidepressant and antipsychotic medication will be needed. A history of previous positive or negative responses to a trial of psychiatric drugs in the patient or in the patient's immediate blood-related family is the main predictor of what will be a current effective treatment.

In addition to the treatment of depression, antidepressant drugs have provided an important model for understanding drug action in the brain in terms of neuroreceptor activity. These investigations have led to a movement toward understanding the biological basis of psychiatric disorders.

CATECHOLAMINE THEORY OF DEPRESSION

The early catecholamine theory of depression proposed by Shildkraut (1982) hypothesized that certain depressive states are caused by a depletion of catecholamines at receptor sites and that elation, or mania, is caused by catecholamines at receptor sites. This theory is quite complex and has been expanded to include not only catecholamines (dopamine), but also indolamine (serotonin), other biogenic amines (acetylcholine and GABA), hormones, and ionic changes. The depletion (or excess) can be caused by blocking reuptake, insufficient release of neurotransmitters, alterations of chemical affinity at the receptor, excessive metabolic breakdown at the synaptic cleft, or failures in the metabolic processes within the pre-synaptic neuron. These include an excess of MAO within the presynaptic cell of norepinephrine, which is hypothesized to lead to increased breakdown of neurotransmitters.

The receptor theory demonstrated by the catecholamine hypothesis has suggested four different neuroregulators functioning in the brain. They are the noradrenergic synapse, the dopaminergic synapse, the serotoninergic synapse, and the gabaminergic synapse. Depressive states have been linked primarily with receptor site excesses and depletions of norepinephrine (noradrenergic), dopamine (dopaminergic), and serotonin (serotoninergic). Neurons emanating from the spinal cord Pi and cranial nerves and nerves innervating peripheral organs transmit widely to various regions.

Tricyclic antidepressants are structurally related to phenothiazines and have similar side effects. In contrast to the phenothiazines, which act in dopamine receptors, the tricyclic antidepressants and venlafaxine block the re-uptake of norepinephrine and serotonin by the pre-synaptic neurons in the CNS. In contrast, the SSRIs block the reabsorption of serotonin to differing degrees, and bupropion blocks re-uptake. Since re-uptake terminates amine activity, inhibition of re-uptake enhances activity at the receptor site. These effects appear to play a role in the antidepressant activity of these agents.

Current thinking underscores that a cogent theory of depression must integrate various levels of observations. Observations need to be made at the chemical, anatomic, and behavioral levels. Even with regard to chemical considerations, although changes in monoamines may be significant, a variety of relationships among the parts of the central nervous system and their unique physiology must be considered.

DOSAGE CONSIDERATIONS AND CLINICAL TREATMENT OF DEPRESSION

Agents that are employed in the clinical treatment of depression are tricyclics, MAO inhibitors, SSRIs, and a number of new miscellaneous agents (Table 42–9). These agents have demonstrated effectiveness in the treatment of major depression and bipolar depression, with emerging evidence for treatment of dysthymic disorder. Although the exact mechanism of the antidepressant effect has not been identified, effective activity has usually been associated with the "biogenic amine hypothesis." It is felt that the antidepressant agents favorably affect the dysfunctional activities of the monoamines, thereby normalizing their biogenic activity. This theory does not totally explain the antidepressant activity of all compounds, and other, as yet unfound, mechanisms may play a part in their activity.

Recent trends have shown that the SSRIs and newer agents (miscellaneous agents) are the most widely prescribed antidepressants. This is primarily due to the different side effect profiles that these agents possess. This does not imply that these medications are without any adverse reactions. Another advantage to the SSRIs and newer antidepressants is their relative safety from overdose compared with tricyclic antidepressants and MAO inhibitors. Thus, the first line of medication treatment for the patient with major depression is likely to be one of the newer agents.

In the situation where a person fails to respond adequately, the next choice may be a different SSRI, one of the newer agents, a tricyclic antidepressant, or the addition of another agent (e.g., lithium, thyroid medication, or another low-dose antidepressant) to augment the action of the drug. For patients who are treatment resistant and have failed several antidepressant trials, MAO inhibitors or electroconvulsive therapy (ECT) may be used. Because of the potential high risk of hypertensive crisis when certain foods and drugs are combined with them, MAO inhibitors are generally not used as the initial treatment.

If drugs do not work or if there are severe cardiac problems or other endangering physical disorders, the safest and most effective intervention for depression is ECT. This method is useful in the elderly and has become increasingly safe with the use of proper relaxant drugs and adequate control over voltage and recovery. If ECT is used, however, the individual needs to be withdrawn from most antidepressant medications.

When initiating the dosage of most antidepressants, the objective is to move slowly to a dose that can be tolerated by the patient. Usually doses are given in the morning for drugs that tend to lead to insomnia and in the evening for drugs that tend to have sedative effects. It is useful to arrange an increase so that a single dose can be administered; however, some antidepressants require multiple dosing (bupropion, venlafaxine, and nefazodone). Doses of bupropion, because of the risk of developing seizures, may not exceed 150 mg at any given time. Thus, most patients taking bupropion generally receive tid doses. Venlafaxine has a relatively short half-life, and therefore, is given bid to tid, depending on the daily dose. Similarly, nefazodone is usually given in bid doses.

Assessments and tests help determine and monitor antidepressant intervention. A careful review is necessary of other medications being used by the patient. To guard against suicide, there must be a cooperative and safe interpersonal context in which to start drug intervention. Overdose can be fatal. The physical examination should include an ECG to check for both ventricular arrhythmias and evidence of cardiac abnormalities, tonometry to check for glaucoma (for tricyclics), assessment for prostatic disease in men, tests for thyroid disease, and comprehensive blood work.

Once medical clearance is given, a schedule of medication must be drawn up with gradually incremented doses. This is particularly true when starting patients on drugs that have moderate to very high anticholinergic effects.

Usually, the first approach for initiating tricyclics has been to start out with 25 mg at bedtime and 25-mg increments every day or every few days, depending on how the patient tolerates the medication, until the maximum dose has been reached. It will take approximately 2 to 3 weeks, once the maximum dose has been reached, to achieve drug effect. It is this time lag that is dangerous with the depressed and suicidal patients. For the SSRIs, an initial dose of 10 to 20 mg in the morning is common for fluoxetine, 25 to 50 mg for sertraline, and 10 to 20 mg for paroxetine, with weekly increases. For bupropion, the person is generally started at 75 mg once or twice daily, with increases of 75 mg every day or every few days, until either the symptoms resolve or the maximum dose is attained. No single dose may exceed 150 mg for bupropion. For venlafaxine, the common starting dose is 37.5 mg once or twice daily with increases of 37.5 every few days, until the maximum dose is achieved. Nefazodone is generally begun at 50 mg bid and increased by 50 mg to the maximum dose.

The SSRIs are generally prescribed once daily, in the morning. Dosage increases may occur every week to 2 weeks, particularly for fluoxetine, which has a long half-life. This also has substantial implications for drug interactions and discontinuation, as the medication will remain in the person's system for weeks, if they have been taking it consistently.

■ NURSING MANAGEMENT OF PATIENTS TAKING ANTIDEPRESSANT DRUGS

NURSING INTERVENTIONS WITH TREATMENT: EMERGENT SIDE EFFECTS

Beginning Treatment

Cardiovascular symptoms, such as postural hypotension, dizziness, tachycardia, and palpitations, are usual in the beginning of the use of tricyclics and MAOIs. Teaching the patient to avoid sudden movements helps deal with these symptoms. Any cardiac symptom or ankle edema must be evaluated immediately. If the patient is under 60 years of age, the following steps are recommended:

1. Take a baseline blood pressure before medication and 1 hour later.
2. Have the patient lie down to measure blood pressure.
3. Repeat with the patient standing up after waiting 2 minutes.

If the systolic pressure drops 30 mm Hg or more or the diastolic drops 20 mm Hg or more, postural hypotension is present, and the doctor should be consulted as to whether to start the drug or not. Blood pressure must be checked weekly for tricyclics, MAO inhibitors, and venlafaxine until stabilization.

Gastrointestinal system symptoms can include nausea and heartburn. Symptomatic treatment and taking drugs after meals may reduce symptoms. Increased appetite and weight gain are important side effects that need early intervention. Frequent monitoring of weight and helping the patient begin an exercise and dieting program are essential nursing interventions. Monitoring of weight is also necessary to determine any significant weight loss. Offering a stool softener and milk of magnesia for the patient with constipation can help the patient cope with these symptoms.

Internal anxiety and akathisia are side effects that are generally difficult for the patient to tolerate. Helping the patient identify and distinguish between these two states is an important nursing intervention. Akathisia is a physical restlessness, characterized by increased motoric movements (e.g., leg shaking or pacing) and the need to keep moving. Other suggestions include offering prn antianxiety medication (e.g., lorazepam) or beta blocker (for akathisia).

It is also important to discuss with the patient their baseline sexual functioning and to assess the nature and severity of any sexual dysfunction (e.g., decreased libido, impotence or lack of orgasm, or decreased performance). Discuss with the prescribing clinician the possibility of pharmacological treatment or the need to consider alternative antidepressants if sexual dysfunction has arisen due to medication.

If insomnia arises, suggest that the medication be ordered and taken in morning doses. If daytime sedation occurs, however, suggest that the medication be given in a nighttime dose. It is also helpful to distinguish whether these effects are related to the medication or may be a worsening symptom of the person's illness. Other nursing interventions include instructing the patient about the importance of good sleep hygiene, which includes regular sleep and rising times, nighttime rituals, and not remaining awake in bed for longer than 30 minutes. Prn medication (e.g., sedative or hypnotic, trazodone) may be necessary for persistent insomnia.

For the patient who describes headaches, first assess the frequency, quality, and severity of symptoms. Frequently depressed patients have somatic complaints as part of their symptom presentation. Offer prn medication (e.g., Tylenol). For hand tremor, assess the degree of interference with writing or other tasks, and notify prescriber if severe (may require treatment with a low-dose beta-blocker).

Dermatologic symptoms may arise with any of these medications and may include the uncommon side effect of a rash. Photosensitivity requires the use of protective clothing and care when exposed to the sun.

The possibility exists that the person treated with an antidepressant may develop symptoms of mania. This serious condition is oftentimes not recognized by the patient because of feelings of euphoria and increased energy. Patients and their families should be instructed about the development of mania, even if no previous episodes have occurred. Antidepressants have the ability to induce symptoms of extreme euphoria, decreased sleep, increased energy, and other symptoms of a manic state. In addition, patients should notify their prescriber if suicidal ideation emerges or worsens. Rare reports of antidepressant-induced suicidal ideation suggest that this may indicate a serious adverse reaction or worsening of an underlying depression (Teicher et al., 1993). For both situations, dose adjustment or discontinuation may be necessary.

Overdose is a serious problem with tricyclics, MAO inhibitors, and bupropion, and depressed patients should not be given large amounts of their prescription because of the possibility of overdose. With most antidepressants, particularly the tricyclics, special precaution must be used with patients with urinary retention, narrow-angle glaucoma, or signs of increased ocular pressure. Cardiovascular disorders and diseases of the thyroid, liver, and prostate are other conditions in which special care must be taken for those who are prescribed antidepressants. Patients with convulsive disorders and organic brain syndrome must be monitored carefully.

The safe use of any antidepressant medication with pregnant or lactating women has not yet been established. When a patient has been on the drug for 2 months or more, withdrawal should be made slowly.

Assessment of Side Effects

A major role for the psychiatric nurse is the assessment of side effects that develop as a consequence of treatment. Although newer antidepressants have been developed with the expectation that their side effects and toxicity will be less than that of the tricyclics and MAO inhibitors, nursing activities, as well as medical practices, are most important. The heterocyclics and the MAO inhibitors, compared to antipsychotic drugs, have a higher incidence of severe anticholinergic and adrenergic effects on the body systems. The newer agents and SSRIs may lead to substantial anxiety, agitation, or insomnia, which can be very disruptive to the person's daily functioning. These reactions can be serious; therefore, it is imperative that a physical examination be carried out before prescribing a drug. A differential diagnosis is required regarding the type of depression, since underlying bipolar and schizophrenic states can be exacerbated. Table 42–11 lists the major side effects related to three major classes of antidepressants, while the side effects of specific recent medications follow.

Trazodone (Desyrel) causes sedation, headache, dizziness, and priapism. Priapism, a sustained erection, is an emergency. If it is not treated successfully, it may result in irreversible impotence. Notify the patient of the possibility of sustained erections and that he must alert staff if this occurs. The immediate intervention is to withhold the medication dosage and notify the prescriber immediately. Because dizziness may occur, administer the medication on a full stomach to attempt to minimize this effect. Trazodone, in low doses (50 to 100 mg), may sometimes be used to treat insomnia related to depression, or insomnia as a consequence of medication treatment.

Bupropion (Wellbutrin) may cause nausea, anorexia, or weight loss; agitation or anxiety; insomnia; or the induction of seizures. This medication is contraindicated in persons with eating and seizure disorders and should be used cautiously in those with head injuries. Bupropion should be administered in doses of 150 mg or less, at intervals of at least 4 hours, to minimize the risk of seizures.

Venlafaxine (Effexor) may cause nausea, anorexia, or weight loss; agitation or anxiety; insomnia; or a slight increases in blood pressure.

Nefazodone (Serzone) side effects include nausea, anorexia, or weight loss; agitation or anxiety; and sedation.

Since treatment will usually extend over a period of years, the medical examination should be repeated every 6 months on people over 60 and at least once a year for those who are younger. Persons with a moderate depression who are suffering from symptoms for the first time should be asymptomatic for at least 6 to 9 months prior to discontinuation of medication. The majority of people with more severe depressions or chronic depressions will require long-term treatment or risk the possibility of a relapse. During discontinuation, the medication should be decreased cautiously, and the patient closely observed for increasing signs of depression.

Since antidepressants are often used with the elderly, certain precautions need to be taken. The elderly may respond to both therapeutic and adverse drug effects because of their slower metabolism and excretion rates. Thus, they need smaller doses and increments, and there is an increased possibility of drug interaction issues. Also, older people often take drugs for other rea-

TABLE 42–11. MAJOR SIDE EFFECTS OF SELECTED ANTIDEPRESSANT DRUGS

Antidepressant	Anticholinergic	Relative Side Effects Anxiety	Insomnia	Sedation
Tricyclic antidepressants (TCAs)				
Desipramine	Mild	Mild	Rare	Mild
Nortriptyline	Mild	Mild	Rare	Mild
Amitriptyline	Moderate	Rare	Mild	Moderate–severe
Imipramine	Mild	Mild	Mild	Moderate–severe
Clomipramine	Moderate	Moderate	Mild	Severe
Serotonin re-uptake inhibitors (SSRIs)				
Huoxetine	Rare	Moderate	Moderate	Mild*
Fluvoxamine	Rare	Moderate	Moderate	Mild*
Sertraline	Rare	Moderate	Moderate	Mild*
Paroxetine	Rare	Moderate	Moderate	Mild*
Atypical antidepressants				
Trazodone	Rare	Mild	Rare	Moderate–severe
Bupropion	Rare	Moderate	Moderate	Mild
Venlafaxine	Rare	Moderate	Moderate	Mild
Nefazodone	Rare	Mild	Rare	Moderate
MAO inhibitors				
Phenelzine	Mild	Mild	Moderate–severe	Moderate–severe
Tranylcypromine	Mild	Mild	Moderate	Moderate–severe

*Increased levels of sedation have been reported with higher doses.

Adapted from Teicher et al., 1993.

sons. Furthermore, anticholinergic drugs are to be avoided because confusion and arrhythmias are likely to occur in this population.

DETERMINING BLOOD LEVELS

Antidepressant drug levels are generally obtained only for those antidepressants that show a relationship between response to the drug and therapeutic level (desipramine, nortriptyline, imipramine). Blood levels of the newer antidepressant agents generally show no correlation to clinical improvement. Plasma levels are determined on a sample of blood drawn 10 to 14 hours after the last dose of the antidepressant. Determining plasma levels of antidepressant drugs will assist the clinician to

- Identify those patients who develop very high plasma levels on low doses.
- Document the therapeutic plasma level in an individual patient at the time of clinical response as a guide to treating future episodes.
- Document compliance or possible short-term metabolic changes in patients who respond and then relapse on a given dose.
- Explore causes for failure to respond to a standard dose of an antidepressant drug.
- Investigate possible causes for the occurrence of pronounced side effects of small drug doses.

Amitriptyline, nortriptyline, imipramine, desipramine, and doxepin have been evaluated with regard to plasma levels.

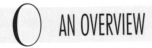

AN OVERVIEW

Antidepressant Drugs

- Antidepressant drugs are most useful in moderately to severely depressed patients, especially when management of suicidal potential is essential.
- Out-patients need to be monitored carefully and frequently to decrease the chances of lethal overdosage, particularly with the tricyclics and MAO inhibitors.
- For those patients who are suicidal, only 1 week's supply of antidepressants should be prescribed at a time.
- Decreasing the dosage or changing the drug may be suggested to the prescriber if any side effects become intolerable.

■ ANTIANXIETY AGENTS

IDENTIFYING ANXIETY DISORDERS

Like depression, anxiety is a human experience that touches everyone to a lesser or greater degree (Chapter 14). It is part of the human condition and is associated with change and stress. It is part of learning, play, joy, and adversity. As a state, it has subjective characteristics (of the person) as well as bodily responses to the tension. Most often we experience anxiety as an unpleasant uneasiness, tension, or apprehension. Bodily signs are extensive and, as such, require scrutiny as to more definitive reasons for the tension. For example, clinically thyrotoxicosis has signs and symptoms that parallel an anxiety state (including feeling jittery, keyed up, muscle tightness, palpitations, tremulousness, dread, and emotional lability, to name a few).

As in psychosis and depression, a framework for assessment is essential for understanding drug interventions. In general, anxiety that is severe (panic) and that may be associated with certain physical problems needs to be reduced. Antianxiety and antidepressant drugs are most important in the reduction of these states. It is essential to recognize the basis of the anxiety and address the causal factors. Antianxiety drugs are beneficial and their effectiveness is often immediate. They may reduce immediate aspects of anxiety, such as narrowed perception, disruption of thinking, and distracting muscular and autonomic symptoms of tension that interfere with the person's taking charge of his or her situation. In the case of anxiety associated with physical illness, reduction is essential so that more specific interventions can have a chance to work. For example, when an individual has a heart attack, fear associated with the attack and excitability over what is going on around the person do not permit the relaxation and rest necessary for the heart muscle to regain its equilibrium. Antianxiety drugs may prove useful at these critical times.

Recognizing the general characteristics of anxiety states and intervention, the following principles must be understood in assessing anxiety:

- Anxiety is an essential dimension of the human condition.
- Symptoms associated with anxiety can be understood as emanating from social or psychological events, somatic events, and psychological reactions to somatic or biological events.
- Anxiety of an intense nature generally is one symptom of a major psychiatric disorder. It must be reduced by some effective means because it is disruptive to rational thinking and problem solving.

- Treatment of anxiety disorders with medication may require long-term treatment in some persons. Other interventions, such as cognitive restructuring (changing thought patterns) and behavior therapy, are often necessary strategies to combine with pharmacotherapy. Frequently, both therapies are used and enhance the other's effectiveness. Psychotherapy is often useful for those persons suffering a major response to a major trauma. Understanding the nature and severity of anxiety can offer a framework for more enduring intervention.
- Continued use of drugs to manage anxiety continues to confront many health professionals with ethical considerations because these drugs can be abused and, in some cases, can lead to addiction.

ANXIOLYTICS

Antianxiety drugs are also called anxiolytics. With the development of newer compounds, however, antidepressants have also been demonstrated to be effective in the treatment of some anxiety disorders. Traditionally, benzodiazepines have been the mainstay of treatment for various anxiety disorders and are indicated for the treatment of panic disorder, generalized anxiety disorder, transient symptoms of anxiety, acute alcohol withdrawal, skeletal muscle spasms, seizure disorders, and for preoperative sedation.

Some of the antidepressant agents have also demonstrated efficacy for panic disorder and obsessive-compulsive disorder. Several tricyclic antidepressants (e.g., imipramine), monoamine oxidase inhibitors, and selected SSRIs are indicated for the treatment of panic disorder. Clomipramine, fluoxetine, paroxetine, and fluvoxamine have demonstrated efficacy in the treatment of obsessive-compulsive disorder. Dosages commonly used to treat anxiety disorders are listed in Table 42–12. For details about these medications see the section on antidepressant agents.

Sedative or hypnotic agents are generally used short term for the relief of insomnia. As needed, doses of sedatives or antianxiety agents are used to quell agitation emanating from a myriad of conditions or to control the symptoms of mania while awaiting the effects of the mood stabilizer.

Antianxiety drugs are beneficial in treating acute or chronic distress. The true usefulness of these agents depends, to a large degree, on the patient's general atti-

E CASE EXAMPLE

Young adults, such as Helen, age 27, present the type of situation in which severe depression can mask additional complex problems.

Helen had been seen at age 25 for short-term counseling because she had broken up with her boyfriend. Helen wanted short-term rather than long-term counseling. She did report that her father had been institutionalized years before for mental illness and that she had many issues regarding her family but did not want to deal with them. She did well in counseling. She found a new job and started dating, at which point she terminated the counseling.

Six months later she contacts the nurse, profoundly depressed. The precipitants are a request to get married and the stress of a new job. She is evaluated in a mental health clinic for drug intervention and possible hospitalization. She refuses to consider the latter. She has her boyfriend, mother, and brother as support, and everyone agrees they will help her at home.

She is started on a serotonin re-uptake inhibitor. She has changed jobs and is working as a service operator for an automobile towing service. Her depression lifts somewhat, but she begins to complain that she can not sleep well at night and is unable to perform sexually. Helen takes herself off the drug. By this time, her thinking process tends to be more concrete. She becomes suspicious and irritable, as well as frightened. With great difficulty, arrangements are made to admit her to the day hospital. While in the hospital and no longer on the drugs, although they are prescribed, she becomes much more aggressive, grandiose, and deluded. She leaves the hospital against medical advice but does agree to come to the clinic. One week later, she comes in, very excited, claiming that she is a borderline patient and hypomanic. She bolts from the room and goes to the streets. For the next week, the staff hear indirectly from her. Other clinics in the city hear from her as well. She is deluded, seeking help and treatment, and then rejecting the efforts. Eventually, she is placed on an antipsychotic drug and lithium.

In the initial drug evaluation, there was concern that Helen's personality was such that, although she did not have a prior history of psychosis or manic episodes, there was the possibility of an underlying bipolar disorder. This proved to be true.

The complexity of Helen's situation underscores how a working relationship is essential, given the possibility that underlying disorders are initially not apparent because of profound states of depression. If such disorders are exacerbated, the relationship becomes the important link to the management of a treatment change.

TABLE 42–12. ANTIANXIETY DRUGS AND ANTIDEPPESSANTS USED TO TREAT ANXIETY DISORDERS

Chemical Group	Generic (Trade) Names	Average Daily Dosage
Benzodiazepines	Alprazolam (Xanax)	0.75 to 6 mg
	Adnazolam	
	Chlordiazepoxide (Librium)	15 to 100 mg
	Clonazepam (Klonopin)	1 to 4 mg
	Diazepam (Valium)	5 to 40 mg
	Halazepam (Paxipam)	60 to 160 mg
	Lorazepam (Ativan)	2 to 6 mg
	Oxazepam (Serax)	30 to 120 mg
	Prazepam (Centrax)	10 to 60 mg
Nonbenzodiazepine anxiolytic	Buspirone (Buspar)	15 to 60 mg
Antidepressants	Fluoxetine (Prozac)	5 to 80 mg
	Sertraline (Zoloft)	25 to 200 mg
	Paroxetine (Paxil)	10 to 50 mg
	Fluvoxamine (Luvox)	50 to 200 mg
	!mipramine	50 to 300 mg
	Clomipramine	25 to 250 mg
	Phenelzine (Nardil)	30 to 90 mg

Adapted from Schatzberg, and Nemeroff, 1995.

tude toward the use of drugs. For obsessive-compulsive disorder, virtually no response is seen when patients are given placebo treatment, and the effectiveness of pharmacological treatment is only partial for some.

Choice of an Antianxiety Agent

In the choice of an antianxiety agent, the diagnoses of the patient are usually the deciding factor. Numerous benzodiazepines and antidepressant agents have therapeutic effects. These drugs, however, differ greatly in their levels of side effects, degree of dependence (psychological or physical), margin of safety, and interactions with other ongoing therapies. Benzodiazepines have hypnotic and muscle-relaxant qualities, and one in particular, clonazepam, possesses anticonvulsant properties. The benzodiazepines and SSRIs are far safer for the potentially suicidal patient than past medication regimens and clomipramine because of its wider margin of safety (e.g., toxic versus therapeutic dose). For the person with panic disorder who has a past or present history of substance or alcohol abuse, antidepressants are preferred because of benzodiazepine's addictive potential.

Antianxiety Drug Action

Antianxiety drugs act at all levels of the CNS, particularly in the limbic system and reticular formation. Benzodiazepines increase the effects of the powerful inhibitory neurotransmitter GABA in the brain, thereby producing a calming effect. In addition, in contrast to many other psychotropic medications, benzodiazepines work acutely to treat anxiety. All levels of CNS depression can be effective, from mild sedation to hypnosis to coma.

While GABA has been identified as a major neurotransmitter involved in the etiology of anxiety and anxiety disorders, the development of newer agents has suggested that the mechanism of action of anxiolytics is associated with other effects. Both buspirone and the benzodiazepines decrease the turnover of serotonin, another major neurotransmitter associated with the development of anxiety (Teicher, 1985). Similarly, antidepressants affect serotonin, and thus, serotoninergic neurotransmission may contribute to anxiety.

General Precautions and Contraindictions

Antianxiety drugs are contraindicated for patients with hypersensitivity to any of the drugs within the classification (i.e., anxiolytics) or group (e.g., benzodiazepines). They should not be taken in combination with other CNS depressants and are contraindicated in pregnancy and lactation, narrow-angle glaucoma, shock, and coma.

Administering these agents to elderly or debilitated patients and those with hepatic or renal dysfunction should be done cautiously; dosages are generally lower, and careful monitoring is necessary to prevent toxicity. Persons with present or past substance or alcohol abuse are not prescribed benzodiazepines or sedatives or hypnotics because of their potential for addiction. Reports of increased aggression or behavioral disinhibition have arisen when benzodiazepines were given to those with borderline personality disorder. Increased irritability or excitement can be due to a paradoxical reaction. Furthermore, these medications should be used cautiously in persons who are very depressed or suicidal.

BENZODIAZEPINES

Benzodiazepines are beneficial in treating the symptoms of panic disorder and generalized anxiety disorder, and generally some symptomatic relief is noticed short term. They are safe drugs if one is concerned with overdose, toxic effects are rare, and benzodiazepines are usually tolerated well. Because benzodiazepines are so widely used, drug interaction must be watched for as well as tolerance and subsequent addiction.

SIDE EFFECTS

- Drowsiness, confusion, lethargy (most common side effects).
- Tolerance: physical and psychological dependence (does not apply to buspirone).

- Potentiates the effects of other CNS depressants.
- Paradoxical excitement or disinhibition.
- Dry mouth.
- Alteration of sleep, particularly the stages of sleep.

Because the benzodiazepines can cause sedation, it is important to instruct the patient not to drive or operate dangerous machinery while taking the medication. Part of the nurse's role is to teach that tolerance to sedation often develops within a few days of beginning the medication or increasing the dose. When prescribed for a period of time, a physical dependence develops. This does not mean that the person is addicted, however. Abrupt discontinuation may lead to serious effects that last as long as 2 weeks. Discontinuation is potentially life threatening. Symptoms of withdrawal include increased anxiety, palpitations, sweating, insomnia, depression, abdominal and muscle cramps, and vomiting, and may progress to convulsions or delirium. Addiction occurs when the person develops drug-seeking behavior in order to increase the dose and achieve the same or a greater euphoric effect.

Because the benzodiazepines potentiate the effects of other CNS depressants and alcohol, people should not drink alcholic beverages or take other medications that depress the CNS while taking a benzodiazepine. An essential part of the nursing role is to continue to assess the patient's potential for alcohol and substance abuse.

In some situations, people with certain other disorders (e.g., borderline personality disorder or post-traumatic stress disorder) may respond paradoxically to benzodiazepines; they may experience excitement or disinhibition or become overly aggressive. If this occurs, the medication should be withheld temporarily, the patient should be monitored closely, and the prescribing clinician notified. Benzodiazepines, like many psychiatric medications, affect the stages of sleep. Thus, the nurse should assess the quality of the person's sleep and identify possible signs of an underlying sleep disorder (e.g., snoring or daytime fatigue).

Benzodiazepines have several advantages in the reduction of anxiety, including rapid relief of symptoms, high tolerability, and few serious side effects. Nonetheless, their low lethal potential from overdose, the lower risk of physical dependency, and their lower interference with the metabolism of other drugs can lead to the potential for careless or cavalier use.

Specific issues need to be considered with the use of benzodiazepines. First, these drugs, break down in the liver, tend to have a long half-life. Their metabolites are stored in the liver. The long-acting effects of the drug accumulate and are not rapidly excreted from the body. This is most important with the elderly because the drugs can become toxic. It is therefore, preferable that older people be treated with lorazepam or oxazepam, which have no active metabolites and are quickly excreted.

Effect is not what distinguishes one benzodiazepine from another; rather, it is duration of action. Short-acting drugs include alprazolam, lorazepam, and oxazepam; diazepam and clonazepam are relatively long-acting drugs. Short-acting antianxiety drugs have to be given in divided doses for effect, whereas the others can be given once or twice a day.

BUSPIRONE

Buspirone, when first introduced, was studied in comparison to diazepam (Valium) for the treatment of generalized anxiety disorder. The results demonstrated that the drug was just as effective in treating the anxiety symptoms without the potential for addiction or interaction with alcohol. Unfortunately, in clinical practice the effectiveness of buspirone has seemingly not lived up to expectations. One reason may be that the drug takes up to 4 weeks to effectively relieve anxiety. Thus, if patients are prescribed buspirone, they should understand that they will not see immediate effects, unlike the benzodiazepines. In addition to the drawback of delayed onset of action, buspirone may cause sedation, headache, nausea, and lightheadedness. Because sedation is a potential side effect, the patient should not drive or use dangerous equipment if experiencing sedation. If headache develops, part of the nursing role is to assess the frequency, quality, and severity of the complaint. This effect may subside with time, and prn medication (e.g., Tylenol) may be necessary. To minimize gastrointestinal distress, instruct patient to take the medication with food to treat nausea.

For information about side effects of antidepressants used to treat anxiety disorders, see the section on antidepressant agents.

RESEARCH IN TREATING ANXIETY DISORDER

No laboratory tests determine which medication is the most effective in treating anxiety disorder. Studies of infusions of sodium lactate or inhalation of carbon dioxide have found an increase in panic attacks in people with panic disorder. These studies are currently being pursued to develop an understanding of the biological underpinnings of panic disorder.

Examination of a neuropharmacological basis to obsessive-compulsive disorder (OCD) has focused on the serotonin system. Because patients with OCD respond effectively to SSRIs, studies have looked at the pre- and post-synaptic receptor changes using challenge studies. In these paradigms, subjects are given a medication that acts like serotonin (serotonin-agonist), and then the mood, behavior, and chemical effects at the synapse are examined. In a review of the use of pharmacologic challenge studies, Wolfe (1994) noted that m-chlorophenylpiperazine (m-CPP), a serotonergic drug acting at the post-synaptic receptor site, increases obsessive-compulsive symptoms. This suggests that post-synaptic serotonin receptors are involved in the regulation of obsessive-compulsive behavior.

O AN OVERVIEW

- Principles of neuroregulation and the hypotheses of how alterations in neuroregulation influence motor, affective, and cognitive behavior are the foundation of clinical pharmacology.

- Because all psychotropic agents have the potential for noxious to dangerous physiological effects, the nurse is in a critical position to educate patients and families about the expected effects of drug intervention.

- The patient's and family's cooperation in drug therapy enhances maintenance, and cooperation helps ensure that serious toxic reactions and side effects will be responded to readily.

- Other treatment modalities are generally used in conjunction with drug therapy.

- Behaviors affected by drugs are not always specific to the major disruptive symptomatology. The risk of adverse reactions to long-term drug intervention must be understood by the nurse, patient, and family.

- Informed consent in drug therapy is essential; clearly understanding why a drug is being given is the only way the ethical consideration can be addressed.

- The mainstay of antianxiety agents, also called anxiolytics, are the benzodiazepines, which are indicated for the treatment of panic disorder, generalized anxiety disorder, transient symptoms of anxiety, acute alcohol withdrawal, skeletal muscle spasms, seizure disorders, and for preoperative sedation.

- The numerous benzodiazepines and antidepressants (particularly clomipramine and the selective serotonin re-uptake inhibitors) are effective as antianxiety agents; however, they differ greatly in their levels of side effects, the degree of psychological and physical dependence they provoke, their margin of safety, and their interactions with other therapies.

- Because benzodiazepines are generally well tolerated and widely used to treat symptoms of panic disorder and generalized anxiety disorder, tolerance and subsequent addiction may result.

- Alcohol or other central nervous system depressants should not be taken while a patient is receiving a benzodiazepine.

- Patients with characterological problems, such as borderline personality disorder or post-traumatic stress disorder, may respond paradoxically to benzodiazepines and become excited, disinhibited, or overly aggressive. Consequently, antianxiety drugs should be used cautiously in these instances.

- Buspirone is effective is treating anxiety symptoms without the potential for addiction or interaction with alcohol seen with the use of benzodiazepines; however, the drug takes up to 4 weeks to effectively relieve anxiety.

- Antianxiety agents are most effective in anxiety disorders with acute to severe symptoms and in treating anxiety associated with somatic diseases.

TD TERMS TO DEFINE

- akathisia
- anticholinergic agents
- anticholinergic syndrome
- anticonvulsant
- anti-Parkinsonian agents
- antipsychotic drugs
- anxiolytics
- benzodiazepine
- bioavailability
- biotransformation
- buspirone
- choreoathetoid movements
- discontinuance syndrome
- dyskinesia
- dystonia
- extrapyramidal symptoms (EPS)
- idiosyncratic effect
- lithium
- medication effects
- Parkinsonism syndrome
- pharmacodynamics
- pharmacokinetics
- steady state
- tardive dyskinesia

Q STUDY QUESTIONS

1. Describe two important principles of drug action.

2. How is neurotransmission within the central nervous system carried out?

3. Discuss tardive dyskinesia.

4. Identify common and severe side effects of overdose with antipsychotic drugs.

5. List the drugs and dosages commonly prescribed for:
   a. depressive states including the schizophrenia-related depressive disorders, bipolar disorders, and unipolar disorders
   b. psychotic states
   c. anxiety states

6. Name the four cardinal symptoms of neuroleptic malignant syndrome.

7. Name three predisposing factors to neuroleptic malignant syndrome.

■ REFERENCES

American Psychiatric Association. *DSM IV.* Washington, DC: American Psychiatric Association; 1994.

Arana G, Hymen S. *Handbook of Psychiatric Drug Therapy.* 2nd ed. Boston: Little Brown; 1991.

Baldessarini RJ. *Chemotherapy in Psychiatry.* rev. ed. Cambridge, Mass: Harvard University Press; 1985.

Ballenger JC, Post RM. Carbamazepine in manic depressive illness: A new treatment. *Am J Psych* 1980; 137:782–789.

Bassuk E, Schoonover S, Gelenberg A. *The Practitioners' Guide to Psychoactive Drugs.* 2nd ed. New York: Plenum Medical; 1983.

Benet LZ, Mitchell JR, Sherner LB. Pharmacokinetics: The dynamics of drug absorption, distribution and elimination. In: Gilmna AG, Rall TW, Nies AS, Taylor P, eds. *The Pharmacologial Basis of Therapeutics.* New York: Pergamon Press; 1990.

Bernstein JG. *Handbook of Drug Therapy in Psychiatry.* 2nd ed. Littleton, Mass: PGS Publishing; 1988.

Birkhimer L, De Vane C. The neuroleptic malignant syndrome: Presentation and treatment. *Drug Intell Clin Pharm* 1984; 18:462–465.

Caroff S. The neuroleptic malignant syndrome. *J Clin Psych* 1980; 41:79–82.

Chin AC, Shaw KA, Ciaranellor RD. Molecular neurobiology. In: Schatzber FA, Nemeroff CB. *The American Psychiatric Press Textbook of Psycophharmacology.* Washington DC: American Psychiatric Press; 1995.

Dalby MA. Behavioral effects of carbemazepine. *Advances in Neurology,* Vol. 11. New York: Raven Press; 1986:331–341.

DiMascio A. *Drugs and Behavior: An Introduction to Psychopharmacology.* Television Lecture Series produced at Boston College, Chestnut Hill, MA.

Endicott J, Spitzer RL, Fleiss JL, Cohen J. The global assessment scale. *Arch Gen Psych* 1976; 33:766–771.

Ereshefsky L, Watanabe MD, Tran-Johnson TK. Clozapine: A novel antipsychotic agent. *Clin Pharm* 1989; 8:691–709.

Gratz S, Levinson D, Simpson G. Neuroleptic malignant syndrome. In: Kane J, Lieberman J, eds. *Adverse Effects of Psychotropic Drugs.* New York: The Guilford Press; 1992:266–284.

Greenblatt DJ. Principles of pharmacokinetics and pharmacodynamics. In: Schatzber AF, Nemeroff CB. *The American Psychiatric Press Textbook of Psychopharmacology.* Washington, DC: American Psychiatric Press; 1995.

Henderson V, Wooten G. Neuroleptic malignant syndrome: A pathogenic role for dopamine blockade? *Neurology* 1981; 31:132–137.

Hestbech J, Hansen HE, Amdisen A, Olsen S. Chronic renal lesions following long term treatment with lithium. *Kidney Internat* 1977; 12:205–213.

Hirsch SR. Clinical treatment of schizophrenia. In: Bradley PB, Hirsch SL, eds. *The Pharmacology and Treatment of Schizophrenia.* Oxford/New York/Tokyo: Oxford University Press; 1986:286–339.

Hollister LE. Psychiatric disorders. In: Melmon KL, Morreeli HD, Hoffman BB, Nierenber DW, eds. *Clinical Pharmacology: Basic Principles in Therapeutics.* New York: McGraw-Hill; 1992.

Jefferson JW. Genitourinary effects of psychotropic drugs. In: Kane JM, Lieberman J, eds. *Adverse Effects of Psychotropic Drugs.* New York: The Guilford Press; 1992:431–444.

Kahn A, Jeffe JH, Nelson W. Resolution of neuroleptic malignant syndrome with dantrolene sodium: Case report. *J Clin Psych* 1985;46;244–46.

Kane JM. Newer antipsychotic drugs: A review of their pharmacology and therapeutic potential. *Drugs* 1993;46(4):585–93.

Kane JM, Lieberman J. Tardive dyskinesia. In: Kane JM, Lieberman J, eds. *Adverse Effects of Psychotropic Drugs.* New York: The Guilford Press; 1992:235–245.

Levenson JL. Neuroleptic malignant syndrome. *Am J Psych* 1985; 142:1137–1144.

Lieberman J, Kane J, Johns C. Clozapine: Guidelines for clinical management. *J Clin Psych* 1989; 50:329–338.

Mansour A, Chalmers DT, Fox CA, et al. Biochemical anatomy: Insights into the cell biology and pharmacology of neurotransmitter systems in the brain. In: Schatzberg AF, Nemeroff CB. *The American Psychiatric Press Textbook of Psychopharmacology.* Washington DC: American Psychiatric Press; 1995.

Marsden CD, Mindham RHS, Mackay AVP. In: Bradley K. and Hirsch SR, eds. *The Psychopharmacology and Treatment of Schizophrenia.* Oxford/New York/Tokyo: Oxford University Press; 1986:340–402.

Meuller PS. Neuroleptic malignant syndrome. *Psychosomatics* 1985; 26:654–662.

Munetz MR, Benjamin S. How to examine patients using the abnormal involuntary movement scale. *Hosp Comm Psych* 1988; 39:1172–1177.

Overall JE. The brief psychiatric rating scale: Recent developments in ascertainment and scaling. *Psycholog Bull* 1988; 24(1):97–100.

Overall JE, Gorham DP. The brief psychiatric rating scale. *Psychol Rep* 1962; 10:799–810.

Post RM, Uhde TW, Putnam FW, et al. Kindling and carbemazepine in affective illness. *J Nervous Mental Disorders* 1982; 170:717–731.

Preston J, O'Neal JH, Talaga MC. *Handbook of Clinical Psychopharmacology for Therapists.* Oakland, Calif: New Harbbinger Publications; 1994.

Schatzberg AF, Nemeroff CB, ed. *The American Psychiatric Press Textbook of Psychopharmacology.* Washington, DC: American Psychiatric Press; 1995.

Schatzberg A, Cole JO. *Manual of Clinical Psychopharmacology,* 2nd ed. Washington DC: American Psychiatric Press; 1991.

Shildkraut JJ. Biochemical discrimination of subgroups of depressive disorders based on differences in catecolamine metabolism. In Hanin I and Usdin E. (eds.), *Biological Markers in Psychiatry and Neurology.* New York, Pergamon Press; 1983:22–23.

Seeman P. Schizophrenia as a brain disease: The dopamine receptor story. *Arch Neurol* 1993; 50(10):1093–1095.

Smego R, Durack D. The neuroleptic malignant syndrome. *Arch Intern Med* 1982; 142:1183–1185.

Spiegle R. *An Introduction to Pharmacology.* 2nd ed. New York: Wiley; 1990.

Teicher MH, Baldessarini RJ. Selection of neuroleptic dosages. *Arch Gen Psych* 1985; 42:636–637.

Teicher MH. Biology of anxiety. *Med Clin of NA.* 1988; 72: 4: 791–814.

Teicher MH, Glod CA, Cole JO. Antidepressant drugs and the emergence of suicidal tendencies. *Drug Safety* 1993; 8:186–212.

Wilcox RE, Gonzales RA. Introduction to neurotransmitters, receptors, signal transduction, and second messengers. In: Schatzberg AF, Nemeroff CB. *Textbook of Psychopharmacology.* Washington, DC: American Psychiatric Press; 1995.

Wolfe BE. The use of challenge studies in biobehavioral nursing research. *Archives of Psychiatric Nursing,* 1994; 8:145–149.

Yehuda R, McFarlane AC. Conflict between current knowledge about posttraumatic stress disorder and its original conceptual basis. *Am J Psych.* 1995; 152:1705–1711.

Zulbenko G, Pope HG. Management of a case of neuroleptic malignant syndrome with bromocriptine. *Am J Psych* 1983; 148:1619–1620.

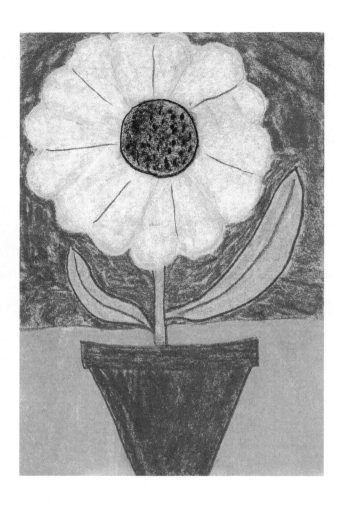

A long pull, and a
strong pull, and a
pull all together.

Charles Dickens,
David Copperfield

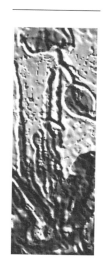

43
Critical Pathways for Mental Health and Planning Care

Kathleen Andolina

After a nursing assessment and diagnosis are completed, the next step is to formulate a plan of care. The patient and nurse together will recognize behaviors that are manifested, determine which need improvement or change, which strengths are available to bring to bear on the process and what resources are needed. Critical pathways will provide the framework for implementation of Standards of Care III, IV, V, and VI.

Standard of Care III: Outcome Identification

In this standard of care, the psychiatric-mental health nurse identifies expected outcomes individualized to the patient. Within the context of providing nursing care, the ultimate goal is to influence health outcomes and improve the patient's health status.

Standard of Care IV: Planning Care

The psychiatric-mental health nurse develops a plan of care that prescribes interventions to attain expected outcomes. A plan of care is used to guide therapeutic intervention systematically and achieve the expected patient outcomes. Identify and prioritize nursing diagnoses with patient needs. Include strengths and assets relevant to nursing interventions and recommend interventions.

Standard of Care V: Implementation of the Nursing Care Plan

The psychiatric-mental health nurse implements the interventions identified in the plan of care. In implementing the plan of care, psychiatric-mental health nurses use a wide range of interventions designed to prevent mental and physical illness, and promote, maintain, and restore mental and physical health. Psychiatric-mental health nurses select interventions according to their level of practice.

Standard of Care VI: Evaluation

As with any hypothesis or intervention, continued evaluation and reassessment is essential to determine if the desired effects are occurring.

■ PATHWAYS FOR MENTAL HEALTH

Critical pathways are a contemporary framework for planning, implementing, and evaluating patient care. The following are common questions and answers about critical pathways for mental health practice.

WHAT IS A PATHWAY OR MAP?

A pathway has several functions that are useful for the care and treatment of psychiatric patients. First, the pathway is often used as the basis of a treatment plan for the clinical care of patients with a given psychiatric diagnosis. A pathway can also be used to describe the care processes used for patients admitted to a level of care within a continuum, for example an in-patient setting or partial hospital setting. The pathway is designed to replace single-discipline care plans, like the nursing care plan or occupational therapy plan of care, with a multidisciplinary plan of care. Other pathway functions relate to cost and quality management, including continuous quality improvement and provider process improvement. The CareMap®, a form and system developed by The Center for Case Management, is an ideal framework for developing pathways in psychiatric–mental health (Table 43–1). The elements of the CareMap® tool include a problem list, outcomes and suboutcomes, a time line, task categories, and a variance coding system.

The CareMap® tool derives from the innovations of Karen Zander and Kathleen Bower at New England Medical Center Hospital, Boston in the mid-1980s. Together they used a critical pathway concept to predict resource use and results of health care interventions in medically ill populations. The tool proved to be successful and multipurpose. The CareMap® became useful as a care planning form, guide for communication, continuous quality improvement device, and predictor model for outcomes and resources, all at the same time. The process used to develop the map proved valuable as well. This process emphasized the use of expert knowledge, consensus techniques, provider accountability, care continuity, guideline validation methods, and cost-measurement technologies.

When the map is used as the care plan, it describes the typical care approach for the average patient in a case type (i.e., major depression, dual diagnosis, psychosis). Interventions, process tasks, and expected outcomes are described in relation to each other across time. Table 43–2 (page 799). displays the pathway concept in the form of a CareMap® tool.

The map is continuously updated by the map design committee until there is sufficient confidence in the content and care processes described. Maps at this stage approximate "best practice." Map systems rely on a dynamic process of continuous improvement.

WHY MIGHT MENTAL HEALTH SYSTEMS USE PATHWAYS AND MAP SYSTEMS?

The trends within mental health care delivery systems demand that systems respond with coordinated care management and outcome measurement systems. Payer consolidation, public and private integration, continuity of care management, outcome measurement, the practice guideline movement, and consumer informatics are only some of the forces influencing the climate today. All patients deserve to be managed efficiently and effectively. Pathway tools and systems are strategies for achieving care coordination in mental health systems.

Reviewing the following checklist will help organizations evaluate the need for additional strategies to cope with industry trends. Is the organization seeking to:

- Address performance improvement criteria from Joint Commission on Accreditation of Health Organizations (JCAHO)
- Provide outcome measurement data for employer purchasers of health care?
- Establish a method of continuous performance improvement and quality management?
- Improve clinical management and care processes?
- Define outcomes and provide evidence of measurement?
- Know the payment per case?
- Lower costs?
- Document by exception?
- Manage risks better?
- Allocate resources appropriately and efficiently?
- Keep pathway programs vital?
- Maintain or enhance market position?
- Become more fiscally sound and business savvy?

If the organization is involved in one or more of these, pathways can be used to manage some aspect within each area.

WHAT ARE SOME OF THE BENEFITS TO USING PATHWAYS?

The benefits to using pathways or map systems in mental health are many. These can include

- Stabilized lengths of stay with the proper levels of care.
- Consistent care approaches and processes for care management.
- Having a method for implementing quality changes.
- Process improvement, such as improved consistency in assessments, discharge planning, patient education, and team communication.

The pathway itself and the data yielded from variance provide a practical method for demonstrating evidence of outcome management, quality management, and performance improvement. As pressures increase for mental health care-givers to describe and provide evidence of their impact on patient outcomes, pathways become essential strategies. Pathways serve the needs of both administrators and clinical providers. Administrators like paths because they provide the medium to keep clinicians responding to industry changes. Clinicians like them for the support of the provider as the patient advocate and treatment evaluator. Pathways offer the best opportunity yet to inject provider-controlled self-regulation, discipline, and multidisciplinary outcome management into daily practice.

ARE PATHWAYS DEVELOPED BY PSYCHIATRIC DIAGNOSIS?

Pathways, when not used exclusively for care process coordination, are often developed for "case types." Case typing is the activity of describing characteristics common to a population. Psychiatric population characteristics include the psychiatric diagnosis, age/gender groupings, medical needs, complexities, and other information that details the patient who will fit into the case type. The path describes the problems, outcomes, and suboutcomes across time, detailing the care-giver tasks and interventions used along the way that support

E CASE EXAMPLE

Male or female patient over age of 18, presents with psychosis, depression, poor coping, or having medication adjustment problems. Meets the criteria for acute inpatient admission, requires daily management of symptoms, an evaluation period, medication adjustment, and intensive discharge planning.

TABLE 43–1   PARTIAL COPY OF A CAREMAP® FOR ADOLESCENTS WITH DEPRESSION

Problems/Focus or Outcomes	Day 1	Day 2
1. Axis I Concerns: Diagnostic assessment: clarification, neurological, major MI or other developmental disorder. Safety: SI/HI, impulse dyscontrol Mood: depression, anxiety, veg.s/s. Behaviors: rejection of authority, limit testing, regression, noncompliance, poor socialization, poor adaptation, impulse dyscontrol.	Meets team, discusses safety plans, states understanding of rights and responsibilities, no behavioral incidents or injury.	Participates in treatment planning, groups, individual counseling. Completes assignments with assistance, as necessary. No behavioral incidents or injury.
2. Axis II: Character or personality traits effecting depression.	Begins MMPI.	Identifies staff to whom they are able to talk.
3. Axis III: Co-existing medical conditions; medical management.	Patient/family share medical history. Completes health activities or medical testing as prescribed.	Completes health activities or medical testing as prescribed.
4. Axis IV: Psychosocial stressors: Family, school, or community service provider (CSP) issues.	Discusses recent stressors and supports or lack of supports.	Discusses emotional response to stressors in group/individual meetings.
5. Axis V: GAF, other scores.	GAF:_____	Other scores:_____
Assessments/consults.	Physical examination, psycho-social–behavioral assessment, vital signs (VS), weight, mental status exam (MSE), safety/suicide risk assessments, pediatrician, OT/RT, education, neurological, psychological.	Assess: MSE, VS, adjustment to milieu, safety behaviors, degree of participation in care, family/significant other (SO) involvement, visits, OT/RT, psychology.
Specimens/tests.	Adolescent screens, U/A, toxic screen, drug levels.	GAF: 1 to 50, Hamilton, BPRS, BSI, ASI, or other.
Safety, containment, milieu management and treatment.	Unit restriction until first team meeting, precaution checks as necessary, discuss safety contracts, counseling within groups and individually.	Form activity schedule; Develop coping plans: anger, depression, behaviors, increase priviledges as appropriate. Identify motivators; encourage strengths.
Medications.	Obtain medical history; meds as ordered.	Evaluate for prn or standing doses.
Nutrition/diet.	Diet as tolerated	Monitor intake.
Teaching.	Orientation to unit layout and routines, staff, team, rights, responsibilities.	Teaching re: coping skills, anger management, substance use, meds, school.
Discharge planning.	Family/SO identified, agrees to be involved; CSP or other agencies contacted.	Team meeting, family meeting scheduled.

From Andolina K. The Center for Case Management, 1996. *The CareMap®Tool and System.* Copyright The Center for Case Management, South Natick, Mass.

the achievement of outcomes. An example of a psychosis case type in mental health may be described in the case example on page 793.

It is important to note that the psychosis care type for one community or setting may be different from another. Pathways, therefore, are not always importable to other organizations, simply because it is named for a psychiatric diagnosis. The case type must be carefully developed to reflect the nature of the patients within the community served.

HOW IS THE PATHWAY A SYSTEM?

A pathway must have policies and procedures for development, implementation, and evaluation. The CareMap® System described by The Center for Case Management includes six components used around the clock to organize and sequence care-giving at the direct care level. The pathway provides for continuity of plan between all disciplines and departments concerned with the case type or patient. All providers using the

Day 3	Day 4	Day 5
Participates in treatment planning, groups, individual counseling. Completes assignments with assistance, as necessary. States +/− gains. No behavioral incidents or injury.	Participates in treatment planning, groups, individual counseling. Completes assignments with assistance as necessary. States +/− gains. No behavioral incidents or injury.	Participates in treatment planning, individual counseling. Completes assignments with assistance, as necessary. States +/− gains. No behavioral incidents or injury.
Continues to form working relationships with staff.	Continues to form working relationships with staff.	Continues to form working relationships with staff.
Completes health activities or medical testing as prescribed.	Completes health activities or medical testing as prescribed.	Completes health activities or medical testing as prescribed.
Identifies steps to take to cope with stressors.	Uses coping plans as able.	Uses coping plans as able.
Other scores:_____	Other scores:_____	Other scores:_____
Assess: MSE, VS, adjustment to milieu, safety behaviors, degree of participation in care, family/SO involvement and patient's response to the involvement, school functioning.	Assess: MSE, VS, adjustment to milieu, safety behaviors, degree of participation in care, family/SO involvement and patient's response to the involvement, school functioning.	Assess: MSE, VS, adjustment to milieu, safety behaviors, degree of participation in care, family/SO involvement and patient's response to the involvement, school functioning.
As ordered.	As ordered.	As ordered.
Encourage activities per plan, strengths, use of coping plans: anger, depression, behaviors, increase privileges as appropriate. Identify and use appropriate motivators.	Encourage activities, strengths, use of coping plans: anger, depression, behaviors, increase privileges as appropriate. Identify and use appropriate motivators.	Encourage activities, strengths, use of coping plans: anger, depression, behaviors, increase privileges as appropriate. Identify and use appropriate motivators.
Prn or standing doses.	Prn or standing doses.	Prn or standing doses. Best med plan determined.
Monitor intake.	Monitor intake.	Monitor intake.
Teaching re: coping skills, anger management, substance use, meds, school.	Reinforce teaching as necessary. Continue school/ tutoring schedule.	Reinforce teaching as necessary. Continue school/ tutoring schedule.
Team meeting, include CSP in DCP discussions.	Case conference (include CSP, patient if possible).	Team meeting.

path are bound to use the processes established for use of the map. The elements that make the CareMap® a system include the maps, data management processes (variance analysis), and communication strategies. Pathway system designs are unique in many ways to each organization, but each must accomplish the same goal of provider-controlled managed care for its patients. The elements of the CareMap® System are

- CareMap® tools.
- Variance analysis.
- Communication systems.

- Case consultation.
- Health care team meetings.
- Continuous quality improvement (CQI) (via variance analysis).

A variance is the difference between what was planned as stated on the map and what actually occurred. Typically, variances fall into four categories: patient related, provider, system, and community variances. Variances in mental health tend to be more patient related and function to alert care-givers to patient changes, enhance team work, and provide a consistent information base. Examples of patient variances are restraint/seclusion, adverse side effects from medications, or patient nonparticipation in care.

Variance data is neither good nor bad; it is simply information. It is used to prompt providers what to pay attention to when expected processes of care or patient benchmarks are not occurring. Variance data can be numerically coded for computer analysis and displayed in a number of different formats. Care-givers use the data to improve organizational performance, design action plans, provide evidence of aggregate clinical outcomes, and problem solve for quality concerns.

Reasons for variance can be coded for easier tracking.

1. Patient and Family
   Condition
   Decision
   Availability
   Resources
   Other
2. Care-giver
   Order
   Decision
   Response time
   Other
3. System
   Appt/bed availability
   Supplies, equipment, or information availability
4. Community
   Transportation availability
   Home care availability
   Other

HOW ARE PATHWAYS USED TO MANAGE QUALITY?

When paths or maps are revised, they provide a track record of improvements made. For example, when variance data indicates that the outcome of patient involvement in care planning is low, the path design group details specific actions to improve the outcome. Actions, such as earlier patient teaching, patient–family involvement in treatment team meetings, and weeknight family groups, become integrated into a new version of the path. These interventions are tested when patient involvement outcomes actually improve after implementing the new path. This is an example of retrospective continuous quality improvement (CQI). Concurrent CQI occurs when care-givers implement corrective actions to manage variances detected day-to-day. For example, if a patient requires restraint or seclusion to reestablish safety, then the path for restraint and seclusion is implemented, providing evidence that the standard of care was adhered to for that procedure.

Pathway systems provide a method for quality management that is consistent with many accrediting bodies, including the Joint Commission on Accreditation of Health Organizations (JCAHO). JCAHO often reviews systems using pathways and rates those that demonstrate helpfulness in clinical management, performance improvement, and outcomes management highly.

WHAT IS THE RELATIONSHIP OF CLINICAL CASE MANAGEMENT TO PATHWAYS?

Kathy Bower, coprinciple of The Center for Case Management, defines clinical case management as a

> clinical system that focuses on the accountability of an identified individual or group for coordinating a client's care (or group of clients) across an episode or continuum of care; insuring and facilitating the achievement of quality, clinical and cost outcomes; negotiating and procuring and coordinating services and resources needed by clients/families; intervening at key points for individual clients; addressing and resolving issues that have a negative quality-cost impact; and creating opportunities and systems to enhance outcomes (Bower, 1993).

Case management roles in mental health often concern themselves with coordinating or gatekeeping functions. While these are necessary functions, they represent a limited concept of the role. Advanced practice nurses, social workers, or highly skilled clinicians who assume case management roles often take on complex case management functions that approximate the definition described by Bower.

Clinical case managers may or may not use pathways to help them manage complex cases. Often, case managers are called to assist in the management of a patient on a pathway that has become complex. Clinical case managers may facilitate the writing of a map, collect data from and for path development or rely on paths to document case management outcomes.

WE ALREADY HAVE A GOOD SYSTEM OF CARE MANAGING PATIENTS. WHAT MORE COULD A PATHWAY HELP WITH?

The pathway is helpful in providing evidence of care. Communicating expected results is becoming more important, not only to patients and their families, but to care-givers across shifts, departments, and settings; payers; cost managers; and administrators. The path is the common denominator that cuts across disciplines, services, and administrative levels. In addition, pathways are effective information management systems and can be designed to provide information without going through tedious chart reviews.

HOW DOES THE PATIENT OR FAMILY BENEFIT FROM A PATHWAY?

When patients and their families see the path, they view it as a contract for care that communicates, first and foremost, that there is a care plan. In addition, it controls expectations, allowing care-givers to negotiate the context and results of care in the absence of an emotionally charged environment. Additionally, paths increase patient satisfaction and reduce risk of litigation by providing numerous fail-safe mechanisms for proactive care planning. For example, prompts are written on to the path suggesting appropriate patient education or team meetings to discuss findings and assessments. The path prevents extemporaneous care planning and provides a complete documentation of care in chronological order. The variance analysis process improves clinician quality by tying performance variance to peer review mechanisms. Finally, paths describe a consensus of clinical management thought and are aimed at reducing any unnecessary variation in clinical practice. This helps to reduce patient and staff frustration and confusion by reducing variant practice approaches.

WHAT HAPPENS IF THE PATIENT HAS TOO MANY COMPLICATIONS AND DOES NOT FIT WITH THE PATH?

Depending on how general or specific the pathway is, there may be a great deal of variance. The intention of the map is not to substitute for the complete assessment of the individual, but to describe the minimum program of care and desired results for an average individual as part of a population of patients. In order to customize the care to the patient, the care-giver changes or adds statements as required, switches to a more appropriate map, or removes the patient from the map if it no longer fits. Some paths start with a generic admission framework, and clinicians add predefined problems and outcomes as necessary. Other paths include common complications, and then clinicians "opt-in" or "opt-out" of the problems as assessment indicates (for example, substance abuse as an opt-in on the depression or psychosis pathway).

ARE THERE ANY PATIENTS OR SITUATIONS WHERE A PATH WOULD NOT BE APPROPRIATE?

Perhaps, if there is an extremely complex patient or the actual patterns of care are not yet apparent. Case managers, as care evaluators, provide the best opportunity to discover the coordination and care management issues and develop the plan of care accordingly in these cases. In some instances, case managers develop pathways after they have worked with a population long enough to discover practice patterns.

Another instance where paths are not the first or best strategy is where intense unit restructuring is occurring or where the unit approach to care is being reformulated. Once care approaches are stabilized, pathways are implemented to establish the best care approach.

HOW CAN DATA BE OBTAINED FROM A PATHWAY?

Three methods exist for retrieving data from pathways and variance reports. First, the pathway itself can serve as a data collection tool. Indicators, clinical results, or patient variance can be recorded directly onto the map and collected by retrospective audit for analysis. Second, a separate variance tracking form can be used to preprint indicators, document the variance, collect, and analyze the data. Third, data can be obtained from automated computer systems. When map documentation is online, data elements can be defined, selected, aggregated, and statistically analyzed by computer.

HOW DO PATHS FIT INTO THE PRACTICE GUIDELINE MOVEMENT?

Practice guidelines are more extensive descriptions of the care of populations, diagnoses, or conditions. Some are developed by national consensus building efforts, such as those from the Agency for Health Care Policy and Research (AHCPR). Other practice guidelines, or standards, are internally developed within each organization. Elements, such as population definition, rationale for the guideline, management of the population and complications, quality indicators, data sets, and definition of terms, are part of the guideline publication. The pathway is often included with the practice guideline and illustrates the process of care for the population. Practice guidelines are not the day-to-day management tools that pathways are, but they provide the context and data that back up the content within the pathway tool.

WHAT IF SEVERAL DISCIPLINES FUNCTION IN A GENERIC CLINICIAN ROLE? HOW IS A PATHWAY DIFFERENT IN APPROACHING THAT ROLE?

Pathways begin to get all care-givers "on the same page" by focusing on patient-centered results. Part of the effort involves having care-givers define their special contribution to care, establishing ownership for their contribution, and clarifying it at the same time. In mental health, however, it is important to remember that it is often not a single discipline's contribution that makes a difference, but the cumulative effect of consistent care-giver actions. To that end, accountability for outcomes is often shared among professional providers, and in some instances, outcomes may be documented

E CASE EXAMPLE

Day 7. Expected Outcomes:

Patient states medication schedule postdischarge.

Patient states intention to continue taking meds.

Mr. A states what makes him stop taking meds and agrees to follow up home visits from home care for med monitoring.

Under the Treatment Approach Standard, care must be individualized to the pa-

tient's needs. Statements on the pathway must be added to reflect that care is individualized. To illustrate, in the admission assessment of Mr. A, it is discovered that within short periods of time after his discharge, Mr. A stops all his medication. A new outcome is added (individualized expected outcome is written in italics).

If additional care-giver tasks and actions are required to achieve this outcome, then these are written into the staff task part of the pathway.

---

by any professional care provider unless noted otherwise.

WHAT IF THERE IS SOME PRESSURE TO SHOW COST AND QUALITY RESULTS OF CARE? WILL PATHWAYS IN MENTAL HEALTH HELP?

Because pathways describe results in outcomes language, it will help to show these results. Outcomes by definition are measurable and objective. Although patient progress is often a subjective measurement experience in mental health, some standard quality issues can be defined (i.e., patient participation, access to care, appropriate discharge planning). Organizations who contract with employer-owned health care plans will also be subjected to requests for information or report cards. Report cards will increasingly be used by employers looking to purchase the best, most affordable health plans for employees. The National Committee for Quality Assurance has developed the Healthplan Employer Data and Information Set (HEDIS) Project. The HEDIS framework is used to acquire data from organizations to publish in report cards. The HEDIS standards for mental health reflect the following criteria:

- Ambulatory patient followup within 30 days of hospitalization.
- Standards for triage, treatment approach, case management, alternative treatment settings, outcomes measurement, benefit design, access, quality management, prevention, education, and early intervention.

WHAT ABOUT MENTAL HEALTH WORKERS? CAN THEY DOCUMENT ON A MAP?

Nonprofessional staff are an integral part of mental health management. So are *per diem* professional work-

ers. Both groups rely on pathways to be informed about the day-to-day management, as well as the big picture; however, even the most talented nonprofessionals are no substitute for the professionally trained care evaluator. While nonprofessional staff will document tasks completed, the outcomes of care remain within the realm of professional assessment and are signed off only by professional staff.

IS IT ALWAYS POSSIBLE TO DEFINE AN APPROACH IN BEHAVIORAL OR PSYCHIATRIC—MENTAL HEALTH IN TERMS OF THE CATEGORIES STATED ON THE PATHWAY? HOW CAN THESE APPROACHES BE STATED ON THE MAP?

The care task categories on the pathway can be changed to better reflect the facility environment. Many facilities, while using the classic eight categories of care (assessments/consults, medications, etc.) may also dedicate separate rows to disciplines (psychology, RT/OT, social work, etc.) or treatment modalities (milieu, group program, relational model, etc.). Sometimes categories are reduced to assessments, treatment, and discharge planning as the only essential categories for care.

THE REASONS THAT A PATIENT OR FAMILY REQUESTS HELP OR IS HOSPITALIZED ARE VARIABLE. ARE PATHWAYS FLEXIBLE ENOUGH TO ADDRESS THIS?

Although patient presentations vary, the rationale for admission to a given level of care is becoming less variable all the time. Managed care requires that facilities develop utilization criteria (level of care criteria). This criteria can form the basis of a generic pathway for a designated setting. Once the outcome expectations for a setting are known, the accountability for comprehensive sets of outcomes becomes more clear. Acute in-patient settings are no longer capable of managing all out-

TABLE 43–2. PATHWAY CONCEPT

Outcomes/ Problems/Focus	Time
1.	Patient/family outcomes, goals written progressively across time.
2.	Outcomes: patient/family participation, knowledge, behaviors, skills, agreements, etc.
	Example **Staff Tasks and Processes for Care**
1. Assessments	Vital signs, OT assessment, nursing assessment, mental status assessments.
2. Specimens/tests	Toxic screens, blood tests, psychiatric testing.
3. Treatments	Milieu therapy, one-to-one counseling, therapeutic approach, group programs.
4. Medications	Medical protocols, MD medication preferences, standing orders, medical consents.
5. Nutrition/diet	Diet orders, monitor intake.
6. Safety/activity	Privileges, precautions.
7. Teaching	Coping, anxiety management.
8. Discharge planning	Contact community providers, refer to home care, family meetings, team meetings, etc.

comes. Some outcomes, such as medication compliance, are better left to be managed in ambulatory settings, such as out-patient, partial hospital, or community settings. While it seems that the scope of care is being reduced in each setting, responsible care across the continuum is increasingly becoming a focus of most organizations and payer entities. Shifting costs and responsibilities to other settings is now a matter of negotiation not patient dumping. The best organizations are interested in forming affiliations with a number of diverse settings (public–private integration) in order to support the highest level of wellness and prevention for psychiatric patients within their community. This is good news for patients who will require long-term care management.

O AN OVERVIEW

- Critical pathways provide a framework for implementing ANA Standards of Care III, IV, V, and VI: outcome identification, planning care, implementing the nursing care plan, and evaluation.
- The CareMap®, an ideal framework for developing pathways in psychiatric nursing, in-

cludes a problem list, outcomes and suboutcomes description, a time line, task categories, and a variance coding system.

- A variance is the difference between what was planned as stated on the map and what actually occurs.
- The map is continuously updated by the interdisciplinary map design committee until there is sufficient confidence in the content and processes described.
- Pathway system designs are unique in many ways to each organization, but they must accomplish the same goal of provider-control managed care for patients.
- Clinical case management is defined as a clinical system that focuses on the accountability of an identified individual or group for coordinating a patient's or group of patients' care across an episode or continuum of care; ensuring and facilitating the achievement of quality, clinical and cost outcomes; negotiating, procuring, and coordinating services and resources needed by patients and families; intervening at key points for individual patients; addressing and resolving issues that have a negative quality-cost impact; and creating opportunities and systems to enhance outcomes.
- Patients and families view their path as a contract for care.
- Practice guidelines are more extensive descriptions of the care of populations, diagnoses, or conditions; they are not the management tools that pathways are, but they provide the context and data that backup the content with the pathway tool.
- Among the benefits of using pathways are stabilized lengths of stay, consistent care and management approaches, a method for implementing quality changes, and process improvement, such as improved consistency in assessment or patient education.

TD TERMS TO DEFINE

- best practice
- CareMap® System
- case managers
- case types
- continuous quality improvement (CQI)
- critical pathway
- Healthplan Employer Data and Information Set (HEDIS)
- outcome identification
- practice guidelines
- variance

Q STUDY QUESTIONS

1. Define the benefits of pathway programs from the point of view of each of these stakeholders. Site examples of the specific benefits.
   Nurse Managers
   Physicians
   Chief Financial Officers
   Directors of Quality Management
   Hospital Administration
   Bedside Caregiver on the weekend night shift

2. Caregivers without the skills, poor leadership, and lack of organizational response to pathway data are barriers that yield poor results in pathway programs. Describe strategies to overcome these barriers and how they would be implemented in your system of care.

3. Construct your own version of a pathway form for any of the following levels of care:
   Crisis Evaluation—Emergency Department
   Acute Care Inpatient
   Day Treatment/Partial Hospital
   Home Care
   Outpatient (Office Visits)

   How will you set up the time intervals (shift, day, hour, visits, etc . . .)? What care categories (assessment, tests, treatments, medications, etc.) will you use?

4. Describe the characteristics of a population for pathways. What resources (human and material) would you use to assist you?

5. Using the case type below, practice writing outcomes:

   Male or female patient over age of 18, presents with psychosis, depression, poor coping, or having med- ication adjustment problems. Meets the criteria for acute inpatient admission, requires daily management of symptoms, an evaluation period, medication adjustment and intensive discharge planning.

   a. Write 3 outcomes expected by discharge (inpatient setting).
   b. Write 3 *intermediate* outcomes (expected to be met prior to discharge).
   c. Write a cost outcome related to length of stay.
   d. Write a quality outcome related to an expected provider activity.

■ REFERENCES

Andolina K. CareMap® development and implementation. In: Zander K, (ed.) *Managing Outcomes Through Collaborative Care.* Chicago: American Hospital Publishing, 1995; 115–130.

Andolina K. The Automation of Critical Paths/CareMap® Systems. In Ball MJ, Hannah KJ, Newbold SK, Douglas JV, eds. *Nursing Informatics: Where Caring and Technology Meet.* 2nd ed. New York: Springer-Verlag, 1995; 167–183.

Andolina K. *Psychiatric CareMaps®.* Published by The Center for Case Management since 1991 and updated yearly.

Bower KA. Case management: Work redesign with patient outcomes in mind. In: *Patient-Centered Hospital Care: Reform From Within.* Ann Arbor, Mich: Health Administration Press; 1993.

Southwick K. Montclair Baptist and AtlantiCare break new ground with care paths for psych patients. *Strategies for Healthcare Excellence* February 1995; 8(2):1–8.

Zander K. *Managing Outcomes Through Collaborative Care: The Application of CareMapping and Case Management.* Chicago: American Hospital Publishing, 1995.

Zander K. CareMaps: The core of cost/quality care. *The New Definition.* Fall, 1991; 6(3):1–3.

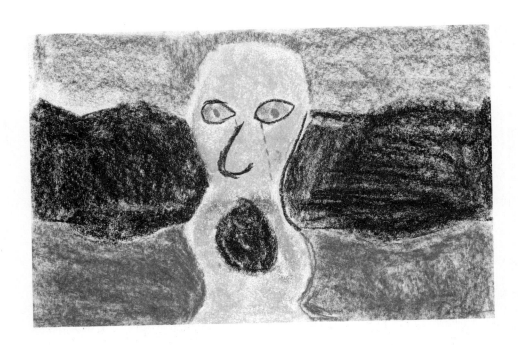

Economic distress will teach men, if anything can, that realities are less dangerous than fancies, that fact-finding is more effective than fault-finding.

Carl Lotus Becker (1873–1945)

Progress and Power, 1935

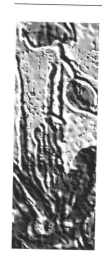

44

Case Management

Kathleen Andolina

Recent trends in health care delivery systems pose new challenges for psychiatric nurses. As care shifts from institutional to community-based systems, psychiatric nurses are required to adapt to expanded role expectations and, at the same time, preserve psychiatric nursing knowledge. Changes in health care delivery also suggest that professionals will work less as individual care providers and more as part of a multidisciplinary team, focusing on an entire episode of illness, rather than the most acute part. Multidisciplinary teams will work in collaborative practices that are unprecedented in their scope and authority in health care delivery. In order to realize effective collaborative practices, care-givers will require information that is reliable, accurate, and instantaneous, making computer technology a valuable part of everyday practice. The emphasis will be on patient-centered care that is coordinated and outcome focused.

Case management, as a coordinating and care evaluation strategy, was first practiced in health care settings in the 1980s, with nursing taking the lead in establishing case management programs for patients within certain diagnostic groups. These clinical case management initiatives, with nurses in the fore, began to demonstrate dramatic results in cost stabilization, quality improvement, *and understanding of realistic care processes for populations of patients. For the first time, nurses were given due credit for their individual and collective contribution to sustaining patient care outcomes. These early experiences with case management in large institutional settings crystallized the collaborative practice trend and continue to drive it.*

■ IDENTIFYING ROLES

Case management programs can be understood as having a role in assisting team members with role adaptation. Bower (1993) incorporates role aspects in the definition of case management as:

> a clinical system that focuses on the accountability of an identified individual or group for coordinating a patient's care (or group of patients) across a continuum of care; ensuring and facilitating the achievement of quality clinical and cost outcomes; negotiating, procuring and coordinating services and resources needed by the patient/family; intervening at key points (and/or at significant variances) for individual patients; addressing and resolving patterns in aggregate variances that have a negative quality–cost impact; and creating opportunities and systems to enhance outcomes.

Case manager activities emphasize achieving and sustaining patient-centered outcomes. The above definition underscores providing expertise or oversight for proactive care planning, resource coordination, daily facilitation of care, and taking actions to reduce problems that interfere with effective care. More simply put, the case manager assesses, plans, intervenes/coordinates and monitors/evaluates (Zander, 1995). Case management roles assumed by psychiatric nurses present another opportunity, other than primary nursing, to apply professional skill and clinical reasoning to psychiatric and mental health nursing practice today. Historically, nurses have always been positioned at the juncture where patient needs, societal demands, and resources intersect. Psychiatric nurses, working independently and as members of a team, coordinate, match, and direct how care resources are used, based on assessments of patients' needs and resources. Bridging, matching, and coordinating resources with patient needs is a familiar component of the psychiatric nursing role, although often unacknowledged. For example, when a young

mother who requires treatment for substance abuse and depression is discharged from the acute care setting, the psychiatric nurse has likely investigated the availability of self-help meetings in the patient's community, worked with the patient and family to procure day care and transportation, and evaluated the obstacles that interfere with maintaining the treatment plan. The nurse case manages the patient toward outcomes, effectively using the nursing process beyond the immediate setting focus and into the immediate future.

The psychiatric nurse is cognizant of the need to support the attainment of outcomes beyond the immediate acute setting. Comprehensive assessment of the patient leads the nurse to anticipate both practical and clinical barriers to treatment success. If psychiatric nurses are relegated to time spent in inefficient assessments that are not geared toward detecting pertinent data or if the professional role is wasted on herding patients from one treatment to another or narrowly focusing practice on medication administration, then the nurse effectively becomes a "task completer," not an "outcome manager." The absence of a practice model that promotes collaborative, outcome-based practice dooms achievement to mere chance.

■ OPPORTUNITIES TO CASE MANAGE

Patients and their families want the results of their care to be predictable and the type of care compatible with their values and resources.

Clinical case management performed by psychiatric nurses familiar with the patient and his or her history is a powerful mechanism for early mobilization of resources and episode prevention. Although many care outcomes cannot be predicted, perhaps more is foreseeable than has been assumed. Case management services offer a framework for beginning to learn about managing care across a continuum of settings. Nurses, as continuum spanners and clinical professionals, are

E CASE EXAMPLE

When Mr. P, a 72-year-old man recovering from a life-threatening episode of depression, was discharged from acute psychiatric care following a series of successful electroconvulsive treatments (ECT), his family reported that he had been referred to a psychiatrist for follow-up in a town not accessible by public transportation. Mr. P, not known for his patience with medical care, threatened to stop taking his medication and began talking about not attending appointments. Consequently, mental health home care visits were established to assess Mr. P's coping and establish continuity of care. Through the therapeutic relationship with both the patient and family, the psychiatric nurse was able to establish a four-way working relationship between the psychiatrist, patient and family,

nurse and home care agency, and the community transportation services. Over a period of months, Mr. P recovered fully from the depression that had almost claimed his life. During that time, he and his family recounted the humiliation of requiring full restraints, police and ambulances to get him to the hospital, the weight loss and poor personal care, the confusion and utter loss of privacy. Upon review of Mr. P's psychiatric treatment history, the health care team discovers that Mr. P had successfully been managed on medication in the past, but after a series of medical problems, was taken off his medication and never followed for long-term outcomes. His wife angrily stated, "This depression never needed to happen."

---

in an excellent position to coordinate care and manage outcomes. Figure 44–1 illustrates the opportunities for psychiatric nurses to span the continuum beyond acute care settings. It is important that psychiatric nurses not think of care within hospital settings only. Taking advantage of the variety of work available within nursing and across the continuum of services, will broaden the experience and knowledge of nurses providing clinical case management services as part of the mental health provider role.

■ FRAGMENTED COST AND QUALITY MANAGEMENT

Until recently clinical care providers have not tracked both cost and quality results. Traditionally, such information was split among the care providers, support services, and payer systems. This separate management fragmented the picture of cost and quality. For example, team leaders, physicians, or program directors were accountable for achieving discharge outcomes and maintaining that information. Support services, such as departments of quality management, risk management, information systems, and medical records, collected and reported information related to traditional quality indicators. Payers, public or private, assumed ultimate fiscal responsibility and were the only ones who knew long-term care costs.

The pressure to contain costs in mental health services arose after many years of unchecked growth and after questions of value were posed. Subsequently, payers began efforts to contain costs through limitations in reimbursement and through level or reduced funding. As a result, health care facilities established cost cutting practices of their own, such as privatization initiatives, staff reductions, and facility downsizing. In general, a managed care philosophy has emerged within health care facilities that emphasizes symptom-based care and systems stabilization verses etiology-based care approaches. Yet, without the connection to clinical reality and without effective, simultaneous cost and quality management, these cost-containment efforts, while bringing budgets into balance, have thrown care-delivery systems into chaos. Systems of care delivery are needed that preserve quality clinical practice, emphasize outcome attainment, and contain costs accordingly.

In actuality, all care requires managing. When care is not managed, fragmentation, miscommunication, and disjointed care planning are the norm. The patient's and family's experiences are often more disjointed than care providers realize. Patients and their families or caretakers have often managed themselves through the episode of illness as well as through the system that oversees their care. Clinical case management

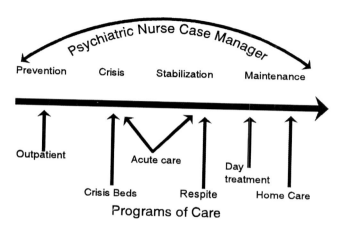

FIGURE 44–1. Opportunities for case management.
Reproduced from Andolina K, The Center for Case Management. 1995.

as a strategy for managing care positions the professional care provider as the source of accountability for coordinated and outcome-based care. When care is managed, care is proactively planned, thereby results are anticipated and interventions not left to chance. In short, care providers using a system of case management have a method for paying attention to the process and the results of care.

■ CASE MANAGEMENT AS A ROLE, SYSTEM, AND PROGRAM

Various programs of case management have been designed. For example, case management initiatives designed at a facility level refer to a system-wide approach to cost and quality accountability and may exist in several forms: a Department of Case Management with its own case management staff; a Case Management Project with a project manager; or an integrated provider model where certain care-givers, through new job descriptions, perform case management functions. In the latter model, psychiatric nurses who enact case management as a distinct, yet integrated part of their role, assess, plan, intervene, coordinate, evaluate, and monitor the patients' responses to care and achievement of health outcomes. Another design involves case management initiatives at a unit (or local) level, which is usually a modest first step toward a fully developed, facility-wide program. These first initiatives are often guided by the positive energy of a few individuals, groups, or providers, who form a well-defined project with specific goals in mind. Some goals for case management include:

- Increase coordination of complex processes and case type needs.
- Link actual costs to care.
- Define and measure outcomes.
- Decrease costs while stabilizing or improving quality.
- Enhance collaborative practice.
- Improve patient satisfaction.
- Operationalize continuous quality improvement at the care management level.
- Clarify accountability for processes and outcomes.

■ CASE MANAGEMENT RESPONSIBILITIES

Psychiatric nurses who will undertake case management responsibilities require that the role be clearly defined. Because the needs of the patient population and health care facilities are not static, job descriptions vary among models and facilities. Job descriptions are based on activities required for both program and population-specific goals (Table 44–1). Zander (1995) describes a "short and long list" of possible responsibilities of a case manager, acknowledging that the long list is a compilation from various models and not recommended in its entirety.

Short List

- Assess.
- Plan.
- Intervene and coordinate.
- Monitor and evaluate.

Long List

- Facilitate development of paths and maps.
- Facilitate collaborative practices.
- Conduct daily utilization review.
- Discharge planning.
- Nursing assessments.
- Join physician rounds.
- Negotiate with payers and insurers.
- Record and collect variances.
- Consult with staff as variances occur.
- Coach staff.
- Teach patients and families.
- Collect and prepare statistics and reports.
- Give direct care to help out.
- Have shift and home care assignment.
- Do follow-up phone calls.
- Participate in peer consultation.
- Keep financial records.
- Arrange placements.

In the instance where all responsibilities are desirable, case management may be a shared role, with the psychiatric nurse assuming accountability for the clinical aspects of care coordination. In coordinating care within complex or in-patient facilities, disciplines and departments may share case management by taking the following actions:

- Merge department staff roles (utilization review and continuous quality improvement, social work, discharge planning and clinical care-giver roles) based on the goals of specific case management programs and populations.
- Spell out expected role description and behaviors.
- Define regular case management planning meetings, peer review, and peer consultation.
- Define indicators for health care team meetings and case consultations.
- Establish who care-givers can go to when there is an accountability issue.
- Increase the frequency and quality of the meetings in proportion to the need for a daily unit-based management system.

TABLE 44–1. SAMPLE CASE MANAGEMENT JOB DESCRIPTION

General Role Description

Coordinates, negotiates, procures and manages the care of complex patients to facilitate achievement of quality and cost outcomes.

Works collaboratively with interdisciplinary staff internal and external to the organization.

Participates in quality improvement and evaluation processes related to the management of care.

Role functions:

Identifies patients for case management services.

Develops a network of the usual services and disciplines required by a typical patient in the case type.

Establishes a coordinating system of care spanning each geographic area of care.

Establishes methods for tracking patient progress across the continuum of care.

Maintains a working knowledge of payer requirements for the case type.

Maintains a working knowledge of community resources available for patients and families.

Demonstrates flexibility and creativity in identifying resources to meet patient and family needs.

Establishes a collaborative communication system with MDs, payers, administrators, and other team members.

Explores, implements, and documents strategies used to decrease length of stay and resource consumption.

Evaluates the effects of case management on the target population.

Introduces self to the patient and family, explains the case manager role and provides written information.

Tracks and assesses patients within the caseload to identify and confirm care plan.

In collaboration with the patient, team, payer, and available resources forms, implements, evaluates, and revises plan of care.

Manages each patient transition through the system and transfers accountability to appropriate persons or agencies on discharge from case management services.

Maintains appropriate documentation of care and progress.

Coordinates, negotiates, and procures needed services and disciplines.

Communicates with other members of the health care team re: patient needs, plan, and responses to care.

Works collaboratively with team.

Identifies need for health care team meetings when necessary to facilitate coordination of complex services or resources.

Educates health care team colleagues about case management, including the role and unique needs of the case type population.

As a member of a case management practice seeks and provides peer consultation about problem cases, consistently attends meetings of the practice group and participates in them, participates in regular peer review, participates in quality review and case management evaluation processes, and arranges for and participates in coverage during long, short, and unexpected absences of self and other case managers.

Reviews pertinent literature about case types and shares with peers.

Adapted from Zander K, 1995.

Another important aspect of case management is to define when and to what populations case management efforts are to be assigned. While it is true that all care needs managing, not all patient care requires case management. For example, case managers are often assigned to the most complex patients. In addition, they may be assigned to patients within a certain case type because the population is high volume and high cost. Table 44–2 illustrates examples of populations often targeted for case management initiatives.

A successful case manager is usually a highly skilled clinician with good clinical judgment who is highly re-

TABLE 44–2. MENTAL HEALTH CASE TYPES TARGETED FOR CASE MANAGEMENT INITIATIVES

High Cost	Unpredictable	Significant Variance	Repeat Admits	High Risk	Program Mission	Complex Care: Multiple MDs, Units
Psychosis	Axis II	AWA (Absent Without Authority)	Axis II	Bipolar (rapid cyclers)	Affective disorders	Medical psychiatric patients
Depression	Dual diagnosis	Gesture		Anxiety/panic	Women's program	Chronic schizophrenia
Dual diagnosis	Alcohol/drug abuse	Restraint/seclusion		Males: dysphoric, angry		
Axis II		Major socioeconomic problems				
		Med nonresponsive				
		Medical psych				

Adapted from Andolina K, The Center for Case Management, 1995

garded by colleagues. Being delegated the authority to coordinate services for patients is based on a high degree of trust. In addition, case managers are knowledgeable about systems, are creative, and appreciate the culture of patient care. They are good communicators, critical thinkers, evaluators, and problem solvers, and they are skilled negotiators.

■ STANDARDS OF PSYCHIATRIC AND MENTAL HEALTH NURSING PRACTICE AND CASE MANAGEMENT

Several statements outlined in the Standards for Psychiatric and Mental Health Nursing (American Nurses Association, 1994) III and V support and take on greater emphasis in psychiatric nursing case management.

Standard III refers to the identification of outcomes and the importance of individualizing them to patients. In addition, identifying outcomes is important to the ultimate goal of improving the patient's health status. Outcomes must be realistic and evaluated for costs and benefits, and they must estimate the time required for attainment, provide direction for continuity of care, and reflect current scientific knowledge in mental health care. Standard III reminds psychiatric nurses that they play a pivotal role in individualizing outcomes to the actual patient need and especially for case-managed patients, who may be managed using predefined care plans (i.e., automated nursing care plans, standards of care, practice guidelines, critical path and CareMap® tools) as part of a population-based care approach.

Under Standard V (f), Concerning Implementation, rationale and measurement criteria for case man-

agement are presented. Standard V (f) states that the psychiatric nurse "provides case management to coordinate comprehensive health services and ensure continuity of care." Case management services are based on a comprehensive assessment approach that matches the patient's needs and considers the accessibility, availability, quality, and cost-effectiveness of care. Nurse case managers negotiate for health-related services for patients and seek specialized care services, such as transportation, family treatment, or educational–vocational services, as determined through the nursing assessment process. The psychiatric nurse case manager ensures continuity by maintaining a relationship with agencies and providers within the network of services the patient is using. Psychiatric nurse case managers are now integrating areas that were previously separately and strictly maintained. As one community therapist recently stated, "Now, I almost always receive a call that my patient is in the hospital. Five years ago, the only time I knew that a patient was hospitalized was if my patient called me or told me why they had missed the last few appointments."

Psychiatric nurse case managers are central communicators and processors for information relevant to patient progress. Yet, jurisdictions of care are defined differently for individual patients, and psychiatric nurse case managers will encounter different continuity situations. For example, when one case manager encounters another, decisions about who is accountable for what outcomes will require discussion and decision making about who will follow and coordinate those outcomes. In addition, the patient's and family's decisions about care and treatment will continue to require support through psychiatric nursing case management. Standard V (f) defines case management as an integral com-

E CASE EXAMPLE

Mr. and Mrs. C both have psychiatric diagnoses. They reside in a metropolitan area surrounded by health care facilities. Mrs. C is diagnosed with paranoid schizophrenia and suffers from somatic delusions, including fears that she has cervical cancer. She constantly makes appointments with specialists and surgeons, frequently calls ambulances to take her to the emergency room, and regularly argues with her care providers about what her physical problems are. Her husband is mildly retarded and becomes concerned and anxious when his wife complains of pain. He urges her to use the medical services available. The services provided to the couple are split and unplanned, with little communication between all the care providers involved. In addition, the couple are receiving

bills that they are unable to understand or pay for, increasing their anxiety and disorganization.

Mr. and Mrs. C require case management services from clinically skilled professionals who understand both the mechanics of coordinating care and the psychosocial interventions required to stabilize the couple. A psychiatric nurse in a community care setting, with case management skills is in a good position to stabilize the care-giving process and define realistic psychiatric, cost, and quality goals, as well as evaluate and monitor the achievement of these goals.

ponent of psychiatric nursing practice. The standard emphasizes patient-centeredness (i.e., matching resources to need and respect patient wishes) and extending nursing accountability beyond narrow care settings (acute or community) by urging negotiation for added services, maintaining relationships with agencies, individual providers, and ensuring continuity.

WHEN TO INITIATE CASE MANAGEMENT

Defining when case management strategies are required is key to timely implementation of case management as a coordinating and evaluation service. The following service definition of case management offers a broad approach for determining case management implementation:

> Case management is a service for coordinating multiple resources, such that if these were *not* coordinated, patient outcomes would be at risk.

Other methods to help clarify when case management is required include clear criteria for activating case management services, such as those based on admission to a facility or program or by the nature of the case type itself. For example, according to Miriam Aaron, Executive Director of the New York State Nurses Association and co-developer of the Statewide Peer Assistance for Nurses (SPAN) program, case management is required automatically for the addicted nurse population due to the complex nature of addiction, the multiple treatment options, and complex back-to-work issues. Case management is implemented at the point that the patient self-refers to the program or is employee referred.

In in-patient settings, the point at which case management begins is the point where care becomes excessively complex. This is often defined as the point where three or more serious complications, variances, or unanticipated problems are identified. In the absence of specific case type criteria for case management intervention, general rules about complications are helpful in determining when to initiate case management services.

TOOLS FOR PSYCHIATRIC CASE MANAGEMENT

Critical pathways, an innovation in care planning technology (see Chapter 43), are a means of defining and communicating standards of care and clinician interventions commonly used to address the needs of a population. Figure 44–2 illustrates the critical pathway and its usual grid format.

Critical pathways represented a breakthrough in care management because, for the first time, actual care could be linked directly to the specific care standards being followed. In addition, the concept of "variance" was introduced in pathways as a means to formally track care along its path and identify its departure from the stated plan. Variance could be attributed to sources, some the agency could control (e.g., care processes, clinician actions, system services, or routines), and others it could not (e.g., patient conditions and community or collateral systems issues). With this knowledge, care-givers can proactively plan an approach to commonly measured variances (e.g., restraint and seclusion) and anticipate how often these might occur.

Table 44–3 illustrates typical mental health variance situations that are identifiable in day-to-day practice. In addition, as critical paths become more refined

Care Category	Time ⟶
1. Assessments/Consults	
2. Specimens/Tests	
3. Treatments	
4. Medications	Caregiver tasks and interventions
5. Diet	
6. Safety/Activity	
7. Teaching/Support	
8. Discharge planning/Coordination	

FIGURE 44–2. The critical pathway.

TABLE 44–3. ILLUSTRATION OF VARIANCE DOCUMENTATION IN ACUTE MENTAL HEALTH PRACTICE

Date	Description of Variance	Reason Code	Corrective Action	Resolution	Initials
1/3/94	Goal: Unit safety/no injury. Substantial risk to others, has positive history, means. Target and expressed verbal intent to harm.	A1	Restraint required	Agreed to room program and contract for safety, released after 2.5 hours.	KMA
1/4/94	Goal: Discharge to home. Family states they do not wish patient to return home: cite fear and anger with patient	A3	Social worker notified. Alternate placements explored with patient. Conditions for return to family home discussed.	⅙ Family meeting held. Family described conditions for patient to return home. Agreed to adjusted discharge date.	RDF

to reflect actual care and best practice, the actual costs of care can begin to be determined. Critical pathways take the guesswork out of the cost of care, something only approximated in the past.

CareMap® tools (Figure 44–3), another advance in case management, measure outcomes as they relate to the tasks and interventions provided (see Chapter 43). The CareMap® format in Table 44–4 illustrates a portion of a grid outlining statements that reflect Standard III outcome criteria. Outcome statements need to be realistic, timed, provide direction for continuity of care, and reflect current scientific knowledge in mental health care.

■ CAREMAP® TOOLS, NURSING DIAGNOSES, AND THE NURSING PROCESS

Nursing diagnostic language has provided psychiatric nurses with descriptive authority to plan care appropriately. Nursing diagnoses become part of the CareMap®

form as the problem statements (or sub-statements in multidisciplinary language maps). Once the nursing diagnoses are determined, the focus of care is clear, shared nurse-client outcomes are identified and the nursing process is used to continuously evaluate the effectiveness of the interventions on the outcomes.

A CareMap® tool provides an opportunity for the entire nursing process to be described in relation to a case management population (Figure 44–4). In addition, the CareMap® and variance analysis are tools for hypothesis testing, as there is an implied predictive or causal relationship between the nursing diagnosis, interventions, and patient outcomes. Research questions can be posed in a manner that the CareMap® tool spatially illustrates, making the assumptions about care approaches and results clear and findable.

Communication systems must be designed to support the flow of information acquired from the critical pathways and the CareMap® tools. For example, formal meetings of the multidisciplinary health care team are often led by the nurse case manager after learning of a serious variance that will affect cost or quality outcomes.

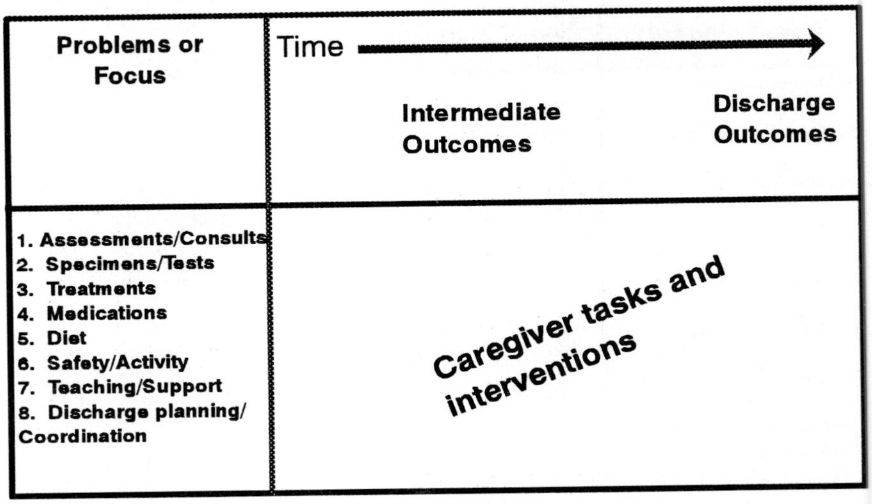

FIGURE 44–3. The CareMap® tool.
CareMap® is a registered trademark and concept of The Center for Case Management.

TABLE 44–4. PARTIAL SAMPLE: BIPOLAR AFFECTIVE DISORDER CAREMAP® TOOL (296.44) DRG 430.

Case type: bipolar affective disorder, 296.44. Description: dysphoric manic episode with psychotic features, high safety risk, may be rapid cycler (>4 episodes per year), requires medication evaluation, may present with noncompliance, financial, legal, or family problems. Length of stay: 10 days.

Problem/Focus	Emergency Room to Admission to Unit/Day 1	Day 2	Day 3	Day 4
1. Reason for admission (individualize)				
2. Pathological coping: safety, impulse control, difficulty functioning, maintaining roles	No injury to self/others; self-destructive impulses managed w/assist. Fam/SO has appts, phone #'s of unit and care-givers for contact. Cooperates with initial behavioral/medical management plan. Accepts meds.	No injury to self/others. Self-destructive impulses managed w/assist. Accepts meds.	No injury to self/others. Self-destructive impulses managed w/assist. Accepts meds.	No injury to self/others. Self-destructive impulses managed w/assist. Accepts meds.
3. Physiological: sleep, appetite, weight loss, increased motor activity	Cooperates with sleep, rest, activity plan w/assistance.	Cooperates with sleep, rest, activity plan w/assistance.	Follows sleep, rest, activity plan.	Follows sleep, rest, activity plan. Physical status stabilized.
4. Delusions (grandeur), denial	Shares thoughts, perceptions as appropriate with staff.	Shares thoughts, perceptions as appropriate with staff.	Shares thoughts, perceptions as appropriate with staff.	Stabilized or diminished psychotic features.
1. Assessment/consults	MD: H & P, med hx. RN: VS BID, Ht, Wt, assess health, nutrition, activity patterns, mental status, strengths, coping. Family/support hx. Nutrition consult prn. Medical consult prn. Psychopharm consult prn.	MD: evaluate for ECT.		
2. Specimens/tests	Routine admission labs, toxic screen, med levels.			
3. Treatments: Groups prescribed as appropriate for reasons for hospitalization	Destimulation program; compensatory health, diet, rest interventions.	Destimulation program. Compensatory health, diet, rest interventions. Groups as tol.	Destimulation program. Compensatory health, diet, rest interventions. Groups as tol.	Destimulation program. Compensatory health, diet, rest interventions. Groups as tol.
4. Medications	MD: med hx. RN: Collect meds brought in.	Med hx available, target s/s identified, initial antimanic regimen begun.		
5. Nutrition/diet: push fluids, finger foods unless contraindicated	Diet.	Diet.	Diet.	Diet.
6. Safety/activity	Unit restrict, routine checks, safety and impulse contracts negotiated. Introduce verbal and behavioral strategies.	Assess for level 1 privileges.	Level 1 privileges.	Level 1 privileges.
7. Teaching/support	Orient to room, staff, unit rules, boundaries. Offer support and consistency (avoid excessive verbal interventions until mania subsides).	Review/reinforce information as necessary. Orient to room, staff, unit rules, boundaries, meds. Offer support and consistency (avoid excessive verbal interventions until mania subsides).	Review/reinforce info as necessary: unit rules, boundaries, meds. Offer support and consistency (avoid excessive verbal interventions until mania subsides).	
8. Discharge planning	Contact w/fam/SO, information given	Contact out-patient care-givers.		Collaborative team meeting.

SO = Significant Other
H & P = History and Physical
VS = Vital Signs
Andolina K., Copyright CCM (1994)

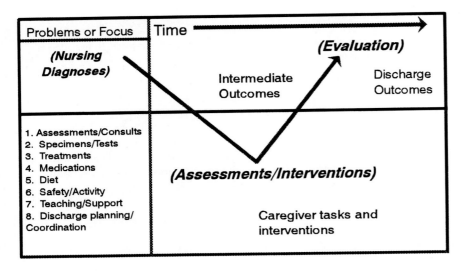

FIGURE 44–4.   The CareMap® tool and the nursing process. CareMap® is a registered trademark and concept of The Center for Case Management.

Case consultation, as a formal or informal method for problem solving, is used by the psychiatric nurse who seeks collaborative input from a peer or colleague.

■ MANAGERIAL LEADERSHIP AND SUPPORT

Managerial leadership and support for psychiatric nurse case managers is pivotal to full realization of the role. Psychiatric nurses do not require excessive supervision, making them efficient and cost-effective care providers, but they will require assistance in the areas that are not their expertise or where administrative assistance is required. Supports such as secretarial assistance, follow-up phone tracking, printing or copying services are often required by nurse case managers. If the case managers are given no resource allocation au-

thority, nurse managers are critical to seeing that these supports are given to case managers as needed to fulfill the requirements of the job. In addition, continuing education requirements for case managers must be planned and implemented as needs dictate. It is essential that nurse managers see themselves as coaches, critical evaluators, standard bearers and innovators for the nurse case managers they are supervising and for the case management programs they may be overseeing.

■ ASPECTS OF THE PSYCHIATRIC CASE MANAGEMENT ROLE

ACCOUNTABILITY

Psychiatric nurse case managers face simultaneous accountability issues for cost, quality, and advocacy. For ex-

E CASE EXAMPLE

Kim, an adolescent, is admitted to an in-patient setting from a residential facility. She was acutely suicidal and behaviorally disruptive at the residential facility, precipitating the inpatient admission. Care planning, however, slows to a stop when it is discovered that the residential facility time line for care planning evaluation is conducted every 30 days. This conflicts with the in-patient facility's continuous care evaluation strategy and requires quick intervention from the psychiatric nurse case manager. The nurse case manager calls a health care team meeting, invites residential staff, obtains input from Kim and quickly establishes realistic goals. The goals include setting a new discharge

date, determining intermediate goals, and organizing timed treatment interventions at key points along the way. Prior to clinical case management, accountability for negotiating appropriate discharge planning and in-patient treatment goals would have been assumed by various members of the treatment team, with perhaps little cohesive follow-up and follow-through from 1 day to the next. The nurse case manager, in this example, uses all the requisite skills to establish a realistic care plan that defines specific accountabilities and leads to realistic outcomes for the patient.

ample, they are accountable to the patient and family for outcomes and to the system that employs them to be responsible cost managers. Case managers understand that while there may be no unrealistic outcomes, only unrealistic time frames, the reality is that patient outcomes are often the result of an extensive negotiation. To successfully navigate the hazards associated with unrealistic expectations, all negotiated outcomes must be made clear to all care providers and supported. The case manager is the person to identify conflicting agendas and then act to address the conflict as early as possible.

PSYCHOTHERAPY ROLE CONFLICT

Nurse therapists who provide psychotherapy may experience role conflict when case management services are required. In providing psychotherapy services, the relationship of the psychiatric nurse therapist to the patient and family is as a provider of therapeutic interventions. Case management is a different service than psychotherapy. Case management involves the nurse on one level as a broker, procurer, linkage, and continuity manager and on another level, as a translator, negotiator, and evaluator of appropriate and realistic outcomes. Case management services are required at the point where linkage to psychotherapy is required or when the patient requires treatment changes.

Nurses who are not comfortable switching roles may choose to set up a referral relationship with other case managers who can provide that service when required. In inpatient settings, the most similar relationship to modern day case management was the therapist–administrator split. In this relationship, the patient was provided with a separate person (the case administrator) to deal with issues related to time, resources, and satisfaction. Similar to clinical case managers of today, the role was activated only when the care process became complex. Therapist–administrator splits were a strategy for severe regression, patient acting out, or when multiple, competing family issues were evident. Despite its contrary image, the therapist–administrator split was not really a split at all. Indeed, the therapist and case administrator worked collaboratively to keep the treatment moving forward in a manner that preserved the patient and family relationship with the care providers and kept the treatment focused on results.

PARAMETERS OF THE ROLE

Some of the most thorny issues in defining a psychiatric nurse case manager role have to do with determining the parameters of the role. Nurses today are more accustomed to wearing multiple hats in the course of a day. It would not be unusual for the psychiatric nurse to be the primary care nurse for some patients, a group psychotherapist within the treatment community, a psychotherapist for some, and a case manager for others. Keeping the roles straight in the nurse's own mind becomes as much of a challenge as communicating which role is being enacted at any one time. Nevertheless, case management is enacted and defined in different ways. In most instances, the responsibilities of case management are provided by one person acting in the role; however, when case management responsibilities are divided between different providers, the role is shared. In shared role case management, communication strategies are even more important and require formal definition.

SCOPE OF THE ROLE IN THE CONTINUUM

In addition to defining who functions in the role and in what capacity, psychiatric nurse case managers must define the scope of their role as well. Cohen and Cesta (1993) described case management as "within-the-walls" and "beyond-the-walls" models. Within-the-walls case management models have been developed using different frameworks, such as primary nursing, unit based, clinical ladder programs or nurse-technician partnered models. Beyond-the-walls case management models focus on the role of the community-based nurse case manager as both a care coordinator and provider of prevention and health maintenance services. The ability of within-the-walls case managers to continue to case manage patients beyond-the-walls of the facility may be based more on the nurse's desire than on the facility intent. Case management beyond traditional geographic boundaries incurs costs that must be anticipated in order to provide a case management service that truly spans the continuum.

ENHANCED COLLABORATIVE PRACTICE

Case managers, by possessing the skills that enable them to perform the role in a high-quality manner, bring added value to team functioning. Collaborative practices are enhanced when psychiatric nurse case managers address issues in practice that interfere with getting patients to outcomes. Through effective use of the health care team meetings and case consultations, team functioning is strengthened.

STRENGTHENED CARE EVALUATION

Nurse case managers with nursing process skills provide the link between problem detection and critical evaluation of results. Psychiatric nurse case managers track the results of care through formal reporting mechanisms, such as indicator tracking, variance analysis, or outcome measurements. Nurse case managers are able to define the results of the treatment process in language that is understood by both patients and families and clinicians. Once patient outcomes are measured and tracked over time, nurse case managers as cost and quality leaders are able to identify strategies that sustain results and support care approaches that consistently succeed.

OPPORTUNITIES FOR RESEARCH

In order for psychiatric nurses to thrive in this role, its impact on patient outcomes and the nursing profession must be researched. Many role studies exist in the nursing literature that provide qualitative and quantitative methods for studying role theory, adaptation, evolution, and enhancement. The psychiatric nurse case manager role could be studied through these methods of nursing research. Descriptive studies, including case studies, that describe the characteristics and attributes of psychiatric nurse case managers offer a grounding point for identifying how prevalent the role is in practice today. Correlation studies that link role functioning with sustained cost, quality, and patient access outcomes represent another level of research, as well as studies that test effectiveness of case management tools and strategies that enhance and support the role. Studies are needed that connect psychiatric nursing case management specifically to cost benefits. In addition, descriptive studies on characteristics of recipient populations, complex care individuals, and the correlating nursing diagnoses will clarify characteristics of patients who benefit the most from psychiatric nursing case management. Psychiatric nursing case management requires research to test its scope, application, and limits as a potential model that bridges population-based care to individual-based care.

○ AN OVERVIEW

- Case manager activities emphasize achieving and sustaining patient-centered outcomes.

- The absence of a practice model that promotes collaborative, outcome-based practice dooms achievement to mere chance.

- Critical pathways and CareMaps® are tools that the nurse uses to define and communicate standards of care and health care team interventions.

- Psychiatric nurses who practice case management, whether as a distinct role or as a value-added aspect to the professional nursing approach, use it to integrate clinical art with practical necessity.

- Patient-centered, outcome-focused case management offers the best opportunity for psychiatric nurses to act as patient advocates and work with multiple systems and providers to establish cost-effective systems in which quality care is delivered.

- When psychiatric nurses add case management to their skill inventory, they establish themselves as highly visible, effective care managers.

- Psychiatric nurse visibility in emerging care delivery systems will be critical for the systems to thrive.

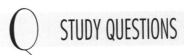

TD TERMS TO DEFINE

- care coordination

- case consultation

- case manager

- patient-centered outcomes

- population-based care

- therapist-administrator split

Q STUDY QUESTIONS

Liz is a 42-year-old single white female with major mental illness subject to exacerbations that occasionally require hospitalization. She resides in a residential facility and presently is in an acute care setting for striking a staff member following a disagreement about limits. She denies depression and psychosis, and is not delusional. As the assigned RN, you notice that Liz is typical of many patients admitted to acute care these days. The reason for admission is not based on psychiatric need, but rather on the side effects of having a major mental illness: poor judgment, insight, social skills, and behavioral control.

1. What complexities does Liz and her situation present that may lend themselves to a case management approach?

2. What cost concerns does Liz present as a patient with chronic mental illness?

3. Why would a nurse be appropriate as a case manager for Liz?

4. Name three outcomes that case management would focus on for Liz and patients like her.

5. What specific skills would be useful for a nurse case manager to have in case managing chronically mentally ill patients?

6. How would a nurse case manager monitor the progress Liz is making, and how far past discharge would case managers wish to follow Liz or anyone from a similar case type?

7. Describe the network of resources that would be appropriate to coordinate during this episode of care. How would you interact with those resources where you have no formal jurisdiction, such as the residential setting and the staff who work the night shift there?

8. Describe how the nurse will obtain support in the case management role. To whom should the nurse case manager report? How should the nurse case manager be evaluated and on what skills?

■ REFERENCES

American Nurses Association. *A Statement on Psychiatric-Mental Health Clinical Nursing Practice and Standards of Psychiatric and Mental Health Clinical Nursing Practice.* Washington, DC: American Nurses Publishing; 1994:23–31.

Bower KA Case management: Work redesign with patient outcomes in mind. In *Patient-Centered Hospital Care: Reform from Within.* Ann Arbour, Mi: Health Administration Press, 1993.

Cohen EL, Cesta TG. *Nursing Case Management: From Concept to Evaluation.* St. Louis: Mosby; 1993:36–46.

Zander K. *The New Definition.* South Natick, Mass: The Center for Case Management; 1995:1–2.

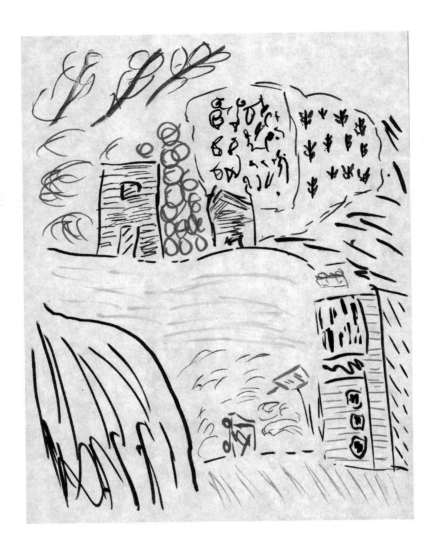

It was one of those delightfully irregular houses where you go up and down steps out of one room into another, and where you come upon more rooms when you think you have seen all there are, and where there is a bountiful provision of little halls and passages. . . .

Bleak House, Chapter 6
Charles Dickens, 1812–1870

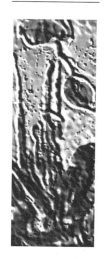

45

Psychiatric Home Health Care

Verna Benner Carson

It has long been known that at home, surrounded by family and possessions, an individual may respond to health care interventions with a more peaceful spirit and greater willingness of mind and body (Benner, 1992; Casserta, 1993; Carson, 1994b; Carson, 1995). Yet formalized psychiatric care in the home did not begin until 1979 when Medicare agreed to reimburse home care agencies for providing psychiatric home care. Prior to this time, community health and home care nurses did assist new families and patients suffering from medical disorders to cope with the psychological stresses caused by situational depression and anxiety, grief, bonding, and parenting issues, but the seriously mentally ill were more than likely cared for in large state facilities.

When Medicare began to reimburse patients for psychiatric home care, the deinstitutionalization movement was well under way. As more patients were moved into the community, psychiatric providers became increasingly aware that many communities and families were woefully ill prepared to welcome the mentally ill into their midst. Models of community-based care were developed that moved individuals into less restrictive settings. Psychiatric home care emerged to ensure that the continuum of care was truly comprehensive.

■ WHAT IS PSYCHIATRIC HOME CARE?

Psychiatric home health care provides a bridge to ease the transition of patients leaving the hospital and moving back into their homes, as well as an anchor to assist the patient to remain in the home when stress threatens to destabilize the patient's situation (Carson, et al., 1994; Carson, 1995). Generally, psychiatric home care is viewed as intermittent and transitional, rather than continuous or long term.

■ WHAT ARE THE GOALS OF PSYCHIATRIC HOME CARE?

The overall goals of psychiatric home care are to shorten or prevent expensive hospitalizations, improve the patient's quality of life, and maximize the patient's potential to live at home (*Home Care Guidelines*, 1981; Duffy et al., 1993; Frisch, 1993; Harris, 1993; Carson et al., 1994; Carson, 1995). Specific interventions to achieve these goals include

- Support of the individual and family to assist them to cope with the symptoms of a psychiatric illness.
- Provide respite to families and responsible caretakers from continuous care of psychiatrically impaired persons.
- Act as an educational resource to the patient, family, or significant other on such issues as medication and diet regimens, interpersonal and communication strategies, and individual coping techniques.
- Intervene psychotherapeutically to maintain patients at their maximal functional level and retard further deterioration.
- Assist the patient to develop appropriate social interaction skills.
- Assist the patient to develop appropriate diversional activities.
- Provide support and follow-up services to patients residing in their own home or with a family member.
- Coordinate the needed services of other community-based health and social services.
- Facilitate the transition of emotionally and psychiatrically impaired individuals from acute and long-term facilities to family care or to other community-based living arrangements.
- Assist the homebound patient to achieve a spiritual sense of well-being by finding purpose in his or her present situation and by accessing spiritual resources within the environment.
- Define the mental health needs of patients to the nonpsychiatric medical community.

- Collaborate with nursing schools to provide educational experiences for future mental health professionals.

Collaborative strategies are implemented within the home care system to increase the patient's level of independence and decrease the effects of existing disabilities. Noninstitutional therapeutic and supportive services are used (Holland, 1993; Klebanoff and Casler, 1986; Carson et al., 1994; 1994b; 1995).

■ A MODEL FOR PSYCHIATRIC CARE

Several authors have suggested models for psychiatric home care, including crisis intervention (Aguilera, 1990) and Orem's (1991) self-care models; however, neither is adequate for psychiatric home care. A more appropriate model—**Carson's Model of Psychiatric Home Care**—uses the structure of a home to illustrate this type of care.

The foundation of the home model is a moral or spiritual one. The nurse approaches the patient as a person of worth, deserving of care and respect, and in full recognition that the patient is not only a biopsychosocial person but a person with spiritual needs that must be attended to. These needs include the patient's desire to relate to an ultimate other, to make sense out of the illness, and to answer questions, such as "Why am I here?" "What is my purpose?" "Does my life matter?" and "Do I make a difference?" (Pellegrino, 1985; Benner, 1992; Carson et al., 1994).

The walls of the home are constructed with relationship and assessment skills. A detailed, focused assessment (described later in this chapter) is performed when care begins, and it continues as long as the nurse is involved in the patient's life. The development of a relationship is one of the nurse's primary goals in the beginning stages of working with the patient. An alliance, or therapeutic connection, is critical to patient compliance with home care interventions. A relationship in which no alliance has been established between the patient and nurse makes other interventions inconsequential.

The second floor of the home consists of medication issues. There, the nurse must address the following concerns:

- Patient compliance.
- Patient knowledge about prescribed medications.
- Administration of parenteral medications.
- Drawing blood samples to determine the serum levels of medications, such as Tegretol, lithium, and nortriptyline.

The roof of the home is composed of teaching or psychotherapeutic interventions and case management skills. As has been stated, several steps are implemented before teaching, counseling, supportive therapy, and case management begin. A patient's strengths and deficits have been assessed; a relationship has been developed that is built on trust, caring, empathy, and mutual respect; and the patient has been assisted in establishing a regimen of care.

In case management, the patient is linked with a support system of other people, care is coordinated with other providers, and inefficiencies in care are eliminated. In addition, the nurse helps to create an order in the patient's life—a life that has often been chaotic.

This model of care is comprehensive and oriented to caring and maximizing the patient's potential. It gives the nurse direction in providing psychiatric care; the patient feels cared about, more stable within the confines of a psychiatric illness, and more connected to a community of support.

■ WHO PROVIDES PSYCHIATRIC HOME CARE?

Psychiatric home care is provided through state-licensed and Medicare-certified home care agencies. In addition, some states allow agencies to offer a single service, such as psychiatric home care. These single service agencies are not Medicare certified and cannot serve the Medicare population.

The exact number of agencies that offer psychiatric home care is unknown. Medicare combines all types of nursing under the category of skilled nursing, and neither the Medicare intermediaries (Blue Cross/Blue Shield, Prudential, Aetna, etc.) who process Medicare claims nor the Health Care Financing Administration (HCFA) maintain statistics relative to the specialty of psychiatric nursing. It is clear, however, from the growing number of home care conferences that include significant content on psychiatric home care and from the increasing body of literature focused on this specialty that there is growing interest among home care providers to add psychiatric nursing to their home services.

■ WHAT IS DRIVING THE INTEREST IN PSYCHIATRIC HOME CARE?

Three forces have increased the numbers of psychiatric patients among those individuals receiving home health care. The first of these forces is the increased public awareness of the benefits of home health care. **The National Alliance for the Mentally Ill (NAMI)** has been especially effective in lobbying state legislatures, as well as Congress, to provide a wider range of care alternatives for the mentally ill. In Maryland, NAMI was instrumental in having a mental health parity bill passed in the summer of 1994. This bill will ensure that psychiatric patients receive equal insurance coverage as patients with other, nonpsychiatric disabilities.

Second, the population needing home health services, and specifically psychiatric services, such as the dependent elderly, is growing dramatically.

The third and most important trend is the cost-containment pressures that have led to patients being discharged from in-patient units "quicker and sicker." Home care, specifically psychiatric home care, is a bargain; a rule of thumb is that the cost of four home visits is the equivalent of the cost of room and board for one inpatient day.

The population using psychiatric home health care is quite varied in age and needs; consequently, a broad range of professional and supportive services should be available. Professional services include direct nursing care provided by a psychiatric nurse to patients with primary DSM-IV Axis I psychiatric diagnoses or emotional problems that develop secondary to a medical diagnosis (for example, depression secondary to a cardiovascular accident). It also includes access to medical nursing skills; dental care; pharmaceutical and social services; physical, speech, and occupational therapies; laboratory testing; and nutritional advice.

Supportive home care services include the provision of a homemaker, home health aide, and durable medical equipment and supplies (Holland, 1993).

■ WHO PAYS FOR PSYCHIATRIC HOME CARE?

For patients meeting the eligibility criteria, psychiatric home care is reimbursed 100% under Medicare and Medicaid. The criteria included in **reimbursement policies** are:

- The patient must be psychiatrically homebound, which does not mean bedbound or physically immobile. Instead, it means that the patient has a significant psychological vulnerability that interferes with the patient's ability to independently and consistently access psychiatric follow-up. Diagnoses that might define patients as psychiatrically homebound are severe depression; agoraphobia; schizophrenia; dementia with psychotic features, depressed moods, or both; or bipolar illness, depressed or manic type.

- The patient must have a DSM-IV psychiatric diagnosis.
- The patient must require the skills of a psychiatric nurse.
- The patient must be under the care of a physician.

Phrases describing **homebound status** are

- Mobility impaired.
- Unable to leave home without assistance from others.
- Leaves home on rare occasions or leaving home requires taxing effort.
- Confused, disoriented, or lacks judgment.
- Psychomotor retardation due to severe depression.
- Altered perception or cognition.
- Altered thought processes.
- Potential for self-harm or harm to others.
- Poor impulse control.
- Impaired social interactions.
- Excessive fear, anxiety, or both.

Since Medicare began reimbursing charges for psychiatric services, other funding sources have developed. Although some states have eliminated their Medicaid benefits for home care, Medicaid follows criteria similar to Medicare's to determine eligibility for services, as well as qualifications for nurse providers. Funding is also available from the Veterans Administration (VA). The VA's guidelines governing eligibility for services and qualifications of psychiatric nurses are similar to those used by Medicare. Each VA field office, however, must be contacted to verify approval for psychiatric home health care prior to initiating a service.

Third-party reimbursement varies widely, and each insurance company must be contacted to verify its policies regarding reimbursement for psychiatric home care. Because insurance companies reimburse (partially or completely) charges for the services of a psychiatric nurse who is certified as a clinical specialist, some home health care agencies have set up a professional organization for their psychiatric nurse providers and allow them to bill private insurance companies. The resistance of private insurance companies to reimburse for psychiatric home health services is dissipating as research continues to document the cost effectiveness of home- versus hospital-based psychiatric care.

Increasingly, managed care companies are using psychiatric home care, especially for patients who have traditionally been frequent users of in-patient services. Although managed care companies may oversee the care provided to Medicare and Medicaid patients, the companies are not bound by the same eligibility criteria imposed by Medicare and Medicaid. The primary criteria for managed care is that the patient has failed traditional modes of psychiatric care and uses a significant amount of health care dollars. Psychiatric home health care services are also available to patients who pay for the service. Service is usually initiated by obtaining a contract signed by the patient indicating the patient's willingness to assume the cost of skilled nursing visits.

■ WHO CAN PROVIDE PSYCHIATRIC HOME CARE?

Medicare states that psychiatric nursing care must be delivered by "a psychiatrically trained nurse who has special training and/or experience beyond the standard curriculum for an R.N. Referral can come from any physician." (Health Care Financing Administration: Home Health and Hospice Manual Regulations and Guidelines {HIM-11}, 1996). Medicare reviews the resumes of every psychiatric nurse before certifying the nurse as qualified to deliver psychiatric services. Medicare requirements for psychiatric nurses are

- A registered nurse with a master's degree in psychiatric or community mental health nursing.
- A registered nurse with a BSN degree and 1 year of related work experience in an active treatment program for adult or geriatric patients in a psychiatric health care setting.
- A registered nurse with a diploma or AD degree and 2 years of related work experience in an active treatment program for adult or geriatric patients in a psychiatric health care setting.
- Certification by the American Nurses Association in psychiatric or community health nursing.
- Other qualifications may be considered on an individual basis.

Managed care companies require a credentialing process for the home care agency as a whole and for each nurse provider. These companies usually limit credentialing of nurses to those who hold advanced nursing degrees.

■ WHO BENEFITS FROM PSYCHIATRIC HOME CARE?

THE ELDERLY

Most referrals for psychiatric home health services are for the elderly. It is the largest subpopulation in the United States using home care services. In the last two decades, the population of persons older than 65 years has increased more than twice as fast as that of persons younger than 65 (Rice and Feldman, 1983; Research

E CASE EXAMPLE

Mrs. Clark has cardiac bypass surgery. After surgery, she develops a depression that is diagnosed as an adjustment disorder.

While still in the hospital, Mrs. Clark is started on Prozac, an antidepressant. At the time of discharge, she is still very sad and not motivated to engage in the cardiac rehabilitation program offered by the hospital. A psychiatric home health nurse begins working with her. The nurse's focus is to help Mrs. Clark resolve her feelings of sadness and despair, facilitate Mrs. Clark's integration of this experience into the totality of her life story, support Mrs. Clark in her rehabilitation program, and monitor Mrs. Clark's compliance with and response to the Prozac.

Initially, Mrs. Clark is seen by the nurse three times a week with visits gradually decreasing to once every other week. After 4 months, Mrs. Clark is discharged from home health care, fully engaged in her cardiac rehabilitation, actively participating in a local senior center, and completely free of depression.

News, 1984; Eliopoulos, 1991, 1993). As people live longer, they use health services more to contend with the demands and limitations imposed by chronic illness. It is estimated that over 80% of the elderly have chronic diseases, and at least 50% of that number suffer physical and social limitations as a result. Many will face multiple hospitalizations to treat exacerbations of chronic conditions. This population is the primary beneficiary of all types of home health care services, including psychiatric services (Lesseig, 1987; Harris, 1993).

A major concern of the elderly is that they will become unable to cope with their conditions at home and be forced into institutions. This fear could be alleviated by providing the elderly with home health care support. Such support allows the elderly to continue to derive a sense of meaning and purpose from their lives even though their activities may become more restricted.

PATIENTS WITH ACUTE PSYCHIATRIC DISORDERS

Another group benefiting from psychiatric home health services are patients who have been treated in an acute care facility (Lehman and Kelley, 1993; Rice, 1993) but no longer require the 24-hour supervision of a hospital. They do, however, need intense monitoring once they return home. They may be seen daily by a psychiatric nurse who will assist them in making the transition from hospital to home.

THE SERIOUSLY AND PERSISTENTLY MENTALLY ILL

The seriously and persistently mentally ill are another group who benefit from home health care services. Research has demonstrated that home health care decreases the total number of days that the chronically mentally ill are hospitalized and presumably improves the quality of their adjustment to the home and community (Stein and Diamond, 1985; Goering et al., 1988; Raschko, 1988; Wasylenski, et al., 1985; Dickstein et al., 1988; Bush et al., 1990). Other studies document the cost effectiveness of home versus hospital psychiatric care (Fenton et al., 1979, 1982). A central home health services department may be established within a hospital to provide continuity of care between the inpatient unit and the patient and patient's family. The case example of Mr. Johnson on page 822 illustrates the effectiveness of psychiatric home care.

THE AIDS PATIENT

A relatively new group of home care patients are those with AIDS, who require not only intensive medical supervision but also psychiatric therapy as they deal with depression, anxiety, grief, and AIDS-related dementia (Barrick, 1988; Carson et al., 1994; 1994a; 1994b; 1994c; 1994d; and 1995). The case example of David on page 822 illustrates this type of patient.

THE YOUNG CHILD

Children are a small but growing number of home health care recipients. They are seen in their homes for continued individual therapy and to help their families deal with problematic behaviors in the home environment. Usually, when children require treatment for acute psychiatric problems, the hospital stay is not long enough for the family to learn workable strategies for dealing with difficult behaviors. During visits, the psychiatric nurse can work directly with the child and family to develop communication and behavioral techniques that will be effective within their life situations, and can assist the family to discover a sense of meaning and significance in their efforts to raise a healthy child.

E CASE EXAMPLE

Mr. Johnson, who is 35 years old, is treated repeatedly for acute episodes of chronic paranoid schizophrenia. His psychiatric history includes multiple admissions usually precipitated by exacerbations of his illness where he became verbally and physically threatening to his elderly mother and father. His parents usually obtain an involuntary admission to force Mr. Johnson into much needed treatment. After a brief stay where he is stabilized, he is returned to his parents. He continues to take his medication for 1 or 2 months, then abruptly stops. His use of follow-up mental health appointments has a similar pattern.

After this scenario has been repeated five times, the hospital staff refers Mr. Johnson for psychiatric home health care. The nurse assesses Mr. Johnson's primary needs would require the nurse to encourage medication compliance and psychiatric follow-up, increase Mr. Johnson's involvement in diversional activities, and teach his parents more effective coping strategies.

Home health care continues for 6 months. At that time, Mr. Johnson is still out of the hospital, involved in an adult day treatment center three times a week, compliant with taking his medications, and getting along fairly well with his mother and father. In addition, his network of family support expresses a sense of their own importance to the welfare of Mr. Johnson as a result of the nurse's focus on providing them with support.

■ THE PRACTICE OF PSYCHIATRIC HOME CARE

The entry level psychiatric home care nurse is guided by the 1994 Standards of Psychiatric Practice, which encompass the nursing process (Coalition of Psychiatric Nursing Organizations, 1994). The standards are discussed in detail in various chapters, but a synopsis of the standards of psychiatric nursing practice follows.

    I. Assessment.
   II. Diagnosis (DSM IV and NANDA).
  III. Outcome identification.

   IV. Planning.
    V(a). Counseling.
    V(b). Milieu maintenance.
    V(c). Improving skills in activities of daily living.
    V(d). Psychobiological interventions.
    V(e). Health teaching.
    V(f). Case management.
    V(g). Health promotion and health maintenance.
   V(i)–V(j). Apply to advanced practice psychiatric nurses.
   VI. Evaluation.

E CASE EXAMPLE

David, a 25-year-old man diagnosed with AIDS, was being treated the fifth time for *Pneumocystis carinii* pneumonia (PCP). It was during this admission that David's significant other and the nursing staff became aware of behavioral and cognitive changes in David. He was forgetful, irritable, displayed emotional lability, and expressed profound sadness about his impending death and his sense that he "counted for nothing." On one occasion, he became angry when a nurse asked what he had eaten from his breakfast tray. He stated, "I can't remember. . . . Just stop asking me these stupid questions!" The medical staff, after a thorough neurological evaluation, determined that David is suffering from AIDS-related dementia and depression. David's significant other expresses serious concern regarding his ability to continue to manage David at home. As part of the discharge plan, the healthcare team refers David for psychiatric home care.

The nurse who visits David identifies the need for several interventions: to monitor David's safety and his ability to comply with his medication regimen; to work with his significant other to ensure that David's environment is safe given his deteriorating cognitive capabilities; to assist David to find meaning and value in his life; and to help the significant other, David's primary care provider, to continue responding to David in the most helpful, loving manner. The nurse augments her visits with the services of a home health aide who provides daily physical care to David. In addition, the nurse arranges to have a hospital bed provided for David so that he can remain on the first floor of his home. This care continues for 3 months, at which time David is readmitted with another bout of PCP.

David dies during this admission; however, David's care provider expresses gratitude to the psychiatric nurse for helping him make David's last days of life more meaningful.

Although the standards are the same across nursing settings, nurses' approaches may differ. Within the hospital, the nurse has greater authority and control; whereas in the home, the nurse is the patient's guest, which may influence how a nurse assesses a patient or recommends treatment. To be able to work in what is an atypical clinical setting, the nurse must be more innovative and flexible. For example, the patient's home may be crowded, dirty, and noisy, and interruptions may be frequent. The nurse may not be able to change these situations but will instead have to work around them.

ASSESSMENT OF THE PATIENT'S NEEDS

In the home, the nurse is usually the only health care practitioner present; therefore, the nurse must be able to perform a holistic assessment of the patient. In addition to a physical assessment of, for example, vital signs, weight, heart and breath sounds, the nurse evaluates the patient's mental status (Frisch, 1993; Carson et al., 1994; 1994a) as to:

- Orientation.
- Judgment.
- Insight.
- Ability to abstract.
- Recent and remote memory.
- General level of knowledge.
- Attention and concentration.
- Thought content.
- Suicidal or homicidal ideation, intent, or lethality.

To assess family dynamics is also critical for the psychiatric home care nurse. While providing care within the home setting, the nurse is better able to develop a collaborative relationship with the family. To capitalize on this collaborative opportunity, the nurse must understand the many ways that families respond.

Social support is important for the nurse to consider. People who have adequate social support systems are able to deal with stress more constructively. Social support benefits people in two ways: First, it is a buffer that reduces the stress of a crisis; and second, it has a direct effect in that self-esteem and confidence are increased when a person is a member of a socially cohesive group (Carson, et al., 1994). Also, who is available to assist the patient with activities of daily living? With finances? With emotional support? With companionship? With transportation?

Whether or not the patient is able to perform daily chores is assessed. The ability to perform tasks usually corresponds with the severity of cognitive impairment documented in testing. A discrepancy between the testing and actual functioning may occur, however (Wein-

traub, et al., 1985). For example, a depressed elderly person may perform tasks well in the structured, supportive testing environment, but lack the motivation to perform daily chores. Formal testing of cognitive functioning sheds little light on exactly how real-life activities are impaired. For example, a patient's inability to dress her- or himself may be related to apathy, a spatial defect, or inability to sequence the necessary steps. The nurse's assessment of the nature of the impairment has important implications for management.

A natural extension of the assessment of the patient's functional abilities is whether or not the patient can live safely at home alone. If the answer is no, options other than institutionalization are worth exploring. They include a homemaker service and supervised housing arrangements.

The patient's physical needs are assessed by the nurse. The services of a nurse specialist, a physical therapist, and a home health aide may all be warranted. The nurse making the assessment writes an order for these services. The order is reviewed and signed by the referring physician. The case study about Mrs. Brandt is an example of a patient with such needs on page 824.

Standardized assessment tools to measure depression, anxiety, psychotic symptoms, movement disorders, and spiritual well-being are used by the psychiatric home care nurse. At the time a patient is admitted to home care, the tools are used to obtain a score that serves as a concrete baseline measure. Their continued use allows the nurse to track patient changes in psychiatric symptomatology that occur throughout care. The tools also facilitate communication between the home care nurse and the psychiatrist, as well as between the home care nurse and the third party payer.

DIAGNOSIS

The diagnostic step involves understanding the DSM-IV and the nursing diagnosis system (NANDA). Psychiatric home care nurses compare the assessment data that they collect with what they know from the DSM-IV. Sometimes a patient's behaviors do not match the criteria of the DSM-IV diagnosis that the patient has received. In such cases, nurses share the findings with the referring psychiatrist; frequently, the psychiatrist modifies the diagnosis to coincide with the nursing observations.

The DSM-IV is a guide for labeling and categorizing specific symptoms, but it sheds no light on the individual patient's or family's particular coping styles, suffering, unique problems in dealing with the DSM-IV diagnosis, or strengths in the midst of turmoil and pain. The DSM-IV criteria, however, is not sufficient ba-

E CASE EXAMPLE

Mrs. Brandt is referred for psychiatric home care because she is depressed with multiple physical problems. Her medical concerns are left-sided weakness from a previous stroke, legal blindness from diabetic retinopathy, a history of cardiac bypass surgery, the fear of impending gastrointestinal surgery, and chronic back pain. In assessing Mrs. Brandt, the nurse discovers that Mrs. Brandt fell from her wheelchair twice in the previous 2 weeks. Following her stroke, Mrs. Brandt did not receive physical therapy and did not know safe transfer techniques. In addition, her knowledge regarding the management of her

diabetes is inadequate. Given this data, the psychiatric nurse orders the services of a physical therapist to teach Mrs. Brandt safe transferring techniques and a home health nurse to teach the patient about diabetes, insulin administration, and adherence to a diabetic diet. By recognizing the needs of Mrs. Brandt other than her psychiatric needs and seeking appropriate resources, the psychiatric nurse helps ensure comprehensive care for the patient. In addition, the psychiatric nurse is able to focus on Mrs. Brandt's depression.

---

sis for nurses to determine a plan of action. NANDA diagnoses, on the other hand, address the individuality of the patient and family and provide direction for nursing care.

For example, Tom Young is diagnosed with schizophrenia, chronic paranoid type. He can be expected to display certain behaviors as outlined by the DSM-IV. No information is provided regarding Tom's supportive family, his perseverance in maintaining a job, nor his involvement in a community mental health support group. The death of Tom's father has precipitated Tom's most recent relapse. A nurse working with Tom might identify a nursing diagnosis as:

Ineffective grieving related to inability to adequately express feelings of sadness and loss as evidenced by delusional thoughts of having killed his father.

Contrast Tom's situation with that of Margie Wallace, an elderly patient who suffers from dementia and lives alone with little social support. The nurse in analyzing data identifies a major safety issue that may necessitate the involvement of community services, including Adult Protective Services, an agency charged with protecting vulnerable adults from harm. One of the nursing diagnoses for Margie Wallace might be:

High risk for self-harm related to memory impairment for recent events as evidenced by repeatedly leaving the stove on and taking twice the amount of prescribed medication because patient forgot that she had taken previous dose.

OUTCOME IDENTIFICATION

Outcome identification is becoming increasingly important to third-party payers who demand to know what the results of psychiatric interventions will be. They are no

longer willing to pay for "improving a patient's ability to express feelings" or "to increase insight regarding early trauma." They are considered "soft issues" and not measurable. Soft outcomes, however, can be restated in concrete terms that are measurable. For example, an outcome statement might read "the patient will state three reasons for expressing negative feelings," and "the patient will, on at least three consecutive occasions, express his feelings rather than act out his feelings in a violent manner" are both acceptable outcomes. Psychiatric home care nurses usually establish outcomes that focus on what the patient, care provider, and family has learned and what the patient, care provider, and family can demonstrate through behavior.

PLANNING

When planning care, the psychiatric home care nurse works with the patient, other care providers, and the family to establish short-term goals. Through collaboration, priorities for care are determined, aspects of the patient's care delegated, and referrals made. Decisions are also made as to how the patient's care should be managed. In one patient situation, for example, the nurse may have assessed that a 77-year-old man diagnosed with a stroke is unable to independently complete the activities of daily living (ADLs) of meeting hygiene needs and preparing simple meals. These needs have a high priority because of their potential threat to his physical well-being. The nurse delegates the ADLs care to a home care aide, who is instructed to encourage a family member to supervise the patient completing these two daily functions. The nurse also makes a referral for Meals on Wheels to ensure that the patient receives adequate nutrition. The nurse manages the patient's care by coordinating the services of the home care aide and the Meals on Wheels providers with the psychiatric care that the nurse is directly providing to the patient.

INTERVENTIONS

Many different types of interventions may be carried out by the psychiatric home care nurse.

- **Counseling:** supportive interventions, such as teaching problem-solving skills, behavior modification, assertiveness training, relaxation skills, coping skills, and stress reduction strategies.
- **Milieu Maintenance:** ensuring that the home environment is safe and that the patient is not victimized physically, financially, or emotionally.
- **Improving Patient Self-Care:** having a home care aide assist the patient in the performance of ADLs or an occupational therapist assist the patient in structuring his or her day; direct nursing interventions to teach the patient the importance of self-care activities to overall well-being.
- **Medication and Other Psychobiological Interventions:** monitoring or administering medications. Most third-party payers, including Medicare, do not reimburse the nurse to administer oral medications; however, administering a parenteral medication, such as Haldol Decanoate or Prolixin Decanoate, is considered a reimbursable nursing intervention. Drawing serum levels for medications, such as lithium, Tegretol, or Clozaril is considered an essential part of medication monitoring. Care given following electroconvulsive therapy is an acceptable psychobiological intervention. As the physiological basis for psychiatric disorders is increasingly understood, so will our nursing repertoire of psychobiological interventions also increase.
- **Health Teaching:** teaching patients how to take medications, the reasons for taking medications, their side effects and how to deal with them.
- **Case Management:** forging links for the patient with the community, such as arranging transportation or negotiating with a patient's landlord to establish an acceptable rent payment schedule (Maurin, 1990; Carson, 1994a).
- **Health Promotion and Health Maintenance:** linking the patient with necessary medical treatment and facilitating the patient's connection with other health care providers (Newton and Brauer, 1989).

EVALUATION

Evaluating the care plan is more than deciding whether a nursing intervention was effective or not. Evaluation takes the nurse through the whole nursing process. For example, if the nurse is teaching about a medication and discovers the patient cannot read, a deficit in the initial assessment is suggested. If the nurse makes a nursing diagnosis of knowledge deficit and the patient is so focused on receiving his social security disability payment that he cannot learn what the nurse is teaching, then the evaluation reveals deficits both in establishing a nursing diagnosis and in planning care that considers the patient's priorities. An evaluation that reveals deficits in the nursing process suggests the need for modifications.

Evaluation also involves looking at the specific outcomes that were identified earlier. Were they achieved in a timely, cost-effective manner? Was the patient satisfied with the care? The answers to these questions are important for the nurse to consider.

■ DOCUMENTATION ISSUES IN PSYCHIATRIC NURSING

Psychiatric home care documentation is similar to, yet different from, the documentation that is done in a hospital setting (Carson, et al., 1994; 1994a; 1994b). The rules for documentation include that every note stand by itself. Every note, therefore, must provide a current assessment of the patient, a statement of the patient's homebound status, goals for that particular visit, specific measurable interventions, the response of the patient to the interventions, and an evaluation of goal achievement.

Notes are always written in the negative, meaning that the nurse must indicate what deficits the patient still has that justify home care. Phrases, such as "patient is stable," "patient is doing well," and "patient is much improved," are red flags to the Medicare reviewers who peruse the notes, and most likely will lead to a denial of reimbursement. Rather than focusing on the patient's improvement, the nurse indicates the goals that still must be met. For example, an acceptable notation is, "Patient achieved part of goal; could state reason for taking Prolixin, but remains unsure of side effects or schedule."

Every visit is documented separately, and all communication about the patient (interdisciplinary, nurse to family/community, or nurse to physician) is documented.

All verbal physician orders are documented as verbal orders. These orders are then sent to the physician for review and signature.

Lastly, interventions and outcomes must be written in concrete language. Most of the Medicare reviewers are medical-surgical nurses who may have little understanding or who place little value on psychiatric nursing. Therefore, the language of the psychiatric nurse must be understandable to the reviewer. It is important to avoid phrases such as "providing support to the

E CASE EXAMPLE

Bill Blane is 35 years old and diagnosed with chronic paranoid schizophrenia. He is referred for psychiatric home care after he experiences a seizure, falls, and fractures his right leg. The seizure results from his taking Clozaril. Because of the fractured right leg, Bill is homebound and unable to get to the clinic to receive his Prolixin Decanoate injection. Sally West, a baccaluareate prepared nurse with 1 year of in-patient adult psychiatric experience, is assigned to care for Bill. On her first visit she administers the Brief Psychiatric Rating Scale and assesses that Bill is experiencing delusional thinking; he has not received any neuroleptic medication for the past 2 weeks; he is unable to independently manage his activities of daily living; he has almost no food in his home; and he is self-medicating the delusional thinking by taking his girlfriend's prescription for Valium. Sally makes several nursing diagnoses, including:

- Patient at high risk for self-harm related to improper medication for delusional thinking as evidenced by taking his girlfriend's prescription of Valium.
- Patient's nutritional requirements being inadequately met related to his inability to manage this part of his life, evidenced by lack of food in home.
- Patient's coping abilities impaired related to immobility caused by fractured right leg and inadequate medication control of schizophrenic symptoms, evidenced by delusional thinking and neglect of ADLs.

Because Bill's thinking is not totally rational at the time of Sally's assessment, he is unable to fully participate in goal setting. Consequently, Sally establishes the expected outcome for Bill's care:

> At the end of 9 weeks of care, Bill will be free of delusional thinking, his score on the Brief Psychiatric Rating Scale will be significantly improved, and he will be able to handle his ADLs with increased independence.

Sally's first priority is to ensure that Bill has food to eat. She calls a food bank in her community and requests an emergency delivery of food, which arrives while she is with Bill. Sally prepares a few simple meals so that Bill will be able to eat until her next visit.

Sally then contacts the referring physician to give an immediate report and request authorization for the services of a home health aide to assist with ADLs; an occupational therapist to help teach Bill to be functional while in a leg cast; a physical therapist, as soon as Bill is able to use crutches; and finally, an order for a neuroleptic. The physician concurs with Sally's requests to order the ancillary home services and orders administration of Prolixin Decanoate, 18.75 mg, intramuscularly once every 2 weeks; the physician also orders Cogentin, 1 mg, bid. The medication orders are called into a pharmacy, which delivers the medication to Bill's apartment. Sally administers the Prolixin Decanoate and begins teaching Bill about his medications. She installs the home health aide and instructs the aide about helping Bill to become increasingly independent in performing activities of daily living. Sally also communicates with the occupational therapist regarding Bill's needs and contacts the agency's social worker for assistance obtaining Meals on Wheels for Bill. Sally informs the physical therapist that physical therapy will begin as soon as Bill is allowed to ambulate on crutches. Once Sally organizes the care, she begins to focus on the direct provision of nursing care, which includes medication teaching, administration, and monitoring; illness teaching and management; increasing Bill's diversional activity within the confines of his apartment; counseling Bill regarding the dangers of self-medicating his symptoms with his girlfriend's Valium; and maintaining ongoing coordination of the various services being provided to Bill.

By the end of 9 weeks, Bill is using crutches to ambulate; his delusional thinking is gone; he has learned to care for his own ADLs; he states the reasons for taking his Prolixin and Cogentin and the side effects of each, and is compliant in taking his medications; he no longer uses his girlfriend's Valium; he describes the symptoms of schizophrenia and states coping mechanisms to deal with these symptoms; and he is willing to return to the day treatment center he attended prior to his seizure and leg fracture. Sally discharges Bill with goals met.

---

patient" or "encouraging expression of feelings." Such phrases as "continued assessment for suicidal ideation," "teaching regarding medication management," and "teaching regarding symptoms of depression" are concrete and represent acceptable interventions. Likewise, patient outcomes must be expressed in concrete terms.

■ PSYCHIATRIC HOME CARE: WHAT DOES IT LOOK LIKE?

The on page 824 case example examines what the nurse with entry level skills would do during a home visit.

 AN OVERVIEW

- Psychiatric home care is a promising treatment modality because it recognizes that, in addition to being a cost-effective modality, patients frequently do better when they remain within the comforts of their own home.

- The largest group using psychiatric home care is the elderly; however, the chronically mentally ill, and persons with acute psychiatric illnesses, AIDS, and children also receive home care.

- The primary payers in psychiatric home care are Medicare and Medicaid; consequently, they have established standards that have had major influences in psychiatric home care. For example, Medicare and Medicaid require that nurses providing psychiatric care have additional training, education, or both in psychiatric nursing; patients must be homebound; and patients must have a DSM-IV diagnosis designated by a psychiatrist.

- Nurses who provide psychiatric home care find that they have a great degree of autonomy in the home but not the power and authority that accompanies hospital nursing.

- Because the home care nurse is the patient's guest, a different approach is taken to assessment and intervention.

- The primary interventions used by the psychiatric home care nurse are defined by the 1994 Standards of Psychiatric Practice; they include counseling, milieu maintenance, health teaching, case management, and health promotion and maintenance.

TD TERMS TO DEFINE

- Carson's Model of Psychiatric Home Care
- homebound status
- National Alliance for the Mentally Ill (NAMI)
- psychiatric home health care
- reimbursement policies
- supportive home care services

Q STUDY QUESTIONS

Short Essay

1. Describe psychiatric home care.
2. How does psychiatric home care act as a bridge to the community?
3. What three driving forces contribute to the growth of psychiatric home care?
4. List the eligibility criteria for patients to receive psychiatric home care under Medicare.

5. What four groups benefit most from psychiatric home care?

Multiple Choice

6. Psychiatric home care is
   a. short term and intermittent.
   b. long term and continuous.
   c. crisis oriented.
   d. brief and periodic.

7. Psychiatric home care does NOT include which of the following interventions:
   a. Teaching the patient regarding medication issues
   b. Assisting the patient to find appropriate diversional activities
   c. Providing custodial care in a cost-effective manner
   d. Teaching the patient appropriate social skills

8. The foundation of Carson's model of psychiatric home care is
   a. medication issues.
   b. relationship building.
   c. moral and spiritual needs.
   d. case management.

9. Mrs. Smith is a 72-year-old woman who recently suffered a cardiovascular accident with secondary depression. Her physician ordered psychiatric home care. During the initial visits the nurse will assess which of the following areas?
   a. Functional status
   b. Affect
   c. Suicidal ideation
   d. All of the above

10. The value of nursing diagnoses is that they
    a. clearly state symptoms of each psychiatric illness.
    b. provide a means for the nurse to classify the patient's symptoms.
    c. identify a patient's problems and responses.
    d. identify the treatment options.

11. Which of the following is an appropriately stated outcome?
    a. Patient will feel less depressed
    b. Patient's score on depression scale will decrease significantly
    c. Patient will have significantly more insight into his or her problems
    d. Patient will feel supported as he or she deals with grief issues

12. Documentation in psychiatric home care is guided by which of the following principles?
    a. Repetition from note to note is avoided
    b. Nursing skills must be documented in concrete terms
    c. Evaluation of care is done at time of discharge
    d. Notes are written in a positive manner

■ REFERENCES

Aguilera DC. *Crisis Intervention: Theory and Methodology.* 6th ed. St. Louis: CV Mosby; 1990.

Barrick B. Caring for AIDS patients. *Nursing 88* 1988; 11:50–59.

Benner P. Lamentations. *J Christian Nurs* 1992; 9:9–11.

Bush CT, et al. Operation outreach: Intensive case management for severely psychiatrically disabled adults. *Hosp Comm Psychiatry* 1990; 41(6):647–649.

Carson VB, Jacik M, Shoemaker N, et al. *Bay Area Psychiatric Home Care Manual.* Baltimore: Bay Area Health Care; 1994.

Carson VB. Doing psych, but talking med-surg language. *Caring* 1994a; 13(6):32–41.

Carson VB. Spiritual care of Evelyn. *Caring* 1994b; 13(12):27–29.

Carson VB. Spirituality and depression: An important relationship. *Smooth Sailing: DRADA Newsletter* 1994c; Jan:3–4.

Carson VB. Caring: The rediscovery of our nursing roots. *Perspect Psych Care* 1994d; 30(2):4–6.

Carson VB. Bay Area Health Care Model of Psychiatric Home Care. *Home HealthCare Nurse* 1995; 13:26–33.

Casserta JE. The mind-body connection. *Home Healthcare Nurse* 1993; 11(2):6.

Coalition of Psychiatric Nursing Organizations. *A Statement on Psychiatric-Mental Health Clinical Nursing Practice and Standards of Psychiatric-Mental Health Nursing Practice.* Washington, DC: ANA; 1994.

Daubert E. Strategic planning in home care. *American J Nurs* 1987; 87(9):1161–1163.

Davis EJ. Home care—What is needed? *Pub Health Nurs* 1987; 4(2):82–83.

Dickstein D, et al. Reducing treatment costs in a community support program. *Hosp Comm Psychiatry* 1988; 39(10):1033–1035.

Duffy J, Miller M, Parlocha P. Psychiatric home care. *Home Healthcare Nurse* 1993; 11(2):22–28.

Eliopoulos C. Development tasks of aging. In: *Long-Term Educator.* Vol. 1. Lesson 6. Glen Arm, Md; Health Education Network; 1991.

Eliopoulos C. *Gerontological Nursing.* 3rd ed. Philadelphia: JB Lippincott; 1993.

Fenton FR, et al. A comparative trial of home and hospital psychiatric care. *Arch Gen Psychiatry* 1979; 36(9):1073–1079.

Fenton FR, Tessier L, Struening E, et al. A comparative trial of home and hospital psychiatric treatment: Financial costs. *Can J Psychiatry* 1982; 27(4):177–187.

Frisch N. Home care nursing and psychosocial-emotional needs of clients. *Home Healthcare Nurse* 1993; 11(2):64–65,70.

Goering PN, et al. What difference does case management make? *Hosp Comm Psychiatry* 1988; 39(3):272–276.

Harris MD. Psychiatric evaluation and therapy. *Home Healthcare Nurse* 1993; 11(2):66–67.

Health Care Financing Administration. *Hm11: Medicare Home Health Agency Manual,* Transmittal 114, Section 204.6; 1996.

Holland L. Mental health supportive home care aides. *Caring* April 1993; 44–48.

Home Care Guidelines. Minnesota Community Health Services, Office of Community Development, Minneapolis, Minn: Minnesota Department of Health; 1981.

Kapust LR, Weintraub S. Home Care for the Elderly. *The Gerontologist* 1988; 28(1):112–115.

Kelley JH, Lehman L. Assessment of anxiety, depression and suspiciousness in the home care setting. *Home Healthcare Nurse* 1993; 11(2):16–20.

Klebanoff N, Casler B. The psychosocial clinical nurse specialist: An untapped resource for home care. *Home Healthcare Nurse* 1986; 4:36–40.

Lehman L, Kelley JH. Nursing interventions for anxiety, depression, and suspiciousness in the home care setting. *Home Healthcare Nurse* 1993; 11(3):35–40.

Lesseig D. Home care for psych problems. *Am J Nurs* 1987; 10:1317–1320.

Maurin JT. Case management: Caring for psychiatric clients. *J Psychosoc Nurs Mental Health Serv* 1990; 28(7):6–12.

Orem D. *Nursing Concepts of Practice.* 4th ed. St. Louis: CV Mosby; 1991.

Pellegrino E. The caring ethic: The relation of physician to patient. In: Bishop AH, Scudder JR, eds. *Caring, Curing, Coping: Nurse, Physician, Patient Relationships.* Birmingham: University of Alabama Press; 1985:8–30.

Pelletier LR. Psychiatric home care. *J Psychosoc Nurs Mental Health Serv* 1988; 26(3):22–27.

Raschko R. Assertive at-home case management for impaired elderly persons. *Hosp Commun Psychiatry* 1988; 39(11):1201–1202.

Research News. Studies on elderly show need for home care. *Caring* 1984; 3(5):11–13.

Rice DP, Feldman JJ. Living longer in the United States: Demographic changes and health needs of the elderly. *Milbank Mem Fund Quart* 1983; 6:362–395.

Rice R. Suicidal thoughts and ideation. *Home Healthcare Nurse* 1993; 11(3):67.

Rusch SC. Continuity of care: From hospital unit into home. *Nurs Manage* 1986; 17(12):39–41.

Stein LI, Diamond RJ. A program for difficult-to-treat patients. *New Directions for Mental Health Services* 1985; 26:29–39.

Warhola C. Planning for home health services—A resource handbook. DHHS Pub No. [HRA] 80–14017. Washington, DC: US Government Printing Office; 1980.

Wasylenski DA, et al. Impact of a case manager program on psychiatric aftercare. *J Nervous Mental Dis* 1985; 173(5):303–308.

Weintraub S, Mesulam MM. Mental state assessment of young and elderly adults in behavioral neurology. In: Mesulam MM, ed. *Principles of Behavioral Neurology.* Philadelphia: FA Davis; 1985.

Suggested Readings

Chapter 1. Beginning the Psychiatric Nursing Experience

Herd F. Studying mental illness. *J Psychosoc Nurs* 1994; 32(6):20–22, 32.

Williams RA, Hagerty BM, Murphy-Weinburg V, Wan JY. Symptoms of depression among female nursing students. *Arch Psychiatric Nurs*, 1995; (IX)5:269–278.

Chapter 2. Psychiatric Nursing

Arbraham IL, Fox JC, Cohen BT. Integrating the bio into the biopsychosocial: Understanding and treating biological phenomena in psychiatric-mental health nursing, *Archi Psychiatric Nurs*, 1992; 6(5): 296–305.

Barker P, Reynolds B. A critique: watson's caring ideology, the proper focus of psychiatric nursing. *Psychoso Nurs*, 1994; 32(5): 17–22.

Dumas RG. Psychiatric nursing in an era of change. *Psychosoc Nurs*, 1994; 32(1): 11–14.

Lowery BJ. Psychiatric nursing in the 1990s and beyond, *Jour of Psychosoc Nurs*, 1992; 30(1): 7–13.

Chapter 4. Brain and Behavior

Harper-Jacques S, Reimer M. Aggressive behavior and the brain: A different perspective for the mental health care nurse. *Arch Psych Nurs*, 1992; 6(5): 312–320.

Chapter 5. Learning and Mental Health Teaching

Trygstad LN. The need to know: Biological learning needs identified by practicing psychiatric nurses. *J Psychosoc Nurs* 1994; 32(2):13–18.

Verhey MP. How do psychiatric nurses learn? Modes of learning and learning self-directedness. *Arch Psychiatric Nurs* 1993; VII(3):139–146.

Chapter 6. Stress, Coping, and Defense Mechanisms

Benham E. Coping strategies: A psychoeducational approach to post-traumatic symptomatology. *J Psychosoc Nurs* 1995; 33(6):30–35.

McCain NL, Smith JC. Stress and coping in the context of psychoneuroimmunology: A holistic framework for nursing practice and research. *Arch Psychiatric Nurs*, 1994; VIII(4):221–227.

Warren CJ, Baker S. Coping resources of women with premenstrual syndrome. *Arch Psychiatric Nurs* 1992; VI(1):48–53.

Chapter 7. Human Growth and Development

Mohit DL. Management and care of mentally ill mothers of young children: An innovative program. *Arch Psychiatric Nurs* 1996; X(1):49–54.

Chapter 9. Culture, Ethnicity and Race in Mental Health and Illness

Campinha-Bacote J. Transcultural psychiatric nursing: Diagnostic and treatment issues. *J Psychosocial Nurs* 1994; 32(8):41–46.

Cravener P. Establishing therapeutic alliance across cultural barriers. *J Psychosocial Nurs* 1992; 30(12):10–14.

Grothaus KL. Family dynamics and family dynamics with Mexican Americans. *J Psychosocial Nurs* 1996; 34(2):31–37.

Worthington C. An examination of factors influencing the diagnosis and treatment of black patients in the mental health system. *Arch Psychiatric Nurs* 1992; VI(3):195–204.

Chapter 10. The Spiritual Aspect of Patient Care

Stepnick A, Perry T. Preventing spiritual distress in the dying client. *J Psychosoc Nurs* 1992; 30(1):17–24.

Chapter 11. Legal and Ethical Issues in Psychiatric Nursing

McDonald S. An ethical dilemma: Risk versus responsibility. *J Psychosoc Nurs* 1994; 32(1):19–26.

Lewin L. Child abuse: Ethical and legal concerns for the nurse. *J Psychosoc Nurs* 1994; 32(12):15–18.

Olsen DP. The ethical considerations of managed care in mental health treatment. *J Psychosoc Nurs* 1994; 32(3):25–28.

Trudeau ME. Informed consent: The patient's right to decide. *J Psychosoc Nurs* 1993; 31(6):9–12.

Chapter 14. Anxiety Disorders

Bille DA. Road to recovery: Post-traumatic stress disorder, the hidden victim. *J Psychosoc Nurs* 1993; 31(9):19–28.

Moyers F. Oklahoma City bombing: Exacerbation of symptoms in veterans with PTSD. *Arch Psychiatric Nurs* 1996; X(1):55–59.

Schweitzer PB, Nesse RM, Fantone RF, Curtis GC. Outcomes of Group Cognitive Behavioral Training in the Treatment of Panic Disorder. *J Am Psychiatric Nurses Assoc* 1995; 1(3):83–91.

Stuhlmiller CM. The construction of disorders. *J Psychosoc Nurs* 1995; 33(4):20–23.

Turner DM. Panic disorder: A personal and nursing perspective. *J Psychosoc Nurs* 1995; 33(4):5–8.

Chapter 15. Dissociative Disorders

Anonymous. Living and working with MPD. *J Psychosoc Nurs* 1994; 32(8):17–22.

Curtin SL. Recognizing multiple personality disorder. *J Psychosoc Nurs* 1993; 31(2):29–33.

Huffman RW. Dissociation and multiple personality disorder: A challenge for psychosocial nursing. *J Psychosoc Nurs* 1993; 31(1):15–20.

Chapter 16. Loss, Grief, and Bereavement

Bateman A, Broderick D, Gleason L, et al. Dysfunctional grieving. *J Psychosoc Nurs* 1992; 30(12):5–9.

Davis JM, Hoshiko BR, Jones S, Gosnell D. The effect of a support group on grieving individuals' levels of perceived support and stress. *Arch Psychiatric Nurs* 1992; VI(1):35–39.

Joffrion LP, Douglas D. Grief resolution: Facilitating self-transcendence in the bereaved. *J Psychosoc Nurs* 1994; 32(3):13–20.

Liken MA. Grieving: Facilitating the process for dementia caregivers. *J Psychosoc Nurs* 1993; 31(1):21–26.

Chapter 18. Issues in Adolescent Mental Health

Brage DG. Adolescent depression: A review of the literature. *Arch Psychiatric Nurs* 1995; IX(1):45–55.

Gary F, Moorhead J, Warren J. Characteristics of troubled youth in a shelter. *Arch Psychiatric Nurs* 1996; X(1):41–48.

Chapter 19. Delirium, Dementia and Aging

Masters JC, O'Grady M. Normal pressure hydorcephalus: A potentially reversible form of dementia. *J Psychosoc Nurs* 1992; 30(6):25–28.

McDougall GJ. A critical review of research on cognitive function/impairment in older adults. *Arch Psychiatric Nurs* 1995; IX(1):22–33.

Richter JM, Roberto KA, Bottenberg DJ. Communicating with persons with Alzheimer's disease: Experience of family and formal caregivers. *Arch Psychiatric Nurs* 1995; IX(5):279–285.

Chapter 20. Mood Disorders

Hagerty BM. Advances in understanding major depressive disorder. *J Psychosoc Nurs* 1995; 33(11):27–33.

US Department of Health and Human Services, Public Health Service, Agency for Health Care Policy and Research. Depression in primary care: Detection, diagnosis, and treatment. *J Psychosoc Nurs* 1993; 31(6):19–28.

Pollack LE. Treatment of inpatients with bipolar disorder. *J Psychosoc Nurs* 1995; 33(1):11–15.

Pollack LE. Striving for stability with bipolar disorder despite barriers. *Arch Psychiatric Nurs* 1995; IX(3):122–129.

Zauszniewski JA. Severity of depression, cognitions and functioning among depressed inpatients with and without coexisting substance abuse. *J Am Psychiatric Nurses Assoc* 1995; 1(2):55–60.

Zauszniewski JA. Potential sequelae of family history of depression. *J Psychosoc Nurs* 32(9):15–21.

Chapter 21. Sexual Issues, Disorders, and Deviations

Lego S. Masochism: Implications for psychiatric nursing. *Arch Psychiatric Nurs* 1992; VI(4):224–229.

Chapter 22. Eating Disorders

Hofland SL, Dardis PO. Bulimia nervosa: Associated physical problems. *J Psychosoc Nurs* 1992; 30(2):23–27.

Irwin EG. A focused overview of anorexia nervosa and bulimia: Part I. Etiological issues. *Arch Psychiatric Nurs* 1993; VII(6):342–346.

Irwin EG. A focused overview of anorexia nervosa and bulimia: Part II. Challenges to the practice of psychiatric nursing. *Arch Psychiatric Nurs* 1993; VII(6):347–352.

Michielli DW. Is exercise indicated for the patient diagnosed as anoretic? *J Psychosoc Nurs* 1994; 32(8):33–35.

Owen SV, Fullerton ML. Would it make a difference? A discussion group in a behaviorally oriented inpatient eating disorder program. *J Psychosoc Nurs* 1995; 33(11):35–40.

Chapter 24. Treating Child Sexual Trauma

Burgess AW, Hartman CR, Clements PT. Biology of memory and childhood trauma. *J Psychosoc Nurs* 1995; 33(3):16–26.

Doob D. Female sexual abuse survivors as patients: Avoiding retraumatization. *Arch Psychiatric Nurs* 1992; VI(4):245–251.

Harper-Jacques S, Masters A. Written communication with survivors of sexual abuse: Use of letters in therapy. *J Psychosoc Nurs* 1994; 32(8):11–26.

Lewin L. Interviewing the young child sexual abuse victim. *J Psychosoc Nurs* 1995; 33(7):5–10.

Ridley PJ. Kaufman's theory of shame and identity in treating childhood sexual abuse. *J Psychosoc Nurs* 1993; 31(6):13–17.

Urbanic JC. Empowerment support with adult female survivors of childhood incest: Part I. Theories and research. *Arch Psychiatric Nurs* 1992; VI(5):275–281.

Urbanic JC. Empowerment support with adult female survivors of childhood incest: Part II. Application of Orem's methods of helping. *Arch Psychiatric Nurs* 1992; VI(5):282–286.

Wingerson N. Psychic loss in adult survivors of father–daughter incest. *Arch Psychiatric Nurs* 1992; VI(4):239–244.

Chapter 25. Victims of Sexual Assault

Mackey T, et al. Factors associated with long-term depressive symptoms of sexual assault victims. *Arch Psychiatric Nurs* 1992; VI(1):10–25.

Chapter 26. Personality Disorders

Gallop R. Self-destructive and impulsive behavior in the patient with borderline personality disorder: Rethinking hospital treatment and management. *Arch Psychiatric Nurs* 1992; VI(3):178–182.

Miller CR, Eisner W, Allport C. Creative coping: A cognitive-behavioral group for borderline personality disorder. *Arch Psychiatric Nurs* 1994; VIII(4):280–285.

Nehls N. Brief hospital treatment plans for persons with borderline personality disorder: Perspectives of inpatient psychiatric nurses and community mental health center clinicians. *Arch Psychiatric Nurs* 1994; VIII(5):303–311.

Simmons D. Gender issues and borderline personality disorder: Why do females dominate the diagnosis? *Arch Psychiatric Nurs* 1992; VI(4):219–223.

Stein KF. Affect instability with adults with borderline personality disorder. *Arch Psychiatric Nurs* 1996; X(1):32–40.

Chapter 27. Child Abuse and Neglect

Devlin BK, Reynolds E. Child abuse: How to recognize it, how to intervene. *Am J Nurs* 1994; March:26–31.

Gill CT. Protecting our children: Where have we gone and where should we go from here? *J Psychosoc Nurs* 1995; 33(3):31–35.

Glod CA. Circadian dsyregulation in abused individuals: A proposed theoretical model for practice and research. *Arch Psychiatric Nursing* 1992; VI(6):347–355.

Glod CA. Long-term consequences of childhood physical and sexual abuse. *Arch Psychiatric Nurs* 1993; VII(3):174–181.

Chapter 28. Violence in Families

Fishwick N. Getting to the heart of the matter: Nursing assessment and intervention with battered women in psychiatric mental health settings. *J Am Psychiatric Nurses Assoc* 1995; 1(2):48–53.

Robinson CA, Wright LM, Watson WL. A nontraditional approach to family violence. *Arch Psychiatric Nurs* 1994; VIII(1):30–37.

Chapter 29. Schizophrenia

Baker C. The development of the self-care ability to detect early signs of relapse among individuals who have schizophrenia. *Arch Psychiatric Nurs* 1995; IX(5):261–268.

Buccheri R, Trygstad L, Kanas N, et al. Symptom management of auditory hallucinations in schizophrenia. *J Psychosoc Nurs* 1996; 34(2):12–26.

Buchanan J. Social support and schizophrenia: A review of the literature. *Arch Psychiatric Nurs* 1995; IX(2):68–76.

Hamera EK, Peterson KA, Young LM, Schaumloffel MM. Symptom monitoring in schizophrenia: Potential for enhancing self-care. *Arch Psychiatric Nurs* 1992; VI(6):324–330.

Kirkpatrick H, et al. Hope and schizophrenia. *J Psychosoc Nurs* 1995; 33(6):15–19.

Mann NA, Tandon R, Butler J, et al. Psychosocial rehabilitation in schizophrenia: Beginnings in acute hospitalization. *Arch Psychiatric Nurs* 1993; VII(3):154–162.

Natale A, Barron C. Mothers' causal explantations for their son's schizophrenia: Relationship to depression and guilt. *Arch Psychiatric Nurs* 1994; VIII(4):228–236.

O'Connell KL. Schizoaffective disorder: A case study. *J Psychosoc Nurs* 1995; 33(10):35–39.

Chapter 30. The Homeless and Chronic Mentally Disabled

Bennett JB, Scholler-Jaquish A. The winner's group: A self-help group for homeless chemically dependent persons. *J Psychosoc Nurs* 1995; 33(4):14–19.

Chafetz L. The experience of severe mental illness: A life history approach. *Arch Psychiatric Nurs* 1996; X(1):24–31.

Murray R, Baier M, North C, et al. Components of an effective transitional residential program for homeless mentally ill clients. *Arch Psychiatric Nurs* 1995; IX(3):152–157.

Smith MK, Harty KM, Riggin OZ. Working with the patient with a chronic mental impairment. *J Psychosoc Nurs* 1996; 34(2):27–30.

Wallsten SM. A portrait of homelessness. *J Psychosoc Nurs* 1992; 30(9):20–24.

Warren BJ, Menke EM, Clement J, Wagner J. The mental health of African-American and Caucasian-American women who are homeless. *J Psychosoc Nurs* 1992; 30(11):27–30.

Chapter 31. Substance Abuse

Clement JA, Williams EB, Waters C. The client with substance abuse/mental illness: Mandate for collaboration. *Arch Psychiatric Nurs* 1993; VII(4):189–196.

Montgomery P, Johnson B. The stress of marriage to an alcoholic. *J Psychosoc Nurs* 1992; 30(10):12–16.

Minicucci DS. The challenge of change: Rethinking alcohol abuse. *Arch Psychiatric Nurs* 1994; VIII(6):373–380.

Wing DM. Applying the "Model of Recovering Alcoholics' Behavior Stages and Goal Setting" to nursing practice. *Arch Psychiatric Nurs* 1993; VII(4):197–202.

Wing DM, Hammer-Higgins P. Determinants of denial: A study of alcoholics. *J Psychosoc Nurs* 1993; 31(2):13–15.

Chapter 32. Managing Suicidal Patients

Bonnivier JF. Management of self-destructive behaviors in an open inpatient setting. *J Psychosoc Nurs* 1996; 34(2):38–42.

Cugino A, et al. Searching for a pattern: Repeat suicide attempts. *J Psychosoc Nurs* 1992; 30(3):23–26.

Rickelman BL, Houfek JF. Toward an interactional model of suicidal behaviors: Cognitive rigidity, attributional style, stress, hopelessness and depression. *Arch Psychiatric Nurs* 1995; IX(3):158–168.

Chapter 34. HIV Positive Persons and Their Families

Hall BA. Overcoming stigmatization: Social and personal implications of the human immunodeficiency virus diagnosis. *Arch Psychiatric Nurs* VI(3):189–194.

Kavanaugh KH, Harris RM, Hetherington SE, Scott DE. Collaboration as a strategy for acquired immunodeficiency prevention. *Arch Psychiatric Nurs* 1992; XI(6):331–339.

McShane RE, Bumbalo JA, Patsdaughter CA. Psychological distress in family members living with human immunodeficiency virus/acquired immune deficiency syndrome. *Arch Psychiatric Nurs* 1994; VIII(1):53–61.

Regan-Kublinski MJ, Sharts-Engel N. The HIV-infected woman: Illness cognition assessment. *J Psychosoc Nurs* 1992; 30(2):11–16.

Swanson B, Cronin-Stubbs D, Zeller JM, et al. Characterizing the neuropsychological functioning of persons with human immunodeficiency virus infection; Part I. Acquired immun-odeficiency syndrome dementia complex: A review. *Arch Psychiatric Nurs* 1993; VII(2):74–81.

Swanson B, Cronin-Stubbs D, Zeller JM, et al. Characterizing the neuropsychological functioning of persons with human immunodeficiency virus infection: Part II. Neuropsychological functioning of persons at different stages of HIV infection. *Arch Psychiatric Nurs* 1993; VII(2):82–90.

Chapter 35. Conceptual Models as Guides for Psychiatric Nursing Practice

Armstrong MA, Kelly AE. More than the sum of their parts: Martha Rogers and Hildegard Peplau. *Arch Psychiatric Nurs* 1995; IX(1):40–44.

Johnston N, Baumann A. A process-oriented approach: Selecting a nursing model for psychiatric nursing. *J Psychosoc Nurs* 1992; 30(4):7–12.

Montgomery CL, Webster D. Caring, curing, and brief therapy: A model for nurse–psychotherapy. *Arch Psychiatric Nurs* 1994; VIII(5):291–297.

Morrison EG. Inpatient practice: An integrated framework. *J Psychosoc Nurs* 1992; 30(1):26–29.

Chapter 36. Therapeutic Nurse–Patient Relationship

Byrne CM, Woodside H, Landeen J, et al. The importance of relationships in fostering hope. *J Psychosoc Nurs* 1994; 32(9):31–34.

Forchuk C. Uniqueness within the nurse–client relationship. *Arch Psychiatric Nurs* 1995; IX(1):34–39.

Heifner C. Positive connectedness in the psychiatric nurse–patient relationship. *Arch Psychiatric Nurs* 1993; VII(1):11–15.

Miles M, Morse J. Using the concepts of transference and countertransference in the consultation process. *J Am Psychiatric Nurses Assoc* 1995; 1(2):42–47.

Pilette PC, Berck CB, Achber LC. Therapeutic management of helping boundaries. *J Psychosoc Nurs* 1995; 33(1):40–47.

Vincent M, White K. Patient violence toward a nurse: Predictable and preventable? *J Psychosoc Nurs* 1994; 32(2):30–32.

Chapter 37. Therapeutic Milieu

LeCuyer EA. Milieu therapy for short stay units: A transformed practice theory. *Arch Psychiatric Nurs* 1992; VI(2):108–116.

Warner S. The milieu enhancement model: A nursing practice model: Part I. *Arch Psychiatric Nurs* 1993; VII(2):53–60.

Chapter 38. Clinical Assessment and Nursing Diagnosis

Abraham IL, Smullen DE, Thompson-Heisterman AA. Assessing geropsychiatric patients. *J Psychosoc Nurs* 1992; 30(9):13–19.

Acorn S. Use of the Brief Psychiatric Rating Scale by nurses. *J Psychosoc Nurs* 31(5):9–12.

Eppard J, Anderson J. Emergency psychiatric assessment. *J Psychosoc Nurs* 1995; 33(10):17–23.

Gabriel SR. The developmentally disabled, psychiatrically impaired client: Proper treatment of dual diagnosis. *J Psychosoc Nurs* 1994; 32(9):35–39.

O'Connor FW, Eggert LL. Psychosocial assessment for treatment planning and evaluation. *J Psychosoc Nurs* 1994; 32(5):31–41.

Chapter 39. Crisis Intervention

Nugent E. Try to remember: Reminiscence as a nursing intervention. *J Psychosoc Nurs* 1995; 33(11):7–14.

Ragaisis KM. Critical incident stress debriefing: A family nursing intervention. *Arch Psychiatric Nurs* 1994; VIII(1):38–43.

San Blise ML. Crisis intervention: Aftershocks in the quake zone. *J Psychosoc Nurs* 1994; 32(5):29–30.

Chapter 40.   Treatment Modalities—Crisis, Behavioral, Relational, and Insight
Hill L, Oliver N. Technique integration: Therapeutic touch and theory-based mental health nursing. *J Psychosoc Nursing* 1993; 31(2):18–22.

Rittman M. Social organization of length of stay of psychiatric patients. *J Psychosoc Nurs* 1993; 31(5):21–27.

Merchant DJ, Henfling PA. Scheduled brief admissions: Patient "tuneups." *J Psychosoc Nurs* 1994; 32(12):7–10.

Wilson JH, Hobbs H. Therapeutic partnership: A model of clinical practice. *J Psychosoc Nurs* 1995; 33(2):27–30.

Chapter 41.   Therapeutic Groups
Clark WG, Vorst VR. Group therapy with chronically depressed geriatric patients. *J Psychosoc Nurs* 1994; 32(5):9–13.

Klose P, Tinius T. Confidence builders: A self-esteem group at an inpatient psychiatric hospital. *J Psychosoc Nurs* 1992; 30(7):5–9.

Pearlman IR. Group psychotherapy with the elderly. *J Psychosoc Nurs* 31(7):7–10.

Wood A, Seymour LM. Psychodynamic group therapy for older adults: The life experiences group. *J Psychosoc Nurs* 1994; 32(7):19–24.

Chapter 42.   Pharmacotherapy
Coudreaut-Quinn EA, Emmons MA, McMorrow MJ. Adherence and accuracy: Self-medication during inpatient psychiatric treatment. *J Psychosoc Nurs* 1992; 30(12):32–36.

Fishel AH, Ferreiro BW, Rynerson BS, et al. As-needed psychotropic medications: Prevalence, indications and results. *J Psychosoc Nurs* 1994; 32(8):27–32.

Talley S, Brooke PS. Prescriptive authority for psychiatric clinical specialists: Framing the issues. *Arch Psychiatric Nurs* 1992; VI(4):71–82.

Zind R, Furlong C, Stebbins M. Educating patients about missed medication doses. *J Psychosoc Nurs* 1992; 30(7):10–14.

Chapter 43.   Critical Pathways for Mental Health and Planning Care
Delaney K, Pitula CR. Seven days and counting: How inpatient nurses might adjust their practice to brief hospitalization. *J Psychosoc Nurs* 1995; 33(8):36–39.

Dunn J, Rodriguez D, Novak JJ. Promoting quality mental health care delivery with critical path care plans. *J Psychosoc Nurs* 1994; 32(7):25–29.

Chapter 44.   Case Management
Connolly PM. What does a nurse need to know and do to maintain an effective level of case management? *J Psychosoc Nurs* 1992; 30(3):35–39.

Van Dongen CJ, Jambunathan J. Pilot study results: The psychiatric RN case manager. *J Psychosoc Nurs* 1992; 30(11):11–14.

Chapter 45.   Psychiatric Home Care
Krach P, Yang J. Functional status of older persons with chronic mental illness living in a home setting. *Arch Psychiatric Nurs* 1992; VI(2):90–97.

Ripich S, Moore SM, Brennan PF. A new nursing medium: Computer networks for group intervention. *J Psychosoc Nurs* 1992; 30(7):15–20.

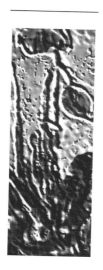

Appendix

North American Nursing Diagnosis Association (NANDA) Approved Nursing Diagnoses

Pattern 1: Exchanging
  1.1.2.1 Altered nutrition: More than body requirements
  1.1.2.2 Altered nutrition: Less than body requirements
  1.1.2.3 Altered nutrition: Potential for more than body requirements
  1.2.1.1 Risk for infection[b]
  1.2.2.1 Risk for altered body temperature[b]
  1.2.2.2 Hypothermia
  1.2.2.3 Hyperthermia
  1.2.2.4 Ineffective thermoregulation
  1.2.3.1 Dysreflexia
  1.3.1.1 Constipation
    1.3.1.1.1 Perceived constipation
    1.3.1.1.2 Colonic constipation
  1.3.1.2 Diarrhea
  1.3.1.3 Bowel incontinence
  1.3.2.1 Altered urinary elimination
    1.3.2.1.1 Stress incontinence
    1.3.2.1.2 Reflex incontinence
    1.3.2.1.3 Urge incontinence
    1.3.2.1.4 Functional incontinence
    1.3.2.1.5 Total incontinence
  1.3.2.2 Urinary retention
  1.4.1.1 Altered (specify type) tissue perfusion (renal, cerebral, cardiopulmonary, gastrointestinal, peripheral)
  1.4.1.2.1 Fluid volume excess
    1.4.1.2.2.1 Fluid volume deficit
    1.4.1.2.2.2 Risk for fluid volume deficit
  1.4.2.1 Decreased cardiac output
  1.5.1.1 Impaired gas exchange
  1.5.1.2 Ineffective airway clearance
  1.5.1.3 Ineffective breathing pattern

    1.5.1.3.1 Inability to sustain spontaneous ventilation
    1.5.1.3.2 Dysfunctional ventilatory weaning response (DVWR)
  1.6.1 Risk for injury[b]
    1.6.1.1 Risk for suffocation
    1.6.1.2 Risk for poisoning[b]
    1.6.1.3 Risk for trauma[b]
    1.6.1.4 Risk for aspiration[a]
    1.6.1.5 Risk for disuse syndrome[b]
  1.6.2 Altered protection
    1.6.2.1 Impaired tissue integrity
    1.6.2.1.1 Altered oral mucous membrane
    1.6.2.1.2.1 Impaired skin integrity
    1.6.2.1.2.2 Risk for impaired skin integrity[b]
  1.7.1 Decreased adaptive capacity: Intracranial[a]
  1.8 Energy field disturbance[a]

Pattern 2: Communicating
  2.1.1.1 Impaired verbal communication

Pattern 3: Relating
  3.1.1 Impaired social interaction
  3.1.2 Social isolation
  3.1.3 Risk for loneliness[a]
  3.2.1 Altered role performance
    3.2.1.1.1 Altered parenting
    3.2.1.1.2 Risk for altered parenting[b]
    3.2.1.1.2.1 Risk for altered parent/infant/child attachment[a]
    3.2.1.2.1 Sexual dysfunction
  3.2.2 Altered family processes
    3.2.2.1 Care-giver role strain
    3.2.2.2 Risk for care-giver role strain[b]
    3.2.2.3.1 Altered family process: Alcoholism[a]

3.2.3.1 Parental role conflict
3.3 Altered sexuality patterns

Pattern 4: Valuing
4.1.1 Spiritual distress (distress of the human spirit)
4.2 Potential for enhanced spiritual well-being[a]

Pattern 5: Choosing
5.1.1.1 Ineffective individual coping impaired adjustment
  5.1.1.1.2 Defensive coping
  5.1.1.1.3 Ineffective denial
5.1.2.1.1 Ineffective family coping: Disabling
5.1.2.1.2 Ineffective family coping: Compromised
5.1.2.2 Family Coping: Potential for growth
5.1.3.1 Potential for enhanced community coping[a]
5.1.3.2 Ineffective community coping[a]
5.2.1 Ineffective management of therapeutic regimen (individuals)
  5.2.1.1 Noncompliance (specify)
5.2.2 Ineffective management of therapeutic regimen: Families[a]
5.2.3 Ineffective management of therapeutic regimen: Community[a]
5.2.4 Effective management of therapeutic regimen: Individual[a]
5.3.1.1 Decisional conflict (specify)
5.4 Health seeking behaviors (specify)

Pattern 6: Moving
6.1.1.1 Impaired physical mobility
  6.1.1.1.1 Risk for peripheral neurovascular dysfunction[b]
  6.1.1.1.2 Risk for perioperative positioning injury[a]
  6.1.1.2 Activity intolerance
  6.1.1.2.1 Fatigue
6.1.1.3 Risk for activity intolerance[b]
6.2.1 Sleep pattern disturbance
6.3.1.1 Diversional activity deficit
6.4.1.1 Impaired home maintenance management
6.4.2 Altered health maintenance
6.5.1 Feeding self-care deficit
  6.5.1.1 Impaired swallowing
  6.5.1.2 Ineffective breastfeeding
  6.5.1.2.1 Interrupted breastfeeding

6.5.1.3 Effective breastfeeding
6.5.1.4 Ineffective infant feeding pattern
6.5.2 Bathing/hygiene self-care deficit
6.5.3 Dressing/grooming self-care deficit
6.5.4 Toileting self-care deficit
6.6 Altered growth and development
6.7 Relocation stress syndrome
6.8.1 Risk for disorganized infant behavior[a]
6.8.2 Disorganized infant behavior[a]
6.8.3 Potential for enhanced organized infant behavior[a]

Pattern 7: Perceiving
7.1.1 Body image disturbance
7.1.2 Self-esteem disturbance
  7.1.2.1 Chronic low self-esteem
  7.1.2.2 Situational low self-esteem
7.1.3 Personal identity disturbance
7.2 Sensory/perceptual alterations (specify) (visual, auditory, kinesthetic, gustatory, tactile, olfactory)
7.2.1.1 Unilateral neglect
7.3.1 Hopelessness
7.3.2 Powerlessness

Pattern 8: Knowing
8.1.1 Knowledge deficit (specify)
8.2.1 Impaired environmental interpretation syndrome[a]
8.2.2 Acute confusion[a]
8.2.3 Chronic confusion[a]
8.3 Altered thought processes
8.3.1 Impaired memory[a]

Pattern 9: Feeling
9.1.1 Pain
  9.1.1.1 Chronic pain
9.2.1.1 Dysfunctional grieving
9.2.1.2 Anticipatory grieving
9.2.2 Risk for violence: Self-directed or directed at others[b]
  9.2.2.1 Risk for self-mutilation[b]
9.2.3 Post-trauma response
  9.2.3.1 Rape-trauma syndrome
    9.2.3.1.1 Rape-trauma syndrome: Compound reaction
    9.2.3.1.2 Rape-trauma syndrome: Silent reaction
9.3.1 Anxiety
9.3.2 Fear

[a] New diagnoses added in 1994 classified at level 1.4 using new Criteria for Staging.
[b] Diagnoses with modified label terminology in 1994. (Changes recommended by the NANDA Taxonomy Committee and adopted to remain consistent with the ICD.)
Source: North American Nursing Diagnosis Association, Nursing Diagnoses, Definitions and Classification 1995–1996. 1994.

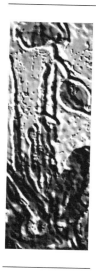

Index

list of, 777t
nursing management with, 779–782
overdose with, 780
plasma levels of, 782
side effects of, 306, 306t, 780–781, 781t
use for major depression, 334
use of in older adults, 305–307
Anti-Parkinsonian agents
and anticholinergic syndrome, 763, 764
effect of on disease states, 764
interaction with antipsychotic drugs, 765
overdose management of, 764
as therapy for EPS, 763
Antipsychotic drugs
dosage, 756, 766
drug action of, 755–756
drug interactions with, 765, 774t
and extrapyramidal symptoms, 756–758
list of, 755t
metabolism of, 756
overdose with, 763
preconditions for use of, 754–755
and psychiatric nursing practice, 765–766
side effects of, 758–759
treatment duration of, 766–767
Antisocial personality disorder
critical pathway for, 451–452
definition of, 442
Anxiety. See also Anxiety disorders
AIDS-associated, 617
versus akathisia, 762
authority, 734–735
biochemical theory of, 203
definition of, 80, 202
genetic theory of, 202
interpersonal theory of, 202–203
levels of, 80–81
peer, 735
psychodynamic theory of, 202
symptoms of, 80
Anxiety disorders. See also Anxiety
characteristics of, 782–783
DSM-IV criteria for, 204
and gamma aminobutyric acid, 50
medication for, 783–786
research in, 785–786
separation. See Separation anxiety disorder
types of, 203–204
Anxiolytics. See Antianxiety drugs
Anxious avoidant attachment, 94
Anxious pattern of symptoms, 416
Anxious resistant attachment, 94
Apathetic withdrawal, as defense mechanism, 87

Apgar score, 93
APNA. See American Psychiatric Nursing Association
ARC. See AIDS-related complex (ARC)
Arousal disharmony, 413
Art therapy, 31
Asian Americans, mourning rituals of, 246
Assertive community treatment (ACT), and the seriously mentally ill, 522
Assessment. See Nursing assessment
Assisted living, 667, 668t
Attachment theory, 241t, 721
Attachment, types of, 94
Attempted suicide
definition of, 564t
pattern of messages with, 572t
Attention deficit hyperactive disorder (ADHD), 261–262
case example of, 263, 265
epidemiology of, 261
nursing assessment of, 261–262
Authority anxiety, among adolescents, 735
Autism, 262–263
case example of, 265
nursing assessment of, 263
Autistic fantasy, as defense mechanism, 86
Auto-eroticism, 351
death resulting from, 363, 364
Auto-intoxication, 372
Automatic behavior, 393
Autonomic nervous system, 44, 46, 47
definition of, 55
divisions of, 47
Autonomic responses, as communication clues, 171–172
Autonomy
of older adults, 319
versus shame and doubt stage, 443
Autopsy, psychological, 564t
Autoreceptors, definition of, 55
Aversive therapies, consent for, 157
Avoidance learning, 62
Avoidance phase of mourning, 246–247, 247t
Avoidant pattern of symptoms, 416
Avoidant personality disorder
critical pathway for, 454–455
definition of, 442
Axon, 38, 38f, 753
definition of, 55
AZT. See Zidovudine (AZT)

Bailey, Harriet, 14
Bargaining mode of transaction, 114, 115f
Baring, Elizabeth, 31

Basal ganglia, 43
Basic level of psychiatric nursing, 20
BASK model of dissociation, 227
Bateson, Gregory, 110
Battered women, 488, 492
Bayley Scales of Infant Development, 262t
Beck Depression Inventory, 301t, 302
use for suicide screening, 570t
Bedlam, 12
Beery Visual Motor Integration Test, 262t
Behavioral change, 721
case example of, 716
definition of, 716
Behavioral System Model. See Johnson's Behavioral System Model
Behavioral therapy, during bereavement, 252
Behaviorism, history of, 721
Behavior modification
of addiction, 556
definition of, 61
Behavior, normal versus abnormal, 79
Bellevue Hospital School of Nursing, 14
Bender Visual Motor Gestalt Test, 262t
Benzodiazepines
abuse of, 546, 547t
dosage, 784t
interactions of, 775t
side effects of, 784–785
as treatment for anxiety, 784
withdrawal from, 547
Bereavement, 102. See also Grief
definition of, 240
versus depression, 303–304
drug therapy during, 253
epidemiology of, 243
group counseling during, 252–253
integrative theory of, 242t
and nursing assessment, 246–248
services in hospices, 252
treatment strategies for, 251t, 251–253
Berg, Henry, 486
Betrayal, in child sexual abuse, 477
Bibring, Edward, 331
Bicetre, 13
Binge eating
definition of, 381
epidemiology of, 381
nursing assessment of, 381
treatment for, 382
Bini, Lucio, 341
Bioavailability, of drugs, 750
Biofeedback, 716
Biological death, 242
Biotransformation factor, in pharmacokinetics, 751